P. Reimer · P. M. Parizel · F.-A. Stichnoth (Eds.)

Clinical MR Imaging

A Practical Approach

P. Reimer · P. M. Parizel · F.-A. Stichnoth (Eds.)

Clinical MR Imaging

A Practical Approach

Second, completely revised and updated edition

With 494 Figures and 141 Tables

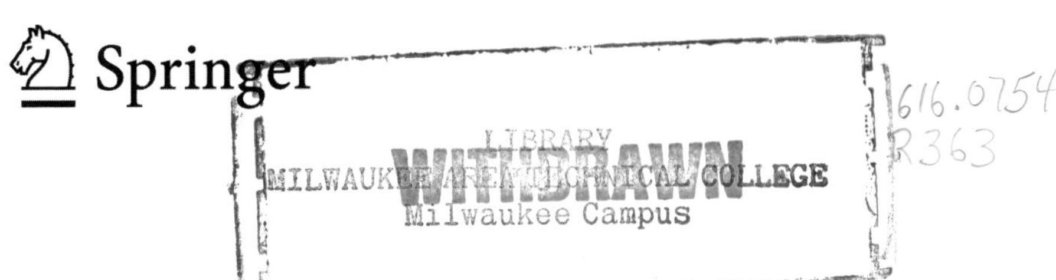

Prof. Dr. PETER REIMER
Department of Radiology
Klinikum Karlsruhe
Moltkestr. 90
76133 Karlsruhe, Germany
e-mail: P.Reimer@web.de

Prof. Dr. PAUL M. PARIZEL
Department of Radiology
Universitair Ziekenhuis Antwerpen
Wilrijkstraat 10
B-2650 Edegem, Belgium
e-mail: parizel@uia.ua.ac.be

Dr. FALKO-A. STICHNOTH
Radiologie München Ost
Wasserburger Landstr. 274–276
81827 München, Germany
e-mail: StichnothFA@t-online.de

2nd edition hardcover ISBN 3-540-43467-4 Springer Berlin Heidelberg New York

ISBN-10 3-540-31530-6 Springer Berlin Heidelberg New York
ISBN-13 978-3-540-31530-8 Springer Berlin Heidelberg New York

Library of Congress Control Number: 2005938673

Published in the medico-scientific book series of Schering as hardcover.

The book shop edition is published by Springer Berlin Heidelberg New York.

Where reference is made to the use of Schering products, the reader is advised to consult the latest scientific information issued by the company.

Typesetting: K. Detzner, 67346 Speyer, Germany
Cover design: Erich Kirchner, Heidelberg, Germany

Printed on acid-free paper 21/3150 5 4 3 2 1 0

Foreword

Since the introduction of magnetic resonance imaging in the early 1980s, unprecedented developments have taken place that have catapulted this imaging modality to the forefront of modern medical imaging. During this development, complex novel techniques have been introduced, including diffusion imaging, perfusion imaging, functional MR imaging, and basic innovations in pulse sequence design and system hardware. Despite the myriad of publications and developments, it is frequently difficult for the practicing radiologist to stay ahead of the game and translate advances into clinical protocols and improvements.

The current book by Drs. Reimer, Parizel, and Stichnoth is an exercise in marrying technological advances and clinical radiology. The book has 17 chapters: basic, contrast agents, hemorrhage, head, ENT, spine, pelvis, abdomen, retroperitonium, vessels, joints, soft tissue, chest breast, cardiac, pediatrics, and interventional imaging. All the chapters have the same structure, including subchapters on coils, pulse sequences, imaging protocols, anatomy, and clinically relevant pathology. Each chapter also contains a succinct reference list. Overall there are over 500 pages with illustrations to highlight key concepts.

The authors have done a fine job and the current work certainly enriches the armamentarium for the clinical radiologist. The editors and contributors are to be commended for their efforts in achieving a clear synthesis of technological and clinical issues. This volume clearly represents an important contribution to the field of medical imaging.

Ralph Weissleder, MD, PhD
Professor of Radiology
Massachusetts General Hospital, Boston, MA, USA

Preface

Magnetic resonance (MR) imaging has become the leading cross-sectional imaging method in clinical practice. Since the 1980s, continuous improvements in hardware and software have significantly broadened the scope of applications. At present, MR imaging is not only the most important technique in neuroradiology and musculoskeletal radiology, but has also become an invaluable diagnostic tool for abdominal, pelvic, cardiac, breast and vascular imaging.

Due to ongoing technical developments, the complexity of MR imaging has increased markedly. This often represents an obstacle not only to beginners (who find it difficult to get started), but also to more experienced users (who find it hard to keep up). Information about MR imaging can be found in many excellent textbooks and reference works, several of which have become encyclopaedic in scope and sheer volume. As editors and authors of this book, we have endeavoured to use a different approach. As a starting point for the first edition, we had taken into consideration that routine diagnostic questions account for more than 90% of examinations. This implies that by adopting a practical protocol-based approach the workflow in a MR unit can be streamlined considerably, which is critical in today's economic environment. We have aimed to provide the reader with such information, based on our combined experience.

The second edition of this book offers practical guidelines for performing efficient and cost-effective MR imaging examinations in daily practice. The authors and editors have reviewed all chapters, included new techniques, added new figures and replaced older ones. As editors, we hope that this work will lead to a better practical understanding of MR imaging and that new sequences and protocols will contribute to solving clinical problems. As such, we believe this book will continue to help beginners to advance their starting point in implementing the protocols and will aid more experienced users in updating their knowledge.

The editors:
P. Reimer, *P. M. Parizel*, and *F.-A. Stichnoth*

Contents

List of Contributors

Dr. THOMAS ALLKEMPER
Institute of Clinical Radiology, Westfälische Wilhelms-Universität,
Albert-Schweitzer-Str. 33, 48129 Münster, Germany

Dr. THOMAS BALZER
Schering AG, Clinical Department, Diagnostics, MR and Ultrasound Contrast Media,
Müllerstr. 178, 13353 Berlin, Germany

Dr. MATTHIAS BOOS
Institut für Radiologie und Nuklearmedizin, Krankenhausstr. 70,
85276 Pfaffenhofen, Germany

Dr. MARTIN BREITENSEHER
Osteologie und MR, Universitätsklinik für Radiodiagnostik,
Allgemeines Krankenhaus (AKH), Währinger Gürtel 18–20, 1090 Wien, Austria

Dr. CHRISTOPH BREMER
Institute of Clinical Radiology, Westfälische Wilhelms-Universität,
Albert-Schweitzer-Str. 33, 48129 Münster, Germany

Dr. GIANPIERO CARDONE
Department of Radiology University "La Sapienza", Policlinico Umberto I,
Viale Regina Elena 324, 00161 Rome, Italy

Dr. JAN W. CASSELMAN
Department of Radiology, A.Z. St. Jan, Ruddershove 10,
8000 Brugge, Belgium

Dr. CARLO CATALANO
Department of Radiology, University "La Sapienza", Policlinico Umberto I,
Viale Regina Elena 324, 00161 Rome, Italy

Prof. Dr. ARTHUR M. DE SCHEPPER
Universitair Ziekenhuis Antwerpen, Department of Radiology,
Wilrijkstraat 10, 2650 Edegem, Belgium

Dr. FRANCESCO FRAIOLI
Department of Radiology, University "La Sapienza", Policlinico Umberto I,
Viale Regina Elena 324, 00161 Rome, Italy

Prof. Dr. Stefan Grampp
Osteologie und MR, Universitätsklinik für Radiodiagnostik,
Allgemeines Krankenhaus (AKH), Währinger Gürtel 18–20, 1090 Wien, Austria

Dr. Paul A. M. Hofmann
Department of Radiology, University Hospital Maastricht, P.O. Box 5800,
6202 AZ Maastricht, The Netherlands

Prof. Dr. Herwig Imhof
Osteologie und MR, Universitätsklinik für Radiodiagnostik,
Allgemeines Krankenhaus (AKH), Währinger Gürtel 18–20,
1090 Wien, Austria

Prof. Dr. Franz Kainberger
Osteologie und MR, Universitätsklinik für Radiodiagnostik,
Allgemeines Krankenhaus (AKH), Währinger Gürtel 18–20,
1090 Wien, Austria

Dr. Birgit Kammer
Röntgenabteilung, Dr. von Haunersches Kinderspital, Klinikum Innenstadt,
LMU München, Lindwurmstr. 4, 80337 München, Germany

Prof. Dr. Hans-Ulrich Kauczor
Abt. für onkologische Diagnostik und Therapie,
Deutsches Krebsforschungszentrum, Im Neuenheimer Feld 280,
69120 Heidelberg, Germany

Dr. Claudia M. Keser
Institut für Anästhesiologie, Klinikum Großhadern und Klinikum Innenstadt,
LMU München, Nußbaumstr. 20, 80336 München, Germany

Priv.-Doz. Dr. Christiane Kuhl
Radiologische Universitätsklinik Bonn, Sigmund-Freud-Str. 25,
53105 Bonn, Germany

Dr. Markus G. Lentschig
Radiologische Praxis St. Jürgenstrasse, Prager Str. 11, 28211 Bremen, Germany

Dr. A. Laghi
Department of Radiology, University "La Sapienza", Policlinico Umberto I,
Viale Regina Elena 324, 00161 Rome, Italy

Dr. David MacVicar, MA, MRCP, FRCP
The Royal Marsden NHS Trust, Department of Diagnostic Radiology,
Downs Road, Sutton, Surrey SM2 5PT, Great Britain

Dr. Jim Meaney
MRI Department, St. James's Hospital, St. James's Street, Dublin 8, Ireland

Dr. A. Napoli
Department of Radiology, University "La Sapienza", Policlinico Umberto I, Viale Regina Elena 324, 00161 Rome, Italy

Dr. Wolfgang Nitz
Siemens A.G. Medical Solutions Magnetic Resonance Division, Henkestr. 127, 91052 Erlangen, Germany

Dr. Karsten Papke
Klinikum f. Radiologie und Neuroradiologie, Klinikum Duisburg, Zu den Rehwiesen 9, 47055 Duisburg, Germany

Prof. Dr. Paul M. Parizel
Department of Radiology, Universitair Ziekenhuis Antwerpen, Wilrijkstraat 10, 2650 Edegem, Belgium

Dr. Federica Pediconi
Department of Radiology University "La Sapienza", Policlinico Umberto I, Viale Regina Elena 324, 00161 Rome, Italy

Dr. Thomas Pfluger
Institut für Radiologische Diagnostik, Klinikum Innenstadt, LMU München, Ziemssenstr. 1, 80336 München, Germany

Dr. Thomas Rand
Osteologie und MR, Universitätsklinik für Radiodiagnostik, Allgemeines Krankenhaus (AKH), Währinger Gürtel 18–20, 1090 Wien, Austria

Prof. Dr. Peter Reimer
Klinikum Karlsruhe, Department of Radiology, Moltkestr. 90, 76133 Karlsruhe, Germany

Dr. Patrick Revell, BSc, DCR
Siemens House, Oldbury, Bracknell, Berkshire RG12 8FZ, Great Britain

Prof. Dr. Karl Schneider
Röntgenabteilung, Dr. von Haunesches Kinderspital, Klinikum Innenstadt, LMU München, Lindwurmstr. 4, 80337 München, Germany

Dr. Mirjam I. Schubert
Institut für Radiologische Diagnostik, Klinikum Innenstadt, LMU München, Ziemssenstr. 1, 80336 München, Germany

Dr. Falko-A. Stichnoth
Radiologie München-Ost, Wasserburger Str. 274–276, 81827 München, Germany

Dr. Hervé Tanghe
Department of Radiology, Academisch Ziekenhuis Rotterdam, Dr. Molewaterplein 40, 3015 GD Rotterdam, The Netherlands

Dr. Bernd Tombach
Institute of Clinical Radiology, Westfälische Wilhelms-Universität,
Albert-Schweitzer-Str. 33, 48129 Münster, Germany

Dr. S. Trattnig
Osteologie und MR, Universitätsklinik für Radiodiagnostik,
Allgemeines Krankenhaus (AKH), Währinger Gürtel 18–20, 1090 Wien, Austria

Dr. Edwin van Beek
Section of Academic Radiology, Floor C, Royal Hallamshire Hospital,
Glossop Road, S1O 2JF Sheffield, Great Britain

Dr. Luc van den Hauwe
Dept. of Radiology, AZ KLINA, Augustijnslei 100, 2930 Brasschaat, Belgium

Dr. Jan van Gielen
Universitair Ziekenhuis Antwerpen, Department of Radiology,
Wilrijkstraat 10, 2650 Edegem, Belgium

Dr. Johan W. M. Van Goethem
Department of Radiology, Universitair Ziekenhuis Antwerpen,
Wilrijkstraat 10, 2650 Edegem, Belgium

Dr. Anja van der Stappen
Universitair Ziekenhuis Antwerpen, Department of Radiology,
Wilrijkstraat 10, 2650 Edegem, Belgium

Abbreviations

ADC	analog to digital converter
B0	main magnetic field strength in Tesla (T)
B1	magnetic component of the RF field
CE-T2-FFE	contrast-enhanced T2-W FFE sequence
CE-FAST	contrast-enhanced FAST sequence
CEMRA	contrast-enhanced magnetic resonance angiography
CHESS	chemical shift selective pulse
CISS	constructive interference steady-state sequence
CNR	contrast-to-noise ratio
CSF	cerebrospinal fluid
DESS	double-echo steady-state sequence
EPI	echo planar imaging
FAME	fast-acquisition multi-echo sequence
FAST	Fourier acquired steady-state sequence
FFE	fast-field echo sequence
FISP	fast imaging with steady-state precession sequence
FLASH	fast low-angle shot sequence
fMRI	functional magnetic resonance imaging
FOV	field of view
FSE	fast spin-echo sequence
FSPGR	fast spoiled GRASS sequence
GMR	gradient motion rephasing
GRASE	gradient and spin echo sequence
GRASS	gradient recalled acquisition in the steady state sequence
GRE	gradient echo sequence
HASTE	half Fourier acquired single-shot turbo spin-echo sequence
HASTIRM	half Fourier acquired single-shot turbo spin-echo sequence using inversion recovery and only the signal magnitude
IR	inversion-recovery sequence
IRM	inversion-recovery sequence that utilizes only the magnitude of the signal
MIN	minimum intensity projection
MIP	maximum intensity projection
MPGR	multi-planar GRASS sequence
MPRAGE	magnetization-prepared rapid acquired gradient echo sequence
MR	magnetic resonance
MRA	magnetic resonance angiography
MT	magnetization transfer
MTC	magnetization transfer contrast

MTS	magnetization transfer saturation
PC	phase contrast
PSIF	a backwards-running FISP sequence
RAM-FAST	rapidly acquired magnetization-prepared FAST sequence
RARE	rapid acquisition with relaxation enhancement
RF	radio frequency
SAR	specific absorption rate
SE	conventional spin-echo sequence
SNR	signal-to-noise ratio
SPGR	spoiled GRASS sequence
SSFP	steady-state free-precession sequence
SSFSE	single-shot fast spin echo sequence
STIR	short tau inversion recovery sequence
T1	tissue-specific spin-lattice relaxation time
T1-W	contrast is weighted by the T1 relaxation time
T2	tissue-specific spin-spin relaxation time
T2*	relaxation time T2 plus additional dephasing mechanism (signal decay) due to local field inhomogeneities or chemical shift
T2-W	contrast is weighted by the T2 relaxation time
TE	echo time
TFE	turbo field echo sequence
TGSE	turbo gradient and spin-echo sequence
TIR	turbo inversion recovery sequence
TIRM	turbo inversion recovery sequence that utilizes only the magnitude of the signal
TOF	time of flight
TONE	tilted optimized non-saturating excitation
TR	repetition time
TSE	turbo spin-echo sequence

Principles of Magnetic Resonance Imaging and Magnetic Resonance Angiography

1

W. Nitz

Contents

1.1
Basic Principles of Magnetic Resonance Imaging

This chapter is written as a practical approach to clinical magnetic resonance (MR) imaging. With most scanners available today, images can be generated without knowledge of the basic principles, mostly by pushing buttons and executing suggested imaging protocols. However, in the event there is a need to change an imaging protocol or use another type of sequence, it is very helpful to have a good understanding of the underlying basic principles. This knowledge might also be very helpful for improving the signal-to-noise ratio (SNR) of an image or for the interpretation of potential artifacts.

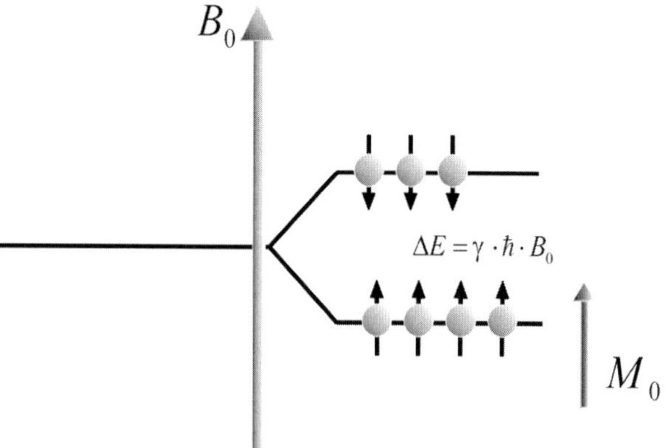

Fig. 1.1. The macroscopic magnetization or 'spin': Exposed to an external field, the magnetic moment of the spin causes a preferred orientation, correlated with a consumption of energy if forced into the less convenient position. Since the preferred position of a parallel alignment shows a higher population, a macroscopic magnetization builds up

1.1.1
Signal Source and Image Formation

1.1.1.1
Magnetic Resonance: What Is Resonating? What Is Spin?

The quantum mechanical description of a subatomic particle such as the proton implies that it has a quantized angular momentum, called a spin. Associated with the spin is a magnetic moment. Because the hydrogen atom has only one proton as a nucleus, this spin property can be observed by looking at hydrogen. Hydrogen is an atom present in water and fat; since the human body consists mostly of water and fat, we have a potential medical application. This spin or, better, its magnetic moment aligns itself to an external field B_0. Another possible position is alignment in the opposite direction, although this is less convenient and causes energy consumption (Fig. 1.1). The energy difference between these two possible positions can be written as the quantized energy of a photon

$$\Delta E = \gamma \cdot \hbar \cdot B_0 = h \cdot \nu$$

with ν being the frequency of an electromagnetic field and h Planck's constant. Unfortunately, we are dealing at this point with the inconvenient quantum uncertainties of a single proton. Fortunately, we are not facing a single proton, but rather a large number of similar protons. The term 'spins' is used to refer to these large groups, also called a spin isochromat. The behavior of this spin isochromat can be considered equivalent to a quantum average or expectation and, fortunately, can be treated

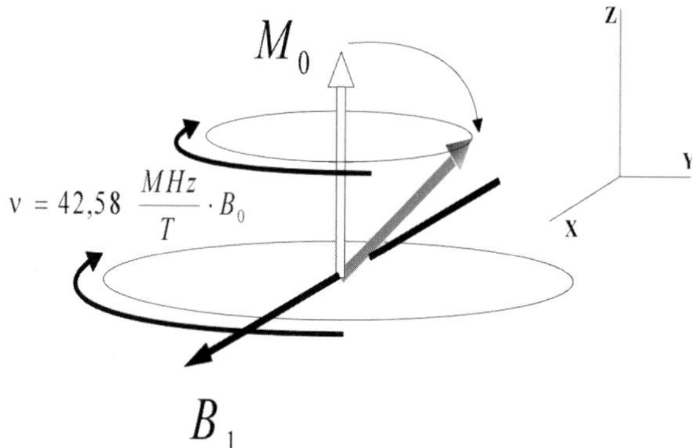

Fig. 1.2. The 'resonance' phenomenon: A B_1 field perpendicular to the main field (z-direction) causes the macroscopic magnetization to flip towards the x-y plane. Any attempt to turn the macroscopic magnetization away from the direction of the main magnetic field will cause a rotation around the z-direction. If the B_1 component of the electromagnetic field is rotating at the same frequency, the situation is called 'on resonance' and the B_1 field will continue to turn the macroscopic magnetization

as a macroscopic magnetization M_0 following the laws of classical electrodynamics. As illustrated in Fig. 1.2, hydrogen nuclei will provide a macroscopic magnetization when exposed to an external magnetic field, aligned in the direction of the main static field, usually referred to as the z-direction. This magnetization rotating is called longitudinal magnetization. Applying a

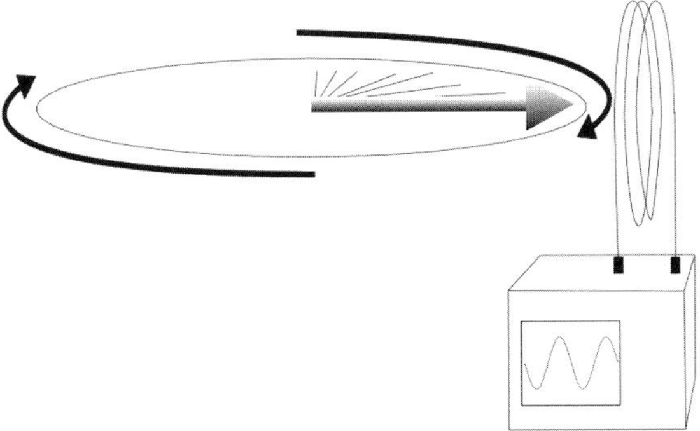

Fig. 1.3. The induction of the MR signal: If the macroscopic magnetization is not aligned with the direction of the main field, the magnetization continues to rotate around the *z*-axis and will induce a signal in a nearby coil

magnetic field perpendicular to the main static magnetic field will cause a rotation of the macroscopic magnetization. Any attempt to turn the macroscopic magnetization towards the *x-y* plane will cause the vector of the magnetization to rotate around the main direction with a frequency of 42.58 MHz/T, similar to a gyroscope. This frequency is also called the Larmor frequency. This magnetization rotating in the *x-y* plane is called transverse magnetization." If the applied electromagnetic field uses the same frequency, one magnetic component of this field rotates with the macroscopic magnetization (being in resonance), mimicking a constant so-called B_1 field. For this so-called in-resonance situation, the macroscopic magnetization can be turned around any angle, depending on the amplitude and duration of the B_1 field. Such a process is called a radio frequency (RF) excitation. With the B_1 field switched off, the macroscopic magnetization continues to rotate with the specific frequency of 42.58 MHz/T and will induce a signal in a nearby coil, as indicated in Fig. 1.3. This is the basic source of the MR signal.

1.1.1.2
Relaxation and Tissue Differentiation

1.1.1.2.1
Pd, T1 and T2 Relaxation Times

The amplitude of the induced signal is proportional to the number of protons involved in the excitation process (proton density). Usually, several excitations are necessary to collect enough information to reconstruct an image. Each time the actual longitudinal magnetization is flipped and thus converted to a signal inducing rotating transverse magnetization. The amplitude of the induced signal depends on the actual amount of longitudinal magnetization 'flipped' into the transverse plane. The actual longitudinal magnetization is a function of the tissue-specific relaxation rate, the time needed for the realignment of the magnetization with the main magnetic field. That time is called the T1-relaxation time. The rotating transverse magnetization is the result of a significant number of individual magnetic moments of hydrogen nuclei, each pointing in the same direction. The dipole-dipole interaction between all

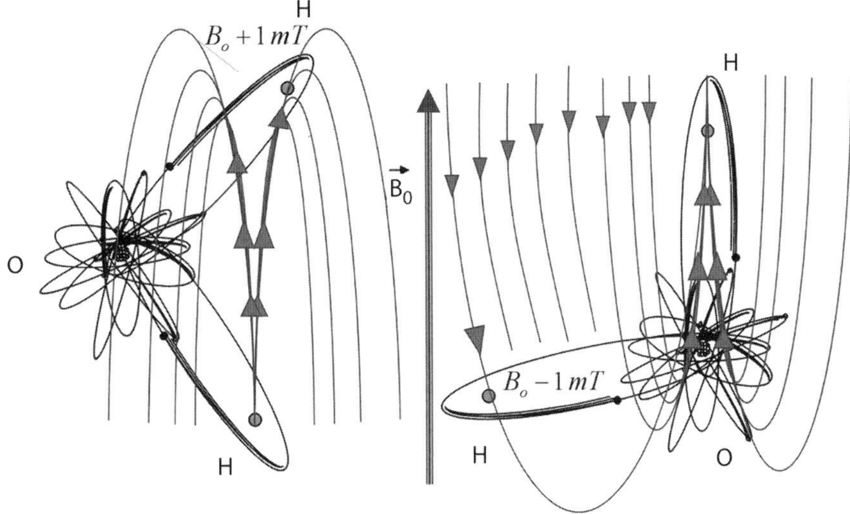

Fig. 1.4. The dipole-dipole interaction as a main source for relaxation: Intramolecular dipole-dipole interactions are the dominant factors for T1 and T2 relaxation times. The spin of a single hydrogen nuclei, aligned parallel to an external field B_0, has a correlated magnetic moment indicated by the field lines. That field is superimposed on the external field experienced by the neighboring hydrogen nuclei. Depending on the orientation of the water molecule within the external field, the effective field is diminished or increased. This will lead to significant differences in resonance frequencies on the molecular level

these magnetic moments will cause a 'dephasing' of the transverse magnetization. The slower the data are acquired after the initial excitation, the lower the induced signal detected. The relaxation rate assigned to the phenomenon of this 'dephasing' is tissue-specific and is called T2-relaxation. The simple dipole-dipole interaction is illustrated in Fig. 1.4. Depending on the orientation of the two protons relative to the main magnetic field B_0, the field of the first proton may either augment or oppose the main magnetic field at the location of the second proton. The difference in field strength can be approximately as high as 2 mT. Such a difference in field strength on a molecular level would lead to a difference in resonance frequencies of approximately 85 kHz, and the transverse magnetization would dephase within 12 µs. Current acquisition schemes allow about 1 ms as a minimum time between excitation and signal acquisition; thus, the signal of a 'frozen' arrangement of water molecules cannot be observed. In the vicinity of macromolecules, the attached immobile water molecules are not visible by MR imaging and are often called 'invisible water pool'. Fortunately, the majority of water molecules in human soft tissue are highly mobile, tumbling around, and the averaging over the fluctuating fields leads to a slower dephasing of the transverse magnetization. The time for the dephasing process, the T2-relaxation time, is also called the transverse relaxation or spin-spin relaxation time. As a rule, the higher the mobility of the water molecules (the 'squishier' the tissue), the longer the T2-relaxation time.

As described for the excitation process, in order to 'flip' or turn the magnetization, the generated B1-field has to be 'in resonance' with the magnetization. The same rule applies for the relaxation process aiming for the realignment of the magnetization with the main magnetic field B_0, the 'recovery' of the longitudinal magnetization. For tissue, where the 'tumbling' water molecules causing field fluctuations close to the Larmor frequency, the T1-relaxation time will be short. If the molecules are very small and mobile (free water), the tumbling frequency will be higher than the Larmor frequency, causing a slow T1-relaxation process. If the water molecules are motion restricted, the tumbling frequency may be below the Larmor frequency, and the result will be the same, a slow T1-relaxation process. The time for the recovery process, the T1-relaxation time, is also called the longitudinal relaxation time or spin-lattice relaxation time, since it depends on how fast the stored energy (of the spin system) can be returned to the surrounding environment (the 'lattice'). As a rule, the higher the mobility of the water molecules

Table 1.1. Relaxation parameters for various tissues

Region		Longitudinal relaxation times T1 (ms)			Transverse relaxation times T2 (ms)
		1,5 T	1,0 T	0,2 T	
Brain	Gray matter (GM)	921	813	495	101
	White matter (WM)	787	683	390	92
	Cerebrospinal fluid (CSF)	3000	2500	1200	1500
	Edema	1090	975	627	113
	Meningioma	979	871	549	103
	Glioma	957	931	832	111
	Astrocytoma	1109	1055	864	141
	Misc. tumors	1073	963	629	121
Liver	Normal tissue	493	423	229	43
	Hepatomas	1077	951	580	84
	Misc. tumors	905	857	692	84
Spleen	Normal tissue	782	683	400	62
Pancreas	Normal tissue	513	455	283	
	Misc. tumors	1448	1235	658	
Kidney	Normal tissue	652	589	395	58
	Misc. tumors	907	864	713	83
Muscle	Normal tissue	868	732	372	47
	Misc. tumors	1083	946	554	87

(the 'squishier' the tissue), the longer the T1-relaxation time.

Since the Larmor frequency depends on field strength whereas the 'tumbling' frequency of common water molecules within human tissue remains the same, T1-relaxation times are field strength dependent, as listed in Table 1.1.

The majority of MR contrast agents utilize the paramagnetic properties of gadolinium (Gd). Gadolinium has a powerful magnetic moment and is chelated to a reasonably mobile ligand. The magnetic moment interacts with the resonating magnetizations of the hydrogen nuclei, allowing the magnetizations to relax more rapidly – leading to a significant shortening of T1-relaxation times.

Although the simple dipole-dipole interactions are the most important processes for the T1- and T2-relaxation process, a variety of other mechanisms may be important in certain tissues. Sophisticated theories have been developed to explain the relaxation properties of even simple solutions. Figure 1.5 illustrates a three-compartment model, and even this more complicated perspective is only a crude approximation of 'reality'.

In conventional spin-echo imaging, a 90° RF pulse is used to convert the longitudinal magnetization M_z to the transverse magnetization M_{xy}. This initial pulse is also called the excitation pulse. The induced signal amplitude depends on how much longitudinal magnetization there was, and how much had recovered since the last excitation. The time between excitations is called the repetition time TR. The T2-relaxation immediately following the RF excitation will cause a dephasing of the transverse magnetization M_{xy}, leading to a decreased signal the later the data are acquired. Leaving ample room between excitations (long TR), the magnetizations of all tissues will be realigned with the main magnetic field, and no differences in T1-relaxation will be observed.

The time between the center of the excitation pulse and the magnetization refocusing point within the data-acquisition window is called the echo time TE. The shorter the TE, the shorter the influence of the T2-related dephasing mechanism. A long TR, short TE generated image is called proton-density weighted (Pd-W), since that is the main tissue parameter influencing the contrast (Fig. 1.6). In conventional Pd-W spin-echo imaging, CSF usually appears hypointense compared with GM or WM, due to a TR of the order of 2.5 s. In fast spin-echo imaging, the TR is usually longer than 3 s, leading to a correct hyperintense appearance of CSF following Pd-W imaging protocols. In order to differentiate tissues based on their T1-relaxation times, the TR has to be reduced, with the TE kept short, to acquire T1-weighted images. In that case, the contrast is strongly influenced by the T1-relaxation time of the different tissues. CSF and 'squishy' tissues with long T1-relaxation times will appear hypointense on T1-weighted (T1-W) images (Fig. 1.7). A T2-weighted (T2-W) contrast is achieved by using a long TR, similar to the Pd-W approach, but instead of using a short TE, a long TE will provide a stronger signal amplitude dependence on the T2-relaxation time of the various tissues. CSF and

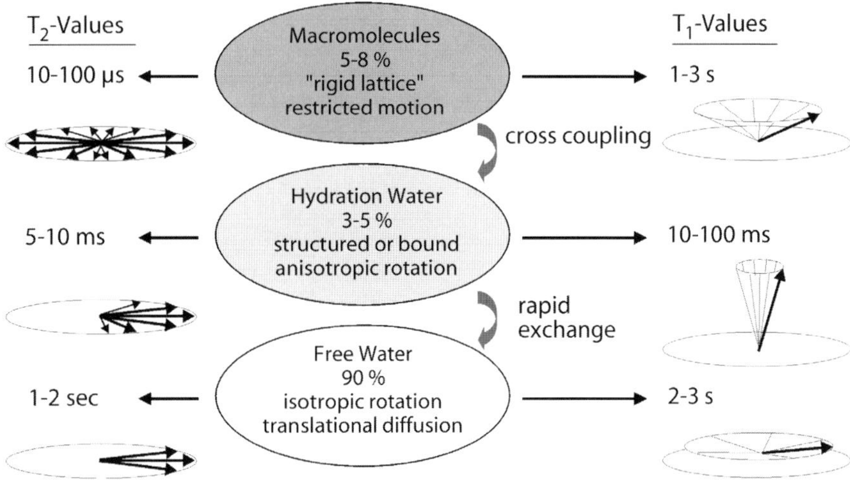

Fig. 1.5. A three-compartment model as an example for approximation of T1- and T2-relaxation times for different tissue hydrogen fractions

'squishy' tissues with long T2-relaxation times will appear hyperintense on T2-weighted (T2-W) images (Fig. 1.8).

1.1.1.2.2
Chemical Shift

The behavior of mobile fatty acids is slightly different compared to the oxygen-bounded hydrogens previously discussed. For the water molecule, the oxygen demands the single electron of the attached hydrogen, thus 'deshielding' the proton. The carbon-bounded hydrogen nuclei are more 'shielded' by the circulating single electron, thus experiencing an effective lower field than the water-bounded hydrogen nuclei. As a result, the Larmor frequencies of mobile fatty acids are below the water frequency. This phenomenon is called chemical shift (Fig. 1.9). The difference in resonance frequency scales with the strength of the main magnetic field and is approximately 3.5 ppm. Molecules containing aliphatic lipid protons are intermediate in size, and their motions are close to the Larmor frequency, causing short T1-relaxation times. Fat appears bright on T1-W images. On the other hand, there are only a few 'static' contributions in adipose tissue to allow a rapid dephasing due to T2-relaxation. As a result, fat also appears bright on T2-W images. Fat is the only tissue for which a long T2-relaxation time is not correlated with a prolonged T1-relaxation time.

1.1.1.2.3
T2 Relaxation Time, BOLD and Perfusion*

As tissue is exposed to an external field, it becomes 'magnetized'. The parameter indicating the ability to become magnetized is called '(magnetic) susceptibility'. There is often a significant 'susceptibility gradient' across tissue boundaries, causing local inhomogeneities of the magnetic field. Field inhomogeneities cause a rapid dephasing of the transverse magnetization. The relaxation time taking into account the dephasing due to T2-relaxation as well as the local field inhomogeneities is called T2*:

$$\frac{1}{T_2^*} = \frac{1}{T_2} + \gamma \cdot \Delta B$$

γ is the magnetogyric ratio, ΔB represents the field inhomogeneity across half a pixel

Local field inhomogeneities are usually fixed in location and consistent over time and are refocused in spin-echo imaging. For all gradient-echo imaging, it is T2* that is observed rather than T2.

Imaging of susceptibility differences is utilized in the evaluation of hemorrhagic lesions and in functional MR imaging based on the blood oxygenation level-dependent (BOLD) contrast. Deoxyhemoglobin is paramagnetic, while oxyhemoglobin demonstrates diamagnetic properties. A relative decrease of the deoxyhemoglobin level, as an 'overcompensation' reaction to oxygen consumption, will lead to a diminished microscopic susceptibility effect and is measured as a small increase in signal intensity – for imaging sequences sensitive to susceptibility gradients.

The majority of MR contrast agents utilize paramagnetic properties which, along with a reduction in T1-relaxation times, also create local field inhomogeneities in perfused areas. The observable signal decay due to shortened T2* relaxation times in those areas can also be used to quantify tissue perfusion.

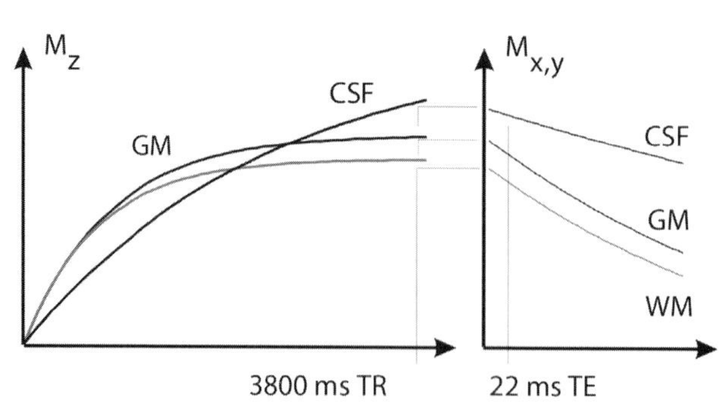

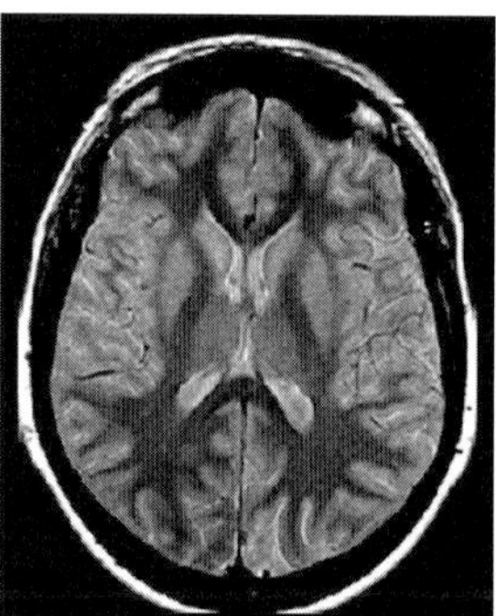

Fig. 1.6. Proton density-weighting: The *left graph* illustrates the recovery of the longitudinal magnetization (M_z) following excitation. The *right graph* demonstrates the dephasing of the generated transverse magnetization ($M_{x,y}$) due to the T2-decay. Cerebrospinal fluid (*CSF*) has a higher proton density than gray (*GM*) or white matter (*WM*) and should appear hyperintense on truly proton-density weighted (Pd-W) images

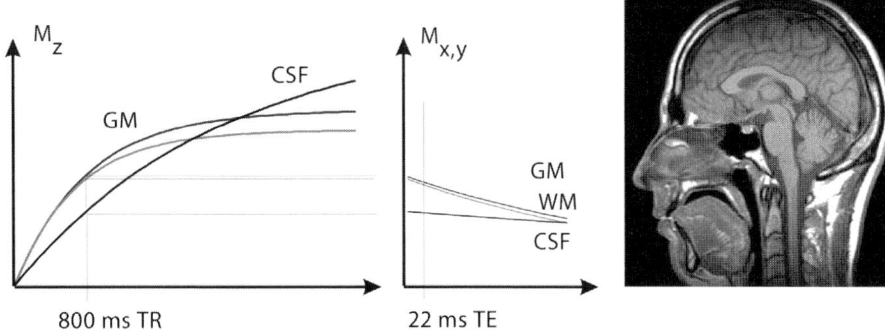

Fig. 1.7. T1-weighting: The *left graph* illustrates the recovery of the longitudinal magnetization (M_z) following excitation. The *right graph* demonstrates the dephasing of the generated transverse magnetization ($M_{x,y}$) due to the T2-decay. For a 1.5-T system, the optimum TR for gray matter–white matter differentiation is 800 ms. The selected TE has to be sufficiently short in order to minimize the influence of the T2-relaxation

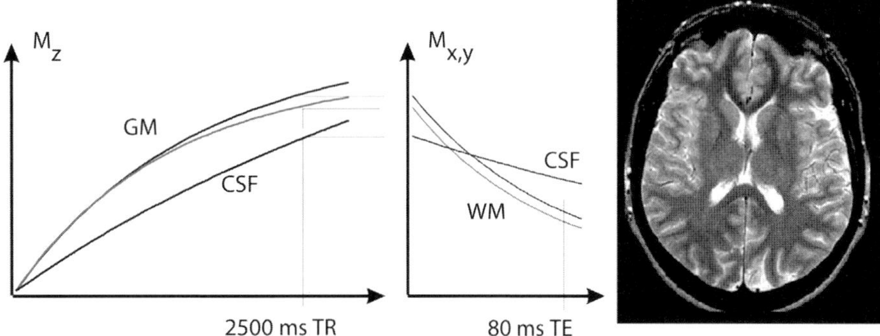

Fig. 1.8. T2-weighting: The *left graph* illustrates the recovery of the longitudinal magnetization (M_z) following excitation. The *right graph* demonstrates the dephasing of the generated transverse magnetization ($M_{x,y}$) due to the T2-decay. A long TR and long TE protocol will result in a T2-W image. Image contrast is dominated by the contribution of proton density and T2-relaxation of the various tissues

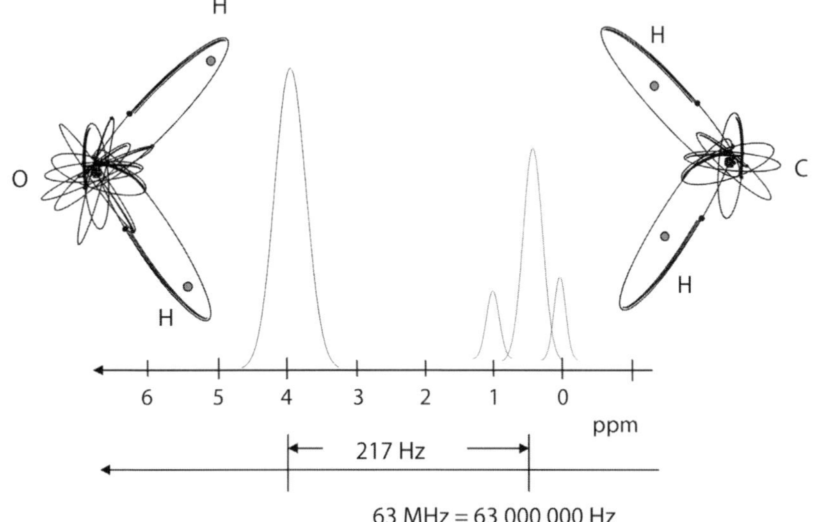

Fig. 1.9. Chemical shift: The electrons of oxygen-bounded hydrogen atoms are more drawn towards the oxygen atom than the electrons of carbon-bounded hydrogen. Hydrogen nuclei in adipose tissue are more 'shielded', leading to a lower resonance frequency than free water. The term describing the effect of an electronic environment on the Larmor frequency is called 'chemical shift'

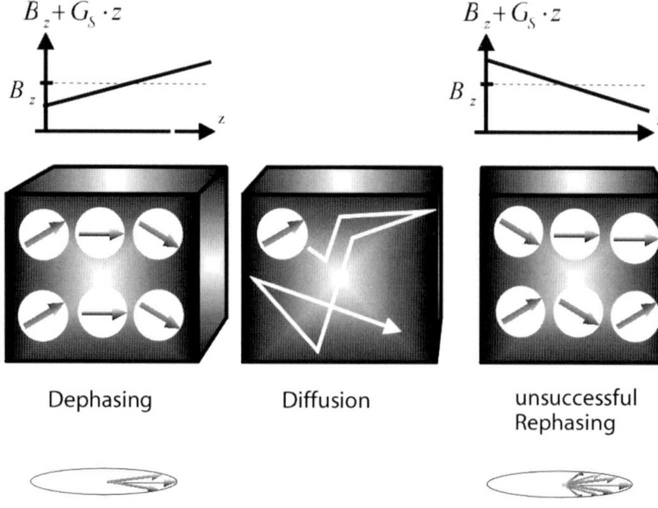

Fig. 1.10. Diffusion weighting: The transverse magnetization can be prepared for diffusion-weighted imaging using large bipolar gradients. Applying a positive gradient after a negative gradient using the same duration and the same amplitude has no effect on stationary tissue. The transverse magnetization is refocused. If the macroscopic magnetization changed position due to motion, flow, perfusion, or diffusion, the refocusing will be unsuccessful. The unsuccessful rephasing will cause a signal void in diffusion-weighted images for regions with increased diffusion

1.1.1.2.4 Diffusion

The ability of water molecules to perform random translational motion within a given tissue is described by the diffusion coefficient. The application of a magnetic field gradient for a short duration will cause a temporary change in resonance frequencies and a correlated dephasing of the transverse magnetization. Applying the same gradient for the same duration but of opposite polarity will result in a 'rephasing' of the transverse magnetization – for stationary tissue. For molecules which have changed position in the meantime, the rephasing of the transverse magnetization will be incomplete (Fig. 1.10). Tissue or tissue areas with an increased diffusion will appear as hypointense areas in diffusion-weighted imaging. Diffusion weighting involves the application of large magnetic field gradients in addition to the field gradients used for spatial encoding. A diffusion-weighted image in which the signal attenuation does not depend on the directionality of diffusion is also called trace-weighted image or isotropic diffusion-weighted image.

1.1.1.2.5 Flow and Motion

Flow and bulk motion can be considered an extreme form of diffusion. Since magnetic field gradients are used for the purpose of spatial encoding, as will be discussed in the next chapter, the positions of the transverse magnetizations, also referred to as 'phase', are altered depending on the velocity or acceleration of the moving tissue. The 'phase' information is actually utilized to measure velocities in MR flow quantification and can also be used to visualize vasculature (also called phase-contrast MR angiography, PC-MRA). Special gradient arrangements can be applied to make an imaging sequence insensitive to flow (and motion), also called flow compensation or gradient motion rephasing, GMR. One extreme form of flow is the replacement of saturated blood (short TR sequences causing a very low longitudinal magnetization of the affected blood and the stationary tissue of the affected slice) with unsaturated (fully relaxed longitudinal magnetization). This phenomenon is utilized in the so called time-of-flight angiography (ToF-MRA). The 'artificial shortening' of the T1-relaxation time due to replacement of 'saturated' spins with 'unsaturated' spins can be bypassed by intravenous injection of T1-shortening contrast agents, as is done in the so-called contrast-enhanced MR angiography, ceMRA.

1.1.1.2.6 Magnetization Transfer

Macromolecules have a layer of 'bound' water. Since static or slow changing magnetic fields are dominant in the vicinity of macromolecules, the associated hydrogen pool has a very short T2. The correlated fast

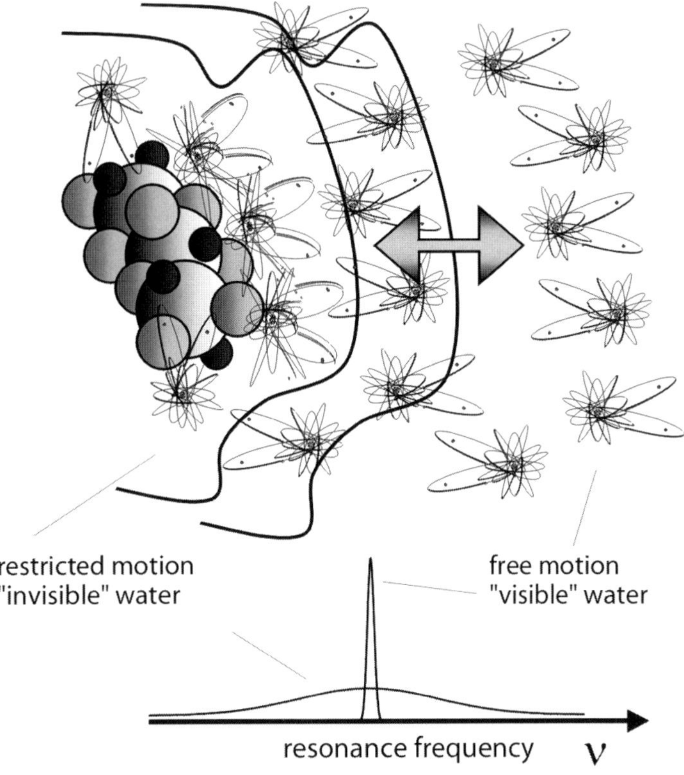

Fig. 1.11. Magnetization transfer: Water molecules that are closely associated with proteins and other macromolecules are restricted in motion. The resulting static dephasing mechanism leads to a very short T2, making these water molecules 'invisible'. A short T2 is also synonymous for a very broad range of resonance frequencies. In contrast, the 'visible' water pool has a very narrow frequency range. Mechanisms like cross-relaxation between protons within the 'invisible' water pool and protons within the 'visible' water pool are called 'Magnetization Transfer' (MT) mechanisms. Saturating the 'invisible' water pool will result in a diminished signal within the 'visible' water pool as a consequence of this magnetization transfer

dephasing of the transverse magnetization causes this pool of water to be 'invisible'. However, the magnetization of that 'invisible' water pool is transferred to the visible pool of 'free' water via various mechanisms like chemical exchange or cross-relaxation (Fig. 1.11). The term for these processes is called 'magnetization transfer', MT. Cross-relaxation is a special form of dipole-dipole interaction in which a proton on one molecule transfers its spin orientation to that of another molecule. A short T2 or fast dephasing is synonymous for a broad range of resonance frequencies, whereas a long T2 is indicative of a narrow range. If there are applicable magnetization transfer mechanisms within the tissue, a saturation of the 'invisible' water pool will affect the 'visible' water pool.

1.1.1.3 Image Formation and Image Contrast

As mentioned at the very beginning, the macroscopic magnetization will be affected if the RF field is 'in resonance'. Creating a small field gradient along one direction and applying a RF pulse covering a specific frequency range, only the macroscopic magnetization of that particular frequency will be affected, as illustrated in Fig. 1.12. This procedure is identical for small flip-angle excitations, as well as the refocusing pulses that

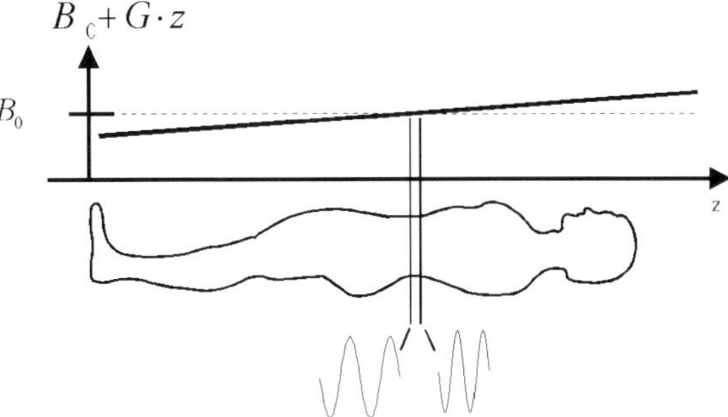

Fig. 1.12. Slice selection gradient: Creating a magnetic field gradient along one direction and applying a RF pulse of a specific bandwidth will enable the rotation of the macroscopic magnetization of a slice, where the resonance frequency of the macroscopic magnetization matches a frequency of the applied bandwidth

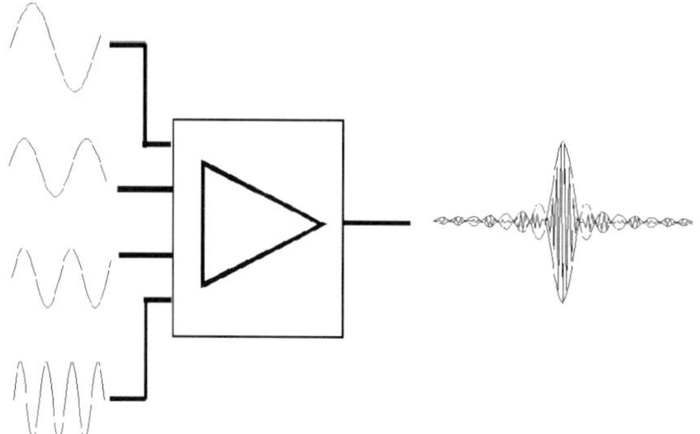

Fig. 1.13. The 'sinc' function: Summing up frequencies will result in a so-called sinc-function, relevant for slice-selective excitation and slice-selective refocusing and dictating the necessary length of the RF duration

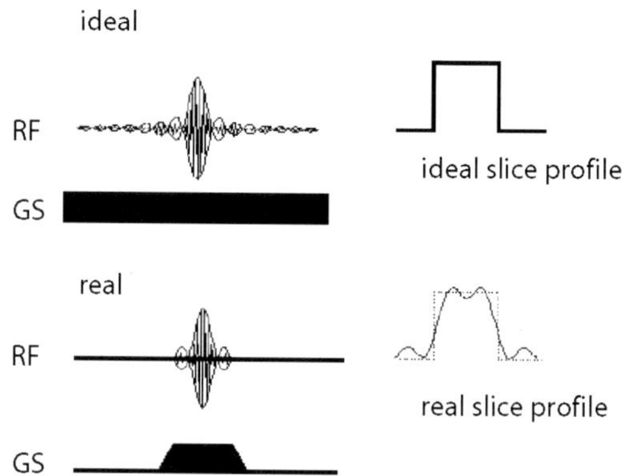

Fig. 1.14. The slice 'profile': A slice-selection gradient (GS) is established in order to have a dependency of the resonance frequency along the direction of slice selection. A RF pulse with no beginning and no end, containing all the frequencies of a desired slice, would lead to a perfect slice profile. In reality, RF pulses have a limited duration, leading to a compromised slice profile. This knowledge is helpful in understanding the necessity of a gap between slices for certain applications, and the limitation for fast, slice-selective imaging

will be described later. Summing up the frequencies to be covered will produce a so-called sinc envelope around the center frequency, as illustrated in Fig. 1.13. This sinc function is infinite, but the most important information is contained within a relatively small time frame, the center of the sinc envelope. There is a minor practical aspect with respect to the duration of this RF pulse. Fast imaging sequences are trying to be fast, keeping everything as short as possible, including the duration of the excitation pulse. In order to get the RF duration as short as possible, there are two possibilities: (1) either the sinc envelope has to shrink, or (2) it has to be truncated. In order to shrink the sinc envelope, the frequency range covered must be increased. For the same slice thickness, this can be done by increasing the gradient field. The latter requires a good strong gradient system. In order to turn the magnetization in less time also requires a larger amplitude for the RF pulse. Therefore, a robust RF system is also needed. An RF pulse is capable of generating heat in tissues as a consequence of resistive losses. This exposure is quantified with a specific absorption rate (SAR). With an increased frequency range for excitation and with an increased RF amplitude due to the short RF duration, the SAR for the patient is increased as well and is, in fact, the limiting factor in faster imaging with a good slice profile. The other solution is truncation of the sinc envelope. In this case, reduction of the overall measurement time happens at the expense of the slice profile. Truncating the sinc envelope will lead to a compromised slice profile as illustrated in Fig. 1.14. A poor slice profile will even lead to an improvement of the SNR since more tissue is contributing to the signal and the edges of the slice will experience a low flip-angle excitation, with the latter causing an increase in the signal contribution. The effect of a low flip-angle excitation is discussed in more detail in Sect. 1.1.2.2. Of course, a poor slice profile compromises the spatial resolution in the direction of slice selection, with a potential increase of partial volume artifacts.

The next step to be discussed after the concept of slice-selective excitation is the concept of spatial encoding. As the local dependence of the resonance frequency in a magnetic field gradient is utilized for slice-selective excitation, the same phenomenon is used for spatial encoding. A magnetic-field gradient is established, usually perpendicular to the direction of slice selection, in order for the resonance frequencies to be different for positions along the so-called read-out direction or frequency-encoding direction. A sampling of the signal at that time will allow the identification of the spatial location of the signal sources in one direction, as illustrated in Fig. 1.15. The frequency range for the selected field of view (FoV) is called the bandwidth of the measurement. In order to be able to display the information as pixel intensity on a screen, the excited slice is split into a number of voxels, where the pixel intensity on the screen corresponds to the signal magnitude received from each voxel. The magnetic field causes a frequency

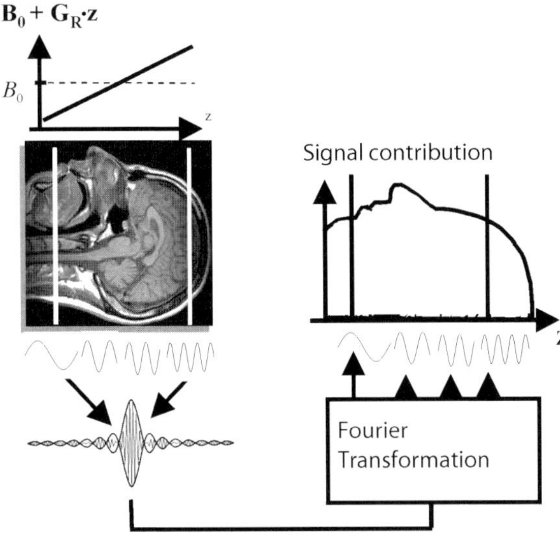

Fig. 1.15. The 'frequency' encoding: All resonance frequencies resulting from a magnetic field gradient being switched on during data sampling are detected simultaneously. Sampling the signal while a field gradient is switched on will provide information on the location of the signal sources in one direction. The information will be later displayed as the signal intensity of a pixel on a monitor, corresponding to the signal magnitude received from a single voxel within the excited slice

range over the FoV, which is now split into columns of voxels. Each voxel covers the same small frequency range, also called pixel bandwidth or simply bandwidth. The bandwidth of a sequence dictates the duration of the sampling window and influences the SNR. A high bandwidth will allow a short sampling window, but will also give a poor SNR. A low bandwidth will dictate a long sampling window, causing the sequence to be more sensitive to artifacts such as chemical shift and local susceptibility gradients or motion, but will provide a better SNR. Since fat- and water-bounded hydrogen atoms experience a different electronic environment, their resonance frequencies differ by approximately 3.5 ppm, that is 217 Hz on a 1.5 T system. Since the frequency information is also used as spatial information, the fat image and the water image have a slightly different position. For a sequence with a pixel bandwidth of 130 Hz, this chemical shift corresponds to a pixel shift of less than two pixels. The missing overlap on one end and the additional overlap on the other end cause hypointense and hyperintense lines at fat-water boundaries and are called chemical-shift artifacts (see also Section 1.4.1.1 Chemical Shift).

The encoding of a second or third direction is approaching the weak point of MR imaging. The only tool available for encoding seems to be switching a gradient field to cause a difference in resonance frequencies. Encoding in the second dimension is actually carried out prior to frequency encoding. A gradient field is switched on for a short duration in which the field direction is perpendicular to the direction of frequency encoding and the direction of slice selection. This gradient field will cause a phase shift, which is a shift in position of the macroscopic magnetization within the transverse plane as a function of location. In order to differentiate between two adjacent voxel rows in the direction of phase encoding, the amplitude and the duration of the phase-encoding gradient must be high enough to cause a phase difference of 180°, as illustrated in Fig. 1.16. Unfortunately, doing so will place the macroscopic magnetization of every other voxel in the same phase position. The signals from voxel 'columns' 1, 3, 5... all have the same phase position and cannot be separated. In order to identify these voxel 'columns', the

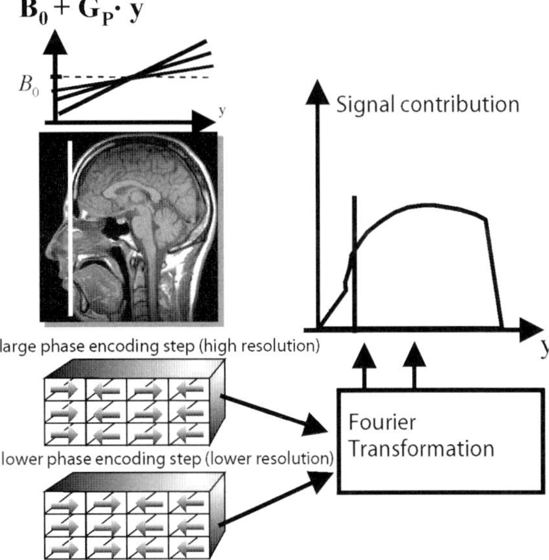

Fig. 1.16. The 'phase' encoding: In order to be able to distinguish the signal of two adjacent voxels, the gradient amplitude and duration of a phase-encoding pulse has to be high enough for the macroscopic magnetization of two adjacent voxels to have a phase difference of 180°. Since the macroscopic magnetization of every other voxel has the same orientation, the phase-encoding steps have to be repeated with reduced phase-encoding amplitudes to create n-equations for the calculation of the signal intensities within n voxel rows.

phase-encoding gradient amplitude is lowered for an additional measurement to have e.g. voxel 'columns' 1+2 and 3+4 pointing approximately in opposite directions. To identify *n* voxel columns in the direction of phase encoding, *n* phase-encoding steps are needed, and this is the annoying, time-consuming part of MR imaging.

The signal that can be detected immediately following an excitation pulse is referred to as a free induction decay. Besides the previously discussed T2 decay, there are other dephasing mechanisms, such as the global field inhomogeneity of the main magnetic field or the local susceptibility gradients within the patient himself, leading to the already discussed faster decay or dephasing, characterized by the T2*-relaxation time. Since most of these latter effects are consistent over time and fixed in location, they can be refocused. Within an inhomogeneous field, there is a component of the transverse magnetization that is rotating faster, due to a higher resonance frequency, and another component that is slower due to an experienced lower resonance frequency. Both phenomenon cause a phase shift, a dephasing between the two extreme components. In order to get a useful signal, this dephasing is refocused using a so-called refocusing pulse. A 180° RF pulse as illustrated in Fig. 1.17 rotates the faster component behind the slower component. Starting with the excitation, the faster component leaves the slower component behind. With the refocussing pulse, the faster component will now be behind the slower component, and at the time it is about to overtake the slower component, a so-called spin echo is formed. At this point, all components of the macroscopic magnetization are again pointing in the same direction, inducing a strong signal in a nearby coil. This is the magnetization refocusing point.

The basic spin-echo sequence is shown in Fig. 1.18 with the slice-selective excitation, phase-encoding, refocusing, and frequency-encoding elements. The signal from a single source is detected as an induced oscillating current over time. The assignment of this oscillating value to a frequency value is called a Fourier transformation. The following explanation is to show the simi-

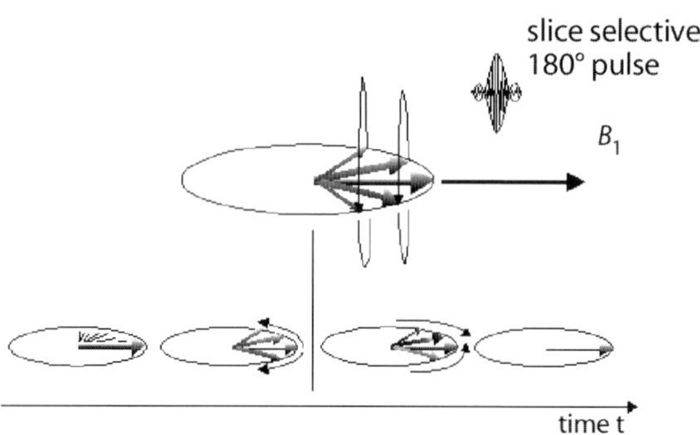

Fig. 1.17. The 180° refocusing pulse: The macroscopic magnetization within a voxel will not only undergo a dephasing due to spin-spin interaction (T2 decay) but will also experience a difference in resonance frequencies due to local variation of susceptibility, due to magnet inhomogeneities, or due to chemical shift. Most of these effects are fixed in location and stable over time. There will be components of the magnetization that experience a lower resonance frequency – falling behind in a rotating group of magnetizations – and there will be components that experience a higher field, a higher resonance frequency – speeding ahead. A 180° radiofrequency refocusing pulse will put the faster component behind the slower and vice versa. Since the effect remains that the faster component will still correspond to a higher magnetic field, the magnetization will be refocused, forming a so-called spin echo

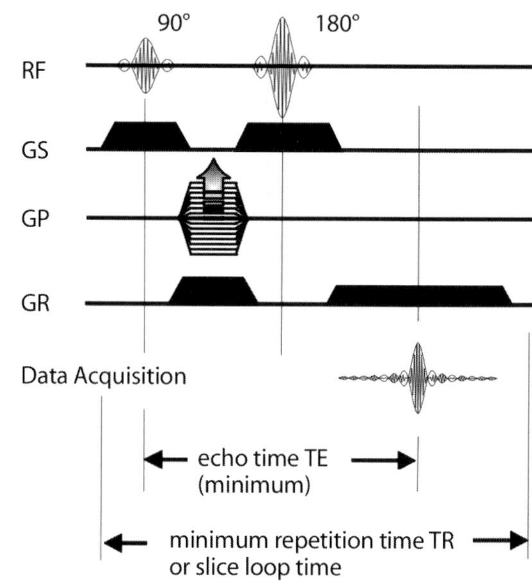

Fig. 1.18. The spin-echo sequence design: The sequence starts with ramping up the slice-selection gradient (GS) to establish a difference in resonance frequencies along the direction of slice selection. A slice-selective (center frequency and bandwidth according to the desired location and slice thickness) 90° radiofrequency (RF) pulse will turn the longitudinal magnetization into the transverse (x-y) plane. After the excitation, the phase encoding is performed with the phase-encoding gradient (GP). For each phase-encoding loop, the amplitude is changed (except for averaging loops). At the same time, the readout gradient (GR), also called the frequency-encoding gradient, is compensating for the later expected dephasing during the readout period. The length of the data acquisition is given by the desired bandwidth per pixel and usually dominates the timing of the sequence. The time between the center of the excitation pulse and the center of the spin echo is known as the echo time (*TE*). *TR*, repetition time

larity between frequency-encoding and phase-encoding. The induced signal in the presence of a frequency-encoding gradient is the sum of all signals for each "frequency column". The signal within each "frequency column" is proportional to the proton-density within each voxel along the "frequency column" and proportional to the other tissue specific parameters within each voxel of the column as previously discussed. The transverse magnetization within each "frequency column" is speeding ahead or falling behind compared to adjacent "frequency columns", depending on the difference in resonance frequency as given by the local field strength. This speeding ahead or falling behind is described as a phase shift ϕ_R. If, as an example, the frequency-encoding gradient is in the x-direction, the phase change for each "frequency column" would be:

$$\phi_R = \gamma \cdot GR_x \cdot t_r \cdot x = k_x \cdot x$$

The frequency difference is given as a function of location $\Delta\nu \approx GR_x \cdot x$ and the phase difference between "frequency columns" is a function of the sampling time t_r. The product of gyromagnetic ratio γ, magnetic field gradient in the read-out direction GR_x and sampling time t_r is denoted as k-value $k_x = \gamma \cdot GR_x \cdot t_r$. The data sampled in the presence of a frequency-encoding gradient are stored along a data vector that has a k-index.

If, as an example, the phase-encoding gradient is in the y-direction ϕ_P, the phase change for each "phase-encoding row" would be:

$$\phi_P = \gamma \cdot GP_y \cdot T_P \cdot y = k_y \cdot y$$

The duration T_p of the phase-encoding gradient is usually not altered, but each „phase-endoding row" is characterized by a different phase-encoding gradient amplitude GP_y.

At this point it is obvious that, if we can apply a Fourier transformation along the k, data columns in order to assign signal contributions to the various "frequency columns", the same approach can be done for the k_y direction in order to achieve an assignment to the different "phase-encoding rows". In fact, prior to a Fourier transformation all "raw-data" can be dumped into a raw data buffer called k-space (Fig. 1.19), which is characterized by the k_x and k_y indizes.

The concept of lines and columns of an acquired image matrix is often misleading and misunderstood. As discussed earlier, in order to acquire the information from two adjacent voxels, it is necessary to switch on a large phase-encoding gradient. This measured line is stored at the beginning of k-space and contains the high spatial frequency information of the object. As the phase-encoding gradient is lowered, the next line contains a lower spatial frequency. The line where no phase-encoding gradient is switched on contains the projection; the very coarse structure of the object. This line is stored in the center of k-space. For standard imaging, the lower part of k-space is again filled with information from higher spatial frequencies. It is important to remember that measured lines do not correspond to a row of tissue within the selected slice, but to the composition of spatial frequencies of the scanned object. The Fourier transformation applied to a few lines around the center of k-space will provide coarse information of the object scanned, indicating at the same time the contrast of the image (Fig. 1.20).

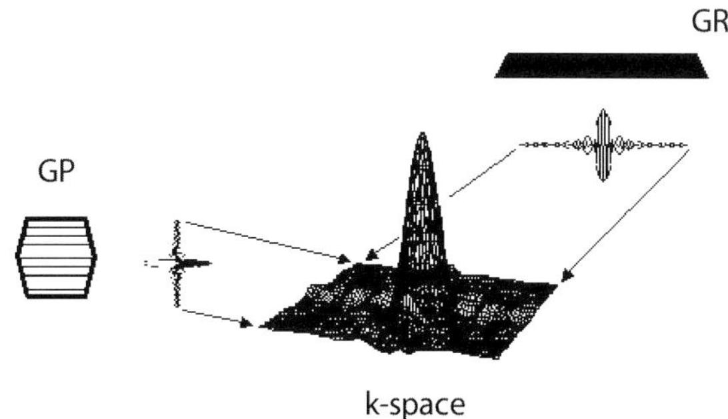

Fig. 1.19. The k-space. Prior to image reconstruction, each measured Fourier line (frequency-encoded data for each phase-encoding step) is stored in a raw data memory. The information stored into this raw data memory is similar to the information a mathematician would expect within the so-called k-space. Since currently all MR imaging techniques use the principle of Fourier encoding, the k-space is a convenient location to discuss methods, advantages, and potential pitfalls. The center of the k-space contains the information about the coarse structure of the object, whereas the information about the details are to be found in the outer regions of the k-space. *GP*, phase-encoding gradient; *GR*, readout gradient

Time is needed in order to provide the information of different frequencies contained in the time course of an oscillating signal. The duration of a selective pulse is usually around 2.5 ms. For the phase encoding, time is needed for ramping the gradient up and down, again 3.8 ms as a typical example. Selective refocusing also takes 2.5 ms, and a reasonable bandwidth requires an acquisition window of 7.7 ms. The shortest possible echo time (TE) for a standard spin-echo (SE) sequence is, therefore, about 12 ms. Considering the other half of the acquisition window and the time necessary for

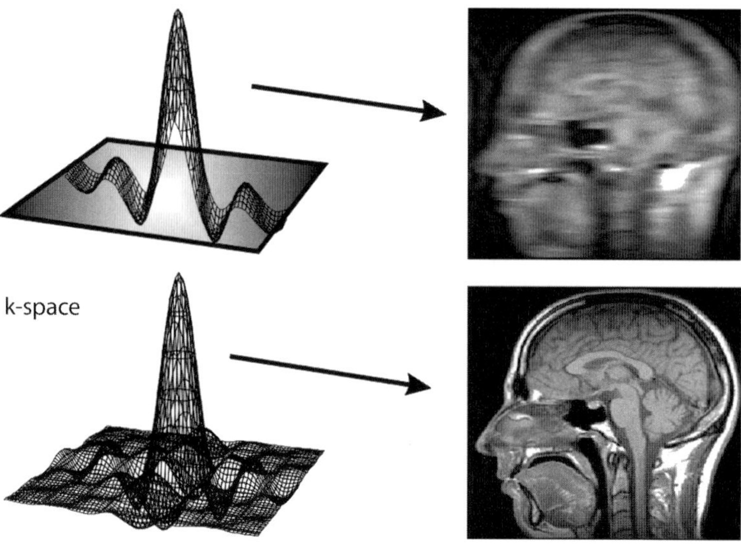

Fig. 1.20. The *k*-space: The center of *k*-space contains the coarse structure of the object. The information about the object details are to be found in the outer regions of the *k*-space

spoiling, the shortest possible repetition time is approximately 18 ms. This time is usually referred to as the 'slice loop time' since this is the minimum time needed to measure one slice.

For SE imaging, it doesn't make sense to excite immediately after 18 ms as there is almost no magnetization recovery during that time. In order to get a nice T1-W contrast, a repetition time of 300–800 ms is reasonable. The time in between excitations of the same slice is utilized to excite and read out lines for other slices before getting back to the first slice and measuring the next line. This is also called multi-slice imaging. To measure the difference of T2-relaxation times or in proton density, the repetition time (TR) has to be prolonged to 2–3 s. At that time, the T1-relaxation is almost completed, and the measured intensities correspond to the number of protons that participate – assuming there is a very short TE. The contrast achieved with a short TR and a short TE is called T1-W, since tissue with differences in T1 will show a difference in signal intensity. For measurements with a long TR and a short TE, signal intensity differences are based on the proton density of the tissue. Those images are called proton density weighted (Pd-W). To get Pd-W images, the TE has to be as short as possible in order to avoid a signal alteration due to different T2 values. To get the T2 information for the different tissues, the TE is prolonged by adding a delay before and after the refocusing pulse. Those images are called T2-W. The measurement time for a standard SE sequence is the selected TR × the number of Fourier lines to be measured in the direction of phase encoding × the number of acquisitions or averages for improving the SNR.

The rattling noise during the MR examination is due to the similarity in design between a loudspeaker and an MR scanner (Fig. 1.21). The loudspeaker usually consists of a small magnet surrounded by a little solenoid coil that is attached to a paper membrane. Sending a small current through the solenoid will result in a small

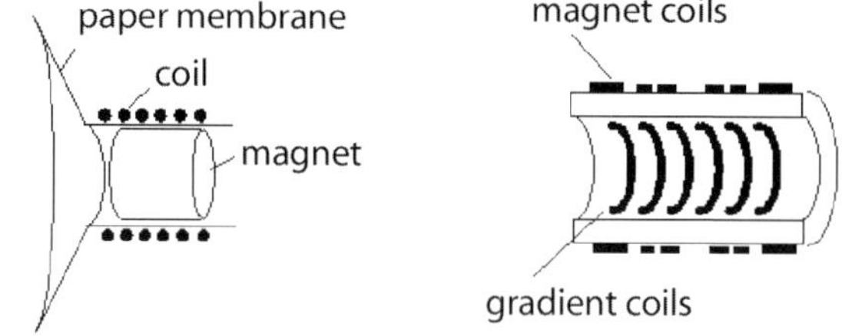

Fig. 1.21. The MR system as a 'noise-maker': Loudspeaker versus magnetic resonance scanner. This is of course an oversimplified drawing, but the effect is unfortunately the same. On the *left side*, we have the loudspeaker, with a little coil glued to a paper membrane, adjacent to a permanent magnet. Depending on the field generated by the current through the coil, a force will try to move the coil and the attached paper membrane, and the oscillation will produce a sound. On the *right side*, the MR scanner is illustrated, and although only the magnetic-field gradients are of interest for the selective excitation and the spatial encoding, the forces are also there, causing the noise during the measurement

magnetic field, which interacts with the field of the permanent magnet. The result is a mechanical force that tries to move the solenoid coil relative to the permanent magnet. Switching this current on and off or changing the polarity will result in different forces, causing the membrane to oscillate. A similar behavior is apparent with an MR scanner. Although the intention is not to produce a sound, the rapid switching of the gradient currents for the purpose of creating a magnetic gradient field will also produce mechanical forces, causing various parts of the system to vibrate. The rattling noise throughout a measurement has its origin in these vibrations. The higher the gradient amplitudes, the louder the rattling noise; the faster the current switching, the higher the pitch.

1.1.1.4 Magnetization Preparation

In addition to the T1 and T2 relaxation times, there are multiple other factors contributing to the contrast, but these are usually specific for the sequence or are targeted with special preparation pulses. The most important preparation pulses are the fat-signal-suppression schemes, the signal nulling of tissue using an inversion pulse, the improvement in T1-weighting using an inversion pulse, the magnetization transfer concept, and diffusion weighting.

1.1.1.4.1 Spectral Suppression of Fat Signal

Fat usually appears hyperintense on proton density-weighted (Pd-W) and T1-WI. The high signal intensity often reduces the dynamic range for windowing the images, or it may obscure lesions. Artifacts due to respiratory motion usually originate within the subcutaneous fat. These are reasons why it is often desirable to eliminate or reduce the signal from fat. As mentioned above, the resonance frequency of fat-bounded hydrogen is approximately 3.5 ppm lower than the resonance frequency for water-bounded hydrogen, i.e., 217 Hz for a 1.5-T system or 147 Hz for a 1.0-T magnet. Applying a spectral saturation pulse prior to the imaging sequence, as indicated in Fig. 1.22, it is possible to suppress the signal from fat. Challenging for this technique is the fact that a good magnetic-field homogeneity is required throughout the imaging volume in order for the resonance frequency of water and fat not to be a function of location. If this condition is not fulfilled, fat may appear unsaturated at one corner of the image and even water may become saturated. In order to obtain a homogene-

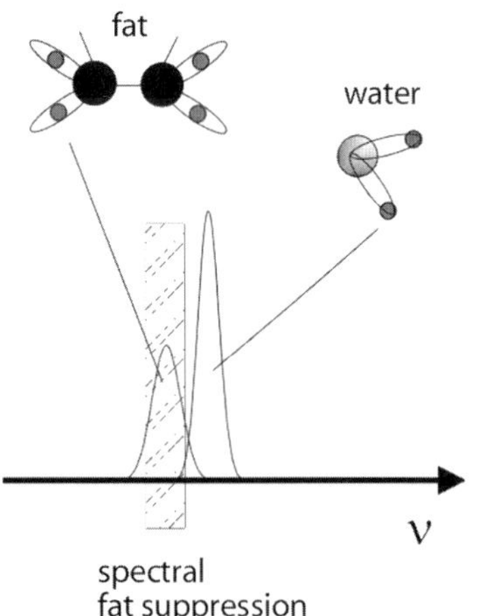

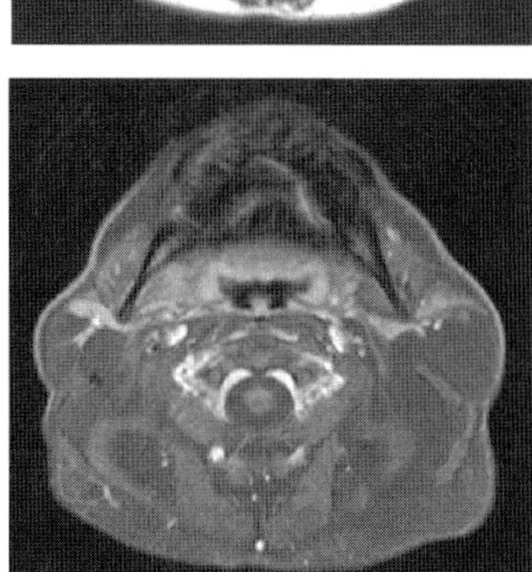

Fig. 1.22. Spectral fat suppression: Since the resonance frequencies of fat and water differ by about 3.5 ppm, a frequency-selective saturation pulse can be used to reduce the signal from fat

ous field, it is often possible to actively 'shim' the magnet. In this case, currents are sent through shim coils, or as an offset, through the gradient coils, in order to have the same magnetic field everywhere within the volume of interest. Field inhomogeneities are also introduced by the various tissue interfaces within the patient. If the inhomogeneity is confined to a small region, it is often impossible to eliminate this variation with 'shimming'.

1.1.1.4.2 Relaxation-Dependent Elimination of Fat Signal

Fat has a very short T1 relaxation time. Using an inversion pulse prior to the measurement, it is possible to apply the excitation pulse of the imaging sequence at the time the recovering longitudinal magnetization of fat is passing through the transverse plane (Fig. 1.23). In this case, fat will not be excited. Such a technique is called STIR (short tau inversion recovery) and is often used in conjunction with faster imaging techniques to be mentioned later. The inversion time for fat suppression on a 1.5-T system is approximately 150 ms when used in conjunction with a conventional imaging sequence. Used in conjunction with faster imaging techniques, the inversion time may have to be prolonged to 170 ms. A disadvantage of this technique is that the inversion pulse affects all tissues, often reducing the SNR dramatically. Since the majority of contrast agents used in MR are T1-shortening agents, it is obvious that STIR techniques should not be used after contrast injection. In the latter case, the tissue of enhancing lesions (T1-reduced) may also be nullified.

1.1.1.4.3 Relaxation-Dependent Elimination of CSF Signal

With the faster imaging techniques to be described later, the discussion of a suitable inversion time in conjunction with a reasonable measurement time becomes obsolete. It is feasible to select an inversion period of, for example, 1.9 s, nullifying the signal of the CSF (Fig. 1.24). This technique is very useful when studying periventricular lesions, often obscured by the bright signal of adjacent CSF spaces. In conjunction with a conventional SE acquisition scheme, this technique has been introduced as FLAIR (fluid-attenuated IR).

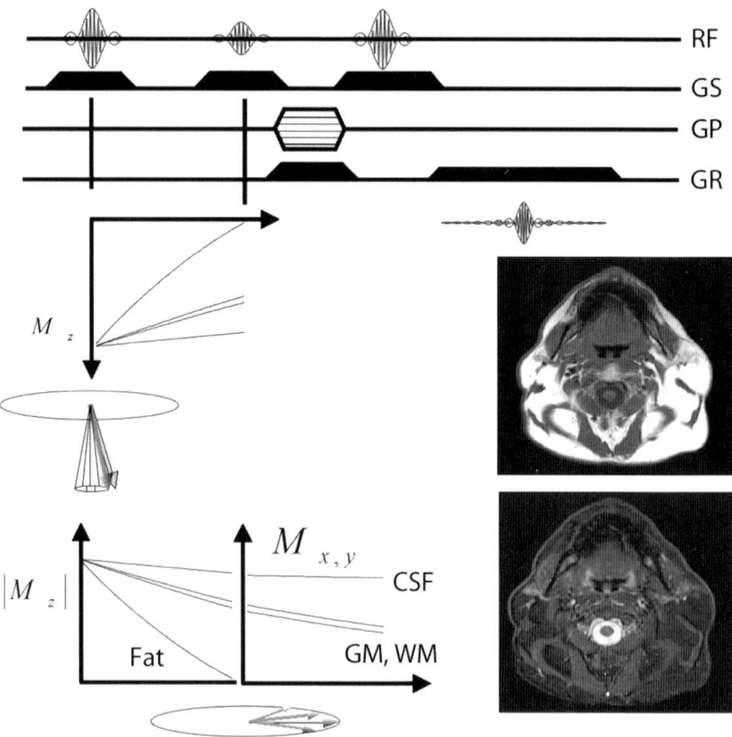

Fig. 1.23. The short tau inversion recovery (STIR) approach used for relaxation-dependent fat suppression. The equilibrium magnetization is inverted at the beginning of the sequence, and the longitudinal magnetization recovers depending on the tissue-specific relaxation time T1. The recovered longitudinal magnetization M_z is turned into the transverse plane, becoming M_{xy} after an inversion time T1. In STIR imaging, TI is the time at which the fat has no longitudinal component, and therefore no transverse component can be generated with the excitation. Fat doesn't appear. Only the magnitude of the longitudinal component is considered, not the direction. *GP*, phase-encoding gradient; *GR*, readout gradient; *GS*, slice-selection gradient; *RF*, radiofrequency; *WM*, white matter; *GM*, gray matter

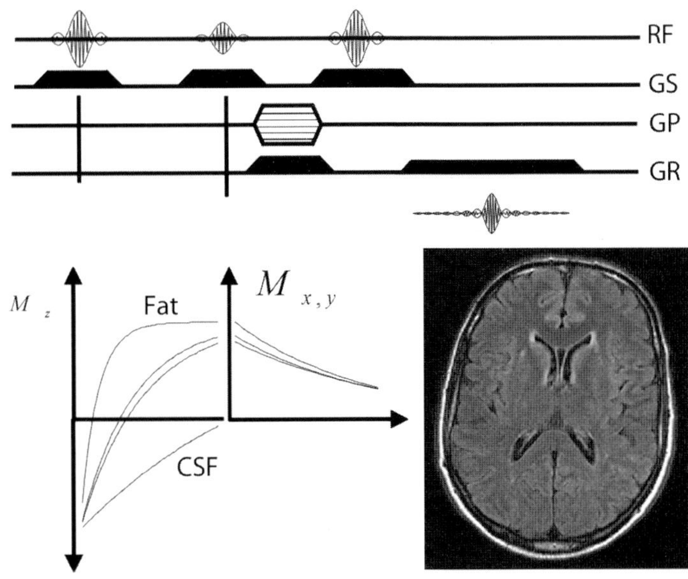

Fig. 1.24. The fluid-attenuated inversion recovery (FLAIR) approach used for relaxation-dependent suppression of the cerebrospinal fluid (CSF) signal. In FLAIR imaging, the inversion time TI is the time at which the CSF has no longitudinal component, and therefore no transverse component can be generated with the excitation. *GP,* phase-encoding gradient; *GR,* readout gradient; *GS,* slice-selection gradient; *RF,* radiofrequency

1.1.1.4.4 RF Inversion of the Magnetization to Improve T1-Weighting

After applying an RF inversion pulse, the macroscopic magnetization recovers with the tissue-specific T1 relaxation rate. As indicated in Fig. 1.25, the contrast between, for example, gray matter and white matter becomes a function of the inversion time and can be maximized. Such an approach is used in some applications, such as pediatric imaging of the brain.

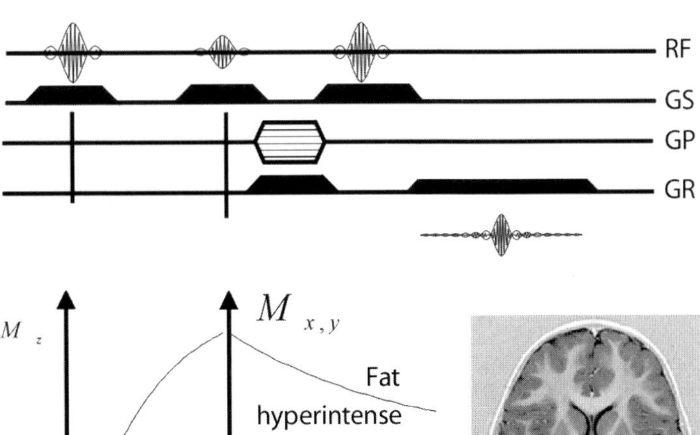

Fig. 1.25. The true inversion recovery technique (TIR). The combination of an IR technique with a TSE sequence provides an impressive differentiation between tissues with a small difference in T1 relaxation times. The magnetization that is still pointing antiparallel to the main field is hypointense. Magnetization that is more recovered and already partially aligned with the direction of the main field is hyperintense. No signal is presented as intermediate gray. *GP,* phase-encoding gradient; *GR,* readout gradient; *GS,* slice-selection gradient; *RF,* radiofrequency

1.1.1.4.5
Magnetization Transfer

Water molecules in the vicinity of macromolecules are called 'bounded' and have a very short T2. A short T2 refers to a large difference in resonance frequencies, causing a rapid dephasing. These water molecules are not directly observable but have a very broad range of resonance frequencies. Applying an RF saturation pulse off resonance, as illustrated in Fig. 1.26, those invisible molecules can be saturated. Since they communicate with their 'free' partners via magnetization transfer, this off-resonance pulse has an effect on the image contrast. The technique is called magnetization transfer saturation (MTS). The contrast achieved with this technique is often referred to as magnetization transfer contrast (MTC). The first and very effective application of MTS pulses was in magnetic resonance angiography (MRA), in which the stationary background is suppressed with this approach.

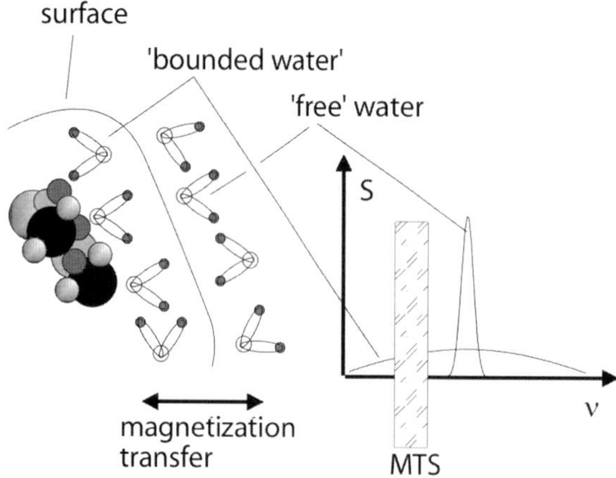

Fig. 1.26. The concept of magnetization transfer: Water molecules in the vicinity of macromolecules are called 'bounded'. They have a very short T2 and are not visible on MR imaging. The short T2 indicates a large difference in resonance frequencies ν, leading to a rapid dephasing. A large difference in resonance frequencies corresponds to a broad line width as indicated here. A magnetization transfer saturation pulse (*MTS*) is an off-resonance pulse, which does not directly affect the appearance of 'free' water but does saturate the invisible 'bounded' water molecules. Magnetization transfer mechanisms provide a transfer of this saturation to the visible pool of 'free' water, leading to a lower signal in areas where 'bounded' water exists in close vicinity to 'free' water

1.1.1.4.6
Diffusion Weighting

Diffusion characterizes the arbitrary motion of water molecules within a given tissue and has recently attracted attention as a tool for the early detection of infarction or brain trauma. A simple (although obsolete) diffusion weighted spin-echo sequence is illustrated in Fig. 1.27. As discussed before, imaging involves the application of gradients, causing a dephasing of the magnetization, followed by a rephasing gradient, refocusing the magnetization again for stationary tissue. If the water molecule has moved between the two gradients, the phase history will be different and the refocusing insufficient, causing a signal loss. In order to enhance this effect, relatively large gradients are necessary. Since physiological or global motion causes changes of magnitude higher than that of diffusion, diffusion-weighted imaging today is solely applied in conjunction with fast or ultra-fast imaging techniques.

1.1.1.5
Imaging Protocols and Image Quality

The progress in MR imaging not only increases the number of imaging sequences designed for specific pathologies, it also provides a significant number of

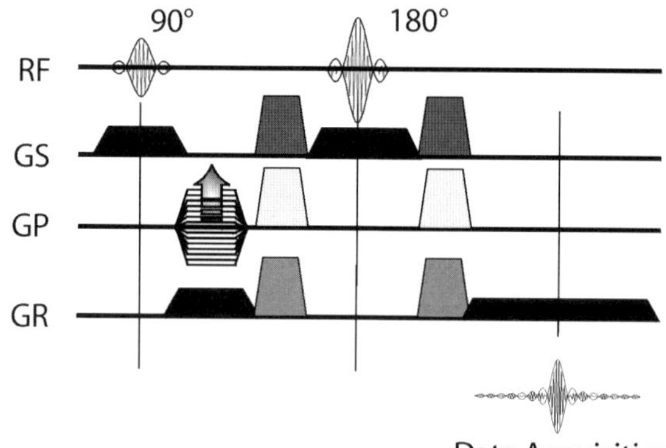

Fig. 1.27. The simple although obsolete Stejskal-Tanner approach for creating diffusion weighted spin-echo images: Applying identical gradients, centered around a 180° RF refocusing pulse, will create a diffusion-weighted image. For molecules that have moved in between or during the switching of the magnetic field gradients, the rephasing (refocusing) remains incomplete. Tissue areas with a higher diffusion will appear hypointense on diffusion-weighted images

imaging parameters that will allow the improvement of the SNR of an image and may speed up the examination time.

- Magnetic field B_0: The higher the field strength, the higher the basic signal. This SNR advantage is decreased due to the higher bandwidth used in high-field imaging. There are other disadvantages for a high-field system, including an increase in costs and an increase of power deposition to the patient.
- Sequence $[(1 - e^{-T_R/T1(B_0)}) \cdot e^{-T_E/T2}]$: The signal contribution corresponds to the sequence type utilized, in this case a SE sequence. To differentiate lesions, it is not enough to have a good SNR; the contrast between two different tissue types is also of importance. The contrast is given by

$$\text{CNR} = \frac{|S_A - S_B|}{\sigma}.$$

  with S_A and S_B being the signal from tissue A and tissue B, and σ being the standard deviation of the noise within the image. The optimization of the contrast depends on the type of image desired. For a Pd-W image, the contribution of a T1 or T2 difference is minimized. The shortest possible TE is usually dictated by hardware limitations. The repetition is usually a compromise between almost no T1 influence and a reasonable measurement time. The same argument serves for the optimization of a T2-WI protocol. Along with the T2-W, a reasonable display of the morphology is also preferred. The theoretical optimization of a T1-W image may lead to a TR which is too short to do a multi-slice measurement with the necessary coverage. The commonly used protocols tend to be a compromise, using as many slices as necessary to cover the region of interest, selecting the shortest possible TR, or using a TR that provides a reasonable measurement time.
- $\sqrt{Acq}$: The number of acquisitions, as they show up in the protocol dialog, contribute proportionally to the square root to the overall SNR. Intuitively, it can be assumed that each acquisition is collecting true signal as well as noise. With an additional acquisition, the signal is collected again, and the received noise may correspond to different frequencies, not remaining at the same location of the previously collected noise. With each acquisition, the probability increases that the noise pattern has similarities with previous measurements, adding up at the same location.

Table 1.2 lists the influence of the TR, TE, and number of acquisitions on SNR and CNR.

- Slice thickness, FoV, and matrix size. This is basically the achieved spatial resolution. The signal intensity emitted by a single voxel depends on the number of protons involved. The latter scales linearly with the slice thickness. The FoV corresponds to the length of the image in the direction of frequency encoding and the length of the image in the direction of phase encoding. With a constant matrix size, the larger the FoV, the bigger the voxel, and the better the SNR. The matrix size dictates into what portions the FoV is to be split up. The lower the matrix size, the better the SNR, and the faster the imaging time. Everything occurs at the expense of the spatial resolution.
- Matrix size, lines, and columns. The basic matrix size dictates the size of the pixel and the number of protons involved. However, each measured Fourier line contains the information of the whole object and can be considered one acquisition. Reducing the number of lines when moving to a rectangular matrix will linearly increase the voxel size, the number of protons involved causing an increase in signal amplitude. However, the number of acquisitions will decrease as well, slightly diminishing the SNR gain achieved with the increase in voxel size.

The effects of the various parameters mainly responsible for spatial resolution and measurement time are listed in Table 1.3.

- Surface coils: The dominant source of noise is the patient. Even though a single slice is excited, a coil will pick up any noise that is within the coil range. The advantage of small surface coils is that they have a limited range and will, therefore, pick up less noise. The disadvantage of small surface coils is that they have a limited range and may not cover the whole area of interest. The solution is that several small coils can be connected with each other in a so-called phase-array concept. A dangerous trap is to select as many coils as possible to ensure that everything is covered at the expense of SNR since more noise is collected, too. So far, we have only considered the

Table 1.2. The optimum repetition time (TR) and echo time (TE) in spin echo imaging for differentiating between two different tissues (gray matter, GM, and white matter, WM)

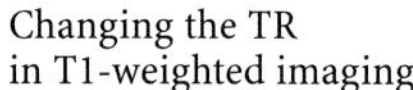

Changing the TR in T1-weighted imaging	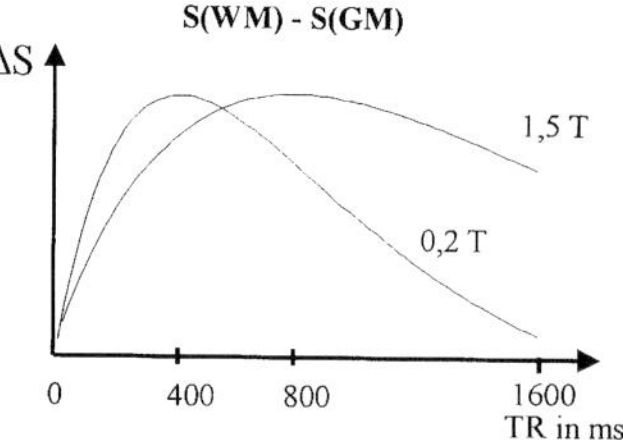	Increasing the TR will increase the overall signal due to recovery. It will allow the acquisition of more slices to the expense of measurement time or to the expense of T1-weighting (signal difference) if selected to be longer than the optimum shown in the left graph
Considering a constant measurement time	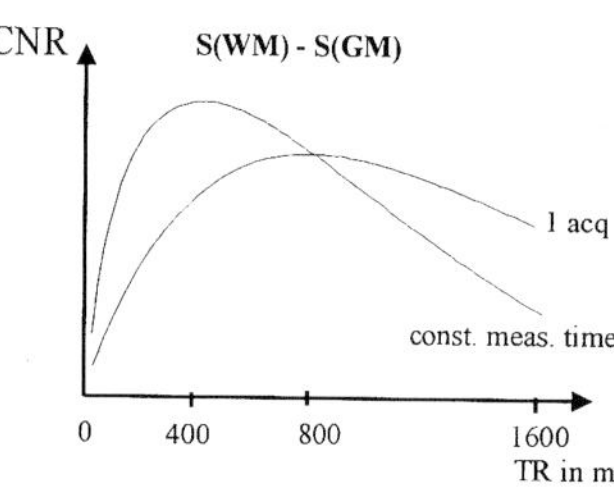	Keeping the measurement time constant, increasing the number of acquisitions when reducing the TR, the optimum CNR is to be found at lower TR. The CNR for T1-weighted imaging optimally differentiating GM from WM is higher for a 400 ms TR with two acquisitions than for a TR of 800 ms with one acquisition (1.5 T system)
Selecting the optimum TE for T2-weighted imaging	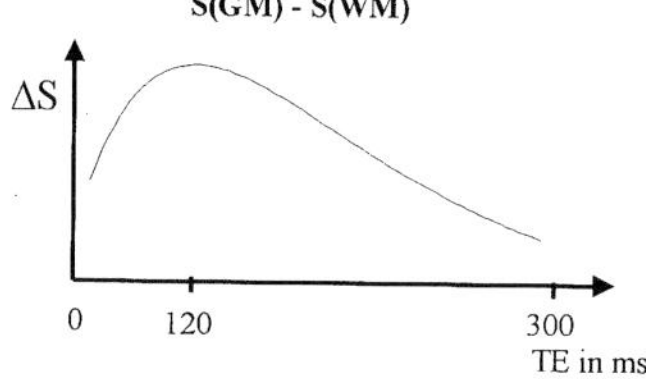	The optimum TE to differentiate GM from WM is approximately 120 ms. The graph to the left shows an exaggerated maximum (optimum). The change in signal difference between 80 ms and 140 ms is almost negligible

T1 Variable for the tissue specific spin-lattice relaxation time; *CNR*, contrast to noise ratio

Table 1.3. Signal-to-noise ratio (SNR), spatial resolution and measurement time as a function of protocol parameters used to specify the spatial resolution, reduce measurement time or avoid wrap in artifacts

	Measurement time	Spatial resolution	SNR
Increasing the slice thickness	↔	↓	↑
Increasing the field of view	↔	↓	↑
Increasing the matrix size	↑	↑	↓
Utilizing a matrix asymmetry, e.g., 256×256→128×256	↓	↓	↑
Using a rectangular field of view, e.g., 8/8→6/8	↓	↔	↓
Utilizing phase oversampling	↑	↔	↑

two-dimensional motion of the macroscopic magnetization, ignoring the existence of a three-dimensional space. Taking advantage of the three-dimensional motion of the macroscopic magnetization will lead to the introduction of circular polarization. The advantage of this concept is that the measurement within an orthogonal plane adds another acquisition without an increase in measurement time, merely due to the coil concept, to the coil design.

- $1/\sqrt{\Delta\nu}$: The frequency range per pixel, also called bandwidth, is a parameter that dictates the length of the data acquisition window and is responsible for the noise that is going to be picked up. Noise is to be found at every frequency. A high bandwidth corresponds to a large frequency range, and more noise is picked up. Similar to the number of acquisitions, the noise level is proportional to the square root of the selected bandwidth. The SNR is, therefore, inversely proportional to the square root of the bandwidth.

1.1.1.6 Basic Elements of a Magnetic Resonance Scanner

As illustrated in Fig. 1.28, some hardware is needed to perform the above-mentioned tasks. In order to generate a macroscopic magnetization, a magnet is needed with a power supply for the initial ramping of the magnet during installation or in the case of major maintenance. In order to reduce the boil-off rate of the cryogen necessary for super-conducting magnets, there is usually a refrigerator system with a cold head. Newer generations of magnets work with helium only. Older generations have a two-chamber construction, the first containing helium and the second nitrogen. Both are within vacuum chambers to avoid thermal contact with the room. Other magnet types produce a magnetic field via an electric current and are called resistive systems, and even fewer have a permanent magnetic field using an assemblage of permanent magnets. For resistive and permanent systems, the field strength is limited to 0.3 T or less. Systems of 0.5 T or more utilize the phenomenon of superconductivity. Residing within the magnet bore are the gradient coils that provide the magnetic field gradient discussed previously. Also within the bore are usually the so-called shim coils. These help to improve the homogeneity of the main field within the region of interest. A body coil is also located within the bore of the magnet, usually serving as a transmit coil; in the worst case it also acts as a receive coil if no other suitable coil is available or if a whole body scout is desired.

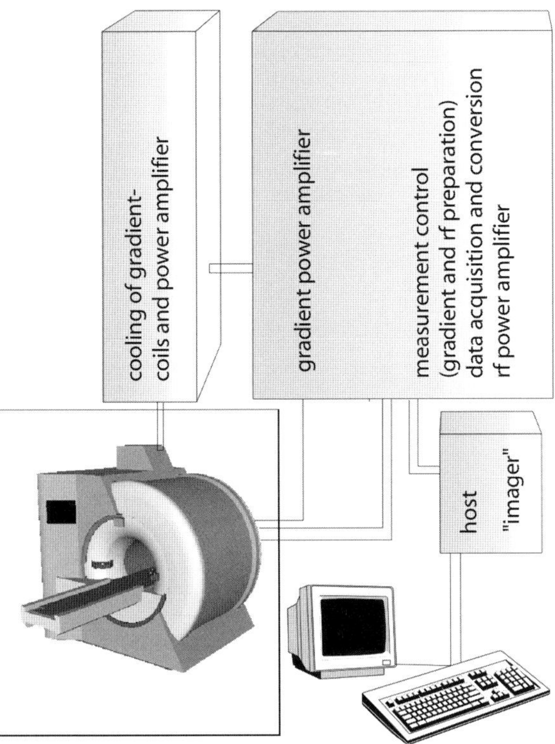

Fig. 1.28. Basic elements of a magnetic resonance scanner. Besides the magnet with the attached patient table, there is the operating console where the protocols are selected and initiated and where the images are viewed and archived. There is usually a so-called host computer handling these tasks. Adjacent to the host is usually a specialized computer called an imager, which does nothing else but image reconstruction and image data administration. The whole measurement is controlled by a so-called measurement control unit which is assigned the task by the host

In order to run the gradient system, a gradient controller and a power amplifier are required. For the RF application, an RF controller and a power amplifier are necessary. A small signal cabinet deals with the incoming signal. A dedicated computer controls the gradient and RF tasks as well as the data reception. Another computer called the 'imager' is usually geared towards image reconstruction. A third computer is called the 'host' and handles the user interface and the management of patient data as well as the imaging sequences and protocols.

A prerequisite for some of the newer fast-imaging sequences has been the progress in hardware development. One of the more dramatic steps has been the introduction of actively shielded gradients for the super-conducting systems built after 1992. Without active shielding, eddy currents induced by the switching gradients were prohibitive in the implementation of faster imaging sequences.

The improvement in hardware that followed was aimed at stronger gradient systems with faster switching times in order to speed up the imaging time or introduce new potential applications. At this point, it seems that the patient rather than the progress in hardware development is the limiting factor in fast imaging. Theoretically, the gradients could switch fast and high enough to cause nerve stimulation and muscle contraction within the patient. Practically, the gradient systems have safety monitors in order to prevent this happening.

More impressive progress has been made with the introduction of circular polarized coils and phased-array technology. Circular polarization takes into account that the excitation as well as the reception are not limited to one dimension but can be extended to two dimensions in order to reduce the SAR during excitation and improve the SNR during reception.

It is well known that a small surface coil will impressively improve the SNR for a targeted region. The biggest source of noise is the patient. With a large coil, a significant volume of potential noise sources is seen, while a small surface coil is sensitive to a confined region. Being limited to a smaller region is also a disadvantage for small surface coils. A solution has been introduced with the phased-array concept. Multiple small surface coils, often circularly polarized, can be used together in a so-called array coil. With this concept, it is possible to cover a larger region and still have the advantage of an improved SNR compared with a body coil. Nevertheless, it must be pointed out that the larger the region covered, the more noise is picked up, reducing the overall SNR. Another disadvantage of the small confined region with a limited depth penetration (which avoids picking up RF noise) is the inhomogeneous signal contribution. Tissue further away from the coil will contribute less signal than the same tissue close to the coil. Although viewing this signal course on the monitor with the flexibility of changing the windowing as desired might not be a problem, it is often difficult to document the result on film. A solution to this obstacle has been introduced with the so-called 'normalization filter' adjustable to specific applications.

1.1.2 Imaging Sequences, Acronyms and Clinical Applications

Fortunately, all of the imaging techniques presently applied, at least the ones currently used in clinical routine, are based on Fourier encoding. The acquired, unprocessed data are stored in a raw data matrix and form the so-called *k*-space. As discussed in the previous chapter and as illustrated in Fig. 1.29, the imaging sequences can be divided into a SE group and a gradient-echo (GRE) group. Within each group, we have the conventional single-echo approaches and the more contemporary multi-echo approaches. Within each of these, we also find applications that require a preparation of the magnetization. We also note two groups in which spin echoes as well as gradient echoes are utilized to generate an image. Table 1.4 presents the pulse

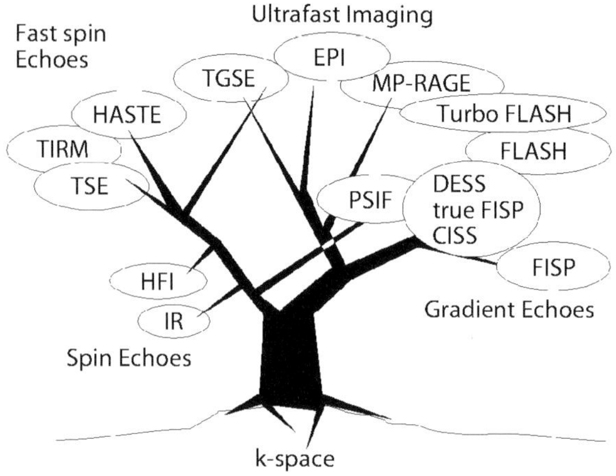

Fig. 1.29. The sequence tree. To keep it from being too confusing, only the acronyms of one vendor (*SIEMENS*) have been illustrated within this sequence tree. The two main branches are the spin-echo branch and the gradient-echo branch. With turbo-gradient spin-echo (TGSE), there is a mixture between gradient echoes and spin echoes, ditto for the echo planar imaging (EPI) approach within a spin-echo envelope. For the steady state techniques (*PSIF*, a backwards running FISP; *DESS*, double-echo steady state sequence; true*FISP*, true fast imaging with steady-state precession), we also find spin-echo contributions within a gradient-echo branch

Table 1.4. Pulse sequence classification

<table>
<tr><th></th><th>Spin-echo sequences</th><th>Gradient-echo sequences</th></tr>
<tr><td>Single-echo techniques</td><td>CSE</td><td>GRE
FLASH
FISP</td></tr>
<tr><td></td><td colspan="2">PSIF
DESS
CISS
trueFISP</td></tr>
<tr><td>Single-echo techniques with magnetization preparation</td><td>IR
IRM
STIR</td><td>turboFLASH (TFL)
MP-RAGE</td></tr>
<tr><td>Multi-echo techniques</td><td>TSE</td><td>segmented EPI</td></tr>
<tr><td></td><td colspan="2">GRASE
TGSE</td></tr>
<tr><td>Multi-echo techniques with magnetization preparation</td><td>TIR, TIRM,
turboSTIR
turboFLAIR</td><td>segmented IR-EPI
segmented DW-EPI</td></tr>
<tr><td>Single-shot techniques</td><td>HASTE</td><td>EPI</td></tr>
<tr><td>Single-shot techniques with magnetization preparation</td><td>HASTIRM</td><td>IR-EPI
DW-EPI</td></tr>
</table>

sequence classification scheme using Siemens sequence acronyms.

1.1.2.1 Conventional Spin-Echo Imaging (CSE)

The basic concept of SE imaging has been introduced in Sect. 1.1.1.3, referring to Fig. 1.18. A slice-select gradient is switched on prior to a slice-selective RF pulse. This is followed by the phase-encoding gradient, during which the dephasing in the direction of read-out is also prepared. The 180° slice-selective refocusing pulse inverts the accumulated dephasing, causing the appearance of a SE, usually in the middle of the acquisition window with the frequency-encoding gradient being activated. This step is repeated with different phase-encoding steps and as often as averages are requested by the user.

1.1.2.2 Magnetization-Prepared Spin-Echo Sequences, the Inversion Recovery Techniques

The IR techniques have already been discussed in Sect. 1.1.1.4. IR techniques use a 180°-inversion pulse prior to the SE imaging sequence to manipulate the contrast. The preparation is repeated prior to each Fourier line measurement. IR techniques that consider the position of the macroscopic magnetization (parallel or antiparallel to the direction of the main field) during image reconstruction are called true IR techniques and are usually utilized to improve the T1-W contrast between gray and white matter. IR techniques that only take the absolute value of the prepared magnetization into account are called IR techniques with utilization of the magnitude of the signal (IRM). Sequences with a short inversion time for fat-suppressed imaging are called STIR techniques and those that attenuate the signal from fluid are called FLAIR techniques.

1.1.2.3 Gradient-Echo Imaging (GRE)

Various imaging techniques have been explored in an effort to obtain images faster. The group of GRE sequences was assigned to the fast imaging techniques at the time they were introduced. Today these are considered 'conventional'. In conventional imaging, the measurement time is given by the TR multiplied by the number of desired Fourier lines times the number of acquisitions. Reducing the TR to speed up the measurement usually generates a SAR problem, at least on a high-field system. Eliminating the RF refocusing pulse, as indicated in Fig. 1.30, will avoid that problem at the expense of dephasing mechanisms contributing to the contrast. The dephasing mechanisms now appearing are fixed in location and stable over time and are refocused with the 180° refocusing pulse in SE imaging. The transverse relaxation time, without the RF refocusing pulse, is referred to as T2*. This includes the dephasing due to T2 as well as the additional mechanisms due to

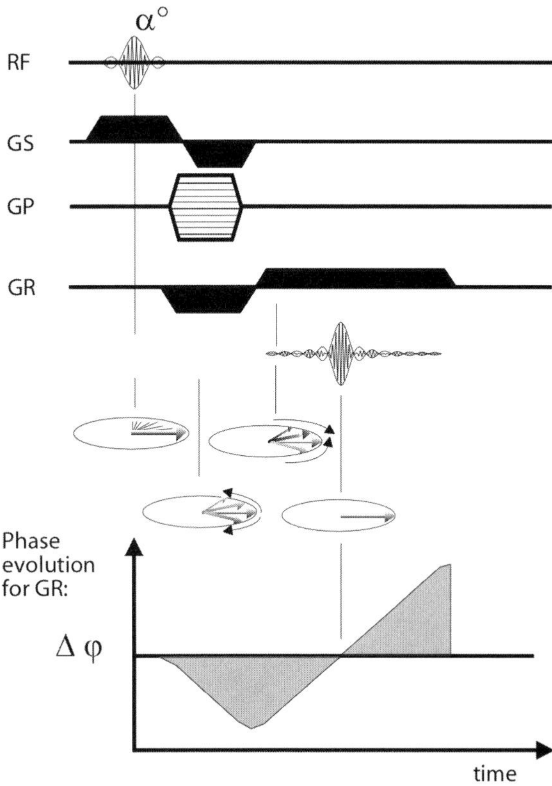

Fig. 1.30. The gradient-echo sequence (GRE). Compared with the spin-echo sequence, the refocusing pulse has been removed. This will lead to a potential shortening of the echo time and repetition time. Since there is a dephasing during slice-selective excitation, a negative lobe has been added for GS to compensate for the dephasing. The order of phase-encoding steps is now reversed, and the gradient lobe for the read-out gradient preparing the dephasing is now also of opposite polarity. The two bipolar lobes of the frequency-encoding gradient GR recall a so-called gradient echo. *GP,* phase-encoding gradient; *GR,* read-out gradient; *GS,* slice-selection gradient; *RF,* radiofrequency

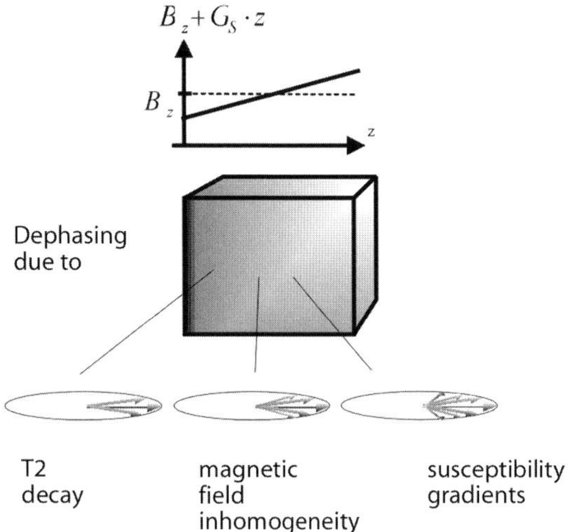

Fig. 1.31. T2* dephasing mechanisms. With gradient-echo imaging, all the dephasing effects that are compensated with the 180° refocusing pulse in SE imaging have to be considered. The T2 decay is identical for both imaging techniques. Any existing magnetic field inhomogeneity will add to the dephasing. The major contribution to T2* comes from the patient, mainly due to local variations of susceptibility. Susceptibility is the ability of tissue to become magnetized

susceptibility gradients, magnet inhomogeneities, etc. as illustrated in Fig. 1.31. This leads to the disadvantage of being sensitive to susceptibility gradients as they are found at bone/tissue or air/tissue interfaces, often leading to a total signal loss in the vicinity of these areas (Fig. 1.32). This increased sensitivity turns into an advantage when looking for hemorrhagic lesions. For ultra-fast imaging, the distortions due to field inhomogeneities turn out to be a major limitation.

Another interesting phenomenon that needs to be mentioned in conjunction with GRE imaging is the so-called in-phase/opposed-phase situation. As previously discussed, the nuclei (protons) of fat and water-bounded hydrogen atoms have a slightly different resonance frequency. Starting with the excitation, the macroscopic magnetization of the water will speed ahead in the transverse plane, while the fat-originated magnetization falls behind. In SE imaging, this is not a problem since the 180° refocusing pulse will place the slower fat component in front of the faster water component. At the time the echo is acquired, they will both be in phase again. In that case, only the shift between the fat and water image remains, depending on the selected bandwidth per pixel. Eliminating the 180° refocusing, the dephasing of the water-originated magnetization and the fat-originated magnetization will continue, starting with the excitation. Depending on the TE, a situation will develop in which the magnetization of fat and water will point in the same direction. This situation is called in-phase. There will also be the other extreme, where the magnetization from fat is pointing in the opposite direction to that from water. This situation is called opposed phase. Depending on the content of fat and water in a single voxel, the residual magnetization from fat and water may be zero, leading to a signal void. The TE-dependent in-phase/opposed-phase situation in GRE imaging is a function of the difference in resonance frequencies between the magnetization of the fat-bounded hydrogen atoms (nuclei) and the water-bounded hydrogen atoms (nuclei). Depending on the type of fat molecule, this difference ranges from 3.2 ppm to 3.5 ppm. Table 1.5 lists the standard suitable TEs to achieve an in-phase or opposed-phase situa-

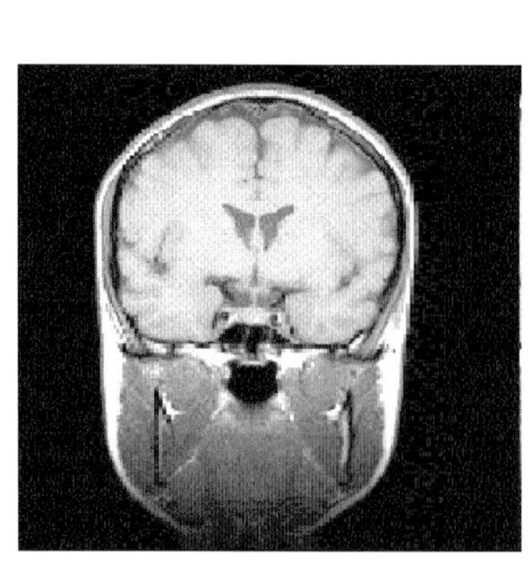

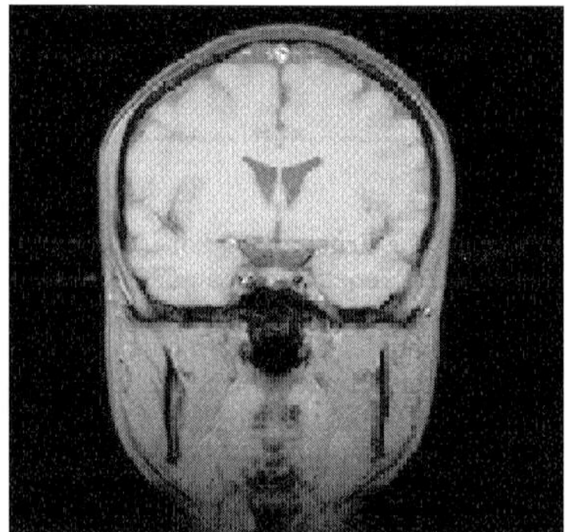

Fig. 1.32. Signal loss in areas of large susceptibility gradients, apparent on gradient-echo imaging. These coronal-head images show an impressive signal loss in the region of the skull base with identical sequence parameters, with the exception of a missing refocusing pulse in the fast low-angle shot sequence (FLASH)

Table 1.5. Echo times for in-phase and opposed-phase situation for different field strength. These are theoretical values based on a water-methylen two component system. For some fat-molecules and fat infiltrated tissue there may be a slight difference compared to these theoretical values leading to a nonperfect in-phase or opposed-phase situation with increasing echo time and may require some tests for selecting the optimal echo time. The first in-phase situation is of course the time immediately following the excitation at a theoretical echo time of 0 ms

Field strength	Difference frequency	First opposed-phase situation at a TE of	Second in-phase situation at a TE of	Second opposed-phase situation at a TE of
0.2 T	29 Hz	17.3 ms	34.5 ms	51.8 ms
0.35 T	51 Hz	9.85 ms	19.7 ms	29.6 ms
0.5 T	72 Hz	6.9 ms	13.8 ms	20.7 ms
1.0 T	144 Hz	3.45 ms	6.9 ms	10.4 ms
1.5 T	217 Hz	2.3 ms	4.6 ms	6.9 ms

tion, depending on the field strength of the MR system used.

Reducing the repetition time will result in a loss of SNR, since the longitudinal magnetization has only a limited time for recovery. Well known from spectroscopy is the fact that excitation angles less than 90° tend to give a higher signal contribution. The excitation angle with a maximum signal response is also called the Ernst angle and is illustrated in Fig. 1.33. A GRE technique in conjunction with a low angle excitation has been named 'fast low angle shot' (FLASH). Various applications of this FLASH technique can be found throughout the book, primarily for musculoskeletal imaging, abdominal breath-hold techniques, dynamic imaging of the heart, studying the temporal course of enhancement after contrast media application, and MRA. With the potential of utilizing short TRs, another application arises: the possibility of acquiring a 3D data set. The image reconstruction software does not care about the direction in which the phase-encoding step has been applied. In order to distinguish two orthogonal phase-encoding directions, the only prerequisite is that for each phase-encoding step in one direction, all the encoding steps in the other direction have to be repeated, as illustrated in Fig. 1.34. The advantage of 3D data acquisition is the gapless coverage of a volume of interest. As there is no gap between adjacent pixels within an image, there is also no gap from one slice to the next for a 3D sequence, in this case referred to as partition instead of slice. The other advantage is that each meas-

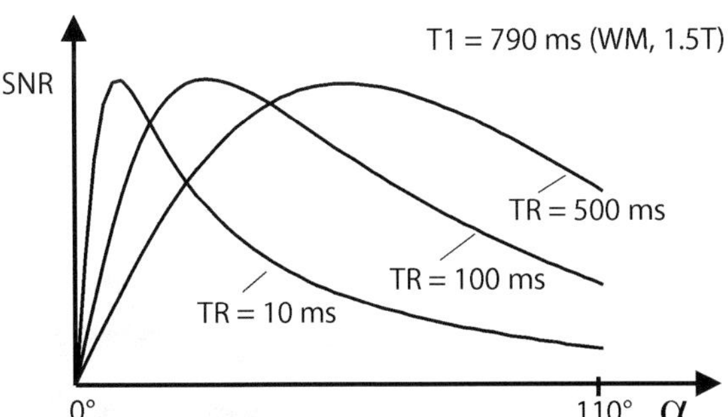

Fig. 1.33. The Ernst angle. For a given tissue (T1 relaxation time) and a given repetition time (*TR*), there is always one excitation angle where the signal response is maximal. This angle is called the Ernst angle. The above curves are normalized to the same measurement time (10 ms TR, 50 acquisitions compared with 500 ms TR, 1 acquisition). For a TR of 10 ms, the optimal angle would be 10°, whereas for the 500 ms TR sequence, the maximal signal response would be achieved with an excitation angle of 58°. This Ernst angle approach is utilized in musculoskeletal imaging as well as for time of flight magnetic resonance angiography. *SNR*, signal-to-noise ratio

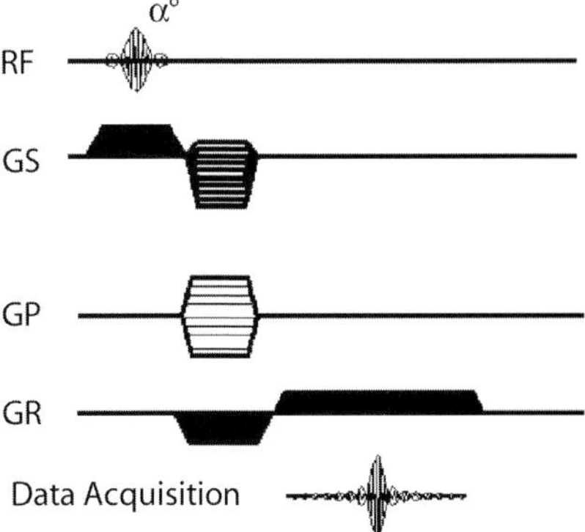

Fig. 1.34. 3D data acquisition. The 2D loop structure is supplemented with a phase-encoding step in the direction of slice selection *GS*. The phase-encoding table is symmetrical, the asymmetric position to the zero line compensates for the dephasing during slice selective excitation. *GP*, phase-encoding gradient; *GR*, readout gradient; *GS*, slice-selection gradient; *RF*, radiofrequency

ured line contains information of the whole object and, therefore, contributes to a better SNR. The only prerequisite for 3D data acquisition is the possibility of a reasonably short repetition time in order to acquire all the necessary phase-encoding steps in a reasonable measurement time.

1.1.2.4 Steady-State Techniques

The FLASH concept evolved while studying steady-state techniques in order to image faster. The steady state for the FLASH concept refers to the longitudinal magnetization. The first excitation pulse will utilize the full magnetization. Since it is a low flip angle, the projection of the tilted magnetization onto the *z*-axis will remain as longitudinal magnetization and will grow pending the recovery or relaxation rate until the next excitation reduces the longitudinal magnetization even further, as illustrated in Fig. 1.35. The more the longitudinal magnetization is reduced, the higher the relaxation rate. After a few excitations, the relaxation rate will be high enough to compensate for the reduction of the longitudinal magnetization caused by the excitation pulse. At that point, a steady state is reached. Utilizing an even lower flip angle, the differences in T1-based recovery can be minimized, achieving a T2*-W impression even with a short repetition time (Fig. 1.36). Using a relatively small excitation angle, the macroscopic magnetization remains close to equilibrium, and the T1 relaxation rate is very small, almost independent of the T1 value. The T1 influence is then suppressed, and the T2* difference will dominate within the image contrast, as desired in T2(*)-WI.

For a larger flip angle, there is the potential of a significant residual transverse magnetization after completion of the Fourier line measurement. In order not to interfere with the next measurement, the transverse magnetization is destroyed using a gradient spoiler or RF spoiling.

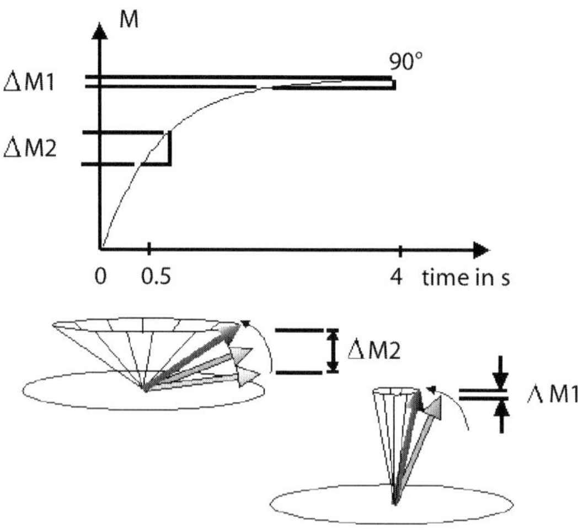

Fig. 1.35. The steady-state concept. The relaxation rate, the amount of recovery per unit time, depends on whether the longitudinal magnetization is far away from the fully relaxed state (ΔM_2) or close to equilibrium (ΔM_1). Between rapid excitations with low flip angle, the magnetization will recover with the relaxation rate at that position of the relaxation curve. If the amount of longitudinal magnetization that is reduced due to a low flip-angle excitation is larger than the recovered magnetization between two excitations, the remaining longitudinal magnetization will be reduced, getting further away from equilibrium. The latter will increase the relaxation rate. This process will continue until the relaxation rate is high enough that the amount of recovered magnetization is identical to the amount of longitudinal magnetization reduced by the low-angle excitation. For each Fourier line, the same magnitude of transverse magnetization is now projected onto the *x-y* plane. That situation is called steady state

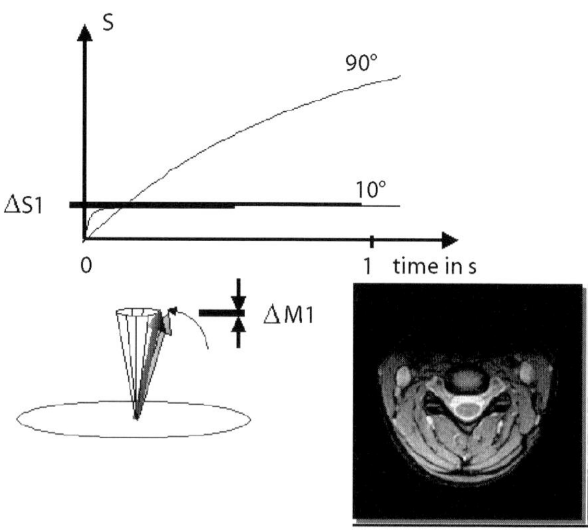

Fig. 1.36. T2*-weighted imaging with FLASH. Working with very low flip-angle excitation, e.g., 10°, the longitudinal magnetization remains close to equilibrium even with TRs as short as 120 ms. Staying close to equilibrium means a small relaxation rate. The T1 influence is suppressed. The same situation is achieved in T2-weighted SE imaging. A long repetition time is selected in SE imaging to avoid the T1 influence in T2-weighted scans. As a consequence, low-angle GRE imaging allows T2*-weighted measurements with very short repetition times. ΔM, the recovered longitudinal magnetization; ΔS, the signal induced by the projection of the longitudinal magnetization onto the *x-y* plane

Another technique uses the residual transverse magnetization by not destroying the magnetization at the end of the measured Fourier line but rephasing the part that has been dephased for the purpose of spatial encoding. Such a sequence is called fast imaging with steady-state precession (FISP) and is illustrated in Fig. 1.37. The original idea was to rephase all three dimensions, the phase-encoding direction, the slice-selection direction, and the frequency-encoding direction. However, the implementation had to be postponed until recent progress was made in hardware development. The implemented sequence based on the original idea is called a trueFISP (Fig. 1.38). In order to get a trueFISP contrast, a large flip angle and a short TR have to be selected. The constructive interference steady-

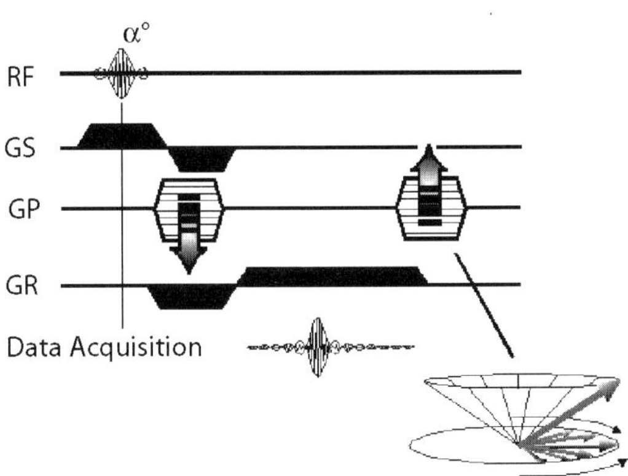

Fig. 1.37. Fast imaging with steady-state precession (FISP). The dephasing with the phase-encoding gradient, done for the purpose of spatial encoding, is rephased after data acquisition. A steady state will build up for the transverse component. Compared with FLASH, an improved signal contribution is achieved for tissue with a long T2*, using a protocol with a short repetition time and a large flip angle. *GP*, phase-encoding gradient; *GR*, read-out gradient; *GS*, slice-selection gradient; *RF*, radiofrequency

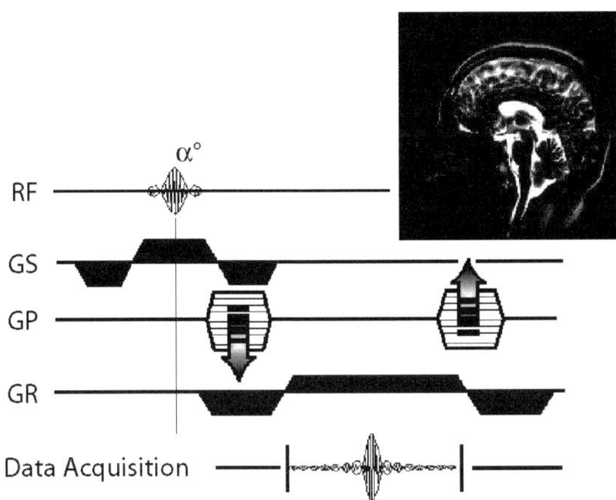

Fig. 1.38. The true fast imaging with steady-state precession (trueFISP) is the originally suggested FISP. Rephasing all components within the direction of slice selection, the direction of phase encoding, and the direction of read out, the contribution of the steady state of the transverse magnetization is maximized. This sagittal image has been acquired within 4 s, using trueFISP. Minor field inhomogeneities will cause a destructive interference pattern. *GP*, phase-encoding gradient; *GR*, read-out gradient; *GS*, slice-selection gradient; *RF*, radiofrequency

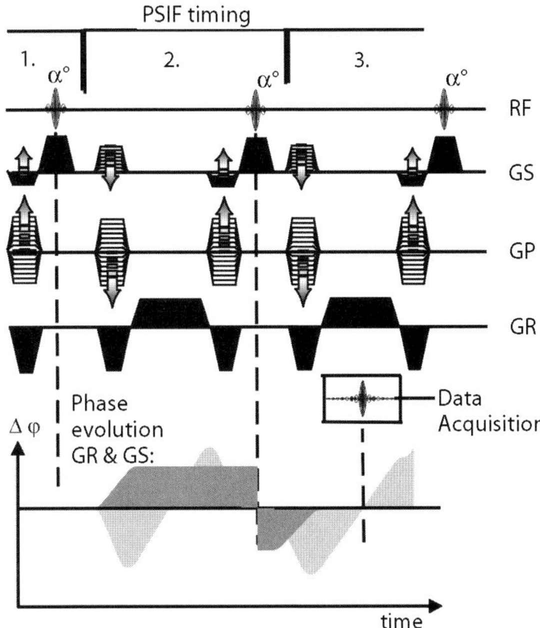

Fig. 1.39. The backward-running fast imaging with steady-state precession (PSIF) technique. The timing for the PSIF (2) sequence looks like a backwards running FISP. This fact is also the explanation for the acronym. First comes the phase encoding, then the data acquisition followed by the excitation – a violation of causality. In order to understand the signal generation, three consecutive loops (1–3) have to be discussed. The transverse magnetization is generated at the end of the first loop (1). For the read-out period of the second loop, the transverse magnetization is dephased by the variable pulse *GS* at the beginning of the sequence. The RF pulse at the end of the second loop operates not only as the excitation pulse, but also as the refocusing pulse. The following variable pulse *GS* refocuses the dephasing in the direction of slice selection, and the *GR* gradient timing of the third loop (3) refocuses the echo in the center of the data acquisition window. Since a radiofrequency pulse has been used for refocusing, this is a spin echo. The echo time for this sequence is almost two repetition times. The sequence provides a heavy T2 weighting. *GP*, phase-encoding gradient; *GR*, read-out gradient; *GS*, slice-selection gradient; *RF*, radiofrequency

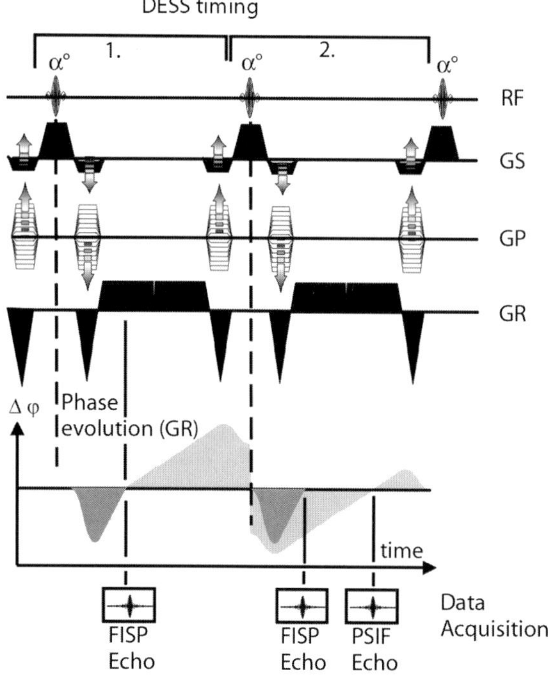

Fig. 1.40. The double-echo steady-state sequence (DESS). DESS combines the fast imaging with steady-state precession (FISP) echo with the backward-running fast imaging with steady-state precession (PSIF) echo, collecting the data out of two directly adjacent acquisition windows. The first loop generates a FISP echo and the transverse magnetization for the PSIF echo, which is refocused with the excitation pulse of the next loop and read out within the second acquisition window. The two images are combined, to add the T2-weighting of the PSIF echo to the FISP image. *GP,* phase-encoding gradient; *GR,* readout gradient; *GS,* slice-selection gradient; *RF,* radiofrequency

state (CISS) sequence is an attempt to eliminate the destructive interference artifacts in a non-perfect trueFISP approach. Utilization of the SE part in steady-state approaches is possible using a PSIF technique (Fig. 1.39). A separate acquisition of the GRE part and the SE part, combining both signal contributions during image reconstruction, is called double-echo steady state (DESS) (Fig. 1.40) and is applied in musculoskeletal imaging. An impressive documentation of the above-mentioned contributions is given in Fig. 1.41. Starting with the FLASH, the transverse component in FISP is adding to the signal of tissue with a long T2*, and DESS increases that signal intensity even further in adding a heavily T2-W SE component.

1.1.2.5
Magnetization-Prepared Gradient-Echo Techniques

The fastest way to acquire an image with a conventional GRE sequence would be to select a high bandwidth, requesting only a small data-acquisition window, selecting a minimum TE, and selecting the shortest possible TR. In order to achieve any signal at all, the Ernst angle needs to be selected. Such a sequence would provide a boring proton density-like contrast. In order to reestablish the contrast, an inversion pulse is used prior to the data acquisition, but not prior to each Fourier line as in IR imaging, rather as a preparation preceding the rapid acquisition of all Fourier lines, as illustrated in Fig. 1.42. With this approach, T1-W can be reintroduced, similar to the improvement achieved in IR imag-

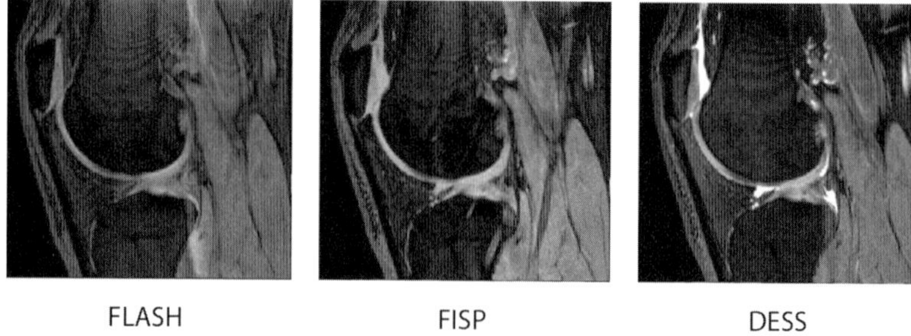

Fig. 1.41. FLASH, FISP, DESS comparison. Sagittal cuts of the knee demonstrate the clinically relevant difference between the fast low-angle shot sequence (FLASH), fast imaging with steady-state precession (FISP), and double-echo steady-state sequence (DESS). Starting with the FLASH, the transverse steady-state component of FISP provides a higher signal intensity for tissue with a longer T2*. The heavily T2-weighted, spin-echo component of the DESS technique that is added to the FISP component acquired simultaneously clearly demonstrates the advantage of this technique. DESS apparently allows a better delineation between fat, cartilage, and joint effusion. *GP,* phase-encoding gradient; *GR,* read-out gradient; *GS,* slice-selection gradient; *RF,* radiofrequency

ing. Each Fourier line, each spatial frequency is measured at a different point in time along the relaxation curve following the inversion. The dominant contrast will be given by the time the low spatial frequencies are acquired. Since the higher spatial frequencies usually contribute significantly different signal amplitudes, turboFLASH images are slightly blurred. This technique is used today as a very fast localizer and is also utilized in tracing the passage of contrast media, monitoring perfusion, or lesion enhancement. The time to acquire a 3D data set is too long for a reasonable contribution of the preparation pulse. The preparation scheme for a 3D approach is, therefore, slightly altered compared with the 2D method and is illustrated in Fig. 1.43. The preparation pulse is placed prior to each depth-encoding loop and repeated after a recovery time for the next depth-encoding loop with a different in-plane phase-encoding step. This technique provides the possibility of achieving a better T1-W than with SE, covering the whole head in about 5 min with no gap. The reason why this sequence did not replace T1-W-SE imaging is the fact that it is a GRE sequence and reacts differently to contrast-media application than SE imaging. The advantage of MPRAGE is that the signal contribution for each phase-encoding step in the plane is constant, presenting an artifact-free image similar to a conventional GRE technique. The signal variation due to the data collection along a relaxation curve is effective along the direction of depth encoding and only visible if a multi-planar reconstruction is performed in that direction. The other advantage of this technique is the control over the T1-weighting via the inversion time, providing a better contrast than possible in SE imaging.

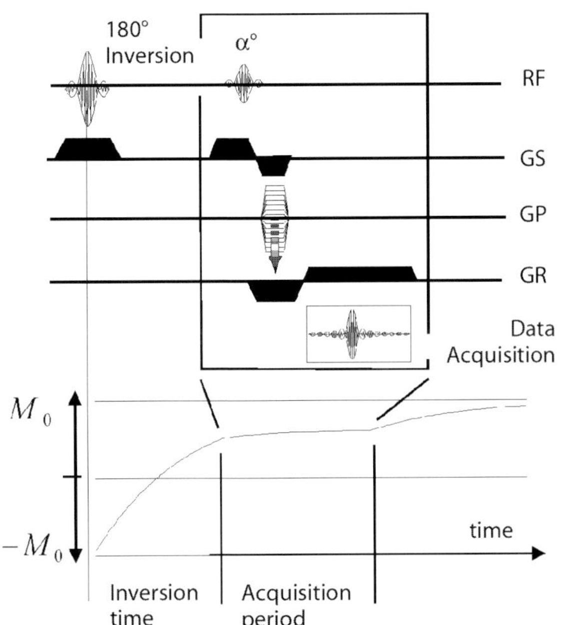

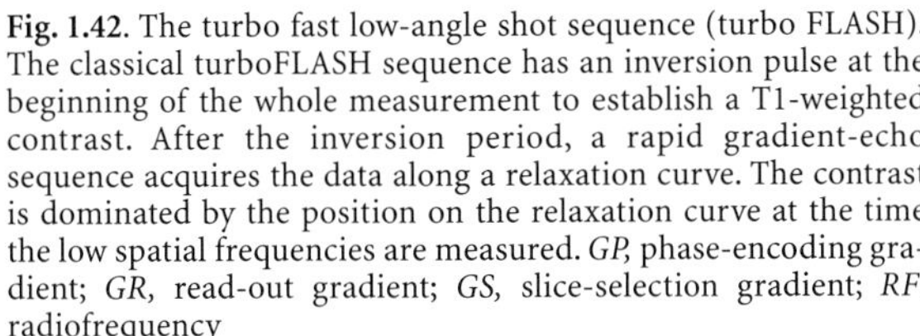

Fig. 1.42. The turbo fast low-angle shot sequence (turbo FLASH). The classical turboFLASH sequence has an inversion pulse at the beginning of the whole measurement to establish a T1-weighted contrast. After the inversion period, a rapid gradient-echo sequence acquires the data along a relaxation curve. The contrast is dominated by the position on the relaxation curve at the time the low spatial frequencies are measured. *GP*, phase-encoding gradient; *GR*, read-out gradient; *GS*, slice-selection gradient; *RF*, radiofrequency

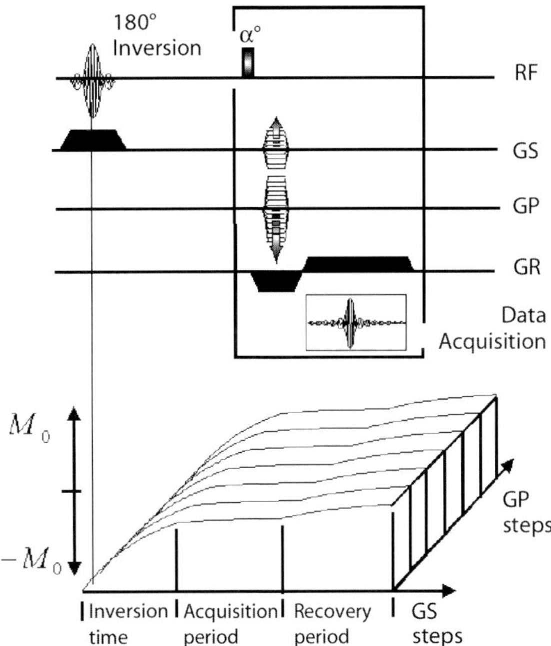

Fig. 1.43. The magnetization-prepared rapid-acquired gradient-echoes (MPRAGE) sequence design. An inversion pulse is placed prior to each *GP* loop. The *GS* loops are then executed, collecting data along a relaxation curve. After a recovery time, the next *GP* value is selected, the inversion pulse applied, and the *GS* loops repeated. The classical MPRAGE sequence uses a nonselective low flip-angle excitation, allowing a further reduction in echo time and repetition time. *GP*, phase-encoding gradient; *GR*, read-out gradient; *GS*, slice-selection gradient; *RF*, radiofrequency

1.1.2.6
k-Space Interpolation and Half-Fourier Imaging

1.1.2.6.1
k-Space Interpolation

The time consuming part in conventional SE or GRE imaging is the 'filling of k-space' in the direction of phase-encoding. On inspecting the k-space, it is observed that the signal content of those lines representing the high spatial frequencies of the object are of very low signal amplitude. Omitting the measurement of these lines corresponds to a loss in spatial resolution in the direction of phase-encoding. The voxel size becomes rectangular. The Fourier transformation of a data set with missing Fourier lines for the higher spatial frequencies will result in a 'blurred' image appearance. The blurring is a consequence of the 'truncation' artifact – missing contributions of the high spatial frequencies of the object. A common approach to 'cheat' involves performing a Fourier transformation after filling in the missing Fourier lines with zero values. This action corresponds to a 'sinc-interpolation' in the direction of phase-encoding (Fig. 1.44). The spatial resolution is not recovered, but the blurring artifacts are smoothed. Since the voxel size is increased, the SNR is improved, and since fewer lines are measured, the measurement time is reduced.

The method of k-space interpolation has been extended to 3D imaging and is hidden behind the acronyms turboMRA and VIBE (volume-interpolated breath-hold examinations). Although k-space interpolation does not alter the partition thickness, it seems to be a common approach to denote the partition thickness as 'half of the actual measured partition thickness after k-space interpolation using zero-filling'. It is incorrect to believe that the images interpolated in this way are identical to what would have been obtained if the object had been scanned with a full k-space acquisition. On the other hand, the zero-filling approach, equivalent to a voxel-shifted interpolation, improves the partial volume effect partially, that is, it does not improve spatial or volume resolution but does reduce the artifacts caused by the shape and size of image pixels. An impressive example of this zero-filling approach is shown in Fig. 1.45.

1.1.2.6.2
Half-Fourier Imaging

In section 1.1.1.3 the concept of phase-encoding was introduced. The first row within the raw data matrix, the k-space, contains the high spatial frequencies of the object. That Fourier line was acquired with a positive phase-encoding gradient high enough and of sufficient duration to cause a 180° phase shift between transverse

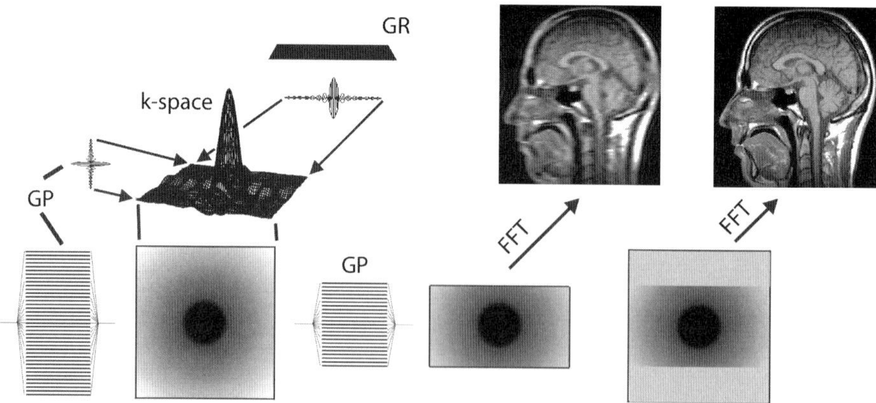

Fig. 1.44. k-space interpolation. The *upper left illustration* indicates the sorting into the raw data matrix ('k-space'): from *left* to *right*, the frequency encoded data; from *top* to *bottom*, the phase-encoded information. For a reduced number of phase-encoding steps, the matrix size is called 'asymmetric', and the pixel size becomes rectangular. The missing Fourier lines cause a 'blurred' appearance of the image due to 'truncation' artifacts. That blurring can be reduced by filling the missing Fourier lines with zero values. The latter has been named 'k-space interpolation'. The illustration is exaggerated in order to exemplify the effect

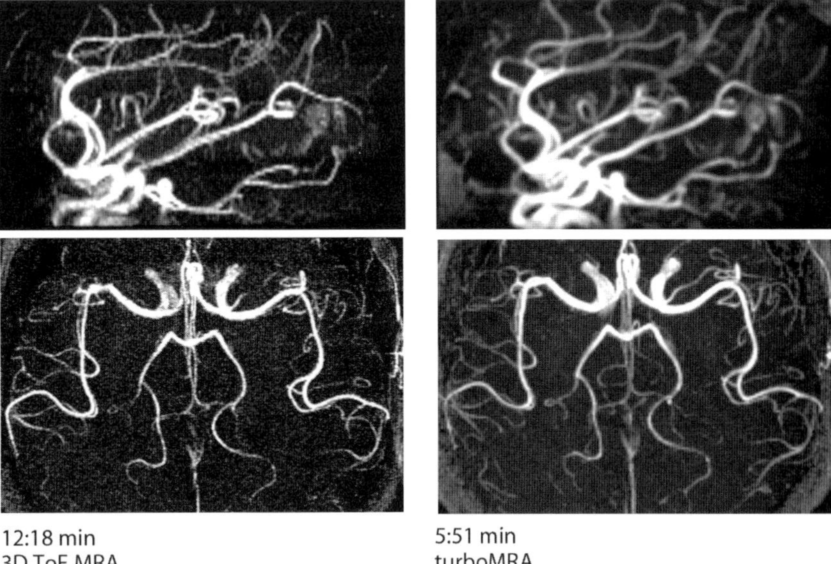

Fig. 1.45. Turbo MRA. The concept of 'k-space interpolation' can be extended to the 'depth' or partition-phase encoding in 3D-ToF-MRA

magnetizations of adjacent voxels. The center of k-space contains the information about the coarse structure of the object, and again the last row within k-space contains the high spatial frequencies of the object collected with a negative phase-encoding gradient high enough and of sufficient duration to cause a 180° phase shift between transverse magnetizations of adjacent voxels. Theoretically, there should not be a difference between a 180° phase shift generated by a positive or by a negative gradient. Theoretically, half of the k-space contains redundant information. In practice, however, there are phase distortions that destroy that symmetry. Since they are assumed to be of low spatial frequency, it is considered sufficient to measure e.g. eight more lines after crossing the center of k-space to correct for these distortions. Such an approach has been named 'half-Fourier' imaging. Although many imaging sequences can be combined with the half-Fourier method, the technique is most relevant in conjunction with a single-shot, multi-echo, spin-echo approach to be discussed in a following chapter. It has to be kept in mind that, although the measurement time can almost be cut in half, there is also a noticeable SNR loss, since each of the measured Fourier lines represents an additional 'acquisition'. Each single Fourier line contains information about the whole object, adding to the number of averages responsible for the SNR.

1.1.2.6.3
Echo Asymmetry

The gradient or spin echoes do not have to be in the center of k-space. In fact, for gradient-echo sequences, it would be a suboptimal alternative to center the echo. If 100% asymmetry is defined as the collection of a free induction decay (maximum echo peak at the beginning of the acquisition window), and no asymmetry would correspond to 0%, then 28% asymmetry would be close to optimal for a flow-compensated or flow-encoded technique (as indicated in Fig. 1.30). In comparison, 0% asymmetry (centering the echo) would require larger gradient amplitudes resulting in prolonged echo times, making the sequence more sensitive to higher-order motion. The consequence would be more ghosting due to motion or pulsatility artifacts. Exceeding the 28% echo asymmetry, the images will start to deteriorate, showing blurring and ghosting.

1.1.2.7
Parallel Acquisition Techniques

The number of phase-encoding steps is one of the factors dictating the length of the measurement time. The number of phase-encoding steps is necessary to spatially encode the signal from an object for a desired field of view (FoV) and a requested spatial resolution. The maximum amplitude and duration of the phase-encoding gradient provide information about the highest spatial resolution causing a phase change of 180° for the transverse magnetization within adjacent voxels. Measuring with as many phase-encoding steps as there are matrix lines in the direction of phase-encoding allows unequivocal assignment to the suitable spatial frequencies. Omitting every other phase-encoding step, as illustrated in Fig. 1.46, corresponds to a reduction of the FoV in the direction of phase encoding by a factor of two. If the object extends beyond that FoV, an aliased image will be the result.

An array of closely packed receiver coils surrounding the object has been suggested to re-establish the unequivocal assignment. As each coil has a defined location and 'sensitivity profile', that information can be used to 'unwrap' the image. Since each coil is separately receiving the signal from the object within the sensitivity region, but parallel to other adjacent coils, these methods are called parallel acquisition techniques. There are multiple strategies for image unwrapping, e.g., the method sensitivity encoding (SENSE) uses the image information for each coil channel, whereas the simultaneous acquisition of spatial harmonics (SMASH) performs the 'unwrapping' within k-space. Other acronyms for different strategies in parallel acquisition reconstructions are 'scissors methods', Roemer method, partially parallel imaging with localized sensitivities (PILS), sensitivity profiles from an array of coils for encoding and reconstruction in parallel (SPACE RIP), and generalized autocalibrating partially parallel acquisitions (GRAPPA).

1.1.2.8 Fast Imaging

The term 'fast imaging' is not well defined. If fast imaging techniques are all methods that provide the information based on Pd-, T1-, or T2-weighting faster than a conventional spin-echo sequence, then fast imaging has already been introduced with the utilization of FLASH, FISP, CISS, DESS, trueFISP, turboFLASH, and MPRAGE.

Recent definitions consider all 'single-echo' methods as conventional imaging as previously described, where the measurement time is calculated by multiplying the TR by the number of acquisitions and by the number of Fourier lines to be acquired. In that case, only multi-echo techniques, to be discussed below, are considered 'fast imaging' techniques.

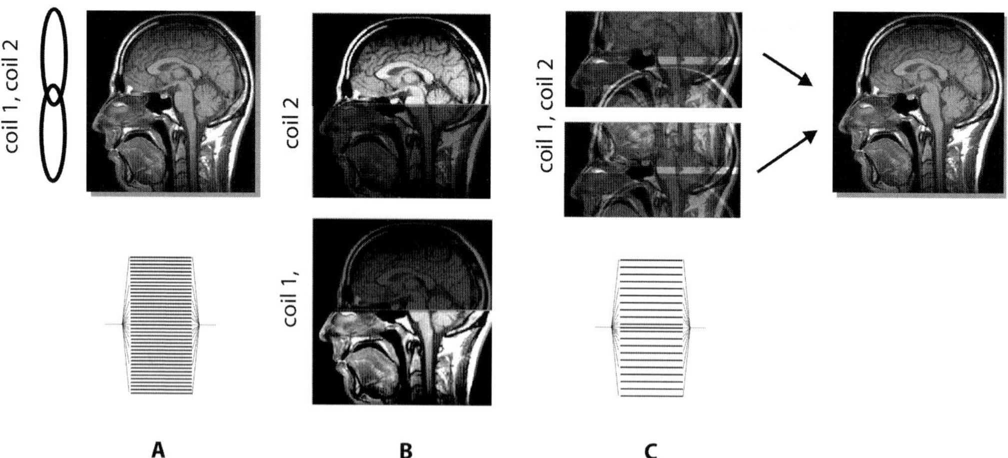

Fig. 1.46A–C. Parallel acquisition techniques. These are graphical illustrations, not actual measurements. **A** A two-coil set-up illustration for the acquisition of a sagittal image with a full k-space matrix. **B** Parallel acquisition and image reconstruction for each of the two coil channels. **C** Undersampling the data corresponds to a rectangular field of view, resulting in aliased images. Notice the aliasing artifact for the neck measured with coil 1 is stronger than the same region detected with coil 2. The aliasing artifact from the upper part of the brain has a stronger signal within the image of coil 2 than the appearance in the image of coil 1. Using this information (the sensitivity profiles of the coils), the image can be 'unwrapped'

1.1.2.8.1 Fast Imaging with Spin-Echo Sequences

Considering a T2-W-SE sequence, it is almost irrelevant whether the TE is 60 ms, 80 ms, or 100 ms. The signal contribution is very similar. The concept of turbo spin-echo (TSE) or fast spin-echo (FSE) is to utilize these echoes, with a new phase encoding, to fill up the required lines in *k*-space as illustrated in Fig. 1.47. This technique has replaced conventional SE imaging in most clinical applications and has only one major disadvantage. Due to the short spacing of refocusing pulses, this sequence is less sensitive in detecting hemorrhagic lesions. Another argument against this technique is the potential loss of small details based on the fact that usually the higher spatial frequencies are acquired with late echoes. Late echoes mean low signal intensities, and the higher spatial frequencies may be underrepresented within the *k*-space. Protocols involving TSE imaging techniques use a longer repetition time for an improved contrast over the SE techniques, and they often utilize a larger matrix size, leading to improved spatial resolution. It has been documented that both parameters overcompensate the potential of missing small lesions. There are two annoying effects in TSE imaging. One already mentioned is the lack of sensitivity to hemorrhagic lesions, the other annoying effect is the hyperintense appearance of fat. The spins in hydrogen atoms bound to fat are coupled. Multiple hydrogen atoms belong to the same molecule, and the corresponding nuclear spins interact with each other via their electromagnetic fields. Such a coupling is referred to as *J*-coupling. This coupling leads to a slow dephasing mechanism, not refocused by the 180° refocusing pulse, and observed with SE imaging. This *J*-coupling is broken with a rapid application of a series of 180° refocusing pulses, as used in TSE imaging. The consequence is a hyperintense appearance of fat compared with the images achieved with SE imaging. Another positive aspect of TSE imaging is the phenomenon of magnetization transfer. The latter has been discussed in Sect. 1.1.1.4. Water molecules in the vicinity of macromolecules are called 'bounded' and have a very short T2. A short T2 refers to a large difference in resonance frequencies, causing a rapid dephasing. They are not directly observable but have a very broad resonance frequency. Applying an RF excitation off resonance, those invisible molecules can be saturated. Since they communicate with their 'free' partners via magnetization transfer, this off-resonance pulse has an effect on the image contrast. Multiple 180° refocusing pulses are used in TSE imaging with a frequency range for one specific slice. Those frequencies act as off-resonance pulses for all adjacent slices and are, therefore, 'MTS' pulses. This is the explanation for the better contrast between gray and white matter in images acquired with a TSE method than those provided by conventional SE techniques. The previously mentioned IR technique combined with the TSE acquisition mode is called TIR or TIRM, similar to the acronym used in SE applications. Due to the potential savings in measurement time using TIRM imaging, the inversion time can be prolonged to more than 2 s to get even the zero crossing of the recovering magnetization within CSF. The latter technique has the potential for a better delineation of periventricular lesions.

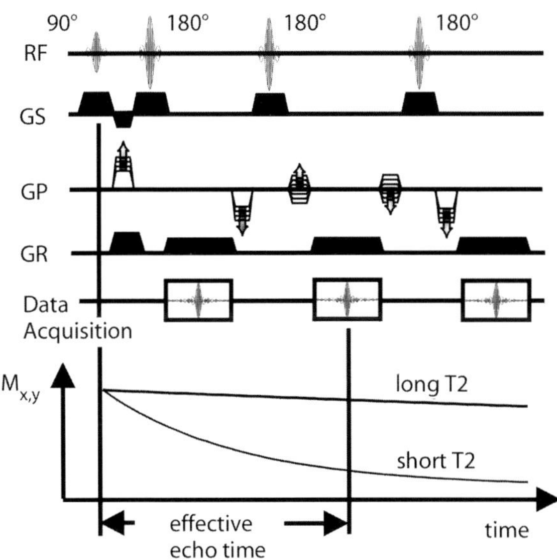

Fig. 1.47. The turbo spin-echo (TSE) sequence design. TSE imaging utilizes multiple echoes to fill the raw data matrix. Each echo has a different phase encoding. The possible reduction in measurement time is directly proportional to the number of echoes used. The effective echo time is given at the time the low spatial frequencies are acquired. Since the data acquisition is along a T2-relaxation curve, there is the potential of image blurring due to signal variation within *k*-space. For T2-weighted imaging, this effect is almost negligible. The illustration above only shows the first three echoes of a sequence design that usually utilizes 15–23 echoes for imaging. *GP*, phase-encoding gradient; *GR*, read-out gradient; *GS*, slice-selection gradient; *RF*, radiofrequency

The half-Fourier technique was mentioned at the beginning of this section. This technique utilizes the theoretical model that the *k*-space should be symmetrical. Theoretically, it should be sufficient to measure only half of the data of what is currently measured. In half-Fourier imaging, the potential perturbations are assumed to be of low spatial frequencies and are eliminated by measuring a little more than half the *k*-space and performing a phase correction prior to image reconstruction. The technique reduces the measurement time almost by a factor of two, but also diminishes the SNR to 70%, since each measured Fourier line contains the information of the whole object and contributes to the SNR. The half-Fourier method combined with a TSE sequence allows an image acquisition within one shot: one excitation pulse and multiple refocusing pulses until all the data are acquired for one slice. This technique is called half-Fourier acquired single-shot turbo spin-echo (HASTE). Of course, this technique can again be combined with a preceding inversion pulse, leading to acronyms such as HASTIRM. In TSE imaging, the 180° refocusing pulse is followed by a phase-encoding step after which the data are collected with a frequency-encoding gradient being switched on. By changing the polarity of the frequency-encoding gradient after data acquisition, another echo, the previously discussed GRE, can be generated. With a phase-encoding 'blip' during the ramp time of the frequency-encoding gradient, this echo can provide the data for another *k*-space line. This technique combines SEs with GREs, as illustrated in Fig. 1.48, and is, therefore, termed TGSE. Since this technique prolongs the distance between RF refocusing pulses, the *J*-coupling pattern is not broken, and fat appears similar to SE images. Since GREs are sensitive to susceptibility differences, the sensitivity to hemorrhagic lesions should also be reestablished.

1.1.2.8.2
Fast Imaging with Gradient-Echo Sequences

The term ultra-fast imaging is currently referred to as echo planar imaging (EPI) techniques. The classical form uses one excitation pulse and multiple phase-encoded echoes to generate an image, as illustrated in Fig. 1.49. With this technique, it is possible to generate an image within 80–120 ms. The major limitations are not only the necessary hardware and the general availability. The classical technique has intrinsic artifacts due to the length of the so-called echo train of GREs as

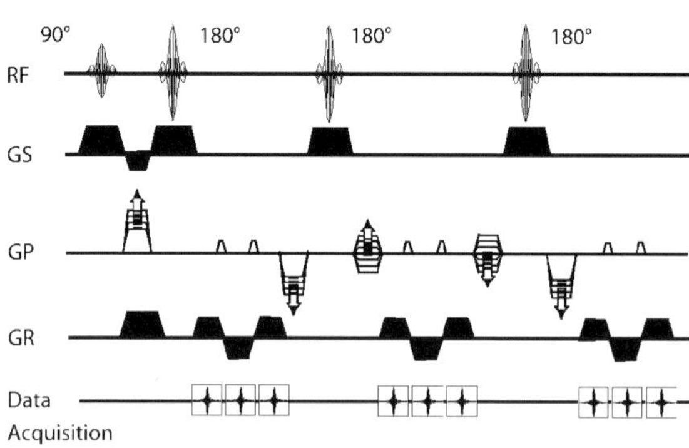

Fig. 1.48. The turbo-gradient and spin-echo sequence (TGSE). Multiple echoes with different phase-encoding steps are used to acquire all the data necessary to fill the raw data matrix. For each spin-echo envelope, multiple gradient echoes (in this case three) are utilized, leading to a further possibility in reducing measurement time compared with the TSE sequence design. Other advantages are the unbroken *J*-coupling (fat appears similar to SE imaging) and the theoretical increase in sensitivity to susceptibility gradients (hemorrhagic lesions should appear similar to SE imaging). *GP*, phase-encoding gradient; *GR*, read-out gradient; *GS*, slice-selection gradient; *RF*, radiofrequency

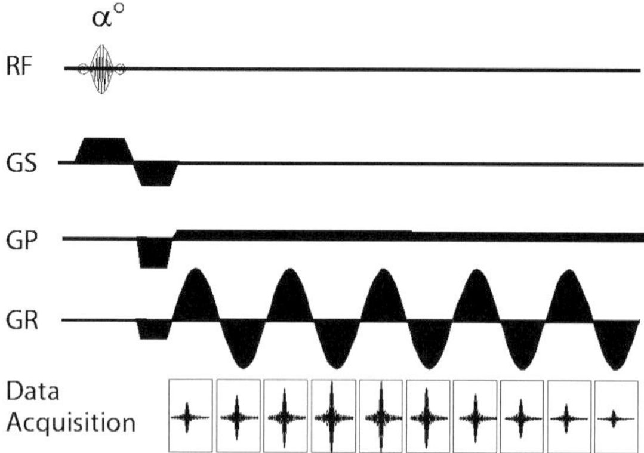

Fig. 1.49. The echo-planar-imaging sequence design. This illustration is only one possible gradient arrangement that would be named echo planar imaging. Following a selective excitation, multiple gradient echoes are generated. In the version reproduced here, a small phase-encoding gradient is on during the whole measurement, providing a progressive phase encoding for the sequence of gradient echoes. The data are collected along a T2* relaxation curve. The effective echo time is the time at which the low spatial frequencies are acquired. *GP*, phase-encoding gradient; *GR*, read-out gradient; *GS*, slice-selection gradient; *RF*, radiofrequency

there are severe geometrical distortions for the regions of large susceptibility gradients such as the facial region or the base of the skull. The other disadvantage is the limited spatial resolution that competes with today's high-resolution TSE imaging. The applied low phase-encoding gradients correspond to a very low bandwidth. Good fat signal suppression is, therefore, a prerequisite for EPI applications, otherwise the fat image will appear as an annoying ghost. Nevertheless, there are a few clinical applications in which EPI will be the only imaging technique of choice. These applications include the utilization of EPI read-out modules for a prepared magnetization that would otherwise be destroyed by a prolonged read-out period. Such preparations include the diffusion weighting in stroke imaging. As indicated in Fig. 1.50, the Stejskal-Tanner approach uses two large gradients around a 180° refocusing pulse. This gradient has no effect on stationary material but produces a sensitivity to flow, motion, and diffusion. Other applications are rapid acquisition of large volumes as needed in functional MR imaging (fMRI) and imaging of the coronary vasculature. The spiral acquisition recently mentioned in conjunction with EPI uses oscillating read-out as well as oscillating phase-encoding gradients, as indicated in Fig. 1.51. In this case, the acquired data follow a trajectory that 'spirals' from the center of *k*-space to the outside. The latter lacks the typical phase-encoding artifacts seen in conventional *k*-space filling, but shows a noise pattern not yet fully understood. The image quality as well as spatial resolution of these techniques will undergo some improvements in the near future, likely at the expense of a prolonged measurement time in multi-shot approaches.

A variety of acronyms has been created by the industry and academic groups, sometimes for the same fast-imaging technique or similar techniques with minor or major modifications. Some acronyms used by different vendors are listed in Table 1.6.

1.1.2.9 Magnetic Resonance Fluoroscopy

MR fluoroscopy is a buzzword used in conjunction with ultra-fast, fast, and even only relatively fast imaging techniques. The basic concept is a continued measurement with a regular update of the actual image, similar to X-ray fluoroscopy. For ultra-fast imaging techniques, the whole *k*-space matrix is usually measured and processed, and the image immediately displayed. For slower imaging techniques, the lower spatial frequencies are measured more frequently than the high *k*-space lines,

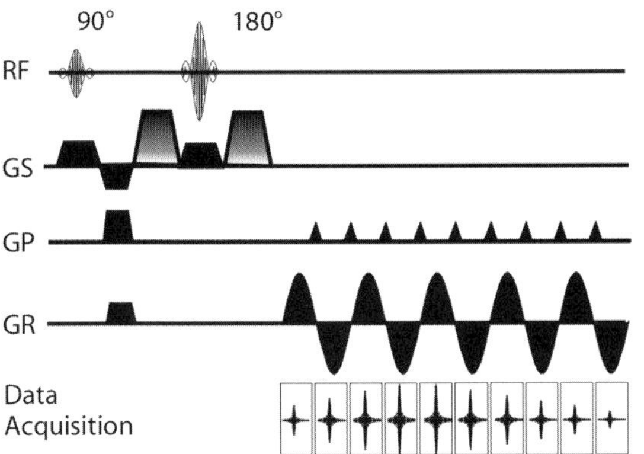

Fig. 1.50. The blipped spin-echo echo-planar imaging (SE-EPI) sequence design with diffusion sensitization. In this example, the gradients providing the diffusion weighting are placed in the direction of slice selection. A spin-echo envelope is generated, containing multiple gradient echoes. In this example, the phase-encoding gradient is 'blipped' between the read-out gradient lobes. *GP*, phase-encoding gradient; *GR*, read-out gradient; *GS*, slice-selection gradient; *RF*, radiofrequency

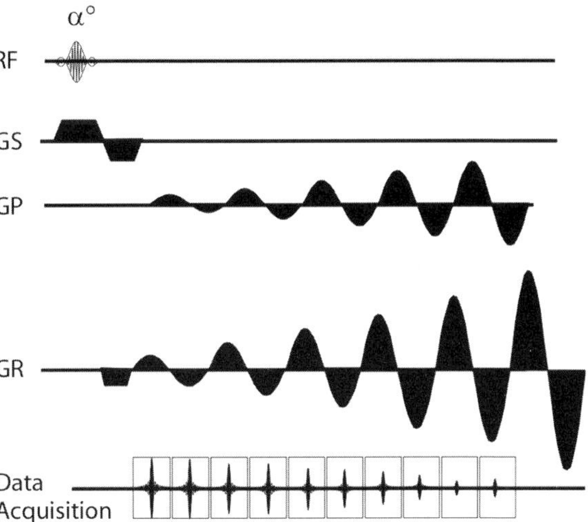

Fig. 1.51. The spiral echo-planar imaging sequence. The read-out gradient as well as the phase-encoding gradient oscillate with increasing amplitude. This causes a data trajectory that 'spirals' through *k*-space, starting in the center of *k*-space with the acquisition of low spatial frequencies. *GP*, phase-encoding gradient; *GR*, read-out gradient; *GS*, slice-selection gradient; *RF*, radiofrequency

Table 1.6. Various sequence acronyms for the same technique used by different vendors

Sequence acronym	Siemens	GE	Philips	Marconi
Spoiled gradient echoes (spoiled GRE)	FLASH	SPGR, MPGR	FFE, T1-FFE	T1-FAST
Steady-state gradient echoes with sampling of the free induction decay (SS-GRE-FID)	FISP	GRASS	T2-FFE	FAST
Steady-state gradient echoes with sampling of the spin-echo component (SS-GRE-SE)	PSIF	SSFP	CE-T2-FFE	CE-FAST
Steady-state gradient echoes with sampling of the free induction decay and the spin-echo component (SS-GRE-FID-SE)	CISS, DESS, trueFISP	FIESTA	Balanced FFE	–
Gradient echoes with magnetization preparation (MP-GRE)	turboFLASH, MPRAGE	FSPGR	TFE	RAM-FAST
Fast spin echo	TSE, TIR, TIRM	FSE	TSE	FSE
Gradient and spin echoes	TGSE	GRASE	GRASE	GSE
Single-shot fast spin-echo technique	HASTE, HASTIRM	SSFSE	SS-TSE	–

while the images are processed and displayed at regular intervals using the whole *k*-space independent of whether lines have been updated or not. In conjunction with a real-time capable interactive slice positioning, MR fluoroscopy is becoming an essential tool for MR-guided interventions.

1.2 Magnetic Resonance Angiography, Techniques and Principles

There are currently three types of MRA techniques. The first group relies on the inflow phenomenon and is, therefore, called the time of flight (ToF) technique. The second group utilizes the fact that the phase behavior of the macroscopic magnetization can be sensitized to motion (phase contrast, PC). The third and recently established group solely relies on contrast enhancement in order to visualize the vasculature (ceMRA). The latter group is based on a 3D GRE sequence with very short TE and TR to produce a very short acquisition time, catching the contrast bolus as it passes through the region of interest. The ToF and PC techniques utilize a feature named gradient motion rephasing (GMR), which deals with the rephasing and the formation of a GRE for flowing structures. The phase of a magnetization characterizes the position within the transverse plane, as illustrated in Fig. 1.52. Switching a field gradient for the purpose of spatial encoding will result in a different phase of magnetization within adjacent voxels. Switching the field gradient in the opposite direction with the same amplitude and duration will move the phase back to the same position for stationary tissue. For moving tissue, the phase history of the voxel that moved will be different than the theoretical phase history of a stationary voxel at the same location (Fig. 1.53). As the phase information is used for spatial encoding, this is an unwanted phenomenon in conventional GRE imaging and ToF techniques and a phenomenon utilized in PC-MRA and flow quantification. It can be shown that with an arrangement of three gradient lobes, a rephasing can be performed at the same location and the same time for the stationary tissue as well as the flowing blood (Fig. 1.54). This method is called

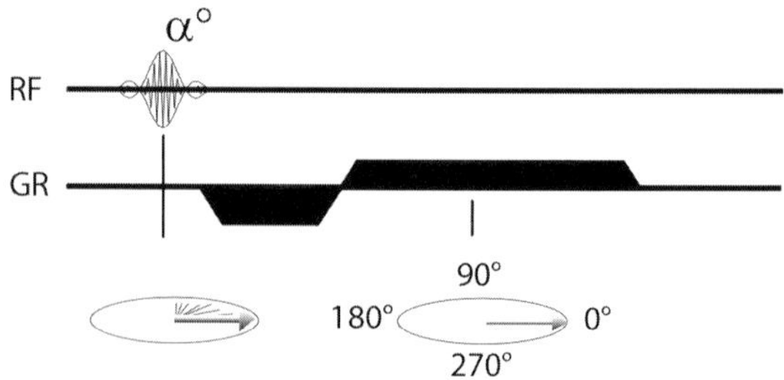

Fig. 1.52. The definition of 'phase'. Phase is the position of the macroscopic magnetization within the *x-y* or transverse plane at any time between excitation and data acquisition. This can be immediately after excitation, at the time the spin echo or gradient echo is generated, or at any other time where a residual vector of magnetization can be identified. *GR*, read-out gradient; *RF*, radiofrequency

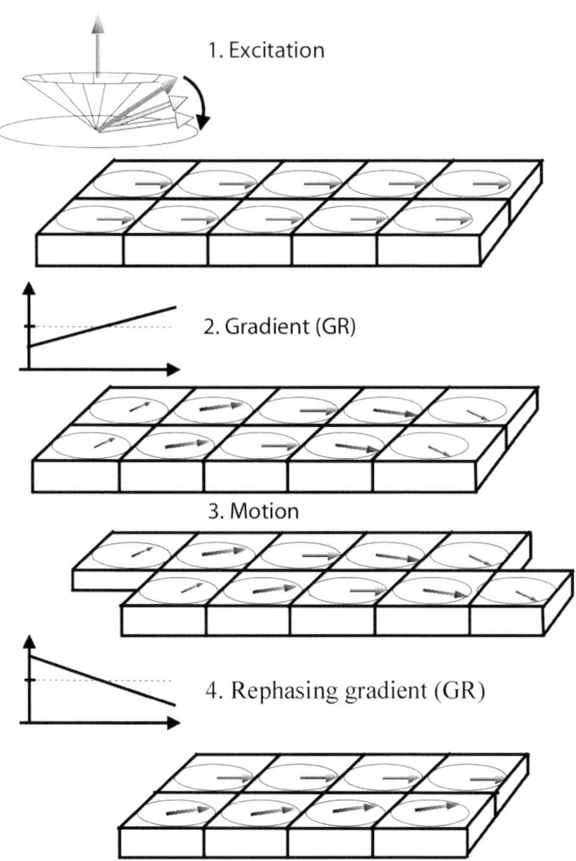

Fig. 1.53. Phase evolution of moving structures. Immediately after the excitation, all macroscopic magnetizations have the same phase position. The gradient *GR* preparing the gradient or spin echo will produce a phase difference in the direction of encoding. At the time the rephasing gradient is applied, parts of the voxel have moved, showing a different phase history as compared with the magnetization of stationary tissue. The rephasing gradient will rephase the magnetization within the stationary tissue, but the magnetization within moving structures will show a different phase. The phase difference may lead to a signal void and thus artifacts, since the phase information is also used for spatial encoding. The phase position can be evaluated to quantify the flow velocity

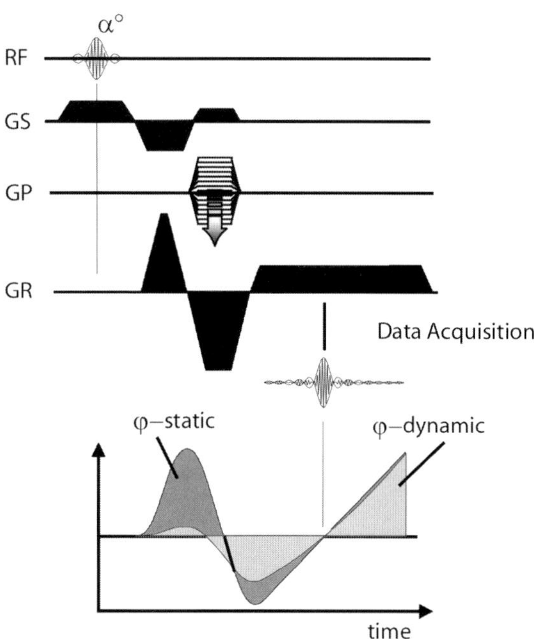

Fig. 1.54. Gradient motion rephasing (GMR). The constant velocity of a moving structure causes the phase evolution to be quadratic in time. It can be shown that with a three-lobe gradient structure, as illustrated here, a rephasing can be achieved at the time of the echo for static tissue as well as for tissue that moves with a constant velocity. This phenomenon is called GMR. *GP,* phase-encoding gradient; *GR,* read-out gradient; *GS,* slice-selection gradient; *RF,* radiofrequency

GMR. Most of the conventional GRE techniques utilize this GMR, with the advantage that the images have fewer artifacts for slices containing vascular structures. The disadvantage of the three-lobe arrangement is a prolonged TE. The GMR implementation into sequences used for ToF-MRA insures a hyperintense signal within the vessel lumen.

1.2.1
3D Time-of-Flight Angiography

The initial version of MRA was based on a ToF effect of unsaturated blood flowing into a 3D imaging volume with primarily saturated stationary tissue. This is illustrated in Fig. 1.55. The unsaturated blood within the vessel appears hyperintense compared with the stationary surroundings. To visualize the vascular tree, projections are reconstructed which assign the highest signal intensity found along a ray of the perspective to the signal intensity of the pixel, as illustrated in Fig. 1.56. Such a projection is called a maximum intensity projection (MIP). The disadvantage of this technique is that small vessels visible on the native slice will be obscured by the higher signal contribution of the noise contained in adjacent slices. Nevertheless, this technique has succeeded so far as a robust method for a fast evaluation of the vascular system. For the evaluation of questionable

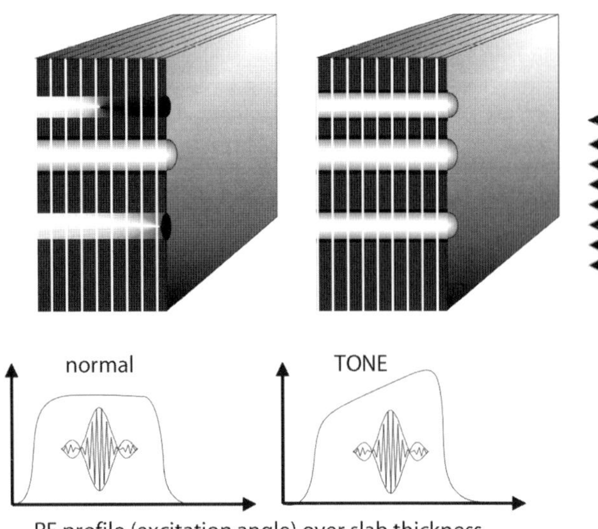

Fig. 1.55. The time-of-flight effect in 3D magnetic resonance angiography (3D ToF-MRA). The contrast is given by the amount of blood that is flowing into the excited slab, replacing the saturated fluid. For a thick slab and slow flow, there is the potential of saturation towards the distal portion of the slab. This effect is reduced by using an asymmetric radiofrequency (*RF*) slab profile, also called TONE (tilted optimized non-saturating excitation). In that case, the excitation angle at the entry point of the vessel is lower than at the exit port. This technique depends on the direction of flow

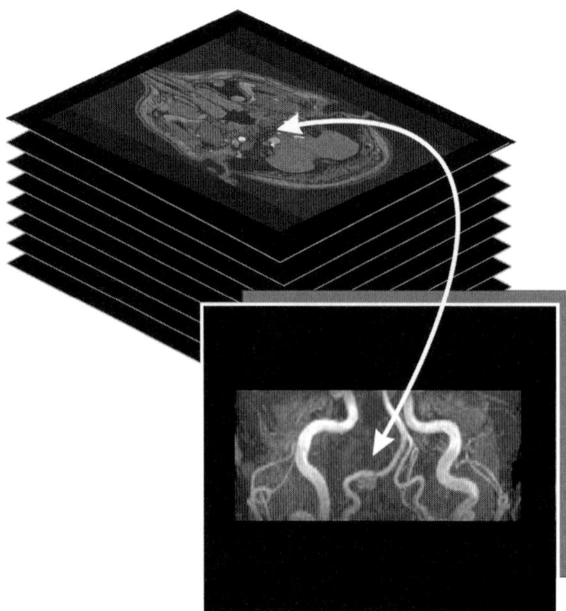

Fig. 1.56. The maximum intensity projection (MIP) projects the maximum intensity found in a stack of images to the pixel intensity on the screen, depending on the view, the perspective, that the user defines. In this example, a transverse 3D ToF-MRA was performed to study the aneurysm in the right vertebral artery. A coronal MIP was applied to these transverse stack of images

areas and for the smaller vessels, there is always the possibility of assessing the native images. This 3D ToF-MRA technique is still used for imaging the intracranial cerebral circulation.

A method to improve the contrast between the vessel lumen and the surrounding brain parenchyma is the application of a MTS pulse as discussed in Sect. 1.1.1.4. The stationary brain parenchyma contains macromolecules which are 'invisible' due to a short T2, bounded water molecules that can be saturated via an off-resonance RF pulse. Via magnetization transfer, this leads to an increased background suppression. The progressing saturation of the flowing blood from the entry point towards the exit point is usually compensated with a linear flip-angle change in the direction of the expected flow: the RF pulse that excites the whole 3D volume is designed to provide a low flip-angle excitation at one side of the 3D slab, the entry point of the vessel, with an increase of flip angle towards the other side of the slab. The aim of this procedure is to achieve a homogeneous signal contribution throughout the 3D volume. Such a technique is also called tilted optimized non-saturating excitation (TONE).

1.2.2 2D Time-of-Flight Angiography

Shortly after the introduction of the 3D MRA method, the 2D technique was presented as being the better method for visualizing the extracranial cerebral circulation and the peripheral arteries. The main source of contrast in 3D ToF-MRA is the inflow of unsaturated blood into the volume. The drawback with the 3D ToF-MRA technique is the progressive saturation of blood that travels through the volume. The idea of the 2D ToF-MRA technique is to make every slice an entry slice as illustrated in Fig. 1.57, improving the contrast dramatically compared with the 3D ToF-MRA technique. One disadvantage of the 2D-ToF technique is the prolonged measurement time or the limited coverage of the sequentially applied slices. These slices have to be

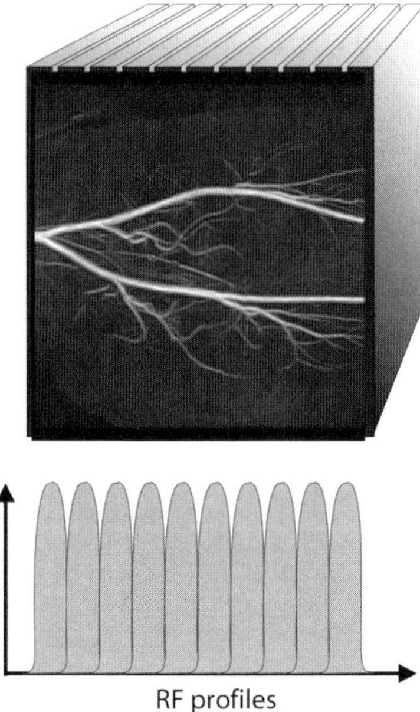

Fig. 1.57. The 2D time-of-flight magnetic resonance angiography technique (2D ToF-MRA) avoids the saturation problem found in 3D applications by acquiring thin 2D slices sequentially. Each slice is therefore an entry slice. The slices are usually acquired with a significant overlap in order to compensate for signal variations at the edges of the slice caused by non-ideal slice profiles. *RF*, radiofrequency

acquired with a significant overlap in order to compensate for the signal distortions at the edges of the slice. Otherwise, a typical 'staircase' pattern is to be observed in the maximum intensity projection (MIP). Another severer limitation of the 2D ToF-MRA technique is the rapid saturation of blood that is coincidentally flowing within the slice or reentering the slice in the case of a vascular loop, mimicking the lack of flow as found after stenoses or occlusions. The evaluation of these data sets are again performed with a MIP technique as discussed in the 3D ToF-MRA section. The 2D ToF-MRA methods are being replaced by the contrast-enhanced MRA techniques, since ceMRA protocols are less complex and much faster, and the resulting images demonstrate fewer artifacts.

1.2.3 3D PC Angiography

MRA techniques based on a velocity-dependent phase shift of the transverse magnetization, the phase-contrast (PC-MRA), use a slightly detuned GMR arrangement. The transverse magnetization within voxels containing flowing blood will have a different phase position than the macroscopic magnetization within the voxel of adjacent stationary tissue. It is usually the 'difference vector' that is utilized for the visualization of the vascular tree (Fig. 1.58). The reference phase is usually acquired with a preceding scan with perfect GMR. In order to obtain all three possible velocity components, the 'detuned' GMR measurements have to be applied to all three possible orientations. The advantages of this technique are the perfect background suppression and the adjustable sensitivity to slow velocities. The major disadvantages of this technique are the relatively long measurement times and the potential selection of an improper flow sensitivity. If the selected sensitivity is too high, corresponding to an underestimated velocity range, the contrast will be poor. If the selected sensitivity is too low, corresponding to an overestimated velocity range, the contrast will be poor. In addition, this technique is sensitive to higher-order motion and apparently not as robust as the ToF techniques. The PC-MRA methods are being replaced by the contrast-enhanced MRA techniques, since ceMRA protocols are much faster, and the results are more consistent.

1.2.4 2D PC Angiography

The 2D PC-MRA technique takes advantage of the same phenomenon. Rather than acquiring multiple 3D partitions, however, only one thick slice is selected. The advantage of such an approach is the relatively short measurement time compared with the 3D method. Another advantage is that the image provided is already the angiogram. There is no need and no possibility of further post-processing, such as the presentation of a different view angle. The latter is a disadvantage of the 2D PC-MRA technique. Another disadvantage is a poorer SNR compared with a 3D acquisition. The fact that the voxel in 2D PC-MRA is highly anisotropic also leads to a potential pitfall of adding the contribution of vari-

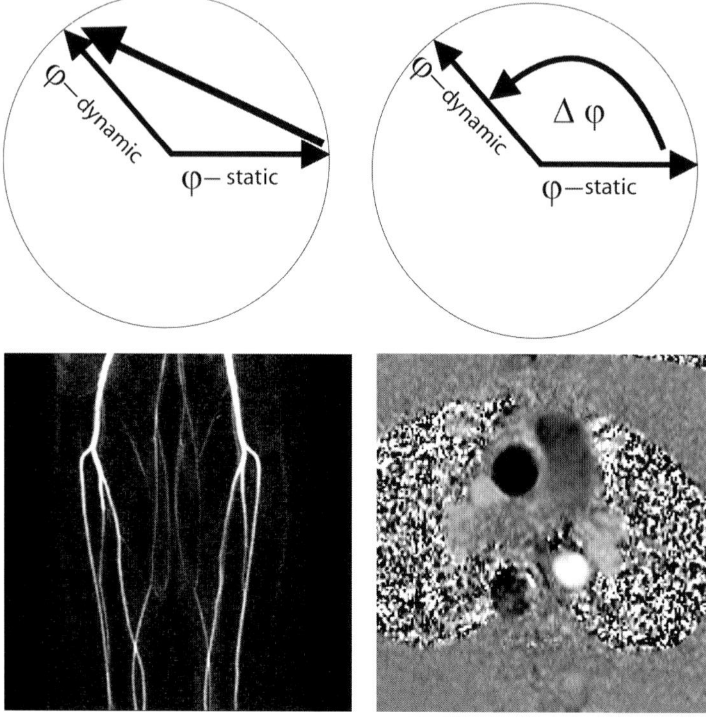

Fig. 1.58. Principles and example of a phase-contrast magnetic resonance angiography (PC-MRA) technique. The *left graph and image* present a so-called PC-MRA of the lower extremity. The length of the vector between the stationary reference and the signal from the moving blood is translated to a pixel intensity within the image. The *right graph and image* demonstrate a so-called phase map (or phase-difference image). The basic sequence structure is identical, but in this case, the phase difference is converted to a signal intensity within the image. The gray scale in this case corresponds directly to a measured velocity. The transverse cut through the aortic arch at the level of the pulmonary artery is shown

ous vessels flowing through the same voxel. 2D PC angiography techniques are usually taken to achieve a fast angiographic localizer.

1.2.5 Contrast-Enhanced Magnetic Resonance Angiography

With the new progress in hardware development and the ability to acquire a 3D MRA within a breath-hold – or the passing of a contrast bolus – the so-called contrast-enhanced MRA techniques have shown a dramatic improvement, especially regarding the abdominal and peripheral vasculature. The technique itself is rather trivial. A GRE technique is applied with the shortest suitable TE selected, the shortest possible TR, and a moderate excitation angle. The aim is to provide an image of a passing contrast bolus. Figure 1.59 demonstrates an example of a so-called time-resolved ceMRA, where the measurement of the transit time is omitted and replaced by multiple sequential acquisitions of the same region. The T1 shortening of the blood as a consequence of administering a paramagnetic contrast agent will allow the imaging of the vascular tree with no saturation effects. There is no entry plane and no concern about saturation. The challenging part for the user is the timing between the injection of the bolus and the start of the breath-hold acquisition, with the goal of acquiring the low *k*-space frequencies at the time the bolus passes through the region of interest. The timing of the measurement depends on the transit time of the bolus to the region of interest, the phase-encoding loop structure of the imaging sequence, and the duration of the injection time. The transit time, the time between intravenous injection of the contrast bolus and the appearance within the region on interest, can be evaluated prior to the ceMRA protocol by using a small test bolus and a turboFLASH technique through the region of interest with an update of 1 image/s. An alternative is usually offered in the form of an interleaved sequence. The user can start a bolus tracking fast 2D technique (e.g., turboFLASH), inject the contrast bolus, and semi-automatically can switch to the (3D) ceMRA technique as soon as the arrival of the bolus is noted within the region of interest (e.g., CARE bolus technique). To cover large regions as required in the ceMRA evaluation of

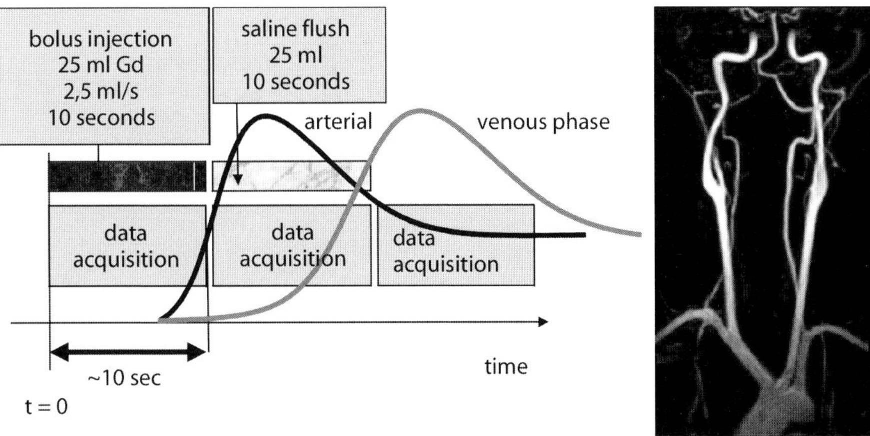

Fig. 1.59. ceMRA Principle. Contrast strongly depends on matching the arrival of the bolus within the region of interest and placing the k-space acquisition accordingly. Time-resolved imaging of the extracranial cerebral circulation will provide the native scan, the arterial phase, and images of the venous phase of the passing contrast media

the peripheral vasculature, protocols are offered that include automatic table feed to cover several vascular stations utilizing one single bolus injection (panoramic table MRA). A more detailed protocol optimization for large vessels and peripheral vessels is discussed in Chapter 13.

1.2.6 Flow Quantification

Since the phase change of a de-tuned GMR is proportional to the velocity of the flowing blood, this phase difference can be used for quantification. Although rarely applied in the clinical routine, it has some future potential in quantifying the flow through a dialysis shunt, investigating valvular insufficiencies, grading of shunts in congenital malformations of the heart, providing information on the extent to which flow in a false lumen supplies vital organs in aortic dissection, and investigating patent CSF channels in patients with hydrocephalus.

1.3 Techniques in Cardiac Imaging

The time-consuming acquisition of multiple Fourier lines usually takes too long to capture the motion of the beating heart. Exceptions are echo planar imaging techniques and recently developed 'real-time' trueFISP sequences. For all other imaging techniques, image acquisition is triggered or gated with physiological signals from ECG electrodes or a pulse sensor. The advantage of the time-of-flight effect of inflowing blood, creating a hyperintense signal appreciated in MRA, turns into a disadvantage for certain cardiac applications and is compensated with a so-called 'dark blood' magnetization preparation scheme.

1.3.1 ECG Gating – Prospective Triggering and Retrospective Cardiac Gating

In order to get a 'frozen' image of the beating heart, the Fourier lines for the slices to be imaged have to be taken at the same point in time within the cardiac cycle. The starting point for a multi-slice measurement of T1-weighted images acquired with conventional spin-echo sequences is estimated prospectively based on the advent of the ECG signal as illustrated in Fig. 1.60. As a practical hint, the acquisition of a stack of slices should be moved towards the end of the cardiac cycle in order to minimize motion artifacts. Conventional spin-echo sequences are usually optimized for cardiac imaging using an additional pair of dephasing gradients in order to dephase the signal from the moving blood. Parallel saturation bands around the stack of slices are used to minimize the inflow effect of unsaturated blood.

With the introduction of fast low-angle shot imaging (FLASH) and other gradient-echo techniques, it became possible to reduce the TR to e.g., 40 ms and lower, allowing the acquisition of time-resolved images of the beat-

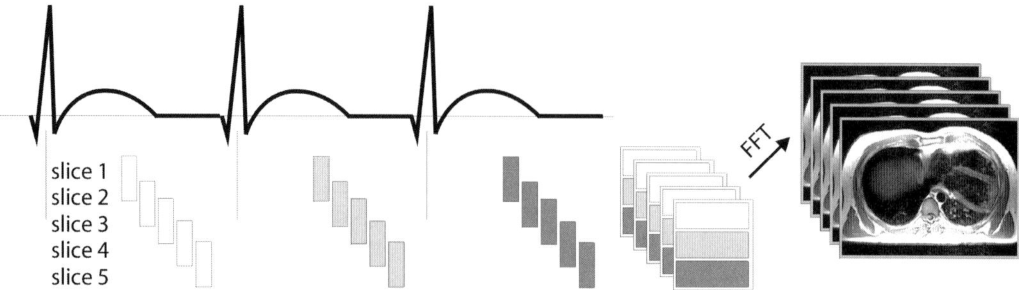

Fig. 1.60. Prospective ECG-triggered multi-slice acquisition. For simplicity, the k-space consists of only three Fourier lines (three different *gray-shaded boxes*) in this illustration. The usual matrix size requires 128 Fourier lines. One Fourier line is measured per heart beat. Multiple slices can be measured within one heart beat. Measurement should take place in end-diastole to minimize motion artifacts

ing heart. Figure 1.61 illustrates the prospective triggering previously described as well as the retrospective cardiac gating approach. For the latter, Fourier lines are measured for the same phase-encoding step with the selected repetition time of the sequence and are stored together with a time stamp of the last ECG event. After completion of one or two cardiac cycles, the phase-encoding amplitude is advanced to measure the next Fourier line. Data are later normalized and resorted, and the user can select the temporal resolution, that is, the number of images that he would like to have calculated for one cardiac phase. The advantage of retrospective cardiac gating is that the cardiac cycle is covered completely, without any gap in time, whereas for prospective triggering there is a gap between the last measurement and the beginning of the next measurement

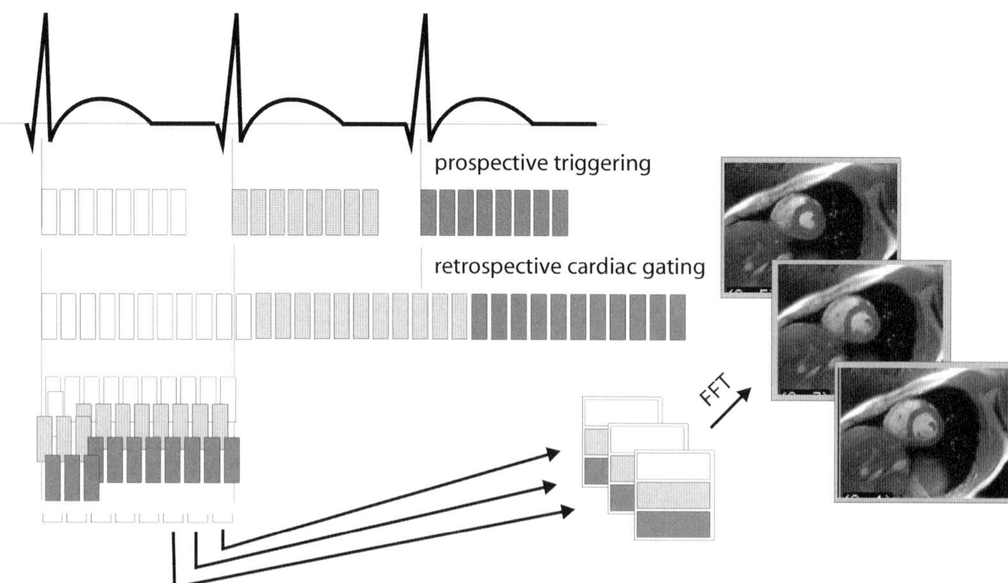

Fig. 1.61. Prospective ECG-triggered single-slice acquisition and retrospective cardiac gating. In this illustration, the k-space consists of only three Fourier lines (three different *gray-shaded boxes*). The usual matrix size requires 128 Fourier lines. In prospective triggering, one Fourier line is measured per heart beat per cardiac phase. In retrospective cardiac gating, the same Fourier line is measured continuously well beyond the time of a cardiac cycle. The Fourier lines are later normalized and resorted. The temporal resolution is given by the number of images per cardiac cycle as selected by the user. Images are reconstructed based on interpolated and weighted Fourier lines measured within the given time segment

with the next ECG event. The disadvantage of retrospective cardiac gating is the sensitivity to extrasystolic events and arrhythmic heart beats. The measurement may become invalid if such an event occurs when the center of k-space is being acquired.

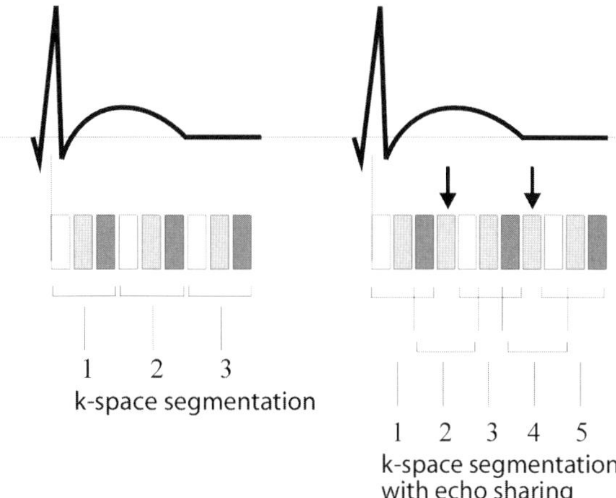

Fig. 1.63. Prospective ECG-triggered 'segmented' acquisition within a breath hold with 'echo sharing'. For reasons of simplicity, the illustration shows a k-space divided into three segments. One additional segment, containing the lower k-space frequencies, is measured in between the k-space segments of adjacent cardiac phases (indicated by the *arrows*). As illustrated, 'sharing' the information contained in the adjacent cardiac phases will allow the reconstruction of an additional cardiac phase, leading to an improved temporal resolution

1.3.2 Segmentation and Echo Sharing

Unfortunately, the heart is not only beating, its position also depends on the breathing cycle. In conventional imaging, two to three averages are used to smooth the artifacts based on respiratory displacement. As a consequence, the measurement time is prolonged, and the outline of the myocardial border becomes soft. In order to reduce the measurement time down to one breath-hold period, the concept of 'segmentation' was introduced. Instead of measuring one Fourier line per heart beat per cardiac phase, multiple Fourier lines are measured (Fig. 1.62). For example, for a 126*256 matrix and a k-space that is split up into 9 segments, 9 Fourier lines are measured per heart beat per cardiac phase, one line for each k-space segment. The measurement time will last one heart beat for the preparation scan, and 14 heart beats are needed to fill up the k-space (14*9=126). Fifteen heart beats are well tolerated for a breath-hold period. The benefit of suspended breathing will result in a crisper representation of the myocardial border, but there is a price to pay. For a gradient-echo sequence with a bandwidth of 195 Hz/pixel, the minimum measurement time for one Fourier line is approximately 9 ms. With 9 segments to be measured, this represents a temporal resolution of 81 ms. In order to re-establish the temporal resolution, the measurement of one segment, the segment containing the low k-space frequencies, is placed between the measurements of adjacent cardiac phases as illustrated in Fig. 1.63, and while sharing the Fourier lines of adjacent measurements, a true image of another cardiac phase can be reconstructed. This leads to an overall temporal resolution of, e.g., 57 ms.

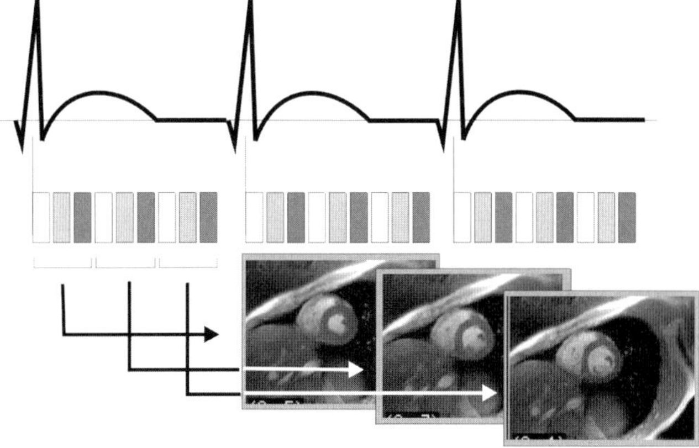

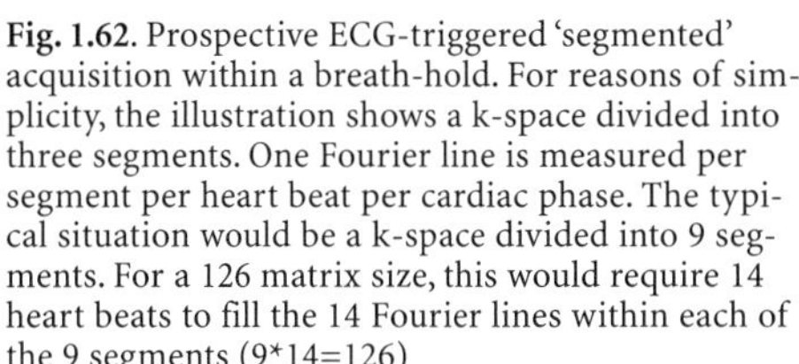

Fig. 1.62. Prospective ECG-triggered 'segmented' acquisition within a breath-hold. For reasons of simplicity, the illustration shows a k-space divided into three segments. One Fourier line is measured per segment per heart beat per cardiac phase. The typical situation would be a k-space divided into 9 segments. For a 126 matrix size, this would require 14 heart beats to fill the 14 Fourier lines within each of the 9 segments (9*14=126)

1.3.3 'Dark Blood' Preparation

The inflow of unsaturated blood into the imaging slice or slab has been utilized in MRA to display the vasculature. In cardiac imaging, the hyperintense blood in conjunction with phase changes due to motion and acceleration causes severe flow artifacts in conventional spin-echo imaging. For T1-weighted conventional spin-echo imaging, these artifacts are suppressed with parallel saturation blocks distal and proximal to the stack of slices and with additional dephasing gradients to cause a signal loss for the moving blood. With the introduction of T2-weighted imaging within a breath hold with fast spin-echo, a more sophisticated solution has been presented and dubbed 'dark blood' preparation. As illustrated in Fig. 1.64, the sequence starts with a nonselective inversion of all the magnetization, followed immediately by a selective re-inversion for the slice to be imaged. This all takes place with the advent of the ECG signal, where the heart is still in end-diastole. During the waiting period to follow, the re-inverted blood is washed out of the slice and is replaced by inverted, saturated blood. As the heart is moving into diastole, the TSE acquisition starts, producing 'dark blood' images. T2-weighted imaging of the beating heart within a breath hold is a single-slice technique.

1.3.4 Coronary Artery Imaging and the Navigator Technique

Coronary artery imaging started with a single-slice gradient-echo imaging approach, using the same effect as utilized in 2D-ToF-MRA. The sequence was triggered and segmented, and the data acquisition was placed in end-diastole, where the heart moves less and where the flow within the coronaries is supposed to be maximal. The usual degree of segmentation allowed data acquisition within 11 heart beats. A further refinement was implemented using variable flip-angles, that is, low flip-angles for the first Fourier lines to be measured per heart beat followed by increased flip-angles for the subsequent k-space segments. This approach compensated for saturation effects during data acquisition. Searching for coronary arteries with a single-slice approach is cumbersome, lengthy, and often not convincing. Questionable areas often remain questionable. A 3D approach is needed for retrospective reconstruction of the coronary vasculature. A 3D approach using similar parameters is too slow to be performed within one breath-hold period. A solution was presented using a so-called navigator technique as illustrated in Fig. 1.65. The 'navigator', a sagittal 2D slice or rod is placed through the liver to monitor the position of the liver/lung interface, and a 3D gradient-echo sequence slab is placed where the proximal parts of the coronary arteries are expected. While the 3D data set is executing the measurement of the same Fourier line multiple times, the data for the 'navigator' is collected immedi-

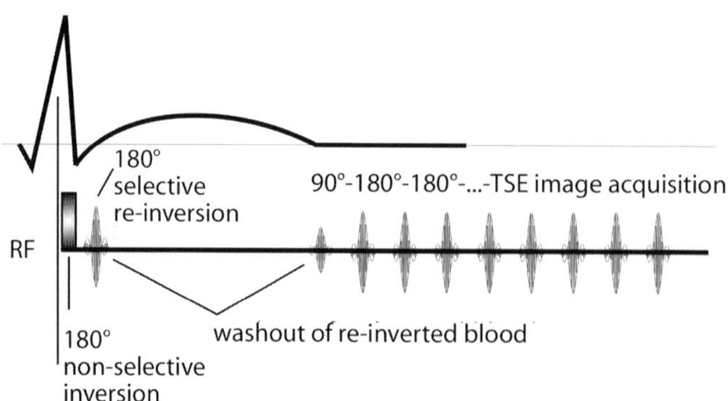

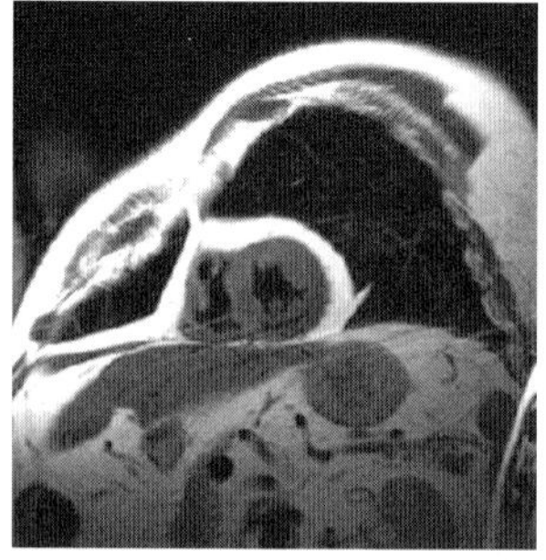

Fig. 1.64. 'Dark blood' preparation scheme. With the detection of the QRS complex within the ECG signal, a nonselective RF inversion pulse is executed, immediately followed by a selective 're-inversion' for the slice to be imaged. During a waiting period, the re-inverted blood is washed out of the slice and is replaced by inverted blood. The TSE image acquisition to follow will produce a 'dark blood' image. Shown is a short-axis perspective of the right and left ventricle surrounded by epicardial fat

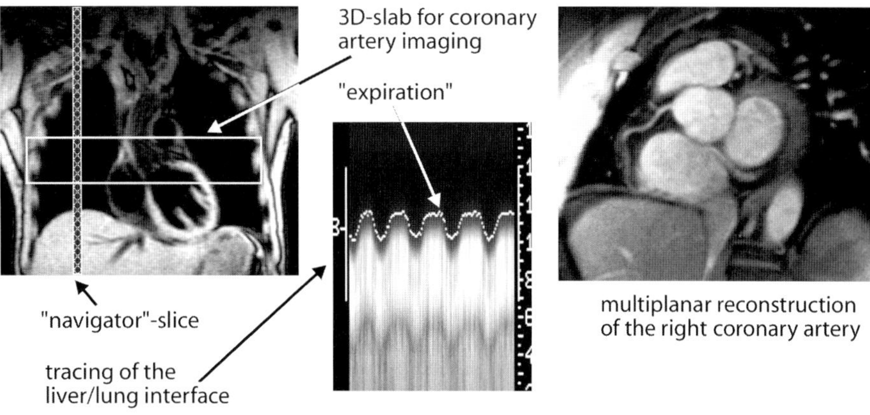

Fig. 1.65. The 'navigator' technique. A 2D-slice or rod is placed across the liver/lung interface to monitor the respiratory cycle. A 3D-ToF-MRA slab is placed across the coronary arteries. The position of the liver/lung interface is evaluated, and the 3D slab is moved prospectively and/or is taken as information to reject/accept the Fourier line for the 3D data set

ately afterwards. If the position of the liver/lung interface indicates 'close to expiration', the Fourier line of the 3D data set is accepted, otherwise it is waived. The position of the liver/lung interface can also be used prospectively to correct the position of the 3D slab (prospective acquisition correction, PACE). Doing so will reduce the measurement time since fewer Fourier lines of the 3D acquisition will be waived.

Recent advances in sequence development show that 3D imaging of the coronary arteries can also be performed within a breath-hold, in conjunction with a T1-shortening contrast agent.

1.4 Artifacts in Magnetic Resonance Imaging

There are three different types of artifacts in MR imaging. The first group is intrinsic to the method or the imaging technique and is almost unavoidable. These artifacts include chemical shifts, the flow and motion artifacts, and the susceptibility gradients within the patient locally destroying the magnetic field homogeneity. The second group of artifacts contains the avoidable artifacts produced by the user him- or herself, which are primarily aliasing artifacts. The third group of artifacts includes those based on compromised system design or system malfunction.

1.4.1 Unavoidable Artifacts

1.4.1.1 Chemical Shift

Since the frequency information is used for selective excitation and spatial encoding, the fact that fat and water have a slightly different resonance frequency will lead to a slight shift between the water image and the fat image. A signal void is created at the fat/water interfaces, where only the water is displayed, and the fat signal is assigned to another pixel based on the lower resonance frequency. Usually, a hyperintense rim is seen at the opposite location of the organ in question, where the fat signal is assigned to a pixel already representing a voxel with the associated water content (Fig. 1.66).

1.4.1.2 Flow and Motion

The phase of the macroscopic magnetization is used as spatial information in the direction perpendicular to the direction of frequency encoding. As discussed previously, flow and motion destroy this phase coherence. Moving and flowing objects often have the wrong phase position, not corresponding to the phase position of stationary tissue at the same location. The consequence is that there might be no signal with a phase corresponding to a certain position. In that case, the pixel representing that location will remain black and/or the phase position of the moving object might correspond to a location outside of the body. In this case, the bright-

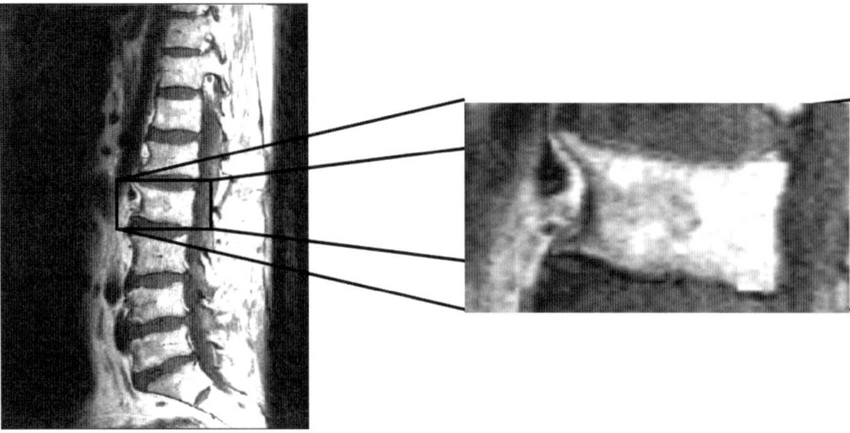

Fig. 1.66. The 'chemical shift' artifact. Frequency encoding is craniocaudal. The fat-containing vertebral body is '-artificially' shifted cranially

ness of the pixel outside of the body reflects the signal intensity matching that phase position. Flow and motion artifacts always propagate in the direction of phase encoding.

In cases of pulsatile flow, the distortions might be periodic during the measurement time. Periodic changes within *k*-space will cause multiple ghosting, e.g., the aorta in transverse cuts is usually apparent as multiple ghosts in the direction of phase encoding (Fig. 1.67).

New artifacts appear with new techniques or applications as shown in this turboFLAIR example (Fig. 1.68). An inflow effect mimics an intraventricular pathology. In turboFLAIR approaches, a selective inversion pulse is used, and, utilizing the fluid-specific relaxation time, an inversion time is selected at which the recovering magnetization of CSF has no longitudinal component. Doing so will attenuate the signal from fluid. Since the inversion is selective, inflow of uninverted CSF will cause the demonstrated hyperintense appearance.

1.4.1.3 Truncation Artifacts

Similar to the discussion about an infinite slice-selective RF pulse, the content of an object would be perfectly measured with an infinite data acquisition. Since there is only limited time for a data acquisition, data are

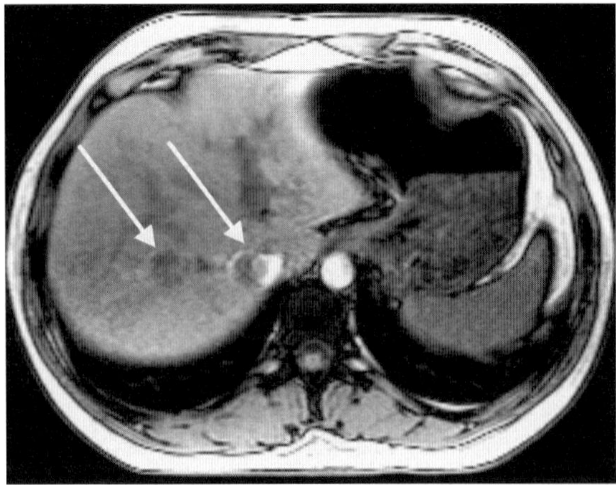

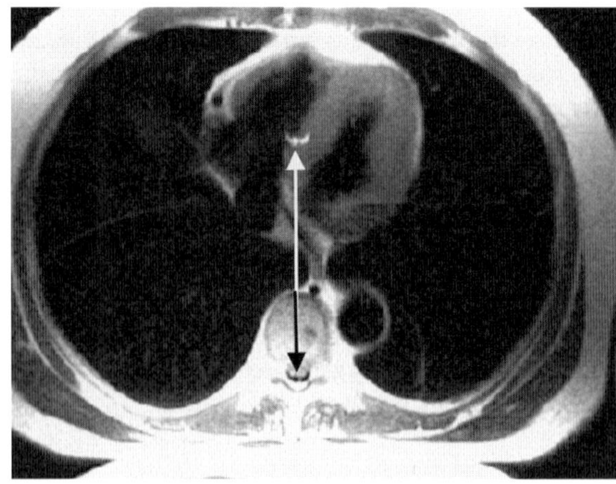

Fig. 1.67. The 'pulsatility' artifact. Periodic pulsatile signal variations during data acquisition manifest themselves as multiple ghosts in the direction of phase encoding

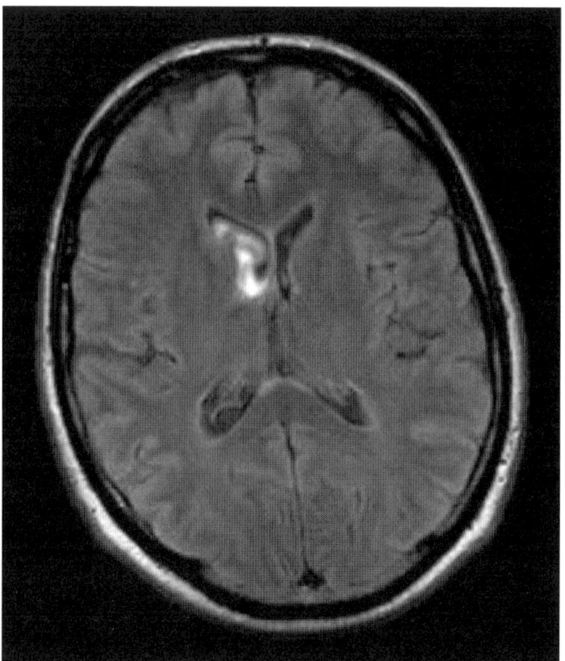

Fig. 1.68. The 'inflow' artifact in turboFLAIR protocols. 'Inverted' CSF is being replaced by 'un-inverted' CSF, causing a hyperintense appearance within an otherwise fluid-attenuated image

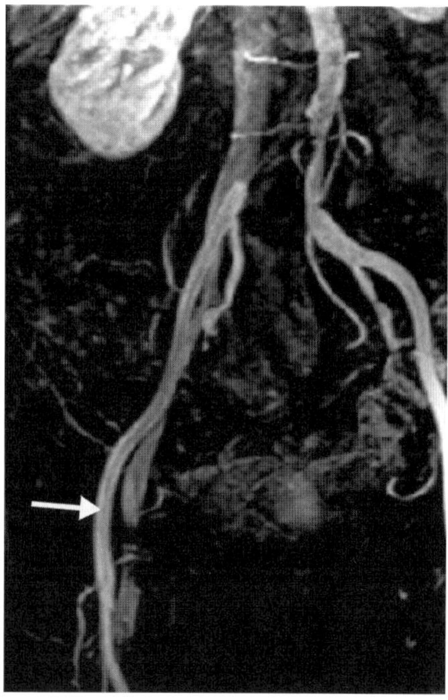

Fig. 1.69. The 'truncation' artifact. A reduced matrix size and a suboptimal timing between bolus arrival and start of the ceMRA measurement may result in a 'truncation' artifact mimicking a dissection

truncated. Imaging high-contrast interfaces will lead to so-called truncation artifacts, also known as Gibbs ringing, since the high spatial-frequency components of that boundary have not been measured, and the step is represented in a similar fashion to the poor slice-profile of a truncated RF pulse. The thin hypointense line in the center of the spinal cord in conjunction with a reduced matrix size is a well-known representation of a 'truncation' artifact. A more recent demonstration is the truncation artifact in ceMRA acquisitions, where the artifact mimics a dissection (Fig. 1.69).

1.4.1.4 Susceptibility Artifacts and RF Shielding Effects

Local inhomogeneities can be introduced with ferromagnetic or nonferromagnetic metallic foreign bodies within the patient, but are also prominent at air-bone-soft tissue interfaces. A local inhomogeneity will cause a nonlinear distribution of resonance frequencies and a nonlinear distribution of the phase information. Since this effect is stable over time and fixed in location, it will be refocused in SE imaging – except for a nonlinear behavior of the resonance frequency during the frequency encoding, the data acquisition period. For GRE imaging, there is usually a dramatic signal void due to the rapid dephasing of the transverse magnetization and a distorted geometry at locations where there is still some signal left but assigned to the wrong location since the Fourier transformation assumes a linear distribution of phases and frequencies. Figure 1.70 shows three typical examples of artifacts caused by ferromagnetic objects for various sequences.

Vascular or biliary stents containing ferromagnetic materials will demonstrate the same dramatic signal void as previously described for foreign bodies. The artifacts resulting from stents made from non-ferromagnetic materials like stainless steel or nickel-titanium alloys are smaller and confined to an adjacent region around the stent itself. As shown in Fig. 1.71a,b, the size of the artifact also depends on the orientation to the main magnetic field. As the stent elements of the Memotherm stent (Angiomed-Bard), for example, are primarily oriented parallel to the main magnetic field,

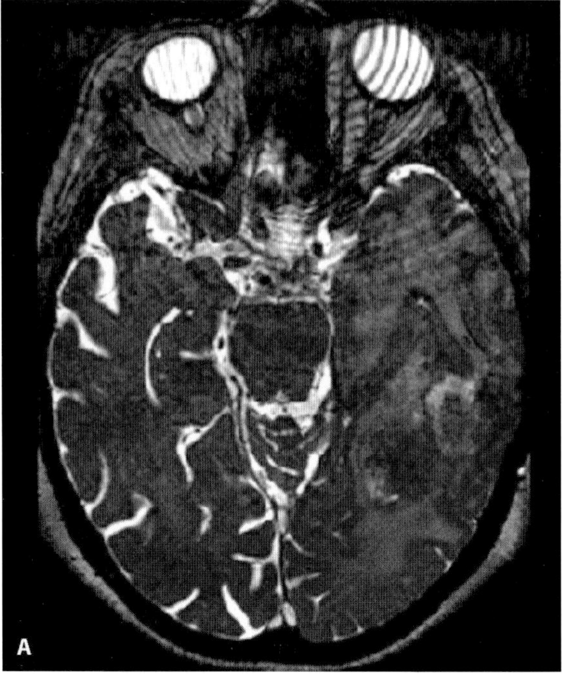

Fig. 1.70A–C. 'Metal' artifacts. **A** For trueFISP techniques, metal does not even have to be inside the imaging slice to cause severe artifacts. The dark lines are results of a destructive interference pattern caused by off-resonance effects due to ferromagnetic objects elsewhere. **B** The total signal void caused by ferromagnetic objects in conjunction with gradient-echo imaging is typical, as presented in this MP-RAGE case. **C** Even in spin-echo imaging, the displacement and distortion due to ferromagnetic components in eye shadow are obvious

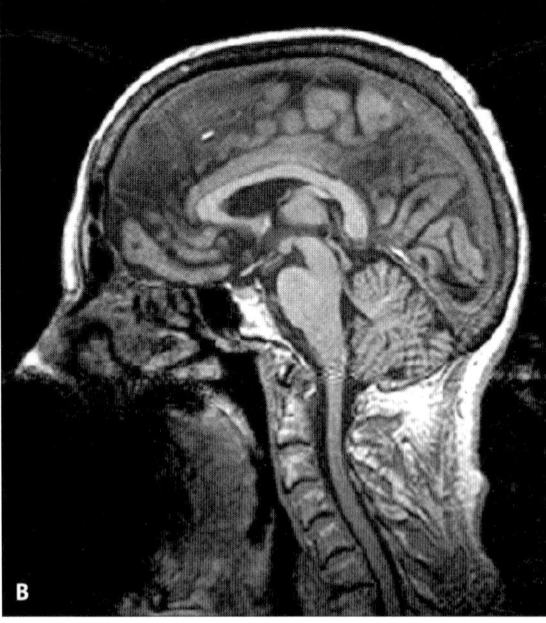

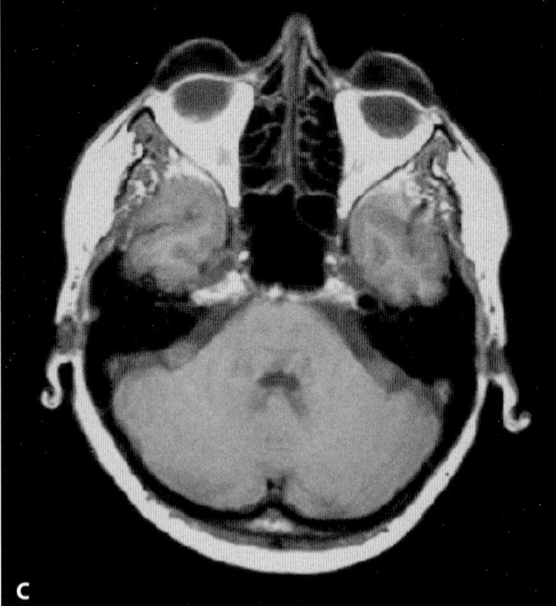

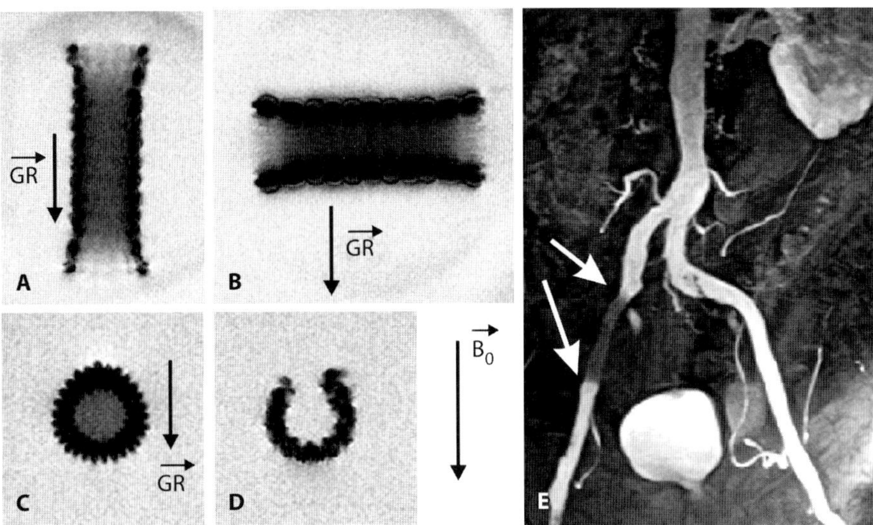

Fig. 1.71A–E. 'Stent' artifacts. **A** High-resolution image of a Memotherm stent (Angiomed-Bard) oriented parallel to B_0 and read-out gradient GR. **B** High-resolution image of the same stent oriented perpendicular to B_0 and read-out gradient. Notice the increased susceptibility artifacts. **C** Transverse cut through the same stent. Notice the hypointense lumen within the stent due to RF-shielding effect. That effect is eliminated for an open (cut-off) stent as illustrated in **D**. **E** ceMRA-MIP of a stented iliac artery showing a hypointense area (*white arrows*) mainly due to the 'shielding' effect of the stent

the artifact is relatively small compared with an orientation perpendicular to the main magnetic field.

In addition to the artifact generated by the susceptibility gradient in close vicinity to the nonferromagnetic stent, there is also an RF-shielding effect pending on the coil design. If there is no insulation between the conductive elements of the stent, the stent operates as a shield for the inner lumen. As a result, the inner lumen will appear hypointense as illustrated in Fig. 1.71c and e.

1.4.2 Avoidable Artifacts

1.4.2.1 Flow and Motion

If the flow is not too fast and not too turbulent, it might help to select a sequence that has GMR. This technique will rephase the dephasing caused by a constant flow or motion. For periodic changes of flow, it will help if the measurement is triggered.

For thoracic and abdominal imaging, the majority of techniques today use measurement times within a breath-hold. Respiratory triggering is also an applicable method to reduce respiratory artifacts. To reduce artifacts due to peristaltic motion, there is only the pharmacological approach.

1.4.2.2 Aliasing

If the FoV is smaller than the object imaged, the excited tissue outside of the FoV will be presented, due to data undersampling, with a phase or frequency information that corresponds to a position at the opposite location within the image. The signal from the tissue outside of the FoV will be assigned to the opposite location within the FoV. This artifact is called aliasing or wraparound (Fig. 1.72a). Going back to the concept of phase encoding, this phenomenon can be easily understood. It becomes more complicated when discussing the frequency encoding. Of course the resonance frequency outside the FoV is higher on one end and lower on the other side of the FoV for the duration of the frequency-encoding gradient. However, it can be shown that depending on the sampling frequency of the analog to digital converter, the signal course of the higher frequency outside the FoV is sampling the same signal

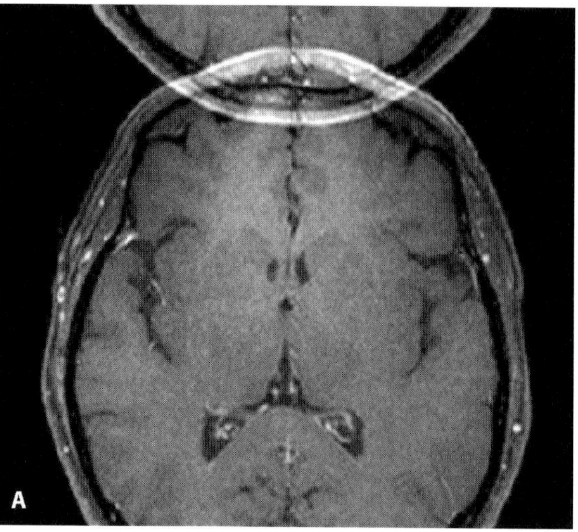

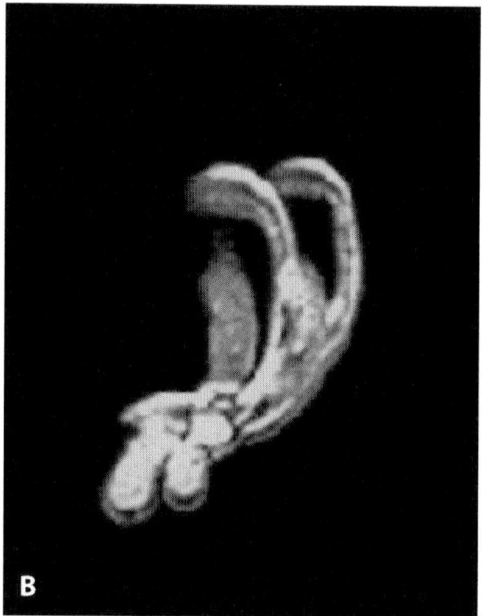

Fig. 1.72A, B. 'Aliasing' artifacts: for a selected FoV being smaller than the object (**A**), for an object that extends beyond the 3D slab of an MPRAGE measurement (**B**, left and right ear show up as wrap-in-artifact into the outer partitions)

course as for the lower frequency within the FoV. The solution is to over-sample the data. There is not a time penalty for over-sampling the data in the direction of frequency encoding. There is, however, a time penalty for over-sampling the data in the direction of phase encoding.

The same argument for wraparound in the direction of phase encoding is also applicable for the wrap in artifacts observed in 3D imaging. The slice profile is never perfect. If the slab profile for the RF-excitation pulse is slightly larger than the encoded 3D partition and if there is still excitable tissue outside of the partitions, the phase outside of the slab will match the phase of an opposite partition within the 3D slab. The solution is either to over-sample or to select a slab thick enough to cover the whole volume. For applications that usually use a nonselective excitation pulse, such as the classical MPRAGE, this approach is mandatory anyway (Fig. 1.72b).

1.4.2.3 Unexpected Software Features

Relatively harmless and avoidable artifacts are caused by software features in unintended use. Figure 1.73 is an example of a normalization filter applied to a 3D gradient-echo data set acquired in coronal orientation, with orthogonal transverse reconstructions. The purpose of the normalization filter is to reduce the brightness within the image for areas close to the surface coil and to increase the brightness in areas further away from the coil. The algorithm has been designed for a brightness normalization within the image, the slice, or the partition. The algorithm has not been written to consider the brightness in adjacent partitions. For orthogonal reconstructions, the corrected brightness within each of the partitions shows up as a staircase pattern.

Fig. 1.73. 'Normalization' artifact. A normalization filter altered the brightness within the slices or partitions of this coronal acquisition. Transverse reconstructions show the staircase pattern as a consequence of different brightness adjustments for the measured partitions

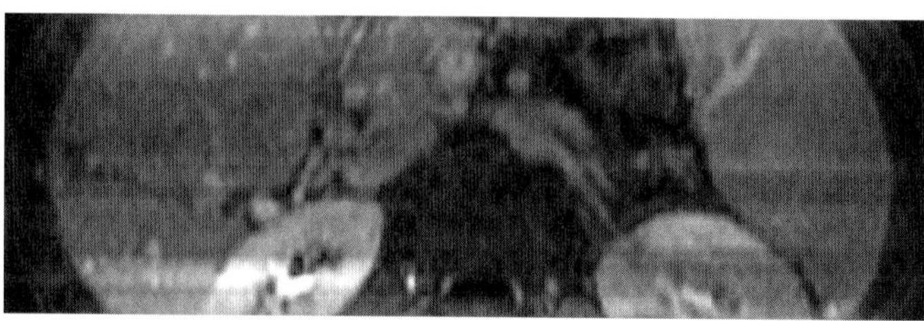

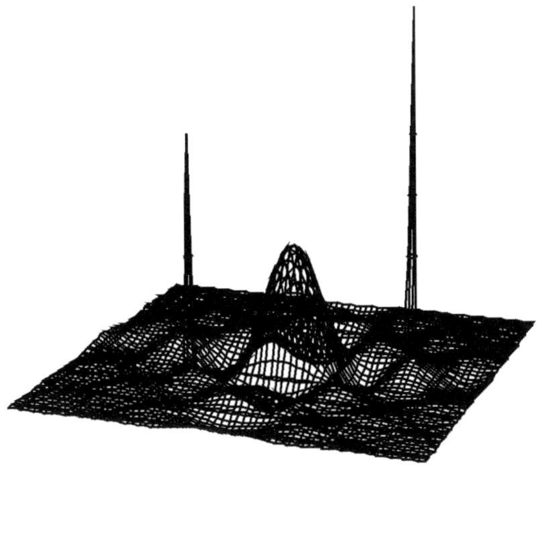

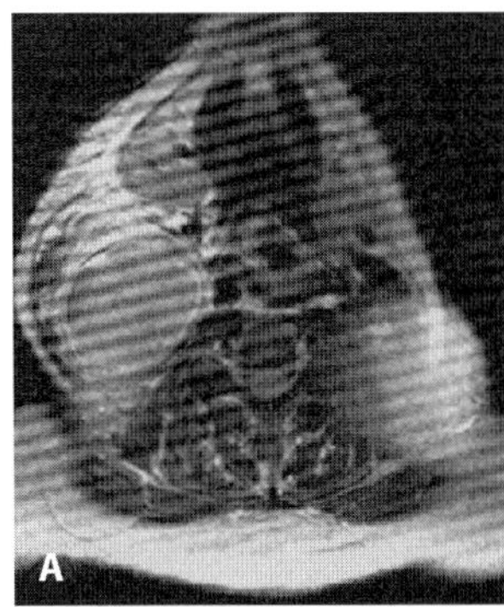

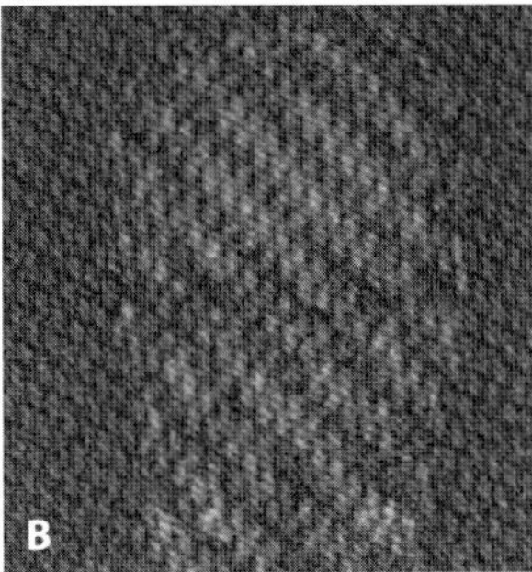

Fig. 1.74A, B. 'Spike' – or herring bone artifacts. **A** Transverse neck study with a 'spike' in the outer region of k-space. **B** Coronal head study with a 'spike' close to the center of k-space

1.4.3 System-Related Artifacts

1.4.3.1 Parasitic Excitation (Third-Arm Artifact)

If a bright coin-shaped or oyster-like object is observed that is not shaped like a pathological enhancement at that location, it may be a parasitic excitation. This usually appears in conjunction with a metallic foreign body within the patient. The magnetic field and the gradient field has to and will drop off outside of the magnet, outside of the gradient coil. The length of the body of the patient exceeds that range. While imaging, e.g., the heart, a small region within the lower legs might have the same resonance frequency during excitation as the slice to be excited within the heart. If the excitation range of the transmitting coil is large enough, it might excite that location. If the reception range of the receiving coil is large enough, it may detect the signal. Since the spatially encoding gradients at that location are usually nonlinear, the excited object is generally not identified, rather the signal is assigned to those pixels corresponding to the frequency and phase information. Transmitting coils of newer generation magnets have a limited range of excitation and reception, minimizing this so-called third-arm artifact.

1.4.3.2 Spikes

Any distortion within *k*-space will cause artifacts within the image. A classic distortion is a single signal peak within the raw data matrix, also called a spike. This spike will cause a crisscross or herring bone artifact within the image (Fig. 1.74). The artifact will be faint if the spike is sitting within a Fourier line containing the higher spatial frequencies of the object. The artifact will make the image unreadable if the spike is sitting close to the center of *k*-space. Spikes can be produced by a discharge of loaded plastic material or a loose connection within the gradient or RF system. They are rarely a sporadic malfunction of the ADC converter. In all cases, they are to be addressed by the vendor's service department.

1.5 MR Safety

It is beyond the scope of this book to elaborate on all safety aspects of MR imaging. There are frequently updated Internet links to MR safety issues, and there are excellent books covering the topic. Nevertheless, there are recent accidents highlighting the importance of the qualification and education of those who operate the MR system – and some basic safety topics shall be mentioned within this book.

1.5.1 Magnetic Force

The fringe field of the static magnetic field will attract ferromagnetic objects. The mass of the ferromagnetic object and the gradient within the fringe field are responsible for the attractive force. In order to confine the fringe field to an area close to the magnet, the magnetic field gradients close to the bore are significant. Calculations show that the attractive force will be in the order of 20 times the gravitational force. A 200 g pair of scissors will suddenly, moved a few centimeters closer to the bore of the magnet, have a 'pulling' weight of 4 kg! For example, at a distance of 1.5 m from the magnet bore, there will be no noticeable attraction. At a distance of 80 cm, the attractive force may be of the same order as the gravitational weight, 200 g. However, at a distance of 78 cm, the pulling weight will suddenly be 4 kg (horizontally into the direction of the bore). A technologist handling a 4 kg oxygen tank will in this case experience a 'pulling' weight of 80 kg! Unfortunately, patients have been killed due to a lack of knowledge, lack of caution, lack of experience, or ignorance. It also has to be pointed out explicitly that a superconducting magnet is 'on field' even when the main power supply to the magnet room is switched off! In case of an emergency, where policemen or firemen are likely to get close to the magnet, there should always be a trained technologist at the site to advice those emergency personnel about the potential danger of the strong magnetic field.

1.5.2 dB/dt – Fast Changes in Magnetic Field Gradient

Progress in hardware development has led to strong gradient systems to allow ultrafast imaging. At this point in time it turns out that the patient is the limiting factor for faster imaging. The dB/dt, the changes in a magnetic field gradient, are capable of inducing currents simulating nerve impulses for muscle contraction. Stimulation monitors precalculate these situations and prevent the execution of such a sequence.

The changes in magnetic field gradients may also induce currents in 'conducting' circles 'built' by the patient himself. Accidents have occurred when parts of the patient's body formed a loop, where the dB/dt changes were able to induce a significant current causing severe burns at locations of high resistance. Possible 'human' loops are the arms with folded hands and the legs with bare feet in contact. A dry towel should be used to isolate legs or arms, to avoid a closed circle of conducting skin or muscle tissue.

1.5.3 SAR and Energy of the RF Pulses

The specific absorption rate is an indicator of the power deposition within the patient; it is well understood and monitored. The guidelines that are followed prevent unnecessary 'heating' of the patient.

In addition, the electric field component of the RF pulses may couple significantly with any conductive straight wire that is longer than 28 cm. This can be a guide wire, a braided catheter, or a low resistance ECG lead. Second- and third-degree burns have been reported for those long conductive structures touching the skin.

Further Reading

Elster AD, Burdette J (2000) Questions and answers in MRI. Mosby Year Book, St Louis

Shellock FG, Kanal E (1996) Magnetic resonance, bioeffects, safety and patient management. Lippincott-Raven, Philadelphia

Stark DD, Bradley WG Jr (2000) Magnetic resonance imaging, 3rd edn. Mosby Year Book, St Louis

Contrast Agents for Magnetic Resonance Imaging

2

T. Balzer

Contents

2.1 Introduction

The alteration of signal intensity in diseased tissue forms the basis for magnetic resonance (MR) imaging in diagnostic radiology. The tissue signal intensity observed in MR images is the result of a complex interaction of numerous factors, which can be classified as those that reflect intrinsic properties of biologic tissues, e.g., T1 and T2 relaxation times and proton density, and those that are equipment related, e.g., field strength or pulse sequences. However, due to a wide biologic variation, the relaxation times of normal and abnormal tissues overlap. This limits the ability of plain MR imaging to detect and, even more, to characterize abnormal tissue. By using very specialized pulse sequences, only some of these limitations can be overcome. An alternative solution is provided by MR contrast agents, which alter the tissue relaxation times and can, therefore, be used to manipulate their signal intensity.

It is mainly contrast agents with so-called paramagnetic or superparamagnetic properties that are used to reduce the T1 and T2 relaxation times. Only those agents that are either already on the market and used in clinical practice or those that are late in clinical trials (phase II/III, with a launch to be expected within the next 2–3 years) will be discussed.

2.2 Mechanism of Action

The underlying principle of contrast media action is a chemical alteration of the proton relaxation time. Certain chemical compounds possess unique magnetic properties that arise from the motion of electrically charged electrons, protons, and neutrons. When protons and neutrons exist in pairs, as in nuclei with an even number of protons and neutrons, their magnetic moments will orient in opposite directions and cancel. However, nuclei with an odd number of protons and neutrons have a nonzero net nuclear magnetic moment, which precesses at the Larmor frequency if placed in an external magnetic field; the surrounding electrons also respond to the applied magnetic field. The resulting magnetic dipole moments arising from the electrons are considerably larger than the nuclear magnetic moments. Thus, if atoms, ions, or molecules with large electronic dipole moments are placed adjacent to protons, their magnetic dipole moments can interact to enhance the relaxation of protons and alter the tissue signal intensity. Therefore, compounds with large electronic magnetic dipole moments may be utilized as contrast agents in MR imaging.

2.2.1 Paramagnetism

Paramagnetism arises in atoms that have unpaired electrons. Placed in an external magnetic field, these atoms show a significant net magnetization because of the preferential orientation of the paramagnetic dipole moments parallel to the applied magnetic field; its magnitude is proportional to the magnitude of the external magnetic field. The most important chemical subgroup of paramagnetic compounds are metal ions (e.g., Mn^{2+} and Fe^{3+}) and lanthanide elements, such as gadolinium (Gd) and dysprosium (Dy). Gadolinium is one of the strongest paramagnetic substances because of its seven unpaired electrons. Paramagnetic agents predominantly shorten both the T1-relaxation time and – especially at higher tissue concentrations – the T2-relaxation time.

2.2.2 Superparamagnetism

Superparamagnetism is induced by smaller ferrimagnetic particles that have only a single magnetic domain. In an external magnetic field, these particles show a magnetization curve like that of paramagnetic agents, but with a much stronger response, and saturation effects are readily attained. The increase in magnetization at a field strength of between 0.3 T and 1.5 T is nonlinear. After removal of the magnetic field, no net magnetization is retained. Superparamagnetic contrast agents are basically small and ultrasmall iron oxide particles that shorten mainly the T2-relaxation time. The smaller particles also shorten the T1-relaxation time.

2.2.3 Relaxation Times, Relaxation Rates, and Relaxivity

The T1 and T2 relaxation times are characteristic times describing how long it takes for the signal mechanism of magnetic resonance to return to the original state or to relax. The time taken to return to the original longitudinal magnetization is described by the T1-relaxation time. The T2-relaxation time refers to the component of the bulk magnetization vector which describes how fast the transversal magnetization vanishes. T1- and T2-relaxation times are not exact measures of the time it takes for relaxation; instead, they are time constants that describe the speed of this process and, in this respect, are comparable to time constants that, for example, describe radioactive decay. Both T1- and T2-relaxation times are tissue specific. A short T1 appears as a bright signal, and a short T2 appears as a dark signal on MR images.

As mentioned earlier, paramagnetic and superparamagnetic contrast agents shorten the T1- and T2-relaxation times or, in other words, increase the relaxation rates (defined as 1/T1 and 1/T2). The ability of a contrast medium to shorten the relaxation times depends both on the contrast medium concentration in the respective tissue and on the intrinsic relaxation time of the tissue. A concentration of 0.1 mM of a paramagnetic Gd chelate is a powerful relaxation enhancer, sufficient to decrease the relaxation times of biological fluids by 50%. However, to influence tissues of shorter intrinsic relaxation times to the same extent, a higher contrast medium concentration is needed. The power or efficiency of a contrast medium to enhance the relaxation rate is called 'relaxivity'. For example, the efficiency of Gd-DTPA at enhancing the longitudinal relaxation in water is expressed as relaxivity R_1=4.5 (mM s)$^{-1}$, whereas the transverse (T'') relaxivity is R_2=6.0 (mM s)$^{-1}$. The R_2/R_1 ratio of 1.3 is typical for paramagnetic contrast media. Because tissue T1-relaxation is inherently slow compared with T2-relaxation, their predominant effect is on T1.

2.3 Extracellular Contrast Agents

The extracellular contrast agents can be divided into low and high molecular-weight agents. The latter will be discussed in Sect. 2.5 due to their blood-pool properties. The low molecular-weight agents belong more or less to the paramagnetic Gd chelates. The prototypical complex of this class of agents is Gd-DTPA (Magnevist, Schering AG, Berlin, Germany), which was the first MR contrast agent introduced into the market in 1988. In the meantime, other agents have been launched or are close to coming to market (Table 2.1).

MultiHance (Gd-BOPTA, Bracco, Milan, Italy) was originally designed as a hepatobiliary contrast agent. However, because about 96% of the compound is excreted renally in humans, it is classified predominantly as an extracellular agent. Another specific feature should be mentioned for Gadovist 1.0 (Gadobutrol, Schering AG, Berlin, Germany): this agent consists of a 1 M concentration instead of the 0.5 M concentration of all other Gd complexes. When compared to other extracellular contrast media, this results in double the concentration and half the injection volume for the same dose, which is advantageous for first-pass imaging examinations, such as perfusion imaging and high-gradient 3D MR angiography.

Apart from these particulars, all Gd complexes basically exhibit the same pharmacodynamic and pharmacokinetic properties, resulting in comparable safety profiles and approvals for nearly the same indications. For detailed information, consult the respective package inserts in the European countries. Therefore, they will be discussed together in the following sections.

2.3.1 Basic Principles and Properties

Because of its strong paramagnetic effect, Gd has been chosen as the metal for all available extracellular MR contrast agents. Due to the high toxicity of free Gd, it has to be firmly bound to ligands, resulting in highly hydrophilic Gd-chelate complexes. The complex stability of all Gd compounds is very high. For example, the in vivo constant for dissociation of Gd-DTPA (Magnevist) is about 10^{23}. This guarantees that the effect of free Gd is not of any toxicological relevance. The molecules of these contrast agents are designed either as a linear (Magnevist, Omniscan, MultiHance, Optimark) or a macrocyclic structure (Dotarem,

Table 2.1. Extracellular contrast agents: overview and registration status

Trademark and generic name	Manufacturer	Chelate structure	Registration status (EU) and dose (mmol/kg)		
			CBS	Body	Children
Magnevist® gadopentetate (Gd-DTPA/dimegl.)	Schering AG	Open chain	0.3	0.3	0.2
Dotarem® gadoterate (Gd-DOTA/megl.)	Guerbet	Macrocyclic ionic	0.2	0.1	0.1
MultiHance® gadobenate (Gd-BOPTA)	Bracco	Open chain ionic	Liver 0.1	Liver 0.05	
Omniscan® gadodiamide (Gd-DTP-BMA)	Amersham	Open chain neutral	0.3	0.1	0.1
ProHance® gadoteridol (Gd-HP-DO3A)	Bracco	Macrocyclic neutral	0.3	0.1	0.1
Optimark® gadoversetamide (Gd-DTPA-BMEA)	Mallinckrodt	Open chain neutral	Submitted	Submitted	
Gadovist® 1.0 and 0.5 gadobutrol	Schering AG	Macrocyclic neutral	0.3	MRA-submitted	

ProHance, Gadovist), which is of minor relevance for their pharmacodynamic and pharmacokinetic properties. The osmolality of these compounds varies from 590 mosmol/kg H_2O (Gadovist 0.5 M) up to 1980 mosmol/kg H_2O (Magnevist). However, due to the low doses of 0.1–0.3 mmol/kg body weight (BW) (0.2–0.6 ml/kg), the amount of osmotically active 'particles' (total osmotic load) is, at the higher doses, even lower than low osmolar nonionic X-ray contrast agents. Consequently, the osmolality of the available contrast agents does not have any effect on the safety or tolerability profile of any of those agents.

While Gd is responsible for the paramagnetic effect of these complexes, the ligand determines the pharmacokinetic behavior. Due to the high hydrophilicity of the Gd chelates and their low molecular weight, they rapidly diffuse into the interstitial space after intravenous injection and a short intravascular phase. The protein binding is negligible. The elimination of the unmetabolized Gd complexes from the body occurs via renal excretion with a plasma half-life of about 90 min. The compounds are completely eliminated after a maximum of 24 h if the glomerular filtration is not diminished. The half-life is prolonged in patients with impaired renal function, but this does not change the safety profile (Sect. 2.3.3.1).

2.3.2 Efficacy

2.3.2.1 Clinical Indications

The extracellular contrast agents have a broad indication spectrum, which will be discussed in more detail in the respective chapters. Mainly for two reasons, about 60%–70% of the contrast-enhanced MRI examinations are performed in CNS indications. The first reason is that, historically, MRI first became clinical routine in those areas for which motion or flow artifacts, due to long-lasting imaging sequences, either did not exist or were of only minor importance. Those areas are predominantly the CNS and the musculoskeletal system, with the latter being the second important indication area in MR imaging.

The second – and probably even more important – reason for CNS being the biggest indication for the use of contrast agents in MR imaging is the existence of a blood-brain barrier (BBB). Therefore, the extracellular agents behave in the normal brain as an intravascular contrast agent that only diffuses into the interstitial space, leading to an enhancement in the case of a BBB-leakage caused by a tumor, trauma, infarction, or inflammatory/demyelinating disease. Metastases do not have a BBB and enhance after the injection of contrast media as well.

As mentioned before, musculoskeletal diseases such as bone tumors or inflammatory diseases are important indications, as are tumors of the kidneys, glands, pelvic organs, breast, and liver. In imaging of the liver, extracellular agents provide important information for the detection of hypervascularized lesions and for lesion characterization in general (using dynamic sequences). Breast imaging has also become a more important indication. However, it should be noted that only for very specific questions, e.g., dense tissue or silicon implants, has MR imaging been accepted as the imaging technique of choice; currently, not enough data from representative populations have been published to justify the use of MR imaging as a routine or even as a screening examination.

A relatively new and very promising indication is 3D MR angiography. This technique requires the use of contrast agents due to the very fast imaging sequences. Most of the examinations can be performed as first-pass imaging using Gd chelates, which provide good image quality. Only a few vessel areas, such as the coronary arteries, venous vessels, or interventional procedures, require an intravascular contrast agent.

2.3.2.2 Dose

The dose which was first established for the use of Magnevist in CNS indications is 0.1 mmol/kg BW or 0.2 ml/kg BW. Although the available pulse sequences and the technology in general have changed significantly during the last decade, the recommended dose for Gd chelates has been widely confirmed and further extended for most of the so-called whole-body indications. Thus, the dose of 0.1 mmol/kg (0.2 ml/kg) can be considered as the accepted standard dose for MR imaging. A few exceptions have to be mentioned: a dose reduction to 0.05 mmol/kg BW (0.1 ml/kg) was discussed for the early detection of hypophyseal microadenomas during a dynamic imaging sequence, and an increase of the dose should be considered for the following:

1. High-gradient 3D MR angiography. This angiography technique was introduced in 1995. At the very beginning, doses of up to 0.5 mmol/kg BW (1 ml/kg) were administered. In the meantime, due to faster sequences and better bolus tracking techniques in particular, the maximum doses are in the range 0.1–0.3 mmol/kg BW (0.2–0.6 ml/kg). A dose of 0.1–0.15 mmol/kg BW (0.2–0.3 ml/kg) seems to be a robust dose providing sufficient and reproducible image quality.
2. Detection and characterization of focal CNS lesions. Several clinical studies have demonstrated that using Gd doses of 0.2 mmol/kg or 0.3 mmol/kg BW (0.4–0.6 ml/kg), additional brain metastases can be detected in about 20% of this patient population compared with the standard dose. A double or triple dose may also allow better characterization of low-grade gliomas, better detection of tumor recurrence, and a more reliable selection of representative biopsy sites in those tumors.
   However, in most of the patients, the additional information does not have any therapeutic consequences. Therefore, the general dosing recommendation is to administer 0.1 mmol/kg BW (0.2 ml/kg) of any Gd chelate and to increase the dose by a further injection of 0.1–0.2 mmol/kg BW (0.2–0.4 ml/kg) only in those patients for whom any additional information would have direct impact on the further therapy.
   Another area which is still under discussion with regard to the necessary Gd dose concerns patients with multiple sclerosis. Many reports suggest that, at a double or triple dose, more enhancing lesions can also be detected. However, the clinical relevance of these findings is not yet fully understood. Consequently, the general dose recommendation is still the standard dose of 0.1 mmol/kg BW (0.2 ml/kg).
3. Brain perfusion. Brain perfusion imaging is normally performed using T2*-W sequences (instead of T1-W sequences) and susceptibility imaging. The optimal dose for this technique depends very much on the sequence used. If brain perfusion imaging is performed with a fast GRE sequence, the optimal dose is in the range of about 0.3 mmol/kg BW (0.6 ml/kg), as shown in a double-blind dose-comparative study with Gadovist 1.0. A lower dose can also be used, but the reproducibility is significantly worse. If the examination is carried out using EPI sequences, the optimal dose is probably slightly lower than 0.3 mmol/kg, due to the higher sensitivity of these sequences for susceptibility effects. As there has been no controlled dose comparison so far, a final recommendation is not yet possible.

2.3.3 Safety

Most of the safety data are based on the published experience with Magnevist, which has been administered intravenously to more than 37 million patients over the last decade. However, on the basis of several comparative clinical trials and the growing experience with the other extracellular Gd compounds, it can be assumed that they all have a comparable safety profile. Overall, this class of contrast agents is by far the safest compared with other contrast agents.

Data from controlled clinical trials and from a pre- and post-marketing surveillance in several million patients show an overall incidence of adverse reactions of 1%–2%. This incidence is about two to three times higher in patients with a history of allergies or in patients with asthma. The most frequent adverse reactions are listed in Table 2.2.

The most relevant adverse reaction which may occur after intravenous (IV) injection of Gd compounds is an anaphylactoid reaction that also occurs with other contrast agents. The incidence of anaphylactoid reactions is about six times lower than with nonionic X-ray contrast agents. Nevertheless, IV injection of Gd complexes should be only performed if emergency equipment is available. As far as is known, there is no relationship between adverse reactions and doses of up to at least 0.3 mmol/kg BW. Based on limited experience, patients given doses of up to 0.5 mmol/kg BW also do not show any further increase in the incidence of adverse reactions.

Table 2.2. Incidence of adverse events after intravenous injection of 0.1 mmol/kg body weight (BW) Magnevist® (*n*=13439)

Type of adverse event	Incidence (%)
Nausea/vomiting	0.42
Local warmth/pain	0.42
Headache	0.26
Paresthesia	0.13
Dizziness	0.10
Urticaria/allergy-like shir reaction	0.10
Focal convulsia	0.03

2.3.3.1 Use in Patients with Impaired Renal Function

In a number of patients, the administration of X-ray contrast agents leads to an impairment of renal function. This is mostly a transient effect, which can be minimized by sufficient hydration of the patient. However, for patients with already impaired renal function, this became a relevant clinical problem that was carefully studied for MR contrast agents as well.

In a study including patients with various degrees of impaired renal function, the short-term effect (24 h) and the long-term effect (up to 120 h) of a single IV injection of 0.1 mmol/kg BW Magnevist on the creatinine clearance was investigated. At no time and in no patient was there an effect on renal function that was attributable to the Gd injection. These results could be confirmed by further retrospective analyses of bigger patient populations, e.g., a meta-analysis of all Magnevist phase-III data. Another result of the above-mentioned study was that the Gd complexes can be removed from the body by hemodialysis in case of acute renal failure. An almost complete elimination is achieved after three hemodialyses. These results were confirmed recently by another controlled clinical study using Gadobutrol 1.0 at doses of 0.1 and 0.3 mmol/kg in patients with different degrees of renal impairment.

2.3.3.2 Use in Pediatrics

From a regulatory point of view, there are two age groups within the category of pediatrics. One group is aged from 2 to 18 years, the other consists of newborns and infants up to 2 years. The four extracellular Gd chelates on the market (Magnevist, Dotarem, Omniscan, and ProHance) are approved for CNS indications in children from 2 to 18 years of age; some are approved for newborns and for whole-body indications as well.

In a clinical study involving 72 children under 2 years of age, a single or repeated injection of 0.1 mmol/kg BW Magnevist was given. Two of the 72 patients experienced an adverse event (2.7%). One adverse event was diarrhea, the other a facial edema, most likely related to a concomitant medication. In a big post-marketing surveillance study of more than 15,000 patients reported by Nelson, more than 900 pediatric patients under the age of 18 years were included. The data confirm a low incidence of adverse reactions in this patient population that was comparable to the incidence in adults. Thus, there is no known age-related specific risk of injecting Gd chelates.

2.4 Tissue-Specific Contrast Agents

The rapid extravasation of the extracellular contrast media leads to a transient but unspecific signal increase in parenchymal organs, e.g., in the liver and spleen. Whereas the characterization of focal lesions can be improved by extracellular agents during the early perfusion phase, the lesion detection of small lesions in particular is not improved significantly. Sometimes lesions are obscured due to the diffuse enhancement (as in CT). Consequently, much effort in contrast-media research went into more specific contrast agents. The most advanced area is the development of liver-specific contrast agents. Another area of interest is improved imaging of lymph nodes – in particular, the question of whether enlarged lymph nodes are metastatic or not. Both areas will be discussed in detail below.

2.4.1 Liver-Specific Contrast Agents

In general, two different approaches or classes of contrast media exist to target the liver: (1) paramagnetic, hepatobiliary T1 contrast media, taken up by the hepatocytes of the liver, and (2) superparamagnetic particles phagocytosed by cells of the reticulo-endothelium system (RES) and acting as T2 contrast agents. The basic idea of both the hepatobiliary and the RES-specific contrast media is that they can only be taken up by liver tissue containing the respective cells. Tissue of nonhepatic origin, such as metastases, does not show any uptake and remains as a bright or dark spot within the liver (Fig. 2.1). In lesions of hepatic origin, the uptake depends on the number and the functional integrity of the hepatocytes or RES cells. The variation between several lesion types and the resulting differential uptake of contrast media provide useful information for lesion characterization.

In general, all liver-specific contrast media that are already on the market or that are currently in late phases of clinical development improve the detection of liver lesions by up to 20%, depending on the patient popula-

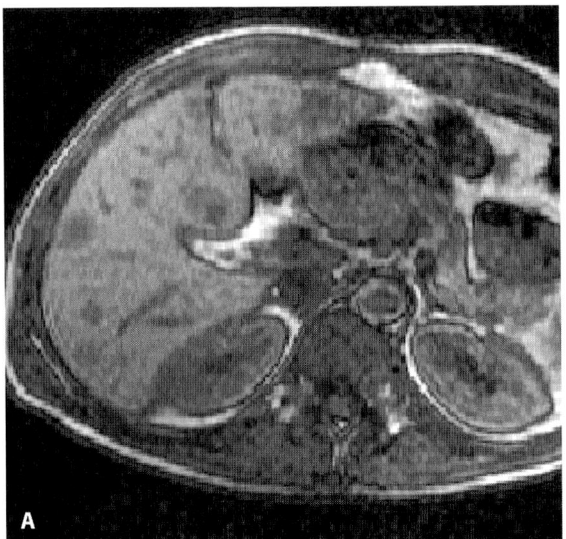

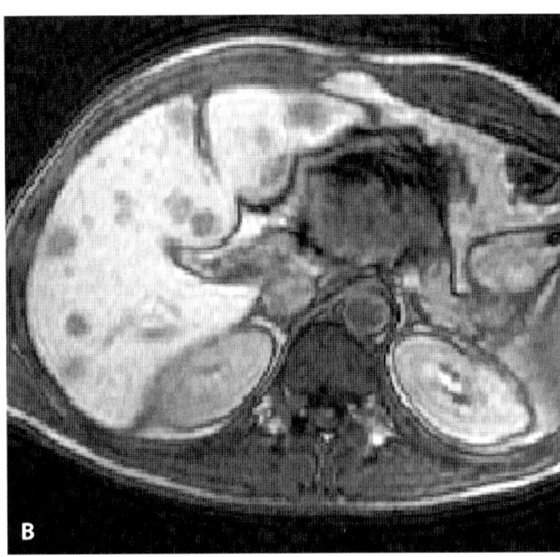

Fig. 2.1A,B. Multiple metastatic lesions at pre- and 20 post-injection of Gd-EOB-DTPA. Distinct signal increase of the normal liver parenchyma but no enhancement within the lesions on T1-GRE sequences (Reimer, Münster, Germany)

tion and how the findings were confirmed by independent procedures. As there are no comparative trials so far, it is not known whether a certain contrast medium or one of the two classes (RES-specific and hepatobiliary CA) is superior with regard to lesion detection.

The ability to characterize lesions depends very much on the capability of a contrast medium to allow dynamic imaging, as important information can be obtained from this early perfusion phase. However, by the principal mechanism of uptake into RES cells and hepatocytes, important information about the integrity of the respective system can be gained.

2.4.1.1 Hepatobiliary Contrast Agents

Three paramagnetic hepatobiliary contrast agents have recently been approved in the USA and Europe or are currently in phase-III clinical development. The three contrast media are given in Table 2.3.

The latter two Gd-based contrast media are chemical derivates of Magnevist in which a carboxyl group is replaced by a lipophilic moiety. This leads to an uptake into hepatocytes by an anionic carrier system, an intracellular binding to transport proteins, and finally, secretion into the biliary system. The degree of specific uptake by the hepatocytes is drug and species dependent. Whereas both Gd-based contrast agents, Eovist and MultiHance, show a distinct uptake in various animal species, in humans only 2%–4% of MultiHance, but about 50% of Eovist are specifically taken up by the liver and excreted into the biliary system. Nevertheless, both agents improve the detection of liver lesions. The contrast media portion not eliminated via the biliary route is excreted via the kidneys, similar to the extracellular contrast agents.

Teslascan is a Mn^{2+}-based chelate. After an in vivo dissociation of the largest portion of the Mn-DPDP complex into free Mn^{2+} and DPDP, free Mn^{2+} is taken up by hepatocytes, whereas a transmetallation with Zn^{2+} could be shown for DPDP. By another, specific carrier mechanism, some of the remaining Mn-DPDP complex is also taken up by the hepatocytes and shows

Table 2.3

1. Teslascan (Mn DPDP, Mangafodipir, Nycomed Imaging AS, Oslo, Norway), which obtained market approval in 1997
2. MultiHance® (Gadolinium BOPTA, Gadobenat, Bracco, Milan, Italy), which has been approved for liver imaging and has also been developed as extracellular contrast agent
3. Eovist® (Gd-DTPA, Schering AG, Berlin, Germany), which completed phase-III development

intracellular dissociation. Whereas DPDP and the still-complete Mn-DPDP complex (15%–20%) are renally eliminated within 24 h, free Mn^{2+} remains in the body for several days and accumulates not only in the liver but to a lesser extent in the pancreas, gastric mucosa, adrenal glands, and some intracerebral structures before it is biliarly or renally eliminated. The half-life therefore is not clearly determined.

2.4.1.1.1 Dose and Mode of Administration

Teslascan is approved for a dose of 5 µmol/kg BW. Whereas this dose is infused in a 10 mM concentration over a period of about 15–20 min, a higher concentration (50 mM) is used for a slow bolus injection (1–2 min) in the USA. However, in both cases, the injection speed does not allow any dynamic imaging. The optimal imaging time point is at 15–30 min after the end of infusion/injection. In some cases, later images at 4 h provide additional information for lesion characterization.

MultiHance is injected as a fast bolus at a dose of 0.05 mmol/kg BW, which provides the opportunity of dynamic imaging. Due to the relatively low uptake of MultiHance (about 2%–4% by hepatocytes), the accumulation of a sufficient amount of contrast medium in the liver lasts longer, and the best imaging time point is therefore about 60–120 min after injection. It could be shown that the signal increase in the liver at that time is comparable to the enhancement after injection of Teslascan.

For Eovist, which can also be injected as a fast bolus for dynamic imaging, doses between 3µmol/kg and 50 µmol/kg BW have been tested in clinical phase-II studies. The recommended dose currently used in phase-III studies is 25 µmol/kg BW, which is sufficient for the combination of dynamic imaging and hepatobiliary phase imaging, as well as for imaging in patients with liver cirrhosis or impaired liver function. The optimal imaging time point for the hepatobiliary phase is about 15–20 min after injection, but the imaging window is at least up to 120 min.

2.4.1.1.2 Safety and Tolerability

All available data indicate a good safety profile for all three agents. It seems that the two Gd-based agents (MultiHance and Eovist) exhibit a comparable pattern and incidence of adverse reactions, as do extracellular Gd compounds. For Teslascan, the rate of adverse reactions depends very much on the dose and injection speed. After a dose reduction from 10 to 5 µmol/kg BW and a slow infusion, the adverse event rate went down to about 7%–10%, without any of the flush symptoms that had been reported in the phase-II studies and in the US studies for which, even in phase III, a slow bolus injection was used. After bolus injection, flush symptoms are reported by more than 70% of the patients. However, these symptoms are transient and of mild intensity and affect the patient's comfort but do not raise a safety concern. For none of the three compounds is any relevant change of laboratory parameters reported.

2.4.1.2 RES-Specific Contrast Agents

One superparamagnetic RES-specific agent or contrast medium has been on the market under the trademark Endorem (AMI 25, Guerbet, France) in Europe since 1996. Another contrast medium, Resovist (Schering AG, Berlin, Germany) has recently received approval in the EU and will be available in most European countries in 2001/2002. Both agents belong to the so-called SPIOs (small iron oxide particles), with hydrodynamic diameters of about 150 nm (Endorem) and 60 nm (Resovist). To avoid in vivo aggregation of the particles and to increase the cardiovascular tolerability in particular, SPIOs have to be coated. This is done with dextran in the case of Endorem and small molecular-weight carboxy-dextran in the case of Resovist.

The two agents are taken up by RES cells (Fig. 2.2) and mainly phagocytosed by Kupffer cells in the liver and to a lesser extent also in the spleen, bone marrow, and lymph nodes. The half-life in plasma before phagocytosis is biphasic. There is a rapid uptake of the bigger particles with a half-life of about 5 min and a slower uptake of smaller particles with a half-life of about 2–3 h. After phagocytosis, the iron goes into the physiological iron pool and the respective physiological iron metabolism.

2.4.1.2.1 Dose and Mode of Administration

The recommended dose range for Endorem in Europe is 15 µmol Fe/kg BW. Endorem has to be prepared

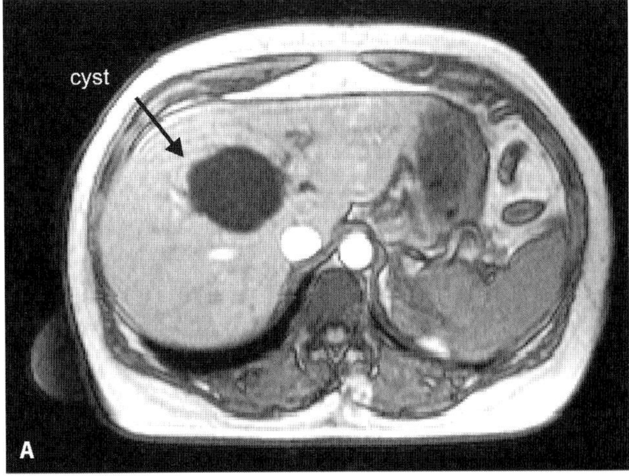

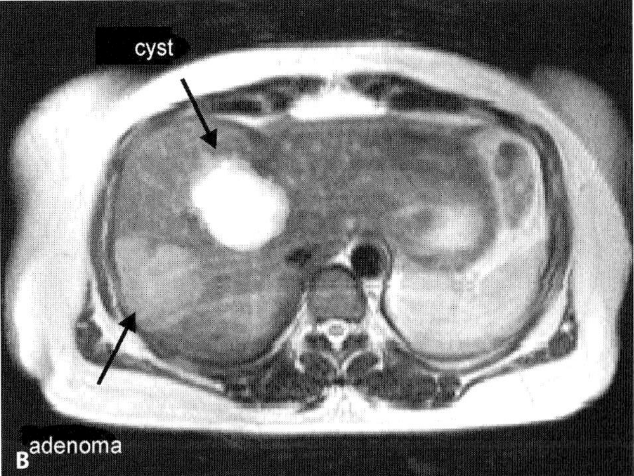

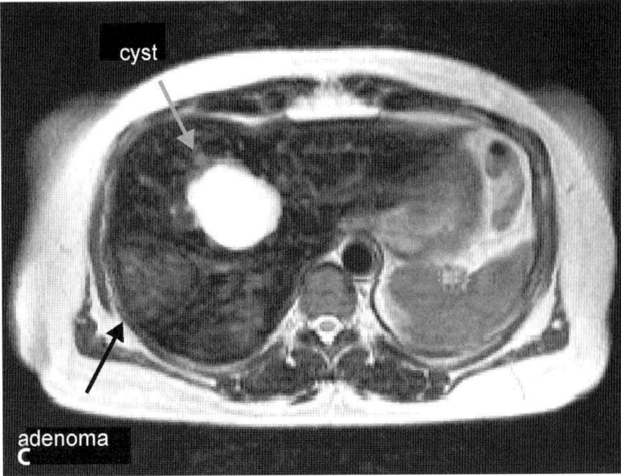

Fig. 2.2A–C. Unenhanced T1 GRE (A) and T2 TSE (B) MR images of a cystic lesion and an adenoma. Signal decrease of the normal liver and of the adenoma on T2 TSE (C) images after intravenous injection of Resovist due to uptake of the iron oxide particles by functioning RES cells. No uptake and no signal decrease in the cystic lesion (Stiskal, Vienna, Austria)

immediately before administration by dissolution in a volume of about 100 ml of 5% glucose. It must be infused over a period of 20–30 min due to some hypertonic reactions in early clinical trials. Imaging can be started after a further 15 min.

Resovist is a ready-for-use suspension that is injected I.V. as a fast bolus, allowing dynamic imaging. The clinical dose is a fixed volume of 0.9 ml per patient with a body weight of 35 kg, but less than 60 kg and 1.4 ml for patients with a body weight of 60 kg and above. These volumes correspond to doses of 6–11 µmol Fe/kg BW.

2.4.1.2.2 Safety and Tolerability

Safety data from more than 800 patients were reported from the phase-III clinical trials with Endorem. The reported incidents of adverse events are between 10.3% in Europe and 15% in the USA. One of the most frequently reported adverse effects is lumbar back pain in more than 4% of the patients. The etiology of this symptom is unknown. In most of the patients, the symptoms disappeared after reduction of the infusion speed; however, in several patients, active treatment was necessary. The remaining adverse reactions are all well-known from other contrast agents and are not of any concern. The reported cardiovascular side effects after rapid injection during the early phase-I studies are not observed when the compound is infused slowly.

Resovist has been administered to more than 1200 patients during clinical phase-II and phase-III trials worldwide so far. No effects on heart rate or blood pressure have been reported after fast bolus injection. The overall incidence of adverse events is about 9%; 5.5% of these were assessed relative to the study drug used by the clinical investigators. Back pain is reported in less than 0.5% of cases and is of mild intensity.

With regard to laboratory parameters, a transient decrease within the normal range of the activity of clotting factor XI has been observed. This does not result in any changes in the overall bleeding time or coagulation tests such as PTT and Quick. As with all other contrast agents, allergoid or anaphylactic reactions can, in principle, occur with both contrast agents.

2.4.2 Lymphographic Contrast Agents

Whereas the bigger iron-oxide particles are mainly phagocytosed in the liver, smaller particles exhibit a blood half-life and are able to penetrate the vascular endothelium. From the interstitial space, they reach the lymphatic system and are taken up by macrophages. One such compound, with the expected trade name Sinerem (AMI 227, Guerbet, Paris, France/Combidex, Advanced Magnetics, USA), is currently under development. The uptake of the iron particles leads to a homogeneous signal decrease in normal lymph nodes, whereas metastatic lymph nodes remain bright and inhomogeneous on T1-W sequences. Sinerem is – comparable to Endorem – infused over about 20 min, at doses of 1.7 mg Fe/kg and 2.6 mg Fe/kg BW. So far, it has been tested in patients with head and neck primaries as well as pelvic tumors. The preliminary first results are promising; however, it has also been reported that there is either no or minimal uptake in inflammatory lymph nodes. This will be a problem in a referential diagnosis of those nodes.

2.5 Blood-Pool Agents

Blood-pool contrast agents are defined by a longer intravasal half-life and are mainly designed for MR angiographic examinations. In principle, the prolongation of blood half-life can be achieved by three different approaches:

- the use of superparamagnetic iron-oxide particles which exhibit an increasing blood half-life the smaller they are.
- the use of paramagnetic Gd compounds which form reversible larger molecules by in vivo protein binding
- the synthesis of paramagnetic Gd-based polymeric macromolecules.

  The latter two approaches have in common that the contrast agents cannot diffuse into the interstitial space due to their macromolecular size.

For all approaches, contrast agents are currently under clinical development. Three of these contrast agents belong to the group of superparamagnetic USPIOs. NC100150 (Clariscan, Amersham) completed phase II in conventional MRA indications. Further trials are ongoing in cardiac as well as in oncologic indications. The safety data known so far do not indicate any relevant problems.

SH U 555 C (Schering AG Berlin, Germany) is about to enter phase-III development in the field of MRA, whereas AMI 7228 (Advanced Magnetics, USA) just started first clinical studies.

MS 325 (Epix Medical, Boston, USA) and B-22956/1 (Bracco, Milan, Italy) are representative of the group of paramagnetic T1 agents with in vivo albumin-binding properties.

Whereas the latter agent is in an early stage of development for which no clinical data have been published, phase-III studies using MS 325 are ongoing. According to published results, the image quality of MR angiograms is excellent, and imaging can be continued for at least 90 min. The safety data indicate a good safety profile of this contrast agent.

For the paramagnetic polymeric T1 agents like Gadomer 17 (Schering AG, Berlin, Germany) and P 792 (Guerbet, Paris, France), also only limited information is available, as both agents are in phase I and phase II of clinical development. Both agents were tested in cardiac indications and seem to provide promising imaging features.

The perspective of all the blood-pool agents is to enable imaging of vessel structures. These agents compete for the standard MR angiography indication with the extracellular Gd compounds. For high resolution MRA, however, a larger imaging window might be advantageous. Furthermore, imaging of the coronary vessels which has not been technically possible with MR imaging so far will most likely require a contrast agent which resides longer in the intravascular space.

Beyond macrovascular imaging, the evaluation of microvascular imaging mainly in tumors might become a promising indication for blood-pool agents in the future.

2.6 Gastrointestinal Contrast Agents

Again, as with the group of IV contrast media, the gastrointestinal compounds can be classified into positive and negative enhancers. Table 2.4 gives an overview of the existing agents.

Table 2.4

Trademark	Manufacturer	Positive/Negative enhancement	Registration status (Europe)
Magnevist enteral® gadopentetate (Gd-DPTP/dimgl)	Schering AG	Positive	Approved
FerriSeltz® OMR (Fe-III-Ammoniumcitrate)	Bracco	Positive	Submitted
Abdoscan® OMP Ferristene)	Amersham	Negative	Approved
Lumirem® AMI 121 (Ferumoxsilum)	Guerbet	Negative	Approved
LumenHance® $MnCl_2$	Bracco	Positive on T1 Negative on T2	Submitted

With regard to clinical efficacy, safety, and tolerability, there is no clear advantage of either positive or negative enhancers. Only a few relative clinical indications exist, such as pancreatic tumors, pelvic tumors, and inflammatory bowel disease. The reported adverse reactions are mainly diarrhea, abdominal pain, and meteorism.

Further Reading

Goyen M, Ruehm SG, Debatin JF (2000) MR Angiography: the role of contrast agents. Review. Eur J Radiol 34:247–256

Helbich TH (2000) Contrast-enhanced magnetic resonance imaging of the breast. Review. Eur J Radiol 34:208–219

Laub G (1999) Principles of contrast-enhanced MR angiography. Basic and clinical applications. Review. Magn Reson Imaging Clin N Am 7:783–795

Lorenz CH, Johansson LO (1999) Contrast-enhanced coronary MRA. Review. J Magn Reson Imaging 10:703–708

Reiser M, Semmler W (2002) Magnetresonanztomographie. 3. Auflage 2002,7 Kontrastmittel. 111–132 H. P. Niendorf, T. Balzer, P. Reimer

Runge VM (2001) Safety of magnetic resonance contrast media. Review. Top Magn Reson Imaging 12:309–314

Schneider G, Altmeyer K (2001) Use of magnetic resonance contrast media in body imaging. Review. Top Magn Reson Imaging 12:265–281

Haemorrhage

T. Allkemper

3

Contents

3.1 Introduction

The identification of haemorrhage with MR imaging is superior to other imaging modalities and may have important implications for the clinical management and outcome of a patient.

Haemorrhage exhibit all possible MR signal patterns, depending on biological factors as well as imaging techniques. Haemorrhage therefore is an excellent tool for understanding the basic principles affecting MR contrast, furthermore allowing us to appreciate the signal characteristics of many other entities. Therefore, it is particularly helpful to gain a basic knowledge of the biological and physical processes underlying the signal changes of an evolving haematoma.

The appearance of haemorrhage mainly depends on the age of a haematoma and the type of MR contrast (T1-W or T2-W). The combination of the MR signal appearance on T1-W or T2-W images defines five temporal stages of haemorrhage which can be distinguished by MR imaging. These signal evolve in an almost predictable temporal pattern within the brain, while the appearance of haemorrhage in other organs may vary. Therefore, MR imaging shows the extent of an intracerebral haematoma and the age of such a lesion.

3.2 Oxidation and Denaturation of Haemoglobin

An important factor influencing the MR appearance of haemorrhage on T1-W or T2-W images is the specific form of haemoglobin within a region of haemorrhage. As the haematoma ages, the haemoglobin passes through several forms (oxy-, deoxy- and methaemoglobin) before red blood cell lysis occurs. To bind oxygen

Table 3.1. Different derivatives during denaturation of haemoglobin

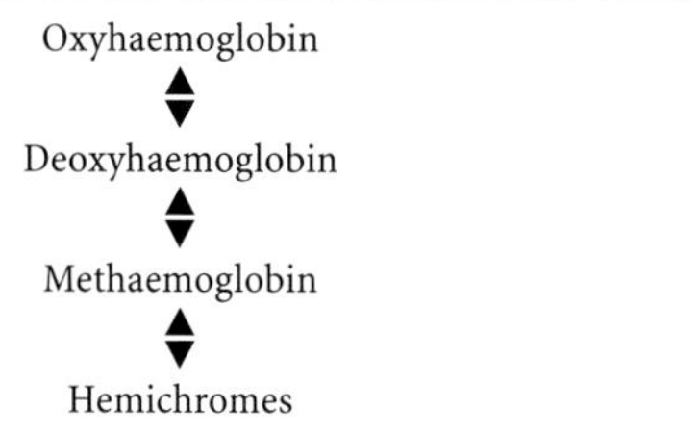

reversibly, the haem iron in the circulating form of haemoglobin (oxy- and deoxyhaemoglobin) must be in the ferrous (Fe^{2+}) state. When removed from the high oxygen level of the circulating blood, haemoglobin is denatured to methaemoglobin, and the haem iron becomes oxidised to the ferric (Fe^{3+}) form. As denaturation and oxidation continue, methaemoglobin is converted to so-called hemichromes. The iron remains in the ferric state, but the tertiary structure of the globin molecule is changed. Later on, the red blood cells become lysed, and the hemichromes are broken down into the haem iron and the globin molecule. After phagocytosis by macrophages or intracranial glial cells, the iron is stored as a derivative called ferritin, which consists of water-soluble ferric hydroxide-phosphate micelles attached to an iron storage protein (apoferritin), which keeps the iron in its hydrophobic centre. If there is a lack of apoferritin, haemosiderin is formed which consists of water-insoluble clumps of ferritin (Table 3.1).

These different oxidation and denaturation stages of haemoglobin have certain magnetic properties which influence the T1- and T2-relaxation times.

3.3 Magnetic Properties in Haemorrhage

Diamagnetism and paramagnetism are two major types of magnetic properties of matter that are most relevant to the MR appearance of biological substances. Most substances consist of elements in which the electrons are paired in atomic and molecular orbitals. Such materials generate a magnetic field opposed to the applied magnetic field. The magnitude of the magnetic field within the material is reduced below that of the applied magnetic field. These materials are called diamagnetic.

Substances containing unpaired electrons have different magnetic properties due to resulting magnetic dipoles. If these dipoles are randomly oriented and separated, the resulting magnetisation is zero. This is changed by application of a magnetic field which causes dipoles to align in a parallel or antiparallel manner depending on the temperature of the material. At physiological temperatures most electrons align parallel to the applied field, causing a magnification of the magnetic field. Materials without an intrinsic magnetic field that show an enhancement of an applied magnetic field are therefore called paramagnetic.

Oxyhaemoglobin and hemichromes are diamagnetic (the haem iron contains paired electrons), whereas deoxy- and methaemoglobin are paramagnetic because of unpaired electrons within the haem iron.

3.4 Relaxation Mechanisms

3.4.1 Diamagnetic Effects

Changes of the T1- or T2-relaxation times of an anatomical structure result in an altered MR appearance. There are several mechanisms that may cause a T1 and T2 shortening in haemorrhage.

3.4.2 Protein Binding

Free water has very high motional frequencies resulting in a very long and inefficient T1-relaxation of substances with a high water content like cerebrospinal fluid (CSF). Addition of protein results in an attraction of polar water molecules to charged protein groups, building a hydration layer. 'Protein-bound-water' is almost prevented from free motion and has shorter T1-relaxation times than pure CSF, and therefore the T1-relaxation time of proteinaceous, diamagnetic oxyhaemoglobin is much shorter than that of CSF and is almost comparable to brain parenchyma.

3.4.3 Paramagnetic Effects

Paramagnetic substances offer considerably greater T1 shortening than that provided by protein-binding effects. This is caused by dipole-dipole interactions between paramagnetic substances with unpaired electrons and the surrounding aqueous solution.

The magnitude of these effects depends mainly on the interaction of water molecules and haemoglobin – the hydrogen nuclei must be able to approach the haem iron, because the interaction falls off as the sixth power of the distance between them. Since the water molecules are not able to approach the haem iron closely enough, methaemoglobin shows paramagnetic T1 shortening while deoxyhaemoglobin does not.

The amount of T1 shortening also depends on the number of unpaired electrons a substance has: the greater the number of unpaired electrons, the greater the paramagnetic effect.

If sufficient amounts of water are bound by the proteinaceous solution, forming an almost mucinous gel, visible T2 shortening occurs. A similar mechanism for T2 shortening is encountered due to an increasing haematocrit as water is resorbed from the haemorrhage.

3.4.4 Susceptibility Effects

Much greater T2* and T2 shortening occurs due to magnetic susceptibility effects resulting from compartmentalisation of paramagnetic deoxy- or methaemoglobin inside intact red blood cells.

The term magnetic susceptibility describes how magnetised a substance becomes when placed in a magnetic field, giving the ratio between the applied and the induced magnetic field.

Compartmentalisation of paramagnetic substances with high magnetic susceptibility inside intact red blood cells causes a nonuniformity of the magnetic field in the imaging volume if the induced magnetic field inside the red blood cell is greater than that outside in the nonparamagnetic plasma. This results in significant T2* shortening due to rapid spin dephasing and signal loss on T2*-W GRE images. Water protons diffuse through these nonuniform regions and lose phase coherence, also resulting in decreased signal intensity on T2-W images.

The magnitude of phase coherency loss depends on the time interval between two successive echoes (interecho time) and increases proportionally with increasing interecho times. Sequences using shorter interecho times than CSE, like TSE sequences, provide a decreased sensitivity to susceptibility effects. The decrease is proportional to the echo train length (ETL) of such sequences.

Susceptibility effects are increased when increasing the applied field strength because the induced field and therefore the induced nonuniformity are proportional to the applied magnetic field.

To summarise, the sensitivity to magnetic susceptibility increases from TSE to CSE to GRE, from T1 to T2 or T2* weighting and from lower to higher field strengths.

3.5 Evolving Parenchymal Haemorrhage

Considering the above-mentioned signal changes, the combination of T1-W and T2-W images allows the definition of five stages of haematoma evolution: hyperacute (intracellular oxyhaemoglobin, first few hours), acute (intracellular deoxyhaemoglobin, 1–3 days), early subacute (intracellular methaemoglobin, 3–7 days), late subacute (extracellular methaemoglobin, older than 14 days) and chronic (intracellular haemosiderin and ferritin, older than 4 weeks) (Table 3.2). The exact times may vary.

3.5.1 Hyperacute

During the initial state, the haematoma consists of a liquid suspension of intact red blood cells containing a mixture of oxy- and deoxyhaemoglobin. Later on water is resorbed, forming a more solid conglomerate of intact red blood cells. These few hours old haematomas mainly consist of oxyhaemoglobin (95%) because most non-traumatic intracranial haemorrhages result from arterial bleeding (e.g. aneurysms). This stage of haemorrhage is very rarely seen on MR imaging.

These 'hyperacute' haemorrhages often have a higher water content than normal brain tissue, which contributes to an iso- to hypointense signal behaviour due to longer T1 times of water on T1-W images and a hyperintense signal behaviour on T2-W images.

Table 3.2. Sequential signal intensity (*SI*) changes of intracranial haemorrhage on MR imaging (1.5 T)

	Hyperacute haemorrhage	Acute haemorrhage	Early subacute haemorrhage	Late subacute haemorrhage	Chronic haemorrhage
What happens	Blood leaves the vascular system (extravasation)	Deoxygenation with formation of deoxy-Hb	Clot retraction and deoxy-Hb is oxidised to met-Hb	Cell lysis (membrane disruption)	Macrophages digest the clot
Time frame	<12 h	Hours – days (weeks in centre of hematoma)	A few days	4–7 days – 1 month	Weeks – years
Red blood cells	Intact erythrocytes	Intact, but hypoxic erythrocytes	Still intact, severely hypoxic	Lysis (solution of lysed cells)	Gone; encephalomalacia with proteinaceous fluid
State of Hb	Intracellular oxy-Hb (HbO_2)	Intracellular deoxy-Hb (Hb)	Intracellular met-Hb (HbOH) (first at periphery of clot)	Extracellular met-Hb (HbOH)	Haemosiderin (insoluble) and ferritin (water soluble)
Oxidation state	Ferrous (Fe^{2+}) no unpaired e–	Ferrous (Fe^{2+}) 4 unpaired e–	Ferric (Fe^{3+}) 5 unpaired e–	Ferric (Fe^{3+}) 5 unpaired e–	Ferric (Fe^{3+}) 2,000×5 unpaired e–
Magnetic properties	Diamagnetic	Paramagnetic	Paramagnetic	Paramagnetic	FeOOH is superparamagnetic
SI on T1-weighted images	≈ or ↓	≈ (or ↓)	↑↑	↑↑	≈ (or ↓)
SI on T2-weighted images	↑	↓	↓↓	↑↑	↓↓ T2 PRE

Hb, haemoglobin; *e–*, electrons; *FeOOH*, ferric oxyhydroxide; ↑, increased SI relative to normal grey matter; ↓, decreased SI relative to normal grey matter

Oxyhaemoglobin is diamagnetic and unable to cause significant T2 shortening. For this reason, hyperacute haemorrhage without a higher water content may exhibit signal intensities on T2-W images which cannot be distinguished from normal brain tissue.

It is important to remember that CT may be more sensitive during the first few hours, because highly oxygenated haemorrhages with a low water content may be undetectable on MR images.

3.5.2 Acute

After 24 h almost all oxyhaemoglobin has been deoxygenated to deoxyhaemoglobin, while the red blood cells are still intact. As thromboses progress, clot retraction occurs, and an increasing haematocrit is observed, resulting in a progressive concentration of intact red blood cells, which causes further T2 shortening.

As noted earlier, deoxyhaemoglobin is not able to cause significant T1 shortening. This results in signal intensities of the haemorrhage that cannot be distinguished from surrounding brain tissue, as water is resorbed from the haematoma.

The compartmentalisation of deoxyhaemoglobin, which is magnetically susceptible, within intact red blood cells creates local nonuniformities in the magnetic field, resulting in T2 shortening due to dephasing of water molecules which diffuse in and out of intact red blood cells. Both effects, increasing haematocrit due to clot retraction and increasing susceptibility due to compartmentalisation of deoxyhaemoglobin, lead to T2 shortening and apparent signal loss on T2-W images during the acute stage, while T1-W images may be slightly hypointense or show almost no signal change (Fig. 3.1, pictograms represent simplified schemes of signal behaviour).

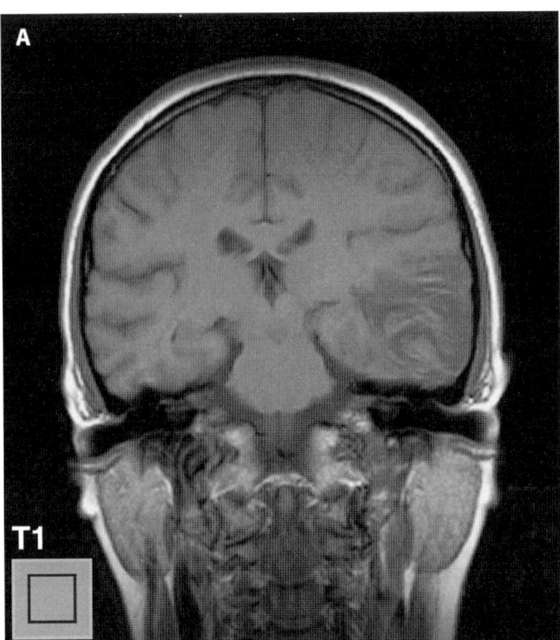

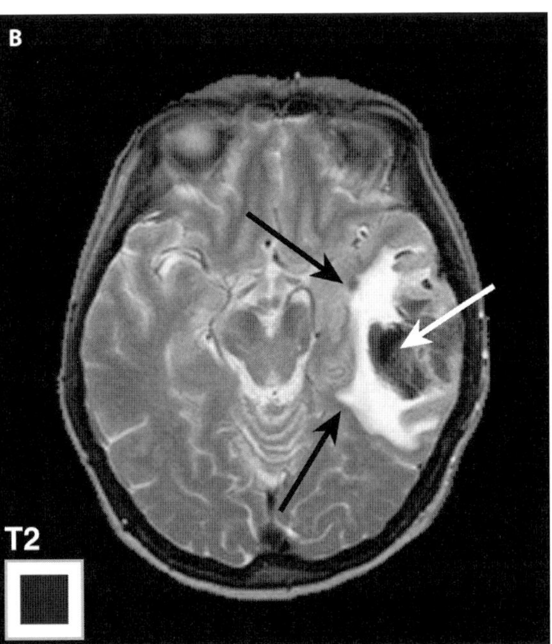

Fig 3.1A,B. Acute haematoma in a 50 year old woman with a 3 day history of thrombosis of the left sinus sigmoideus. The T1-W coronal CSE image (TR 500, TE 15) demonstrates a slightly hypointense area compared to brain. The T2-W axial CSE image (TR 2000, TE 90) demonstrates the hypointense centre (white arrow) with a hyperintense surrounding oedema (black arrows). The combination of T1-W and T2-W findings indicate that this haematoma mainly consists of intracellular deoxyhaemoglobin

3.5.3 Early Subacute

In the early subacute stage, the red blood cells are still intact, but deoxyhaemoglobin undergoes permanent oxidisation to methaemoglobin. The dipole-dipole interaction between these paramagnetic molecules causes severe T1 shortening, resulting in increased signal intensity on T1-W images. The oxidisation of methaemoglobin starts peripherally, because oxygen levels in the normal surrounding brain tissue are higher than in the centre of the haemorrhage. Later on, central deoxyhaemoglobin becomes oxidised as well.

Since a great proportion of the red blood cells is still intact, the centre of these cells becomes more magnetised than the surrounding plasma due to magnetically susceptible methaemoglobin. These magnetic nonuniformities also cause severe T2 shortening, with strong signal loss on T2-W images.

Since methaemoglobin has five unpaired electrons and deoxyhaemoglobin four unpaired electrons, these effects should be less apparent in acute than in early subacute stages of a haematoma. However, the best way to distinguish between these two stages remains the hyperintense signal behaviour of methaemoglobin in the early subacute stage on T1-W images (Fig. 3.2).

3.5.4 Late Subacute

The red blood cells undergo further degeneration by membrane lysis. Methaemoglobin is now no longer compartmentalised, and T2 shortening based on compartmentalisation is attenuated.

Late subacute stage haematomas are bright on T1-W and T2-W images as well. T2-W imaging is necessary to distinguish between early and late subacute haemorrhage (Fig. 3.3).

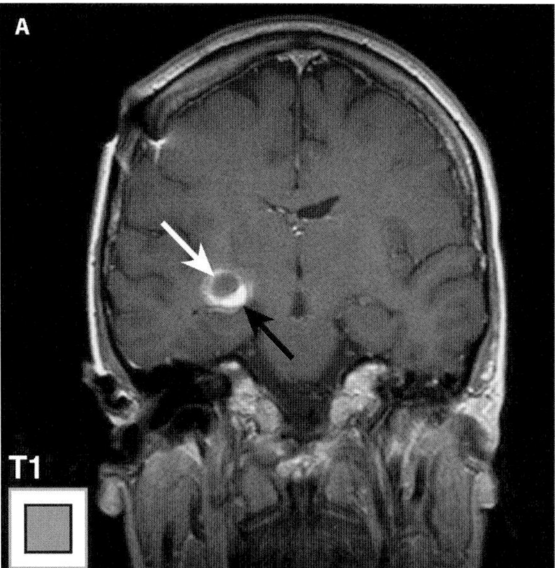

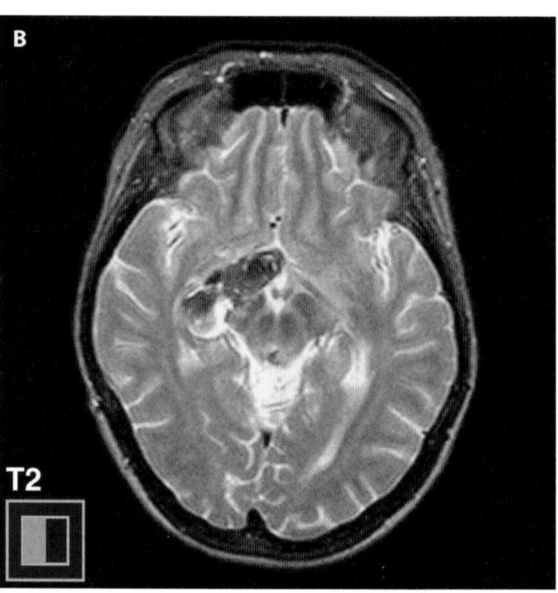

Fig. 3.2A,B. Early subacute haematoma in a 35 year old woman with a glioblastoma after radiotherapy. The T1-W coronal CSE image (TR 500, TE 15) demonstrates an isointense central (white arrow) area with a hyperintense rim (black arrow). T2-W CSE imaging (TR 2000 TE 90) shows the hypointense to isointense centre. These findings are typical for the early subacute stage and show the beginning oxidisation of deoxyhaemoglobin to methaemoglobin at the rim

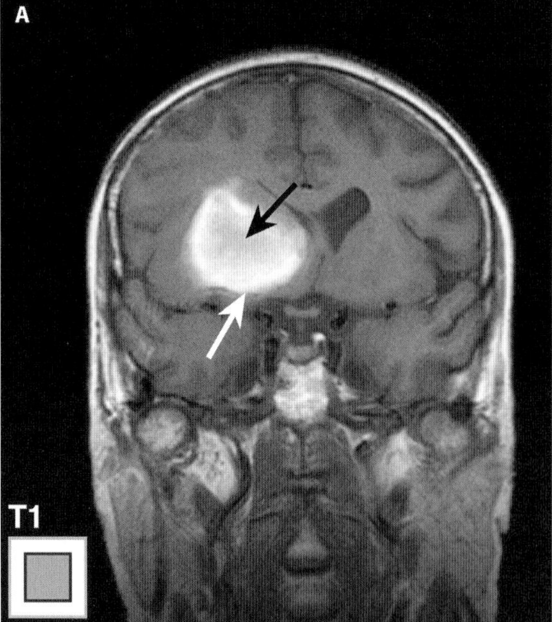

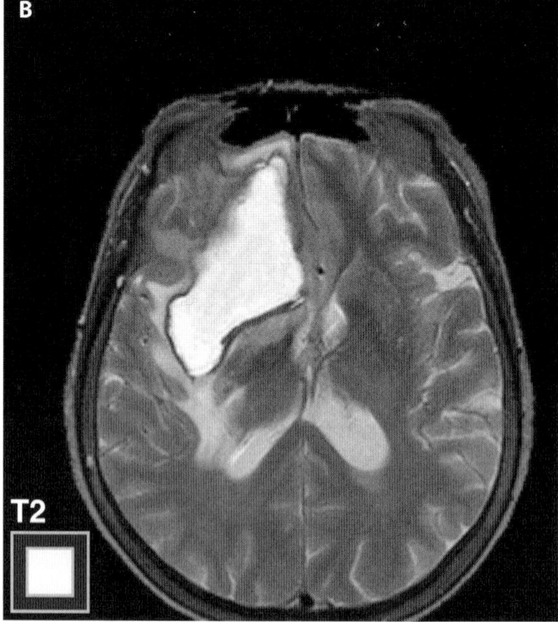

Fig. 3.3A,B. Late subacute haematoma in a 74 year old woman, 3 weeks after spontaneous haemorrhage. The T1-W coronal CSE image (TR 500 TE 15) demonstrates an isointense central area (black arrow) with a hyperiniense rim (white arrow). T2-W CSE imaging (TR 2000 TE 90) shows the hyperintense centre with a slightly hypointense rim (white arrow) caused by beginning phagocytosis of methaemoglobin and production of hemichromes. These findings are typical for the late subacute stage and show the prolonged T2 due to methaemoglobin that is no longer compartmentalised within red blood cells

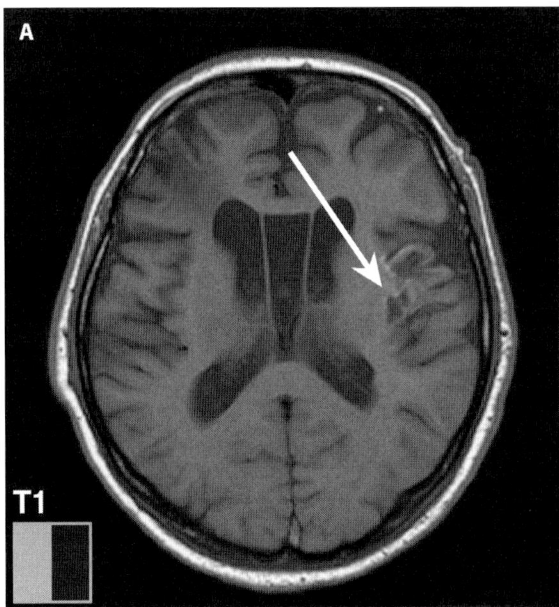

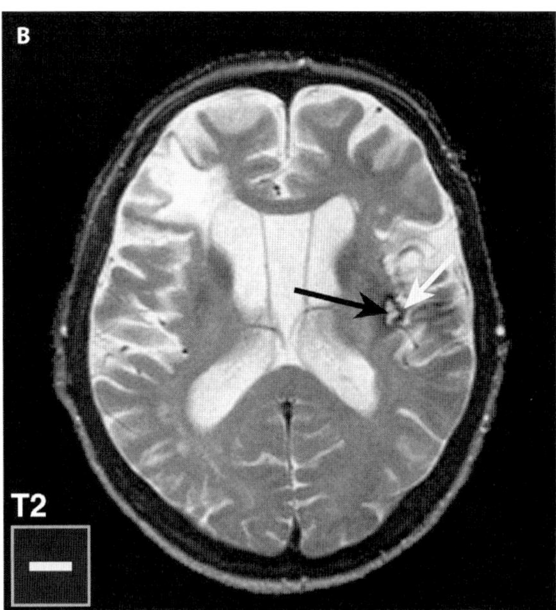

Fig. 3.4A,B. Chronic haematoma in a 71 year old man, 5 months after stroke in the left A. cerebri media territory. The T1-W axial CSE image (TR 500, TE 15) demonstrates an hypointense to isointense central area (white arrow). T2-W CSE imaging (TR 2000 TE 90) shows the hyperintense centre (black arrow) with a hypointense rim (white arrow) caused by susceptibility effects of phagocytised haemosiderin. These findings may stay for a long time with an eventually further collapse of the lesion over years

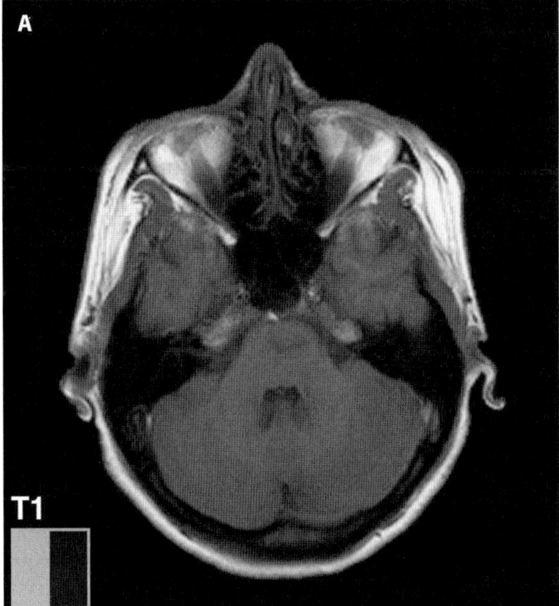

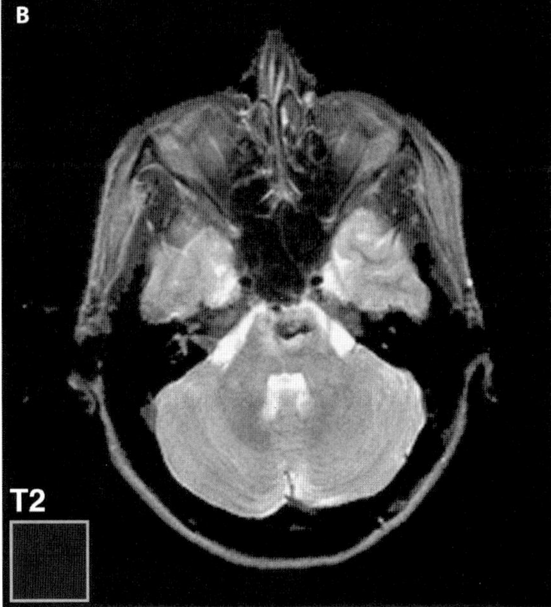

Fig. 3.5A,B. Late chronic haematoma in a 31 year old woman with a history of haemorrhage in the pons during childhood due to an AV malformation. T1-W axial CSE imaging (TR 500, TE 15) demonstrates an hypointense to isointense central area. T2-W CSE images (TR 2000 TE 90) show the collapsed, hypointense haematoma with susceptibility effects. These findings may remain for a lifetime.

3.5.5 Chronic

After red blood cell lysis, paramagnetic haemosiderin and ferritin with high magnetic susceptibility are formed and stored inside macrophages surrounding the haematoma. The compartmentalisation of these susceptible substances produces strong T2 shortening at the rim of a haematoma while the centre is filled with non-phagocytised and therefore not susceptible methaemoglobin, which appears bright on T2-W images.

These hemichromes have little or no effect on T1-W images. They appear almost isointense or slightly hypointense, caused by great magnetic nonuniformities due to strongly susceptible hemichromes, resulting in T2 shortening and prolonged T1-relaxation times (Fig. 3.4).

During a long time (in general years) haematomas may be completely resorbed or transformed into a collapsed scar, which may remain for a lifetime as a small, completely hypointense lesion (Fig. 3.5).

3.6 Sub- and Epidural Haemorrhage

Epidural and subdural haematomas evolve in five stages almost like parenchymal haemorrhage. In contrast to parenchymal haemorrhage, however, they show a slower progression to the next stage, caused by the very well vascularised dura.

The first four stages evolve in a similar pattern, but the chronic stage normally shows no dark rim due to missing tissue macrophages. Since no phagocytosis takes place, no susceptibility effects caused by compartmentalisation of hemichromes are visible. The chronic stage of sub- and epidural haematomas is characterised by continued oxidative denaturation of methaemoglobin, which causes an increase of T1 times. Therefore, the signal intensity of chronic subdural haematoma may be somewhat lower than during the subacute stage.

Recurrent bleeding can sometimes cause a ‘haemosiderin staining’ which resembles haemosiderin surrounding a parenchymal haematoma in the chronic phase.

Epidural haematomas are distinguished from subdural haematomas by classic morphology, i.e. concave versus convex shape, and by the low signal intensity of the dura mater between the haematoma and normal brain tissue.

3.7 Subarachnoid and Intraventricular Haemorrhage

Subarachnoid and intraventricular haemorrhages have high ambient oxygen levels and therefore age more slowly than sub- and epidural haematomas. Acute subarachnoid and intraventricular haematomas may provide higher signal intensities due to mixture with CSF.

Sometimes red blood cells may be resorbed; therefore, the anticipated T1 shortening may not be seen. In chronic, repeated subarachnoid haemorrhages, haemosiderin may stain the meninges, causing a hypointense T2 appearance (superficial siderosis).

3.8 Intratumoral Haemorrhage

Intratumoral haemorrhage may evolve more slowly due to lower oxygen tensions. Delayed evolution of haematoma is therefore visible at high oxygen levels (methaemoglobin is deoxidised to deoxyhaemoglobin by the methaemoglobin reductase system) and comparatively low oxygen levels (deoxyhaemoglobin is not oxidised to methaemoglobin).

Intratumoral haemorrhage builds haemosiderin membranes like parenchymal haemorrhage, but these membranes may become disrupted with renewed tumour growth. This sign is not necessarily tumour specific since any other rebleeding can cause a membrane rupture, too.

3.9 Technical Considerations

3.9.1 Operating Field Strength

Since the degree of para/diamagnetic and susceptibility effects depends directly on the applied field strength, the operating field strength of an imaging unit has an important influence on the signal behaviour of a haemorrhage. Changing the operating field strength mostly affects the sensitivity of T2-W images to susceptibility effects, causing a signal loss on T2-W images.

Acute haemorrhage on T2-W images may not be detected at low field-strength systems using spin-echo sequences. In vitro studies of deoxygenated erythrocytes show a quadric dependence of T2 times on magnetic field strength, demonstrating that the minimal concentration of deoxyhaemoglobin that produces visible T2 shortening mainly depends on the applied field strength (Fig. 3.6).

With low field strength systems every stage seems to be prolonged since more time is required to form appropriate amounts of deoxy-, methaemoglobin or haemosiderin.

Generally speaking, imaging with low field strength systems will provide less lesion contrast and cause a virtual prolongation of the ageing process of a haematoma.

3.9.2 Sequence Types

MR contrast of an intracerebral haemorrhage depends greatly on the pulse sequence applied. Image acquisition protocols generally use three different pulse sequences: GRE, CSE and TSE.

Gradient-echo sequences use a gradient reversal to rephase spins for echo generation, providing a very high sensitivity for susceptibility effects. Although sensitivity to paramagnetic constituents of the haematoma and magnetic susceptibility effects is increased, other zones of altered susceptibility (for example, interfaces between air and tissue) produce strong signal loss and geometric distortions, decreasing visualisation of large regions of the brain. It is sometimes difficult not to interpret these artefacts as real pathology. These dephasing effects are voxel size dependent and can be reduced to a certain degree by reducing the voxel size, which reduces the magnitude of magnetic gradients between two voxels.

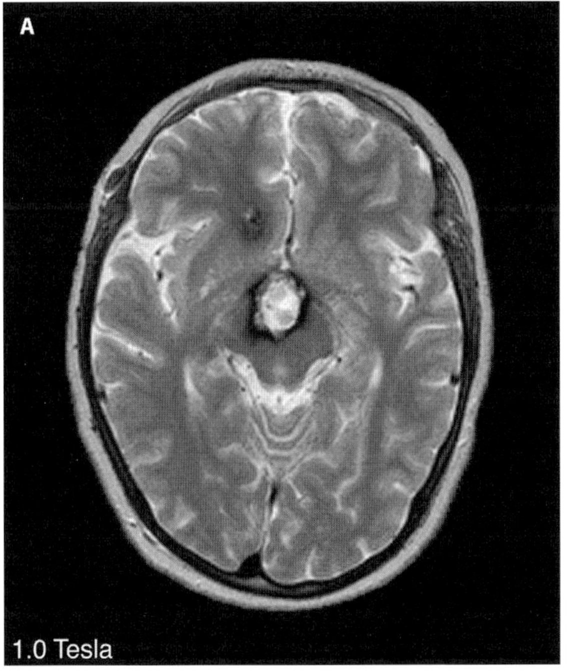

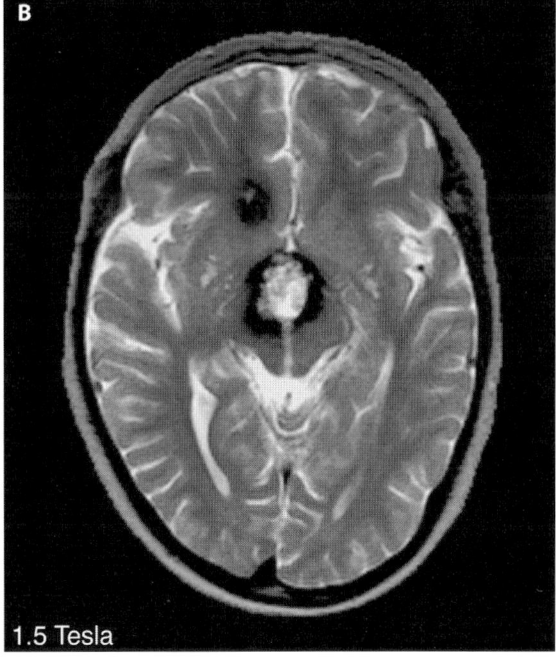

Fig. 3.6A,B. T2-W CSE images (TR 2000, TE 90) of a 17 year old patient with two cavernomas, acquired at the same level, but with different operating field strengths (left: 1.0 Tesla, right: 1.5 Tesla). Susceptibility effects due to phagocytised hemichromes within macrophages are much more pronounced at higher field strengths and make the areas of haemorrhage appear bigger

GRE sequences are very sensitive to the detection of mild intracerebral haemorrhage, but often show anatomical misregistrations. Gradient-echo sequences should therefore preferably be used at lower field strengths. They may also serve as a sequence type for the very sensitive detection of mild or small intracranial haematomas, if other sequence types fail to detect them (Fig. 3.7).

CSE sequences generate echoes in a different manner. They use a 180° radiofrequency pulse to refocus the dephasing transversal magnetisation to generate an echo. Due to this sequence design they are able to correct the distorting effects of magnetic field inhomogeneities that normally cause rapid signal loss. However, if the lesion itself is identified by these distortions, as in haematomas, the required contrast for detection of these lesions is also diminished.

Despite this, effects resulting from the diffusion of water through local field gradients are not considerably diminished unless the echo time TE is made very short in relation to the correlation time of water diffusion, which means that no significant dephasing can occur.

TSE sequences differ from CSE sequences by generating multiple spin-echoes per repetition time (TR), called an echo train. The number of spin-echoes per excitation cycle is also called the echo train length (ETL). In combination with a shortened interecho time, this sequence design significantly shortens the total acquisition time.

The use of multiple spin-echoes in combination with a shortened interecho time results in a lower sensitivity of TSE sequences for magnetic susceptibility and diffusion effects compared with CSE. Sensitivity towards these effects is proportionally reduced with increasing ETL.

If TSE images are acquired for the detection of intracerebral haemorrhage, only TSE sequences with a short ETL (e.g. 5–8 echoes per echo train) should be used (Fig. 3.8).

Gradient- and spin-echo (GRASE) sequences, which are also called turbo-gradient spin-echo (TGSE)

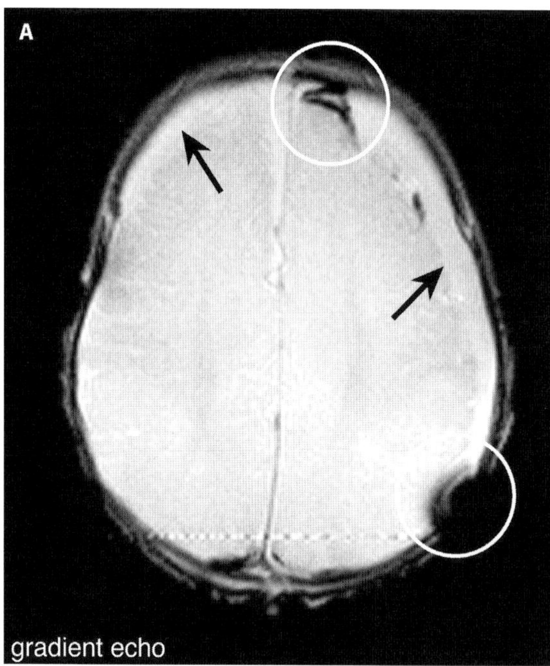

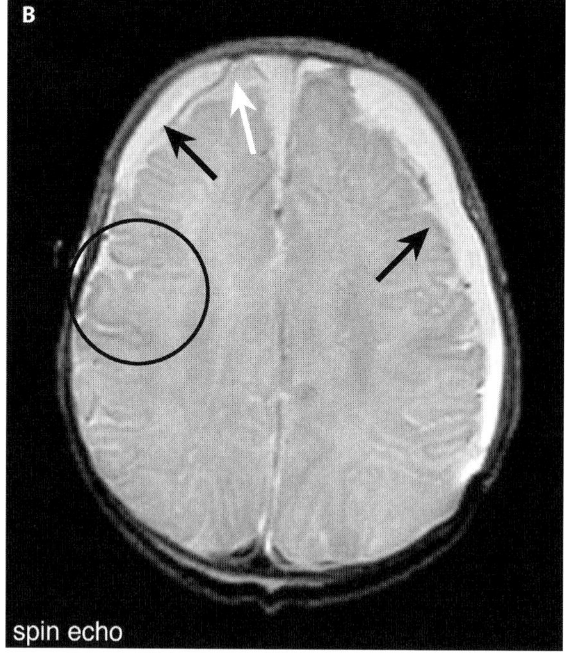

Fig. 3.7A,B. T2-W images of the same level of a 8 month old boy, suspicious for a battered child syndrome, with subdural fluid (black arrows), acquired with different sequence types (left: GRE, TR 150, TE 4.1; right: CSE, TR 2000, TE 90). CSE images provide much more anatomical information (e.g. oedema in right frontal lobe (white arrow), differentiation between white and grey matter (black circle)), whereas susceptibility effects ('haemosiderin staining'), which proof the existence of haemorrhage, are much more pronounced on gradient echo images and almost invisible on spin echo images (white circles).

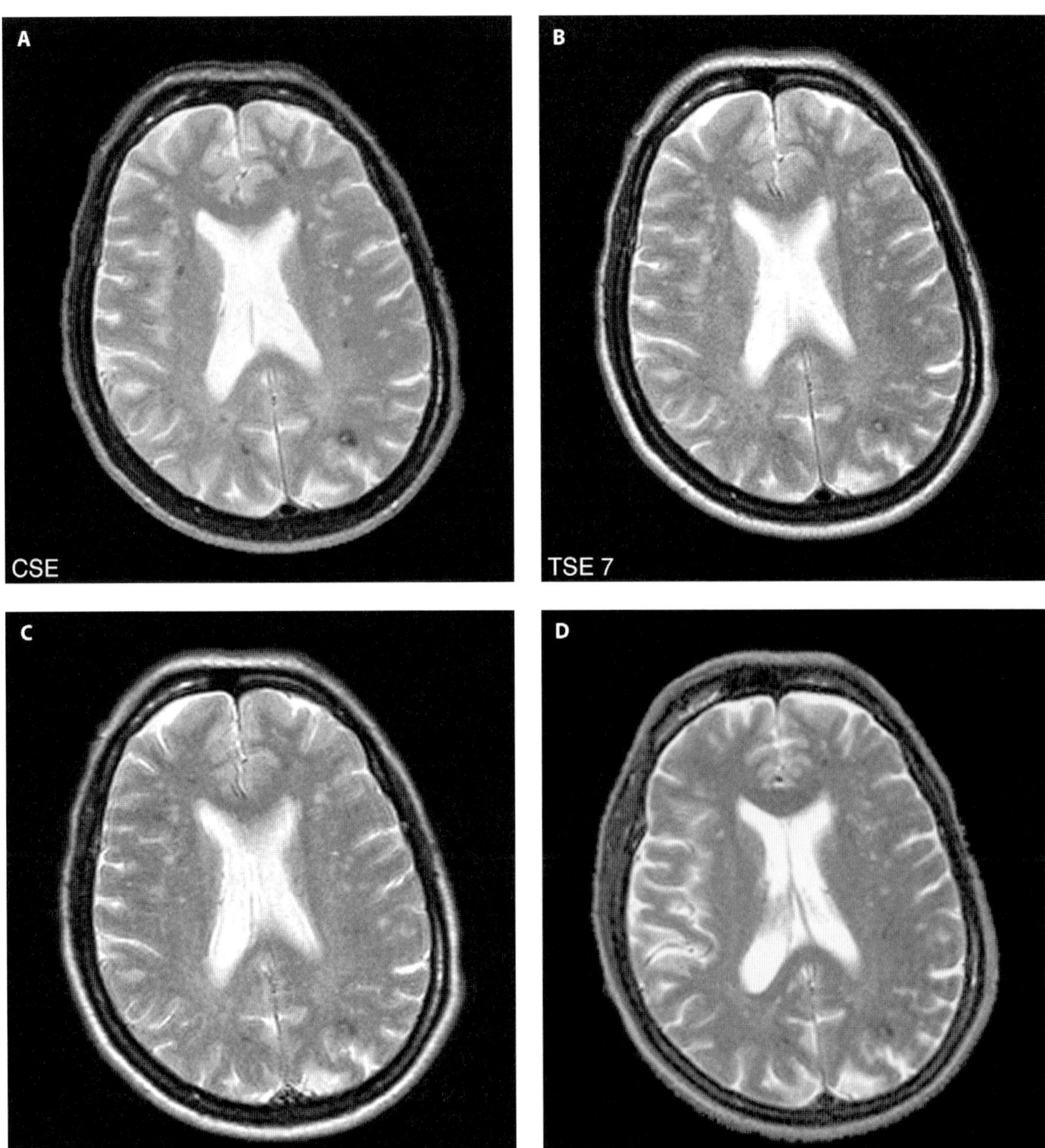

Fig. 3.8A–D. Four T2-W images of a 54 year old woman with multiple small haemorrhagic lesions, acquired at almost the same level, but with different sequence types (upper left: CSE, upper right: TSE with an ETL of 7, TSE with an ETL of 15, GRASE with an ETL of 21). These images demonstrate the decreased susceptibility based contrast of small haemorrhagic lesions with increasing number of echoes per echo train because of decreasing sensitivity to susceptibility effects. This also accounts for the GRASE 21 sequence, although this sequence type should theoretically provide an increased susceptibility contrast compared to the TSE 7 counterpart. Conventional spin echo demonstrates strongest susceptibility contrast, whereas some smaller lesions are not detectable on TSE and GRASE images

sequences, are a kind of hybrid technique mixing gradient- and spin-echoes (see Chapter 1). A GRASE sequence with an ETL of 21 is derived from a TSE sequence with an ETL of 7 by adding a gradient-echo before and after a spin-echo, forming an echo triplet.

GRASE was expected to provide higher sensitivity to susceptibility effects because of its gradient-echo content in combination with good anatomical resolution due to the spin-echo content, but several studies showed that TSE sequences are still more sensitive to susceptibility effects. GRASE sequences require very short acquisition times but are unable to provide proper detection of small parenchymal lesions (Fig. 3.8).

In conclusion, SE and TSE sequences with short ETLs are the sequence types of choice for the detection and classification of haemorrhage, although they are more time consuming than GRE or GRASE sequences.

Further Reading

Bradley WG (1993) MR Appearance of Hemorrhage in the Brain. Radiology 189:15–26

Hardy PA, Kucharczyk W, Henkelman RM (1990) Cause of signal loss in MR images of old hemorrhagic lesions. Radiology 174:549–555

Jones KM, Mulkern RV, Mantello MT et al. (1992) Brain hemorrhage: evaluation with fast spin-echo and conventional dual spin-echo images. Radiology 182:53–58

Parizel PM (1999) Intracranial hemorrhage. European Radiology 9:57–58

Stark DD, Bradley WG (/eds) (1992) Magnetic resonance imaging. Mosby, St. Louis

Magnetic Resonance Imaging of the Brain

4

P. M. Parizel, H. Tanghe, P. A. M. Hofman

Contents

4.1 Coils and Positioning

4.1.1 Coil Choice and Patient Installation

Magnetic resonance (MR) imaging examinations of the brain can be performed with several coil types, depending on the design of the MRI unit and the information required.

- The vast majority of brain examinations are performed with circularly polarized (CP) head coils. These volume coils are closely shaped around the head of the patient. At best, CP coils provide a signal-to-noise ratio (SNR) gain of $\sqrt{2}$ compared with non-CP coils. In superconducting systems, they usually have a 'bird-cage' configuration.
- A interesting new development is the use of phased-array head coils, which contain independent coil elements in an integrated design which surrounds the head (e.g., 8-channel head coil). Because the SNR is non-uniformly distributed throughout the volume to be examined, a 'normalization' process is required to compensate for SNR differences between the peripheral and central parts of the brain. The major advantage of a multichannel, phased-array head coil is that it allows the application of parallel acquisition techniques (PAT), which can be used to speed up MR imaging. The concept is to reduce the number of phase-encoding steps by switching a field gradient for each phase-encoding step. Skipping, for example, every second phase-encoding line accelerates the acquisition speed by a factor of two. This is called the acceleration or PAT factor. The trade-off for this increased imaging speed is a decrease in SNR. Image reconstruction with PAT techniques is more complicated, and two major algorithms have been described, depending on whether image reconstruction takes place before (SMASH, GRAPPA) or after (SENSE) Fourier transform of the image data.
- In MR imaging systems where the direction of the B_0 field is oriented perpendicular to the long axis of the body, e.g., open-design resistive or permanent magnet systems, solenoid head coils are used. By diagonally crossing two solenoid wire loops, a CP head coil can be created to improve SNR.
- Surface coils are rarely used for brain imaging and are usually reserved for 'special' applications: high-resolution imaging of the orbits or the temporomandibular joints (double-doughnut surface coil).

For MRI examinations of the brain, the patient is placed in a supine position. Before the table is entered into the magnet, the patient should be correctly positioned in the head coil. Most MRI systems provide laser crosshairs to assist in patient positioning. The narrow nature of the head coil may induce anxiety. Therefore, it is important that the patient feel comfortable. A pillow placed under the shoulders may be helpful. Sedation may be required and should be individually tailored.

4.1.2 Imaging Planes

The actual MRI examination begins with one or more fast localizer scans (syn. scout or survey images). For this purpose, we use fast-gradient sequences (obtained in seconds), with slices in the orthogonal imaging planes. On the basis of the initial localizer images, additional localizer scans are set, if needed, until the radiologist is satisfied that imaging sequences can be started in true sagittal, coronal or axial planes. On the coronal localizer image, a single slice fast mid-sagittal acquisition is positioned. We set out our first series of axial scans on this image. Modern MRI scanners often provide software that allows the user to position slices simultaneously on three localizer images. This permits multiple oblique slice orientations and obviates the need to obtain several sequential localizer scans.

The positioning of sagittal images is obvious, due to the symmetry of the brain. Sagittal images are placed on a coronal localizer image if the head is not rotated. An axial plane can also be used, provided there is no left-right tilt of the head. In clinical practice, the positioning of sagittal images is self-explanatory. Ideally, on the midsagittal image, the following anatomical landmarks should be identified: corpus callosum (over its entire length), aqueduct of Sylvius, fourth ventricle, cervical spinal cord.

The plane of axial images should be parallel to the bicommissural line (linking the anterior to the posterior commissure) (Fig. 4.1). Sometimes this line is difficult to identify on a low-resolution localizer image. There are two alternative solutions: (1) position the center of the slice group at the inferior borders of the genu and splenium of the corpus callosum or (2) use a plane parallel to a line linking the floor of the sella turcica to the fastigium of the fourth ventricle, which is easier to identify. In many patients, these imaging planes differ by only a few degrees. It is important, however, to set a standard imaging plane, so that images obtained in follow-up examinations can be compared with the baseline study.

For coronal images, we typically choose a tilted plane, perpendicular to the long axis of the temporal lobes. This can be obtained by positioning the coronal slices on a midsagittal image, parallel to the posterior part of the brainstem. For pituitary studies, the coronal images should be perpendicular to the sellar floor or tilted slightly backward (parallel to the pituitary stalk).

The choice of imaging planes must be determined by the clinical questions to be answered. For example, in a patient with optic neuritis, thin coronal fat-suppressed images through the orbits are useful for comparing the right and left optic nerves. To rule out hippocampal sclerosis in patients with intractable partial complex seizures, tilted coronal slices perpendicular to the long axis of the hippocampus are preferred; axial scans tilted parallel to the hippocampal axis may also be helpful. In a patient with multiple sclerosis, subependymal white-matter lesions perpendicular to the ventricular

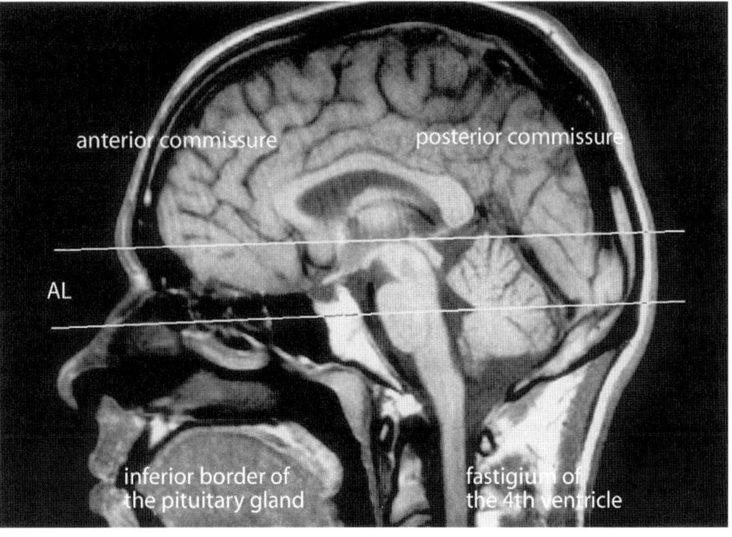

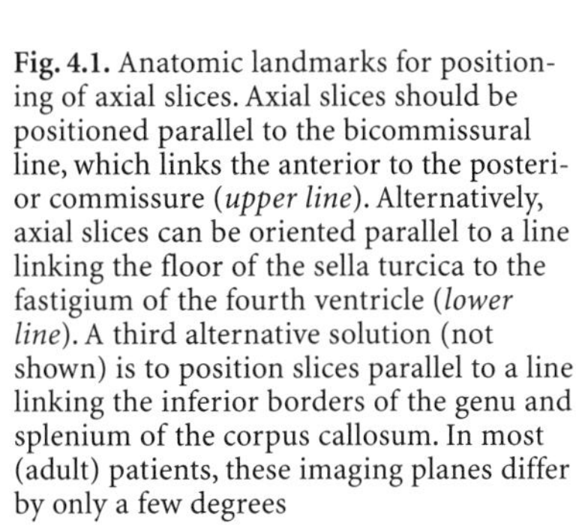

Fig. 4.1. Anatomic landmarks for positioning of axial slices. Axial slices should be positioned parallel to the bicommissural line, which links the anterior to the posterior commissure (*upper line*). Alternatively, axial slices can be oriented parallel to a line linking the floor of the sella turcica to the fastigium of the fourth ventricle (*lower line*). A third alternative solution (not shown) is to position slices parallel to a line linking the inferior borders of the genu and splenium of the corpus callosum. In most (adult) patients, these imaging planes differ by only a few degrees

surface ('Dawson's fingers') are particularly well seen on sagittal images. Lesions within the corpus callosum are well depicted on sagittal or coronal sections and may be difficult to see on axial scans.

4.1.3 Protocol for Routine MR Imaging of the Brain

Ideally, imaging protocols for the brain should be as short as possible and focused on the clinical questions. Protocols should be standardized to ensure continuity over time. Because the diagnosis is based on experience, frequent changes in protocols should be avoided; moreover, frequent protocol changes may be confusing to the technologists operating the MRI equipment. Finally, imaging protocols should be adapted to the equipment available.

As a general rule, MR imaging studies of the brain should include at least two imaging planes and two 'weightings'. Tables 4.1 and 4.2 show the 'traditional' and 'modern' protocols for MR imaging of the brain.

In the traditional screening protocol, the long TR sequence can be obtained with either a spin-echo (SE) or turbo spin-echo (TSE) technique. This sequence provides proton-density weighted images (PD-WI) and T2-W images (T2-WI). They are used to detect intraparenchymal signal abnormalities. Most pathological processes in the brain result in increased water content (vasogenic edema, cytotoxic edema, necrosis, or cyst formation) and are therefore readily identified on T2-WI.

Small high-signal intensity (SI) lesions adjacent to the ventricles or subarachnoid spaces, e.g., periventricular white matter and cortical gray matter, may be missed on T2-WI because they cannot be differentiated from the cerebrospinal fluid (CSF), which is also hyperintense. These lesions are better appreciated on PD-WI, where the lesions are hyperintense but the SI from CSF is diminished. A more modern alternative is to use a T2-W sequence with dark CSF signal, such as fluid-attenuated inversion recovery (FLAIR) (Table 4.2). In this T2-W sequence, the signal of CSF is attenuated by the use of a long inversion time, typically around 2000 ms. FLAIR provides excellent contrast resolution at brain-CSF interfaces and improves the conspicuity of small white-matter lesions. Thus, in the modern imaging protocol, FLAIR and TSE T2-W sequences are used instead of the dual-echo PD-W and T2-W sequence (Table 4.2).

The short repetition time (TR)/short echo time (TE) or T1-W sequence is used to evaluate the gross anatomy and structure of the brain. Moreover, T1-WI are often

Table 4.1. Traditional screening protocol for MR imaging of the adult brain. For routine studies, we prefer 19 or 20 slices. In this way, all images of one sequence can be fitted on one film, together with a localizer when needed. If the head cannot be covered with 19 or 20 slices, the number should be increased; alternatively a slice thickness of 6 mm can be used. For brain imaging, a 512 matrix should be preferred, especially when TSE sequences are used. When not available, or when the signal-to-noise ratio is critical, a smaller matrix, e.g., 256, can also be used. It should be remembered that anatomic definition is determined by pixel size, which depends not only on the matrix, but also on the field of view (FOV). A rectangular FOV (recFOV) is used only in transverse and coronal slice orientations. For these imaging planes, the preferred phase encoding direction is left to right. The additional coronal sequence is not needed for most screening examinations. Instead of performing a single-echo T2-W TSE sequence, a dual echo PD- and T2-W sequence is used in some institutions

Pulse sequence	WI	Plane	No. of sections	TR (ms)	TE (ms)	TI (ms)	Flip angle	Echo train length	Section thickness (mm)	Matrix	FOV	recFOV	No. of acq.
1. Axial PD- and T2-W sequence (double echo)													
SE or TSE	PD-T2	tra	19	2000–5000	15–30/ 90–130	–	90/180	1 (SE) –15 (TSE)	5	256 or 512	230–240	75	1–2
2. Sagittal T1-W sequence													
SE	T1	sag	19	500–700	10–20	–	90/180	–	5	256 or better	230–240	100	1–3
3. Coronal T2-W sequence (optional; not necessary for most screening examinations)													
TSE	T2	cor	19	3000–6000	90–130	–	90/180	7–15	5	256 or better	230–240	75	1–2

Abbreviations: *WI* weighted image; *TR* repetition time (ms), *TI* inversion time (ms), *TE* echo time (ms); *TD* time delay (sec); *no part* number of partitions; *Matrix* (phase × frequency matrix); *FOV* field of view (mm) *recFOV* % rectangular field of view

Table 4.2. Modern screening protocol for MR imaging of the adult brain. In the modern screening protocol for MR imaging of the adult brain, TSE T2-W and turbo-FLAIR sequences are substituted for the traditional dual-echo PD- and T2-W sequence. The inversion time (TI) should be shorter at 1 T field strength (1800 ms) than at 1.5 T field strength (2200 ms). The diffusion-weighted sequence is can be added for its increased sensitivity to cytotoxic edema. When looking for hemorrhagic lesions, a GRE sequence should be added, because of its increased sensitivity to susceptibility artifacts

Pulse sequence	WI	Plane	No. of sections	TR (ms)	TE (ms)	TI (ms)	Flip angle	Echo train length	Section thickness (mm)	Matrix	FOV	recFOV	No. of acq.
1. Axial T2-W sequence (single echo)													
TSE	T2	ax	19–25	3000–6000	90–130	–	90/180	7–15	5	512	230–240	75	1–2
2. Axial T2-W turbo FLAIR sequence													
Turbo FLAIR	T2	ax	19	6000–10000	100–150	1800–2200	180	7–11	5	512	230–240	75	1–2
3. Sagittal T1-W sequence													
SE	T1	sag	19	600	10–20	–	90/180	–	5	256 or better	230–240	100	1–2
4. Axial SE-EPI diffusion-W sequence (optional)													
SE-EPI	diffusion	ax	12–15	∞	100–140	–	90/180	–	5	128	230–300	75	1

Abbreviations: *WI* weighted image; *TR* repetition time (ms); *TI* inversion time (ms) *TE* echo time (ms); *TD* time delay (sec); *no part* number of partitions; *Matrix* (phase × frequency matrix); *FOV* field of view (mm); *recFOV* % rectangular field of view

better for the anatomical definition of an underlying lesion (the increased signal of an intraparenchymal area of edema on T2-WI may obscure the underlying lesion). Following intravenous injection of a paramagnetic contrast agent, T1-WI in two orthogonal planes should be obtained. Alternatively, a three-dimensional (3D) volume acquisition can be used, which permits reconstructions in multiple planes. Unenhanced and gadolinium (Gd)-enhanced images with the same thickness, positions and parameters should be available for comparison in at least one imaging plane.

The effect of contrast agents can be potentiated using spectral fat-suppression techniques (e.g., in the orbit) or magnetization-transfer contrast techniques for background suppression (e.g., in multiple sclerosis). On most modern MRI equipment, magnetization transfer is a push-button option that is frequently used for most Gd-enhanced brain scans, except when thin slices are required, e.g., for the pituitary gland or internal auditory canal.

4.1.4 Spatial Resolution

Spatial resolution in an MR image is determined by slice thickness, field-of-view (FOV), and matrix size. These parameters define the size of a voxel (volume element). The slice thickness for routine MR imaging of the brain is usually 5 mm, with an interslice distance of 0.5–1.5 mm (distance factor: 0.1–0.3). In this way, complete coverage of the brain can be obtained with approximately 20 slices in axial or sagittal planes. When quantitative assessment of the number of lesions is being performed, as in multiple sclerosis trial protocols, a slice thickness of 3 mm is usually advocated. Since a greater number of slices are needed to cover the brain, this implies that the examination time is prolonged accordingly. In specific anatomic regions (pituitary gland, CP angle, and internal auditory canal), thin slices (1–3 mm) must be used. With 3D volume acquisitions, the data set consists of a much larger number of thin slices (thickness ≤1.5 mm), e.g., magnetization-prepared rapid acquired gradient-echoes (MP-RAGE).

In-plane resolution is determined by FOV and matrix size. For routine adult MR imaging of the brain, we use a FOV of 230 mm (range 220–250 mm, depending on the size of the patient's head) and a matrix of 256. However, images with 512 matrix are progressively replacing 256 matrix images, because of their improved spatial resolution. It appears likely that in the near future, the matrix size will be further increased to 1024 for selected applications. Images with higher in-plane spatial resolution can be obtained by increasing the

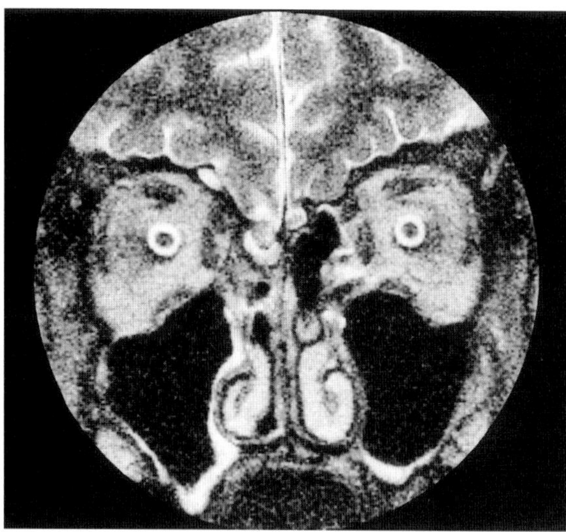

Fig. 4.2. High-resolution imaging. In this patient with a recurrent right frontal meningoencephalocele herniating through the cribriform plate, this coronal turbo spin-echo, T2-weighted image (TSE T2-WI) with a 130-mm field-of-view (FOV) and 256 matrix provides high in-plane spatial resolution. The trade-off is a decreased signal-to-noise ratio (SNR); the image appears grainy. The same spatial resolution could be obtained using a 512 matrix with a 260-mm FOV

matrix size (with constant FOV) or by decreasing the FOV (with constant matrix); however, increasing the spatial resolution results in decreased SNR, due to the smaller pixel size (Fig. 4.2).

Rectangular FOV is routinely used in cerebral MR imaging in the axial and coronal imaging planes (*not* in the sagittal plane). In axial images, phase encoding is chosen left to right, to avoid superimposition of phase artifacts from eye movement on the temporal and occipital regions.

4.1.5 Signal-to-Noise Ratio

SNR is determined to a great extent by the field strength of the magnet and the intrinsic quality of the head coil. CP head coils generally provide a satisfactory SNR. For a given magnet and coil, SNR is also proportional to the pixel size (FOV/matrix), slice thickness, number of excitations (NEX), and is inversely proportional to the receiver bandwidth.

SNR can be improved by increasing NEX. SNR increases with $\sqrt{\text{NEX}}$, whereas acquisition time increases linearly with NEX. Thus, after increasing to 4 NEX, it becomes relatively inefficient in terms of improving SNR. Moreover, the probability of patient motion increases with longer imaging times.

SNR for a particular examination can be optimized using sequences with a narrow bandwidth. This is commonly done at lower field strengths, where chemical-shift artifacts are less of a problem. At higher field strengths, mixed bandwidth sequences are useful with multi-echo sequences. The bandwidth for the second echo of a long TR sequence (T2-WI) is lower than for the first echo (PD-WI). This improves SNR on the longer TE images, where it is most needed.

Spatial resolution can be traded in for improvements in SNR. The larger the voxels, the better SNR is obtained. Therefore, in each MR examination, there is a trade-off between spatial resolution (slice thickness, FOV, matrix size) and SNR. The goal should be to find a voxel size that provides adequate SNR for contrast resolution yet is small enough to provide the spatial resolution necessary.

With phased-array head coils, SNR is non-uniformly distributed throughout the volume examined, and a 'normalization' process is required to compensate for SNR differences between the peripheral and central parts of the brain. When phased-array head coils are used in conjunction with PAT, the imaging speed increases, but SNR decreases by the square root of the acquisition time (Fig. 4.3). Furthermore, the image reconstruction process for a phased-array head coil with PAT may further reduce SNR.

4.2 Congenital Disorders and Hereditary Diseases

Clinical suspicion of a developmental anomaly of the central nervous system (CNS) is a frequent indication for performing an MRI examination of the brain. For a more complete discussion of developmental abnormalities, the reader should consult Chapter 16 (see section 16.2.3.1). In the following paragraphs, we shall focus on practical guidelines for interpreting MRI studies in adult or adolescent patients with suspected congenital disorders.

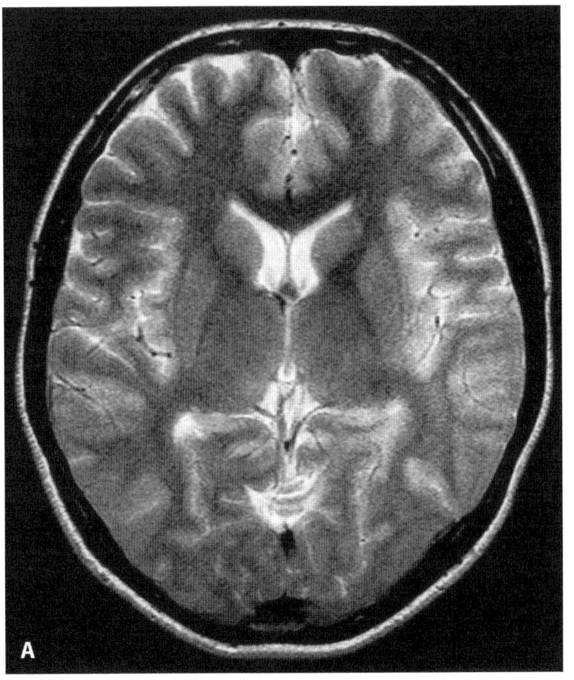

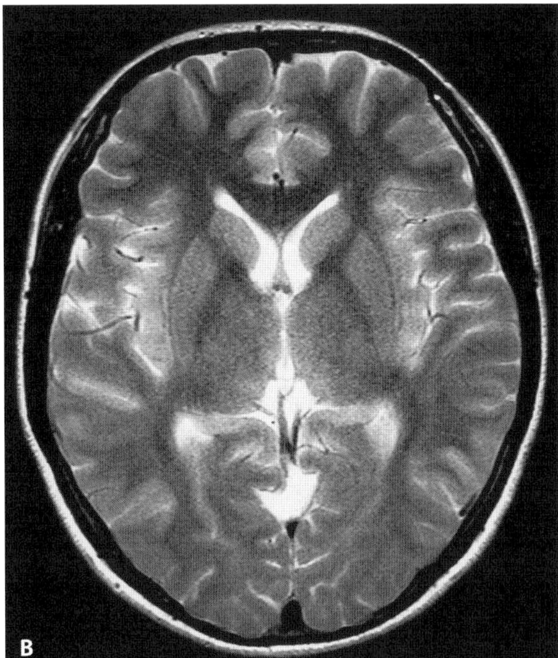

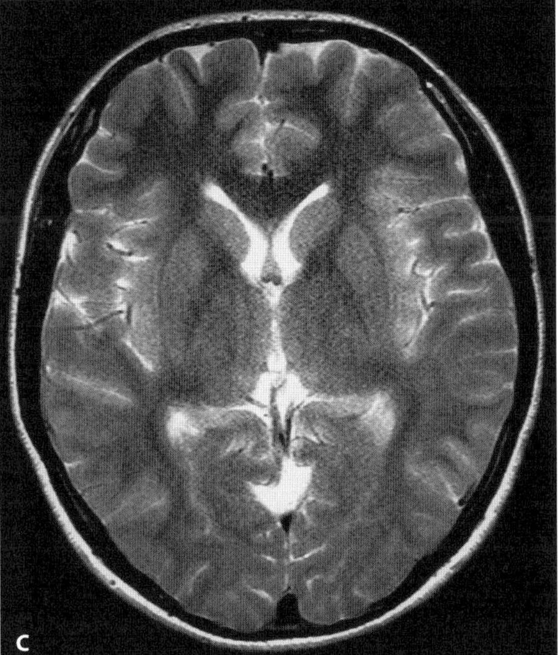

Fig. 4.3A–C. Comparison of SNR obtained with a standard circularly polarized birdcage coil (**A**), and an integrated 8-channel phased array coil, used without (**B**) and with (**C**) parallel acquisition techniques (PAT). Axial slices were obtained in each case with the same TSE T2-WI sequence. In **B**, the noise is more prominent in the deep parts of the brain than on the surface; this reflects the non-uniform SNR obtained with a phased-array head coil. The image in **C** was obtained in half the imaging time with PAT, but the SNR is worse. The increased imaging speed of PAT is associated with a decrease in SNR by the square root of the acquisition time

4.2.1
Craniocervical Junction

The craniocervical junction (CCJ) is best appraised on sagittal images. Sagittal (T)SE T1-WI constitute an essential part of the imaging protocol, although sagittal T2-WI are also acceptable. Coronal sections are useful as a second imaging plane for the CCJ.

On a midsagittal image, the level of the foramen magnum can be identified by drawing a line from the *basion* (lowermost portion of the clivus, anterior border of the foramen magnum) to the *opisthion* (free margin of the occipital bone, which constitutes the posterior margin of the foramen magnum). Normally, the inferior pole of the cerebellar tonsils lies above or not more than 3 mm below this line. Chiari type I malformation is defined as a downward displacement of the cerebellar tonsils through the foramen magnum into the upper cervical spinal canal. When the tonsillar herniation is 5 mm or less, this condition is described as 'tonsillar ectopia'. In the true Chiari I malformation, tonsillar herniation is more than 5 mm. Sagittal MR images show a low position of the cerebellar tonsils with a wedge-like configuration of the most inferior aspect. The cisterna magna is obliterated. Chiari I malformation is commonly associated with syringohydromyelia (40%–70%) and hydrocephalus (10%–30%). The 4th ventricle is normal in size and position. In 20%–30% of cases, there is an associated osseous abnormality of the CCJ (platybasia or basilar invagination) (Fig. 4.4).

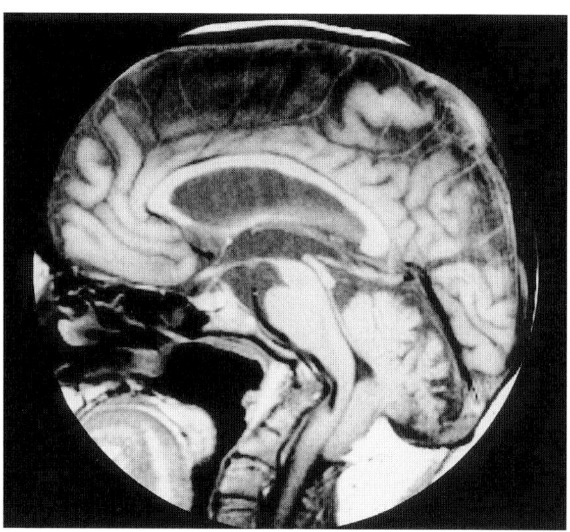

Fig. 4.4. Chiari I malformation. This sagittal SE T1-WI shows downward displacement and peg-like configuration of the cerebellar tonsils. There is an associated osseous malformation of the skull base. The tip of the odontoid is projected above the level of the foramen magnum

Chiari II malformation is a complex hindbrain-mesodermal malformation involving the entire neuraxis, most likely caused by a congenitally small posterior fossa (Fig. 4.5). The main imaging findings are: small posterior fossa with low tentorial attachment, compression of the hindbrain, indentation of the lower cerebellum by the foramen magnum or C1 and indentation of the upper cerebellum by the tentorium, abnormality of the midbrain with tectal 'beaking'. Chiari II malformation is almost invariably associated with myelomeningocele. Hydrocephalus and a variety of other intracranial abnormalities are common.

Osseous abnormalities of the CCJ can be congenital (basilar invagination) or acquired (basilar impression). Primary developmental craniocervical dysgenesis includes conditions such as basiocciput hypoplasia, occipital condyle hypoplasia, abnormalities of C1–C2, Klippel-Feil syndrome, etc. Acquired basilar impression results from softening of the skull base, e.g., Paget's disease, osteomalacia, rheumatoid arthritis. Achondroplasia is characterized by narrowing and deformation of the foramen magnum, short and vertical clivus, stenotic jugular foramina, hydrocephalus, and macrocephaly which occurs secondary to impaired venous outflow.

4.2.2
Posterior Fossa

The gross anatomic relationships of the posterior fossa contents are best evaluated on sagittal images. On a midsagittal image, the following anatomic landmarks should be recognized: mesencephalon, pons, medulla oblongata, fourth ventricle, cerebellar vermis, foramen magnum, as defined by the line linking the basion to the opisthion.

Vermian-cerebellar hypoplasia is characterized by a small vermis and cerebellum with a prominent folial pattern, a large fourth ventricle, a large cisterna magna, and a wide vallecula. It can be complete or partial. Vermian and/or cerebellar hypoplasia can be an isolated anomaly or occur in association with malformative syndromes.

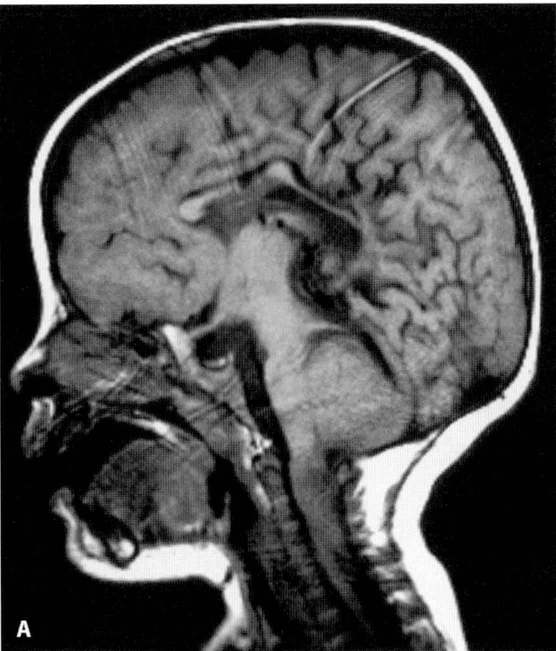

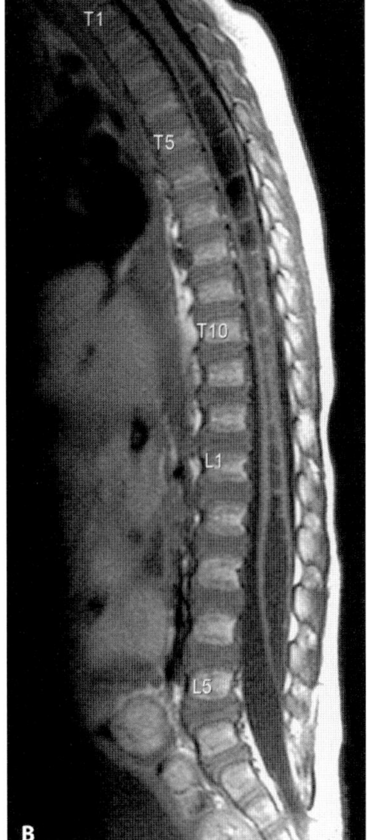

Fig. 4.5A,B. Chiari II malformation. **A** Midsagittal SE T1-WI through the brain. **B** Midsagittal SE T1-WI through the thoraco-lumbar spine region. The patient is an 1-year-old boy after surgical repair of a myelomeningocele. At the level of the posterior fossa and craniocervical junction, the typical features of a Chiari II malformation are seen: beaking of the midbrain, small posterior fossa with low tentorial attachment, inferior displacement and narrowing of the fourth ventricle, downward displacement of the pons and medulla, peg-like protrusion of the vermis with cervicomedullary kinking.The spinal cord is tethered by scar tissue, and is widened by a segmented syringohydromyelia extending down to the low-lying conus medullaris

Cystic malformations of the posterior fossa range from megacisterna magna, retrocerebellar arachnoid cyst, Dandy-Walker malformation, and Dandy-Walker variant. These entities may represent a continuum of posterior fossa developmental anomalies. They are sometimes referred to as the Dandy-Walker complex.

Megacisterna magna is a large CSF space posterior and inferior to the cerebellum, which is normally developed. There is no mass effect. It cannot be differentiated from a retrocerebellar arachnoid cyst (Blake's pouch), which is a collection of CSF not communicating with the fourth ventricle (Fig. 4.6). It is most commonly situated in the midline, behind the vermis. The thin membrane surrounding the cyst is usually not seen on imaging. The cerebellar hemispheres and vermis are normally developed, but may be compressed from behind. The inner table of the occipital bone may be scalloped. The size of the posterior fossa, the position of the tentorium and straight sinus are normal. However, the cyst, when large, may show a diverticulum-like extension through the splayed tentorium. In most instances, a retrocerebellar arachnoid cyst is an incidental imaging finding. The condition is usually asymptomatic.

Dandy-Walker malformation (Fig. 16.8) is characterized by three key features: (1) dysgenesis or agenesis of the cerebellar vermis, (2) cystic dilatation of the 4th ventricle, which balloons posteriorly, and (3) enlargement of the posterior fossa, with high position of the tentorial insertion ('torcular-lambdoid inversion'). Additional imaging features include scalloping of the inner table of the occipital bone and hypoplasia of the cerebellar hemispheres. Associated findings are: hydrocephalus, corpus callosum dysgenesis, and heterotopic gray matter.

The term Dandy-Walker 'variant' covers a heterogeneous group of atypical cystic posterior fossa malfor-

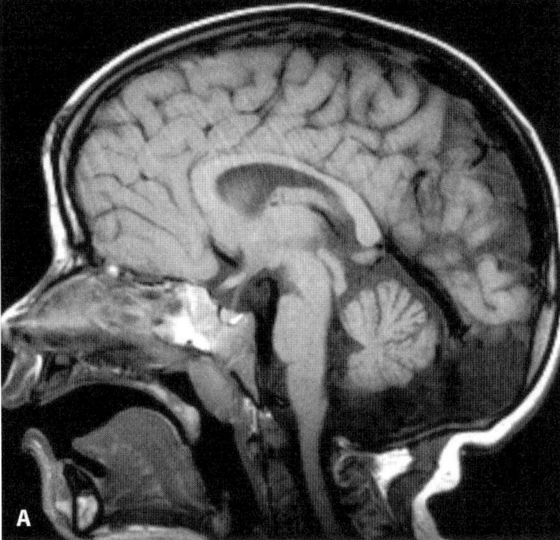

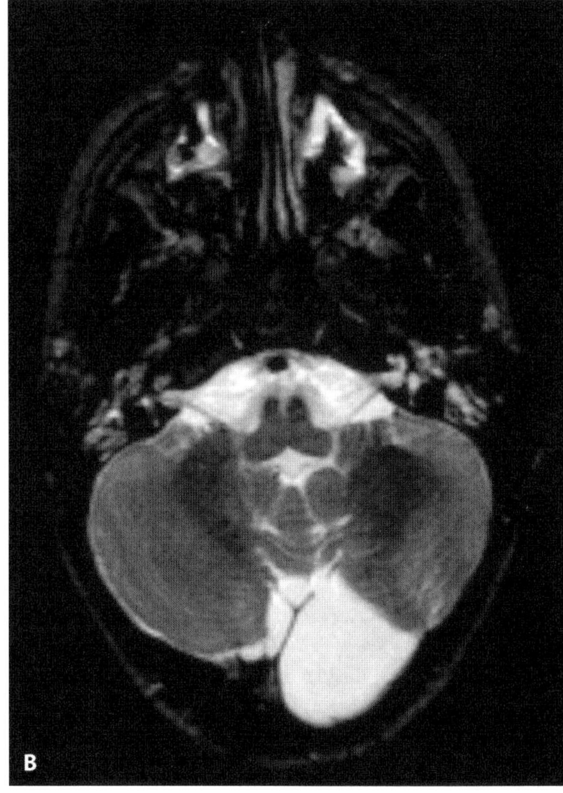

Fig. 4.6A,B. Megacisterna magna or retrocerebellar arachnoid pouch. **A** Midsagittal SE T1-WI. **B** Axial SE T2-WI. The normally developed vermis and cerebellar hemispheres are associated with an enlarged cisterna magna, or retrocerebellar arachnoid pouch, which causes some scalloping of the inner table of the occipital bone and mild enlargement of the posterior fossa. There is an incomplete and bifid falx cerebelli

mations, for which common MRI findings include: cystic dilatation of the fourth ventricle, dysgenesis or hypoplasia of cerebellar hemisphere(s) and/or vermis. However, the posterior fossa is not enlarged, and the torcular is not elevated.

4.2.3 Supratentorial Midline Structures

On the midsagittal image, the corpus callosum should be identified. It is the largest interhemispheric commissure and the most concentrated bundle of axons in the brain. It contains myelinated fibers linking the left and right cerebral hemispheres. The corpus callosum is an extremely firm structure and helps the ventricles maintain their normal size and shape. Anatomically, on the midsagittal image, four elements constituting the corpus callosum should be identified: rostrum, genu, body (or truncus), and splenium. Embryologically, the corpus develops in anterior to posterior fashion (genu first, then body, then splenium), with the exception of the rostrum which forms last.

Agenesis of the corpus callosum can be partial or complete (Fig. 4.7). Axons that would normally cross the midline instead run along the medial wall of the lateral ventricles, and thereby form the bundles of Probst. MR imaging findings of corpus callosum agenesis include:

- Partial or complete absence of the corpus callosum (midsagittal image)
- Radial orientation of the gyri on the medial surface of the cerebral hemispheres (sagittal images) and eversion of the cingulate gyrus (coronal images)

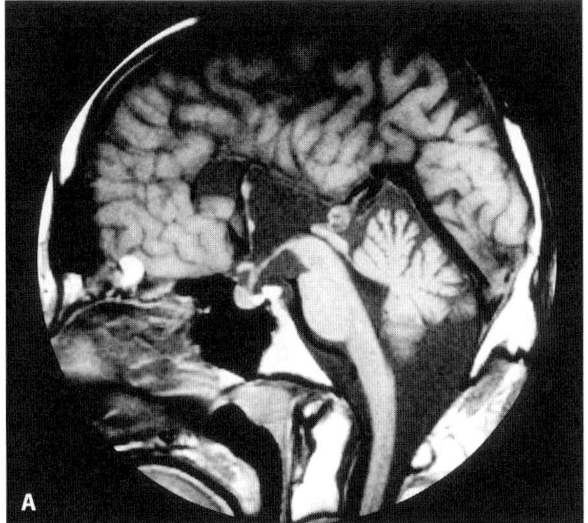

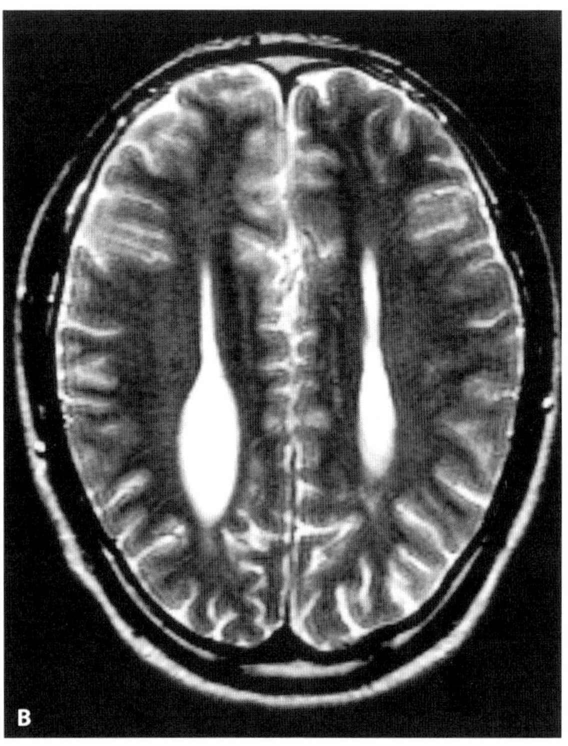

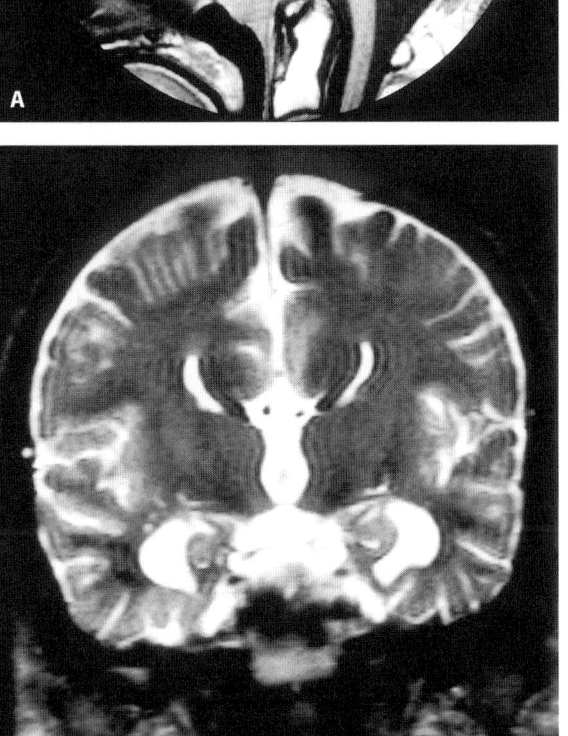

Fig. 4.7A–C. Agenesis of the corpus callosum. **A** Midsagittal SE T1-WI. **B** Axial SE T2-WI. **C** Coronal SE T2-WI. There is a complete absence of the corpus callosum. In the axial imaging plane, there is a parallel orientation of the widely spaced lateral ventricles. Note the widening of the posterior section of the lateral ventricles; this is termed colpocephaly. In the coronal plane, the high-riding third ventricle is in continuity with the interhemispheric fissure. The lateral ventricles are indented medially by Probst's bundles

- Parallel orientation of the lateral ventricles (axial images)
- Longitudinal white-matter tracts (Probst bundles) indent the superomedial walls of the lateral ventricles (axial and coronal images)
- Colpocephaly, i.e., dilatation of the trigones and occipital horns
- Superior extension of the third ventricle between the lateral ventricles (coronal images)
- Crescent-shaped ('bull's horn') frontal horns

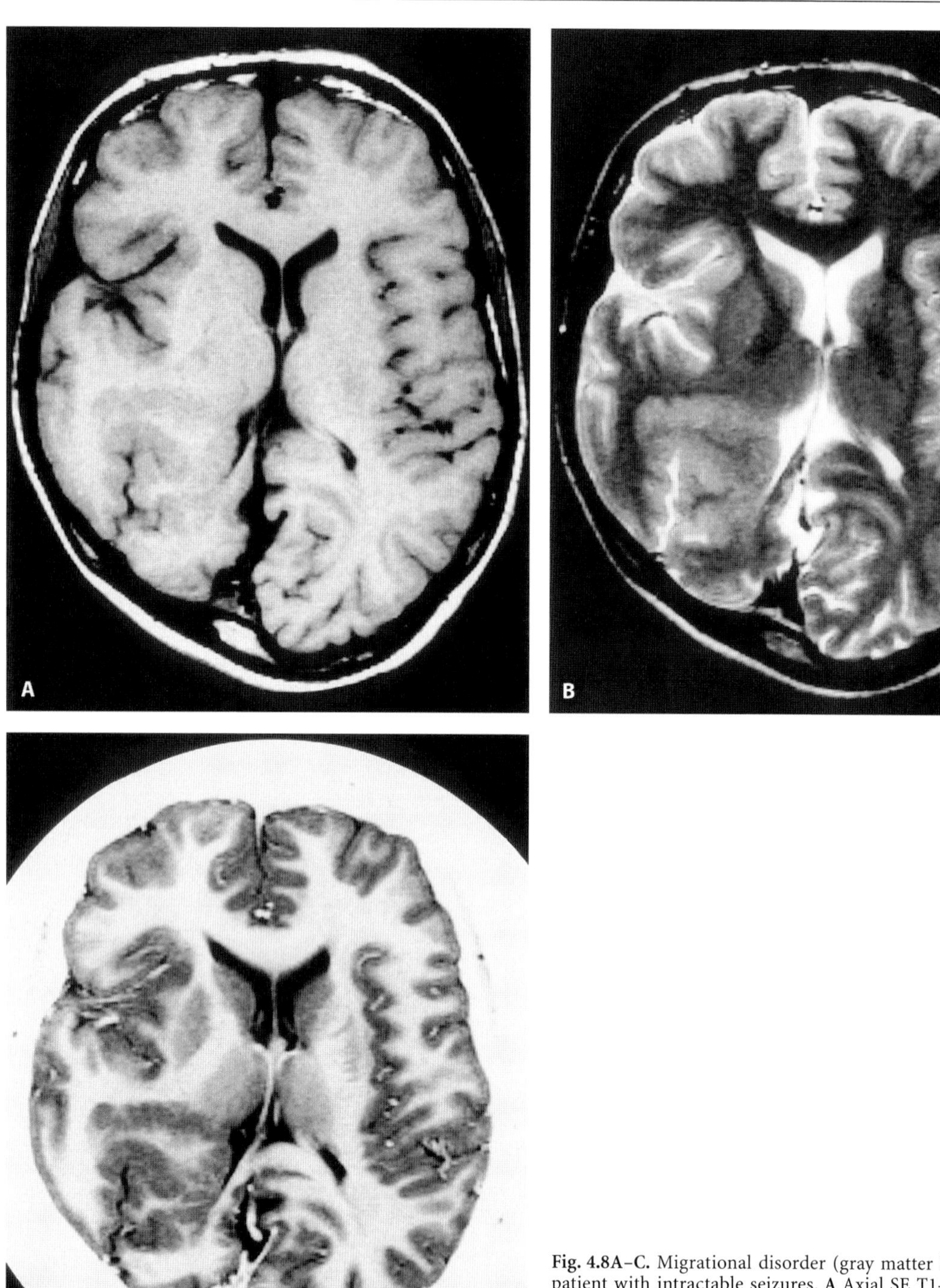

Fig. 4.8A–C. Migrational disorder (gray matter heterotopia) in a patient with intractable seizures. **A** Axial SE T1-WI. **B** Axial TSE T2-WI. **C** Axial TIR T1-WI. The right occipital lobe contains dysplastic, disorganized gray matter. The heterotopic gray matter indents the right lateral ventricle. On all sequences, the heterotopic gray matter is isointense to cortex. TIR images provide the best contrast between gray and white matter and can be very helpful in the characterization of migrational disorders

- Hypoplastic or dysgenetic anterior commissure and hippocampal formation

Agenesis of the corpus callosum can occur as an isolated finding but is often associated with other congenital anomalies of the brain, including Chiari II, Dandy Walker, interhemispheric cysts, migration disorders, and lipoma. Other midline structures that should be identified on the midsagittal image include the anterior commissure, the posterior commissure, the pineal gland, the pituitary and pituitary stalk, the aqueduct, the quadrigeminal plate, and the floor of the anterior fossa.

4.2.4 Cerebral Hemispheres

The symmetry of the cerebral hemispheres is best appreciated on axial and/or coronal scans. A sequence providing high contrast between white and gray matter is preferred. Our choice is a 'true' turbo inversion recovery (IR), heavily T1-W sequence (Fig. 4.8). In these MR images, gray matter appears 'gray' and white matter appears 'white'. These images are well-suited for the detection of cortical lesions and neuronal migrational disorders. Embryologically, these conditions result from the abnormal migration of neurons from the germinal matrix to the brain surface. These disorders include lissencephaly, cortical dysplasias, heterotopias, schizencephaly, and megalencephaly, and are discussed in greater detail in Chapter 16.

When evaluating complex malformations of the brain or cystic lesions (Fig. 4.9), imaging should be performed in the three orthogonal planes to show the extent and anatomic relationships of the lesion accurately. Alternatively, a 3D sequence can be employed. IR images are also of value in following the process of myelination and in the diagnosis of myelin disorders. Fast FLAIR images are an alternative for the detection of white-matter diseases.

4.3 Mass Lesions

4.3.1 Introduction

Many patients with focal neurological deficits, e.g., hemiparesis, hemianopia, and seizures, are referred for MR imaging to rule out an intracranial mass lesion; the symptoms depend on the location of the lesion. Some of these patients have had a prior computed tomography (CT) scan of the brain. If the CT scan shows a mass lesion, MR imaging should be performed to look for additional lesions, to characterize the mass and to plan the treatment. If the CT scan is negative but there is strong clinical suspicion of an intracranial mass, MR imaging should also be performed. Administration of contrast material is essential. MR imaging has now become the method of choice for all types of intracranial mass lesions. For the initial diagnostic screening of a suspected intracranial mass, we suggest the imaging protocol shown in Table 4.3.

When confronted with an intracranial lesion, the radiologist should be able to answer the following questions:

1. Is the lesion a tumor?
2. What is the location of the lesion? (supra- or infratentorial? intra-axial or extra-axial?)
3. What is the amount of mass effect and edema?
4. What is the most likely diagnosis, keeping in mind the patient's age?

4.3.2 Tumor or Not?

The clinical and MRI diagnosis of an intracranial mass lesion can be challenging. In most cases, the initial clinical symptoms are nonspecific and result only from mass effect, local pressure, and distortion of adjacent structures. Not all mass lesions are tumors. Tumors are usually characterized by a gradual onset of symptoms, preferential involvement of white matter with sparing of cortical gray matter, round or infiltrating shape, and are not confined to a specific vascular distribution. Some of the major differential diagnostic considerations include: recent infarct, abscess, encephalitis, developmental anomaly. The use of intravenously injected contrast agents does not always solve the issue.

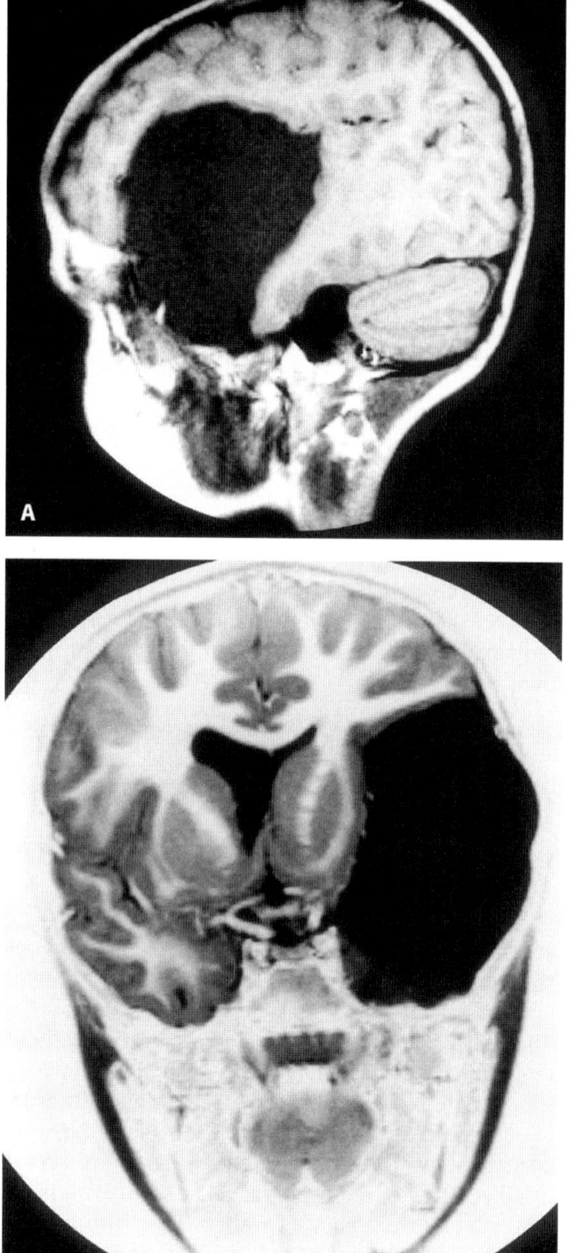

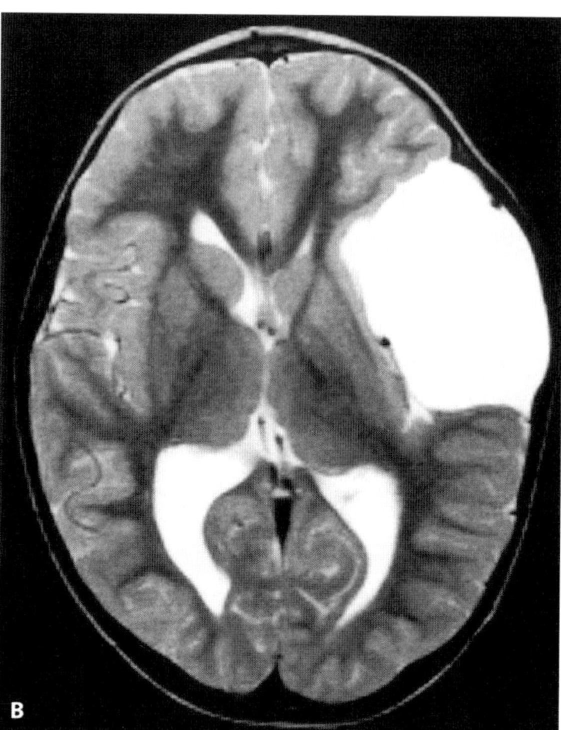

Fig. 4.9A–C. Arachnoid cyst. **A** Sagittal SE T1-WI. **B** Axial TSE T2-WI. **C** Coronal TIR image. These images illustrate the typical appearance of a middle cranial fossa arachnoid cyst. Cyst contents are isointense to CSF. Branches of the middle cerebral artery, seen as small areas of flow void, are displaced medially. Note that there is some outward bulging of the skull overlying the cyst (this 5-year-old boy presented with a growing 'bump' on the head). The cyst is lined by displaced cortical gray matter (coronal image)

Table 4.3. Protocol for intracranial mass lesions and infections. Imaging planes should be adapted in function of the location of the lesion(s). Magnetization transfer (MT) is switched on for most gadolinium (Gd)-enhanced MR imaging; ideally, the precontrast T1-W sequence is also performed with MT. When cerebral metastases are suspected, the use of double dose contrast has been advocated. For the purpose of comparison, we recommend to perform SE T1-W images with the same parameter settings (imaging plane, thickness and position) before and after Gd administration. When needed, subtraction images can be calculated from the pre- and postcontrast images. The final sequence can also be a T1-W 3D gradient echo sequence (MP-RAGE, SPGR) with multiple thin slices. Reformated images can be generated in other imaging planes from the 3D data set

Pulse sequence	WI	Plane	No. of sections	TR (ms)	TE (ms)	TI (ms)	Flip angle	Echo train length	Section thickness (mm)	Matrix	FOV	recFOV	No. of acq.
1. Axial T2-W sequence (single echo)													
TSE	T2	ax	19–25	3000–6000	90–130	–	90/180	7–15	5	512	230–240	75	1–2
2. Axial T2-W turbo FLAIR sequence													
Turbo FLAIR	T2	ax	19	6000–10000	100–150	1800–2200	90/180	7–11	5	512	230–240	75	1–2
3. Axial (or sagittal) T1-W sequence (MTC optional)													
SE	T1	ax	19	600–800	10–20	–	90/180	–	5	256 or better	230–240	75	1–2
Intravenous contrast injection													
4. Axial T1-W sequence (MTC optional)													
SE	T1	ax	19	600–800	10–20	–	90/180	–	5	256 or better	230–240	75	1–2
5. Coronal and/or sagittal SE T1-W sequence, choice of imaging plane at the discretion of the radiologist and/or technologist performing the examination													
SE	T1	cor or sag	19	600–800	10–20	–	90/180	–	5	256 or better	230–240	75	1–2

Abbreviations: *WI* weighted image: *TR* repetition time (ms); *TI* inversion time (ms); *TE* echo time (ms): *TD* time delay (sec); *no part* number of partitions: *Matrix* (phase × frequency matrix); *FOV* field of view (mm); *recFOV* % rectangular field of view

Some tumors do not enhance (e.g., low-grade astrocytoma), whereas intense enhancement is sometimes observed in nontumoral conditions (e.g., enhancement in recent stroke due to blood-brain barrier breakdown, ring-like enhancement of an abscess). The amount of enhancement is not directly related to the degree of malignancy.

4.3.3 Lesion Location

Intracranial lesions can be classified as supra- or infratentorial, depending on their position relative to the tentorium cerebelli. Infratentorial tumors are more frequent in the pediatric age group. Some tumors occur in different topographical compartments, depending on the patient's age. A typical example are choroid plexus papillomas; in infants, they tend to occur supratentorially (lateral ventricles), whereas in adults they are more common infratentorially (fourth ventricle). Other tumors preferentially occur in one compartment, e.g., hemangioblastoma is almost exclusively an infratentorial tumor.

Perhaps even more important for the differential diagnosis is to determine whether the site of origin of the lesion is intra-axial or extra-axial, depending on whether the neoplasm originates in the brain parenchyma or from the coverings of the brain. The prognosis and surgical approach for the two types differ. Extra-axial tumors can be of meningeal origin (meningioma, leptomeningeal seeding, lymphoma), nerve-sheath origin (schwannoma of N. VIII, V, VII), or osseous origin (chordoma, eosinophilic granuloma). In the broad sense of the definition, extra-axial tumors also include maldevelopmental cysts and tumors (arachnoid cyst, (epi)dermoid cyst, lipoma). The cardinal feature of extra-axial tumors is that they are separated from the brain surface. The diagnosis depends primarily on the identification of anatomical boundary layers, which are interposed between the brain surface and the extra-axial tumor, e.g., CSF cleft, vascular cleft, dural cleft. Most extra-axial tumors are benign. Because they are located outside of the brain, they do not possess a blood-brain barrier. When an extra-axial tumor enhances after intravenous injection of a contrast agent, it is because of its intrinsic tumor vascularity. Enhancement often helps to define the anatomic compartmentalization of extra-axial tumors. Contrast enhancement is highly characteristic of some extra-axial tumors (meningioma, schwannoma), whereas others almost never enhance (epidermoid, dermoid).

The most common supratentorial extra-axial tumors are meningiomas and metastases. Meningioma is the most common primary nonglial intracranial tumor (13%–19% of all operated brain tumors) (Fig. 4.10). Meningioma capillaries lack a blood-brain barrier, and therefore, the tumor enhances strongly with Gd. Calvarial invasion is common. Some meningiomas are intraventricular. Extra-axial metastases are most commonly caused by breast carcinoma (most common primary tumor). Metastasis may involve the skull, the pachymeninges (dura mater), and the leptomeninges (arachnoid-subarachnoid metastases, pial metastases). Other supratentorial extra-axial tumors include lymphoma, sarcoidosis, and chordoma.

Infratentorially, extra-axial tumors occur predominantly in the cerebellopontine angle (CPA). In decreasing order of frequency, they include acoustic schwannoma (80%), meningioma (13%–18%), epidermoid tumor (5%), and other lesions (schwannoma of N. V, VII, foramen jugulare tumors, chordoma, arachnoid cyst, aneurysm of basilar artery, exophytic glioma).

Intra-axial tumors originate within the substance of the brain. They can be subdivided into primary and secondary tumors. The most common primary brain

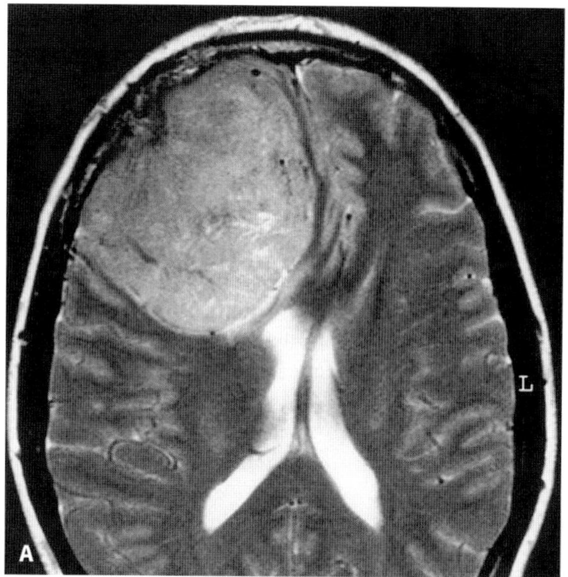

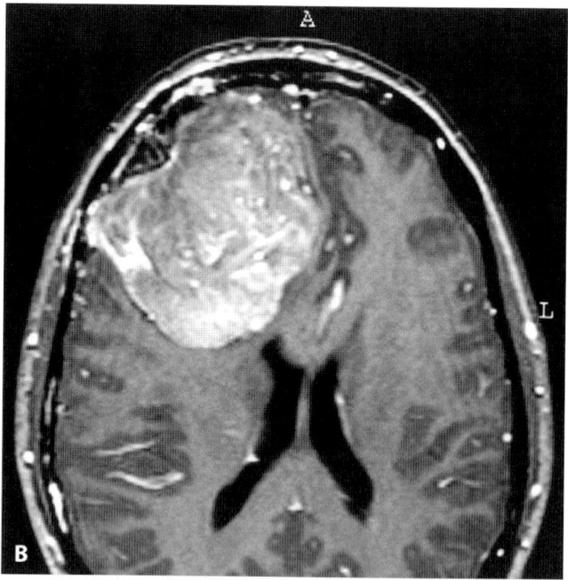

Fig. 4.10A,B. Frontal convexity meningioma. **A** Axial TSE T2-WI. **B** Axial gadolinium-enhanced gradient-echo 3D FT T1-WI. The T2-WI reveals a large tumor which is isointense to cortical gray matter. The lesion is well demarcated. Displaced vessels and CSF clefts are visible in the brain-tumor interface, indicating the extra-axial nature of the tumor. There is no perifocal edema. The tumor enhances inhomogeneously. Numerous intratumoral vessels are present. Note the pathognomonic enostotic spur and the accordion sign at the posterior margin of the lesion

tumors are of glial cell origin. Gliomas account for 40%–50% of all primary intracranial tumors. Examples of intra-axial tumors include astrocytoma (low-grade, anaplastic, glioblastoma multiforme), oligodendroglioma, ependymoma, DNET (dysembryoplastic neuroectodermal tumor), and lymphoma. However, metastases are still the most frequent intra-axial tumors in the supratentorial compartment. Intra-axial tumors can enhance because of blood-brain-barrier breakdown (e.g., high-grade astrocytoma) or because of their intrinsic tumor vascularity (hemangioblastoma). The degree of enhancement may play a role in differentiating high-grade from low-grade gliomas. Table 4.4 provides an overview of intracranial tumors depending on their location. Some tumors are located in the ventricles. Table 4.5 provides a differential diagnostic list for intraventricular mass lesions.

Table 4.4. Topography of intracranial tumors

	Intra-axial	Extra-axial
Supratentorial	**Primary:** glioma (astrocytoma, GBM, oligodendroglioma, ependymoma, DNET/PNET, lymphoma)	**Primary:** meningioma, pituitary adenoma, epidermoid, dermoid, bone tumors
	Secondary: intraparenchymal metastases	**Secondary:** leptomeningeal metastases
Infratentorial	**Primary:** astrocytoma, medulloblastoma (PNET), ependymoma, brainstem glioma, hemangioblastoma	**Primary:** schwannoma, meningioma (epi)dermoid, chordoma, leptomeningeal metastases
	Secondary: intraparenchymal metastases	**Secondary:** leptomeningeal metastases

Table 4.5. Intraventricular tumors

- Ependymoma
- Astrocytoma
- Colloid cyst
- Meningioma
- Choroid plexus papilloma/carcinoma
- Epidermoid/dermoid
- Craniopharyngioma
- Medulloblastoma (PNET)
- Metastases (CSF seeding)

4.3.4 Edema and Mass Effect

MR imaging is more sensitive than CT in detecting intracranial mass lesions because the associated edema is easily observed on FLAIR and T2-WI. In many instances, the peritumoral edema is more conspicuous than the tumor itself. Three types of edema can be discerned.

Vasogenic edema is caused by a breakdown of the blood-brain barrier, which allows excessive fluid to pass from the capillaries into the extracellular space. Vasogenic edema extends along white-matter tracts and generally spares the cortical gray matter. Vasogenic edema is associated with primary and metastatic tumors, contusion, inflammation, hemorrhage, and the subacute stage of cerebral infarcts (Fig. 4.11).

Cytotoxic edema is most often due to ischemia. When the blood supply to a cell is decreased, the production of ATP is reduced, and the Na/K pump fails. This results in cellular swelling and a decrease in the volume of the extracellular spaces. Cytotoxic edema is typically seen in (hyper)acute ischemic infarction, and it involves both gray and white matter. If damage to the blood-brain barrier follows, vasogenic edema may ensue in addition to the cytotoxic edema.

Interstitial edema results from transependymal migration of CSF into the periventricular white matter. It is due to a pressure gradient in acute forms of hydrocephalus.

All types of edema result in an increased water content of the tissues and are therefore hyperintense on FLAIR and T2-WI. Interstitial edema results in diffuse periventricular hyperintensity along the lateral ventricles. Newer techniques such as diffusion-weighted MR imaging are important for the early detection of (cytotoxic) edema, which may be detected within minutes after an acute cerebral infarct.

The amount of edema determines to a great extent the amount of intracranial mass effect. The mass effect may lead to brain herniation. This is important to recognize because it can lead to severe neurological dysfunction and is more commonly the cause of death than the tumor itself. Four types of internal **brain herniation** are distinguishable.

1. Subfalcine herniation. The cingulate gyrus is pushed under the falx. This is best seen on coronal MR images.

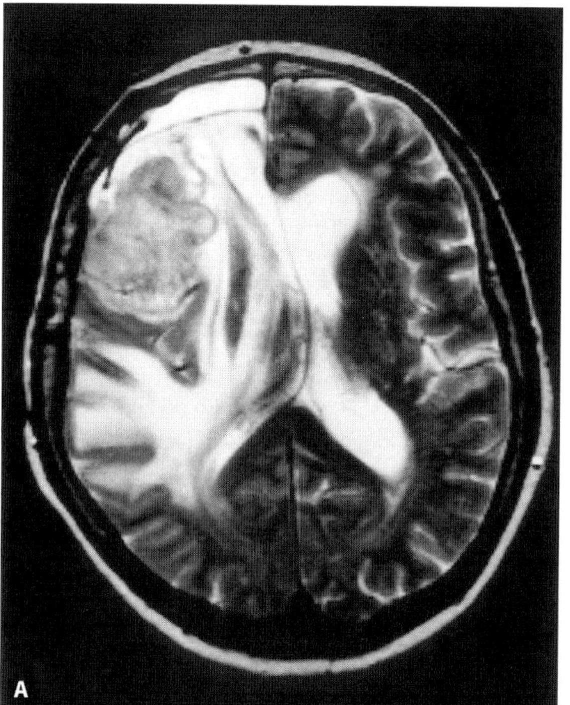

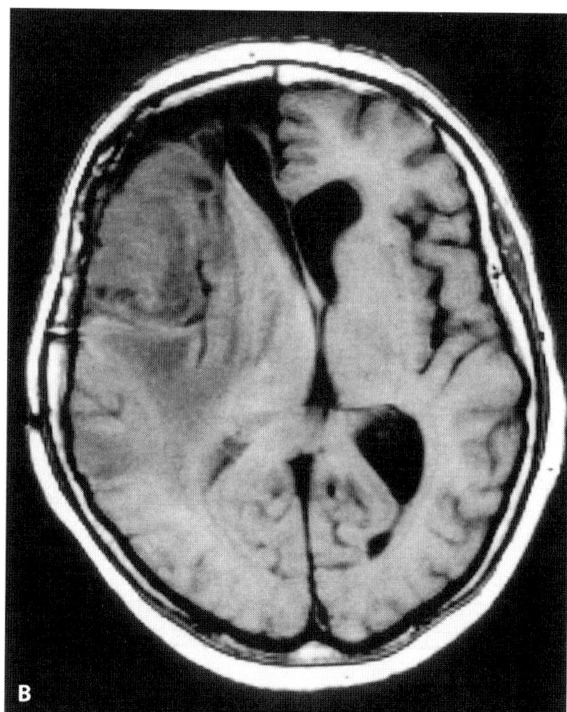

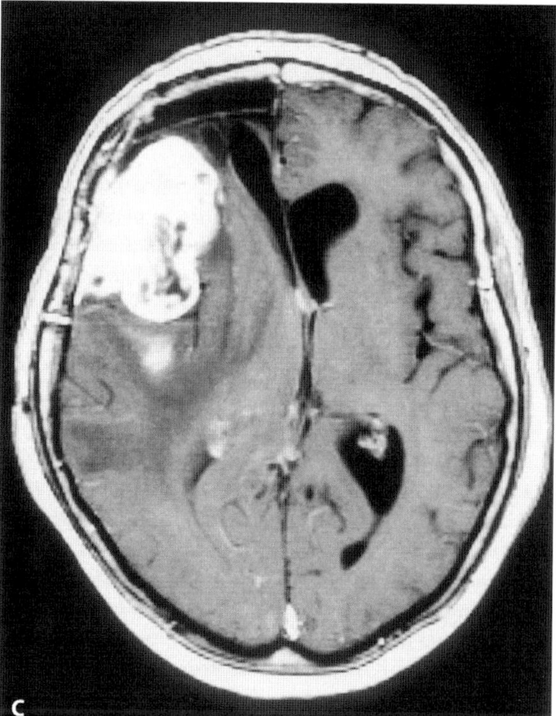

Fig. 4.11A–C. Recurrent glioblastoma multiforme with vasogenic edema. **A** Axial TSE T2-WI. **B** Axial SE T1-WI. **C** Gadolinium-enhanced axial SE T1-WI. In this patient with recurrent right frontal glioblastoma multiforme, the axial TSE T2-WI shows extensive vasogenic edema. The vasogenic edema extends along white matter tracts. The mass effect is caused predominantly by the perilesional edema. Note that the claustrum is outlined by edema in the capsula externa and extrema. The digitiform extensions of the edema are much better seen on the T2-WI than on the T1-WI. After gadolinium injection, the tumor enhances inhomogeneously and contains necrotic sections

2. Descending transtentorial herniation (uncal herniation, hippocampal herniation). The uncus and/or hippocampal gyrus of the temporal lobe are pushed medially into the tentorial incisura. Displacement of the medial temporal lobe is best seen on coronal images, but the compression of the brainstem is best observed on axial T2-WI.
3. Ascending transtentorial herniation. Upward displacement of the vermis and cerebellum through the incisura due to an infratentorial mass. The sagittal imaging plane is preferred.
4. Cerebellar tonsillar herniation. Downward displacement of the cerebellar tonsils and hemispheres through the foramen magnum behind the cervical spinal cord. Sagittal and coronal imaging planes are preferred.

4.3.5 Lesion Characterization

4.3.5.1 Signal Intensity

Most tumors are hyperintense on FLAIR and T2-WI, and iso- to hypointense on precontrast T1-WI. These MR findings are not helpful in characterizing the lesion. Some mass lesions display unusual signal features, which narrow the differential diagnosis. Table 4.6 lists a differential diagnosis for lesions that are hypointense on T2-WI. Table 4.7 provides a differential diagnostic list for lesions that are hyperintense on T1-WI. Cystic lesions are relatively rare, and their differential diagnosis is listed in Table 4.8.

Table 4.6. Low SI on T2-W images (Atlas SW, 1996)

Paramagnetic effects	• Iron in dystrophic calcification • Old hemorrhage (ferritin, hemosiderin) • Acute hemorrhage (deoxyHb) • Subacute hemorrhage (intracellular metHb) • Melanin (free radicals)
Low proton density	• Calcification • High nucleus/cytoplasm ratio • Dense cellularity
Macromolecule content	• Very high protein concentration • Fibrocollagenous stroma
Intratumoral vessels	• Rapid blood flow (flow voids)

Table 4.7. High S1 on T1-W images (Atlas SW, 1996)

Paramagnetic effects from hemorrhage	• Subacute-chronic blood e.g. methemoglobin
Paramagnetic effects without hemorrhage	• Melanin • Ions associated with necrosis or calcification: Mn, Fe, Cu
Nonparamagnetic effects	• Very high protein concentration • Fat • Flow-related enhancement in vessels

Table 4.8. Cystic lesions

True cyst	• Sharply demarcated, ovoid or round
Signal intensity	• Isointense with CSF on all pulse sequences (e.g. arachnoid cyst, cysts associated with extra-axial masses) • Slightly higher SI than CSF on T1-WI and PD-WI (proteinaceous debris and/or small concentrations of paramagnetic substances)
Enhancement	• Ring enhancement • Mural nodule (e.g. hemangioblastoma)

4.3.5.2 Enhancement Pattern

The presence of contrast enhancement does not necessarily differentiate a tumor from a nontumoral lesion, since many nonneoplastic conditions enhance. The boundary of the enhancing area does not always delimit the tumor extent. This is especially true for gliomatous tumors, which infiltrate beyond the margin of

Table 4.9. Ring-enhancing brain lesions

Neoplasm	• Primary neoplasm (high-grade glioma, meningioma, lymphoma, acoustic schwannoma, craniopharyngioma) • Metastatic tumor
Abscess	• Bacterial, fungal, parasitic abscess • Empyema (epidural, subdural, or intraventricular)
Hemorrhagic-ischemic lesion	• Resolving infarction • Aging hematoma • Operative bed following resection
Demyelinating disorder	
Radiation necrosis	

enhancement. Moreover, the intensity of contrast enhancement is not always correlated with the degree of malignancy of the lesion (pilocytic astrocytomas demonstrate marked enhancement, despite their relatively benign nature). Some specific types of enhancement provide interesting diagnostic gamuts, e.g., ring-like enhancement (Table 4.9).

4.4 Supratentorial Brain Tumors

4.4.1 Introduction

The MR examination for supratentorial brain tumors should consist of a combination of at least two imaging planes and two different weightings. The axial plane is the plane of first choice for the supratentorial compartment; the coronal plane is the second best. In cases of midline lesions, such as pineal region tumors, the sagittal plane must be used.

Intravenous (i.v.) contrast agents, such as Gd-chelates, are frequently necessary for the detection and improved delineation and characterization of the tumor. Without i.v. contrast, it is not possible to differentiate nonspecific high-intensity foci attributed to aging or ischemia from metastasis or lymphoma. Small lesions, such as metastases, can be invisible without Gd. The pattern of contrast enhancement yields important information about the differential diagnosis and the degree of malignancy.

The questions to be answered are: what is the exact location of the tumor, and what is the probable histologic type and degree of malignancy? The radiologist must be aware of other factors of clinical importance: the mechanical effects such as obstructive hydrocephalus and descending transtentorial herniation.

Although intrinsically superior to CT, MR imaging also has its limitations! Neuroradiological examinations do not give the true neuropathological extent of many intra-axial brain tumors. MR imaging is a highly sensitive technique, but there is still a lack of specificity. On T2-WI, high SI lesions from a multiple sclerosis plaque and a metastasis can be very similar. MR imaging is not as sensitive for intratumoral calcifications as CT. Necrosis, a prognostically important factor in brain tumor diagnosis, is not reliably detected by MR imaging.

4.4.2 Basic Neuroradiological Features

4.4.2.1 Description of the Lesion

In an MRI report, the following basic neuroradiological characteristics of an intracranial tumor should appear: location (intra-axial or extra-axial, supratentorial or infratentorial, frontal or temporal, etc.), SI, degree of perifocal edema, space-occupying characteristics, what happens after i.v. contrast, solitary or multiple lesions. Together with other factors, such as the clinical information, the speed of evolution, the age of the patient, and the relative frequency of certain tumors in certain locations, these neuroradiological features should lead to a probable neuropathological diagnosis or differential diagnosis.

4.4.2.2 Intra-axial or Extra-axial Location

The initial question for the radiologist in the presence of an intracranial mass lesion is whether the mass is intra-axial or extra-axial. This is of great clinical importance. The location affects the operative planning and prognosis. Extra-axial tumors are located outside the brain parenchyma and are mostly benign. There are several signs of an extra-axial location (Table 4.10).

4.4.2.3 Signal Intensity

Because of their high water content, most brain tumors exhibit low SI on T1-WI and high SI on T2-W images. However, there are many exceptions to this rule. The SI

Table 4.10. MR signs of extra-axial tumor location

Difference in signal intensity between tumor surface and cortex	Arterial encasement; dural sinus invasion
Elements of a brain-tumor interface	Dural-tail sign
White-matter buckling	Gyral compression: the accordion sign
Osseous changes	Paradoxical cisternal widening
Vascular pedicle	Broad-based dural contact

Table 4.11. Causes of heterogeneous SI

Hemorrhage	Necrosis
Calcification	Cyst
Blood vessels	Inhomogeneous enhancement
Fat	Melanin

Table 4.12. Superficial tumor with homogeneous enhancement

Meningioma
Lymphoma
Anaplastic astrocytoma
Metastasis

Table 4.13. Cyst with enhancing mural nodule

Pilocytic astrocytoma
Hemangioblastoma
Pleomorphic xanthoastrocytoma
Ganglioglioma

of a tumor can be homogeneous or heterogeneous. There are many causes of heterogeneous SI (Table 4.11).

Tumors with a dense cellularity have a relatively low SI on T2-WI. This is a characteristic MR feature of medulloblastoma, pinealoblastoma, neuroblastoma, lymphoma, and mucinous adenocarcinoma metastasis (Table 4.6).

Some tumors exhibit high SI on T1-WI. This characteristic is mainly found in tumors containing fat (lipoma, dermoid), melanin (metastatic melanoma), methemoglobin (hemorrhagic tumors), or high protein concentrations (craniopharyngioma) (Table 4.7).

4.4.2.4 Patterns of Contrast Enhancement

The pattern of contrast enhancement supplies important information about the possible histological type of the tumor (Tables 4.9, 4.12, and 4.13).

4.4.3 Extra-axial Supratentorial Tumors

Extra-axial tumors are located outside the brain parenchyma. Meningioma is the most common tumor in this category. Other extra-axial tumors include schwannoma, arachnoid cyst, epidermoid-dermoid, lipoma, extra-axial metastasis.

Meningiomas arise from meningothelial (arachnoidal) cells along the inner surface of the dura mater. They have a distinct predilection for specific locations: convexity, parasagittal, inner and outer ridge, anterior skull base, cavernous sinus, cerebellopontine angle, etc. (Fig. 4.7). The majority of meningiomas demonstrate a heterogeneous SI pattern. Meningiomas are typically isointense with gray matter on all SE sequences and may, therefore, be missed unless contrast is given. On T1-WI, meningiomas are almost always hypo- to isointense compared with white matter. On PD-WI and T2-WI, meningiomas are can be iso- to hyperintense compared with the adjacent brain. The identification of an anatomic brain-tumor interface is pathognomonic for the extra-axial localization. Three different anatomic interfaces may be identified with MR imaging: pial vascular structures, CSF clefts, and dural margins.

Following Gd administration, meningiomas almost always display intense and homogeneous enhancement. Even heavily calcified meningiomas tend to enhance. Multiplanar imaging is useful for the preoperative delineation of the extent of the meningioma. Dural enhancement adjacent to the tumor is a striking finding in contrast-enhanced MR imaging. It is referred to as the 'dural-tail sign'. It is not specific for meningiomas; it only indicates dural involvement by an adjacent mass.

4.4.4 Intra-axial Supratentorial Tumors

4.4.4.1 Glial tumors

Glial tumors (or 'gliomas') account for 40%–45% of all primary intracranial tumors. They arise from the glial cells, which have a great propensity to malignant transformation. There are three major groups of gliomas, which correspond to the three histologic subgroups of glial cells: astrocytoma, oligodendroglioma, ependymoma. Neoplasms arising from the choroid plexus can also be considered as glial cell tumors, because the choroid plexus contains modified ependymal cells. Gliomas occur predominantly in the cerebral hemispheres, but the brain stem and cerebellum are frequent locations in children, and they can also be found in the spinal cord.

4.4.4.1.1 Astrocytomas

Astrocytic brain tumors can be divided into two major groups: the fibrillary (also known as infiltrative or diffuse) astrocytoma and the circumscribed (localized or non-infiltrative) astrocytoma (Table 4.14.).

Astrocytomas are the low-grade member of the fibrillary or diffuse astrocytomas (Fig. 4.12). Well-differentiated low-grade astrocytomas are relatively rare, affect younger patients, and have a better prognosis than their more aggressive counterparts. On MR imaging, a low-grade astrocytoma is seen as a homogeneous mass lesion, involving gray and white matter. The lesion is typically hypo- or isointense on T1-WI and hyperintense on T2-WI. The tumor may cause a local mass effect with gyral swelling, though perifocal edema is usually absent or slight. MR imaging misleadingly displays these lesions as clearly defined, especially on T2-WI. However, it should be remembered that they belong to the group of diffuse astrocytoma, and tumor tissue can be found outside the MRI visible border of the tumor! In principle, the low-grade astrocytoma shows no contrast enhancement. Moreover, though initially benign, a low-grade astrocytoma can evolve into a higher grade tumor over time. Different parts of the tumor can exhibit varying degrees of malignancy; this makes histological grading from biopsies difficult.

Anaplastic astrocytomas are much more common than their low-grade counterparts. These malignant, aggressive tumors infiltrate the adjacent brain structures, and have a poor prognosis. On MR imaging, anaplastic astrocytomas present a more heterogeneous appearance, both on T1-WI and T2-WI. There is a marked mass effect and perifocal vasogenic edema, which spreads with fingerlike projections along white matter tracts. The tumor may contain hemorrhagic foci. Marked but irregular enhancement is usually present, indicating breakdown of the BBB.

Glioblastoma multiforme (GBM) is the most malignant neuroglial tumor. In the older adult (>50 years), high-grade GBM is the most common intra-axial supratentorial neoplasm. The imaging findings can be pre-

Table 4.14. Classification of astrocytic brain tumors

	Fibrillary (diffuse or infiltrative) astrocytoma			Circumscribed (localized or noninfiltrative) astrocytoma		
Name	**Low-grade astrocytoma**	**Anaplastic astrocytoma**	**Glioblastoma multiforme**	**Pilocytic astrocytoma**	**Giant-cell astrocytoma**	**Pleomorphic xanthoastrocytoma**
Common locations	Cerebral hemispheres, pons (in children)	Cerebral hemispheres, brainstem	Cerebral hemispheres	Cerebellum, diencephalon	Subependymal in lateral ventricle (at the foramen of Monro)	Cerebral hemispheres, superficially located, often temporal lobe
Demographics	4th and 5th decades	Variable	Peak 50–65 years	5–15 years (peak around 10 years)	Children, young adults	Young adults with a history of seizures
Imaging findings	Expansion, no enhancement (intact BBB), follows white matter tracts	Variable appearance, enhancement, no necrosis or cyst formation	Grossly heterogeneous (necrosis, ring enhancement, vasogenic edema, hemorrhage)	Cyst with enhancing nodule	Variable enhancement, associated with other features of tuberous sclerosis	Heterogeneous (cyst with enhancing mural nodule, dural tail due to superficial location)
Malignancy grading (WHO)	Grade II	Grade III	Grade IV	Grade I	Benign	Benign (10% may have malignant degeneration)
Enhancement	Enhancement with Gd-chelates increases with degree of malignancy (breakdown of blood-brain barrier)			Enhancement is not related to degree of malignancy		

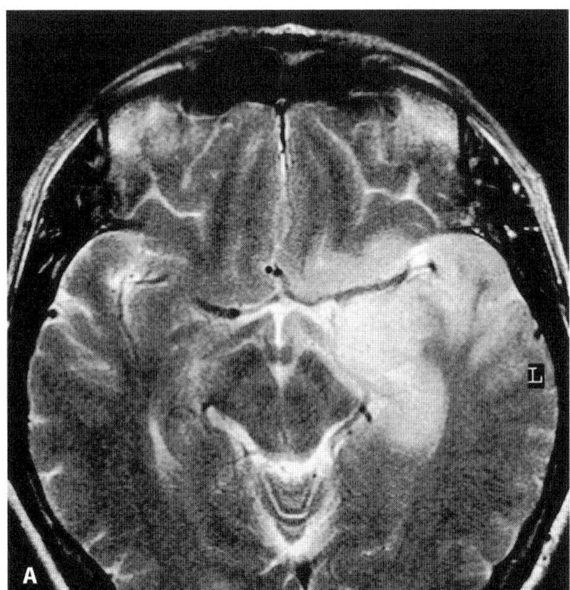

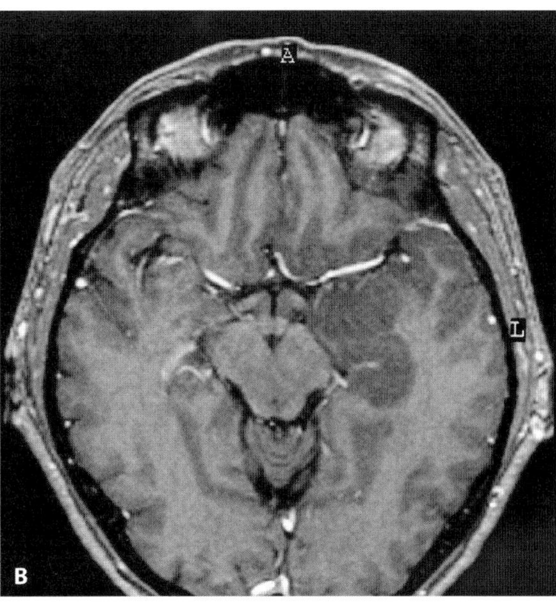

Fig. 4.12A,B. Low-grade astrocytoma. **A** Axial TSE T2-WI through the temporal lobes. **B** Axial gadolinium-enhanced GRE 3D FT T1-WI. An area of abnormal signal intensity involves both gray and white matter of the left frontal and temporal lobes. The SI within the tumor is homogeneous. After Gd injection, there is no enhancement (no disruption of the BBB). The tumor cannot be distinguished from the surrounding edema. There is only a moderate mass effect

dicted from the neuropathologic key features: cell heterogeneity, vascular cell proliferation, necrosis, and infiltration. On MR images, these properties are translated into: heterogeneous SI, cystic areas, perifocal edema (with tumor inside and outside), intratumoral signal void of vessels, extensive mass effect, and inhomogeneous contrast enhancement (Fig. 4.11). Sometimes, these highly vascular tumors may mimic arteriovenous malformations. They often contain intratumoral hemorrhages. Enhancement with contrast is intense and heterogeneous.

Gliomatosis cerebri is an unusual condition in which multiple lobes of the brain are diffusely invaded by contiguous extension of glial tumor cells. It may represent the extreme form of diffusely infiltrating glioma.

The group of circumscribed (localized or noninfiltrative) astrocytomas includes pilocytic astrocytoma, pleomorphic xanthoastrocytoma, and subependymal giant cell astrocytoma..

Pilocytic astrocytomas occur predominantly in children and adolescents. They are also known as 'juvenile pilocytic astrocytomas' (JPA). The most common location for pilocytic astrocytomas is infratentorial (see Sect. 4.5.4.3.), but the tumor can be encountered supratentorially in the optic chiasm or hypothalamus or, less commonly, in the cerebral hemispheres. Optochiasmatic-hypothalamic pilocytic astrocytomas are usually solid tumors, with moderate or even strong enhancement. When large, these tumors may contain cysts or trapped CSF, and should be differentiated from craniopharyngioma. There is an association with neurofibromatosis type 1.

Subependymal giant cell astrocytoma (SCGA) is a slow-growing, indolent, benign tumor and is typically found in a subependymal location at the foramen of Monro. It occurs most commonly in children and young adults. Symptoms are usually secondary to obstructive hydrocephalus. SCGA shows intense and heterogeneous enhancement. The tumor occurs with tuberous sclerosis.

Pleomorphic xanthoastrocytoma (PXA) is a rare and generally benign tumor. It is found predominantly in young adults, who often present with a history of seizures. PXA occurs in the cerebral hemispheres and is often located superficially, with the temporal lobes most commonly affected. On MR imaging, PXA presents as a superficial, partially cystic mass, with an enhancing mural nodule.

4.4.4.1.2 Oligodendrogliomas

Oligodendrogliomas arise from oligodendrocytes. They are less common than astrocytic tumors, and constitute 2%–5% of all primary brain tumors. They tend to occur in adults between the ages of 25 and 50 years, with a peak incidence around 35–45 years. Oligodendrogliomas are the most benign of the gliomas. They are slow-growing and are found predominantly in the frontal lobes and tend to infiltrate the cortex. MR imaging is less sensitive than CT in detecting calcifications, which occur in >70% of cases.

4.4.4.1.3 Ependymomas

Ependymomas are slow-growing neoplasms arising from cells of the ependymal lineage. They comprise 4%–8% of primary brain tumors and are most commonly found in children. Two-thirds of ependymomas occur infratentorially (especially in the fourth ventricle), and one-third are found supratentorially. Of the supratentorial ependymomas, more than half are extraventricular, presumably arising from ependymal cell nests in the cerebral parenchyma. On MR imaging, ependymomas present as a heterogeneous tumor of mixed signal intensities. Calcifications, present in 50% of cases, may be difficult to detect on routine MRI sequences, and the use of a gradient-echo T2*-W sequence can be helpful. After contrast injection, the enhancement is moderate to intense, depending on the vascularization of the tumor.

4.4.4.2 Intracranial Lymphoma

Intracranial lymphoma may be primary or secondary. Primary CNS lymphoma is usually non-Hodgkin's lymphoma (NHL), B-cell type. It is an aggressive tumor with a poor prognosis. In most series, the rate for multiplicity ranges from 11% to 50%, with a higher rate of 60% in acquired immunodeficiency syndrome (AIDS) patients.

MRI findings include (Fig. 4.13):

- Location. The most frequent location is peripherally in the cerebral hemisphere (45%). The central gray matter is a characteristic location, albeit not the most frequent one (23%). Intraventricular and infratentorial lesions are less common. Contact with an ependymal or meningeal surface is another characteristic feature.
- SI. In contradistinction to glioma, primary CNS lymphoma tends to be iso- to hypointense to brain on both T1-WI and T2-WI. The diminished signal on T2-WI may be due to the dense cellularity and relatively decreased water content (high nucleus-to-cytoplasmic ratio) of these tumors. The SI is of course altered in the presence of necrosis, which is a feature frequently found in AIDS patients.
- Contrast enhancement. Primary CNS lymphoma typically enhances intensely. The pattern of enhancement is usually homogeneous. In one series, all lesions enhanced after i.v. contrast, except in patients who had received corticosteroids before the MRI examination. Irregular rim enhancement is rare, except in tumors undergoing central necrosis, as is commonly observed in AIDS patients.

4.4.4.3 Intracranial Metastasis

Intracranial metastases are estimated to account for 20% of all clinically detected brain tumors. Metastases can be located in the skull, epidural space, meninges, and subarachnoid space (meningeal carcinomatosis) but are most frequent in the brain parenchyma.

The most sensitive examination for the detection of intracerebral metastases is i.v. contrast-enhanced MR imaging. A high-dose (0.3 mmol/kg) immediate study is superior to a normal-dose or delayed study in detecting small lesions. The use of magnetization transfer with a 3D GRE sequence improves the contrast between the enhancing lesion and the background.

MRI findings include:

- Location. Can be anywhere but occurs frequently in the cortex or at the corticomedullary junction (hematogenous spread).

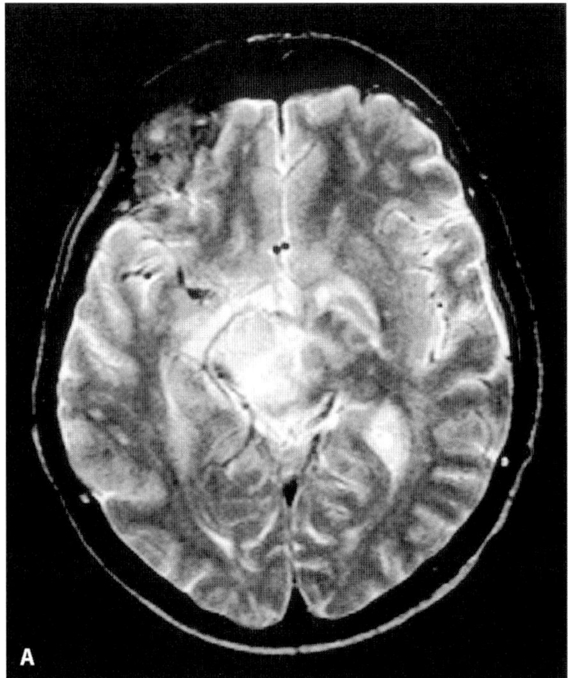

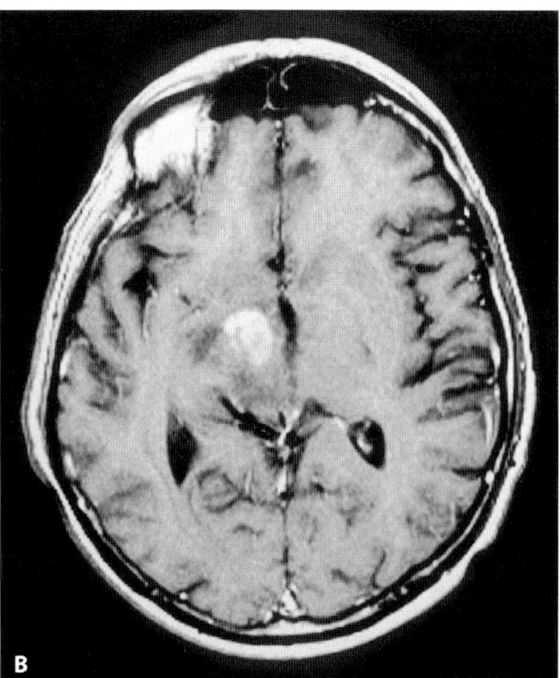

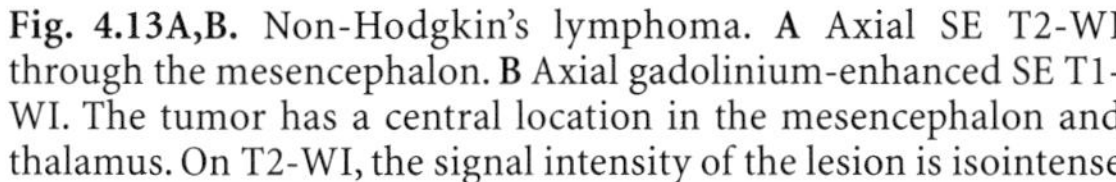

Fig. 4.13A,B. Non-Hodgkin's lymphoma. **A** Axial SE T2-WI through the mesencephalon. **B** Axial gadolinium-enhanced SE T1-WI. The tumor has a central location in the mesencephalon and thalamus. On T2-WI, the signal intensity of the lesion is isointense with cerebral gray matter, reflecting the high cellularity of the mass. After Gd injection, the tumor enhances strongly. The perilesional edema does not enhance

- Morphology. Round and better circumscribed than primary tumors.
- SI. The SI pattern of a metastasis is nonspecific and variable. Several specific pathological changes influence the SI: necrosis, cystic necrosis, intratumoral hemorrhage. Most metastases are slightly hypointense on T1-WI and hyperintense on T2-WI (in part due to vasogenic edema). Some metastases are hyperintense on T1-WI due to the presence of hemorrhage or melanin (paramagnetic effect).
- Contrast enhancement. The pattern of contrast enhancement can be homogeneous, nodular, inhomogeneous, or ring-like (see Table 4.9).

The amount of peritumoral edema is variable. In small cortical lesions, edema may be absent, but in general, the degree of edema is greater with metastatic lesions than with primary neoplasms (Fig. 4.14). There are no pathognomonic MRI features of metastasis. However, the following situations are highly suggestive of metastasis:

- An intracranial, enhancing tumor in a patient with a primary extracranial neoplasm
- A small lesion with prominent peritumoral edema
- Multiple enhancing lesions (Fig. 4.15)
- A solitary, thick-walled, ring-enhancing lesion

4.5 Infratentorial Tumors

4.5.1 Anatomy and Technique

The posterior fossa is bordered anteriorly in the midline by the dorsum sellae and the clivus (body of sphenoid bone, basilar part of occipital bone, separated by the spheno-occipital synchondrosis). The posterior aspect of the petrous bone constitutes the anterior lateral border, while the lateral and posterior borders are formed by the occipital bone, parietal bone, sigmoid,

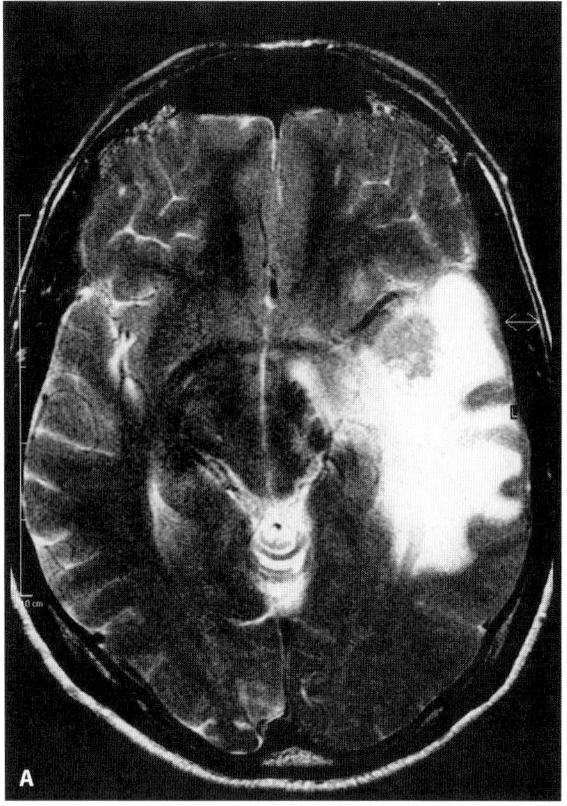

Fig. 4.14A,B. Solitary brain metastasis. **A** Axial TSE T2-WI. **B** Axial Gd-enhanced GRE 3D FT T1-WI. A nodular mass lesion is observed in the anterior part of the left temporal lobe. On T2-WI, the tumor is isointense with gray matter. Relative to the size of the tumor, there is a disproportionately large amount of perilesional edema. After Gd injection, there is intense enhancement. The enhancing tumor can be sharply separated from the surrounding vasogenic edema

and transverse sinus. The tentorium cerebelli and straight sinus compose the roof of the posterior fossa; the foramen magnum and jugular foramen are found in the floor of the posterior fossa.

The posterior fossa contains the brainstem (mesencephalon, pons, medulla oblongata), cranial nerves III–XII, cerebellum (vermis, hemispheres, and tonsils), CSF spaces (fourth ventricle, cisterna magna, prepontine cistern, cerebellopontine angle cisterns), arteries [vertebrobasilar artery and branches: posterior-inferior cerebellar artery (PICA), anterior-inferior cerebellar artery (AICA), superior cerebellar artery (SCA)], veins, and dural sinuses.

For the evaluation of posterior fossa lesions, axial and coronal imaging planes are preferred. Sagittal imaging is useful in fourth-ventricle mass lesions and CCJ abnormalities. When studying cranial nerve lesions, thin slices (1–3 mm) should be obtained. T2-WI are useful for demonstrating edema, cysts, areas of necrosis, and the presence of a CSF cleft in extra-axial tumors. Ultra-thin T2-WI (3D TSE) or T2*-WI constructive interference in the steady state (CISS) are useful for visualizing the CSF within the internal auditory canal and the fluid within the inner ear structures (cochlea, vestibule, semicircular canals). When a tumor is suspected clinically, pre- and postcontrast T1-WI must be obtained.

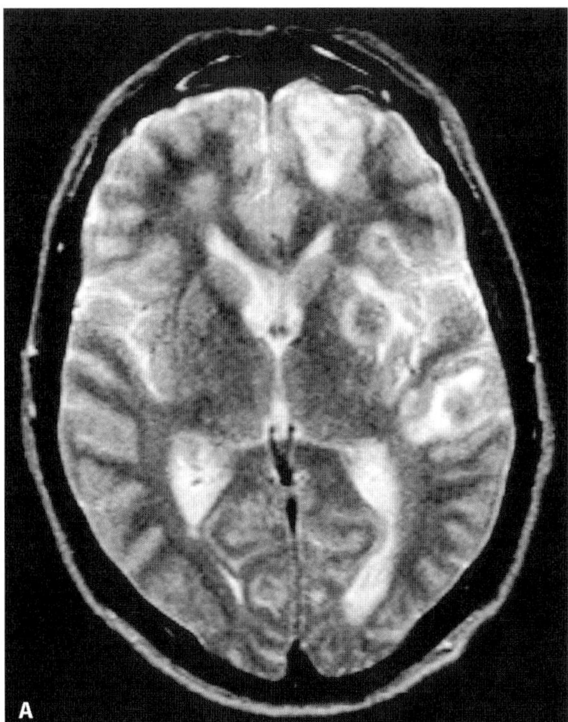

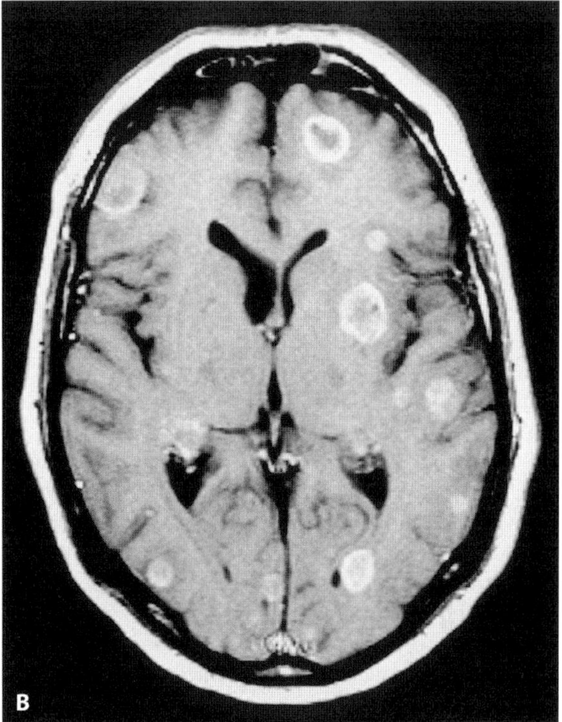

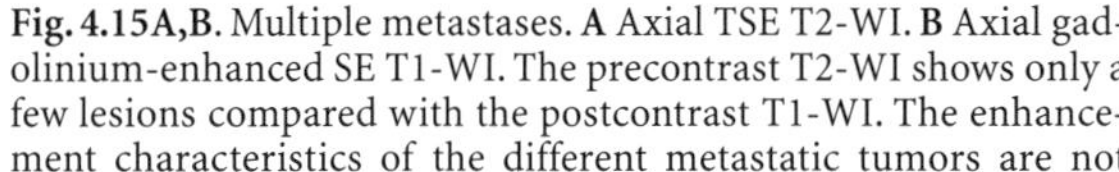

Fig. 4.15A,B. Multiple metastases. **A** Axial TSE T2-WI. **B** Axial gadolinium-enhanced SE T1-WI. The precontrast T2-WI shows only a few lesions compared with the postcontrast T1-WI. The enhancement characteristics of the different metastatic tumors are not uniform; some enhance homogeneously, while other lesions display a ring-shaped enhancement pattern. Also the amount of perilesional edema is variable. Notice the characteristic location of many of the metastatic lesions at the corticomedullary junction

4.5.2 Age-Related Frequency of Posterior Fossa Lesions

In children, posterior fossa tumors constitute the largest group of solid neoplasms. Posterior fossa tumors are second only to leukemia in overall frequency during childhood. They are associated with a high mortality rate, despite recent therapeutic advances. In children over 1 year old, 50% of brain tumors occur infratentorially. Conversely, in infants (<1 year old), supratentorial tumors are more frequent [primitive neuroectodermal tumor (PNET), low-grade gliomas, choroid plexus tumors]. Topographically, posterior fossa tumors can be subdivided into extra-and intra-axial tumors. The latter group can be further split into brainstem, cerebellar, and fourth-ventricle tumors.

4.5.3 Extra-axial Posterior Fossa Tumors

In adults, the most common posterior fossa tumors are extra-axial in nature. The site of predilection is the CPA cistern, which is located between the anterolateral surface of the pons and cerebellum and the posterior surface of the petrous temporal bone. The following imaging signs may be helpful to determine the extra-axial nature of a mass lesion:

- Enlargement of the ipsilateral CPA cistern
- Presence of CSF cleft between the tumor and the cerebellum
- Rotation of the brainstem away from the lesion
- Displacement of the gray matter–white matter interface around the mass

Table 4.15. Mass lesions in the cerebellopontine angle cistern

Connnon	• Acoustic schwannoma (80%) • Meningioma (13–18%) • Epidermoid (5%)
Less common	• Other schwannomas: facial nerve, trigeminal nerve • Vascular: vertebrobasilar dolichoectasia, aneurysm of basilar artery, AVM • Metastases • Paraganglioma • Arachnoid cyst • Lipoma • Foramen jugulare tumors • Chordoma

Mass lesions in the CPA are, in decreasing order of frequency: acoustic schwannoma (80%), meningioma (15%), epidermoid (5%), other schwannomas (facial nerve, trigeminal nerve), vascular (vertebrobasilar ectasia, aneurysm of basilar artery, AVM), metastases, paraganglioma, arachnoid cyst, lipoma, foramen jugulare tumors, chordoma (Table 4.15). Some intra-axial tumors may secondarily extend into the CPA cistern, e.g., exophytic glioma, metastasis, hemangioblastoma, ependymoma.

Acoustic nerve schwannoma is the most common CPA tumor (80%). Clinically, the tumor presents with sensorineural hearing loss, dizziness, and gait disturbance. Many acoustic schwannomas have both an intracanalicular and a CPA component. They may be solid or cystic (in large tumors necrosis occurs secondary to hemorrhage) (Fig. 4.16). In less than 5% of cases, there is an associated CPA arachnoid cyst. The hallmark of acoustic schwannomas on MRI, except for their typical location, is the intense, often heterogeneous, enhancement. Small, purely intracanalicular schwannomas can be detected with thin (submillimeter), heavily T2-weighted images (e.g., 3D CISS or 3D TSE T2), and their presence can be confirmed on Gd-enhanced T1-WI (Fig. 4.17).

Bilateral acoustic schwannomas occur in the setting of neurofibromatosis type 2. This is a neurocutaneous disorder with autosomal dominant inheritance (with high penetrance, linkage to chromosome 22). The occurrence frequency is ±1/40,000. The condition is characterized by bilateral acoustic schwannomas, intracranial meningiomas (convexity, falx), schwannomas of cranial nerves V, VII, IX, and X, spinal cord ependymoma, and astrocytoma. Neurofibromatosis type 2 is sometimes described by the acronym 'MISME' (multi-

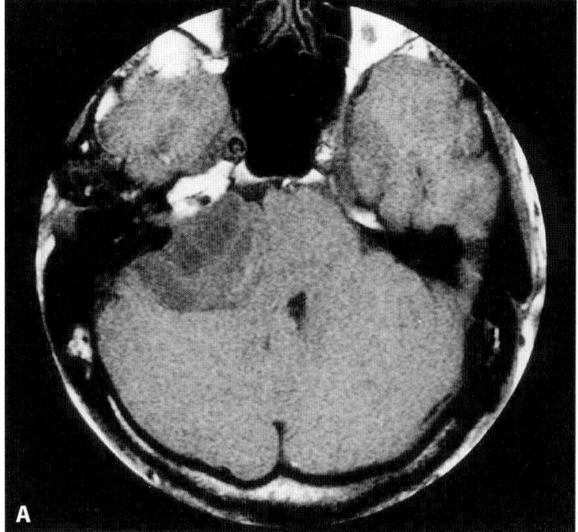

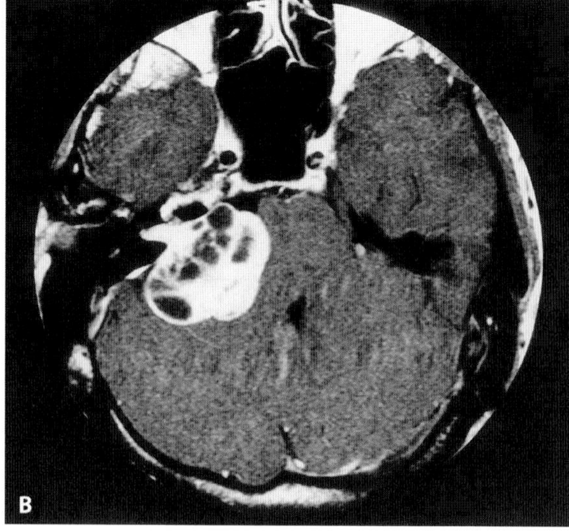

Fig. 4.16A,B. Acoustic schwannoma. **A** Axial SE T1-WI. **B** Gd-enhanced axial SE T1-WI. A large tumor extends from the right internal auditory canal to the cerebellopontine angle cistern. The enhancement pattern is inhomogeneous. The tumor contains numerous cystic areas. The brainstem is displaced, and the fourth ventricle is flattened, due to mass effect. Note that there is some enhancement of the meninges lining the posterior surface of the petrous bone

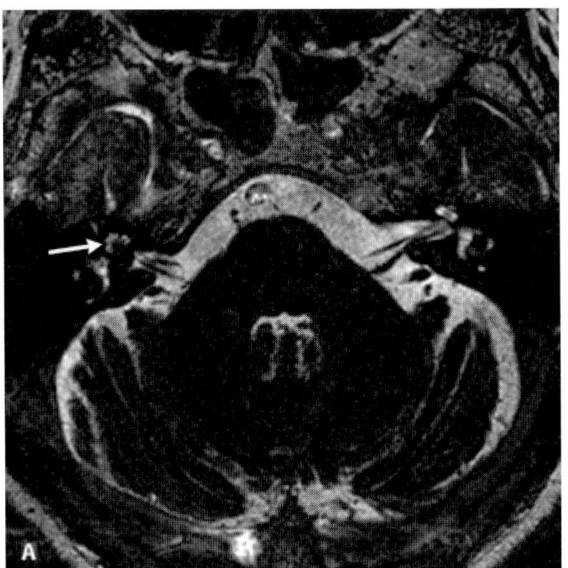

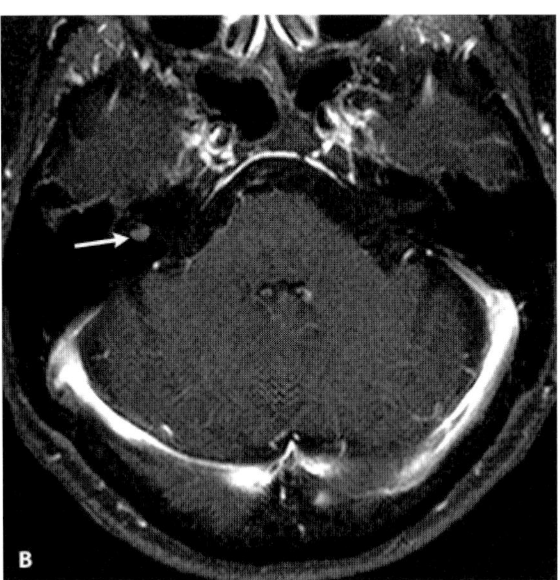

Fig. 4.17A,B. Intracanalicular acoustic schwannoma. **A** Axial CISS T2-WI. **B** Gadolinium-enhanced axial SE T1-WI with fat saturation. On the heavily T2-weighted CISS image, the intracanalicular acoustic schwannoma appears as a 'filling defect', outlined by bright CSF. Enhancement is intense and homogeneous. Fat saturation can be of use to distinguish the enhancing tumor from the bright fatty bone marrow signal of the petrous apex or the walls of the IAC

ple inherited schwannomas, meningiomas, and ependymomas). Cutaneous lesions are less frequent than in neurofibromatosis 1. Symptoms usually develop in the second decade (adolescents and young adults).

Meningioma is the second most common CPA tumor (<10%). Meningiomas show a broad-based dural attachment at the posterior surface of the petrous pyramid. A 'dural-tail' sign is a frequent finding and is an important element in the differential diagnosis with acoustic schwannomas. Meningiomas are eccentric from the internal auditory canal. These tumors may contain (extensive) calcifications, which are difficult to show on MR imaging. After Gd-injection, enhancement can be heterogeneous or homogeneous, depending on the composition of the tumor.

Epidermoid tumor is the third most common CPA tumor. This benign, slow-growing cystic lesion results from an 'inclusion' of epithelium during neural tube closure (3rd to 5th week of gestation). The wall of an epidermoid is composed of a connective tissue capsule (stratified squamous epithelium); the cyst contains desquamative epithelial debris (keratin products) and cholesterol crystals. On MR imaging, SI can be highly variable, but most often the cyst is isointense to CSF. Epidermoids do not enhance; they are avascular in nature. Though the CPA cistern is the site of predilection, epidermoids can also occur in the middle cranial fossa in the parasellar-paracavernous region. Moreover, epidermoids can also be extradural, located within the calvarium, producing well-defined bone erosion.

Other schwannomas include facial nerve schwannoma, trigeminal nerve schwannoma (also known as gasserian ganglion schwannoma), and jugular fossa schwannomas arising from the glossopharyngeal (IX), vagus (X), accessory (XI) nerves. Less common CPA lesions are listed in Table 4.15.

4.5.4 Intra-axial Posterior Fossa Tumors

4.5.4.1 Brainstem

Brainstem gliomas represent 25% of intracranial gliomas in children and young adults compared with only 2.5% of intracranial gliomas in adults. Two distinct histologic subtypes can be discerned:

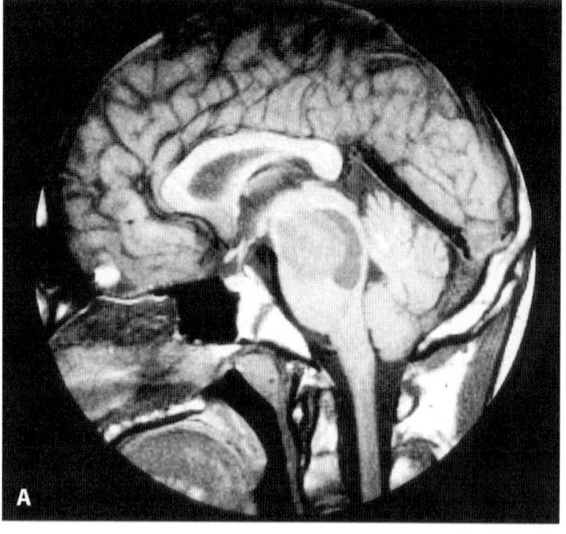

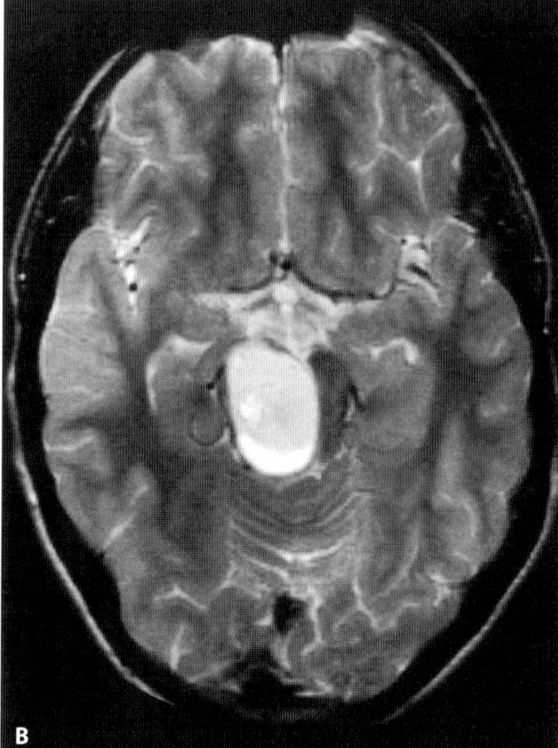

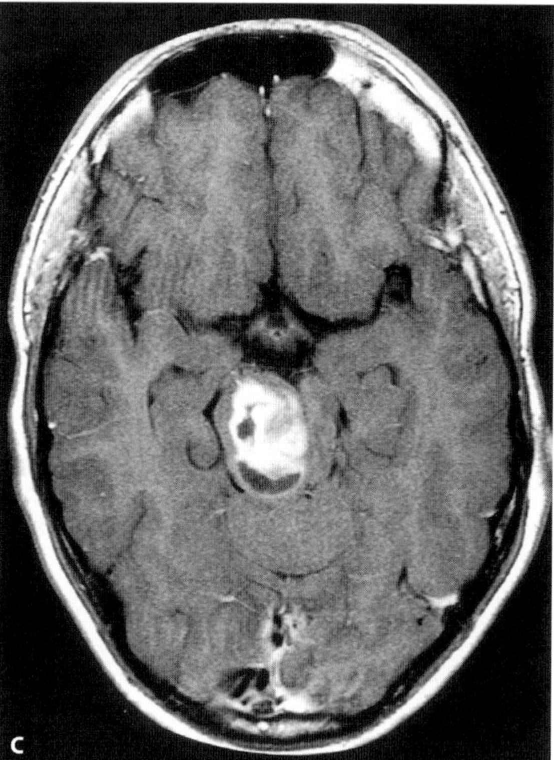

Fig. 4.18A–C. Brainstem glioma. **A** Sagittal SE T1-WI. **B** Axial TSE T2-WI. **C** Gd-enhanced axial SE T1-WI. In this 16-year-old boy with a brainstem glioma, the tumor consists of an anterior solid component and a posterior cystic component. The signal intensity within the cyst is higher that that of CSF, reflecting a higher protein content. Within the solid portion of the tumor, a necrotic area can be discerned. The necrotic portion does not enhance. There is linear enhancement along the walls of the cyst, confirming that this is an intrinsic part of the tumor

- Pilocytic brainstem glioma (exophytic or intrinsic; enhancing; occurs in pons, midbrain or medulla; better prognosis).
- Fibrillary brainstem glioma (intrinsic, diffuse; variable enhancement; poor prognosis with median survival after diagnosis of less than 1 year).

Brainstem gliomas are not resectable. The fourth ventricle is displaced backwards, and its width may be increased (stretching). Patients usually present with cranial nerve symptoms; hydrocephalus is uncommon at the time of initial presentation. The cardinal imaging feature is the characteristic location of the tumor (Fig. 4.18).

Although 90% of cavernous malformations (syn. cavernous angioma, cavernoma, OCVM, CVM) occur supratentorially, they can also occur in the brainstem. Clinical symptoms of brain-stem cavernous malformations include focal motor or sensory changes and are related to the exact location of the lesion. Imaging characteristics are discussed in Sect. 4.7.4.4.

4.5.4.2 Tumors in or around the Fourth Ventricle

Primitive neuroectodermal tumors (PNET) constitute the second most common group of CNS tumors in children (Fig. 16.24). **Medulloblastoma** is the most common representative of this group in the posterior fossa. The peak age range is 5–10 years, with a second, lesser peak between 20 and 30 years. In children, medulloblastoma typically arises in the midline in the posterior vermis (Fig. 16.25). Due to its origin in the roof of the fourth ventricle, obstructive hydrocephalus is common. The presenting symptoms are related to increased intracranial pressure (headache, vomiting). On MRI examinations, these tumors are hypointense on T1-WI and hyperintense on T2-WI. They enhance with Gd-chelates. They have a propensity to leptomeningeal dissemination (metastatic seeding in the subarachnoid space). Therefore, during follow-up examinations, not only the posterior fossa, but the entire neuraxis should be examined. In adults, medulloblastoma typically arises in a cerebellar hemisphere.

Ependymoma represents 10% of childhood brain tumors. There appears to be a bimodal age peak at age 5 years and 34 years. Two-thirds of intracranial ependymomas are located in the infratentorial compartment, especially in children. Ependymomas are often situated in the floor of the fourth ventricle (Fig. 16.27). They have a propensity to extend through the foramina of Magendie or Luschka, and grow into the CPA cistern or cisterna magna. As in medulloblastomas, the presenting symptoms are related to increased intracranial pressure (obstructive hydrocephalus). On noncontrast CT images, calcifications are present in 50% of cases. The MRI appearance of ependymomas is markedly inhomogeneous, due to the presence of calcifications, necrosis, and hemorrhage. Ependymomas are vascular in nature and enhance moderately or intensely with Gd.

Lesions of the choroid plexus can be cysts, papillomas, or carcinomas. Choroid plexus cysts are most often discovered in the lateral ventricles and are infrequent in the fourth ventricle. The MRI appearance is that of a small cystic lesion that is hypointense on T1-WI; there is no enhancement of the cyst contents. The location of choroid plexus papilloma is age-related. In adults, choroid plexus papilloma is found in the fourth ventricle and CPA. In infants, it is found in the trigone of the lateral ventricle. On MRI, choroid plexus papilloma is iso-hypointense on T1-WI and slightly hypointense on T2-WI. The papilloma enhances markedly with Gd. Ventricular dilatation is a frequently associated finding; this can be due to overproduction of CSF by the papilloma, but also to obstruction of CSF pathways by tumor and by repeated episodes of occult hemorrhage.

4.5.4.3 Primary Cerebellar Tumors

Cerebellar astrocytoma is the most common CNS tumor in children and the second most common posterior fossa tumor (PNET is slightly more frequent) (Fig. 16.24); it is much less frequent in adults. Histologically, most cerebellar astrocytomas are low grade and slow growing. They are typically large at diagnosis. Cerebellar astrocytomas arise in the cerebellar hemisphere or vermis. The fourth ventricle is displaced forward and often obliterated; obstructive hydrocephalus is common. The prepontine cistern is narrowed, due to mass effect. Many cerebellar astrocytomas are cystic, often with an enhancing mural nodule (Fig. 4.19). They can be indistinguishable from hemangioblastoma on MR imaging.

A special type of astrocytoma is the **juvenile pilocytic astrocytoma** (Fig. 16.26). It is the most benign histologic subtype of astrocytoma and predominantly

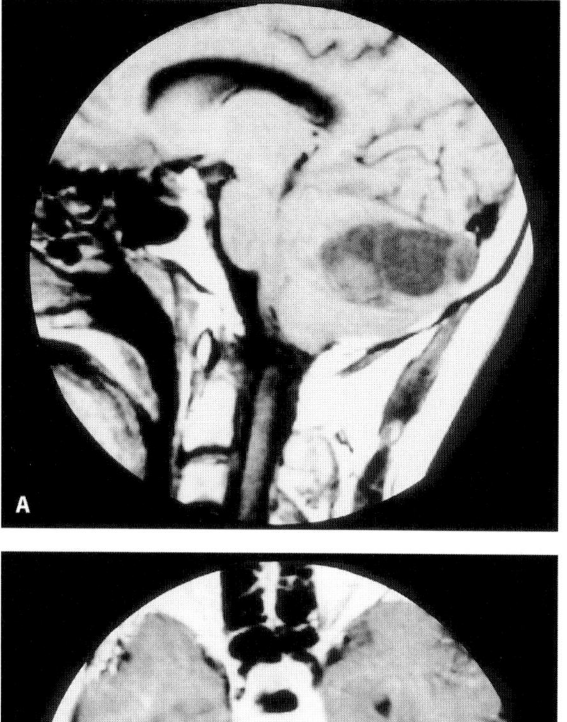

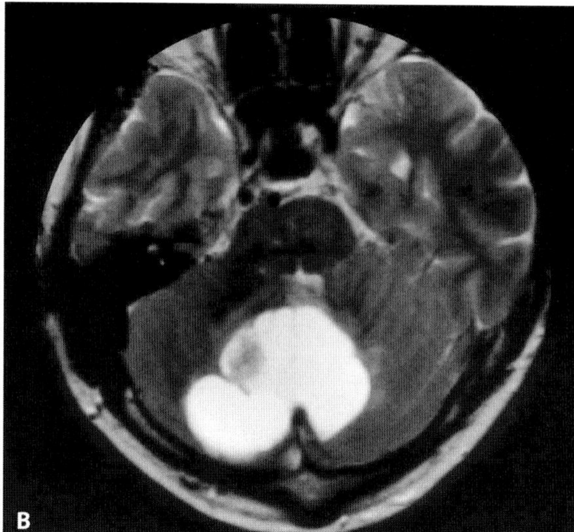

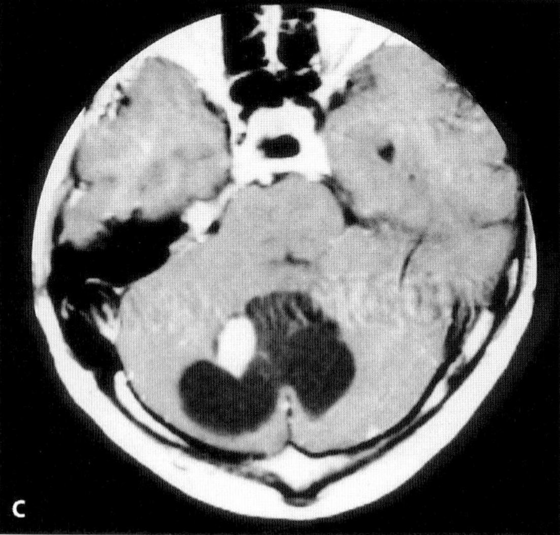

Fig. 4.19A–C. Cystic cerebellar astrocytoma .**A** Sagittal SE T1-WI. **B** Axial TSE T2-WI. **C** Gd-enhanced axial SE T1-WI. There is a cystic-appearing cerebellar mass with a small mural nodule. The fourth ventricle is flattened and displaced anteriorly. The cyst contents are of higher signal intensity than CSF, both on the T1-WI and T2-WI, presumably indicating a higher protein content. After contrast injection, the mural nodule enhances strongly and uniformly. The principal differential diagnosis involves hemangioblastoma, a tumor which can exhibit identical imaging characteristics

affects children and young adults (Table 4.14). The typical appearance on MRI is that of a cyst with an enhancing mural nodule (Table 4.13). The SI of the cyst is higher than CSF on T1-WI and T2-WI due to an increased protein content. However, solid forms are not unusual. On MRI, they are characterized by a heterogeneously increased SI on early Gd-enhanced T1-WI, representing an enhancing matrix; homogeneous enhancement is observed on delayed images.

Hemangioblastoma is the most common primary intra-axial tumor of the adult posterior fossa. It is a benign tumor arising along a pial surface of the cerebellum, brain stem, or spinal cord. The MRI appearance is characterized by a combination of cysts containing proteinaceous fluid and solid mass lesions. A typical appearance is that of a sharply demarcated cyst with an enhancing mural nodule (Table 4.13). Hemangioblastomas can be sporadic or inherited, solitary or multiple (von Hippel-Lindau). Between 4% and 40% of patients with hemangioblastoma match criteria for **von Hippel-Lindau syndrome**. This syndrome is a neurocutaneous disorder. It is defined by the association of two or more CNS hemangioblastomas (cerebellar hemangioblastoma, retinal angiomatosis, spinal cord, cauda equina hemangioblastoma) with multiple visceral organ cysts or neoplasms (kidney, liver, pancreas, epididymis, pheochromocytoma) and a family history of von Hippel-Lindau disease.

4.5.4.4
Secondary Tumors (Metastasis)

Although 85% of metastatic lesions are supratentorial, metastasis is still the most common intra-axial neoplasm of the adult posterior fossa; 15%–20% of all intracranial metastases occur in the posterior fossa. Multiple lesions are the hallmark, but in the posterior fossa there is a high incidence of solitary lesions (25%–50%). Metastases typically are found at gray-white matter interfaces; presumably because tumoral micro-emboli get stuck in the small capillaries. The MR imaging features of metastases have been described in Sect. 4.4.4.3. The MR SI of metastases can be altered by the presence of hemorrhage (methemoglobin, hemosiderin), mucin content (hypointense appearance on T2), melanin (paramagnetic effect), necrosis (high SI on T2-WI, no enhancement in the necrotic areas). Thus the MRI aspect is nonspecific. Abscess, primary glial tumor, and radiation necrosis should be considered in the differential diagnosis. The origin of metastases is in decreasing order of frequency: lung>breast>skin (melanoma)>GIT & GUT. Lung cancer remains the most common source of brain metastases; 50% of lung-tumor patients have CNS metastases. Breast carcinoma is the second most common source of intracranial tumors; 30% of breast carcinomas have associated CNS metastases. Malignant melanoma is the third most common tumor to involve the brain secondarily. Other primary tumors arise from the GIT and GUT.

4.6
Sella Turcica and Hypophysis

4.6.1
Introduction

The pituitary gland consists of two lobes that are physiologically and anatomically distinct: the anterior lobe (adenohypophysis) and the posterior lobe (neurohypophysis). Both are contained within the sella turcica.

The appearance of the pituitary gland depends on the age and the gender of the subject. In neonates (up to 2 months of age), the pituitary gland is normally of high SI on T1-WI. It also appears larger than later in life. In adults, the adenohypophysis is isointense to cerebral white matter, whereas the neurohypophysis is hyperintense on sagittal T1-WI. The higher signal of the posterior lobe is believed to be caused by the presence of neurosecretory granules containing vasopressin. Absent high signal can be associated with diabetes insipidus, but can also occur as a normal finding.

In men, the hypophysis is generally smaller than in women, with a maximum height of 6–8 mm. The pituitary gland decreases in size with aging. In pregnant women, the pituitary gland is spherical or upwardly convex. The anterior pituitary is enlarged, and the height may reach up to 12 mm. It may be hyperintense on precontrast T1-WI. Pituitary lesions associated with pregnancy are lymphocytic adenohypophysitis and Sheehan's syndrome.

4.6.2
MR Imaging Technique

The examination of the sella turcica and hypophysis places high demands on the MRI equipment and sequences. Because of the small volume of the pituitary gland, thin slices must be obtained (2–3 mm). In order to improve in-plane spatial resolution, a small FOV (≤20 cm) and a fine matrix (256 or better) are recommended.

The close proximity of the air-filled sphenoid sinus constitutes an additional difficulty, because susceptibility artifacts may occur. Therefore, SE sequences are preferred; GRE sequences are generally avoided, except when operating at lower field strengths.

A presaturation pulse can be applied to eliminate phase-shift artifacts from the pulsatile flow in the internal carotid arteries. The disadvantage is that the use of a presaturation pulse reduces the number of slices that can be obtained within a given TR interval.

To improve the intrinsically lower SNR in mid- and low-field MRI units, SE sequences with a narrow bandwidth are often used. These sequences have a longer minimal TE value, and therefore, the number of slices (coverage) is lower. However, this is not a problem in pituitary imaging, since only a limited number of slices are needed to cover the area of interest. Another disadvantage is that sequences with narrow bandwidth increase chemical-shift artifacts. This may cause the fatty marrow of the dorsum sellae to overlap the high signal of the posterior pituitary on sagittal T1-WI; this artifact can be avoided by setting the read-out gradient in the anteroposterior direction, so that fat is shifted posteriorly. Similarly, on coronal images, the read-out gradient should be adjusted so that the fatty marrow of the sellar floor is shifted inferiorly. This technique ensures adequate visualization of the inferior part of the pituitary gland. Our standard imaging protocol is given in Table 4.16.

Following i.v. injection of Gd contrast agents, there is an immediate and intense enhancement of the pituitary stalk, adenohypophysis, and cavernous sinus. Enhancement is maximal after 1–3 min. The dynamic process of progressive enhancement of the pituitary gland can be visualized by using sequential T1-WI. In most institutions, dynamic imaging in the coronal plane has become part of the standard imaging protocol for pituitary adenoma. It is generally performed with a TSE T1-sequence, which is repeated every 20–30 s. Key-hole TSE sequences have been advocated for this purpose. Ideally, multiple locations should be imaged to completely cover the anterior pituitary lobe. GRE sequences are to be avoided because of the magnetic susceptibility artifacts caused by the air-containing sphenoid sinus.

Literature data suggest that for dynamic post-contrast pituitary imaging, a half dose of Gd may be sufficient (0.05 mmol/kg body weight). Moreover, a half dose of Gd improves contrast between the pituitary gland and the cavernous sinuses. However, when performing MR imaging of the pituitary at lower field strengths, we recommend a standard dose of Gd (0.1 mmol/kg body weight), because the T1-shortening effect of Gd is less pronounced.

For the post-contrast images, magnetization transfer should not be switched on, because it further reduces the SNR of the thin-section, small-FOV images.

The protocol, as suggested in Table 4.16, should be adapted to the clinical demand. In children with growth-hormone-deficient dwarfism, the imaging protocol can be limited to precontrast sagittal and coronal SE T1-W sequences, which show an ectopic posterior pituitary lobe and absence of the stalk (Fig. 4.20). In patients with central diabetes insipidus, the precontrast T1-WI demonstrate an absence of the posterior pituitary lobe high signal.

Table 4.16. Protocol for MR imaging of the pituitary gland. For pituitary gland imaging, high spatial resolution is required. This implies use of a small FOV (≤200 mm) with a 256 matrix. Alternatively, when a 512 matrix is used, the FOV can be somewhat larger. The key issue is pixel size. For the dynamic sequence, the FOV may need to be incrcased some what, to improve SNR. A limited number of slices is sufficient for a non-enlarged pituitary gland. In cases of pituitary macroadenoma, more slices should be obtaincd to cover the tumor. Slice thickness for the dynamic study may need to be increased to cover the whole mass. For the dynamic TSE coronal T1-W images, a high ETL increases the speed of the sequence, but also increases T2-W of the image, which is an unwanted effect. Therefore, a balance must be found between a short acquisition time (which requires a high ETL) and sufficiently T1-W images (which requires a shorter ETL).

Pulse sequence	WI	Plane	No. of sections	TR (ms)	TE (ms)	TI (ms)	Flip angle	Echo train length	Section thickness (mm)	Matrix	FOV	recFOV	No. of acq.
1. Coronal T1-images													
SE	T1	cor	9–15	400–600	10–30	–	90/180	–	2–3	256	≤200	75	2–4
2. Sagittal T1-W images													
SE	T1	sag	9–15	400–600	10–30	–	90/180	–	2–3	256	≤200	100	2–4
3. Coronal T2-W images													
TSE	T2	cor	9–15	3000–5000	90–120	–	90/180	7–15	2–3	256	≤200	75	1–2
Intravenous contrast injection (half dose)													
4. Dynamic coronal T1-W images (when technically feasible)													
TSE	T1	cor	variable	400–600	min TE	–	90/180	3–8	2–4	256	≤250	75	1
4′. Coronal T1-W images													
SE	T1	cor	9–15	400–600	10–30	–	90/180	–	2–3	256	≤200	75	2–4

Abbreviations: *WI* weighted image; *TR* repetition time (ms); *TI* inversion time (ms); *TE* echo time (ms) *TD* time delay (sec); *no part* number of partitions: *Matrix* (phase × frequency matrix); *FOV* field of view (mm); *recFOV* % rectangular field of view

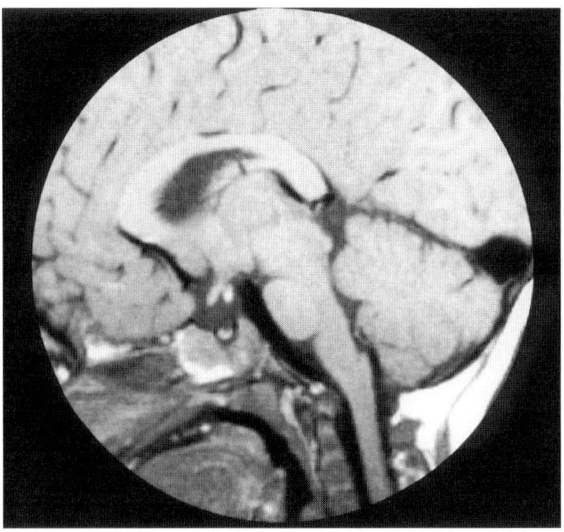

Fig. 4.20. Growth-hormone-deficient dwarfism. In this 3-year-old child with growth-hormone-deficient dwarfism, the sagittal SE T1-WI shows the ectopic posterior pituitary lobe as a focal area of high signal intensity at the proximal infundibulum. The pituitary stalk is absent. This example illustrates that pre-contrast sagittal SE T1-WI constitute an important part of the examination, especially in children and patients with diabetes insipidus

4.6.3 Pituitary Adenoma

Pituitary adenomas are benign, slow-growing neoplasms arising from the adenohypophysis. They represent 10%–15% of all intracranial neoplasms and are the most frequent indication for pituitary MR imaging. On the basis of histology, pituitary adenomas are subdivided into chromophobe (80%), acidophilic or eosinophilic (15%), and basophilic (5%) types. Alternatively, pituitary adenomas can be classified into functioning (prolactinoma, corticotrophic, somatotrophic adenoma) or nonfunctioning lesions. An 'incidentaloma' is defined as a nonfunctioning pituitary adenoma or pituitary cyst. However, there are no imaging features to distinguish between different types of adenomas. For medical imaging purposes, the most useful classification is to categorize pituitary adenomas by size into microadenoma (≤10 mm) or macroadenoma (>10 mm).

Microadenomas are by definition no larger than 10 mm in diameter. In many cases, MR imaging provides direct visualization of the adenoma. Typically, on precontrast or (early) postcontrast scans, the adenoma is seen as a small lesion of low SI relative to the normally enhancing pituitary gland (Fig. 4.21). This is due to

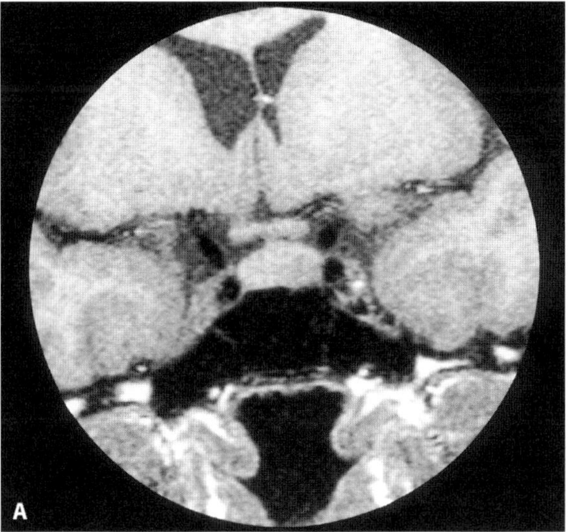

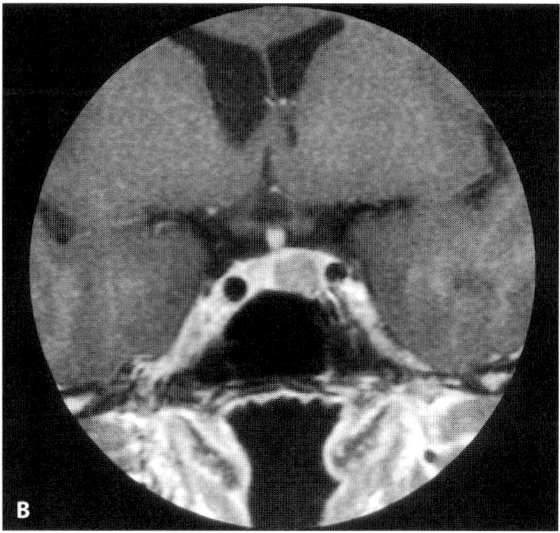

Fig. 4.21A,B. Pituitary microadenoma. **A** Coronal SE T1-WI. **B** Coronal Gd-enhanced SE T1-WI. This 38-year-old woman had elevated serum prolactin levels. The precontrast image shows an asymmetry between the right and left pituitary lobes. On the postcontrast image, the adenoma in the left pituitary lobe is outlined by the normally enhancing pituitary tissue. Thin slices with high spatial resolution are required

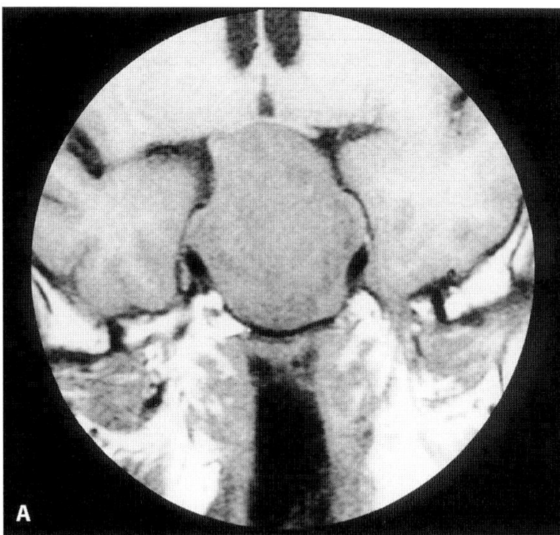

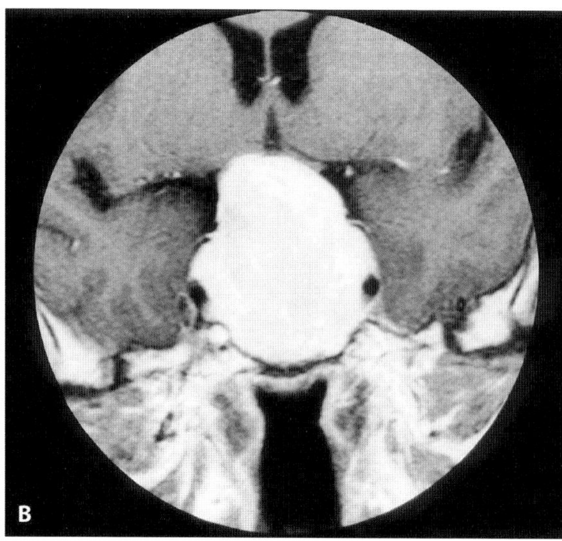

Fig. 4.22A,B. Pituitary macroadenoma. **A** Coronal SE T1-WI. **B** Coronal Gd-enhanced SE T1-WI. This 45-year-old woman presented with progressive visual loss. The images show a typical pituitary macroadenoma. Note the upward displacement of the optic chiasm, which is draped over the top of the tumor. After Gd, the tumor enhances strongly but inhomogeneously

the greater relative enhancement of normal pituitary tissue versus adenoma. Adenomas display a later peak of enhancement, with slower washout. This implies that early postcontrast scans are required for lesion identification. On later postcontrast T1-WI, the adenoma may become isointense to normal pituitary tissue and may even become slightly hyperintense. Indirect signs of the presence of a pituitary adenoma include: focal depression or erosion of the sellar floor, displacement of the pituitary stalk, asymmetrical, focal upward convexity of the hypophysis, and invasion of the cavernous sinus.

By definition, **macroadenomas** are 10 mm or greater in size. Frequently, macroadenomas are nonsecretory. Clinical symptoms are caused by pressure on adjacent structures, especially the optic chiasm (Fig. 4.22). This may lead to visual loss, most commonly bitemporal hemianopia. Compression of normal pituitary tissue may lead to hypopituitarism. The MRI technique is essentially the same, although more (or thicker) slices should be obtained to cover the tumor completely. On T1-WI and T2-WI, macroadenomas are usually isointense to brain tissue. They enhance with contrast; intratumoral cysts or areas of necrosis do not enhance and are hypointense on T1-WI and hyperintense on T2-WI. The use of Gd improves delineation of the mass, especially from the cavernous sinus. Many macroadenomas display enlargement and erosion of the sella, as well as extension into the suprasellar cistern, cavernous sinus, sphenoid sinus, and even the nasopharynx. On sagittal and coronal images, macroadenomas often display a dumbbell configuration, the 'waistline' being caused by a constriction of the diaphragma sellae. Cavernous sinus invasion is common but difficult to ascertain on MR imaging. The most reliable sign is encasement of the internal carotid artery. The differential diagnosis includes suprasellar meningioma, pituitary metastasis, and craniopharyngioma. MR imaging allows reliable differentiation from an aneurysm.

The appearance of a pituitary adenoma changes after treatment. Imaging findings after medical treatment (bromocriptine, cabergoline) include a decrease in the size of the adenoma, hemorrhage, and low SI on T2-WI. After transsphenoidal surgery, the following can be observed: a defect in the anterior floor of the sella, fat and/or muscle plug, secondary empty sella, and herniation of the optic chiasm. After surgery via craniotomy, the FOV should be enlarged to study potential brain damage along the surgical approach route.

4.6.4 Other Intra-, Supra-, and Parasellar Lesions

Empty sella is defined as an extension of the subarachnoid space into the sella turcica. Primary empty sella can be due to a defect in the diaphragma sellae, involution of a pituitary tumor, or regression of the pituitary gland after pregnancy. Secondary empty sella is postsurgical in origin, presumably secondary to disruption of the diaphragma sellae. MR imaging shows an enlarged sella turcica, filled with CSF. The position of the optic chiasm should be noted; visual symptoms may occur if there is downward herniation of the optic chiasm.

Empty sella should be differentiated from a **suprasellar arachnoid cyst**, which is developmental in origin, due to an imperforate membrane of Lillequist. On MR imaging, a suprasellar arachnoid cyst appears as a well-marginated, homogeneous lesion, which is isointense to CSF on all pulse sequences. In the differential diagnosis, epidermoid and craniopharyngioma should be considered.

Enlargement of the pituitary stalk, best seen on coronal and sagittal postcontrast T1-WI, is a nonspecific finding. The differential diagnosis includes: histiocytosis X, leptomeningeal carcinomatosis, metastasis, and granulomatous disorders (sarcoidosis, giant cell granuloma, tuberculosis, syphilis).

Craniopharyngiomas are slowly growing, benign tumors arising from epithelial remnants of Rathke's pouch. They represent 3%–4% of all intracranial neoplasms and are the most common suprasellar mass lesions; 70% are both intra- and suprasellar, whereas 20% are entirely suprasellar. The age distribution is bimodal: the adamantinomatous type is encountered in children (first and second decades), whereas the papillary type occurs in adults (fourth and fifth decades). The pediatric craniopharyngioma (adamantinomatous type) is the most frequently occurring form. It typically contains cystic and solid components, and calcifications are frequent. It often invades the adjacent brain, leading to dense gliosis. Recurrence after surgery is common. The adult variety (papillary craniopharyngioma) is generally solid and often extends into the third ventricle.

Clinical symptoms are related to compression of the optic chiasm (bitemporal hemianopsia), hypothalamus, and pituitary gland (hypopituitarism, diabetes insipidus, growth failure in children). Headaches may be secondary to hydrocephalus and increased intracranial pressure.

MRI typically shows a heterogeneous tumor with cystic and solid components. The cysts display variable SI on T1-WI, depending on their contents (cholesterol, protein, hemorrhage). Most frequently, the cysts are of higher SI than CSF on both T1-WI and T2-WI (Fig. 16.30). The solid components and the rim of cysts display enhancement with Gd. This is helpful in defining the extent of the lesion. Though essentially benign in nature, craniopharyngiomas have a tendency to recur after surgery, and Gd is useful in defining recurrent or residual tumor in the postoperative patient.

Calcifications, which occur in up to 80% of craniopharyngiomas in children (30%–40% in adults) and which are the hallmark of the lesion on plain skull films and CT, are difficult to detect on MR images. In theory, it would be useful to add a spoiled GRE sequence [fast low-angle shot sequence (FLASH), spoiled gradient recalled acquisition into steady state (GRASS), fast-field echo sequence (FFE)] to the imaging protocol, to detect susceptibility effects from calcifications. Unfortunately, this sequence also brings out susceptibility artifacts due to air in the sphenoid sinus and, therefore, is of limited use.

Meningiomas occur in the suprasellar and parasellar region (sphenoid wing and cavernous sinus meningioma). They are usually slow growing but may compress vital structures. Meningiomas are isointense relative to gray matter on T1-WI. On precontrast T1-WI, the sole clue to the diagnosis may be the presence of a dural or CSF cleft. Therefore, post-Gd images should always be obtained: meningiomas enhance intensely and homogeneously with Gd. A dural-tail sign is frequent: extension along the anterior margin/floor of the middle cranial fossa or along the tentorium.

Optochiasmatic and hypothalamic gliomas are discussed together because the point of origin is often undeterminable. They account for 10%–15% of all supratentorial tumors in childhood, with 75% occurring in the first decade (peak age 2–4 years). Histologically, most optochiasmatic-hypothalamic astrocytomas are of the pilocytic type. There is an association with neurofibromatosis type 1. Symptoms include vision loss, diencephalic syndrome, obesity, sexual precocity, and diabetes insipidus. MRI shows a suprasellar, lobulated mass with intense, inhomogeneous contrast enhancement. Hydrocephalus is common, due to obstruction of the foramen of Monro by large tumors.

Germinoma is a highly malignant tumor with a predilection for the suprasellar and pineal region. If, in a child, an enhancing suprasellar lesion is discovered in conjunction with a pineal tumor, germinoma should be the primary diagnosis (Fig. 16.29). Germinoma is histologically similar to seminoma and is characterized by a rapid clinical evolution. It is also called 'ectopic pinealoma'. Germinoma enhances strongly with Gd, due to its highly vascular nature. CSF spread is common, and therefore, the entire neuraxis should be examined for staging and follow-up.

Tuber cinereum hamartoma is not a true neoplasm. It can be sessile or pedunculated and is attached to the hypothalamus between the pituitary stalk and the mammillary bodies. It typically causes precocious puberty. On MR imaging, the hamartoma is isointense to gray matter on all pulse sequences (Fig. 16.31). It does not enhance, because it contains an intact BBB.

An **aneurysm** of the cavernous segment of ICA (extradural portion) must not be missed. Cavernous sinus aneurysm may cause progressive visual impairment and cavernous sinus syndrome (trigeminal nerve pain and oculomotor nerve paralysis). MRI is helpful in showing flow artifacts along the phase-encoding direction. The aneurysm is often of mixed SI and contains different stages of hemorrhage, thrombus, and calcifications.

An infrequent parasellar tumor is **trigeminal schwannoma**, arising from the Gasserian ganglion, in Meckel's cave. It is located in the middle cranial fossa, posterior cranial fossa, or both. On MR imaging, a dumbbell- or saddle-shaped mass of variable SI is seen. Enhancement is inhomogeneous due to necrosis and cyst formation in large tumors. The tumor may erode the petrous tip. Thin slices should be obtained to look for enlargement of contiguous fissures, foramina, canals (extension into the infratemporal fossa through an enlarged oval foramen).

4.7 Cerebrovascular Disease

4.7.1 Stroke

The term stroke refers to a sudden or rapid onset of a neurologic deficit (in a vascular territory) due to a cerebrovascular disease lasting longer than 24 h. If the neurologic deficit lasts for less than 24 h, the term transient ischemic attack (TIA) is used. Two major types of stroke can be discerned: ischemic and hemorrhagic stroke (Table 4.18). In this section, we shall focus on the role of MRI in ischemic stroke. Hemorrhage is covered in Chapter 3 and shall not be discussed here.

The arrival of promising new aggressive therapies aimed at re-establishing the blood flow, reducing the size of the infarction, and protecting the surrounding brain at risk (penumbra) has changed the traditional role of neuroimaging. MR imaging plays a crucial role in the diagnosis, clinical management, and treatment monitoring of stroke. The narrow time window for thrombolytic therapy (up to 6 h after the onset of symptoms) necessitates a rapid and accurate diagnosis. In the patient with acute stroke, the MR imaging protocol should be able to:

- Rule out intracranial hemorrhage. Traditionally, CT has been the gold standard for detecting intracranial blood, but there is growing evidence that MR imaging with susceptibility imaging (e.g., gradient-echo T2* sequence) may be equally valid, for example in ruling out hemorrhagic infarction. FLAIR sequences have been shown to be highly sensitive and specific for the detection of acute subarachnoid and intraventricular blood. The role of FLAIR as compared to CT and gradient-echo T2* sequences has yet to be established.
- Show parenchymal injury. Diffusion-weighted imaging (DWI) can reveal regions of acute cerebral infarction within minutes after onset of symptoms.
- Provide information on tissue blood flow. This is by perfusion-weighted imaging (PWI) can show areas of brain with decreased perfusion
- Indicate areas of potentially salvageable brain tissue. If the PWI deficit is larger than the DWI abnormality (diffusion-perfusion mismatch), there is still brain tissue to be saved.
- Assess vessel patency. MR angiography can reveal vessel occlusion, narrowing, or intracranial stenoses.

4.7.1.1 Large Vessels

The imaging manifestations of cerebral infarction caused by large vessel occlusion vary with time. We can consider four stages: hyperacute (0–6 h after symptom onset), acute (first 4 days), subacute (between 4 days and 8 weeks), and chronic (after 8 weeks).

Table 4.17. Protocol for MR imaging of acute stroke. The SE-EPI and FID-EPI sequences are critically motion sensitive; therefore the patient should be instructed to keep perfectly still. It is important to immobilize the patient's head as much as possible. Scan time for these sequences is <30 s. The sequence parameters are highly dependent on the equipment used. The contrast medium should be injected as a very short bolus, about 10 s after the start of the FID-EPI sequence. An MR-compatible power injector is useful. When evaluating for hemorrhagic stroke, add a partial flip angle spoiled GRE sequence, because of its increased sensitivity in detecting susceptibility artifacts. To evaluate for internal carotid artery dissection, add an axial SE T1-W sequence which includes the upper neck and the skull base.

Pulse sequence	WI	Plane	No. of sections	TR (ms)	TE (ms)	TI (ms)	Flip angle	Echo train length	Section thickness (mm)	Matrix	FOV	recFOV	No. of acq.
1. Axial SE-EPI diffusion-W sequence													
SE-EPI	diffusion	ax	12–15	∞	100–140	–	90/180	–	5	128	230–300	75	1
2. Axial T2-W turbo FLAIR sequence													
Turbo FLAIR	T2	ax	19	6000–10000	100–150	1800–2200	180	7–11	5	512	230–240	75	2–4
3. MRA 3D-TOF through circle of Willis													
GRE 3D-TOF	MRA	ax	64 (1 slab)	40	5–25	–	15–25	–	35–100	512	≤230	75	1–2
4. Axial T2-W sequence (single echo)													
TSE	T2	ax	19–25	3000–6000	90–130	–	90/180	7–15	5	512	230–240	75	1–2
5. FID-EPI perfusion with bolus injection of contrast (10 seconds after the start of the scan)													
TSE	T1	ax	12–15	∞	60–80	–	–	–	5	128	230–300	75	1

Abbreviations: *WI* weighted image, *TR* repetition time (ms); *TI* inversion time (ms), *TE* echo time (ms); *TD* time delay (sec); *no part* number of partitions, *Matrix* (phase × frequency matrix); *FOV* field of view (mm); *recFOV* % rectangular field of view

Table 4.18. Classification of stroke types

1. Ischemic stroke
   - 1.1. Thrombotic stroke
     - 1.1.1. Internal carotid artery disease
     - 1.1.2. Vertebrobasilar disease
     - 1.1.3. Lacunar infarcts
   - 1.2. Embolic stroke (from cardiac or arterial source)
     - 1.2.1. Middle cerebral artery and branches
     - 1.2.2. Anterior cerebral artery
     - 1.2.3. Posterior cerebral artery
     - 1.2.4. Vertebrobasilar distribution
   - 1.3. Hypercoagulable states (including veno-occlusive disease)
     - 1.3.1. Primary (e.g., protein S/protein C deficiency, antithrombin III deficiency)
     - 1.3.2. Secondary (e.g., antiphospholipid antibody syndrome, paraneoplastic)
2. Hemorrhagic stroke
   - 2.1. Intracerebral hemorrhage (e.g., due to hypertension or amyloid angiopathy)
   - 2.2. Subarachnoid hemorrhage
     - 2.2.1. Aneurysm rupture
     - 2.2.2. Arteriovenous malformation

4.7.1.1.1 Hyperacute and Acute Infarction

The pathophysiological changes induced by acute stroke should be understood to interpret the MRI findings. Global cerebral blood flow (CBF) is approximately 60 ml/100 g/min; the blood flow is higher in gray matter than in white matter. A mild decrease in CBF interferes with protein synthesis. A moderate decrease in CBF causes glycolysis, with lactate accumulation and acidosis. When CBF decreases below 20–25 ml/100 g/min, the cellular energy supply starts to fail (ATP is depleted), causing neurological dysfunction. A further decrease of CBF below 10–15 ml/100 g/min impairs active membrane transport. Failure of the ATP-dependent sodium-potassium pump causes an irreversible ion flux across the cell membrane and results in cytotoxic edema (starting minutes after the onset of ischemia). The process of cytotoxic edema ultimately leads to cell death. **Vasogenic edema** occurs 4–6 h after the onset of ischemia and is caused by injury to endothelial cells, disruption of the capillary tight junctions, with breakdown of the BBB. This results in an accumulation of plasma proteins and water in the extracellular space from the intravascular space. Vasogenic edema usually peaks around 3–4 days after the onset of infarction.

Conventional MRI techniques are of limited use in demonstrating hyperacute stroke (<12 h). Two newer MRI techniques – diffusion-weighted MR imaging and perfusion MR imaging – have shown great promise.

Diffusion-weighted imaging (DWI) is an echo-planar imaging (EPI)-based technique that measures the random motion of water molecules (i.e., diffusion) in biological tissues during the application of strong magnetic field gradients. The sensitivity to diffusion is expressed by the '*b* value' of the sequence (in s/mm²).

$$b = \gamma^2 G^2 \delta^2 \left(\Delta - \frac{\delta}{3}\right)$$

g: gyromagnetic constant
G: amplitude of the diffusion gradients
δ: time during which the diffusion gradients are switched on
Δ: time interval between the 2 diffusion gradients

The higher the *b* value, the more dephasing occurs, and the more heavily the signal reflects areas of restricted diffusion. In clinical practice, *b* values around 1000 s/mm² are most commonly used.

The symmetric diffusion gradients are applied in (at least) 3 orthogonal directions. These images can be combined in a so-called 'trace' image, which represents the geometric mean of the individual images. In clinical practice, we obtain 3 images per anatomic slice position (Fig. 4.23):

- *b*=0 image. This is merely a heavily T2-weighted EPI image, with the diffusion gradients switched off.
- *b*=1000 'trace' image. Trace images are the geometric mean of the individual DWI with gradients applied to the slice, read, and phase directions. In regions of acute cerebral infarction (cytotoxic edema), diffusion of water is restricted, causing the lesion to appear bright on DWI.
- apparent diffusion coefficient (ADC) maps. ADC maps are parametric images in which each pixel reflects the 'apparent diffusion coefficient' at that location. Tissues in which water mobility is restricted appear dark on ADC maps (the ADC is lower in the infarcted lesion).

In the case of a complete vessel occlusion, DWI can depict the lesion within minutes, due to the rapid onset of cytotoxic edema. The DWI lesion volume progressively increases up to day 3 or 4; this presumably reflects penumbral tissue infarction, as well as increasing edema. After the 1st week, the volume of the DWI abnormality starts to decrease to a level approaching the T2-defined lesion on day 30. This is explained by the fact that, as cells die, cell membranes and other microstructures restricting diffusion disappear.

Perfusion-weighted imaging (PWI) can be performed using two basic approaches. In arterial spin labeling (ASL), hydrogen protons are labeled outside the head, and the flow of this *endogenous* contrast agent (i.e., tagged spins) through the brain is observed. This technique is not widely used in clinical practice, because it suffers from poor SNR and necessitates long imaging times; it shall not be discussed further. The currently more widespread approach uses injection of an *exogenous* contrast agent (Gd-based chelate) to act as a T2* contrast agent during its first pass through the cerebral vasculature. The contrast agent causes a transient decrease in signal intensity (T2*-shortening susceptibility effect), proportional to the concentration in a given region (Fig. 4.24). The technique is known as dynamic susceptibility contrast (DSC) imaging. Using a rapid imaging sequence (typically EPI), as many as 50 sequential images can be obtained during bolus injection of contrast, covering a time interval of roughly 70 s. Bolus injection of contrast is performed 5–10 s after the start of the imaging sequence, to ensure that an adequate number of baseline images are obtained. We inject a contrast volume of 0.2 mmol/kg body weight (i.e., 30 ml for a 75 kg person) at an injection rate of 5 ml/s (antecubital vein, 18-gauge i.v. catheter). This is followed by injection of 20–30 ml of saline, to flush the gadolinium out of the tubing, arm vein, and lung vasculature. When available, a power injector should be used, although with some experience, adequate results can also be obtained with hand injection (two syringes, containing contrast and saline flush, connected to a bifurcated 'y' check valve system). Sequential images are acquired simultaneously in multiple slice positions. The EPI sequence that we currently use performs 50 chronological images in 12 slice positions, yielding to a total dataset of 600 images. If more slice positions should be required, this would necessitate a longer TR, and this would negatively influence the quality of the sequence.

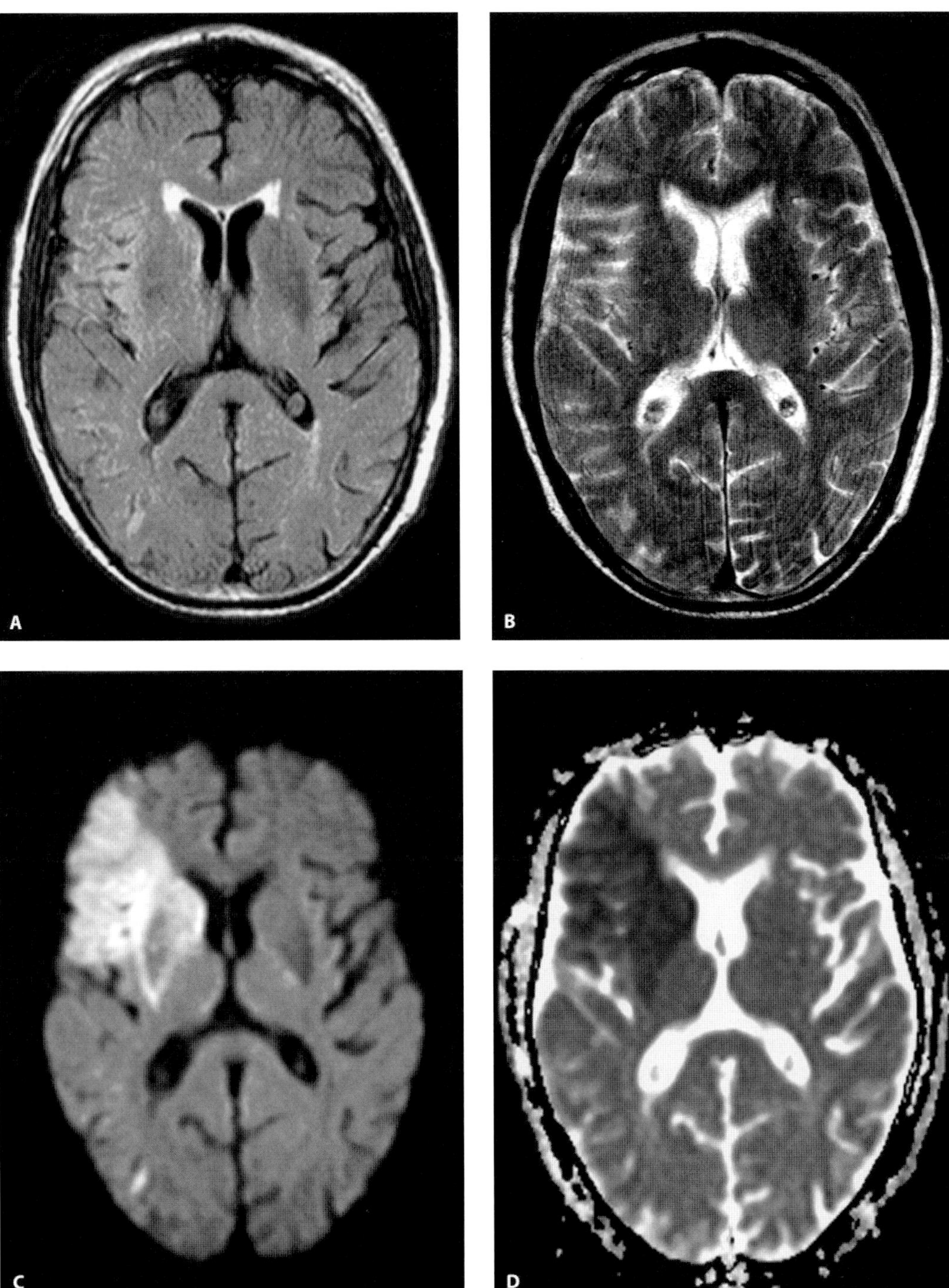

Fig. 4.23 A–D. Diffusion-weighted MR imaging in hyperacute infarction. The patient is a 71-year old man examined within 2 hours after acute onset of left hemiplegia and left facial nerve paralysis. **A** Axial turbo FLAIR image. **B** Axial TSE T2-WI. **C** Axial diffusion-weighted image (DWI), trace image. **D** Axial apparent diffusion coefficient map (ADC). The axial FLAIR and TSE T2-WI are within normal limits. Image quality is somewhat degraded by motion artifacts. The DWI shows a focal area of bright signal intensity in the right operculofrontal and sylvian region. On the ADC map, the area of restricted diffusion is confirmed as a hypointense lesion (decreased ADC). Signal abnormalities in the DWI and ADC maps indicate cytotoxic edema. The findings are consistent with hyperacute infarction of the right middle cerebral artery

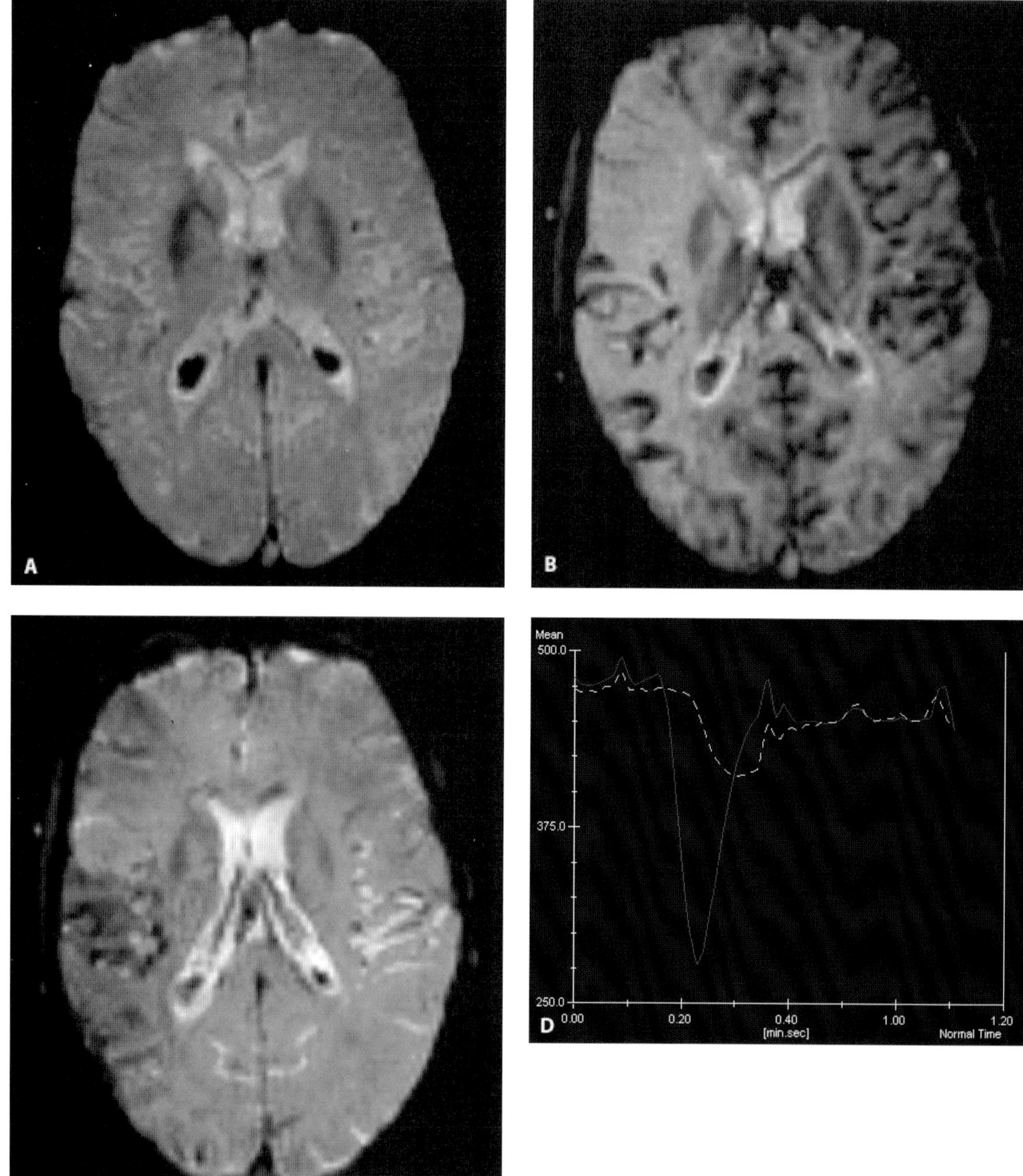

Fig. 4.24A–D. Technique of perfusion-weighted imaging in a patient with hyperacute right middle cerebral artery stroke (same patient as Fig. 4.23). Fast EPI images are obtained during rapid intravenous injection of a contrast bolus (5 ml/sec, antecubital vein, 18-gauge IV catheter). **A** Baseline image before arrival of the bolus. **B** Image during first pass of the contrast bolus. **C** Image after passage of the bolus. **D** Time-intensity plot, covering 70 seconds. The first pass of the contrast agent through the cerebral vasculature causes a rapid and sharp decrease in signal intensity (*large arrow*), which is due to a T2-shortening susceptibility effect. Specific regions-of-interest can be placed on the image to assess local differences in the bolus arrival time

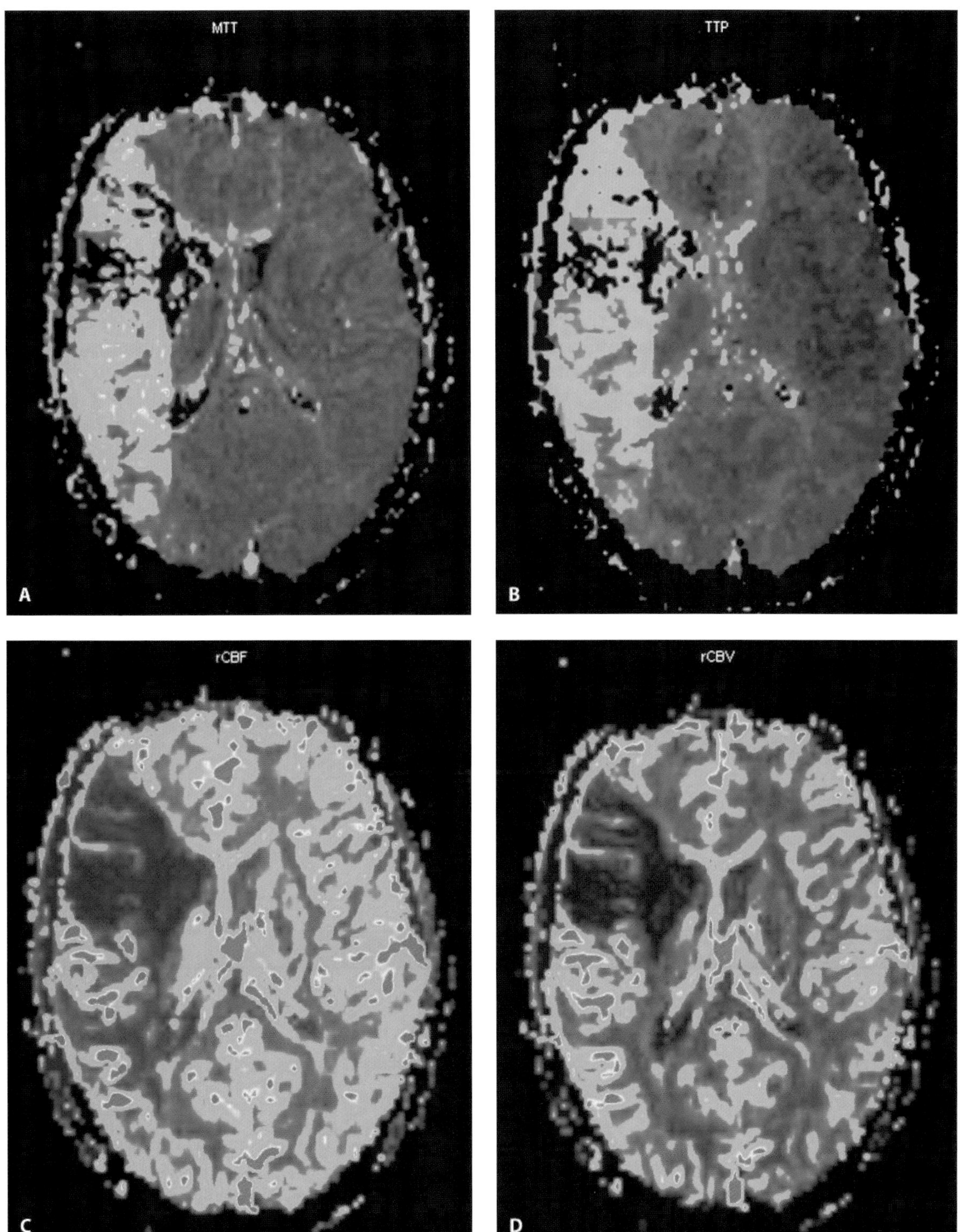

Fig. 4.25A–D. Parametric maps generated by perfusion-weighted imaging (PWI) in a patient with hyperacute right middle cerebral artery stroke (same patient as Fig. 4.23 and 4.24). **A** Mean transit time (MTT) map. **B** Time to peak (TTP) map. **C** Regional cerebral blood flow (rCBF) map. **D** Regional cerebral blood volume (rCBV) map. The hypoperfused area corresponds to the distribution territory of the right middle cerebral artery. The perfusion deficit is much larger than the diffusion abnormality (compare with Fig. 4.23 C and D). This represents a diffusion-perfusion mismatch, and indicates potentially salvageable brain tissue (see text)

These images must then be processed in parameter maps such as Fig. 4.25:

- Time to peak (TTP)
- Percentage of baseline (PBL)
- Mean transit time (MTT)
- Cerebral blood volume (CBV)
- Cerebral blood flow (CBF), which can be calculated using the formula: CBF = CBV/MTT

Perfusion MR imaging is used widely in the setting of (hyper)acute (and subacute) stroke.

■ **DWI/PWI Mismatch.** In patients with (hyper)acute stroke, the volume of ischemic tissue documented by PWI is often greater than the region of parenchymal injury shown by DWI. In this patient population, intravenous thrombolysis with recombinant tissue plasminogen activator (r-TPA) is of proven benefit within 3 h of symptom onset, and intraarterial thrombolytic therapy shows promise within a 6-h window of therapeutic opportunity. The DWI/PWI mismatch has been considered as a possible correlate of the ischemic penumbra (i.e., tissue at greatest risk for infarct progression). The DWI abnormality reflects the area of brain tissue that is irretrievably lost (cytotoxic edema with cell death). The penumbra region indicates an area of decreased CBF, but the threshold for irreversible cell death has not yet been reached. Table 4.19 provides an overview of the theoretical possibilities and clinical implications of comparing PWI and DWI abnormalities.

Even without the use of such advanced techniques as diffusion and perfusion imaging, MRI is more sensitive than CT in the detection of acute stroke. Within the first 24 h, the infarct is visible on standard SE or TSE sequences in 82% compared with 58% with CT. However, in the hyperacute and acute stages of a stroke, the FLAIR sequence is the most sensitive 'conventional' imaging sequence. Early findings on FLAIR images include:

- Hyperintense vessel sign. Arterial hyperintensity, most commonly observed in the middle cerebral artery, may reflect slowly moving or stationary blood or intraluminal thrombus. The presence of the hyperintense vessel sign, together with abnormal findings on DWI, should prompt consideration of revascularization and flow augmentation strategies.
- Hyperintense swollen cortical gyri. These gyriform areas of increased signal intensity on FLAIR images indicate cytotoxic edema of brain parenchyma, which occurs more rapidly in gray matter than in white matter, due to its higher metabolic activity.
- Hyperintense intracranial hemorrhage. FLAIR images are also useful in detecting hyperacute hemorrhagic lesions, including subarachnoid and intraventricular hemorrhage.

Additional early MRI findings include:

- Absence of normal signal void. MRI can detect the alteration in blood flow during acute ischemia immediately. High velocity blood flow is normally seen on MR imaging as an absence of signal. Absence of flow void indicates a significant compromise of arterial blood flow.

Table 4.19. Clinical implications of comparing perfusion-weighted imaging (PWI) and diffusion-weighted imaging (DWI) abnormalities

PWI and DWI findings	Clinical implication
Normal PWI and normal DWI	No stroke
Normal PWI and abnormal DWI	Early reperfusion (the DWI abnormality indicates some cytotoxic edema, but vessel patency has been restored, and PWI is normal)
Abnormal PWI and normal DWI	This situation can be found in chronic vessel stenosis. Alternatively, this could reflect a false-negative DWI.
Abnormal DWI = abnormal PWI	Constituted stroke. The nonperfused brain has evolved to infarction with cytotoxic edema. The involved brain tissue is irretrievably lost, and there is no indication for thrombolysis.
Abnormal PWI > abnormal DWI	Mismatch. The DWI abnormality (core infarct) is surrounds the PWI deficit, reflecting the penumbra. In this case, there is a potential role for thrombolytic therapy, to prevent the penumbra region from evolving to infarction.

- Intravascular contrast enhancement. Arterial enhancement most likely represents slow flow associated with stenosis, or occlusion in the presence of poor collateral circulation.
- MR angiography shows an occluded vessel.

Other later acute (1–3 days) findings include (Fig. 4.26):

- Sulcal effacement, gyral swelling.
- Loss of gray-white matter distinction. The SI changes in infarction involve both white and gray matter. This is an important element in differentiating infarct from tumor. The vasogenic edema associated with a brain tumor involves the white matter and tends to spare gray matter.
- Increased SI of the brain parenchyma on PD-WI and T2-WI (due to increased water content), in a typical vascular distribution pattern.
- Mass effect (maximal 1–5 days after the event).
- Meningeal enhancement adjacent to the infarct.

In addition to the diffusion (and perfusion)-weighted sequences, the MR imaging protocol should consist of a SE sequence with T1-WI and a SE or TSE sequence with PD-W and T2-W images. Pay attention to the presence of normal signal void in all the *major* arteries, especially at the skull base. Use of i.v. contrast allows identification of the abnormal intravascular enhancement. Use of two different imaging planes facilitates identification of the other acute findings. The sagittal plane is more useful as a second plane than the coronal plane for vertebrobasilar stroke. An MR imaging protocol for acute stroke is given in Table 4.17.

Accurate determination of the patency of the internal carotid artery can be difficult with conventional MR imaging. The presence of normal signal void in the carotid siphon does not exclude significant stenosis in the extracranial carotid artery. Isointense signal in the lumen may be due either to occlusion or high-grade stenosis with slow flow. With MR angiography (MRA), we can investigate both the carotid bifurcation and the intracranial circulation. This topic is covered elsewhere.

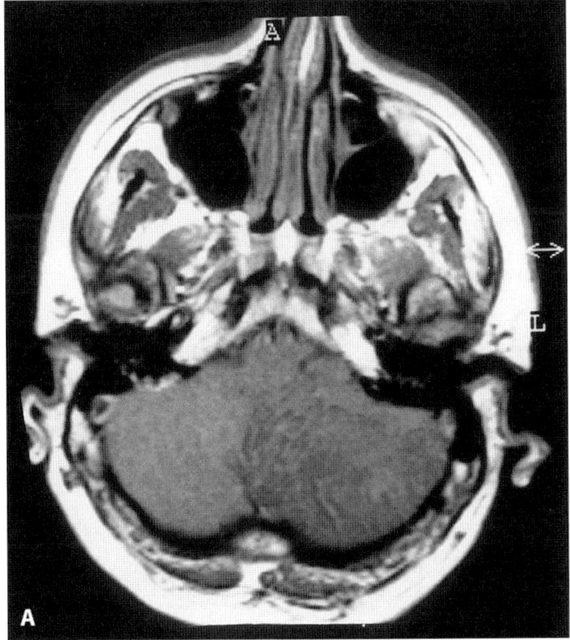

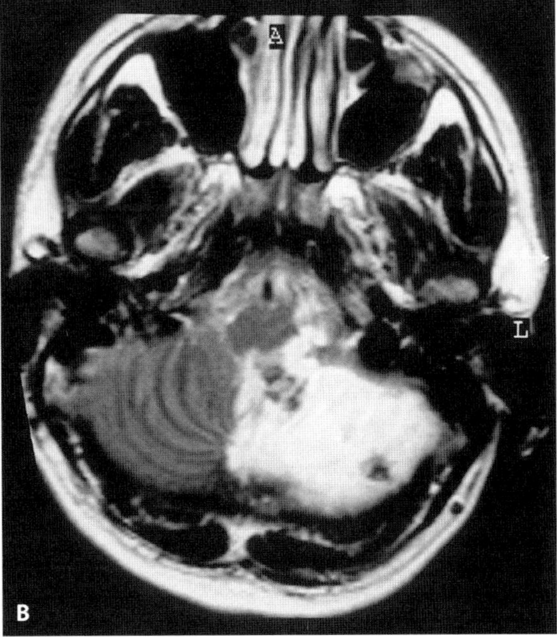

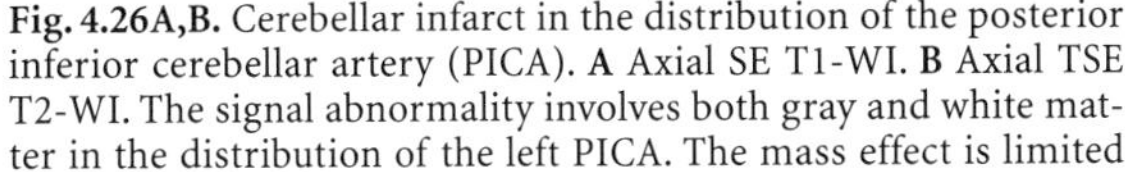

Fig. 4.26A,B. Cerebellar infarct in the distribution of the posterior inferior cerebellar artery (PICA). **A** Axial SE T1-WI. **B** Axial TSE T2-WI. The signal abnormality involves both gray and white matter in the distribution of the left PICA. The mass effect is limited compared with the size of the lesion. There are a few hemorrhagic components, which are isointense on T1-WI and hypointense on T2-WI (deoxyhemoglobin)

4.7.1.1.2
Subacute Infarction (Days to Weeks)

In the early subacute stage, the vasogenic edema becomes more prominent. The mass effect initially increases and then gradually diminishes. Although experimentally disruption of the BBB occurs 6 h after the onset of ischemia, parenchymal enhancement only becomes visible in subacute infarctions, because it requires reestablishment of a certain amount of blood supply. The parenchymal enhancement tends to follow a gyri-form pattern (Fig. 4.27). Hemorrhagic changes are more frequently observed (25%) than with CT. Therefore, it is useful to add a partial nip-angle GRE sequence to the protocol as given in Table 4.17, in order to detect hemorrhagic changes.

4.7.1.1.3
Chronic Infarction (Months to Years)

Prolonged ischemia causes irreversible brain damage. Tissue loss (negative mass effect), encephalomalacia, and replacement of tissue by CSF and/or gliosis are the causes of the SI abnormalities in this stage. Dilatation of the ipsilateral ventricle is common. The encephalomalacic area is sharply demarcated. Absence of normal flow void in major vessels in this stage indicates permanent vascular thrombosis.

4.7.1.2
Small-Vessel Disease

4.7.1.2.1
Lacunar Infarct

The occlusion of small, penetrating end arteries arising from the major cerebral arteries causes deep cerebral

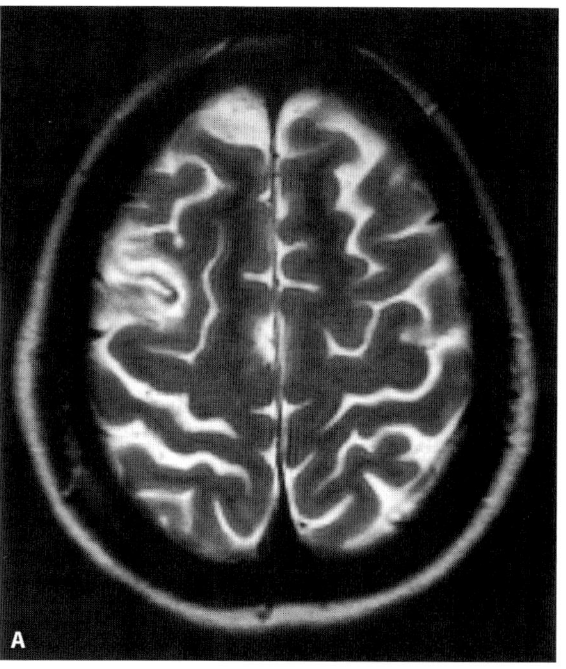

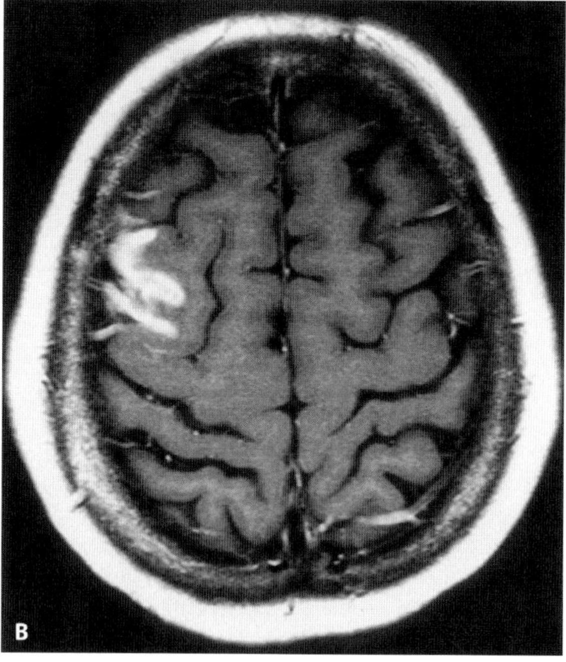

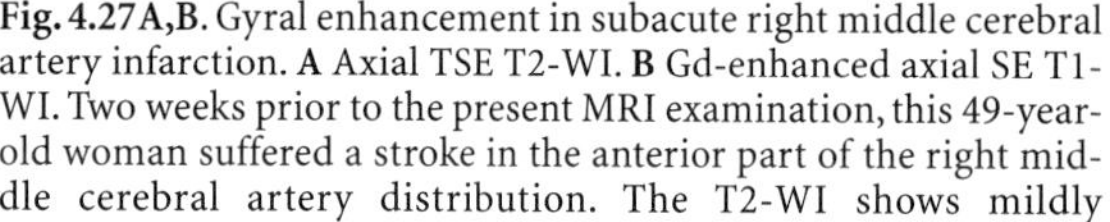

Fig. 4.27 A,B. Gyral enhancement in subacute right middle cerebral artery infarction. **A** Axial TSE T2-WI. **B** Gd-enhanced axial SE T1-WI. Two weeks prior to the present MRI examination, this 49-year-old woman suffered a stroke in the anterior part of the right middle cerebral artery distribution. The T2-WI shows mildly increased signal intensity in the cortical-subcortical region of the right frontal lobe. After Gd injection, the typical gyriform enhancement is seen. This parenchymal enhancement denotes breakdown of the BBB

'lacunar' infarcts. They account for 15%–25% of all strokes and are most frequently associated with hypertension. Lacunar infarcts are often multiple. The most commonly involved locations are basal ganglia, thalamus, internal capsule, and pons. When diagnosing lacunar infarcts on MRI, one should keep in mind that:

- Lacunar infarcts are difficult to see in the first 24 h.
- Lacunar infarcts become visible by the 3rd day as hyperintense, small, rounded lesions in the T2-WI (due to edema).
- In the acute and subacute phase, enhancement is consistently demonstrated following Gd-chelate administration, indicating disruption of the BBB.
- The SI of lacunar infarcts in the chronic stage is equal to CSF on all images.

4.7.1.2.2
Leuko-araiosis

Hyperintense white matter lesions on PD-WI and T2-WI are a frequent finding in routine MR imaging, particularly in elderly people. No mass effect is present, and little or no abnormality is seen in the T1-WI. These lesions may be focal, multifocal, or confluent and extend from the periventricular white matter to the subcortical region. Most of these areas of abnormal SI are now believed to be ischemic in origin, due to atherosclerosis in small arteries of the subcortical white matter. Their clinical significance is not clear. The term leuko-araiosis literally means 'white rarefaction'. Other terms used are subcortical leukoencephalopathy and microangiopathic leukoencephalopathy.

4.7.1.2.3
Normal Hyperintense Areas in the T2-WI

Lacunar infarcts and leuko-araiosis must be distinguished from normal and age-related areas of hyperintense signal in the T2-WI. They include:

- Areas of late myelination in the deep parieto-occipital white matter, adjacent to the ventricular trigone
- Focal breakdown of the ependymal lining with periventricular hyperintense signal anterolateral to the frontal horns
- Decreased myelination in posterior internal capsule
- Perivascular spaces of Virchow-Robin

4.7.2
Subarachnoid Hemorrhage

CT remains the most sensitive imaging method for the detection of acute subarachnoid hemorrhage (SAH). Acute SAH is difficult to detect with MR imaging, unless the SAH is massive. It is believed that the higher oxygen tension in the subarachnoid space impedes the transformation of oxyhemoglobin to paramagnetic breakdown products such as deoxyhemoglobin and methemoglobin. Additionally, pulsatile CSF flow tends to dilute and disperse the red blood cells. Recent reports indicate that FLAIR images are more sensitive than SE or TSE sequences, but in the acute phase, CT should still be the method of choice.

Repeated episodes of SAH may cause ferritin and hemosiderin deposition on the leptomeninges covering the brain. This is termed superficial siderosis. On T2-WI MRI, superficial siderosis is seen as a hypointense line along the surface of the brain, especially the pons, mesencephalon, and cerebellar vermis.

In the postoperative follow-up of a patient after aneurysm clipping, MR imaging is useful because the clip causes fewer artifacts on MR imaging than on CT. Most aneurysm clips currently used are composed of nonferromagnetic material. However, in the past, many patients have undergone aneurysm clipping with ferromagnetic clips. There is a danger of fatal intracranial hemorrhage after movement of a ferromagnetic aneurysm clip in a MR imaging unit. Never scan a patient with an aneurysm clip without identifying the exact type of the clip!

4.7.3
Veno-occlusive Disease

Venous sinus occlusive disease (VSOD) is a serious, potentially lethal (30%–80%) disease; the clinical presentation is often confusing and nonspecific. The goal of neuroradiologic examination is twofold: (1) to prove the existence of a thrombosis and (2) to evaluate the intracranial damage caused by the thrombosis. MRI is the method of choice for both of these tasks.

4.7.3.1 Identification of a Thrombosed Sinus or Vein by MR Imaging

The superior sagittal sinus is the most common site of dural sinus thrombosis, followed by the transverse sinus, sigmoid sinus, and cavernous sinus. Deep cerebral vein thrombosis is less common, but even more dangerous. Cortical vein occlusion usually occurs in association with dural sinus thrombosis and is rarely isolated.

There are three methods of identifying an occlusion of a dural sinus by MR imaging (Fig. 4.28):

1. Conventional MR imaging: careful interpretation of the SI within the lumen of the venous sinus may indicate whether it corresponds to flow or to thrombosis. FLAIR images are especially useful: thrombosis of a dural venous sinus is detected as an intravascular area of high signal intensity.
2. Phase-shift imaging.
3. MRA ('slow flow' technique or magnetic resonance '-venography').

The first method is unreliable. In practice, it is sometimes difficult to decide whether the luminal signal corresponds to flow or to thrombosis. The SI of a clot varies with its age. An acute clot is isointense on T1-WI and hypointense on T2-WI. A subacute clot is hyperintense on both T1-WI and T2-WI. The SI of normal flow in a sinus is also variable. Instead of flow void, a high signal may be observed on T1-WI because of the entry phenomenon, in plane flow or slow flow. In T2-WI, the luminal signal can be high because of even-echo rephasing or slow in-plane flow, accentuated by flow compensation techniques. Therefore, in the imaging protocol for VSOD, you must use an asymmetric first, second echo T2-W sequence without the flow compensation technique. Two rules of thumb almost always apply:

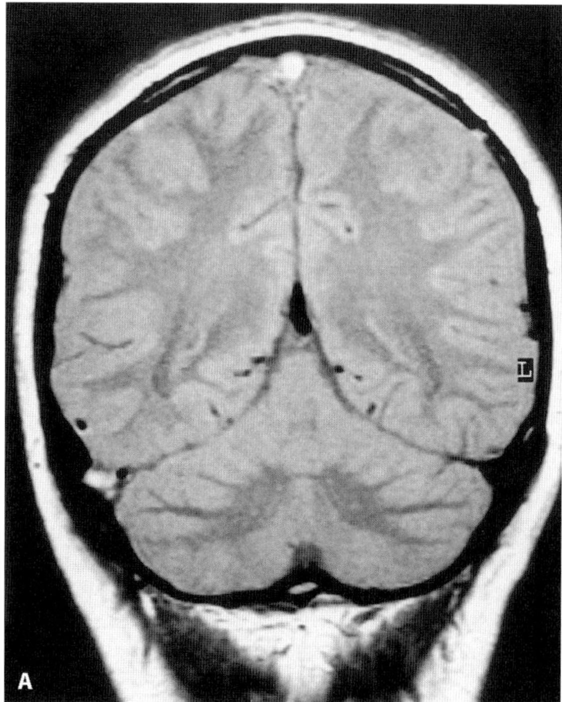

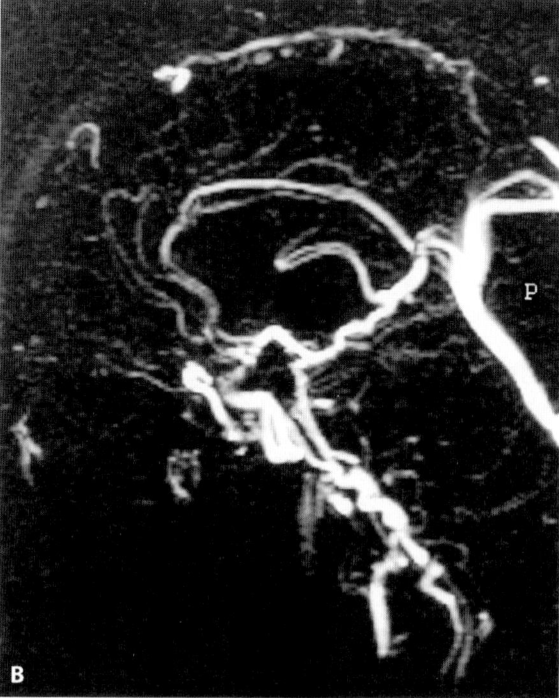

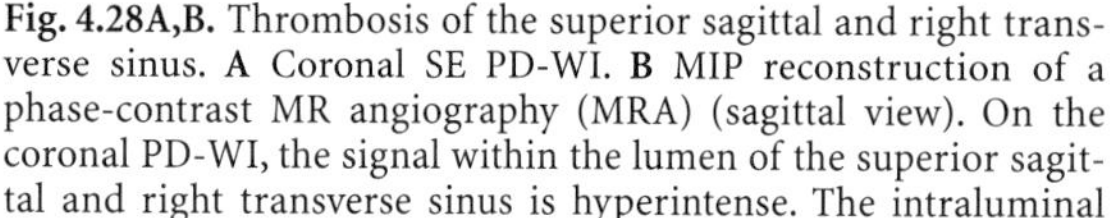

Fig. 4.28A,B. Thrombosis of the superior sagittal and right transverse sinus. **A** Coronal SE PD-WI. **B** MIP reconstruction of a phase-contrast MR angiography (MRA) (sagittal view). On the coronal PD-WI, the signal within the lumen of the superior sagittal and right transverse sinus is hyperintense. The intraluminal signal intensity was also high on the T1-WI and T2-WI (not shown). This signal-intensity behavior is consistent with a blood clot (extracellular methemoglobin). The phase-contrast MRA image reveals an absence of flow within the superior sagittal sinus, thereby confirming the diagnosis of thrombosis

1. High luminal signal on the T1-WI and T2-WI corresponds to extracellular methemoglobin (subacute clot).
2. Enhancement of the lumen after i.v. contrast suggests flow, except in the presence of a chronic fibrotic clot; but this possibility is not important in the acute situation.

In phase-shift imaging, we look at the direction and not at the magnitude of the MRI signal. The direction of the MRI vector is related to the presence or absence of flow. Phase-shift images provide no anatomical information, but their only purpose is to indicate the presence or absence of flow.

The need to perform phase-shift imaging is now lower, due to the availability of MRA. The recommended techniques for MRA in suspected VSOD are:

- Time of flight (TOF) MRA, e.g., oblique coronal 2D TOF (2D FLASH) with saturation of the arterial inflow.
- Phase-contrast MRA, e.g., single-slab phase-contrast angiography (Fig. 4.28).

A more detailed discussion of MRA techniques can be found in Chapter 13.

4.7.3.2 Evaluation of the Intracranial Damage

VSOD can cause intracranial hypertension, hydrocephalus, venous infarction, and hemorrhage. MRI findings include:

- Mass effect, sulcal effacement
- Areas of hyperintense signal in the T2-WI, not corresponding to an arterial territory, frequently bilateral or with involvement of more than one vascular distribution
- Hemorrhagic components

T1-W after i.v. contrast may show:

- Absence of arterial enhancement
- Visualization of the thrombus, as a central area of intermediate SI, surrounded by enhanced rim of dura
- Prominent venous enhancement in dilated cortical venous branches

4.7.4 Vascular Malformations

4.7.4.1 Classification

The four archetypal vascular malformations are (1) arteriovenous malformation (AVM), (2) capillary telangiectasia, (3) cavernous angioma, and (4) developmental venous anomaly (venous angioma). The latter is considered an anatomic variant and not a true malformation.

4.7.4.2 Arteriovenous Malformation

AVMs are congenital disorders. The angioarchitecture of an AVM consists of one or more enlarged feeding arteries, a tangled collection of blood vessels (the nidus), and a tortuous assortment of dilated draining veins. AVMs are a cause of intracerebral hemorrhage; they are also associated with headaches, ischemic or hemorrhagic infarctions, or subarachnoid hemorrhage. The MRI examination is complementary to cerebral angiography for the treatment planning. It must identify:

- Number, location, and identification of the feeding arteries
- Exact delineation of the nidus
- Location of the draining veins, with possible dilated portions
- Parenchymal damage, atrophy
- Presence of hemorrhage and its relationship to the nidus

An important issue of the MR imaging protocol is the accurate anatomic definition of the nidus and its relationship to vital cerebral structures. Therefore, the MRI examination has to include images in three imaging planes (axial, coronal, and sagittal), eventually supplemented by MRA. In at least one imaging plane, T1-WI and T2-WI should be performed. MRI findings in the typical case are:

- Multiple round, linear, or serpiginous areas of signal void
- Little or no mass effect in the absence of recent bleeding
- Atrophy of the surrounding brain, gliosis
- Absence of brain tissue inside the nidus

4.7.4.3
Capillary Telangiectasia

Capillary telangiectasias are vascular malformations which are composed of dilated capillaries with interposed normal brain parenchyma. They are the second most common vascular malformation (second only to venous developmental anomalies). At autopsy, they are frequently found as multiple lesions. The brainstem, especially the pons, is the most typical location, but capillary teleangiectasias can also be found in the cerebellum, spinal cord, and supratentorially. Most of these lesions are clinically silent and are incidentally discovered on imaging studies. Capillary teleangiectasias are invisible on cerebral angiography. On Gd-enhanced MR images, the so-called 'racemose' type of capillary teleangiectasia may be seen as an region of mild, stippled contrast enhancement. The 'cavernous' type presents as hypointense lesions on T2*-weighted images, indicating evidence of old hemorrhage with hemosiderin deposition.

4.7.4.4
Cavernous Malformation (syn. Cavernous Hemangioma)

Cavernous malformations occur in the brain and the spinal cord. The most frequent location is in the cerebral hemispheres, though they also occur in the brainstem. Sporadic and familial forms are possible. Lesions are frequently multiple (20%–30%), with a familial pattern in 10%–15% of the patients. Cavernous malformations may be asymptomatic. When symptomatic, their clinical presentation consists of seizures, headache, hemorrhage, and progressive neurological deficit.

Histopathologically, a cavernous malformation has three components: sinusoidal vascular spaces lined by a single layer of endothelial cells, fibrous septa with calcifications, and a peripheral component of gliotic hemosiderin-laden tissue. There is no brain parenchyma within the lesion. The flow is very slow or absent, with frequent intravascular thrombosis.

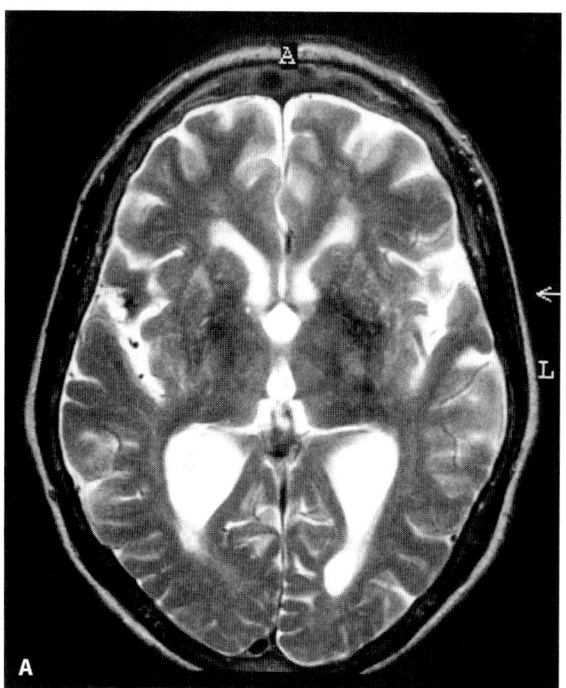

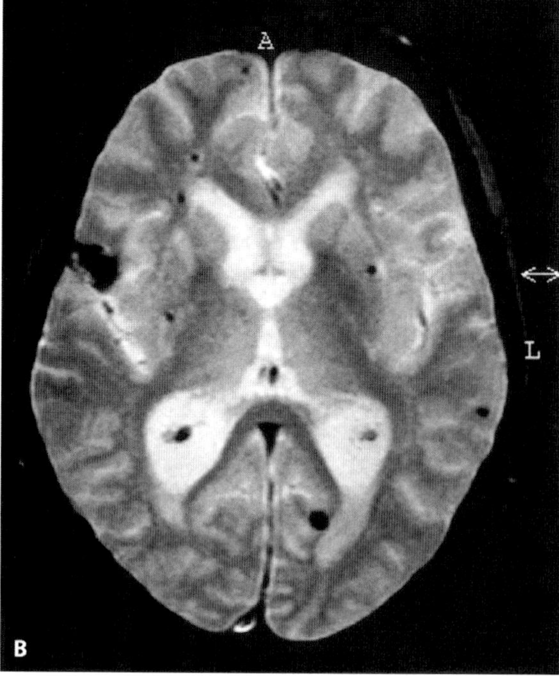

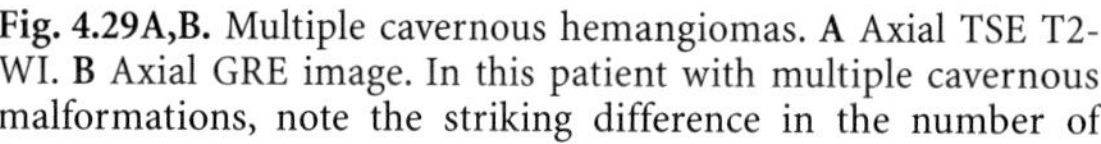

Fig. 4.29A,B. Multiple cavernous hemangiomas. **A** Axial TSE T2-WI. **B** Axial GRE image. In this patient with multiple cavernous malformations, note the striking difference in the number of lesions detected by the partial flip-angle GRE compared with the TSE T2-W sequence. This is due to the insensitivity of the TSE sequence for blood degradation products, such as hemosiderin

Noncontrast CT demonstrates cavernous angiomas as small, rounded, dense foci, often with associated calcification. However, MR imaging is more sensitive and more specific, due to its sensitivity to old blood-breakdown products. In a typical cavernous angioma, MRI findings are:

- Small, well delineated lesion, often with a high SI core on T1-W images
- Reticulated appearance; heterogeneous SI represents blood products of different age; hypointense signal areas (due to blood-breakdown products such as hemosiderin) are more prominent on T2-W and GRE images
- Peripheral closed rim of hemosiderin
- No flow; no arterial feeders, no draining veins
- No mass effect and no perifocal edema, unless a recent episode of bleeding has occurred

The MRI protocol should contain pulse sequences sensitive for old blood products (hemosiderin). The TSE sequence is insensitive and may miss the lesions. A spoiled partial flip-angle GRE sequence with T2-W (FFE or FLASH) is the most sensitive method (Fig. 4.29).

4.7.4.5 Developmental Venous Anomaly

Developmental venous anomalies (DVAs; also known as 'venous malformation' or 'venous angioma') are believed to represent an anatomic variant of the normal venous drainage pattern, and not a true malformation. Most often, they are discovered as an incidental finding. DVAs do not contain an arterial or capillary component. They consist of small tributary veins that drain into an enlarged venous channel. On T1-WI, they are seen as linear or curvilinear flow voids, often perpendicular to the cortex or the ventricular wall. On T2-WI, their SI is variable, depending on the direction and speed of flow, as well as technical factors, such as the entry phenomenon. After Gd injection, the small tributary veins enhance in a stellate fashion, often presenting the shape of a caput medusae. Up to one-third of venous angiomas are only discovered after the injection of Gd.

4.8 White Matter Lesions

4.8.1 Introduction

In the radiological assessment of white matter disease, it is important to consider both the patient's age and the clinical presentation. Most white matter diseases present with similar findings on MRI, with hypointense lesions on T1-WI and hyperintense lesions on T2-WI. Contrast enhancement is an infrequent finding. Subtle differences in the pattern of white matter changes may direct us to the correct diagnosis.

The imaging strategy has to be directed by the expected pathology, which depends on the age of the patient. In the first year of life, periventricular leucomalacia and delayed myelination are frequent findings. In the first decade, the leukodystrophies can be the cause of white matter changes. In the adult population, multiple sclerosis is the most common white matter disease, with an increasing incidence of nonspecific and vascular-related white matter changes with aging. Within certain patient groups, other diseases are more frequent (toxic demyelination, radiation necrosis).

4.8.2 Normal Development

Brain myelination begins in the 5th fetal month. At the age of 2 years, 90% of the myelination is complete. The remainder of the process continues into adulthood. The progression of myelination can be studied with MR imaging, and the visualization of this process depends on the pulse sequence and field strength. Imaging sequences must be heavily T1-W (SE T1: TR$\geq$3000 ms, TE$\geq$100 ms). Early changes ($\leq$6–8 months) are best studied with a T1-W sequence; at a later age (6–18 months), changes are best depicted on T2-WI. The process of myelination follows a distinct pattern. In broad terms, myelination progresses from caudad to craniad, and from posterior to anterior. The myelination process is discussed in greater depth in Chapter 16 (section 16.2.3.2).

The posterior limb of the internal capsule contains an area with different SI than the anterior limb. On T2-WI, this is seen as a focal symmetric area of high SI. Proton density and T1-WI show no difference between the anterior and posterior limb of the internal capsule. These regions probably represent a portion of the pyramid tract (parieto-pontine bundles). This normal finding should not be mistaken for lesions in the internal capsule.

4.8.3 T2-W Sequence

Myelinated structures are hypointense on T2-WI. At birth, the dorsal white matter tracts of the brainstem, the superior and inferior cerebellar peduncles, and the medio-dorsal tracts in the diencephalon are myelinated. Supratentorially, only the posterior limb of the internal capsule and the white matter in the post-central gyrus are myelinated. As the process continues, more cerebral structures become myelinated. At the age of 6 - months, the brainstem has a mature myelination pattern, and the cerebellar hemispheres show central myelination. The optic radiation is fully myelinated, while the internal capsule and the corpus callosum are partially myelinated. The occipital and parietal lobes and the motor areas myelinate earlier than the frontal and temporal lobes. This is also reflected in the myelination of the internal capsule and the corpus callosum. The anterior limb of the internal capsule and the genu of the corpus callosum myelinate 4 months later than the posterior limb and the splenium. The occipital and parietal lobes reach a mature myelination between 6 months and 18 months; the frontal and temporal lobes reach this point between 21 months and 27 months.

4.8.4 T1-W Sequence

Myelinated structures are hyperintense on T1-WI. The myelination process as seen on IR-SE T1-WI proceeds parallel to that seen on T2-WI. However, myelination is seen earlier than on T2-WI. At birth, all three cerebellar peduncles are myelinated, and the optic pathways also show a high SI due to myelination. Not only the post-central but also the pre-central gyrus is myelinated at birth on IR-SE T1-WI. At age 6 months, most of the brain reaches a mature myelination on the IR-SE T1-WI, the frontal and temporal poles are fully myelinated on IR-SE T1-WI after 10 months.

4.8.5 Delayed Myelination

There is a close correlation between myelination and psychomotor development, both in normal and in delayed myelination. In infants with a developmental delay of unknown cause, delayed myelination is present in 10% of cases. The most common causes of delayed myelination are malnutrition, hypoxia-ischemia, infections, congenital heart failure, hydrocephalus, and chromosomal abnormalities (Down's syndrome).

4.8.6 Leukodystrophy

Leukodystrophies constitute a group of disorders that are characterized by an abnormal formation, turnover, or destruction of myelin. The underlying cause is an enzyme deficiency. Most of these disorders are encountered in the pediatric population. White matter changes on MR imaging are often nonspecific, though some are suggestive of certain diseases.

Canavan disease (Fig. 16.18) is rare and results in a diffuse, symmetric, low SI of the white matter on T1-WI. On T2-WI, the supratentorial white matter has a uniformly high SI. In Alexander disease (Fig. 16.19), the abnormal SI is initially located in the frontal lobes. Enhancement after contrast medium administration of the basal ganglia and periventricular white matter has been reported. Adrenoleukodystrophy (Fig. 16.15) affects only boys and results in high SI in the occipital lobes on T2-WI; in due course, these abnormalities advance anteriorly. The anterior rim of the lesion may enhance after contrast medium administration. An almost complete lack of myelination is seen in Pelizaeus-Merzbacher disease (Fig. 4.30). Hyperintense lesions on T2-WI are found in the basal ganglia or thalamus in Krabbe disease, Leigh disease (Fig. 16.16), and methylmalonic acidemia. A more exhaustive discussion of leukodystrophies is presented in Chapter 16 (Section 16.2.3.3).

4.8.7 Multiple Sclerosis

Multiple sclerosis (MS) is an inflammatory demyelinating disease of the CNS. It is the most common demyeli-

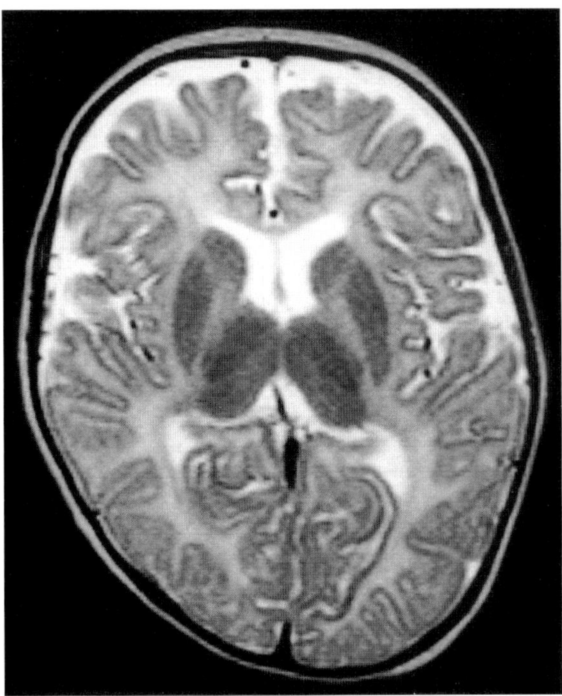

Fig. 4.30. Pelizaeus-Merzbacher disease. This axial TSE T2-WI shows abnormally high signal intensities throughout the white matter in both hemispheres. This finding is consistent with an almost complete lack of normal myelination

nating disease after vascular- and age-related demyelination. MS is characterized by multiple 'plaques' of demyelination in the white matter of the brain and spinal cord. The primary lesions are found in the perivascular spaces along penetrating veins. Though the etiology of MS is not fully understood, the destruction of myelin is most likely caused by an autoimmune process. Initial symptoms sometimes can be triggered by trauma or a viral infection, but a convincing link to the disease has not been made.

The clinical course of MS is variable. The age of symptom onset in MS is usually between 18 and 40 years; onset is uncommon in childhood and after the age of 50 years. There is a female:male ratio of 3:2. The most common presentation is the prolonged relapsing-remitting disease (70% of cases). Symptomatic episodes can last from 24 h to several weeks. As white matter lesions increase over time, the disease frequently becomes chronically progressive. Accumulating neurological deficits ultimately lead to permanent disability. Alternatively, MS can be chronically progressive from the beginning.

Initial symptoms are typically numbness, dysesthesia, double vision, or problems with balance and coordination. Loss of motor function is also a frequent initial presentation. Less commonly, spinal-cord-related symptoms constitute the initial presentation of MS.

4.8.7.1 Diagnostic Criteria

No single clinical or laboratory test is pathognomonic for MS. For this reason, diagnostic criteria have been developed to assess the relative probability of MS. The ones most widely used are the Poser criteria (Table 4.20). Since the introduction of MR imaging, the role of neuroimaging in the diagnosis of MS has changed. In the old days, CT and myelography were used to exclude diseases that could mimic MS. Nowadays, MR imaging is the method of choice. MR imaging is far more sensitive than CT in the detection of white matter disease. Moreover, MR imaging techniques have revealed MS to be a dynamic disease, with

Table 4.20. Poser criteria

I.	Clinically definitive MS	• Two symptomatic episodes ('attacks') and clinical evidence of two separate lesions • Two attacks and clinical evidence of one lesion and paraclinical evidence (MR imaging) of another lesion
II.	Laboratory-supported definitive MS	• Two attacks with either clinical or paraclincal evidence (MR imaging) of one lesion and demonstration of typical CSF findings • One attack, clinical evidence of two separate lesions and typical CSF findings • One attack, clinical evidence of one lesion and paraclinical evidence (MR imaging) of another lesion and typical CSF findings
III.	Clinically probable MS	• Two attacks and clinical evidence of one lesion • One attack and clinical evidence of two separate lesions • One attack, clinical evidence of one lesion, and paraclinical evidence (MR imaging) of another lesion
IV.	Laboratory-supported probable MS	• Two attacks and typical CSF findings

lesions waxing and waning, which was not predicted by clinical methods.

4.8.7.2
MR Imaging Appearance of MS

The characteristic abnormalities of MS in the brain consist of multiple white matter lesions with a high SI on FLAIR, PD-WI, and T2-WI (Fig. 4.31) and low SI on T1-WI. These lesions are seen in 85%–100% of the patients with definite MS according to the Poser criteria (Table 4.20). Lesions are found predominantly in a periventricular distribution and at the callososeptal interface. Additional sites of involvement include other parts of the cerebral white matter such as the optic nerves, corpus callosum, internal capsule, cerebellar peduncles, brainstem, and spinal cord.

Lesions appear smaller on T1-WI than on T2-WI. Occasionally, they show a hyperintense border on T1-WI. Lesions in MS can be small, large, or confluent. The typical configuration is that of an ovoid lesion extending perpendicularly from the ventricular surface (Dawson's finger) (Fig. 4.31). This probably reflects the perivascular inflammation along a penetrating medullary vein. Atypical lesions and mass-like lesions occur with sufficient frequency to cause diagnostic errors.

MS lesions may enhance after contrast administration on T1-WI, depending on the age and activity of the lesion. New and active lesions commonly show contrast enhancement, due to BBB breakdown. New lesions tend to show solid enhancement, whereas reactivated lesions enhance in a ring-like fashion (Fig. 4.32). After 2 months, the integrity of the BBB is restored, and the majority of lesions no longer show contrast enhancement.

As with unenhanced lesions, the contrast-enhancing lesions are smaller than the corresponding lesions on the T2-W scan. The discrepancy between the size of the lesion on T1-WI and T2-WI reflects the different components of the local process: edema, inflammation, and demyelination.

The poor correlation between the MRI findings and the clinical events is demonstrated by the frequent finding of enhancing lesions in clinically stable patients.

4.8.7.3
Lesion Distribution

White matter lesions are abundant in the centrum semiovale, corpus callosum, optic chiasm, and optic nerves. Hyperintense lesions on T2-WI are commonly found in the corpus callosum. Typically, these lesions occur along the inner callosal-ventricular margin, creating an irregular ventricular surface of the corpus callosum. This aspect can be differentiated from callosal atrophy due to the lobar white matter lesions. The existence of

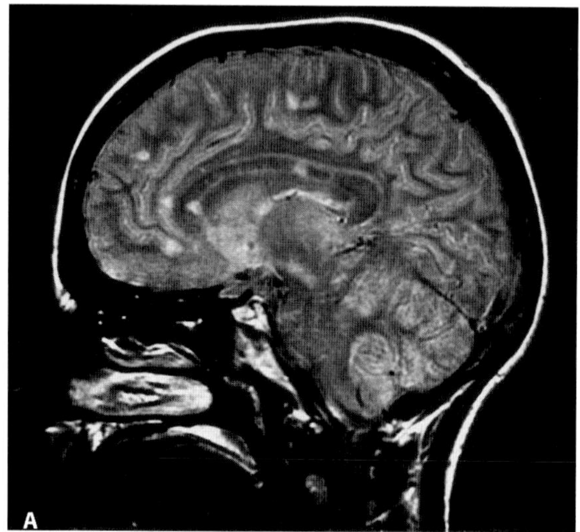

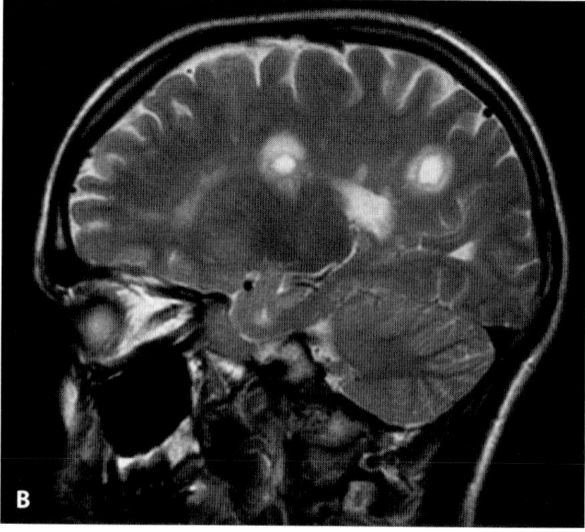

Fig. 4.31A,B. Multiple sclerosis: value of sagittal images. **A** Sagittal TSE PD-WI through the corpus callosum. **B** Sagittal T2-WI through the right lateral ventricle. These sagittal images in a 24-year-old woman with multiple sclerosis show demyelinating lesions in the corpus callosum and periventricular white matter. The typical configuration is that of an ovoid lesion extending perpendicularly from the ventricular surface (Dawson's finger). The perilesional edema is indicative of active plaques

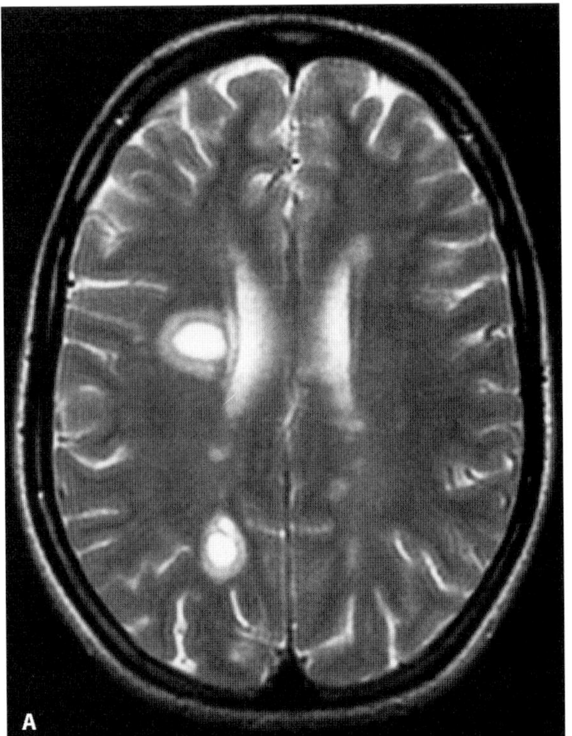

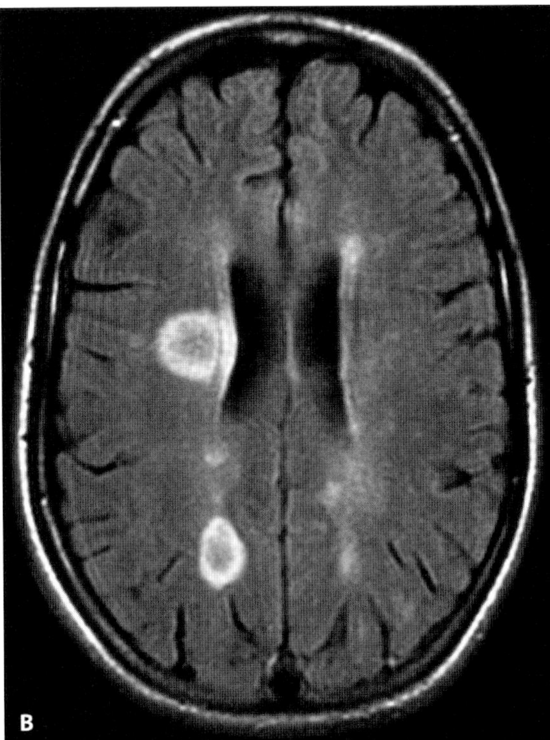

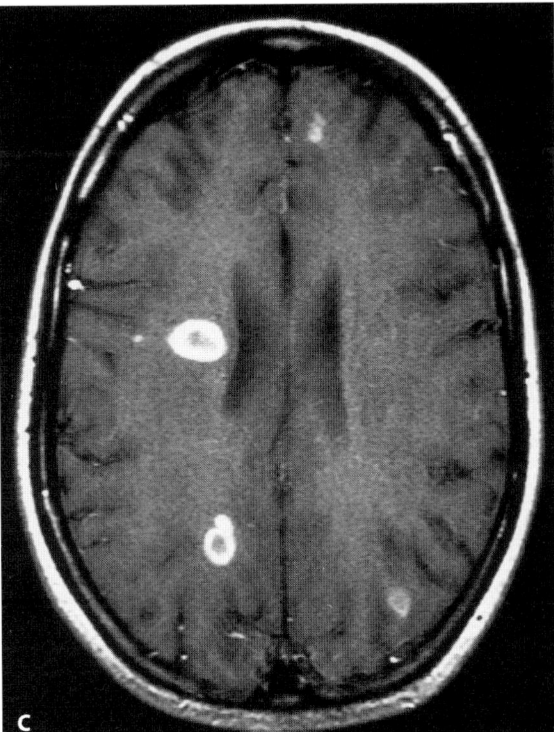

Fig. 4.32A–C. Multiple sclerosis: role of gadolinium. **A** Axial TSE T2-WI and **B** axial TSE Flair through the centrum semiovale. C Gd-enhanced axial SE T1-WI through the centrum semiovale. On the T2-WI, all white matter lesions are hyperintense. Active lesions have basically the same imaging appearance as older lesions. After Gd injection, only a few lesions enhance, indicating disruption of the BBB. In the right parietal lesion, the enhancement is solid (presumably indicating a fresh lesion); ring-like enhancement is observed in the right frontal lesion (believed to represent an older or reactivated lesion)

callosal lesions improves both the sensitivity and the specificity of MR imaging for MS. The absence of callosal lesions renders the diagnosis of MS less likely, but does not exclude it.

A frequent initial presentation of MS is optic neuritis, although there is controversy regarding the likelihood of definitive MS developing in patients who have had an optic neuritis. Brainstem lesions are common, and a lesion in the medial longitudinal bundle affects approximately one-third of MS patients. In patients with clinically possible MS and a normal MR imaging study of the brain, a spinal MRI study should be performed.

Table 4.21. Protocol for "rule out multiple sclerosis". Sagittal images are especially useful for demonstrating lesions within the corpus callosum and at the callososeptal interface. Perivenular extension into the white matter of the centrum ovale is called Dawson's fingers. Thin sagittal turbo FLAIR images with 2-mm to 3-mm slice thickness are used in some centers for high-resolution imaging of the callososeptal region. Slices for the coronal fat-suppression sequences are positioned from the eye globe to the optic chiasm

Pulse sequence	WI	Plane	No. of sections	TR (ms)	TE (ms)	TI (ms)	Flip angle	Echo train length	Section thickness (mm)	Matrix	FOV	recFOV	No. of acq.
1. Axial double-echo PD- and T2-W sequence (or combination of T2-W TSE and turbo-FLAIR, see Table 2)													
SE or TSE	PD-T2	ax	19	2000–5000	15–30/ 90–130	–	90/180	1 (SE) 15 (TSE)	5	256 or 512	230–240	75	1–2
2. Sagittal double echho PD-and T2-W sequence (or combination of T2-W TSE and turbo FLAIR, see Table 2)													
TSE	PD-T2	sag	19–25	3000–6000	15–30/ 90–130	–	90/180	3–25	3–5	256 or 512	230–240	100	1–2
Add-on for 'optic neuritis': fat-suppressed sequence (STIR or spectral fat suppression)													
TSE-fat sat	T2 fat sat	cor	15	4000–5000	90–130		90/180	7–15	3	256	≤200	75	2
STIR	fat sat	cor	15	4000–9000	20–30	100–150	180	7–15	3	256	≤200	75	2

Abbreviations: *WI* weighted image; *TR* repetition time (ms); *TI* inversion time (ms); *TE* echo time (ms); *no part* number of partitions; *effth* effective thickness (mm), *matrix* matrix (phase×frequency matrix), *FOV* field of view (mm); *recFOV* % rectangular field of view; *Acq* number of acquisitions

Table 4.22. Protocol for determining disease activity in multiple sclerosis. This protocol should be used only to monitor disease activity in a patient with known multiple sclerosis

Pulse sequence	WI	Plane	No. of sections	TR (ms)	TE (ms)	TI (ms)	Flip angle	Echo train length	Section thickness (mm)	Matrix	FOV	recFOV	No. of acq.
1. Axial double-echo PD- and T2-W sequence (or combination of T2-W TSE and turbo-FLAIR, see Table 2)													
SE or TSE	PD-T2	ax	19	2000–5000	15–30/ 90–130	–	90/180	1 (SE)– 15 (TSE)	5	256 or 512	230–240	75	1–2
2. Axial T1-W sequence *(MTC optional)*													
SE	T1	ax	19	600–800	10–15	–	90/180	–	5	256 or better	230–240	75	1–2
Intravenous contrast injection (double dose contrast optional). 5 min delay!													
3. Axial T1-W sequence (MTC optional)													
SE	T1	ax	19	600–800	10–15	–	90/180	–	5	256 or better	230–240	75	1–2
4. Sagittal T1-W sequence (MTC optional)													
SE	T1	sag	19	600–800	10–15	–	90/180	–	5	256 or better	230–240	100	1–2

Abbreviations: *WI* weighted image: *TR* repetition time (ms); *TI* inversion time (ms); *TE* echo time (ms); *TD* time delay (sec); *no part* number of partitions; *Matrix* (phase × frequency matrix); *FOV* field of view (mm); *recFOV* % rectangular field of view.

4.8.7.4
Imaging Strategies in MS

4.8.7.4.1
Clinical Question: 'Rule Out MS'

The majority of lesions in MS are found in the periventricular white matter. Therefore, the optimal MRI sequence for the detection of MS lesions should provide: (1) high contrast between lesions and CSF and (2) high contrast between lesions and normal white matter (Table 4.21).

Traditionally, this dual goal has been achieved by a double-echo SE sequence, which provides PD-WI (first echo) and T2-WI (second echo) (Fig. 4.31). On PD-WI, the SI of CSF is almost equal to that of periventricular white matter; this allows excellent detection of periventricular lesions which stand out as high-signal areas. On T2-WI, lesions are markedly hyperintense relative to the cerebral white matter. However, small periventricular lesions may be difficult to separate from the high SI CSF in the ventricles.

The combination of high-lesion CSF and high-lesion white matter contrast can also be achieved by the FLAIR sequence. FLAIR is an inversion recovery technique and typically uses a long inversion time of ±2000 ms (2 s) to suppress the signal of CSF in combination with a long TR/long TE sequence. FLAIR possesses a superior sensitivity for focal white matter changes in the supratentorial brain, but lesions can be missed in the posterior fossa.

In addition to the standard axial imaging plane, long TR sagittal images are particularly useful for the detection of MS plaques at the callosal-septal interface. Moreover, sagittal images demonstrate the radial orientation of plaques, perpendicular to the ventricular margins (Dawson's fingers). This characteristic finding reflects the perivenular inflammation of MS.

4.8.7.4.2
Clinical Question: Disease Activity

MR imaging shows dissemination in place and time of MS lesions (Table 4.22). New and active lesions are associated with BBB breakdown and may therefore enhance after contrast administration. Enhancement tends to be solid with fresh lesions and becomes ring-like when the lesion is several weeks old (Fig. 4.32). Therefore, in the follow-up of a patient with MS, T1-WI before and after contrast medium administration should be part of the imaging protocol (Table 4.22).

A 5-min delay is suggested between contrast injection and the start of the first post-contrast sequence to provide sufficient time for Gd to leak through the BBB. In order to avoid this delay, some authors have proposed the following protocol: axial SE T1-W sequence > contrast injection > axial PD-and T2-W sequence > axial SE T1-W sequence > (sagittal SE T1-W sequence).

The confidence of detecting enhancing lesions can be increased by the use of double-dose contrast or by the application of a magnetization transfer contrast (MTC) pre-pulse. Injection of a double dose has the significant disadvantage of doubling the cost of the contrast. Application of a MTC pre-pulse renders the T1-W sequence more sensitive for contrast enhancement (Fig. 4.33). To avoid confusion between enhancement and an MTC effect, the pre-contrast T1-W sequence should also be performed with a MTC pre-pulse.

Anti-inflammatory medications (e.g., corticosteroids) restore the BBB. Therefore, it is important to perform the MRI examination before medical treatment is instituted. If not, the activity of the disease may be underestimated.

4.8.7.4.3
Clinical Question: (Semi-)quantitative Assessment

For routine imaging of the brain in a patient with suspected MS, an imaging protocol using a slice thickness of 5 mm is usually sufficient. However, when follow-up studies are performed for (semi-)quantitative assessment of the lesion load, thinner slices may be required. Most international trials monitoring the effect of new drugs on the course of MS require MR imaging protocols with contiguous 3-mm slices. This usually implies that 40–50 axial slices are needed to cover the brain from the skull base to the vertex. In practice, each axial sequence is performed twice, to obtain the desired number of slices. In order to improve reproducibility of the quantitative assessment, slices should be carefully positioned according to internal landmarks within the patient, e.g., the bicommissural line (see Sect. 4.1.2).

4.8.7.4.4
Clinical Question: Optic Neuritis

The imaging of optic neuritis is best performed using thin coronal images with fat-suppression techniques

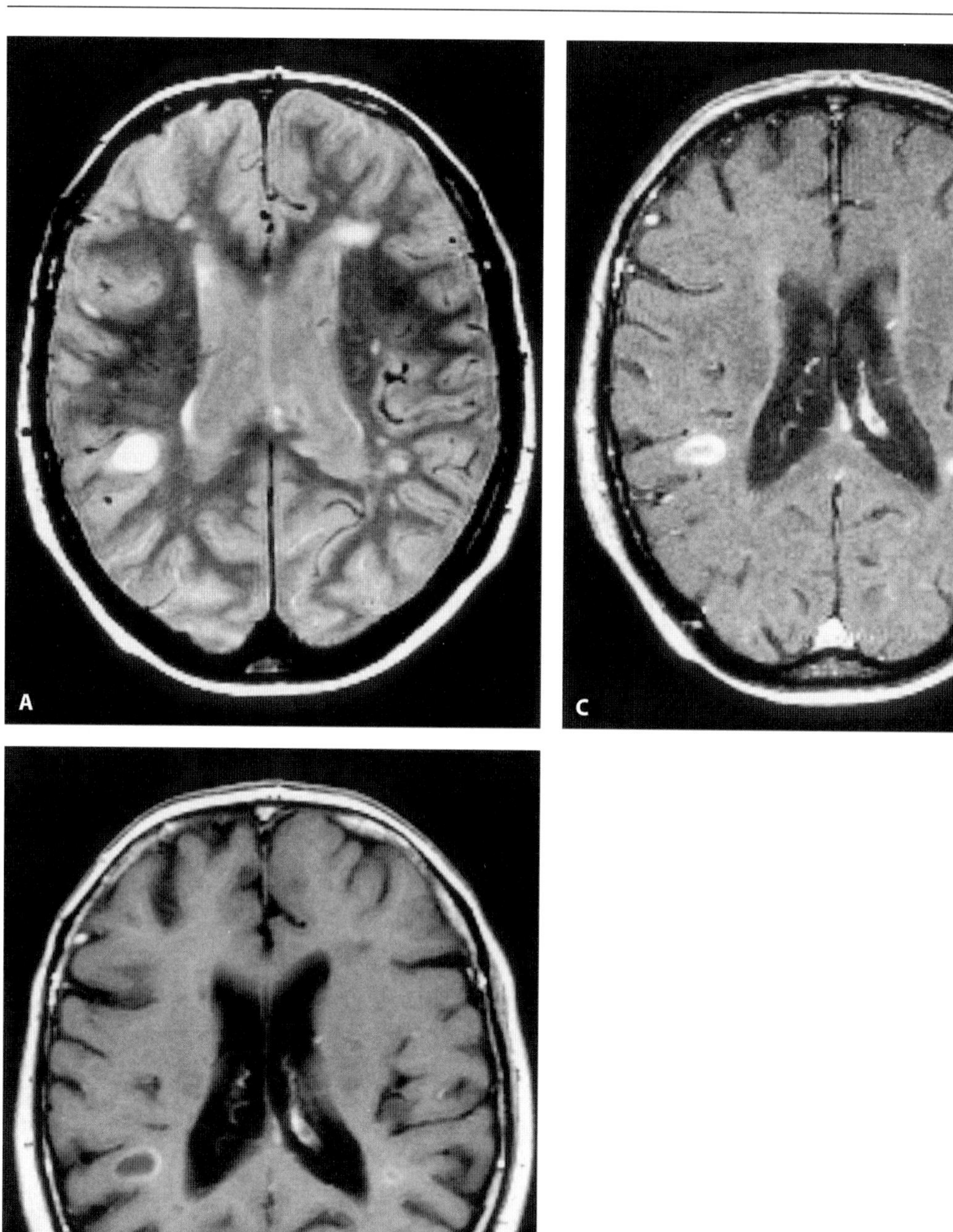

Fig. 4.33A–C. Multiple sclerosis: value of magnetization transfer contrast. **A** Axial TSE PD-WI through the lateral ventricles. **B** Gd-enhanced axial SE T1-WI (same level). **C** Gd-enhanced axial SE T1-WI with MTC (same level). PD-WI shows multiple white matter lesions in both hemispheres. The distribution pattern is consistent with MS. After Gd injection, ring-like enhancement is observed in two lesions. The Gd-enhanced image with MTC shows more intense enhancement. The signal-to-noise ratio is poorer due to background suppression

(inversion recovery or spectral fat saturation) (Fig. 4.34). Coronal images should cover the orbit and include the optic chiasm. On T2-WI, high SI indicating edema of the optic nerve can be seen. Due to swelling of the nerve, the CSF-filled perioptic sheath is compressed, and the normal 'target' configuration of the optic nerve surrounded by CSF, disappears. T1-W sequences after contrast administration may show enhancement of the optic nerve.

4.8.7.5 Differential Diagnosis

There is no single pathognomonic sign of MS on MRI. MS remains a clinical diagnosis which can never be made on an MRI study alone. Overdiagnosis should be avoided, and special care must be taken in the elderly population where the incidence of nonspecific white matter lesions is high. Other conditions, such as Lyme disease, neurosarcoidosis, and vasculitis, may present clinical and MRI findings remarkably similar to MS. Lyme disease can mimic MS on a MRI study, and in endemic regions this treatable disease should be considered in the differential diagnosis. Vasculitis preferentially involves the peripheral, subcortical white matter and gray matter, with focal gray matter atrophy. Acute disseminated encephalomyelitis (ADEM) is a monophasic disease with an MRI appearance indistinguishable from MS. A short list of multifocal white matter lesions is provided in Table 4.23.

Table 4.23. Etiology of multifocal white-matter lesions

Aging
Multiple sclerosis
ADEM
Lyme disease
PML
Metastasis
Trauma
Vasculitis
Hypertension
Migraine

4.8.8 Toxic and Degenerative Demyelination

Radiation therapy and chemotherapy may lead to degeneration of cerebral white matter. T2-WI show focal or diffuse confluent lesions in the lobar white matter. Local mass effect can be present, due to focal necrosis. Peripheral enhancement is often seen after contrast administration. These lesions can therefore mimic recurrent or residual tumor.

Alcohol is also one of the common causes of toxic demyelination. Osmotic myelinolysis is an acute condition classically occurring in alcoholics or after rapid correction of hyponatremia. The most common site is the central pons (central pontine myelinolysis, Fig. 4.35) although myelinolysis is also found in the basal ganglia and the thalamus. Involvement of the pons is seen on T1-WI as well as on T2-WI. Peripheral enhancement may be observed after contrast administration. Chronic

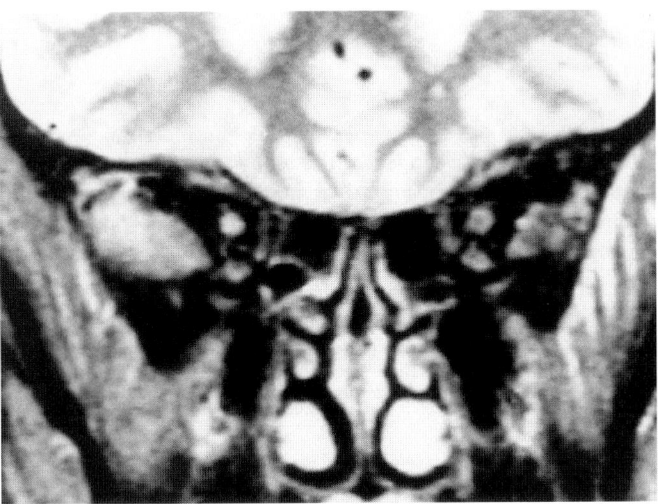

Fig. 4.34. Optic neuritis. This coronal STIR image with fat suppression shows abnormally high signal intensity in the right optic nerve. Note normal 'target' appearance of the left optic nerve, which is outlined by the CSF space surrounding it

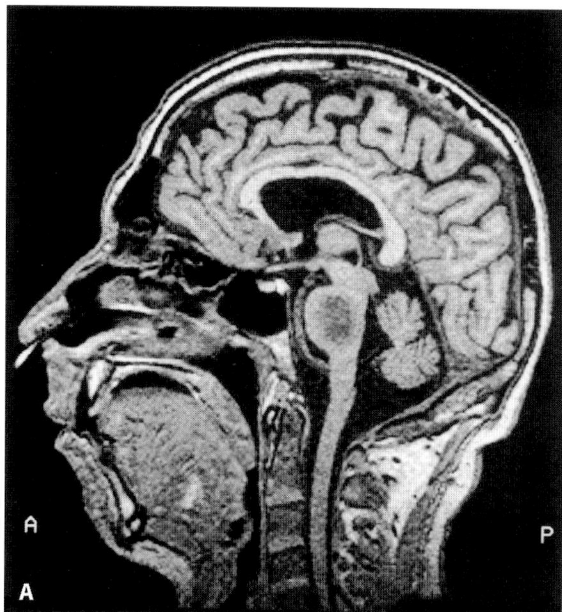

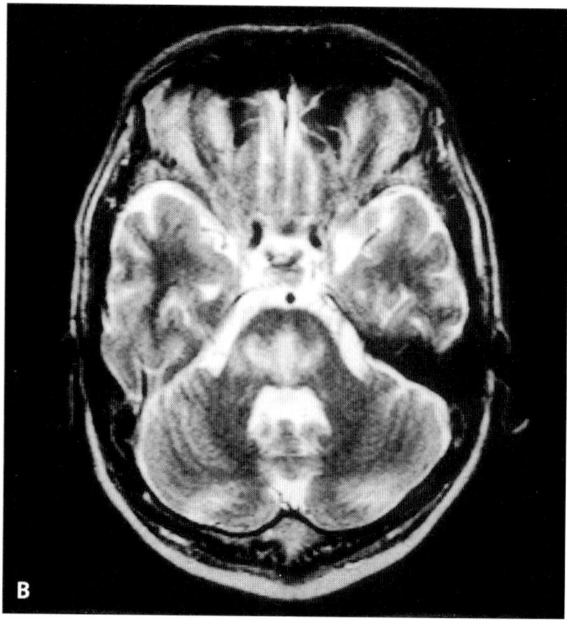

Fig. 4.35A,B. Central pontine myelinolysis. **A** Sagittal SE T1-WI. **B** Axial TSE T2-WI. Within the pons, there is a lesion which is hypointense on the T1-WI and hyperintense on the T2-WI. There is a surrounding rim of normal-appearing pontine parenchyma. On the axial image, the 'trident' shape reflects the position of the corticospinal tracts in the anterior lateral part of the pons

alcoholism can also cause nonspecific deep white matter lesions and periventricular demyelination.

4.9 Intracranial Infection

4.9.1 Imaging Strategy

MRI is superior to CT for the detection of intracranial infections. The pulse-sequences used for the evaluation of intracranial infections are straightforward. Use of a paramagnetic contrast agent is crucial. In most cases, we use the same protocol as proposed for intracranial mass lesions (Table 4.3).

4.9.2 Meningitis

Meningitis is the most common presentation of CNS infection. It can be caused by bacterial, viral, or fungal infection. Clinically, meningitis is an acute febrile illness with severe headache, stiffness of the neck, photophobia, and vomiting. Imaging does not contribute to the diagnosis but is used to monitor the complications of meningeal infections.

Unenhanced scans may show obliteration of the basal cisterns with strong enhancement after contrast-medium administration. In adults, 50% of patients with bacterial meningitis develop complications. The fibropurulent infectious exudate obstructs the CSF flow and leads to hydrocephalus. The infection can spread to the ventricular system, resulting in ventriculitis and choroid plexitis, both showing ependymal enhancement after contrast administration. Subdural effusions are a common complication of meningitis. They are seen as extra-axial fluid collections with smooth contours which displace the cortical veins medially and do not extend into the sulci. They should be differentiated from widened subarachnoidal spaces, where the extra-axial fluid extends into the sulci and does not displace the cortical veins.

An empyema can be caused by meningitis, but the most common cause is sinusitis. MRI shows a lentiform extra-axial fluid collection with strong enhancement of the surrounding pseudomembrane (Fig. 4.36).

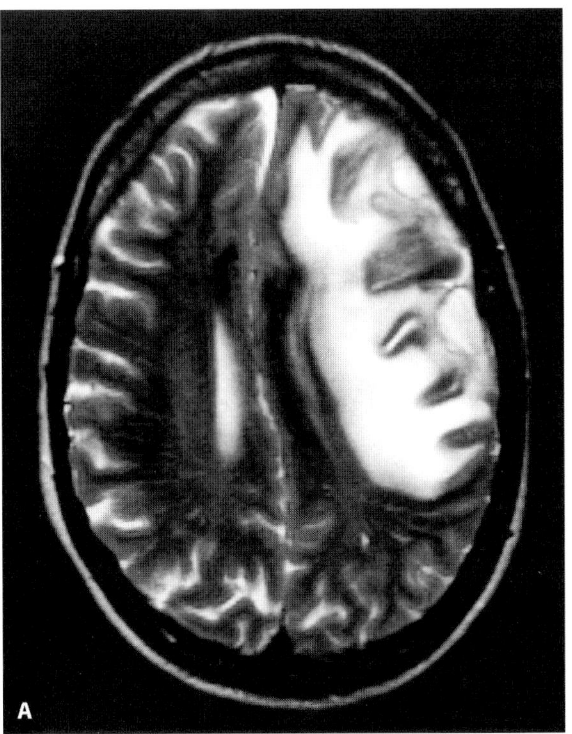

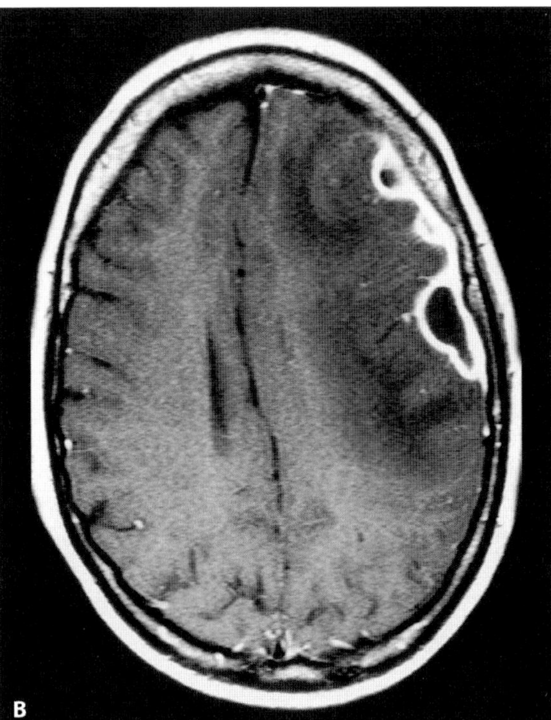

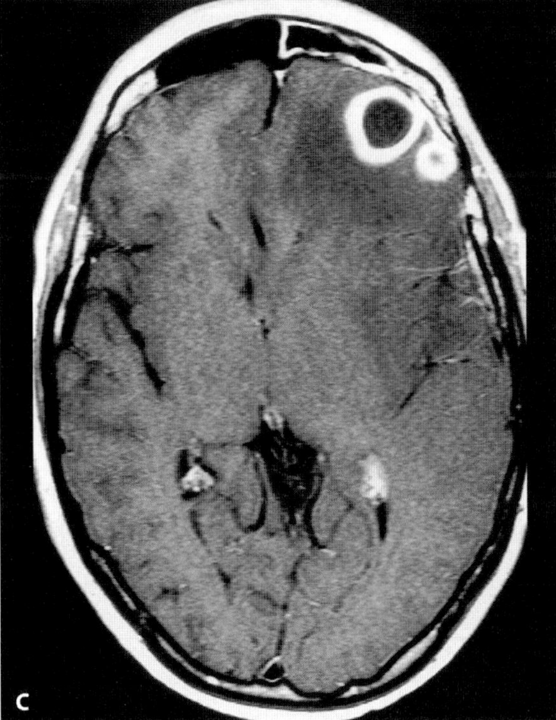

Fig. 4.36A–C. Subdural empyema and intracerebral abscess. **A** Axial TSE T2-WI through the centrum semiovale. **B** Axial Gd-enhanced SE T1-WI (same level as **A**). **C** Axial Gd-enhanced SE T1-WI through the lower frontal lobes. The axial T2-WI shows nodular meningeal thickening over the left frontal convexity; there is extensive vasogenic edema in the white matter of the left cerebral hemisphere. After Gd injection, extra-axial fluid collections are observed. There is strong enhancement of the meninges and surrounding pseudomembranes. In the lower frontal lobe, the pyogenic empyema has spread into the cerebral parenchyma with the formation of an intracerebral abscess, which enhances in a ring-like pattern

Pyogenic meningitis can spread into the cerebral parenchyma causing cerebritis. Hematogenous spread, however, is the most common cause of a cerebritis. MRI shows an ill-defined region of low signal on T1-WI and high signal on T2-WI. Patchy enhancement can be seen after contrast medium administration. When ring enhancement is seen, the cerebritis is evolving into a cerebral abscess (Fig. 4.36). This process of encapsulation may take weeks depending on the organism, immune response, and therapy. An abscess has a thick enhancing wall and surrounding white matter edema. On T2-WI, the wall of the abscess is hypointense. The lesion exerts mass effect. On MR imaging alone, an abscess cannot be differentiated from a brain metastasis or a primary brain tumor (see Table 4.9: ring-enhancing lesions). Because most abscesses result from hematogenous spread of microorganisms, the preferred location is the corticomedullary junction.

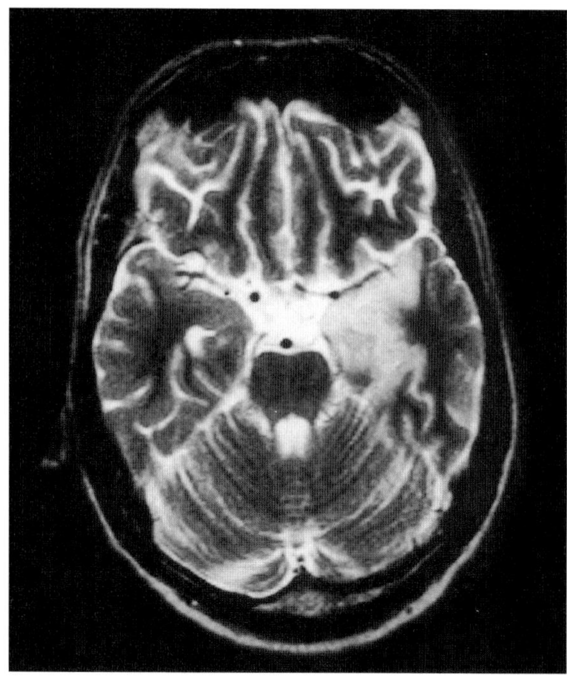

Fig. 4.37. Herpes simplex virus encephalitis. This axial TSE T2-WI was obtained in a patient with Herpes type 1 encephalitis. Note the increased signal intensity of the medial part of the left temporal lobe. There is some mass effect due to edema

4.9.3 Encephalitis

Encephalitis is a diffuse, nonfocal, parenchymal brain infection. The most common causative agents are: herpes simplex virus (HSV), cytomegalovirus, and, in patients with AIDS, the papovaviruses. Most of the encephalitides resemble each other and have few identifying imaging characteristics. Areas of involvement are characterized by mass effect, edema, hyperintensity on T2-WI, and perhaps petechial hemorrhages. A common nonviral cause of encephalitis is toxoplasmosis, especially in immunocompromised patients. ADEM is an autoimmune allergic encephalitis.

4.9.3.1 Herpes Encephalitis

Two types of HSV encephalitis must be distinguished, type I and type II.

HSV type 1 (oral herpes) is the most common cause of sporadic viral encephalitis. It has a predilection for the subfrontal and medial temporal lobes. Although initially unilateral, most patients develop lesions in both hemispheres. The temporal lobe, insular cortex, subfrontal area, and cingulate gyrus are affected. Early MR imaging changes are: gyral effacement due to edema on T1-WI and high signal of the temporal lobe and cingulate gyrus on T2-WI (Fig. 4.37). Bilateral temporal lobe involvement is considered nearly pathognomonic of HSV encephalitis. Later in the course of the disease, T1-WI may demonstrate gray matter hyperintensities in a gyriform pattern (petechial hemorrhages). After contrast administration, gyral enhancement may be observed. HSV encephalitis has a high mortality rate (50%–70%), and those who survive show marked atrophy and encephalomalacia of the temporal and frontal lobes.

The neonatal HSV type 2 (genital herpes) is a diffuse nonfocal encephalitis: panencephalitis. Because the neonatal brain is largely unmyelinated, diffuse edema is difficult to detect with MR imaging. Patchy meningeal or parenchymal enhancement can be seen.

4.9.3.2 HIV Encephalitis and AIDS-Related CNS Infections

The retrovirus that causes AIDS is neurotropic and directly invades the peripheral nervous system and CNS. This virus is the most common pathogen in AIDS patients. Other AIDS-related CNS infections are opportunistic and are caused by *Toxoplasma gondii*, *Cryptococcus neoformans*, and papovaviruses.

4.9.3.2.1
HIV Encephalitis

The HIV virus causes a variety of neurological disorders, including encephalopathy (AIDS dementia complex), myelopathy, and peripheral neuropathy. HIV encephalitis causes marked cerebral atrophy. On T2-WI, confluent or patchy areas of increased signal are observed in the deep white matter, most commonly in the frontal lobes (Fig. 4.38). There is no enhancement after contrast injection.

4.9.3.2.2
Progressive Multifocal Leukoencephalopathy

Progressive multifocal leukoencephalopathy (PML) is a CNS infection caused by a papovavirus. This results in extensive demyelination. Initial T2-WI show multifocal, subcortical, high-signal lesions in the parietal-occipital area. In due course, these lesions become confluent and show central cavitation. Contrast enhancement is a rare finding. Although PML can be unilateral, an asymmetric bilateral distribution is more common. In many cases, the posterior fossa is also affected.

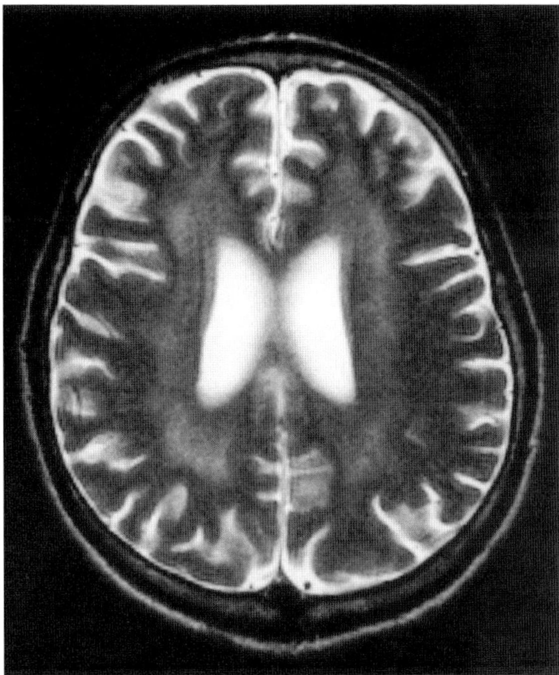

Fig. 4.38. HIV encephalitis. Axial TSE T2-WI in an HIV-infected patient displays confluent areas of increased signal intensity in the deep white matter of both hemispheres. These signal intensity changes are presumed to reflect HIV encephalitis

4.9.3.2.3
Toxoplasmosis

Toxoplasmosis is the most common opportunistic CNS infection in AIDS patients. Most lesions are found on the corticomedullary junction and in the basal ganglia. Lesions are difficult to appreciate on unenhanced T1-WI; after contrast administration, lesions show ring-shaped or nodular enhancement. T2-WI are more sensitive in localizing multifocal lesions. This is of particular importance because multifocality helps to differentiate a toxoplasmosis infection from a primary CNS lymphoma.

4.9.4 Acute Disseminated Encephalomyelitis

Occasionally after a viral infection, a patient develops an autoimmune response to normal white matter resulting in demyelination. ADEM is usually a self-limiting disease and, as opposed to relapsing-remitting MS, is a monophasic disease. Preceding viral infections associated with ADEM include measles, chickenpox, rubella, mumps, pertussis, Epstein-Barr, and viral upper airway infections. Vaccinations are also associated with ADEM. It is mostly a disease of children and young adults, but can be seen in all ages. FLAIR or T2-WI show multifocal subcortical areas of increased SI, with or without involvement of the posterior fossa (Fig. 16.21). Lesions are widely distributed in both hemispheres, usually asymmetrically. After contrast injection, some lesions will enhance on a T1-W sequence. Although most patients recover completely without residual lesions, 10%–20% of patients develop permanent sequelae.

4.9.5 Tuberculosis

Tuberculosis is still a public health problem, not only in developing countries, but also in industrialized nations. CNS tuberculosis results from hematogenous dissemination. Tuberculosis can affect the CNS in two ways:

- Tuberculous meningitis is typically located in the basal cisterns. It causes thickening ('pachymeningitis') and marked enhancement of the basal leptomeninges (Fig. 16.22). The lenticulostriate and thalamoperforating arteries are affected, with infarctions occurring in the basal ganglia and thalami. Hydrocephalus is a common complication. T1-WI after contrast administration show thickening and intense enhancement of the meninges in the basal cisterns.

- Tuberculomas occur in the brain parenchyma, usually in the cortical and subcortical regions near the gray-white matter junction. Most lesions are solitary, which poses a differential diagnostic problem. There are no distinguishing features on unenhanced T1-WI; after contrast administration, parenchymal tuberculomas enhance in a nodular or ring-like fashion.

4.10 The Aging Brain

The morphologic appearance of the brain changes over time. MRI studies reflect the development of the brain. In the neonate, the process of myelination can be followed on T1-WI and T2-WI. Myelination continues into adulthood. Regions of incomplete myelination may persist in the white matter around the trigone of the lateral ventricles, and can been seen well into adulthood as areas with slightly prolonged T1 and T2 relaxation times. In the adult and elderly individual, specific age-related changes occur in the cerebral white matter, CSF spaces, and gray matter.

4.10.1 White Matter Changes in Aging

4.10.1.1 Periventricular Hyperintensities

In almost all adult individuals, one finds so-called 'capping' and 'lining' of the lateral ventricles. The capping regions, which are hyperintense on T2-WI, are found predominantly around the frontal horns of the lateral ventricles. They are usually small, although larger, often symmetric foci can also be found in normal individuals. High-signal rims contiguous with the margins of the lateral ventricles on T2-WI, especially on T2-FLAIR images, are a frequent normal finding. This lining of the ventricular margin is regular and thin in the younger population, but can become thicker and irregular, with extensions into the white matter, in the elderly population. Larger lesions must be differentiated from demyelinating disease and infarcts; the MR imaging appearance can be indistinguishable. Extensive periventricular hyperintensities are also found in hydrocephalus as a result of intraparenchymal leakage of CSF ('interstitial edema').

4.10.1.2 Deep White Matter Hyperintensities

With increasing age, focal hyperintense regions are found in the deep white matter of normal individuals. With the exception of the subcortical U-fibers, they can be found anywhere in the cerebral white matter. These lesions can be small or large and confluent. These foci show high SI on both echoes of a long TR sequence, low SI on T1-WI, and no contrast enhancement or mass effect. There is a correlation between the incidence of these nonspecific white matter lesions and cerebrovascular disease and hypertension. On MR imaging alone, it is often impossible to distinguish these age-related lesions from multifocal disease, although the MR imaging characteristics together with the clinical data usually lead to the correct interpretation.

4.10.1.3 Perivascular Hyperintensities

Perivascular spaces or Virchow-Robin spaces (VRS) are CSF-filled spaces that surround penetrating arteries as they enter the cerebral parenchyma. VRS are found predominantly in the basal ganglia and in the centrum semiovale (Fig. 4.39). On T1-WI, they are seen as punctuate or linear structures with low SI. As VRS are CSF filled, they are not seen on PD-WI, unlike non-specific age-related white matter lesions. On the second echo of a long TR sequence, they have a high SI. VRS follow the signal pattern of CSF on all pulse sequences. The most common location is in the basal part of the putamen and around the anterior commissure, where VRS are an almost constant finding in adults, and a frequent finding in children. Most VRS are small and punctuate, or linear, larger, and more confluent perivascular spaces can occur in the basal ganglia. The occurrence of VRS is age related.

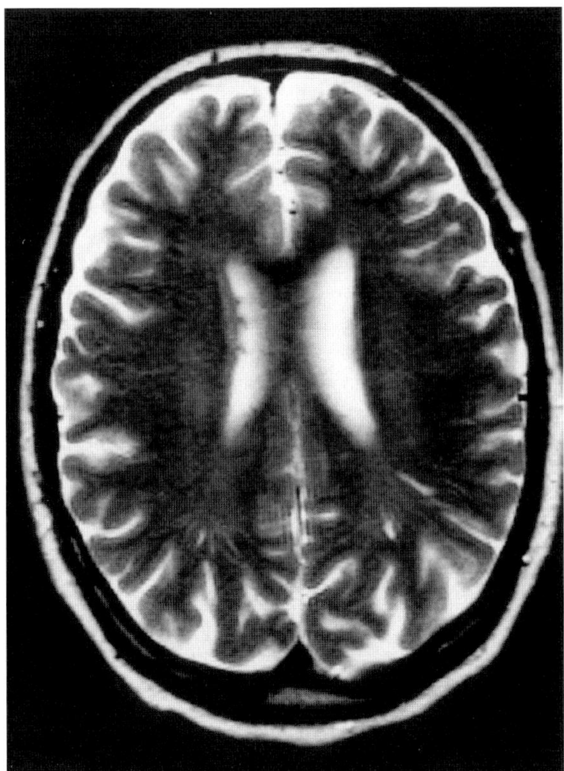

Fig. 4.39. Perivascular Virchow-Robin spaces. This axial TSE T2-WI shows prominent perivascular Virchow-Robin (VRS) spaces in the parietal-occipital white matter of a normal individual. VRS spaces are not visible on PD-W images, because the CSF they contain is isointense to brain on this sequence. On T2-WI, these perivascular spaces are seen as linear areas of increased signal intensity

4.10.2 Age-Related Changes in the CSF Spaces and Cortical Gray Matter

Volume loss of the cerebral parenchyma and subsequent widening of the sulci and cisterns is a normal effect of aging. There is, however, a large overlap with neurodegenerative disease such as Alzheimer-type dementia and Pick's disease. Prominent sulci are also seen in young children up to the age of 1 year. The interhemispheric distance can be as wide as 6 mm in normal neonates.

Widening of the ventricles in elderly patients can be due to atrophy, reflecting central volume loss of the brain. However, ventricular enlargement due to central atrophy may be impossible to differentiate from certain types of hydrocephalus, such as normal pressure hydrocephalus.

4.10.3 Age-Related Changes in Brain Iron

Iron metabolism in the brain is independent of the iron metabolism and storage in the rest of the body. It is an essential element for the maturation and function of the brain. Iron depositions can be detected on MR imaging because of the susceptibility effect. On T2-W scans, iron deposition is seen as hypointense areas. In the first year of life, iron deposition becomes visible in the basal ganglia, substantia nigra red nucleus. In childhood, the dentate nucleus also becomes hypointense on T2-WI. The iron content of the basal ganglia increases with age; the globus pallidus becomes hypointense on T2-WI in the middle-aged and elderly population, and the putamen is hypointense only in the elderly population.

4.11 Craniocerebral Trauma

4.11.1 Acute Trauma

In the acutely traumatized patient, CT remains the initial study of choice. Disadvantages of MRI in the acute situation include:

- Relatively long acquisition times cause problems with regard to patient motion. This disadvantage may be overcome by the use of ultrafast sequences, which are however not always available.
- There are logistic difficulties in installing a traumatized patient in the MR unit. Life support systems, monitoring equipment, and intubation devices should be compatible with the requirements of the MR room.
- The availability of the MR scanner on a stand-by basis may be problematic and interferes with normal patient flow.

For all of these reasons, in most hospitals, CT scanning is the preferred technique in acute trauma patients. Moreover, CT with bone window settings is excellent for the detection of skull fractures.

Acute epidural hemorrhage is a life-threatening situation. Although epidural hemorrhage is seen equally well on MRI and CT, CT remains the preferred technique. CT has the advantage of showing the skull fracture (bone window settings).

Subdural hematoma can be detected equally well with MRI and CT. This is discussed in Chapter 3.

For the detection of acute subarachnoid hemorrhage, CT remains the method of choice. There is, however, increasing evidence that MRI with FLAIR sequences can be used to detect subarachnoid hemorrhage. On FLAIR images, subarachnoid blood appears bright relative to the brain parenchyma. CSF flow artifacts in the basal cisterns constitute a potential pitfall (because they are also bright on FLAIR images) and may lead to erroneous image interpretation (see Sect. 4.7.3).

Acute intracerebral hematoma (<24 h) may be relatively isointense to gray matter and not readily distinguishable from the surrounding brain on MRI scans. The SI changes in intracerebral hemorrhage are discussed further in Chapter 3.

4.11.2 Subacute and Chronic Trauma

Whereas CT is the preferred imaging technique for the evaluation of acute trauma, MR imaging is of great use in the evaluation of trauma patients in the subacute and chronic phases.

Chronic subdural hematomas that are isodense to brain on noncontrast CT are very hyperintense on MR T1-WI because of their methemoglobin content. When a subdural hematoma contains blood of varying ages, due to repeated episodes of bleeding, MRI may show layers of different SI, reflecting varying phases of the blood-breakdown process.

Very small petechial hemorrhages, in the setting of diffuse axonal injury (DAI), are frequently missed on CT but well seen on MR imaging, provided spoiled GRE or echoplanar (EPI) sequences are used (Fig. 4.40). These lesions are the result of shearing injuries due to rotational acceleration and deceleration forces, commonly encountered in motor vehicle accidents and blunt trauma to the head. DAI lesions occur in the cerebral hemispheres (subcortical brain parenchyma, gray-white matter junction, centrum semiovale), corpus callosum, basal ganglia, brainstem, and cerebellum. Whenever there is a history of previous head trauma, a spoiled GRE sequence, which is highly sensitive to blood-breakdown products such as hemosiderin and ferritin, should be routinely added to the MRI scanning protocol. The visibility of hemorrhagic DAI lesions in the chronic stage is improved by strongly T2*-WI on MRI, i.e., imaging at high field strength using sequences with longer TE. DAI lesions are seen as punctate hypointense foci; multiple lesions are frequent. We use a FLASH sequence, with dual TE of 15 ms and 35 ms. More lesions are seen on the longer TE images, but susceptibility artifacts from the air-containing structures in the skull base (mastoid air cells, paranasal sinuses) may mask lesions in the lower frontal lobes and temporal lobes. As an alternative to GRE imaging, an EPI sequence may be employed. EPI scans are also very sensitive to susceptibility artifacts caused by blood-breakdown products. Nonhemorrhagic DAI lesions can be detected with PD or FLAIR images. Our protocol for imaging the patient with a history of trauma is given in Table 4.24.

Post-traumatic encephalomalacia is better appreciated with MR imaging than with CT, because of the absence of bone artifacts and the multiplanar imaging capabilities of MR. Foci of encephalomalacia often result from cortical contusions and should be looked for in the basal frontal and anterior temporal lobes. These regions are vulnerable to deceleration injury. They are seen as areas of tissue loss, which are hyperintense on T2-WI. On PD or FLAIR images, the area of tissue loss is isointense to CSF and is surrounded by a higher SI rim of gliosis.

4.12 Seizures

The primary goal of MRI in the evaluation of epilepsy is to identify and localize the neuropathologic substrate of a partial onset seizure. The diagnosis and localization of the lesion determines the therapeutic possibilities. Many different abnormalities can cause epilepsy (Table 4.25). Most of these abnormalities are dealt with in other chapters; in this section, we will discuss mesial temporal sclerosis and a general imaging strategy for epilepsy.

4.12.1 Mesial Temporal Sclerosis

Temporal lobe epilepsy is the most common type of medically intractable epilepsy. Mesial temporal sclero-

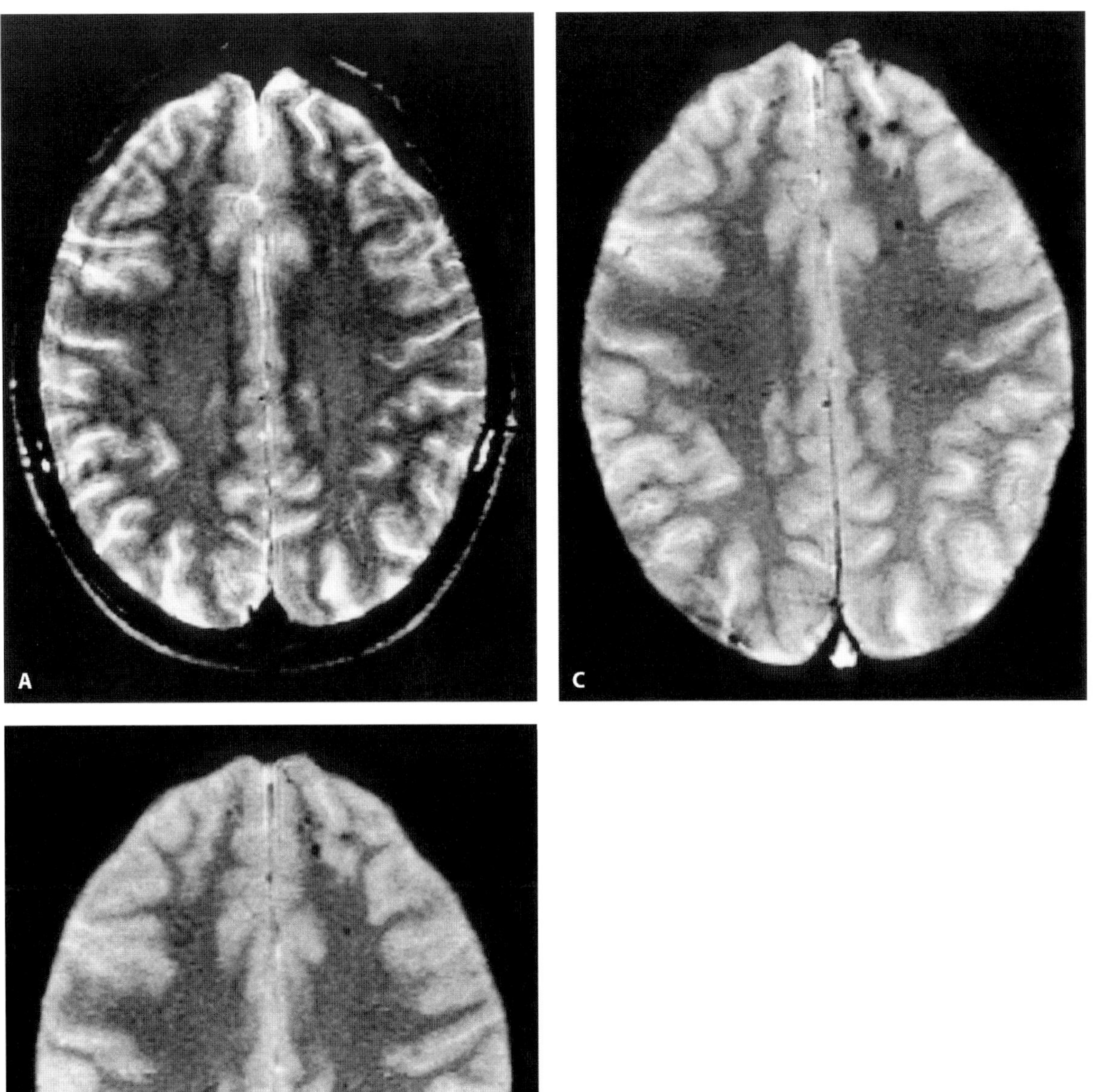

Fig. 4.40A–C. Diffuse axonal injury. **A** Axial TSE T2-WI. **B** Axial partial flip-angle GRE T2*-WI [echo time (TE)=15 ms]. **C** Axial partial flip-angle GRE T2*-WI (TE=35 ms). This 17-year-old man had suffered a motorcycle accident 8 months prior to the present examination. Although the axial TSE T2-WI is mildly degraded by motion artifacts, no signal abnormalities are observed. Conversely, the GRE images show multiple, punctate, hypointense lesions at the corticomedullary junction and in the subcortical white matter. The pattern of distribution is typical for diffuse axonal injury due to shearing stresses. The susceptibility artifact due to old blood-breakdown products (hemosiderin) is more pronounced on the second GRE image, due to the longer TE value

Table 4.24. Subacute and chronic trauma protocol. The sagittal T1-W sequence is used for detecting acute or subacute hemorrhage (methaemoglobin), and for sequelae such as post-traumatic encephalomalacia, The turbo-FLAIR sequence and TSE T2-W sequences are useful for the visualization of cerebral edema, and non-hemorrhagic diffuse axonal injury lesions as well as post-traumatic gliosis. The dual echo GRE (FLASH) sequence is used for the detection of blood degradation products (hemosiderin), The first echo (15 ms) are used for evaluating the basal frontal and temporal lobes, the brainstem and cerebellum. Lesions in the hemispheric gray-white matter junction are better seen on the second echo (35 ms) images.

Pulse sequence	WI	Plane	No. of sections	TR (ms)	TE (ms)	TI (ms)	Flip angle	Echo train length	Section thickness (mm)	Matrix	FOV	recFOV	No. of acq.
1. Sagittal T2-W sequence													
SE	T1	sag	19	600	10–20	–	90/180	–	5	256 or better	230–240	100	1–2
2. Axial T2-W sequence (single echo)													
TSE	T2	ax	19	3000–6000	90–130	–	90/180	7–15	5	512	230–240	75	1–2
3. Axial T2-W turbo FLAIR sequence													
Turbo FLAIR	T2	ax	19	6000–10000	100–150	1800–2200	90/180	7–11	5	512	230–240	75	1–2
4. Axial and/or coronal GRE sequence with 'susceptibility' weighting													
GRE (FLA SH)	sus-cept-ibility	ax/cor	15	750	15 and 35	–	20	–	6	256 or better	230–240	75	1–2
5. Diffusion-weighted SE-EPI sequence (optional)													
SE-EPI	diffu-sion	ax	12–15	∞	100–140	–	90/180	–	5	128	230–300	75	1

Abbreviations: *WI* weighted image, *TR* repetition time (ms); *TI* inversion time (ms); *TE* echo time (ms); *TD* time delay (sec); *no part* number of partitions; *Matrix* (phase × frequency matrix); *FOV* field of view (mm); *recFOV* % rectangular field of view

Table 4.25. Causes of partial-onset seizures (Jack 1995)

Tumors	Astrocytoma Oligodendrogioma Ganglioma DNET Metastasis
Migration disorders	Tuberous sclerosis Focal cortical dysplasia Schizencephaly Nodular heterotophia Laminar heterotoppia Lissencephaly Hemimegaloencephaly
Vascular malformations	AVM Cavernous angioma Sturge-Weber
Mesial temporal sclerosis	
Brain injury	Ischemia Trauma

sis (MTS) is the most common pathological finding in these cases, and the outcome of surgery in this group is excellent. MTS is characterized by local tissue loss in the hippocampus, amygdala, parahippocampal gyrus, mesial temporal cortex, and entorhinal cortex. The terms mesial temporal sclerosis, hippocampal sclerosis, and Ammon's horn sclerosis are used interchangeably, but the extent of the lesion differs for each term. With MR imaging, the main findings are the hippocampal changes, and in these cases, the correct term would be hippocampal sclerosis. The classic form is often associated with a preceding history of febrile convulsions. In the majority of cases, the abnormality is bilateral but asymmetric, and the most affected side is presumed to be the origin of the seizures. The patho-anatomical substrate is cell loss and gliosis with or without local tissue loss. On MR imaging, this can be seen as a focal signal change on T1-WI and T2-WI and as focal atrophy. The abnormalities are best appreciated on coronal slices, preferably orientated perpendicular to the long axis of the temporal lobe. T1-WI show hippocampal atrophy and dilatation of the temporal horn (Fig. 4.41). T2-WI show an increased SI of the hippocampus (Fig. 4.41). The tissue loss in not mandatory; increased SI of the hippocampus is the most reliable sign. FLAIR sequences are more sensitive to the signal changes than (fast) SE sequences. There is no enhancement of the hippocampal sclerosis after contrast medium administration.

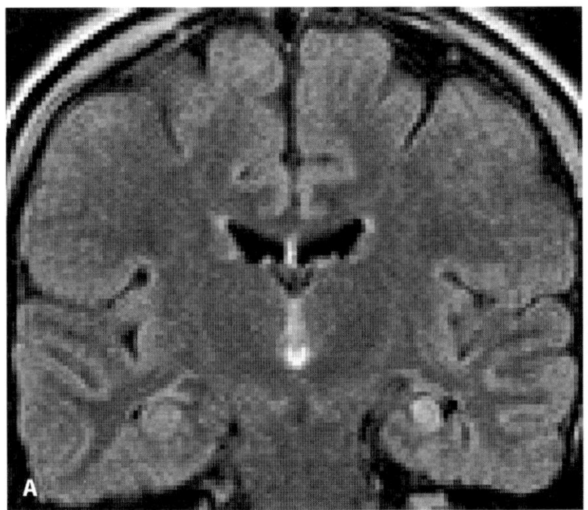

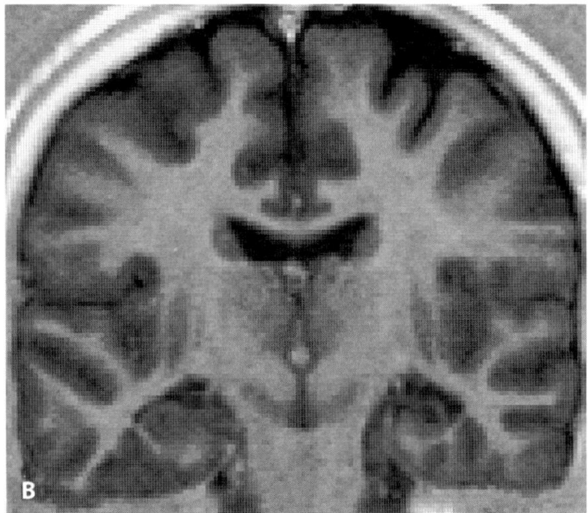

Fig. 4.41A,B. Mesial temporal sclerosis. **A** Coronal FLAIR T2-WI through the hippocampus. **B** Coronal IR-T1-WI (same slice position). On the FLAIR T2-W sequence, there is an area of abnormally increased signal intensity in the left hippocampus. IR T1-WI shows focal tissue loss with widening of the left temporal horn. T1-WI show hippocampal atrophy and dilatation of the temporal horn. T2-WI show an increased signal intensity of the hippocampus

Table 4.26. Seizure protocol. The first three sequences in this protocol provide a general survey of the brain. Their purpose is to rule out tumor, vascular malformations (e.g. cavernous malformations), gross developmental anomalies, infection, etc. The latter three sequences are specifically focused on the hippocampal region, to detect mesial temporal sclerosis. They should be oriented perpendicular to the long axis of the temporal lobe. In a patient with post-traumatic seizures an additional gradient echo sequence must be added in order to rule out diffuse axonal injury sequelae

Pulse sequence	WI	Plane	No. of sections	TR (ms)	TE (ms)	TI (ms)	Flip angle	Echo train length	Section thickness (mm)	Matrix	FOV	recFOV	No. of acq.
1. Sagittal T1-W sequence													
SE	T1	sag	19	600	10–20	–	90/180	–	5	256 or better	230–240	100	1–2
2. Axial T2-W sequence (single echo)													
TSE	T2	ax	19–25	3000–6000	90–130	–	90/180	7–15	5	512	230–240	75	1–2
3. Axial T2-W turbo FLAIR sequence													
Turbo FLAIR	T2	ax	19	6000–10000	100–150	1800–2200	90/180	7–11	5	512	230–240	75	1–2
4. Coronal TSE T2-W sequence with 3 mm slice thickness													
TSE	T2	cor	19–25	3000–8000	90–130	–	90/180	7–15	3	512	≤230	75	1–3
5. Coronal turbo-FLAIR T2-W sequence with 3 mm slice thickness													
Turbo FLAIR	T2	cor	19–25	6000–10000	100–150	1800–2200	90/180	7–11	3	512	≤230	75	1–2
6. Coronal MP-RAGE sequence with thin slices													
GRE (MP-RAGE)	T1	cor	1 slab (160–200 mm)	10	4		12	–	1	256 or better	≤230	75	1

Abbreviations: *WI* weighted image: *TR* repetition time (ms); *TI* inversion time (ms); *TE* echo time (ms); *TD* time delay (sec); *no part* number of partitions; *Matrix* (phase × frequency matrix); *FOV* field of view (mm); *recFOV* % rectangular field of view

4.12.2 MR Imaging Strategy for Epilepsy

Imaging protocols for the diagnosis of hippocampal sclerosis vary widely from center to center. An imaging protocol for epilepsy should be guided by the location of the epileptogenic focus as provided by the clinical presentation and the electroencephalogram (EEG). For general screening, one can substitute axial turbo FLAIR and TSE T2-W sequences for the traditional double-echo long TR sequence (Table 4.26). The imaging protocol should include most cerebral pathologies associated with seizures, including cortical development disorders. Therefore, a coronal T1-W sequence with thin slices should be added, e.g., an MP-RAGE sequence. Cortical alterations, e.g., migration disorders, can be detected on this high-resolution scan, and side-to-side comparison of the hippocampus can be made. A coronal turbo-FLAIR sequence will show signal changes in the hippocampus more clearly than the conventional T2-WI. When there is a suspicion of old hemorrhagic foci or cavernous malformations, a partial flip-angle GRE sequence or EPI sequence should be added. Finally, the imaging protocol must be adapted to the equipment that is available (field strength, gradient performance, available sequences, etc.).

Further Reading

Armed Forces Institute of Pathology (1994) Tumors of the central nervous system. Armed Forces Institute of Pathology, Washington DC

Atlas SW (1996) Magnetic resonance imaging of the brain and spine. Lippincott-Raven, Philadelphia

Barkovich JA (2000) Pediatric neuroimaging, 3rd edn. Lippincott Williams and Wilkins, Philadelphia

Byrd SE, Darling CF, Wilczynski MA (1993) White matter of the brain: maturation and myelination magnetic resonance in infants and children. Neuroimaging Clin North Am 3:247–266

Castillo M (1997) Prethrombolysis brain imaging: trends and controversies. AJNR Am J Neuroradiol 18:1830–1833

Castillo M (guest ed) (1998) New techniques in MR neuroimaging. In: Magnetic resonance imaging clinics of North America 1998, vol 6. Saunders, Philadelphia

Finelli DA, Hurst GC, Gullapalli RP (1998) T1-W three dimensional magnetisation transfer MR of the brain: improved lesion contrast enhancement. AJNR Am J Neuroradiol 19:59–64

Gilman S (1998) Imaging the brain (first of two parts). N Engl J Med 338:812–820

Gilman S (1998) Imaging the brain (second of two parts). N Engl J Med 338:889–896

Hoang TA, Hasso AN (1994) Intracranial vascular malformations. Neuroimaging Clin North Am 4:823–847

Jack CR (1995) Magnetic resonance imaging: neuroimaging and anatomy. Neuroimaging Clin North Am 5:597–622

Lee SH, Rao KCVG, Zimmerman RA (1992) Cranial MRI and CT, 3rd edn. McGraw-Hill, New York

Lufkin RB (1998) The MRI manual, 2nd edn. Mosby-Year Book, St Louis

Osborn AG (1994) Diagnostic neuroradiology. Mosby-Year Book, St Louis

Sorensen AG, Reimer P (2000) Cerebral MR perfusion imaging: principles and current applications. Thieme, Stuttgart

van der Knaap MS, Valk J (1995) Magnetic resonance of myelin; myelination and myelin disorders. Springer, Berlin Heidelberg New York

Addendum. Classification of central nervous system tumors (WHO Classification)

1. Neuroepithelial (neuroectodermal)
   - 1.1. astrocytoma
   - 1.2. oligodendroglioma
   - 1.3. ependymoma
   - 1.4. mixed gliomas
   - 1.5. choroid plexus tumors
   - 1.6. uncertain origin
   - 1.7. neuronal and mixed neuronal/glial
   - 1.8. pineal parenchymal tumors (pineocytoma, pineoblastoma, mixed)
   - 1.9. embryonal (medulloepithelioma, PNET, medulloblastoma, neuroblastoma, retinoblastoma, ependymoblastoma)
2. Tumors of nerve sheath
   - 2.1. schwannoma
   - 2.2. neurofibroma
   - 2.3. malignant (peripheral) nerve sheath tumor
3. Tumors of the meninges
   - 3.1. meningioma
   - 3.2. mesenchymal (benign / malignant / hemangiopericytoma)
   - 3.3. primary melanotic lesions
4. Lymphoma
5. Germ cell tumors
   - 5.1. germinoma
6. Cysts and tumor-like lesions
   - 6.1. Rathke cleft cyst
   - 6.2. epidermoid cyst
   - 6.3. dermoid cyst
   - 6.4. colloid cyst
7. Tumors of the sellar region
   - 7.1. pituitary adenoma
   - 7.2. craniopharyngioma
8. Local extension of regional tumors
9. Metastases
10. Unclassified

Magnetic Resonance Imaging of the Spine

5

J. W. M. Van Goethem

Contents

5.1 Patient Positioning and Coils

5.1.1 Positioning of the Patient

In magnetic resonance (MR) imaging of the cervical and thoracic spine, patients are positioned supine, head first. When imaging the lower thoracic spine, patients can be positioned feet first if they are not too tall. Otherwise, their feet may reach the end of the magnet bore before they are in the correct position. If the magnet is open on both sides, this may not be a problem. Children are positioned feet first for thoracic examinations. We use a knee support for patient comfort, which in turn is favorable for the image quality since patients are less likely to move during the examination.

MR imaging of the lumbar and sacral spine is best performed with the patient in supine position and feet first. This tends to diminish claustrophobic reactions. We do not use a knee support in imaging the lumbar spine, since this reduces the lumbar lordosis and may lead to an underestimation of disc herniations. Only when patients are unable to remain motionless without support of the legs, e.g., patients with substantial back pain, should a knee support be used. In any case, the patient should be positioned as comfortably as possible to minimize movement artifacts. On high field magnets with strong gradients, ear plugs or a headphone should be provided to the patient.

5.1.2 Coils

In general, two types of coils are used in spine imaging: linearly polarized (LP) and circularly polarized (CP) coils. CP coils are constructed to generate more signal and, hence, provide images with a higher signal-to-noise ratio (SNR). Therefore, CP coils are preferred.

Although all coils are designed to receive the signal generated by the patient during imaging, only certain coils are also used to transmit the radiofrequency (RF) pulses used in MR imaging. These so-called send-receive coils tend to produce better images, since the RF transmission is performed closer to the region of interest.

Usually, one type of coil can be used for imaging the thoracic and lumbar spine. It consists of a flat box incorporated in a lumbar (or thoracic) support or directly incorporated into the patient table. Depending on the type of coil and the manufacturer, these coils generate a maximum field-of-view (FOV) of 25–40 cm.

A cervical spine (CS) coil is usually more raised so that it provides better support for the patient's neck. In general, it is made of a lower and an upper part, whereby the latter is fixed in position after the patient is placed on the lower part. The maximum FOV of these coils usually covers the craniocervical junction, the CS, and the cervicothoracic junction. Depending on the coil design and the patient's stature, imaging down to the first to sixth thoracic vertebra may be possible. Some manufacturers also provide circular solenoid coils, which can be placed around the neck. These coils tend to generate a smaller FOV. Flexible coils can be used in patients who cannot be positioned in the normal cervical coil, e.g., patients with large neck collars or extreme thoracic kyphosis.

If the magnet is equipped with phased-array spine coils, they should be used since coil selection and patient positioning in relation to the coil are less critical. The use of several phased-array coils simultaneously allows for a larger FOV. Moreover, new software solutions, known as parallel acquisition technique (PAT) and SENSE, permit a considerable reduction in acquisition time using phased-array coils in spine imaging with a large FOV. If phased-array spine coils are not available and a very large section of the spine, or even the entire spine, needs to be imaged, the built-in body coil should be used. Depending on the homogeneity of the magnetic field outside the magnet center and the length of the gradient coils, 45–50 cm of the spine may be visualized (which is the complete spine in children or small individuals). Indications for imaging the entire spine without use of phased-array coils should be carefully monitored. If the body coil is used, image quality and, in particular, contrast and spatial resolution are not up to par with images generated with local coils. Therefore, subtle lesions may be missed, e.g., smaller disc herniations or intramedullary lesions as in multiple sclerosis (MS). It is, therefore, preferable to perform separate examinations of the cervical, thoracic, and/or lumbosacral segments of the spine in such cases.

5.1.3 Positioning of the Coil in Relation to the Patient

When imaging the thoracic spine, it can be useful to attach one or more markers on the skin of the patient's back prior to starting the examination. These markers simplify the problem of determining the examined levels afterwards, especially in a system in which it is not possible to obtain large FOV (50 cm) localizer images with the body coil while the surface coil is already in place. The use of a console-operated table movement, if available, also facilitates this problem.

When positioning patients in the cervical coil, one must try to place the coil relatively low down so that cervico-thoracic junction is included in the images. To minimize movement, a cervical collar can be used for cervical MR examinations. In patients with a very pronounced thoracic kyphosis and/or stiff CS, normal positioning in the cervical coil may be impossible. Some coils allow imaging without the upper part attached, but one still has to pay attention to be sure the distance between the coil and the neck is not too large. It sometimes helps when cushions are placed under the patient's buttocks and/or legs. In extreme cases, it may be necessary to allow the patient to lay his or her head on a pillow. In these cases, one can use a flexible or collar-like coil or, if this is not available, the body coil. This may also be the case in patients with dyspnea, who are unable to lie completely flat.

For MR imaging of the lumbar spine without phased-array coils, the center of the coil should be positioned about 5 cm above the iliac crest (which is usually at the L4–5 level). The conus medullaris and the sacrum should be included in the FOV. For all examinations, one should try to match the center of the region of interest to the center of the bore of the magnet.

5.1.4
Patient Information

Patients should be cleared for any MR imaging contraindications before they enter the magnet room. They should also be informed of the benefits and potential risks of MR imaging before the examination is performed. In particular, before administering intravenous contrast products, informed consent (written or oral) should be obtained.

The scenario and length of the examination should be explained in understandable terms. It is helpful to keep the patient informed during the examination about the length of each sequence. That way, swallowing and movement can be minimized since patients will have a better idea about the time they must keep still.

As with all MR examinations, the patient should be instructed to lie as motionless as possible. Excessive thoracic or abdominal breathing movements should be prevented when imaging that region. In imaging the CS, the patient must be instructed not to swallow or at least minimize swallowing during the measurements. Since this is very hard for some patients, it may be useful to leave enough time between measurements (more than 15 s) to allow the patient to swallow or cough.

When examining children, we allow a parent(s) to be present in the magnet room. With young children (<6 years), parents are sometimes placed together with their child inside the magnet, lying in pronc position, head to head with the child. With anxious patients, it can be helpful to leave a member of the nursing staff inside the magnet room to calm the patient down when necessary. Anxiolytic medication can be beneficial in claustrophobic patients.

MRI in patients with metallic or electronic implants is discussed further below (see 5.2.3.2 The Postoperative Lumbar Spine).

5.2
Sequence Protocol

5.2.1
General Guidelines

In general, both sagittal and axial images are obtained in spine imaging.

T1- and T2-weighted images (WI) offer different and complementary information.

On T2-WI, normal intervertebral discs are bright. With aging, water loss occurs, the T2 relaxation time shortens, and the discs gradually become darker (degenerative disc disease or 'black disc disease'). However, with longer echo train lengths (ETL) (more echoes sampled after each 90° pulse), normal discs also become darker due to certain physical effects (Fig. 5.1).

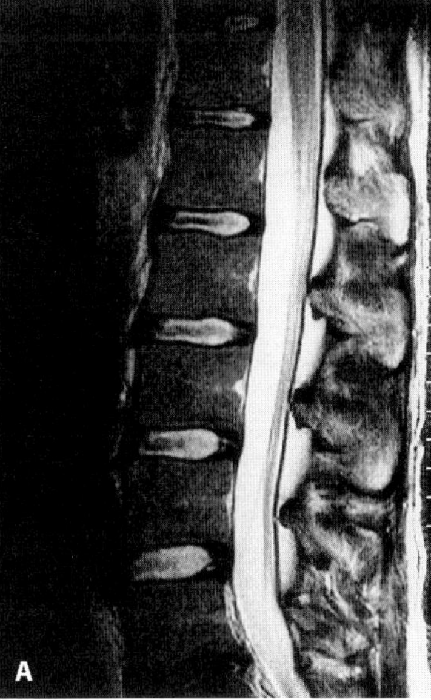

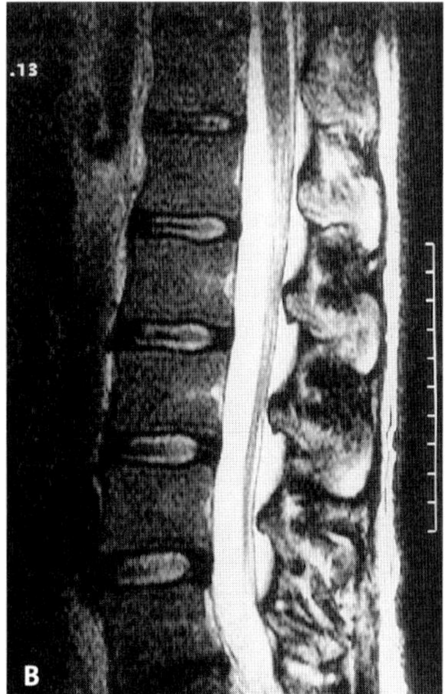

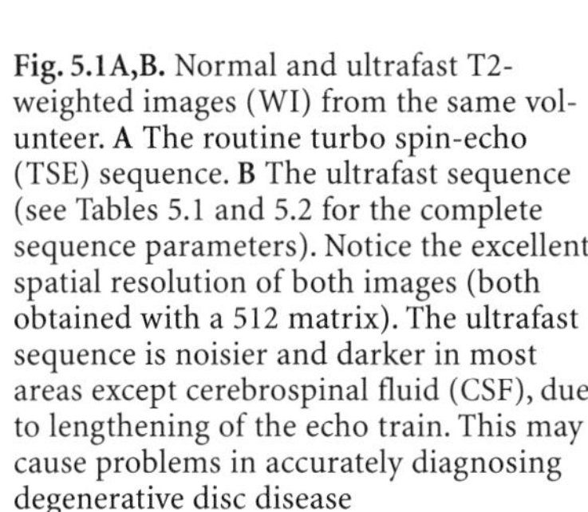

Fig. 5.1A,B. Normal and ultrafast T2-weighted images (WI) from the same volunteer. **A** The routine turbo spin-echo (TSE) sequence. **B** The ultrafast sequence (see Tables 5.1 and 5.2 for the complete sequence parameters). Notice the excellent spatial resolution of both images (both obtained with a 512 matrix). The ultrafast sequence is noisier and darker in most areas except cerebrospinal fluid (CSF), due to lengthening of the echo train. This may cause problems in accurately diagnosing degenerative disc disease

Therefore, in order to diagnose degenerative disc disease, sagittal T2-WI with a relatively short ETL are preferable (e.g., 15). Sagittal T2-WI are also excellent to visualize the spinal cord and cauda equina nerve roots. Finally, spinal canal stenosis and impressions on the thecal sac are most easily recognized on sagittal T2-WI. One should be aware of the fact that turbo spin-echo (TSE) or fast spin-echo (FSE) T2-W sequences are not effective in diagnosing marrow-infiltrating disease, unless fat-suppression techniques are used.

Sagittal T1-WI are more sensitive than conventional nonfat-suppression TSE/FSE T2-WI in detecting bone-marrow disease, e.g., degenerative endplate changes or vertebral metastases, but short T1 inversion recovery (STIR) or other fat-suppression T2-WI are also able to increase the detection of certain bone marrow diseases. Also, the difference between osteophytes and disc material (with or without posterior disc protrusion) is usually better appreciated on T1-WI, especially in the CS.

The epidural fat tissue in the lumbar (and thoracic) spine is very bright on T1-WI and contrasts well with the dural sac and the intervertebral disc. This is why axial T1-WIs are preferred in the (thoraco-)lumbar region. Since acquisition times are substantially shortened with the newer techniques, we also use axial T2-WIs in our standard imaging protocol of the (thoraco-)lumbar spine. This sequence allows excellent visualization of the nerve roots in relation to other structures, especially the intervertebral disc.

In the CS, there is no epidural fat tissue, but an epidural venous plexus. To optimize contrast between the dural sac and the intervertebral discs, axial T2-WIs are preferred. These images are also useful in detecting medullary disease. On conventional spin-echo (SE) and TSE T2-WI, it is difficult to differentiate osteophytes from disc material. On gradient-echo (GRE) images, these can usually be differentiated because bone is markedly hypointense and disc is hyperintense. Moreover, the shorter echo time of gradient-echo T2-W sequences in comparison to spin-echo sequences reduces CSF-induced pulsation artifacts.

5.2.2 Localizer Images

After positioning the patient, mid-sagittal and coronal localizer images (syn. scout images, survey images) are obtained. The type of sequences used for this purpose is of little importance and depends on the manufacturer of the system. The FOV of the localizers should be larger than the FOV of the images desired. The same coil (surface or body) should be used as the one to be used during the actual examination. The coronal localizers are positioned so that they intersect the spine.

When imaging the thoracic spine, extra-large FOV sagittal localizers using the body coil (or phased-array coils) are useful to determine the exact levels to be imaged. Sagittal sequences are positioned parallel to the spine on coronal localizers. Axial images are positioned on sagittal localizers, perpendicular to the spinal canal, rather than parallel to the intervertebral disc space.

5.2.3 Specific Types of Sequences

The sequences used in MR imaging of the spine depend on the kind of pathology (expected to be) found.

5.2.3.1 Degenerative Disc Disease

In imaging patients with degenerative spinal disease, sagittal T1 and T2-W SE or TSE sequences are used for all spine examinations. In the CS, axial T2-W GRE sequences are added, while in the thoracic and lumbosacral region, axial T1-W SE images are applied. In axial T2-WI, GRE sequences are preferable over SE sequences since SE sequences, and especially TSE sequences, tend to be severely degraded by cerebrospinal fluid (CSF) flow artifacts. Also, as mentioned before, GRE sequences are of value in differentiating between disc and bone, e.g., soft disc herniation versus osteophytic spur formation.

For all axial and sagittal T1-WI, TSE is preferable over SE imaging since the imaging time is considerably shorter. The slight blurring or loss in spatial resolution is an acceptable penalty to pay for the shorter imaging time (Fig. 5.2). In choosing a TSE T2-W sequence for sagittal imaging, one should experiment with different ETLs. If a long ETL is chosen (>10), the discs become darker, the contrast with the vertebrae decreases, and only the bright CSF stands out. An ETL should be chosen that is long, but with an acceptable remaining signal of the intervertebral discs to be able to differentiate between normal and degenerative discs (Fig. 5.1). Some

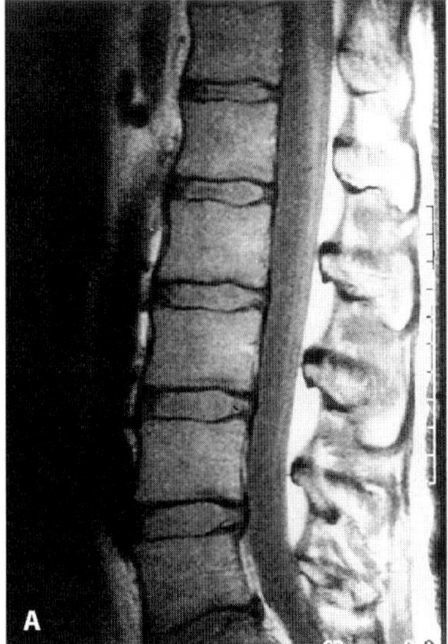

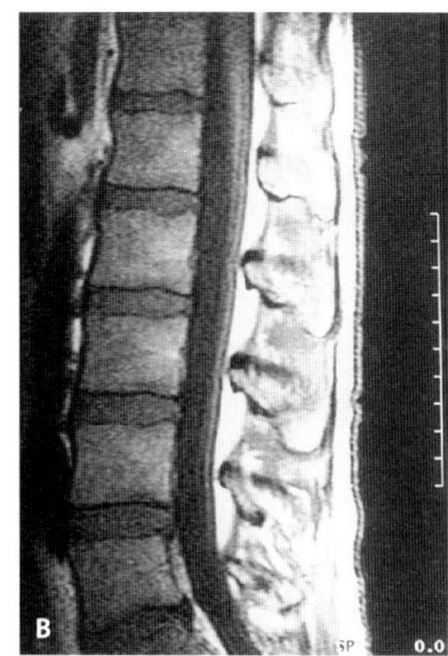

Fig. 5.2A,B. Turbo spin-echo (TSE) and spin-echo (SE) T1-weighted images (WI). Sagittal T1-WI from the same volunteer. **A** The routine TSE sequence (see Table 5.1 for the complete sequence parameters). **B** The SE sequence (TR 500, TE 15, 256 × 512, TA 4'19"). The SE sequence has a lower resolution in the phase direction (anteroposterior) to partially compensate for the longer acquisition time. Image contrast is very similar, but signal-to-noise ratio (SNR) is clearly superior in the TSE image. Therefore, there is no reason for using SE T1-W sequences in normal spine imaging

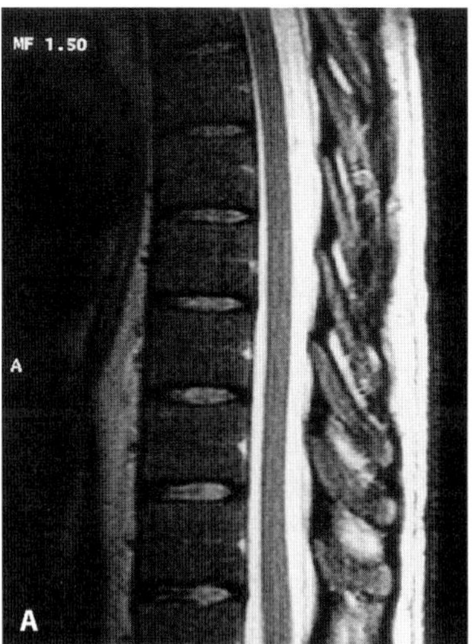

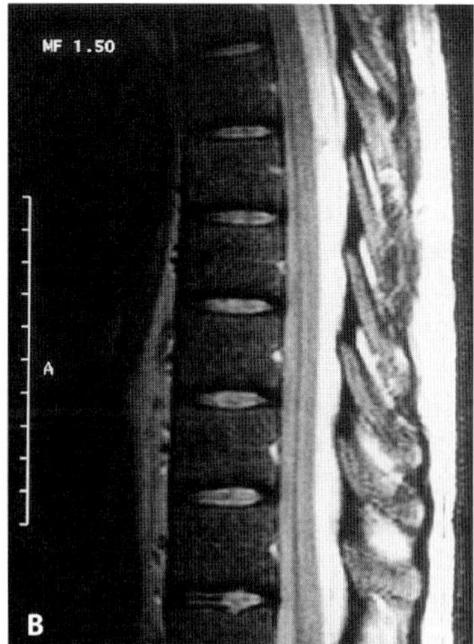

Fig. 5.3A,B. Cerebrospinal fluid (CSF) flow compensation. Sagittal T2-weighted images (WI) of the mid-thoracic spine from the same volunteer. **A** The routine TSE sequence for the thoracic spine. **B** The sequence without CSF-flow compensation (actually the sequence used in the lumbar spine) (see Table 5.1 for the complete sequence parameters). The latter (**B**) is slightly blurred, especially at the level of the thoracic medulla, due to the non-compensated up and downward movement of the CSF (pulsating CSF in the read direction)

sagittal T2-W sequences are flow compensated; this means they are specifically designed for imaging the (cervical and thoracic) spine by minimizing flow artifacts caused by the craniocaudal CSF pulsations. If these sequences are available, they should be used (Fig. 5.3).

In the CS, axial images are usually positioned from C2 down to T1. Since the cervical neural foramina are not visible on sagittal images, axial images should be obtained even if no pathology is discernible on the sagittal images. No examination of the CS is complete without axial images. In the lumbosacral or thoracic spine, axial images should only be obtained at the level(s) of the (most) affected discs (as seen on the sagittal T2-WI). The thoracolumbar neural foramina are much more accurately displayed on sagittal images than on axial images (Fig. 5.4).

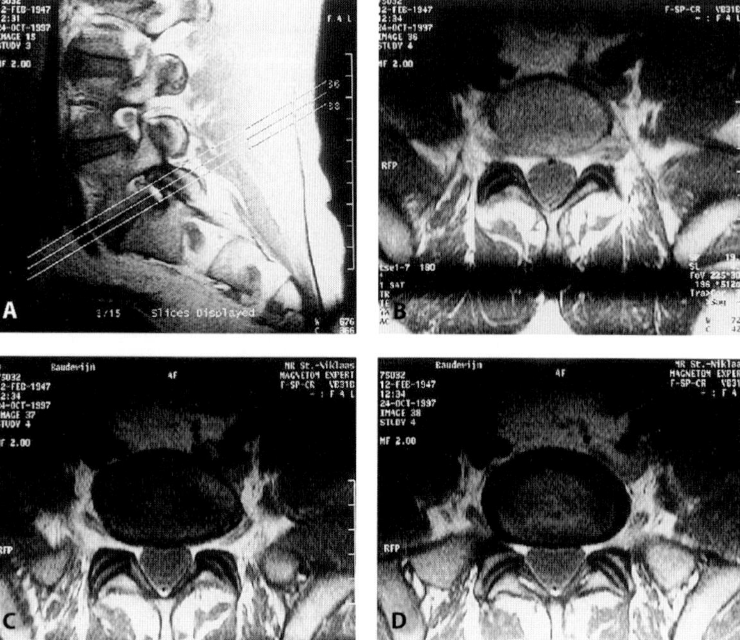

Fig. 5.4A–D. Foraminal stenosis. Foraminal stenosis can be underestimated on axial images. In this figure, three consecutive axial images through the neural foramen are depicted (**B,C,D**) and cross-referenced on the parasagittal image (**A**). Note that only the first of the axial images (**B**, *right upper quadrant*) actually represents the part of the foramen through which the nerve roots pass. Anatomic relationships in the neural foramen are much better depicted on the sagittal image. The slight deformity or compression of the nerve sheath as seen on this image is not visible on the axial images

5.2.3.2
Postoperative Lumbar Spine

Additional axial SE T1-WI after intravenous gadolinium injection should be obtained in patients after lumbar disc surgery. The postcontrast images should be obtained as quickly as possible after gadolinium injection (sequence completed within 5–8 min after injection). The most important use of gadolinium is in differentiating scar tissue from (recurrent or residual) disc herniation, since the latter is generally accepted to be a possible indication for reintervention. Also, the evaluation of enhancement of nerves, meninges, posterior spinal facet joints (i.e., zygapophyseal joints), and perispinal soft tissues is important in some patients. Some authors also stress the usefulness of (T)SE T2-WI or fluid-attenuated inversion recovery (FLAIR) T2-WI in addition to or instead of T1-WI after gadolinium in the differentiation of recurrent disc herniation and epidural fibrosis.

Fat suppression can be used to differentiate enhancing scar tissue from epidural fatty tissue in i.v. gadolinium-enhanced T1-WI of the postoperative spine. However, the detection of abnormal postoperative nerve root enhancement may be more difficult to differentiate from the normal small amount of enhancement usually seen on fat-suppression images. In some rare cases, fat suppression can be helpful in the differentiation between postoperative blood and normal epidural fat.

Metallic implants used for spinal fusion are not a contraindication for MR imaging. However, superparamagnetic materials, e.g., steel, will create severe susceptibility artifacts (Fig. 5.5). TSE sequences are less susceptible than SE sequences, which in turn are less susceptible than GRE sequences (Fig. 5.5). Also, shortening the echo time and increasing the bandwidth of the sequence lessens artifacts. If a particular region is not interpretable due to artifacts, it may be worthwhile trying to swap read- and phase-encoding directions. Nonsuperparamagnetic metals, e.g., titanium, only produce RF artifacts, which are smaller in size.

Spinal stimulators and other electronic implant devices in principle constitute an absolute contraindication for MR imaging. Some types of electronic implants, however, are 'MR-compatible'. This should be checked with the manufacturer and the surgeon or clinician who implanted the device before the patient is brought into the magnet room. In any case, these devices have to be switched off before the MR examination.

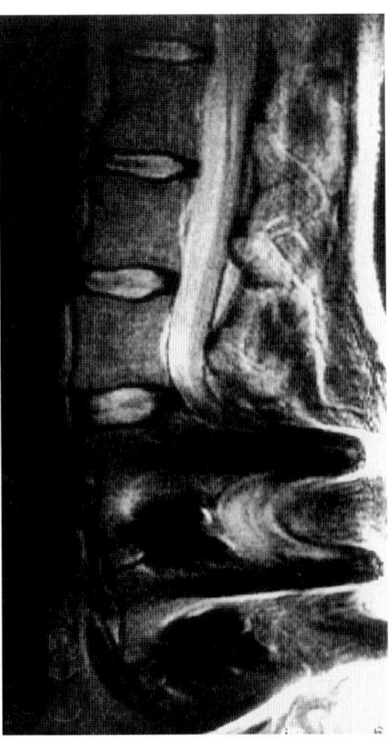

Fig. 5.5. Susceptibility artifacts. Superparamagnetic metal implants (e.g., stainless steel) cause severe susceptibility artifacts. Although these spinal orthopedic implants are not a contraindication for MR imaging in general, they almost always exclude imaging of the involved region. Note, however, that the disc spaces above the fusion are not affected

Patients have to be carefully instructed to signal during the examination when they have the impression the device is turned on again, or in any case when they sense something unusual.

5.2.3.3 Postoperative Cervical Spine

No additional sequences are necessary since the problem of epidural fibrosis is almost nonexistent in the CS. As in the lumbar spine, one should be aware of the susceptibility artifacts on GRE sequences that may be caused by metallic implants (Fig. 5.6). In these cases, SE or, better, TSE sequences are preferred.

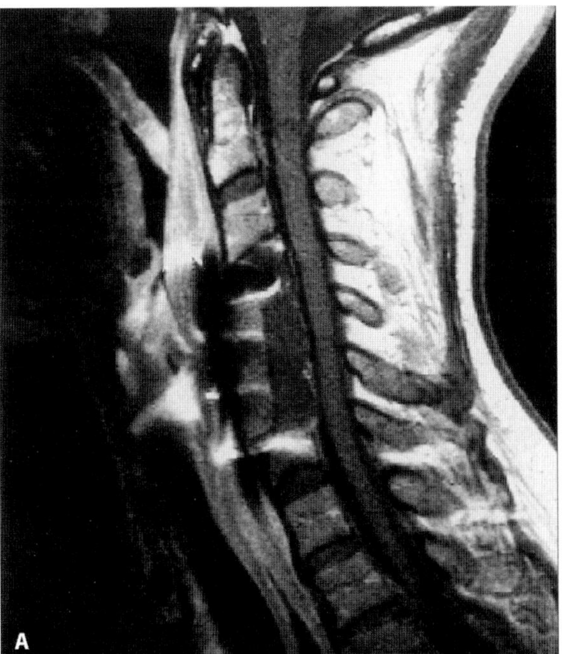

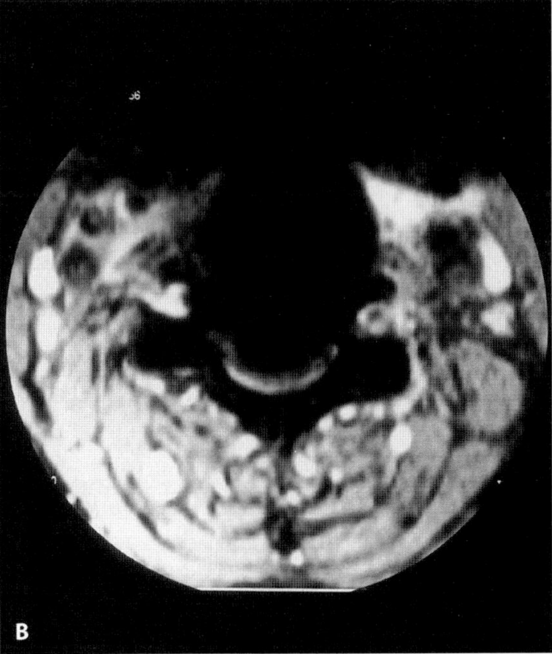

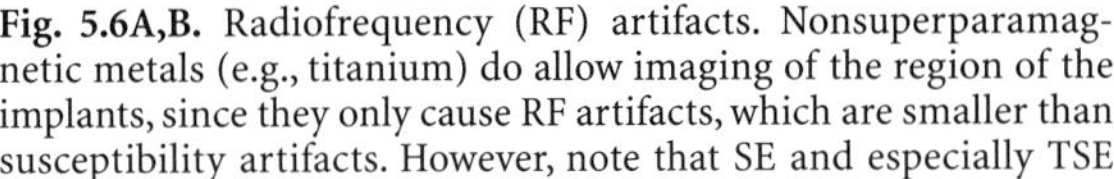
Fig. 5.6A,B. Radiofrequency (RF) artifacts. Nonsuperparamagnetic metals (e.g., titanium) do allow imaging of the region of the implants, since they only cause RF artifacts, which are smaller than susceptibility artifacts. However, note that SE and especially TSE sequences are preferred over gradient recalled echo (GRE) sequences; compare the sagittal TSE T1-W sequence (**A**) with the axial GRE T2-W sequence (**B**). Therefore, in these cases, GRE sequences should be replaced by (T)SE sequences, also in the axial plane

5.2.3.4
Nontumoral Medullary Lesions

When looking for inflammatory (MS) or infectious medullary lesions, one should perform axial GRE T2-WI (instead of T1-WI) in the thoracic spine. In addition, the routine sagittal T1-W and T2-W sequences are performed. Gadolinium-enhanced images may be useful in suspected inflammatory and infectious lesions, especially in nonviral myelomeningitis.

For suspected ischemic medullary lesions, diffusion-weighted imaging (DWI) is very useful, both in the detection and the differential diagnosis. Moreover, DWI allows us to make an assumption about the age of an ischemic lesion (hyperacute, acute, chronic).

5.2.3.5
Intraspinal Tumoral Lesions

In addition to the normal imaging protocol, one should perform axial and sagittal TSE T1-WI after gadolinium injection.

5.2.3.6
Vertebral Metastases

In screening for vertebral metastases, one should perform sagittal TSE T1- and T2-WI. In addition, a sagittal GRE so-called out-of-phase sequence should be used. This is a sequence with a specific echo time (TE) corresponding to the time it takes for water and fat protons to move exactly 180° out-of-phase. This time depends on the field strength of the magnet and is approximately 7 ms for a 1.5-T imager, and 11 ms for a 1.0-T machine. In the normal adult human, the medullary bone of the vertebral bodies contains approximately equal amounts of water and fat protons. In out-of-phase conditions, the signal of both will cancel out, leaving the vertebrae completely black. In the case of vertebral pathology, however, the signal will increase, and as such, vertebral metastases (or other lesions) will clearly stand out (Fig. 5.7).

If a metastasis extends into the spinal canal or neural foramen, additional axial T1-WI after gadolinium injection should be performed.

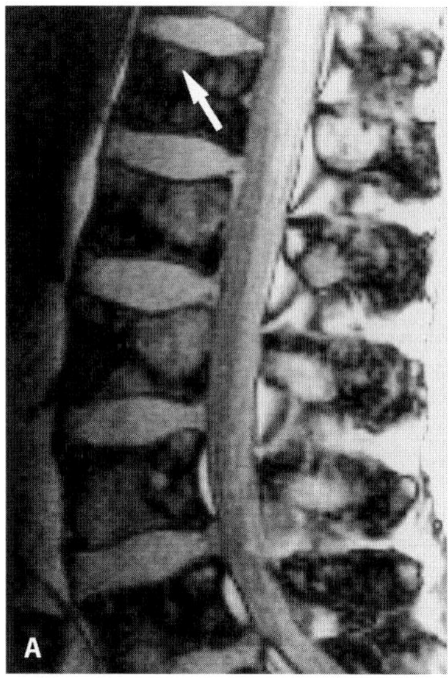

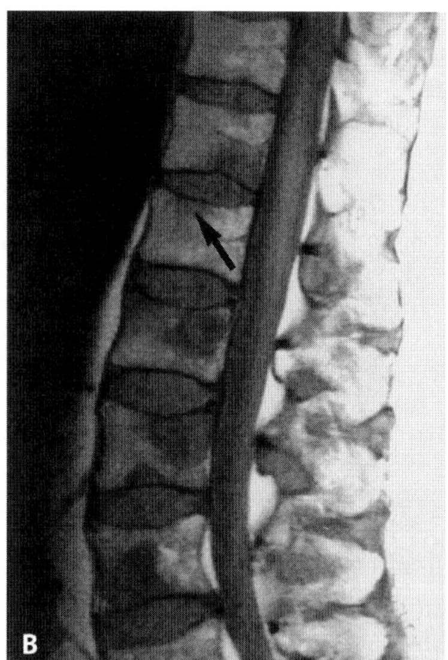

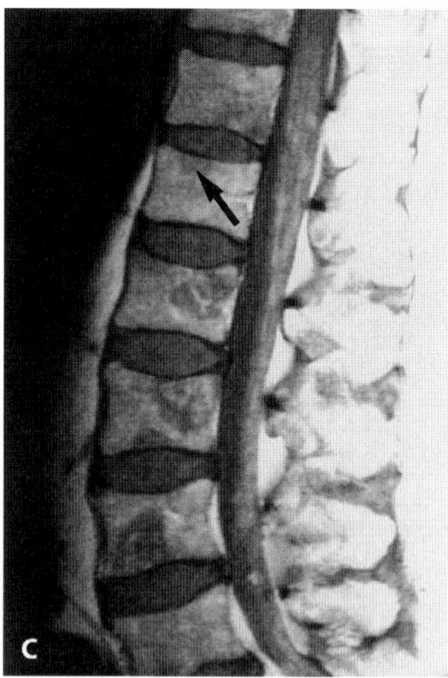

Fig. 5.7A–C. Vertebral metastases. Out-of-phase gradient-echo (**A**), unenhanced (**B**), and gadolinium-enhanced (**C**) TSE T1-weighted images (WI). Out-of-phase sequences use an echo time (TE) that effectively cancels out water and fat signals by imaging at a time when protons of both are in opposed phases (180°). Therefore, structures that contain equal amounts of both water and fat are effectively black on these sequences. This is especially true for vertebral bone marrow in the adult patient. Any pathology of the bone marrow, as in this patient with vertebral metastases, causes an increase in signal, making the involved region clearly stand out (**A**). Therefore, this is a good sequence in the search for vertebral metastases. Also note that hypointense bone-marrow lesions on the T1-WI (**B**) (such as most metastases) become less conspicuous after administration of gadolinium, since enhancement of the lesions renders them isointense to the normal marrow (**C**). Compare, for example, the contrast of the small metastasis subjacent to the superior endplate of L1 (*arrow*)

5.2.4
Sequence Parameters

Table 5.1 lists the standard sequence parameters for MR imaging of the CS, thoracic, or lumbar spine. All matrices of images with a large FOV (lumbar spine) should be at least 512. On some newer machines, even 1024 matrices are possible.

Rectangular field-of-views (RFOV) can be used to shorten the imaging time. However, this can also be achieved by decreasing the number of acquisitions, e.g., a sequence with two acquisitions and 50% RFOV is identical in imaging time and SNR to the same sequence with one acquisition and no RFOV (100%). RFOV, however, may cause infolding (or wrap-around) artifacts. To avoid infolding artifacts in general, oversampling can be used. In the read direction, this can be achieved without lengthening the acquisition. In the phase direction, oversampling linearly increases the imaging time, but SNR also increases. For this reason, 100% oversampling and one acquisition is equal to no oversampling and two acquisitions, both in imaging time and SNR. Therefore, we can state:

- 4 acquisitions + 50% RFOV
- = 2 acquisitions + 100% RFOV
- = 1 acquisition + 200% RFOV
- (100% phase oversampling)

This occurs in both imaging time and SNR, but the latter solution prevents infolding artifacts. There may, however, be an advantage in obtaining more acquisitions with RFOV, since image degradation by motion artifacts decreases when more averages are obtained.

Since motion (respiration, movement, pulsatile blood flow, CSF flow, etc.) usually causes artifacts in the phase-encoding direction, it can be useful to swap the read-out and phase-encoding directions. In the lumbar spine, choosing phase encoding in the craniocaudad direction diminishes artifacts due to CSF pulsations (Fig. 5.8).

5.2.5
Slice Thickness and Orientation

Standard slice thickness for sagittal sequences in the spine is 3–4 mm. One should use an uneven number of slices so that the middle slice is precisely centered on the midpoint of the spinal cord. For axial slices, one can use 3-mm to 4-mm slices in the neck and 4-mm to 5-mm slices in the lumbar region, since lumbar disc spaces are relatively thick and the foramina are large. Thicker slices, although generating a significantly better SNR, are unsatisfactory in depicting small disc herniations due to partial volume effects.

These axial slices should be oriented perpendicular to the spinal canal rather than parallel to the intervertebral disc. Usually, this does not make much difference except in the CS when the discs are angulated downward.

Coverage on the sagittal images should include the neural foramina on either side. At least part of the adjacent anatomic region should be imaged, e.g., the conus medullaris in imaging the lumbar spine or the craniocervical junction in imaging the CS. It is not unusual for

Table 5.1. Suggested sequence parameters for standard MRI of the lumbar and cervical spine. Imaging of the thoracic spine can be done using lumbar spine sequences

Region	Sequence type	Plane	No. of slices	TR (ms)	TE (ms)	Flip angle	Echo train length	Slice thickness (mm)	Matrix	FOV (mm)	Band width (Hz)	No. of acq.	Acq. time (min:s)
Lumbar	TSE T1	Sag	11	835	12	180	5	4	512×410	320×320	195	2	2:19
	TSE T2	Sag	11	4000	136	180	15	4	512×308	320×320	130	1	2:34
	TSE T1	Ax	3×5	570	14	180	7	4	512×308	230×230	130	2	2:34
	TSE T2	Ax	3×5	4000	99	180	15	4	512×308	230×230	130	1	1:38
Cervical	TSE T1	Sag	11	750	10	180	3	3	512×308	280×280	195	2	3:32
	TSE T2	Sag	11	2900	102	180	15	3	512×308	280×280	191	2	2:47
	GRE T2	Ax	19	960	27	30	–	3,5	256×220	200×200	195	1	3:30

Abbreviations: *TR* repetition time (ms); *TE* echo time (ms); *Matrix* (phase × frequency matrix); *FOV* field of view (mm); *Acq* acquisition(s)

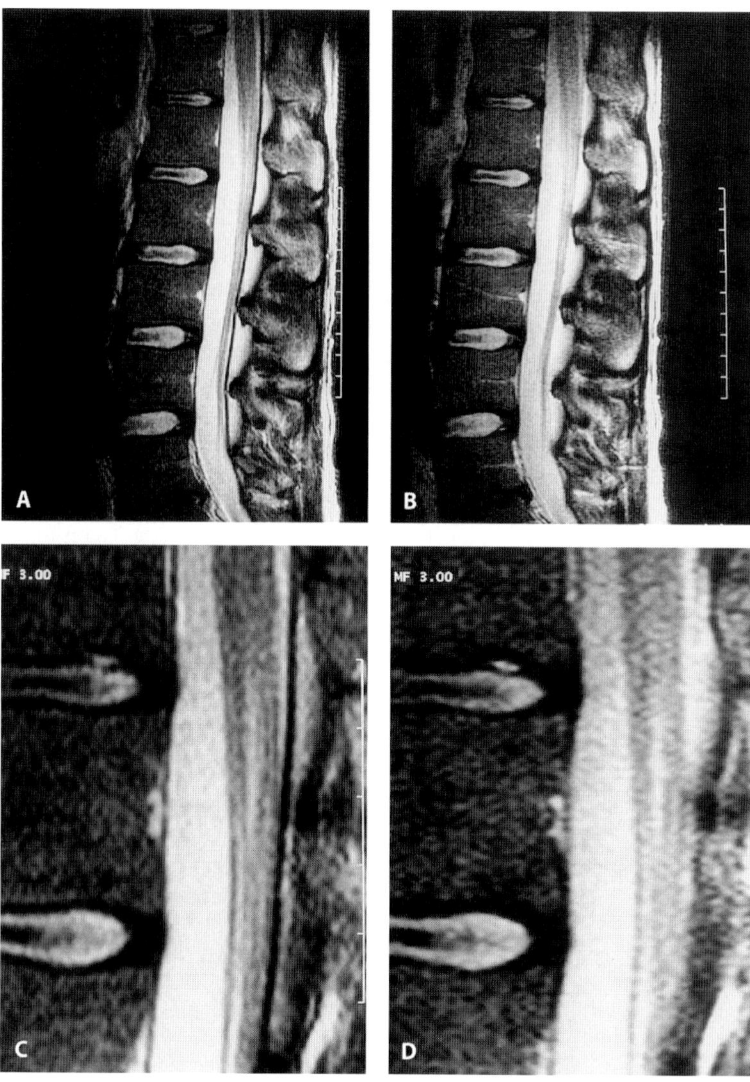

Fig. 5.8A–D. Sagittal T2- WI from the same volunteer. **A** The sequence with swapped phase and read directions (phase direction craniocaudal). **B** The non-swapped sequence. Swapping reduces blurring due to artifacts from the pulsating cerebrospinal fluid (CSF). Magnified views (**C, D**) of the same anatomic region clearly show blurring of the conus medullaris and the nerve roots on the non-swapped image (**D**). Do not use rectangular field-of-views (RFOV) in combination with swapped images since this will create infolding artifacts

a conus medullaris tumor to present clinically as a radiculopathy or low-back pain.

5.2.6 Saturation Zones

Saturation techniques use a selective pulse that is applied to tissues either inside or outside the field of view. Their purpose is to excite (or saturate) moving spins that lie outside the region of interest. They are extremely useful to eliminate motion-induced artifacts arising outside the spine. If possible, all tissues in front of the spine should be saturated. This diminishes the phase-encoding artifacts caused by moving tissues in this region, e.g., breathing, swallowing, cardiac motion, pulsating blood flow, etc. If the saturation is not effective enough, two smaller bands instead of one larger band can be used.

5.2.7 Special Sequences

5.2.7.1 Coronal Images

Coronal images can be useful in evaluating spinal scoliosis. Also, paraspinal extension of processes, such as foraminal neurinomas, are more clearly depicted. Finally, developmental anomalies, such as lumbosacral transitional vertebrae (Fig. 5.9), craniocervical junction abnormalities, or failures of segmentation and fusion of vertebrae, are more readily assessed on coronal images.

5.2.7.2 Large FOV

In some cases, the use of a large FOV can be helpful. In particular, when screening or staging a patient with vertebral metastases, an overview of the spine is sensible. When phased-array coils are available, large segments of the spine can be portrayed with excellent image quality. However, when phased-array coils are not available, the body coil must be used, and the image quality will be suboptimal. For vertebral metastases, this should not pose a major problem, but in screening for more subtle lesions, such as intramedullary lesions in MS, these large FOV images may give false-negative results.

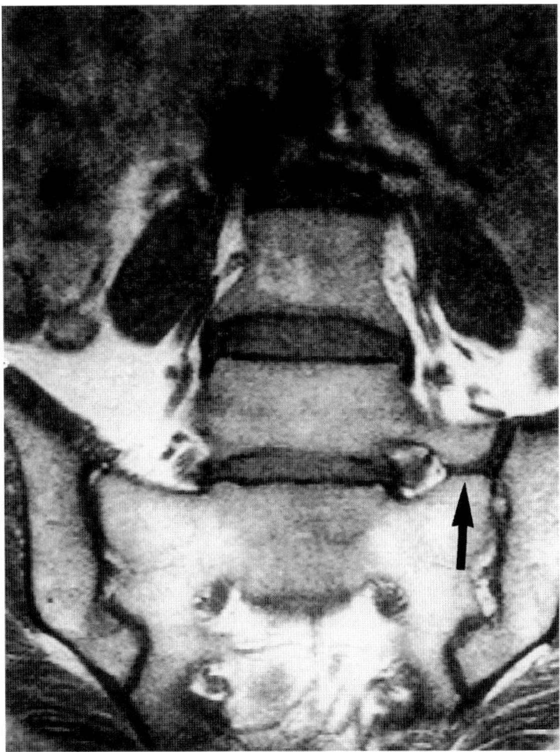

Fig. 5.9. Transitional vertebra. A lumbosacral transitional vertebra can be difficult to detect if only axial and sagittal images are acquired. This (para)coronal image clearly depicts the abnormal articulation of the left L5 transverse process with the sacrum and the ilium, with formation of a pseudarthrosis (*arrow*)

5.2.7.3 Sequences with Fat Suppression

In the CS, no intraspinal fat is present, and fat-suppression sequences are of limited use. In the lumbar spine, fat suppression can be used to differentiate enhancing scar tissue from epidural fat tissue in gadolinium-enhanced T1-WI of the postoperative spine. Nevertheless, the same result can be obtained by subtracting pre- and postcontrast images without fat suppression. In some rare cases, fat-suppression techniques can be helpful in the differentiation between blood and fat.

5.2.7.4 Out-of-Phase Imaging

Out-of-phase or opposed-phase images occur in GRE sequences when the TE equals the time needed for water and fat protons to progress 180° out of phase. In these circumstances, objects consisting of equal amounts of water and fat protons are hypointense (black) on MR images, since the contributions of water and fat protons to the overall signal intensity effectively cancel each other out. During adult life, vertebral bodies consist more or less of equal amounts of water and fat. When a pathologic process disturbs this equilibrium, the vertebrae will show areas of higher signal, which clearly stand out in relation to the normal black background. A frequently used indication involves screening for vertebral metastases. One exception is osteoblastic metastases, which remain dark on out-of-phase images since they are already hypointense due to the lack of mobile protons (Fig. 5.7). Therefore, standard T1-WI should always also be obtained.

5.2.7.5
Ultrafast Imaging

In some patients, it can be useful to shorten the imaging time in order to decrease motion artifacts (children, uncooperative patients, etc.) or to decrease the overall examination time (claustrophobic patients, monitored patients, etc.). In these cases, the sequence parameters listed in Table 5.2 can be used. Although the acquisition time is reduced to 1 min or less, these ultrafast sequences still produce high-quality images or even better images with patient movement (Fig. 5.10). Imaging time is (or can be) further decreased by eliminating saturation zones. SNRs are substantially lower but still sufficient.

5.2.7.6
MR Myelography

MR myelography can be helpful in addition to the normal imaging sequences. Although three-dimensional (3D)-TSE sequences have been proposed, they significantly add to the total imaging time of the examination. Therefore, I prefer single-shot wide-slab T2-W sequences with a very long echo train (Fig. 5.11). Although these allow only one view of the thecal sac at a time, their imaging time is very short, making it possible to obtain different views by running the sequence in different orientations (one frontal view, one sagittal view, and two obliques). This sequence has the added advantage of eliminating postprocessing (no maximal intensity projection is necessary).

5.2.7.7
MR Angiography

Magnetic resonance angiography (MRA) has limited use in spinal imaging. Even arteriovenous malformations or fistulae are hard to image with MRA. Normally, postcontrast T1-W sequences are sufficient (Fig. 5.12).

5.2.7.8
Diffusion-Weighted Imaging

Diffusion-weighted imaging (DWI) is a special technique using very strong magnetic gradients, effectively canceling signal from protons in free moving water, e.g., CSF. Protons that are more restricted in movement, e.g., in intracellular water, still produce a measurable MR signal. The spontaneous movement of protons is known as 'Brownian motion' and results among others in diffusion, hence the term DWI.

This technique is especially useful in detecting cytotoxic edema, where there is cell swelling effectively increasing the amount of intracellular over extracellular water and thereby reducing water diffusion. Since ischemia produces cytotoxic edema very early on (after 1 h), DWI is capable of the early detection of ischemic lesions.

5.2.7.9
Functional Imaging

Functional imaging of the spine consists mainly of semidynamic imaging. Flexion/extension imaging of the CS

Table 5.2. Suggested sequence parameters for ultrafast MR imaging of the lumbar and cervical spine. Imaging of the thoracic spine can be done using lumbar spine sequences

Region	Sequence type	Plane	No. of slices	TR (ms)	TE (ms)	Flip angle	Echo train length	Slice thickness (mm)	Matrix	FOV (mm)	Band width (Hz)	No. of acq.	Acq. time (min:s)
Lumbar	TSE T1	Sag	11	835	12	180	5	4	512×205	320×320	195	1	0:35
	TSE T2	Sag	11	3000	136	180	23	4	512×205	320×320	130	1	0:42
	TSE T1	Ax	3×5	570	14	180	7	4	512×205	230×230	130	1	0:51
Cervical	TSE T1	Sag	11	750	10	180	3	3	512×205	280×280	195	1	0:35
	TSE T2	Sag	11	2900	102	180	23	3	512×205	280×280	191	1	0:41
	GRE T2	Ax	12	610	27	30	–	4	256×120	200×200	195	1	1:03

Abbreviations: *TR* repetition time (ms); *TE* eche time (ms); *Matrix* (phase × frequency matrix); *FOV* field of view (mm); *Acq* acquisition(s)

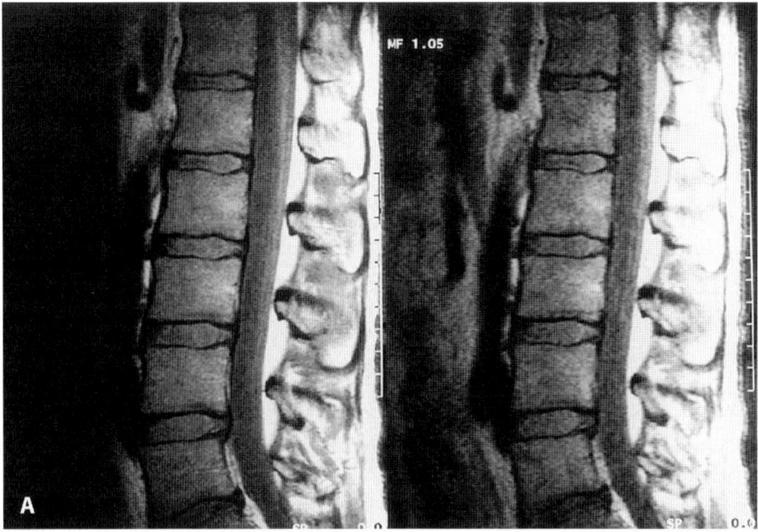

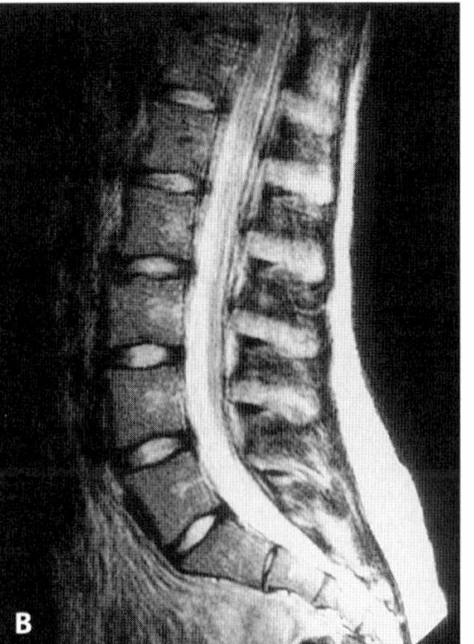

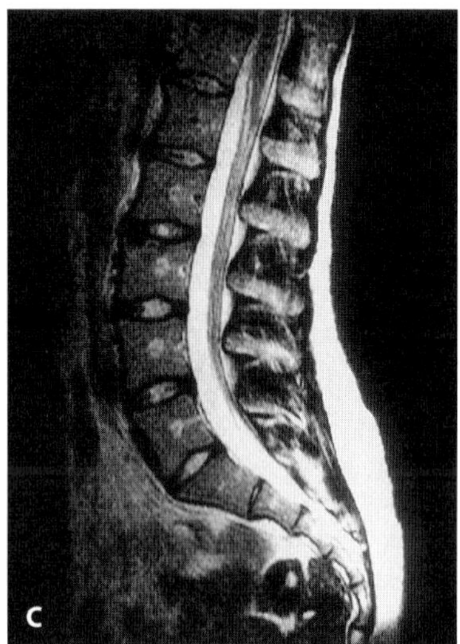

Fig. 5.10A–C. Ultrafast imaging. **A** Sagittal TSE T1-WI from the same volunteer. On the *left* is the routine sequence [repetition time (TR) 1350, echo time (TE) 15, echo train length (ETL) 7, acquisition time (TA) 2 min 28 s], on the right, the ultrafast sequence (TR 1270, TE 15, ETL 7, TA 53 s', see also Tables 5.1 and 5.2 for complete sequence parameters). Notice the comparable spatial resolution of both images (both 512 matrix), but the higher SNR of the routine sequence on the *left*. **B** Routine sagittal TSE T2-W sequence (TR 3000, TE 96, ETL 7, TA 4 min 19 s) in a patient with considerable low-back pain. The image is degraded by motion artifacts, and the quality is unsatisfactory. **C** Ultrafast sequence (TR 3200, TE 128, ETL 23, TA 1 min 7 s; see Tables 5.1 and 5.2 for the complete sequence parameters) in the same patient. Owing to the shorter imaging time, the quality of the ultrafast sequence is clearly better

is relatively easy to perform with fast sequences. The first images are made with the head flexed forward. This can be readily achieved by placing an inflated balloon under the patient's head. By letting air out of the balloon in small amounts, imaging can be performed in different positions between flexion and extension. This way, dynamic relationships between anatomic structures and pathology, e.g., herniated disc, can be assessed. Depending on the coil design, it can be necessary to switch the normal neck coil for a flexible coil or to use the body coil.

Dynamic imaging of the lumbar spine is more difficult because of the limited space available in the magnet; this problem can be solved in two ways. The most simple solution is to image the patient supine and prone, thus simulating extension and flexion. Another possibility is to use specially designed devices and/or balloons or to image the patient in lateral decubitus. These techniques are relatively cumbersome. Flexion-extension views of the spine have also been obtained with the patient in sitting position with a special type of open interventional MR system ('double-doughnut'

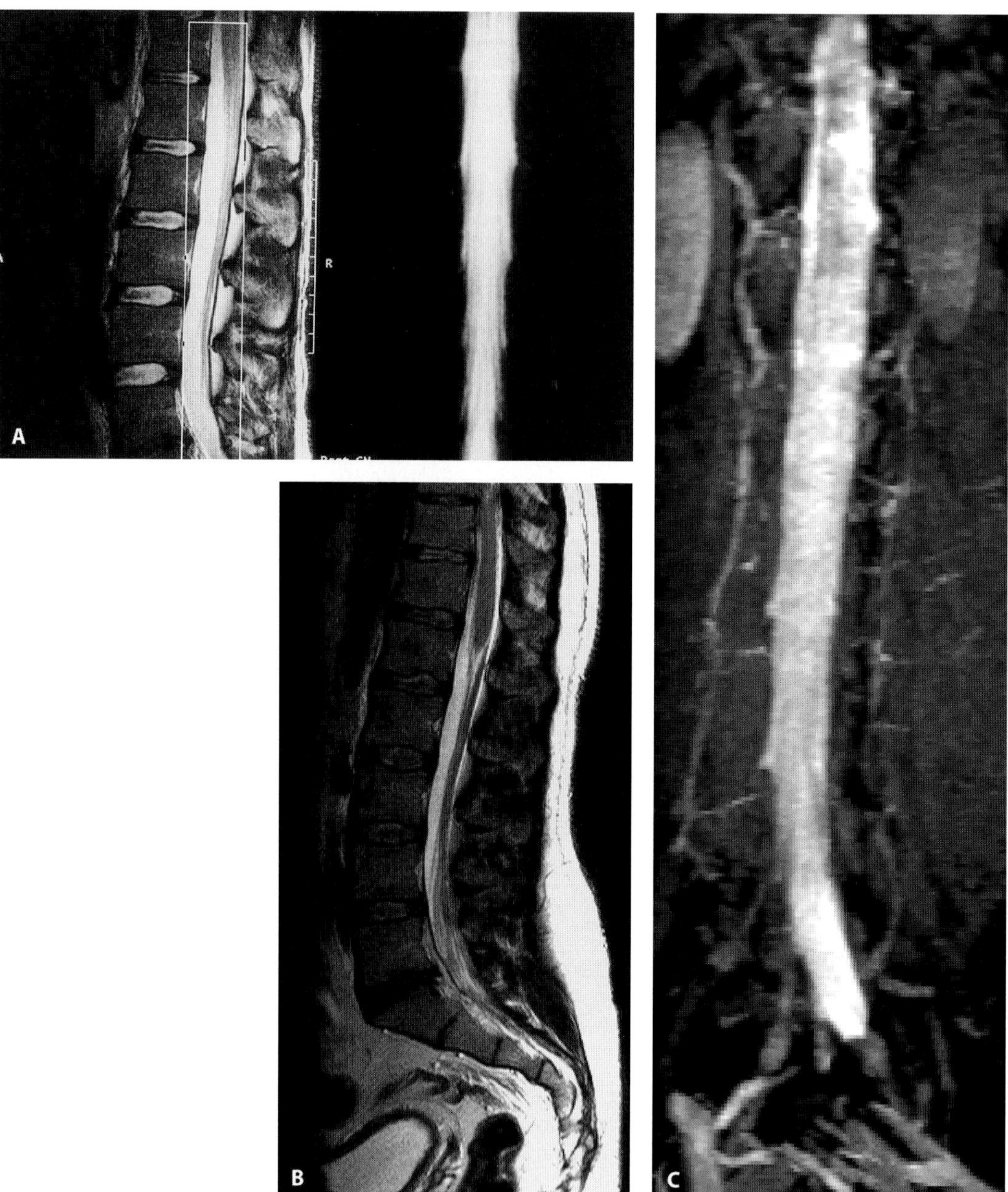

Fig. 5.11A–C. MR myelogram. **A** Routine MR myelogram in a normal volunteer [repetition time (TR) 2800, echo time (TE) 1100, echo train length (ETL) 240, TA 7 s]. In this example, a frontal view MR myelogram (*right*) is obtained by placing the slice on a sagittal image (*left*). Slice thickness should be adjusted to include the complete dural sac and nerve sheaths. Excellent detail with symmetric nerve roots and sheaths. The sequence can be run in different directions to obtain frontal, lateral, or oblique-view myelograms. **B,C** For comparison a 3D TSE T2-W sequence. This sequence has a markedly longer acquisition time but has the advantage of producing multiple views

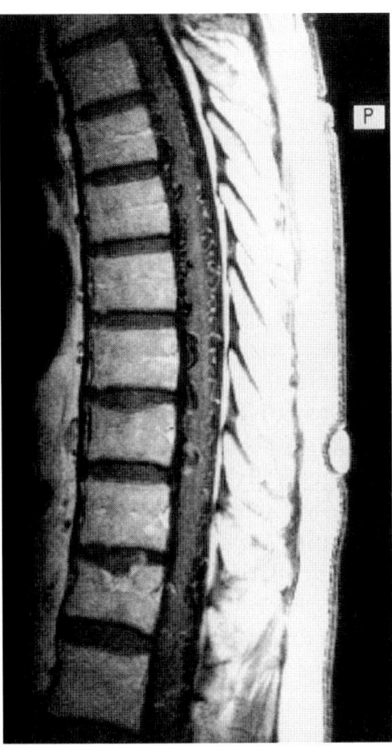

Fig. 5.12. Spinal AV malformation, gadolinium-enhanced T1-WI. Notice the presence of multiple serpiginous blood vessels on the surface of the thoracic cord in this typical example. The small blood vessels with slow flow enhance with gadolinium, and the medium-sized vessels with higher flow do not enhance and are seen as areas of flow void. These gadolinium-enhanced images are typical and sufficient for making the diagnosis. High-quality MR angiography images are difficult to obtain due to the small size and tortuous course of these blood vessels

design). Newer machines allow standing weight-bearing MR of the spine. These have the advantage of imaging the spine under physiological loading, and during bending and rotation.

The term functional magnetic resonance imaging (fMRI) is also used for the detection of neuronal activity. Usually, a special MR technique, called blood oxygen level dependent (BOLD) imaging, is used to detect minute changes in the blood level of deoxyhemoglobin due to neuronal activity and secondary autonomous blood flow adaptation. The technique is mostly used in the brain, since susceptibility artifacts make it very hard to obtain useful images of the spinal cord.

5.2.8 Contrast Media

The use of contrast agents has been discussed in previous sections of this chapter. The most common indications for the use of intravenous gadolinium in the spine are:

1. The postoperative lumbar spine, especially after discectomy (use of gadolinium obligatory)
2. Detection of small tumors, especially neurinomas
3. Imaging of tumors in general
4. MS and other inflammatory diseases

5.3 Clinical Examples

The MR imaging findings in some typical examples of spinal pathology are demonstrated in Figs. 5.13–5.24.

5.3.1 Degenerative Disease

The most frequently encountered pathology in the spine is degenerative disease. Degenerative disc disease is typified by dehydration of the intervertebral disc. This phenomenon is easily recognized on T2-W sequences as black or dark discs. Secondary changes, such as reduced intervertebral space, osteophytic reactions, and bulging disc, are also easily recognized. Sometimes tears of the annulus fibrosus can be detected on T2-WI as a region of high signal intensity near the posterior margin of the disc (Fig. 5.13). These annular tears typically enhance after intravenous gadolinium injection.

Other characteristic findings in degenerative disc disease are alterations in the adjacent vertebral body endplates (Table 5.3.). These endplate changes were first categorized by Modic. Type I endplate changes represent vascularized bone marrow and/or edema and are seen as low-SI changes on T1-WI and high-SI areas on T2-WI. Type II changes represent more chronic alterations with proliferation of fatty tissue and are bright both on T1-WI and T2-WI. Type III changes, also seen on conventional radiographs and computed tomography (CT) images, represent dense, sclerotic bone and are dark on T1-WI and T2-WI. Type I and II changes

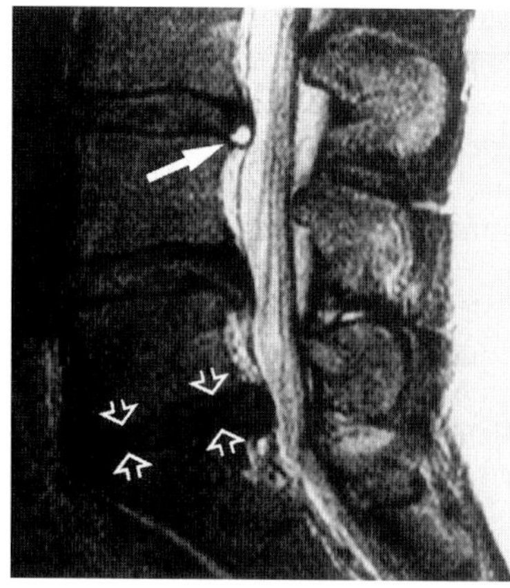

Fig. 5.13. Degenerative disc disease is characterized by T2-shortening of the disc and decreased intervertebral height (*open arrows*), degenerative vertebral endplate changes, bulging disc, and/or osteophytes. A radial tear of the annulus, which is found consistently with the other degenerative changes in the intervertebral disc, involves all layers of the annulus fibrosus. It may be detected by MR imaging as a band of high signal intensity on T2-WI (*arrow*)

Table 5.3. Modic type changes of vertebral endplates in degenerative disease (Modic et al. 1988)

Modic classification	T1-SI changes	T2-SI changes	Represents
I	–	+	Vascularized bone marrow and/or edema
II	+	+	Proliferation of fatty tissue
III	–	–	Sclerotic bone

may enhance with gadolinium, but should not be confused with inflammatory enhancement commonly seen with disc infection.

Degenerative changes of the facet joints may play an important role in low-back pain, but may also cause irradiating leg pain due to secondary foraminal stenosis (Fig. 5.4). Foraminal narrowing, or foraminal pathology in general, is more accurately assessed on sagittal images than on axial images (CT or MRI) (Fig. 5.4).

In the CS, uncovertebral degenerative disease may play an important role in irradiating shoulder or arm pain due to secondary foraminal narrowing. In assessing the cervical neural foramen, one should be aware of the underestimation of the diameter (up to 10%) on MR imaging because of chemical shift artifacts.

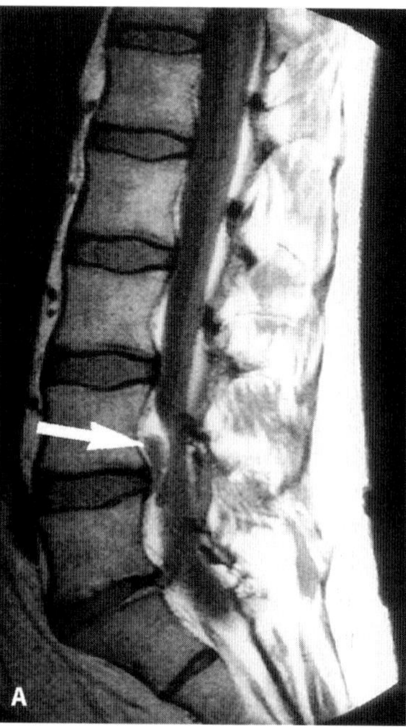

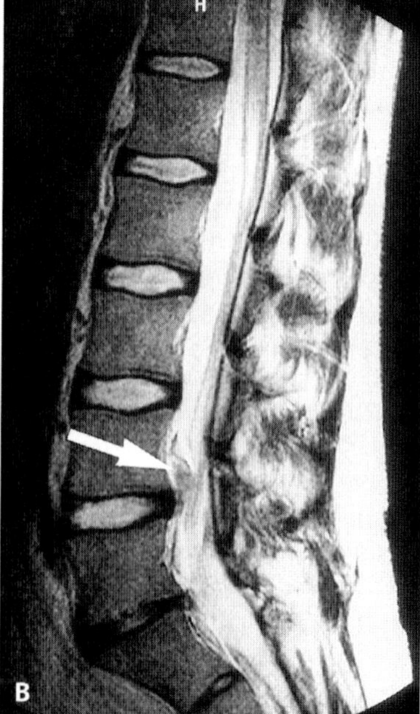

Fig. 5.14A,B. Sequestered disc. Sequestered disc fragments can migrate upward (or less frequently downward) behind the vertebral bodies all the way up to the next intervertebral space. As such, they may be missed on axial computed tomography (CT). Therefore, sagittal imaging is an important advantage of MR imaging. The contrast between the extruded disc fragment and the surrounding epidural fat tissue is better seen on T1-WI (**A**) than on T2-WI (**B**) (*arrows*)

5.3.2 Herniated Disc

Herniated discs are more easily detected with MRI than with CT. First, MR imaging allows visualization of the complete lumbar (or cervical or thoracic) spine in one examination. Second, sagittal images also depict the spinal canal in between intervertebral disc spaces. It is not unusual for a disc fragment to migrate (or extend) into the area behind the vertebral body (Fig. 5.14). Some of these migrated discs can be missed on CT if axial slices are limited to the intervertebral disc spaces examined. Third, the intrinsic tissue contrast is usually better on MR. Especially the cervicothoracic and/or lumbosacral region can be hard to assess on CT due to beam hardening, especially in larger patients.

The terms used to describe or classify bulging or herniated discs are somewhat ambiguous and sometimes misused. Recently, a nomenclature project initiated by the American Society of Spine Radiology has found wide acceptance among radiologists, clinicians, and surgeons (Table 5.4). In this nomenclature, herniation is defined as a localized displacement of disc material beyond the limits of the intervertebral disc space. The disc material may be nucleus, cartilage, fragmented apophyseal bone, anular tissue, or any combination thereof. The term 'localized' contrasts to 'generalized,' the latter being arbitrarily defined as greater than 50% (180°) of the periphery of the disc.

Localized displacement in the axial (horizontal) plane can be 'focal', signifying less than 25% of the disc circumference, or 'broad-based', meaning between 25% and 50% of the disc circumference. The presence of disc tissue 'circumferentially' (50%–100%) beyond the edges of the ring apophyses may be called 'bulging' and is not considered a form of herniation, nor are diffuse adaptive alterations of the disc contour secondary to adjacent deformity as may be present in severe scoliosis or spondylolisthesis.

Herniated discs may take the form of protrusion or extrusion, based on the shape of the displaced material. Protrusion is present if the greatest distance, in any plane, between the edges of the disc material beyond the disc space is less than the distance between the edges of the base in the same plane. The base is defined as the cross-sectional area of disc material at the outer margin of the disc space of origin, where disc material displaced beyond the disc space is continuous with disc material within the disc space. In the craniocaudal direction, the length of the base cannot exceed, by definition, the height of the intervertebral space. Extrusion is present when, in at least one plane, any one distance between the edges of the disc material beyond the disc space is greater than the distance between the edges of the base in the same plane, or when no continuity exists between the disc material beyond the disc space and that within the disc space. Extrusion may be further specified as sequestration, if the displaced disc material has completely lost all continuity with the parent disc (Fig. 5.14). The term migration may be used to signify displacement of disc material away from the site of extrusion, regardless of whether it is sequestrated or not. Because posteriorly displaced disc material is often constrained by the posterior longitudinal ligament,

Table 5.4. Nomenclature of disc herniation

General terminology	Definition	Specification I	Specification II	Definition
Bulging	Displacement over >50% of the periphery of the disc			
Herniation	Localized displacement (<50% of the periphery of the disc)	Focal (<25%) OR broad-based (25%...50%)	Protrusion	No extrusion
			Extrusion	Distance of the edge of the herniated material>disc heigth or hernia base
			Sequestration (=special form of extrusion)	No continuity with parent disc

images may portray a disc displacement as a protrusion on axial sections and an extrusion on sagittal sections, in which cases the displacement should be considered an extrusion. Herniated discs in the craniocaudal (vertical) direction through a break in the vertebral body endplate are referred to as intravertebral herniations.

Disc herniations may be further specifically described as contained, if the displaced portion is covered by the outer anulus, or uncontained when any such covering is absent. Displaced disc tissues may also be described by location, volume, and content.

5.3.3 Inflammatory and Infectious Lesions

The most common inflammatory intramedullary lesions are seen in patients with MS. Most of these lesions are hard to detect on precontrast T1-WI, as are MS lesions of the brain. On T2-WI, lesions are hyperintense (Fig. 5.15) and can be quite large in the acute phase. Sometimes, they also exhibit uptake of gadolinium contrast, which is believed to be a sign of an active lesion. An MRI examination of the brain and the com-

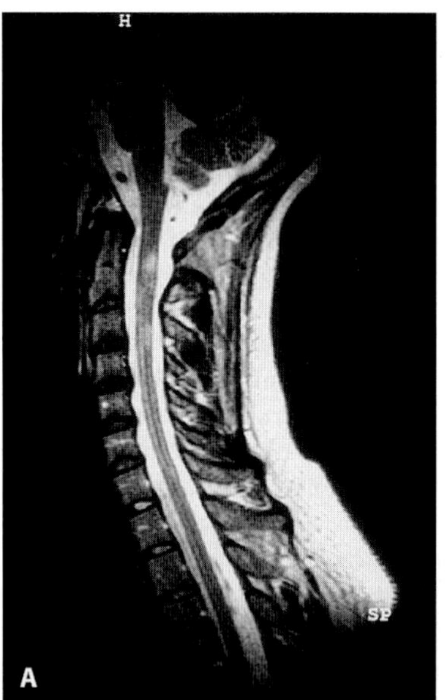

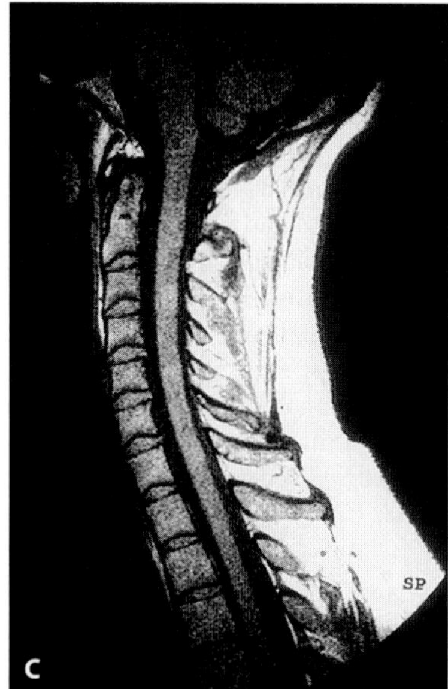

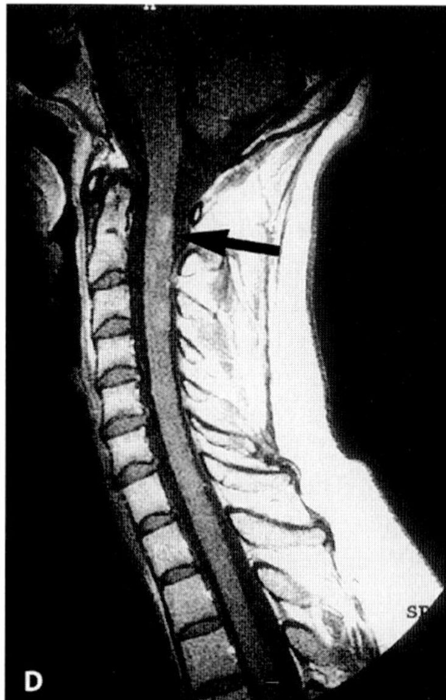

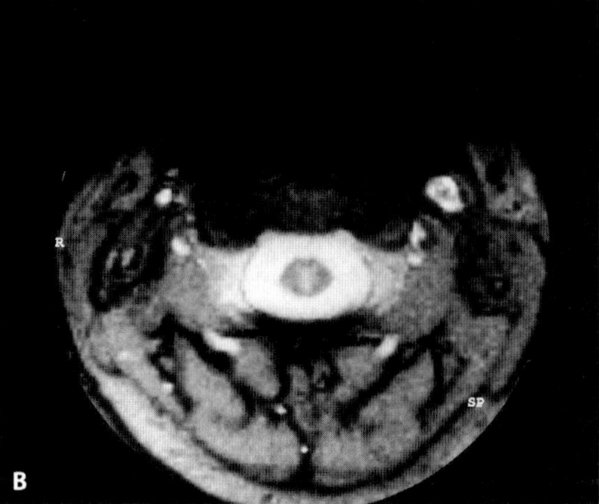

Fig. 5.15A–D. Multiple sclerosis. In this 24-year-old woman with multiple sclerosis, sagittal TSE T2-weighted images (WI) (**A**), axial gradient-echo T2-WI (**B**), and sagittal unenhanced (**C**) and gadolinium-enhanced TSE T1-WI (**D**) were obtained. The signal changes observed with intramedullary multiple sclerosis lesions are comparable to those in the brain. The sagittal T2-WI shows three hyperintense lesions; only one lesion manifests enhancement (*arrow*, **D**). Note that multiple sclerosis can be seen on magnetic resonance (MR) imaging with lesions in the brain and/or the spine. Therefore, when a presumptive diagnosis of spinal multiple sclerosis plaques is made, MR examination of the brain should be performed to confirm the diagnosis, by demonstrating typical brain lesions

plete spinal cord should be performed to search for other lesions. Clinically, one-third of MS patients exhibit spinal symptoms only. The cervical cord is twice as likely to be involved as the lower levels.

Spinal infections can be (intra-)medullary (Fig. 5.16), intraspinal or, more frequently, vertebral and/or discal in location. Spondylodiscitis is frequently caused by bacteria or tuberculosis (Fig. 5.17). Postoperative spondylodiscitis can be difficult to diagnose in the early postoperative phase, since normal (inflammatory) postoperative changes may resemble infectious pathology.

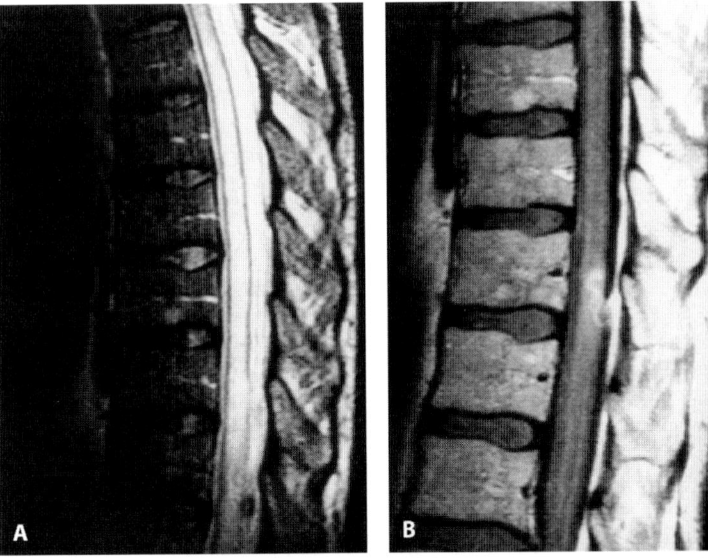

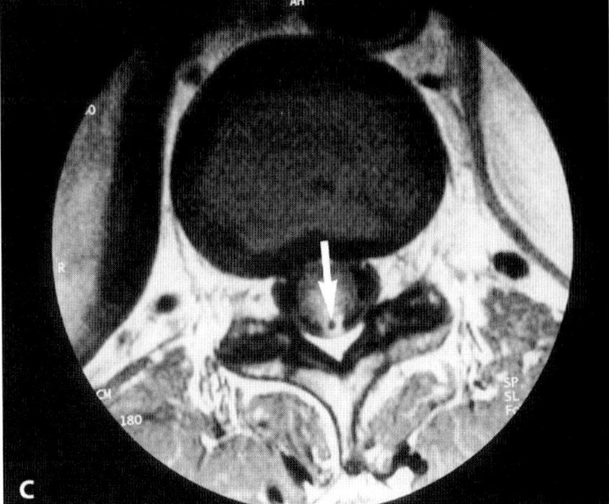

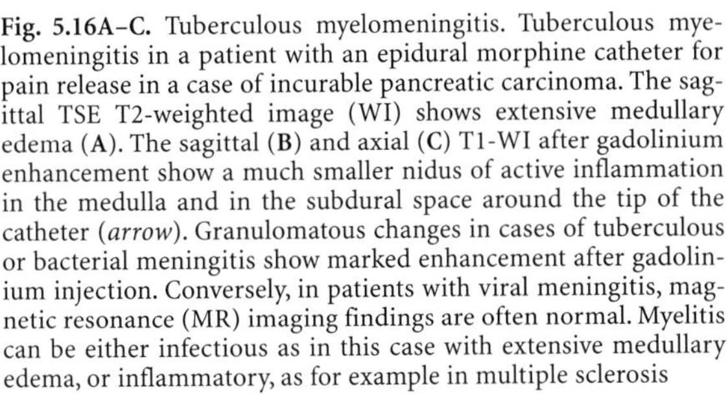

Fig. 5.16A–C. Tuberculous myelomeningitis. Tuberculous myelomeningitis in a patient with an epidural morphine catheter for pain release in a case of incurable pancreatic carcinoma. The sagittal TSE T2-weighted image (WI) shows extensive medullary edema (**A**). The sagittal (**B**) and axial (**C**) T1-WI after gadolinium enhancement show a much smaller nidus of active inflammation in the medulla and in the subdural space around the tip of the catheter (*arrow*). Granulomatous changes in cases of tuberculous or bacterial meningitis show marked enhancement after gadolinium injection. Conversely, in patients with viral meningitis, magnetic resonance (MR) imaging findings are often normal. Myelitis can be either infectious as in this case with extensive medullary edema, or inflammatory, as for example in multiple sclerosis

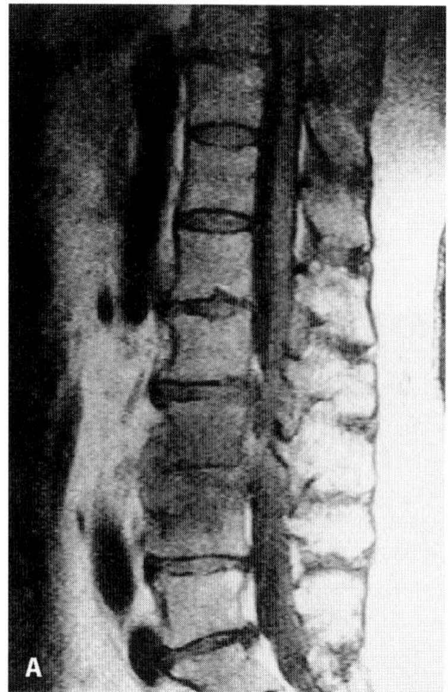

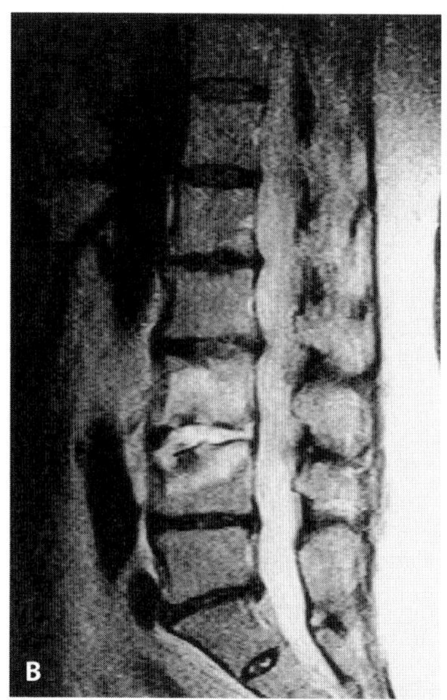

Fig. 5.17A,B. Spondylodiscitis. Spondylodiscitis or disc space infection with osteomyelitis. Note the substantial signal changes both in the vertebral bodies and in the intervertebral disc space. The blurry margins of the vertebral endplates on the T1-WI (**A**) and the high SI of the disc space on the T2-WI (**B**) allow differentiation with degenerative or postoperative changes

5.3.4 The Postoperative Lumbar Spine

As mentioned earlier, MR imaging is capable of differentiating postoperative epidural fibrosis and recurrent disc herniation. This is important since the latter can be an indication for reintervention. On postcontrast T1-WI, herniated disc material shows no or minor enhancement (Fig. 5.18), while epidural fibrosis enhances intensely, especially in the first years after surgery (Fig. 5.19). However, smaller disc fragments or 'older' recurrent herniated discs may progressively show more enhancement due to secondary inflammatory changes.

It is important to note that when the intervertebral disc space narrows after discectomy, secondary foraminal stenosis may occur, causing irradiating pain without recurrent herniation.

5.3.5 Spinal Tumors

5.3.5.1 Intramedullary Tumors

Three primary intramedullary tumors are frequently encountered: astrocytoma, ependymoma, and hemangioblastoma.

The peak incidence of spinal astrocytomas is around the third and fourth decade, and they are most often found in the thoracic cord. Clinical symptoms vary and are sometimes very minor. Most often patients have motor changes with gait difficulties, but pain and bladder disturbances are also possible. In children, sometimes a secondary scoliosis is found. The cord is often enlarged, and most cord astrocytomas are low signal on T1, high signal on T2, and, contrary to brain astrocytomas, show enhancement after gadolinium injection (Fig. 5.20). After gadolinium injection, the delineation of potential cysts is usually more apparent.

Cord ependymomas are usually found in older patients, with a peak incidence around the fourth and fifth decade. It is the most frequent tumor of the lower

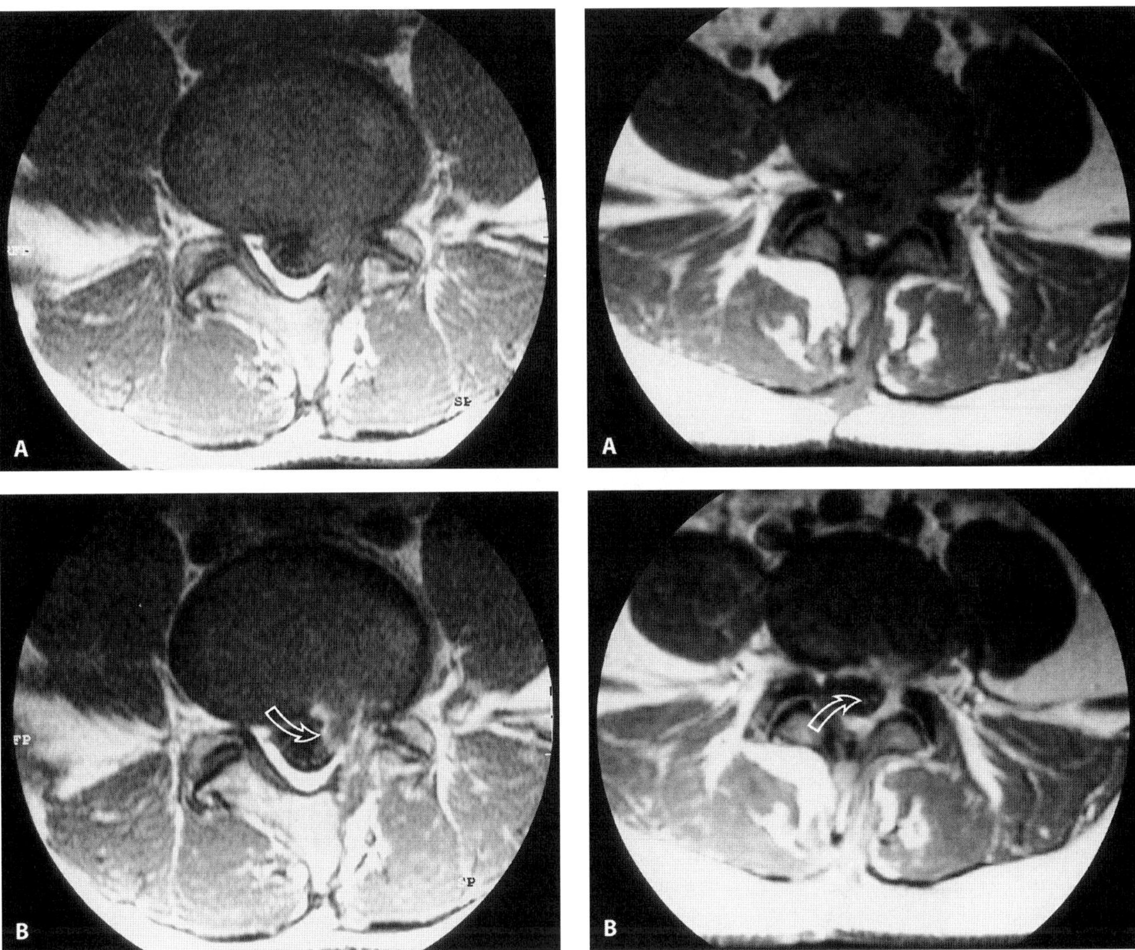

Fig. 5.18A,B. Recurrent disc herniation. Axial T1-WI before (**A**) and after (**B**) gadolinium enhancement in a patient with a large recurrent disc herniation. Differentiating postoperative recurrent disc herniation from epidural fibrosis is important, since the latter is no indication for surgical reintervention. When imaging is performed directly after gadolinium injection, disc material only shows peripheral enhancement (*curved open arrow*)

Fig. 5.19A,B. Postoperative epidural fibrosis. Axial T1-WI before (**A**) and after (**B**) gadolinium enhancement in a patient with postoperative epidural fibrosis. Compare with Fig. 5.18; epidural fibrosis shows complete enhancement after contrast administration. Nerve root enhancement can be seen in asymptomatic patients up to 6 months after surgery (*curved open arrow*). Thereafter, enhancement of the nerve roots is considered abnormal, and a sign of active nerve root damage

thoracic cord and conus medullaris, where they are usually of the myxopapillary type. Clinically, patients with ependymomas more often present with back or neck pain and sometimes radicular pain, but bladder dysfunction and gait problems are also encountered. These lesions also show cord enlargement and tend to be more centrally located than cord astrocytomas. Cord ependymomas are usually hypointense on T1 and hyperintense on T2, but can be more heterogeneous than astrocytomas due to areas of hemorrhage. Ependymomas show strong enhancement after gadolinium injection (Fig. 5.21).

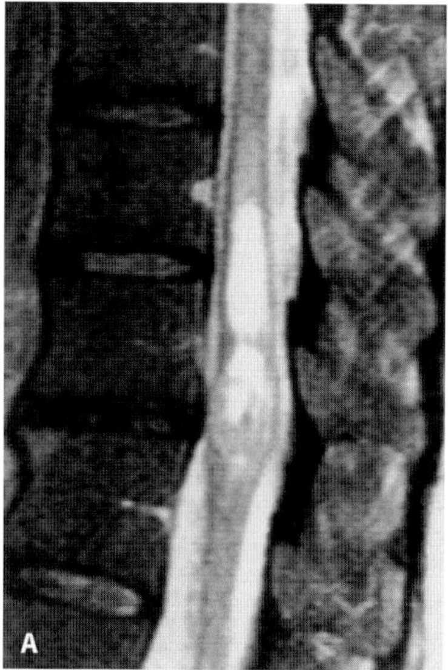
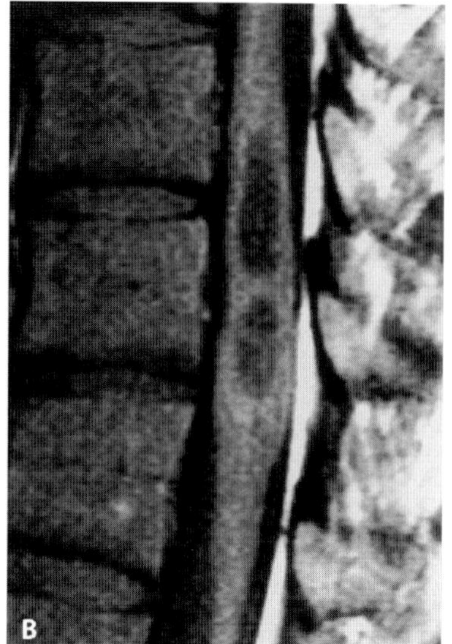
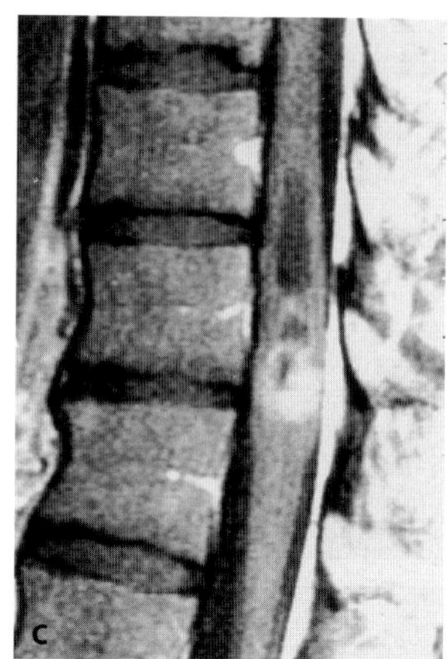

Fig. 5.20A–C. Spinal cord astrocytoma. Astrocytoma of the thoracic spinal cord: sagittal T2-WI (**A**), unenhanced T1-WI (**B**), and gadolinium-enhanced T1-WI (**C**). Because of their infiltrative nature, intramedullary astrocytomas nearly always enhance. Often, there are associated cysts, but the cysts are usually not lined by tumor and do not require excision

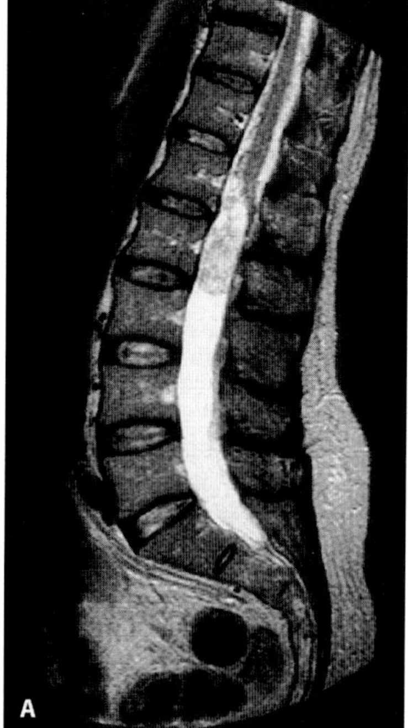
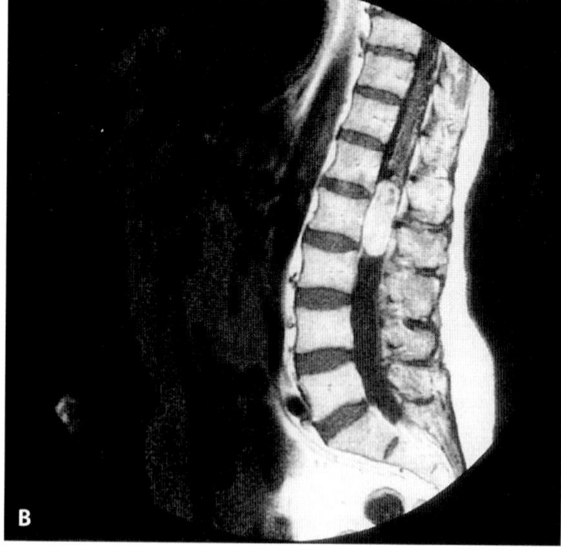

Fig. 5.21A,B. Ependymoma of the conus medullaris. In this patient with an ependymoma of the conus medullaris (myxopapillary type), sagittal T2-WI (**A**) and gadolinium-enhanced T1-WI (**B**) were performed. Ependymomas are usually better delineated than astrocytomas. On histopathologic examination, they are often surrounded by a capsule. Ependymomas usually show intense and homogeneous enhancement. Ependymomas tend to be central and are more frequently hemorrhagic than astrocytomas

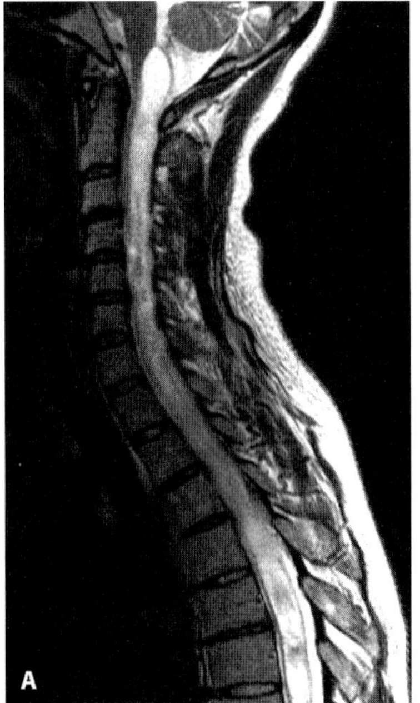

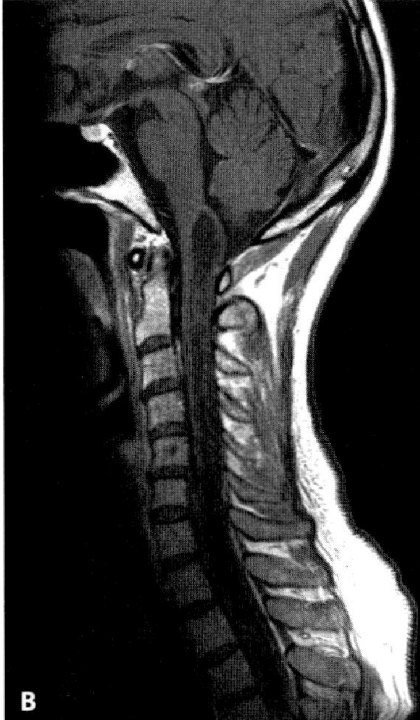

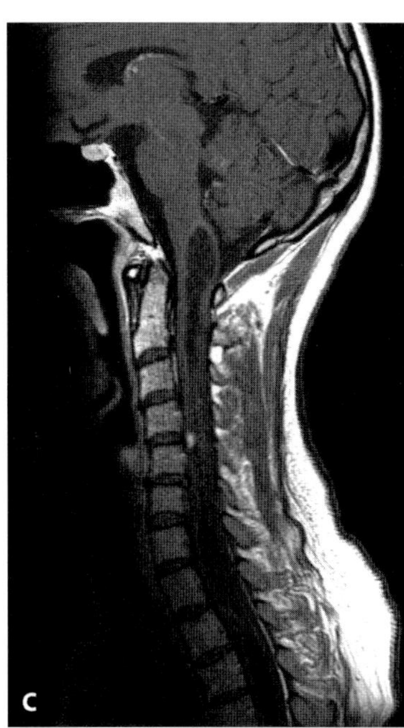

Fig. 5.22A–C. Spinal hemangioblastoma. In this patient with a spinal hemangioblastoma, sagittal T2-WI (**A**), sagittal T1-WI (**B**), and gadolinium-enhanced sagittal T1-WI (**C**) were performed. The typical pattern of this tumor is a small enhancing nodule with a large accompanying cystic lesion and edema. There is marked swelling of the cord, and the lesion is very extensive, especially compared to the small enhancing tumor nodule.

Finally, spinal hemangioblastomas are less common than the two other types of intramedullary tumors. One out of three patients with spinal hemangioblastomas have von Hippel-Lindau syndrome. Spinal hemangioblastomas typically have associated cyst formation and substantial cord edema. Strong enhancement of the tumor nidus after gadolinium injection is always seen in these tumors (Fig. 5.22).

5.3.5.2 Intraspinal Extramedullary Tumors

Two types of tumors are frequently encountered: neurinoma (Figs. 5.23 and 5.24) and meningioma (Fig. 5.25).

Neurinoma, neurofibroma, neurolemmoma, and schwannoma are various names for tumors that arise from Schwann cells or nerve sheaths. Schwannoma, neurinoma, and neurolemmoma are synonyms. Usually, neurinomas (Fig. 5.24) do not envelop the adjacent, dorsal sensory root, while neurofibromas (Fig. 5.23) surround the nerve and are mostly associated with neurofibromatosis, even when single. Nerve sheath tumors are the most frequent intraspinal tumors, and they have a peak incidence around the fourth decade. Patients usually present with radicular pain. These lesions are most often markedly hyperintense on T2-WI, and iso- to hyperintense on T1-WI. After gadolinium injection, there is homogeneous tumor enhancement.

Spinal meningiomas tend to be encapsulated and are attached to the dura. They do not invade the spinal cord, but displace it. They are usually anterior in the cervical region and posterolateral in the thoracic region. Only 3% of spinal meningiomas occur in the lumbar region. Most patients are women, with a peak incidence in the sixth decade. Generally, patients present with radicular, neck, or back pain. Meningiomas are hypo- to isointense on T1-WI, iso- to hyperintense on T2-WI, and show intense, homogeneous contrast enhancement.

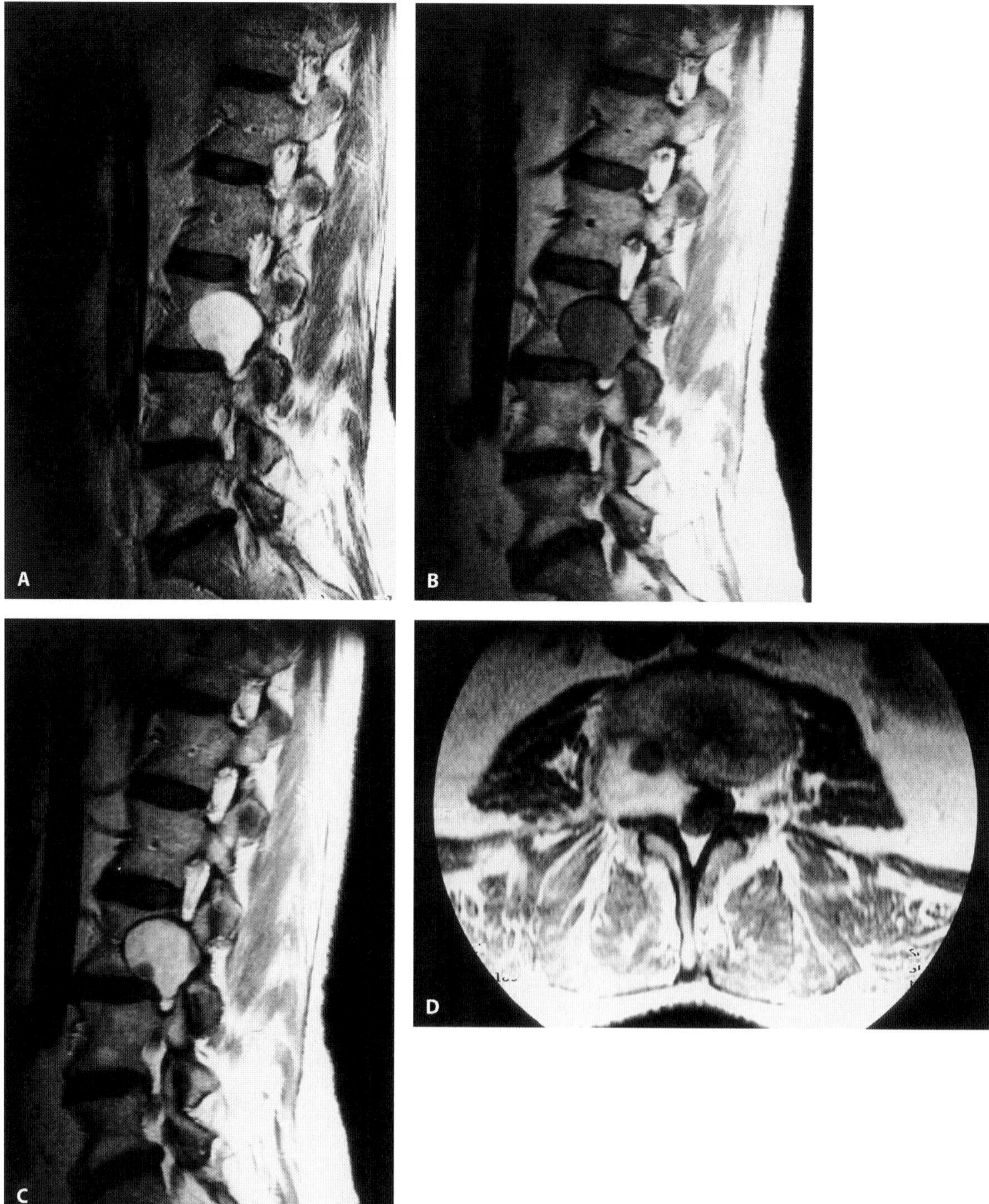

Fig. 5.23A–D. Neurofibroma. In this patient with a neurofibroma in the lumbar region, sagittal T2-WI (**A**), sagittal T1-WI (**B**), and gadolinium-enhanced sagittal (**C**) and axial (**D**) T1-WI were performed. Scalloping of the vertebral bodies and widening of the neural foramen are typical in nerve sheath tumors. The high signal on T2-WI reflects the high water content of the tumor. Enhancement is usually homogeneous, although central fibrous portions may enhance less intensely. Tumors extending through the neural foramen are typically dumb-bell-shaped as in this case (**D**)

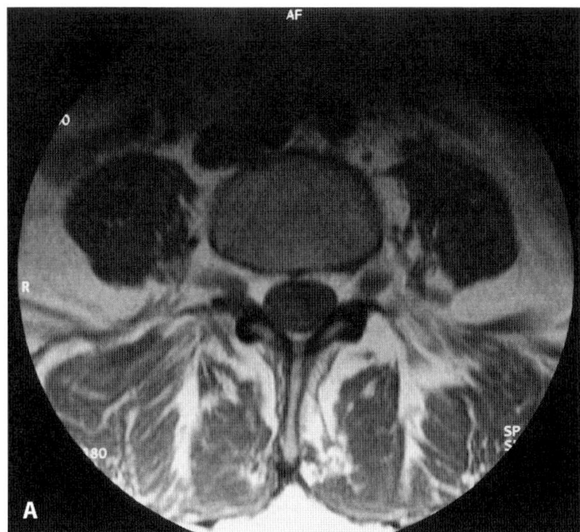

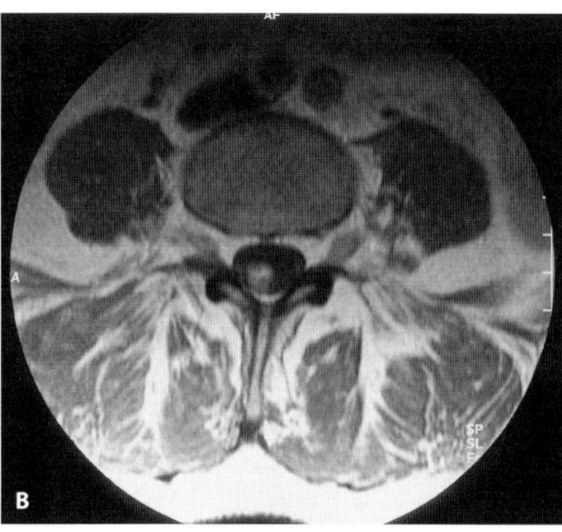

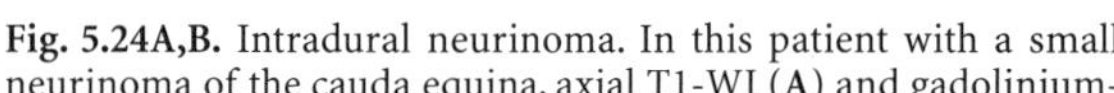

Fig. 5.24A,B. Intradural neurinoma. In this patient with a small neurinoma of the cauda equina, axial T1-WI (**A**) and gadolinium-enhanced T1-WI (**B**) were obtained. Smaller neurinomas may be impossible to detect without gadolinium administration

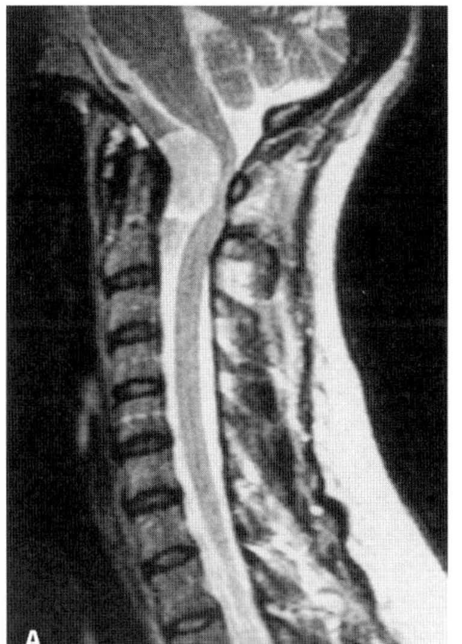

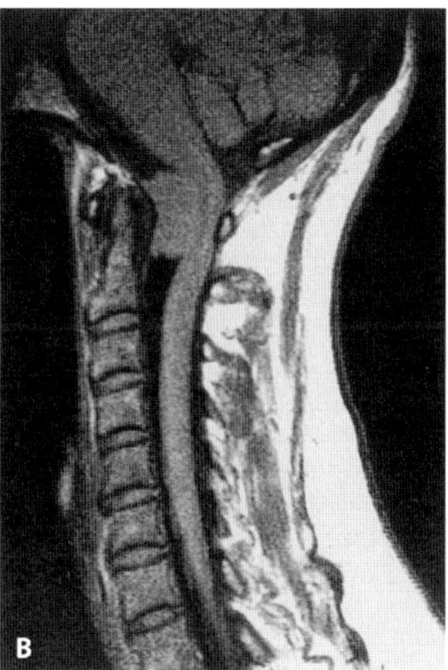

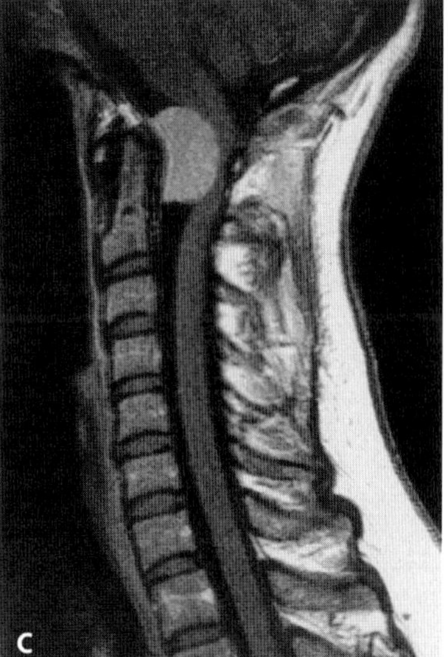

Fig. 5.25A–C. Intradural extramedullary meningioma. In this 65-year-old woman with a meningioma near the craniocervical junction, the following imaging sequences are shown: sagittal T2-WI (**A**), sagittal T1-WI (**B**), and gadolinium-enhanced sagittal T1-WI (**C**). From 60% to 80% of meningiomas are seen in middle-aged to elderly women. The average age at presentation is in the fifth and sixth decades. The lesions are hypo- to isointense to the spinal cord on T1-WI (**B**) and slightly hyperintense on T2-WI (**A**). Intense and homogeneous enhancement is typical (**C**), and the presence of a dural tail indicates the dural-based nature of the tumor

Acknowledgements. I would like to thank Bavo Van Riet, Paul Parizel, Geert Van Hoorde and Chris Goris for their collaboration.

Reference

Modic MT, Steinberg PM, Ross JS, Masaryk TJ, Carter JR (1988) Degenerative disk disease. Assessment of changes in vertebral body bone marrow with MR imaging. Radiology 166:193–199

Further Reading

Atlas SW (2001) Magnetic resonance imaging of the brain and spine. Lippincott-Raven, Philadelphia

Debatin JF, McKinnon GC (1998) Ultrafast MR imaging, techniques and applications. Springer, Berlin Heidelberg New York

Parizel PM, Wilmink JT (1998) Imaging of the spine: techniques and indications. In: Algra PR, Valk J, Heimans JJ (eds) Diagnosis and therapy of spinal tumours. Medical radiology – diagnostic imaging and radiation oncology. Springer, Berlin Heidelberg New York, pp 15–48

Stoller DW (1997) Magnetic resonance imaging in orthopaedics and sports medicine. Lippincott-Raven, Philadelphia

Wiesel SW (1996) The lumbar spine. Saunders, Philadelphia

Magnetic Resonance Imaging of the Head and Neck

6

L. van den Hauwe, J. W. Casselman

Contents

6.1 Temporal Bone

6.1.1 Introduction

The external and middle ear are best examined with computed tomography (CT). However, in patients presenting with sensorineural hearing loss (SNHL), vertigo and tinnitus, one must evaluate the inner ear, the internal auditory canal (IAC), the cerebellopontine angle (CPA) and the auditory/vestibular pathways in the brain and brainstem. Only magnetic resonance (MR) imaging is able to visualize all these structures and detect a sufficient amount of pathology in these patients. MRI also has become the method of choice in the detection and characterization of lesions of the petrous apex (cholesterol granuloma, congenital cholesteatoma) and in the diagnosis of meningo(encephalo)coeles in case of defects in the tegmen of the middle ear.

6.1.2 Coils and Patient Positioning

Patients are examined in the supine position with the head firmly fixed in the head coil. Axial images should be centred on the superior border of the external auditory canal. Multiple coronal localizers may be required

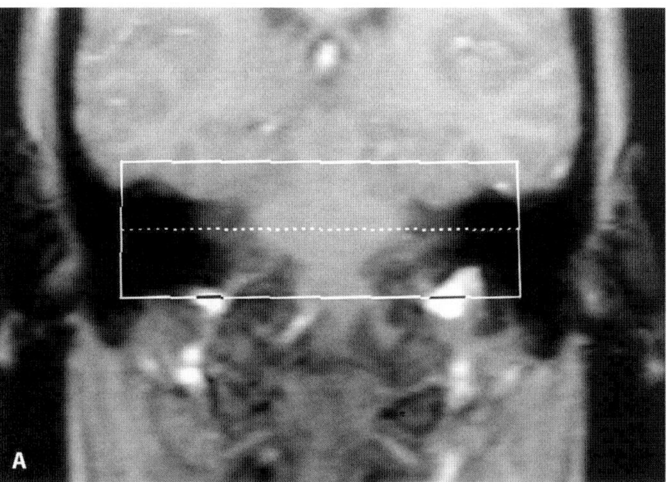

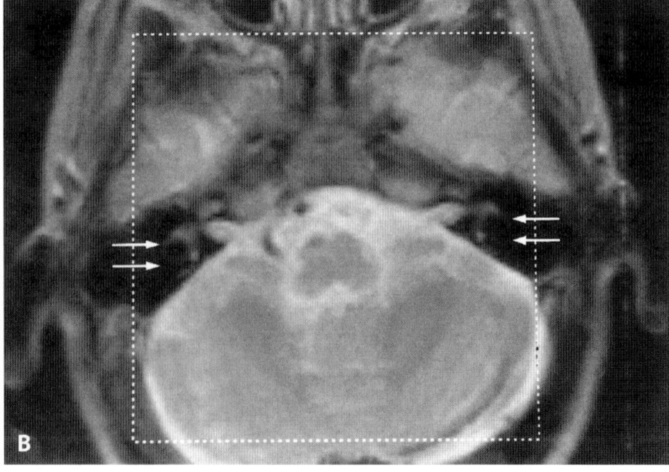

Fig. 6.1A,B. Positioning and orientation of the T2-weighted (T2-W) gradient-echo (GRE) slab on the coronal scout view (**A**) and a transverse spin-echo (SE) T2-weighted image (T2-WI) (**B**). The internal auditory canal (IAC) is not always easy to visualize on the thick and blurred coronal scout views. However, the complete inner ear is included in the study if the slab covers the inferior border of the temporal lobes and reaches the level of the jugular foramen and hypoglossal canal inferiorly. The slab can be angulated to correct for skull or positioning asymmetries (**A**). Transverse T2-WI or T1-WI can be used to verify whether the small field of view (FOV) (95 mm) GRE slab is correctly positioned so that both lateral semicircular canals (*arrows*) are included in the study (**B**)

to correct imperfect positioning (head tilting) or intrinsic asymmetries of the skull (Fig. 6.1). We prefer a standard circularly polarized head coil, because it allows imaging of both temporal bones simultaneously, and the signal remains homogeneous throughout the image. With this type of coil, even the root-entry zone and brainstem can be assessed. Moreover, the same coil can also be used to acquire a T2-weighted (T2-W) brain study, which is mandatory in patients with SNHL, vertigo and tinnitus.

Before positioning the patient in the magnet, hearing aids should be removed. Most cochlear implants are incompatible with MRI. In general, modern prostheses used for ossiculoplasty are not a contraindication for MRI.

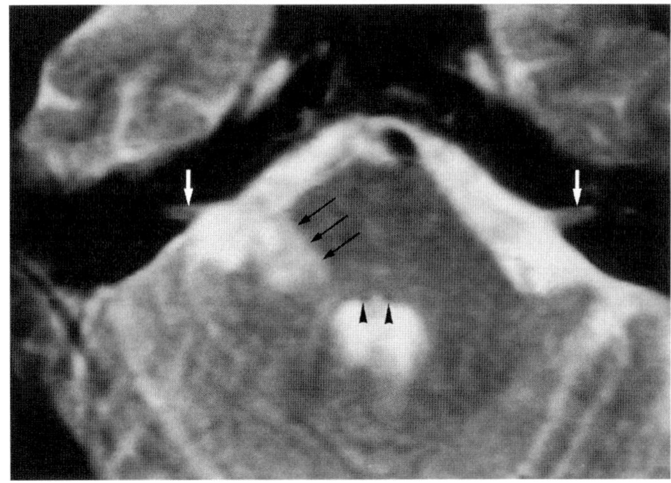

Fig. 6.2. Brainstem infarction. Thin spin-echo (SE) T2-weighted image of the brainstem in a patient with acute sensorineural hearing loss on the right side. A high signal intensity infarction (*black arrows*) can be seen at the level of the right cochlear nucleus in the lower pons. Notice also the low signal intensity of the myelinated medial longitudinal fasciculus on both sides (*arrowheads*). The IAC is also recognizable (*white arrows*)

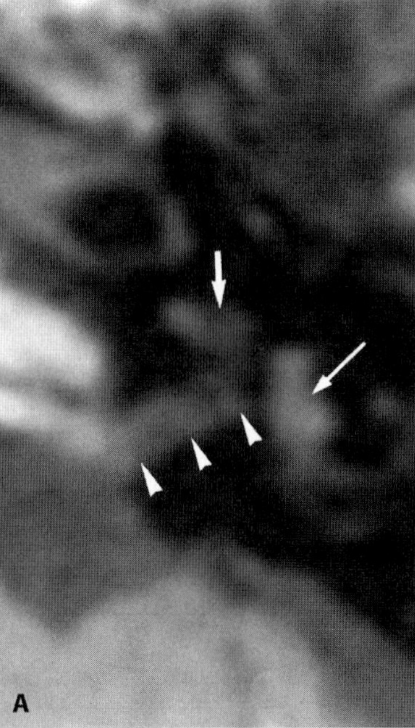

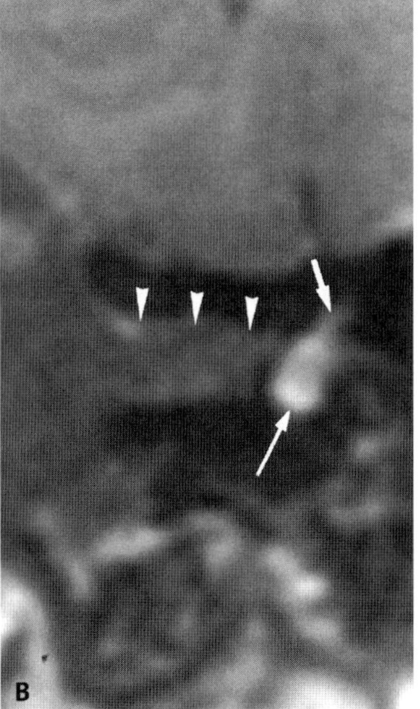

Fig. 6.3A,B. Labyrinthitis. Transverse unenhanced (**A**) and coronal gadolinium (Gd)-enhanced (**B**) SE T1-WI through the left membranous labyrinth in a patient with labyrinthitis. **A** A spontaneous high signal intensity is seen in the vestibule (*long white arrow*) and represents intralabyrinthine fluid with a high protein concentration or fluid mixed with blood. The posterior wall of the IAC (*arrowheads*) and the cochlea (*small white arrow*) are seen. On the Gd-enhanced image (**B**), enhancement is observed in the vestibule (*long white arrow*) and superior semicircular canal (*small white arrow*). The roof of the IAC is indicated by *arrowheads*. The GE T2-WI (not shown) demonstrated the presence of fluid throughout the left membranous labyrinth

6.1.3 Sequence Protocol

1. A routine T2-W brain study, with axial scans from the base of the skull to the vertex, should always be performed in order to exclude a sometimes clinically unexpected central cause of SNHL or vertigo (Fig. 6.2).
2. Axial unenhanced spin-echo (SE) T1-weighted images (T1-WI) are needed to detect intrinsically hyperintense lesions, such as schwannoma, lipoma, blood (trauma), cholesterol granuloma or fluid with a high protein concentration. Without these images, it becomes impossible to differentiate enhancement from spontaneous hyperintensities on the gadolinium (Gd)-enhanced T1-WI. An alternative solution is not to acquire unenhanced images routinely to save time and to re-examine the patient the next day whenever an intralabyrinthine enhancement or high signal, occurring in about 2% of studies, is found.
3. A Gd-enhanced T1-W sequence provides the most sensitive images for detecting pathology in the membranous labyrinth, IAC and CPA (Figs. 6.3 and 6.4). It is, therefore, obligatory to obtain this sequence. Intravenous administration of 0.1 mmol/kg of Gd is sufficient. The axial Gd-enhanced images must be obtained in the same positions (table positions) as the precontrast images so that comparison is possible. Slice thickness of the pre- and postcontrast T1-WI should not exceed 3 mm; 2-mm thin

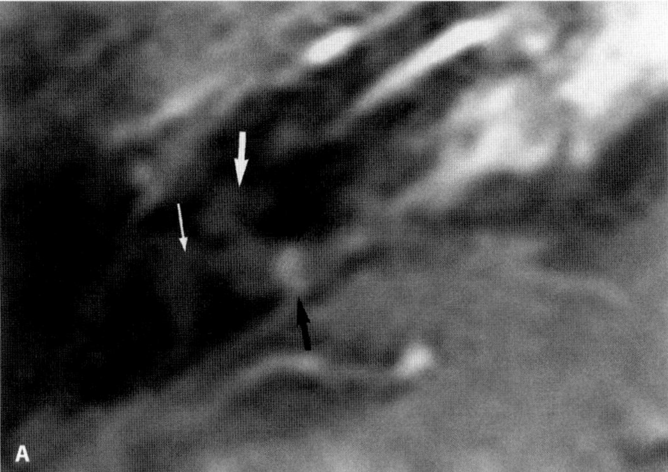

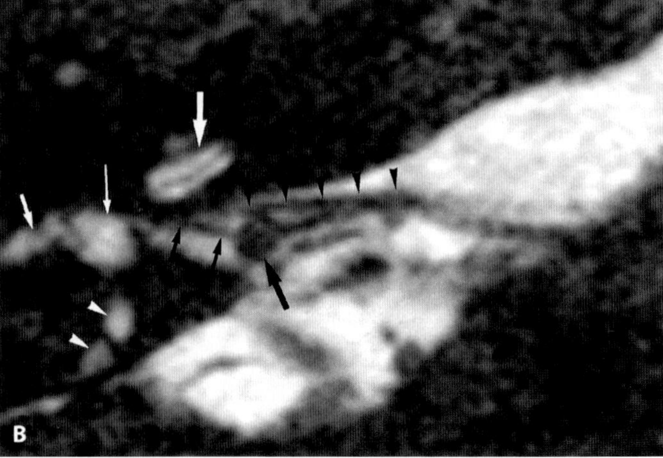

Fig. 6.4A,B. Acoustic schwannoma. Transverse 2-mm-thick Gd-enhanced T1-weighted image (T1-WI) (**A**) and 0.7-mm-thick gradient-echo (GRE) T2-WI (**B**) in a patient with a schwannoma of the superior vestibular branch of the vestibulocochlear nerve. **A** A nodular enhancing lesion (*black arrows*) can be seen in the IAC, but it is impossible to further define the exact position of the lesion on this image. The cochlea (*thick white arrow*) and vestibule (*thin white arrow*) are noticed. On the thin-section T2-W GRE images (**B**), the facial nerve (*black arrowheads*) can be recognized anteriorly in the IAC. A nodular lesion (*large black arrow*) can be seen in the course of the vestibular branch of the vestibulocochlear nerve (*small black arrows*). Notice the cochlea with separate visualization of the scala tympani and scala vestibuli (*large white arrow*), the vestibule (*long white arrow*), the lateral (*small white arrow*) and posterior (*white arrowheads*) semicircular canals

slices are considered state of the art. Slices should be contiguous, i.e., there should be no interslice gap. The same technique should be applied for coronal images, which can be helpful to confirm doubtful or subtle pathology.

4. T1-WI with fat suppression are particularly useful in the postoperative patient to separate residual/recurrent schwannoma from high signal fatty material used by the surgeon. On Gd-enhanced T1-WI, both have a high signal intensity and can be difficult to differentiate.
5. Gradient-echo (GRE) or turbo spin-echo (TSE) T2-WI are required to evaluate the very small structures of the CPA, the four nerve branches in the IAC, and the fluid inside the membranous labyrinth (Figs. 6.4 and 6.5). It is important to obtain the GRE images prior to the administration of Gd to avoid Gd-intensified flow artefacts. When possible, 0.5-mm to 0.7-mm-thick slices should be used; slice thickness should not exceed 1 mm. The slab becomes thinner when submillimetric images are used, and hence, positioning becomes critical in the coronal plane. High-resolution imaging can be achieved with a 512×512 matrix at the expense of increasing the acquisition time and decreasing the signal-to-noise ratio. Alternatively, we prefer to use a very small field-of-view (FOV) of 95 mm with a 256 matrix, which provides a similar in-plane spatial resolution, but without increasing the acquisition time. In most patients, both inner ears will just fit in a FOV of

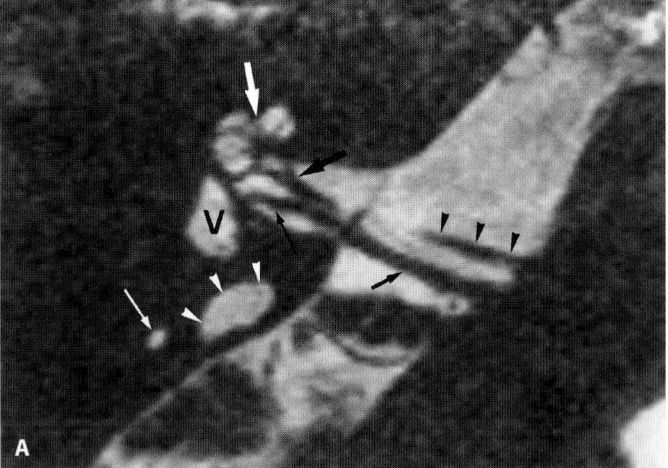

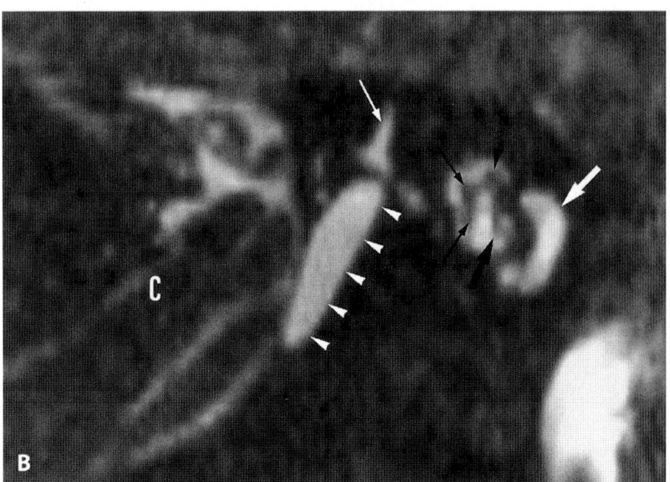

Fig. 6.5A,B. Large vestibular aqueduct syndrome. Transverse 0.7-mm thick GE T2-WI (**A**) and a parasagittal reconstruction (**B**) of the right membranous labyrinth, made from these transverse 0.7-mm-thick images, in a patient with a large endolymphatic duct and sac (large vestibular aqueduct syndrome). The patient had sensorineural hearing loss and was, therefore, referred for MRI. An enlarged, fluid-filled endolymphatic sac can be recognized (*white arrowheads*). The sac is abnormal when the diameter is larger than the diameter of the fluid-filled posterior semicircular canal (*long white arrow*). Fluid-filled vestibule (*V*) and cochlea with separate visualization of the two scalas (*large white arrow*). Facial nerve (*black arrowheads*), common trunk of the vestibulocochlear nerve (*small black arrow*) and its more peripheral cochlear (*large black arrow*) and inferior vestibular (*long black arrow*) branches (**A**). The enlarged, fluid-filled endolymphatic sac (*white arrowheads*) can be followed from the labyrinth to the anterior border of the cerebellum (*C*). Fluid-filled superior semicircular canal (*long white arrow*) and cochlea (*large white arrow*). Facial nerve (*black arrowhead*), cochlear branch (*large black arrow*) and vestibular branches (*long black arrows*) of the vestibulocochlear nerve, surrounded by cerebrospinal fluid (*CSF*) in the fundus of the IAC (**B**)

95 mm, but accurate positioning is crucial, and it is best to use the thin-section axial unenhanced T1-WI or T2-WI to check whether the GRE slab also covers the outer borders of the lateral semicircular canals. Only these GRE T2-WI can discriminate high signal intralabyrinthine fluid from low signal intralabyrinthine fibrosis or tumour.

In acoustic neuroma surgery, these T2-WI will allow us to determine the type of surgery to be performed. If fluid is still present between the schwannoma and the fundus of the ICA, hearing preservation surgery (middle cranial fossa or retrosigmoid approach) is possible. If no fluid is observed, the surgeon has to remove all the tissue up to the base of the cochlea, leaving the patient deaf. In these patients a less invasive translabyrinthine approach is performed. An even more important sign is the signal intensity of the cerebrospinal fluid between the schwannoma and the fundus of the ICA and the signal intensity of the intralabyrinthine fluid. Hearing preservation is achieved four times more often when a normal signal intensity of these fluids is observed (Fig. 6.6).

6. To detect vascular malformations and neurovascular conflicts, 1-mm-thick, high-resolution, time-of-flight

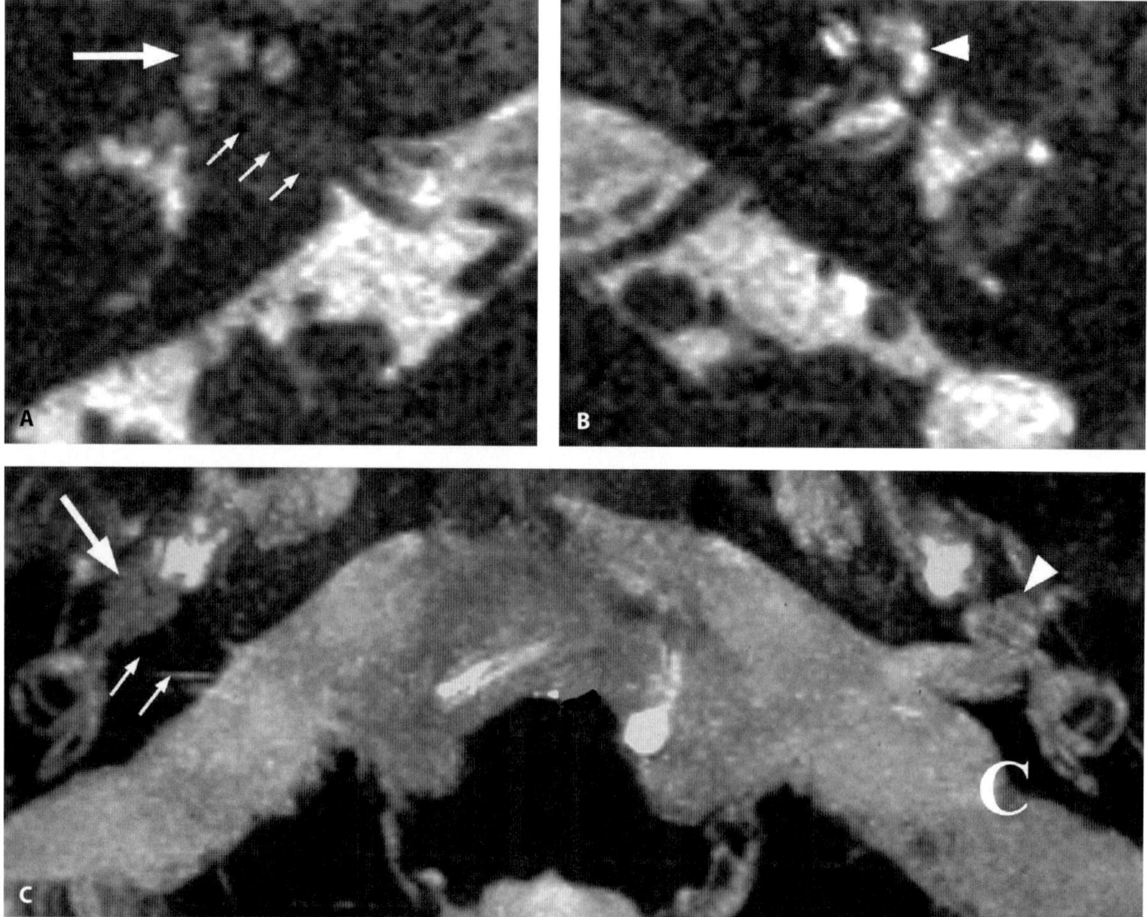

Fig. 6.6A–C. Transverse 0.7-mm-thick GE T2-WI through the right (**A**) and left (**B**) inner ear and projection image of all axial images through both inner ears (**C**). An acoustic schwannoma can be seen in the right internal auditory canal (*small white arrows*), replacing the cerebrospinal fluid (CSF). Normal CSF is present on the left side. The intralabyrinthine fluid and especially the fluid in the right cochlea have lost their high signal intensity (*large white arrow*) in comparison with the fluid in the normal left cochlea (*white arrowhead*). The signal difference is always seen better on the projection image

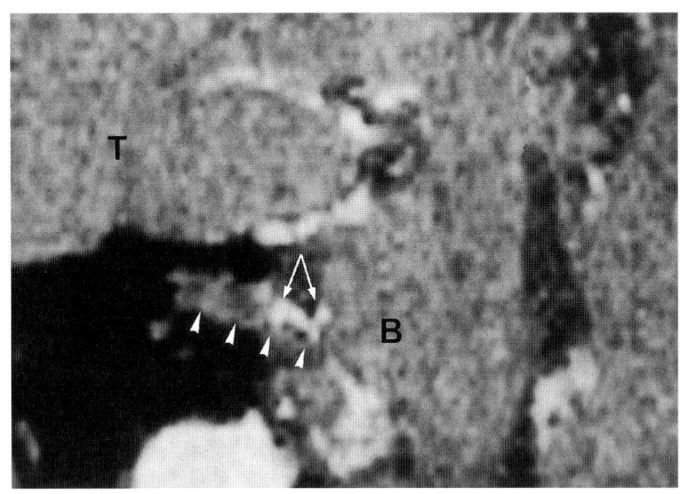

Fig. 6.7. Neurovascular compression syndrome. Paracoronal reconstruction of a set of gadolinium-enhanced MR angiography images in a patient with tinnitus and hemifacial spasm. The neural bundle can be followed in the IAC and cerebellopontine angle (*arrowheads*), and prominent blood vessels are resting on the superior border of the nerves near the root-entry zone (*white arrows*). The brainstem (*B*) and temporal lobe (*T*) are indicated

Table 6.1. Magnetic resonance imaging protocol recommendations for temporal bone examinations

Pulse sequence	WI	Plane	No. of sections	TR (ms)	TE (ms)	Flip angle	Echo train length	Section thickness (mm)	Matrix	FOV	recFOV	BW	No. of acq.	Acq. time (min:s)
SE (T1±Gd)	T1	tra/cor	10	490	20	90	–	2	160×256	230	62.5	65	4	5:17
GRE 3DFT-CISS	T2	tra	46	12.25	5.9	70	–	0.7	192×256	95	–	195	2	7:14
GRE-MRA 3DFT-FISP	–	tra	64	39	7	25	–	1.13	192×512	240	75	81	2	8
SE- (brain stem)	T2	tra	19	1900	12/80	62	–	4	157×256	230	75	195/67	2	10

Abbreviations: *WI* weighted image; *TR* repetition time (ms); *TI* inversion time (ms); *TE* echo time (ms); *TD* time delay (sec); *no part* number of partitions; *Matrix* (phase × frequency matrix); *FOV* field of view (mm); *recFOV* % rectangular field of view; *BW* bandwidth (Hz)

Table 6.2. Overview of imaging protocols for peripheral and central sensorineural hearing loss (SNHL), vertigo and tinnitus. Protocols should always begin with a T2-weighted brain study

Peripheral SNHL and vertigo	General SNHL and vertigo	Tinnitus
1. *Axial unenhanced T1-weighted images*	1. **T2-weighted brain stem sequence**	1. *Axial unenhanced T1-weighted images*
2. **Thin T2-weighted GRE sequence**	2. **Thin T2-weighted GRE sequence**	2. **Thin T2-weighted GRE sequence**
3. **Axial Gd-enhanced T1-weighted images**	3. **Axiai Gd-enhanced T1-weighted images**	3. **Axial Gd-enhanced T1-weighted images**
4. *Coronal Gd-enhanced T1-weighted images*	4. *Gd-enhanced T1-weighted brain study*	4. **Gd-enhanced high resolution MRA**
	5. *Coronal T2-weighted study of the auditory pathways and cortex (SNHL)*	

Bold = necessary: *Italics* = optional, call be omitted. *Gd* gadolinium; *GRE* gradient echo

MR angiography (MRA) images should be used. This sequence is routinely added to the imaging protocol in patients with tinnitus (Fig. 6.7).

7. Selective, 4-mm-thick, SE T2-WI of the brainstem (axial) and auditory cortex (coronal) are used when more subtle pathology along the auditory/vestibular pathway is suspected (Fig. 6.2)

For an overview of the imaging protocols, see Tables 6.1 and 6.2.

6.1.4 Pathology

The most frequent pathology is 'schwannoma'; these tumours can be found in the labyrinth, IAC (Fig. 6.4) and CPA. The second most frequent pathology in the membranous labyrinth is acute/chronic labyrinthitis (Fig. 6.3). Other frequently found lesions causing SNHL, vertigo, tinnitus or a combination of these clinical signs include labyrinthine malformations (Fig. 6.5), other types of CPA tumours such as meningiomas or epidermoids (Fig. 6.8), neurovascular conflicts (Fig. 6.7), brainstem infarctions (Fig. 6.2) or demyelination, etc. MR imaging has become indispensable in patients who are candidates for cochlear implant surgery, as only the GRE T2-WI can inform the surgeon whether the cochlea is filled with fluid and whether a normal cochlear branch of the vestibulocochlear nerve is present. Finally, in the middle ear, MR imaging is the method of choice for the detection of postoperative meningo(encephalo)coeles in patients with defects of the tegmen (Fig. 6.9).

6.2 Eye and Orbit

6.2.1 Introduction

CT scanning still plays an important role in the diagnosis of orbital pathology. The differences in attenuation values of the orbital contents (retrobulbar fat, extrinsic muscles, globe, bone, air and vessels) provide an excellent natural tissue contrast. However, MR imaging is the modality of choice when available. The major advantage of MRI over CT is that the entire visual pathway can be examined in one go with higher sensitivity and specificity. In this manner, MR imaging not only detects orbital lesions, but is also able to demonstrate a wide range of intracranial pathology associated with visual impairment [parasellar lesions, multiple sclerosis (MS) plaques]. At present, CT still remains the imaging modality of choice in the following circumstances: detection of calcifications, trauma patients, primary lesions arising from the bony orbit, or when MRI is not available. A drawback of MRI is that because of the longer examination time, it is more prone to globe and lid motion artefacts. Continuing efforts have been made by the MR vendors to overcome these problems by introducing faster imaging techniques. Fat-suppressed images allow better discrimination between enhancing structures located within the retrobulbar fat (Fig. 6.11).

6.2.2 Coils and Patient Positioning

Prior to performing MR imaging of the eye and orbit, patients must be screened in order to rule out the presence of metallic foreign bodies in or near the orbit, e.g., metallic slivers, fragments, or iron dust in industrial workers. These objects can move under the influence of the magnetic field, with blindness as a possible consequence. Therefore, thorough questioning of the patient is necessary. When in doubt, conventional X-rays should be obtained before positioning the patient in the magnet. Patients are asked to remove their mascara since it may contain ferromagnetic components, causing image degradation due to susceptibility artefacts. It is important to encourage the patient to fix his or her gaze on one point during the examination to avoid motion artefacts, which might arise during blinking.

The MR examination of the orbit can be performed using a circularly polarized head coil or a dedicated surface coil. Surface coils have the advantage of providing a higher signal-to-noise ratio. Ultra-thin slices with a high spatial resolution (small FOV of 40–50 mm and high matrix of 512×512) can, thus, be obtained. This is useful to examine the globe for the presence of tumours (Fig. 6.10). A disadvantage of surface coils is that only the anterior portion of the orbit is depicted (the globe), leaving the remainder of the orbit and the optic pathway unexamined. A second disadvantage is that only one orbit can be visualized, unless binocular surface coils are used.

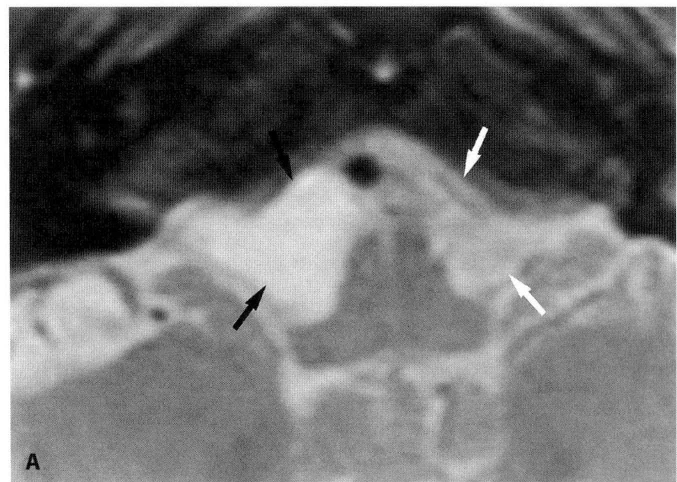

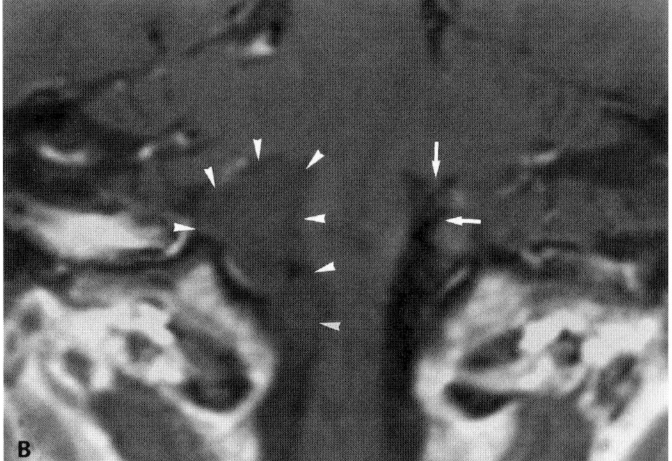

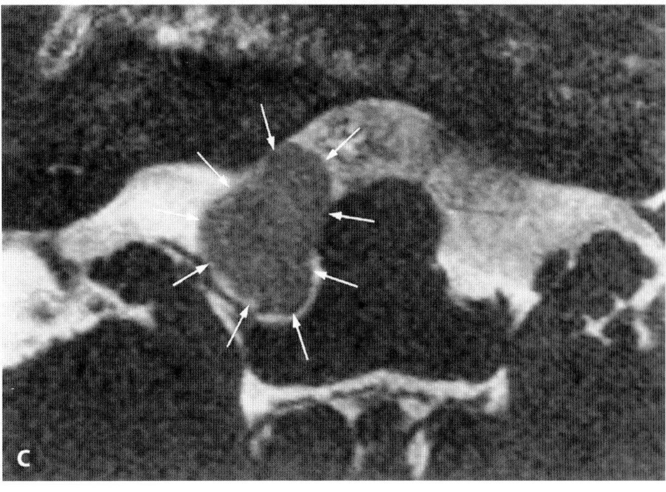

Fig. 6.8A–C. Posterior fossa epidermoid tumour. Transverse SE T2-WI (**A**), coronal Gd-enhanced SE T1-WI (**B**) and transverse GRE T2-WI (**C**) in a patient with an epidermoid tumour in the lower cerebellopontine angle (CPA). A larger lower CPA space is seen on the right side (*black arrows*), and also the signal intensity on the right side is slightly higher than on the left side (*white arrows*) (**A**). The lesion in the right CPA does not enhance (*arrowheads*) and has a slightly higher signal intensity than the normal CSF in the left CPA (*white arrows*) (**B**). Only on the GRE T2-WI (**C**) can the lesion (*white arrows*) be distinguished from the surrounding CSF. The solid nature of the tumour is proved, and a subarachnoid cyst can be excluded

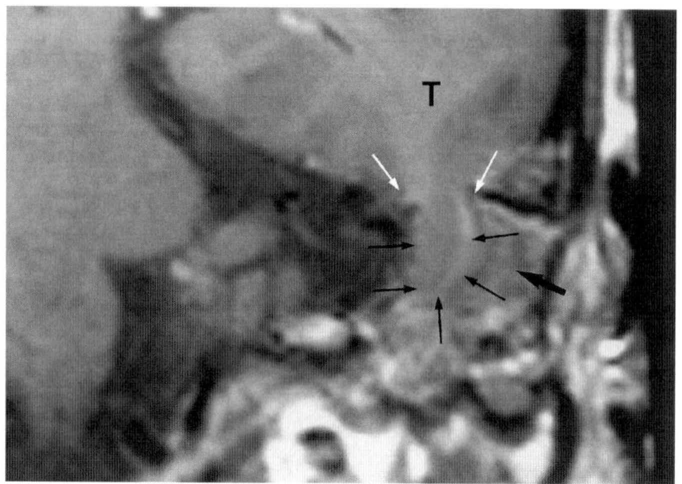

Fig. 6.9. CSF leak. Coronal Gd-enhanced SE T1-WI through the left middle ear in a patient with a CSF leak. A large tegmental defect can be seen (*white arrows*) with herniation of brain (*long black arrows*) into the middle ear cavity. It was impossible to recognize the presence of brain in the completely obliterated middle ear on CT. There is adjacent inflammation and/or granulation tissue in the middle ear/antrum (*large black arrow*). The structure above the tegmental defect is the temporal lobe (*T*)

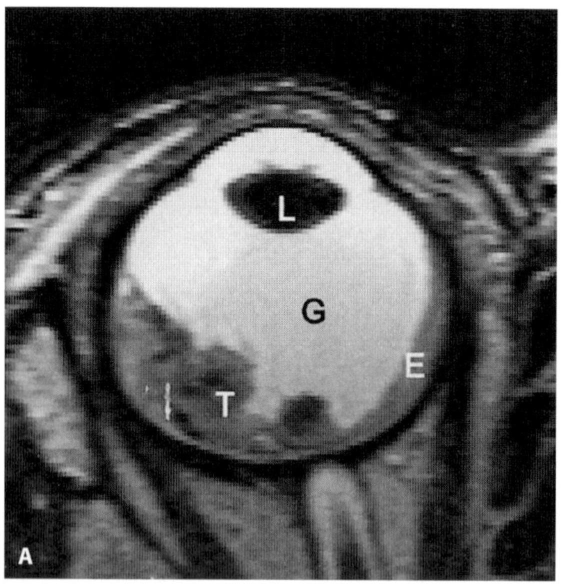

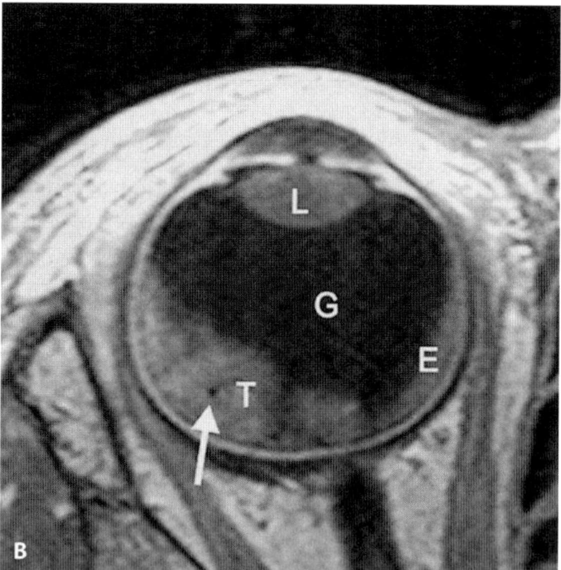

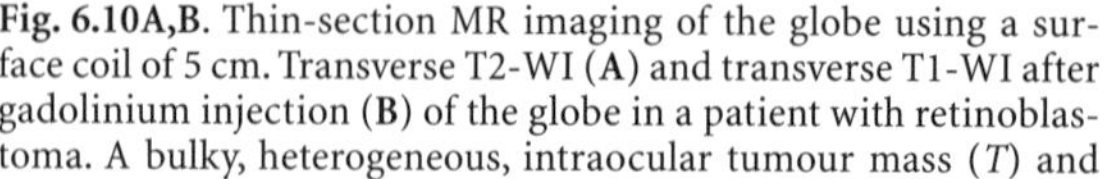

Fig. 6.10A,B. Thin-section MR imaging of the globe using a surface coil of 5 cm. Transverse T2-WI (**A**) and transverse T1-WI after gadolinium injection (**B**) of the globe in a patient with retinoblastoma. A bulky, heterogeneous, intraocular tumour mass (*T*) and accompanying retinal detachment (*E*) are observed. Notice the presence of a small flow void in the tumour, reflecting small calcifications (*arrow*) (**B**) (Courtesy of Dr A. Lemke, Berlin)

Table. 6.3. Magnetic resonance protocol recommendations for imaging of the orbit and visual pathway

Pulse sequence	WI	Plane	No. of sections	TR (ms)	TE (ms)	Flip angle	TI (ms)	Echo train length	Section thickness (mm)	Matrix	FOV	recFOV	BW	No. of acq.	Acq. time (min:s)
SE	T1	tra/cor	15	450	15	90	–	–	2	256×512	200	75	130	2	3:50
STIR	T2	cor/tra	11	2700	19	90	150	–	3	192×256	200	75	130	1	6:39
TSE	T2	tra/cor	15	3000	19–93	90	–	3	3	256×512	360	50	130	2	6:32
spectral	T1	tra/cor	11	650	15	90	–	–	3	192×256	230	75	130	2	4:10
fatsat	–	–	–	–	–	–	–	–	–	–	–	–	FS63		

Abbreviations: *WI* weighted image; *TR* repetition time (ms); *TI* inversion time (ms); *TE* echo time (ms); *TD* time delay (sec); *no part* number of partitions; *Matrix* (phase×frequency matrix); *FOV* field of view (mm); *recFOV* % rectangular field of view; *BW* bandwidth (Hz)

6.2.3 Sequence Protocol

To reduce motion artefacts, the scanning time should be kept as short as possible. This can be achieved by reducing the repetition time (TR) and/or the number of excitations (NEX). Thin slices (thickness of 3–5 mm) and a small FOV are combined to optimize spatial resolution. For the MR protocol for imaging of the orbit and visual pathway, see Table 6.3.

1. High-resolution SE T1-W semiaxial or coronal imaging sequences are performed as the initial screening sequence. Both slice orientations allow comparison of both orbits. The semiaxial slices are oriented along the course of the optic nerve.
2. TSE T2-W and fat-suppressed sequences are added when a lesion is seen, and further characterization is required. Fat suppression is necessary to subdue the bright signal arising from the retrobulbar fat. This causes chemical-shift misregistration artefacts at fat-water interfaces (the margins of the globe) and, furthermore, the bright signal of the retrobulbar fat may overwhelm small structures of intermediate to low signal intensity (the use of fat suppression is mandatory for lesion demonstration in the optic nerve, e.g. optic neuritis). Fat suppression can be obtained by frequency-selective spectral presaturation or by short tau inversion recovery (STIR) techniques.
3. Gd-enhanced SE T1-WI with fat suppression may be required for further differentiation of tumours, optic nerve lesions and orbital masses. After intravenous injection of Gd, spectral fat saturation is the technique of choice (Fig. 6.11). STIR sequences should be avoided for post-contrast MR imaging, because the fat signal will be suppressed as well as the signal arising from enhancing structures. This phenomenon is known as negative enhancement.
4. GRE sequences are of limited use, but may detect changes in susceptibility in the presence of calcifications (retinoblastoma) or haemorrhage.

6.2.4 Pathology

Major indications for MRI of the eye and orbit include tumours (Tables 6.4 and 6.5), such as uveal melanoma

Table 6.4. Ocular tumours

Uveal melanoma
Metastasis
Choroidal haemangioma
Retinoblastoma[a]
Astrocytic hamartoma[a] (tuberous sclerosis, neurofibromatosis)

[a] Intraocular calcifications

Table 6.5. Orbital tumours

Optic nerve glioma
Optic nerve sheath meningioma
Plexiform neurofibroma
Haemangioma (capillary, cavernous)
Lymphangioma
Lymphoma – pseudotumour
Rhabdomyosarcoma
Metastases

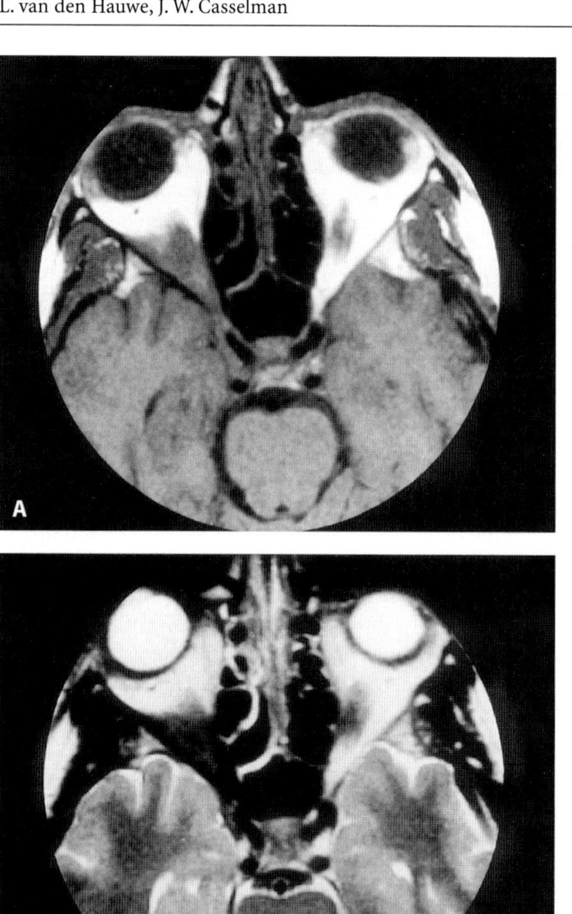

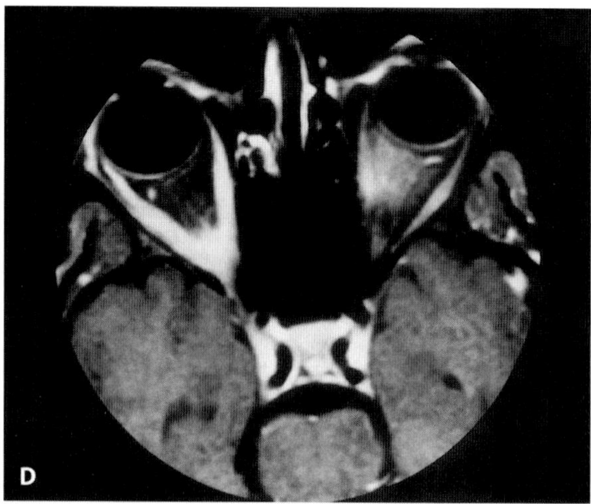

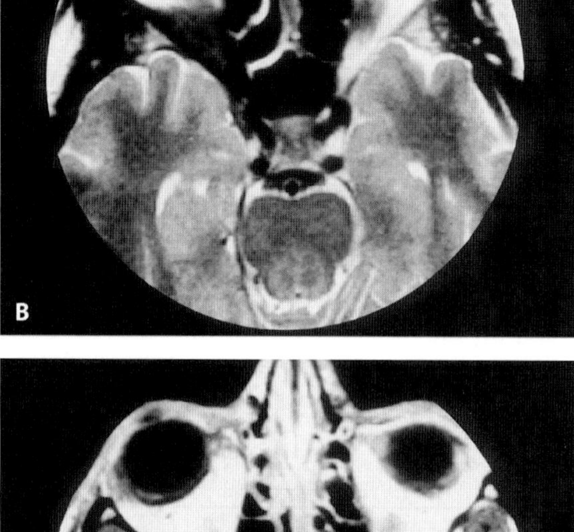

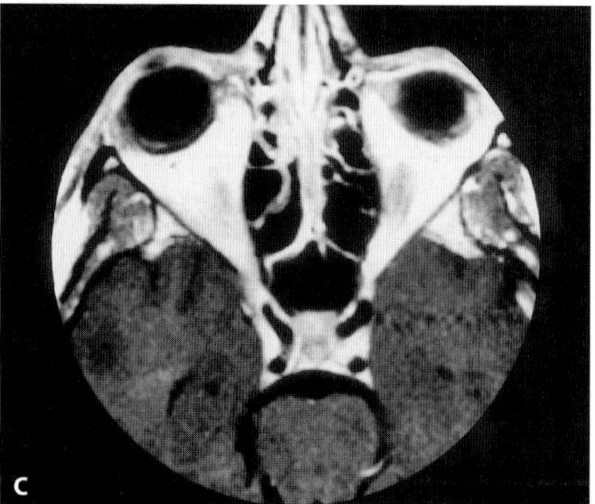

Fig. 6.11A–D. Idiopathic inflammatory pseudotumour. Transverse SE unenhanced T1-WI (**A**), turbo SE (TSE) T2-WI (**B**), SE Gd-enhanced T1-WI without (**C**) and with (**D**) spectral fat suppression in a patient with idiopathic inflammatory pseudotumour of the right orbit. An intraconal mass lesion with signal intensity iso-intense to muscle is noticed in the apex of the right orbit (**A**). The lesion extends into the cavernous sinus. On the T2-W sequence, the lesion displays a low signal intensity, reflecting a high cellular content (**B**). After contrast injection, enhancement of the lesion is difficult to detect because of the high signal intensity of the retrobulbar fat (**C**). A sequence with spectral fat suppression shows enhancement of the lesion located in the orbital apex (**D**). Note also the normal enhancement of the extraocular muscles and of the choroidal layer in the globe

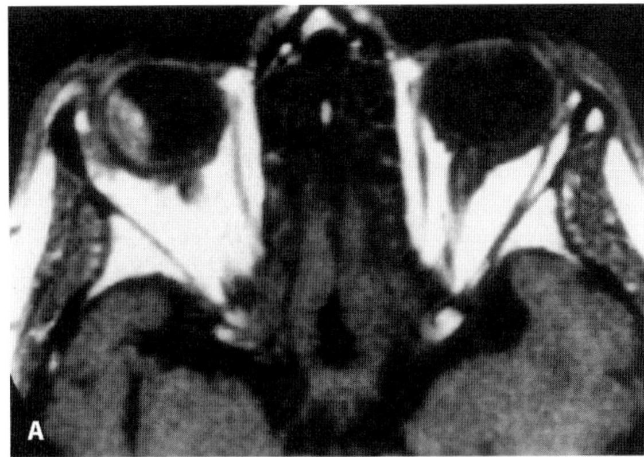

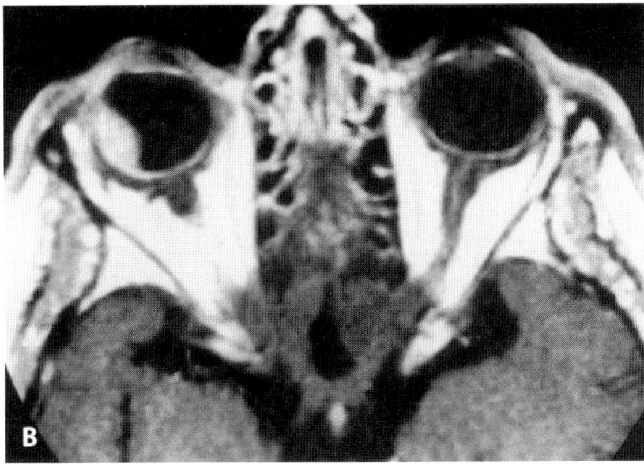

Fig. 6.12A,B. Uveal melanoma. Fat-suppressed transverse SE T1-weighted images (T1-WI) before (**A**) and after (**B**) Gd injection in a patient with an uveal melanoma of the left globe. A fusiform, spontaneously hyperintense, nodular lesion (**A**) is observed in the lateral part of the left eye globe. The high signal intensity on the precontrast image indicates the presence of a paramagnetic substance such as melanin. Intense enhancement of the lesion is observed after Gd injection (**B**)

(Fig. 6.12), retinoblastoma (Fig. 6.10), optic-nerve glioma, optic nerve sheath meningioma (Fig. 6.13), haemangioma (Fig. 6.14) and metastases (Fig. 6.15). Also, inflammatory lesions of the orbit, e.g. idiopathic inflammatory pseudotumour (Fig. 6.11) and inflammatory lesions of the optic nerve (Fig. 6.16), may be demonstrated. Lesions that arise outside the orbit and interfere with the function of the optic pathways can be seen, e.g. pituitary macroadenoma (Fig. 6.17).

6.3 Paranasal Sinuses

6.3.1 Introduction

CT and MRI are complementary techniques for imaging the paranasal sinuses. The bony structures surrounding the air-filled sinus cavities are better seen on CT. Therefore, CT is the preferred imaging modality in trauma patients. Moreover, CT is superior in demonstrating the ostiomeatal complex, which occupies a key position in inflammatory/infectious disease, especially when functional endoscopic sinus surgery (FESS) is planned. The use of MR imaging is advocated in patients with complicated inflammatory sinus disease and in patients with suspected tumoral pathology in this region.

6.3.2 Coils and Patient Positioning

The patient is placed in a supine position in the circularly polarized head coil with the head firmly fixed.

6.3.3 Sequence Protocol

1. The MR examination of the paranasal sinuses starts with coronal unenhanced SE T1-WI and TSE T2-WI . The purpose of these sequences is to discriminate between different soft-tissue structures and retention of serous and mucinous fluid.
2. Contrast-enhanced, high-resolution, axial and coronal SE T1-WI are obtained to further differentiate soft-tissue structures, thereby allowing discrimination between tumoral components from normally enhancing mucosa or polyps (Figs. 6.18 and 6.19). Also, intracranial and/or intraorbital extension of pathology can be better demonstrated in this manner (Fig. 6.20).

For the MR imaging protocol for sinonasal examinations, see Table 6.6.

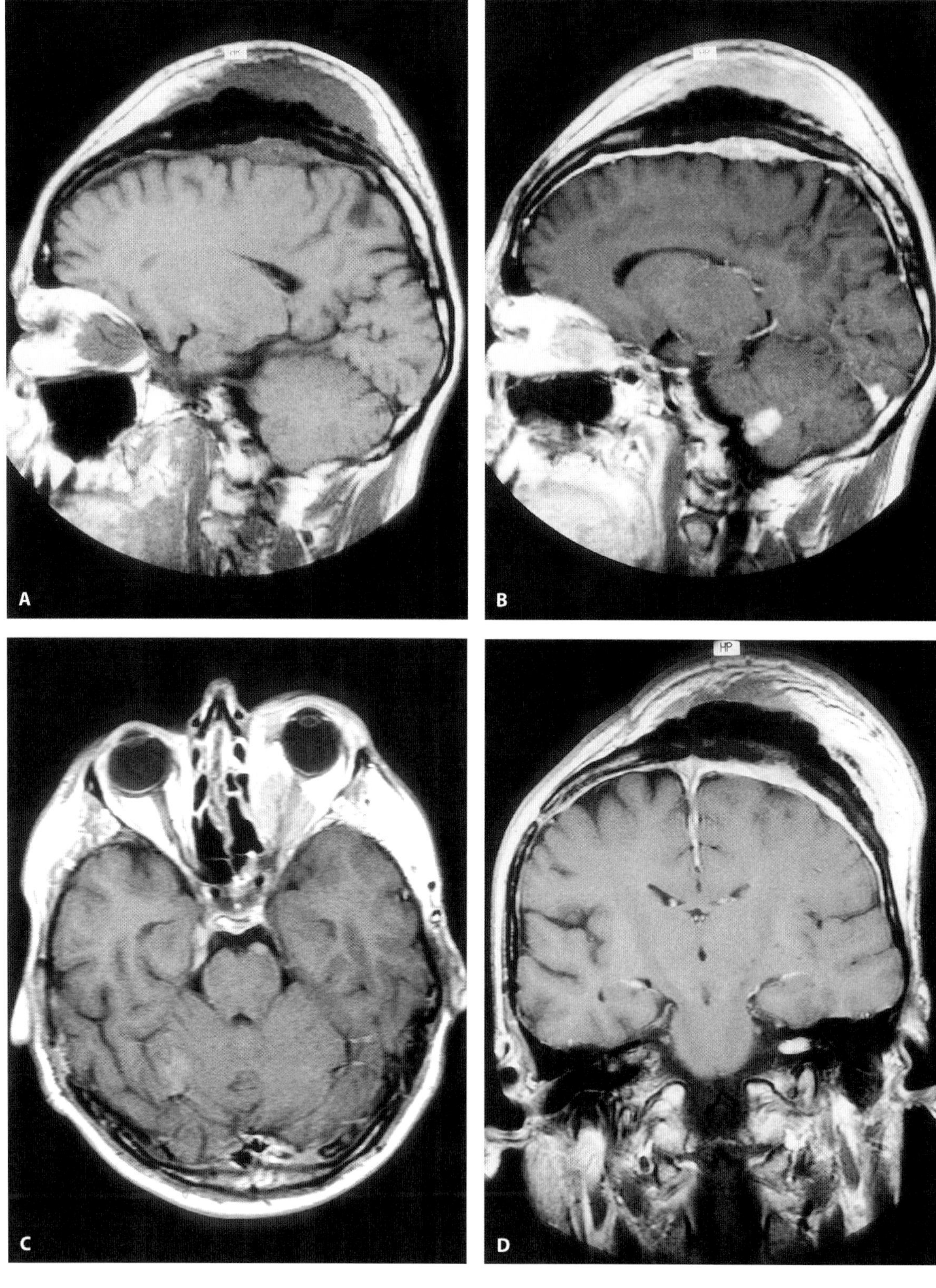
HP
A
B
C
D

Fig. 6.14A–C. Intraconal cavernous haemangioma of the right orbit. Transverse turbo TSE T2-WI (**A**), transverse SE T1-WI with spectral fat saturation before (**B**) and after (**C**) Gd injection in a 27-year-old man presenting with proptosis of the right eye. A heterogeneous, lobulated, retrobulbar mass of the right orbit is observed. On T2-WI, the lesion is markedly hyperintense (**A**). The lesion contains areas of high signal intensity on T1-WI (**B**) that may represent areas of thrombosed vascular spaces. Cavernous haemangiomas always enhance after Gd injection (**C**)

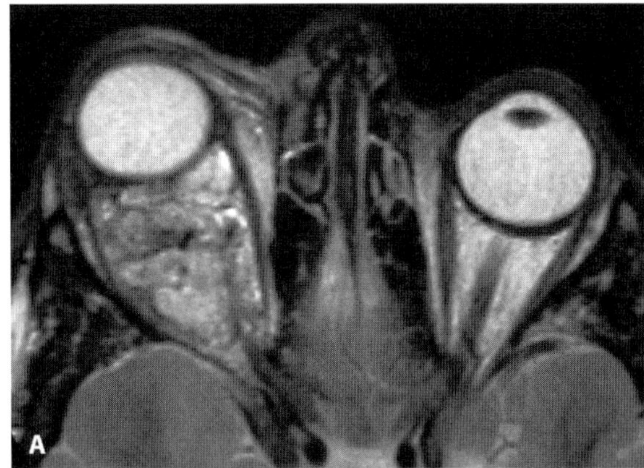

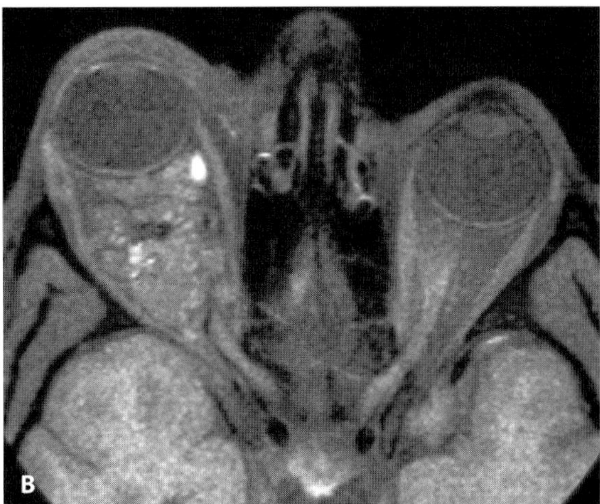

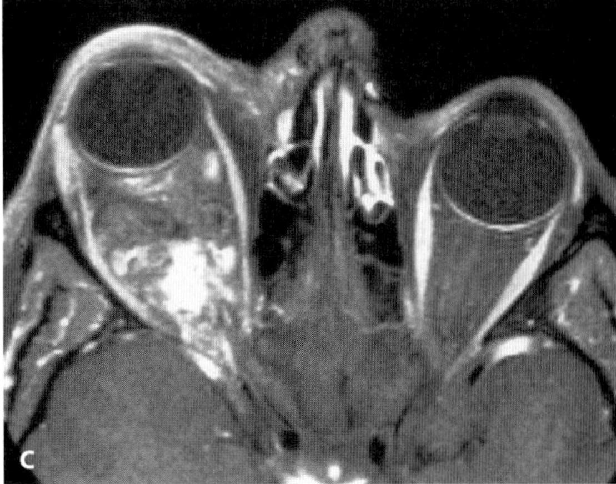

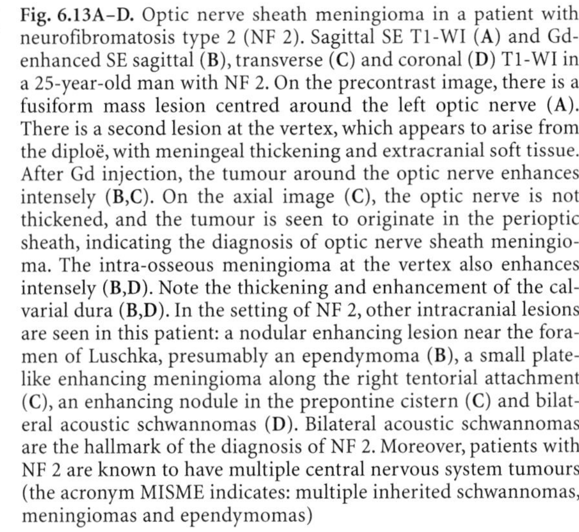

◀ **Fig. 6.13A–D.** Optic nerve sheath meningioma in a patient with neurofibromatosis type 2 (NF 2). Sagittal SE T1-WI (**A**) and Gd-enhanced SE sagittal (**B**), transverse (**C**) and coronal (**D**) T1-WI in a 25-year-old man with NF 2. On the precontrast image, there is a fusiform mass lesion centred around the left optic nerve (**A**). There is a second lesion at the vertex, which appears to arise from the diploë, with meningeal thickening and extracranial soft tissue. After Gd injection, the tumour around the optic nerve enhances intensely (**B,C**). On the axial image (**C**), the optic nerve is not thickened, and the tumour is seen to originate in the perioptic sheath, indicating the diagnosis of optic nerve sheath meningioma. The intra-osseous meningioma at the vertex also enhances intensely (**B,D**). Note the thickening and enhancement of the calvarial dura (**B,D**). In the setting of NF 2, other intracranial lesions are seen in this patient: a nodular enhancing lesion near the foramen of Luschka, presumably an ependymoma (**B**), a small plate-like enhancing meningioma along the right tentorial attachment (**C**), an enhancing nodule in the prepontine cistern (**C**) and bilateral acoustic schwannomas (**D**). Bilateral acoustic schwannomas are the hallmark of the diagnosis of NF 2. Moreover, patients with NF 2 are known to have multiple central nervous system tumours (the acronym MISME indicates: multiple inherited schwannomas, meningiomas and ependymomas)

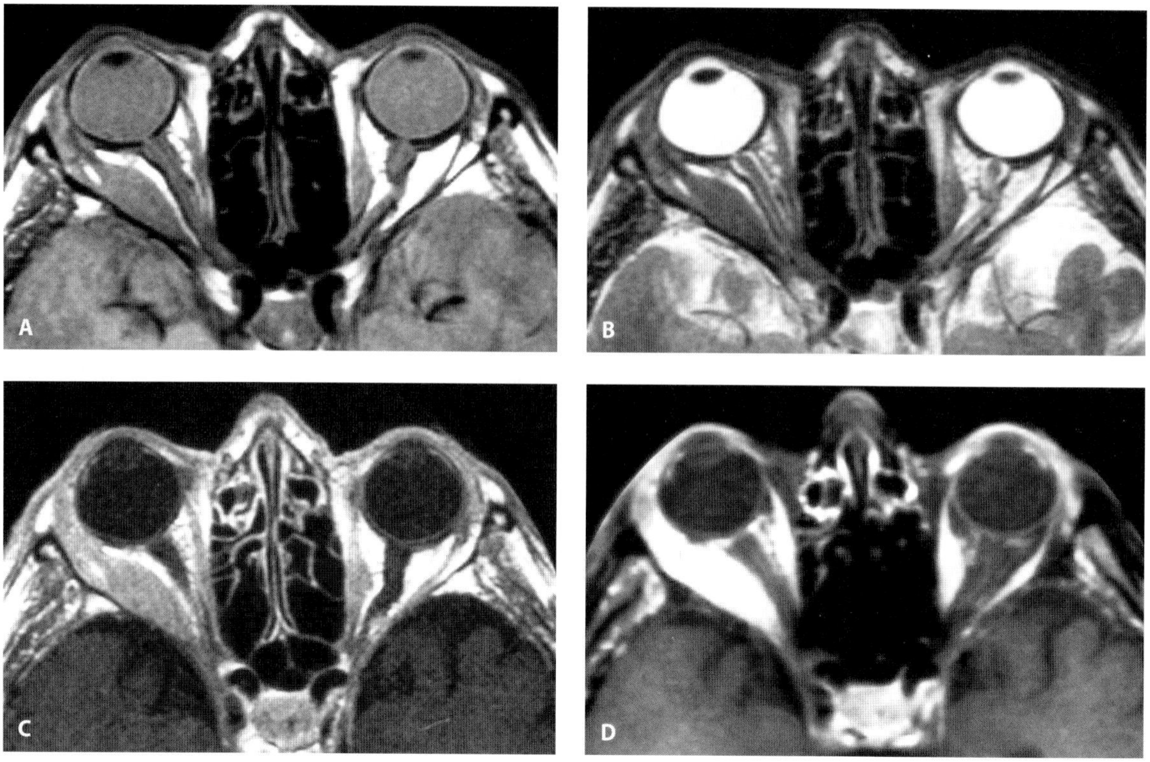

Fig. 6.15A–D. Bilateral rectus muscle metastases. Transverse SE proton density-weighted images (T1-WI) (**A**), transverse TSE T2-WI (**B**) and transverse SE T1-WI (**C**) and transverse fat-suppressed T1-WI (**D**) after Gd injection in a 77-year-old woman with a previous medical history of breast carcinoma. Enlargement of the right lateral rectus muscle and of the left medial rectus muscle is observed. Signal intensities are nonspecific, and without her clinical history, the differential diagnosis should include idiopathic inflammatory pseudotumour, lymphoma and thyroid ophthalmopathy. In children, rhabdomyosarcoma is the most common primary malignant orbital tumour

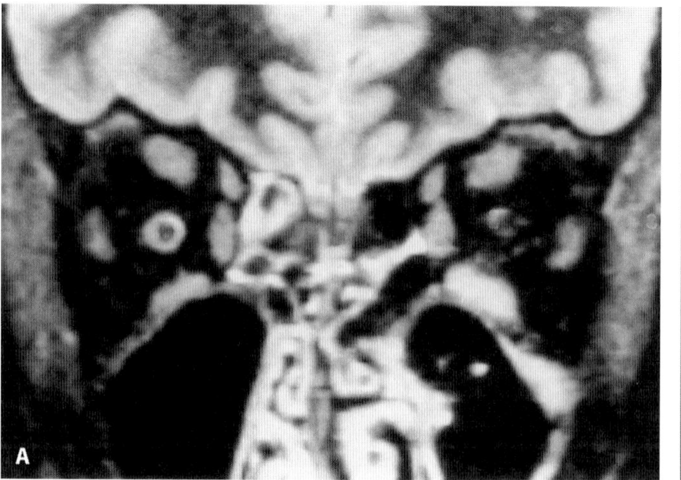

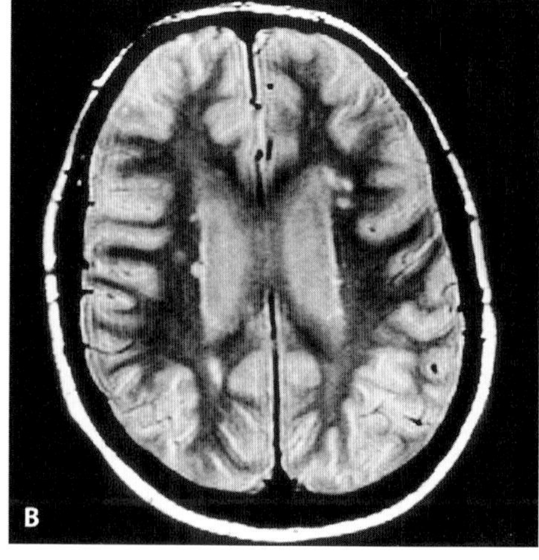

Fig. 6.17A,B. Pituitary macroadenoma. Sagittal SE T1-WI (**A**) and coronal Gd-enhanced SE T1-WI (**B**) through the pituitary gland and parasellar region. The suprasellar component of the pituitary macroadenoma displaces and compresses the optic chasm. The lesion arises from the left lobe of the pituitary gland and invades the left cavernous sinus. There is also extension into the sphenoid sinus

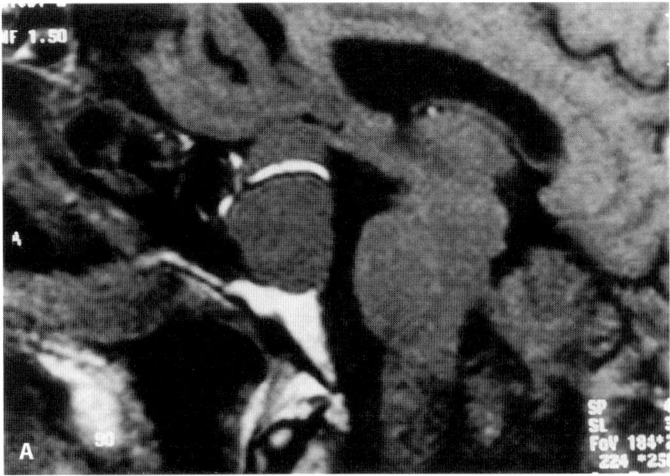

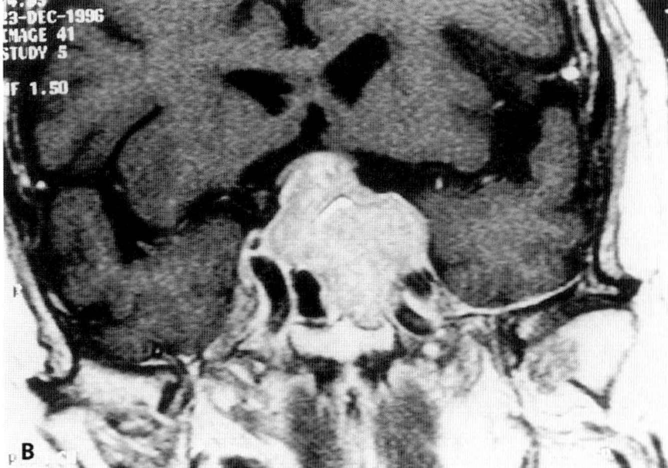

◀ **Fig. 6.16A,B.** Optic neuritis. Coronal short tau inversion recovery (STIR) image through the orbits (**A**) and transverse proton density-WI through the cerebral hemispheres (**B**). On the normal right side, there is a 'target appearance', which is caused by the CSF-filled meningeal sheath surrounding the optic nerve (**A**). On the abnormal left side, the 'target appearance' has disappeared due to swelling and inflammation of the left optic nerve in a patient with relapsing remitting multiple sclerosis (MS) (**A**). The proton density-WI through the brain reveals multiple punctate white matter abnormalities in both hemispheres (**B**). The multifocality, morphology, distribution and location of the lesions suggest the diagnosis of MS

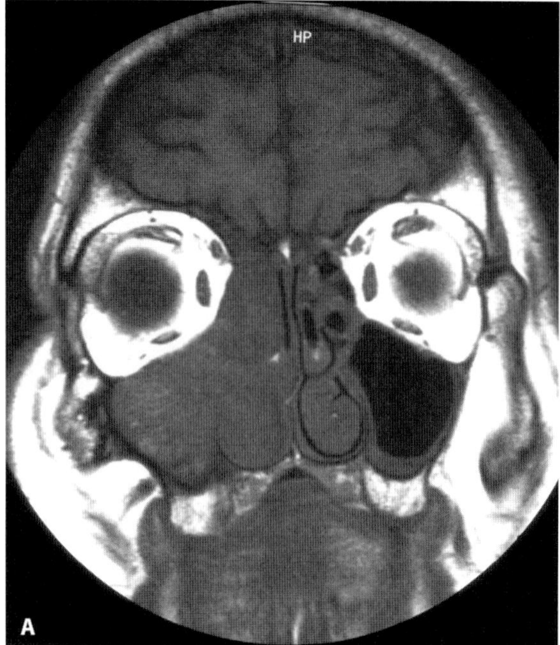

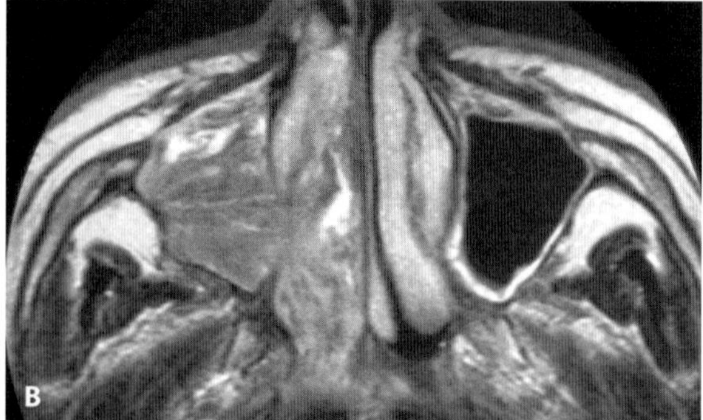

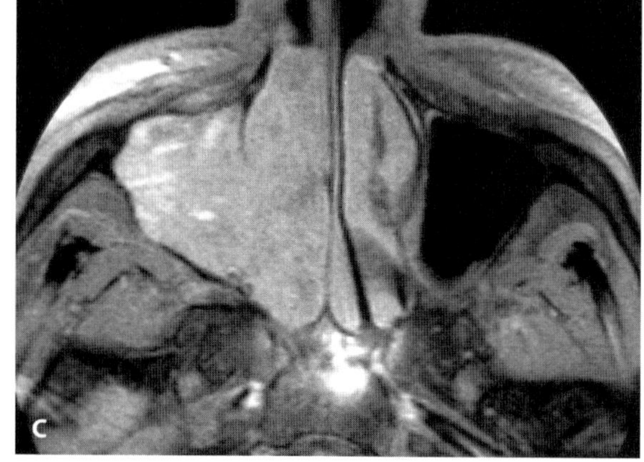

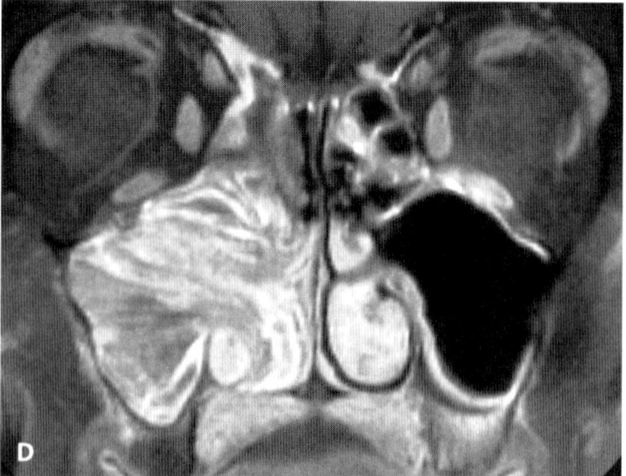

Fig. 6.18A–D. Inverted papilloma. Coronal SE T1-WI (**A**), transverse TSE T2-WI (**B**) and Gd-enhanced SE T1-WI with spectral fat saturation in the transverse (**D**) and coronal planes (**C**) in a 60-year-old man with complaints of nasal obstruction and epistaxis. The lesion appears to arise from the lateral nasal wall near the middle turbinate and extends into the left maxillary sinus (**A**). There is remodelling of the medial wall of the maxillary sinus, without frank bone destruction. Complete opacification of the maxillary sinus is noticed. No differentiation can be made between tumoral tissue, normal mucosa and retention of mucus on the pre-contrast T1-WI (**A**). After Gd injection (**C**,**D**), there is enhancement of the normal mucosa with heterogeneous enhancement of the tumour. No enhancement is noticed in the retained secretions. Biopsy of the lesion demonstrated inverted papilloma

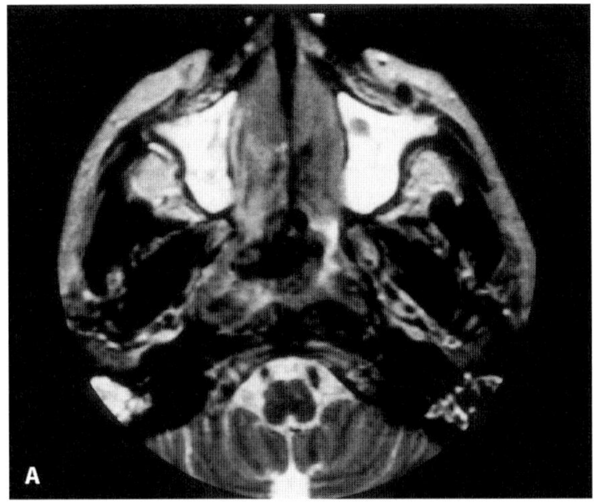

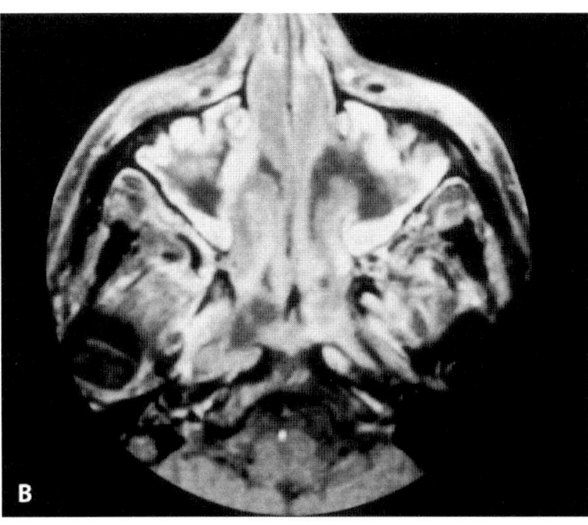

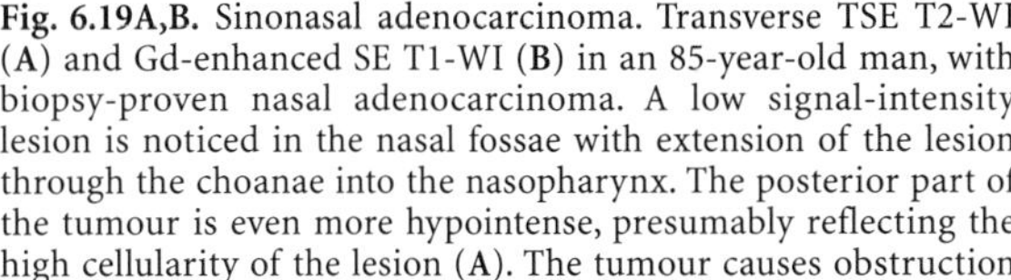

Fig. 6.19A,B. Sinonasal adenocarcinoma. Transverse TSE T2-WI (**A**) and Gd-enhanced SE T1-WI (**B**) in an 85-year-old man, with biopsy-proven nasal adenocarcinoma. A low signal-intensity lesion is noticed in the nasal fossae with extension of the lesion through the choanae into the nasopharynx. The posterior part of the tumour is even more hypointense, presumably reflecting the high cellularity of the lesion (**A**). The tumour causes obstruction of the ostiomeatal complex; the retained secretions in the maxillary sinuses are hyperintense on T2-WI (**A**). After Gd injection, the tumour enhances (**B**). The area of enhancement extends posteriorly in the parapharyngeal spaces and into the right longus colli muscles, indicating tumoral invasion and/or reactive changes. In the maxillary sinuses, the mucosa enhances, whereas the retained fluid does not

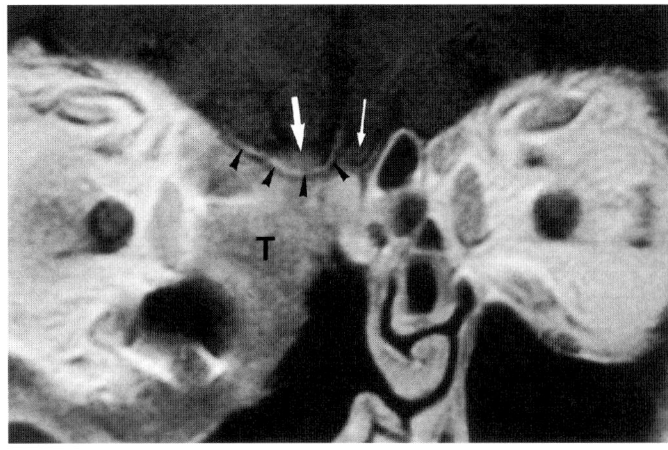

Fig. 6.20. Recurrent ethmoid adenocarcinoma. Coronal Gd-enhanced, high-resolution SE T1-WI through the anterior skull base in a patient with a recurrent ethmoid adenocarcinoma. Tumour recurrence (*T*) can be seen in the right ethmoid region. Enhancement of the meninges can be depicted above the right cribriform plate (*arrowheads*), and enhancement of the olfactory bulb (*large white arrow*), representing tumour invasion, can also be recognized. Compare with the normal low signal intensity of the left olfactory bulb (*long white arrow*)

Table 6.6. Magnetic resonance imaging protocol recommendations for sinonasal examinations

Pulse sequence	WI	Plane	No. of sections	TR (ms)	TE (ms)	Flip angle	Echo train length	Section thickness (mm)	Matrix	FOV	recFOV	BW	No. of acq.	Acq. time (min:s)
SE	T1	cor/tra	19	570	15	90	–	5	192×512	230	75	130	2	3:39
TSE	T2	cor/tra	26	8000	90	90	12	3	240×256	130	–	130	2	5:20

Abbreviations: *WI* weighted image; *TR* repetition time (ms); *TI* inversion time (ms); *TE* echo time (ms);*TD* time delay (sec); *no part* number of partitions; *Matrix* (phase × frequency matrix); *FOV* field of view (mm); *recFOV* % rectangular field of view; *BW* bandwidth (Hz)

6.3.4 Pathology

Complications of inflammatory sinus diseases, such as mucocoele (Fig. 6.21), brain abscess or subdural empyema, cavernous sinus thrombosis, meningitis, etc., are much better demonstrated on MRI than CT. MRI is indicated to demonstrate the exact extent of tumoral lesions and discriminate them from normal mucosa and secondary retention of fluid, whereas on CT only opacification of the sinuses will be seen. Tumoral lesions (Table 6.7) include both benign (inverted papilloma, juvenile angiofibroma, fibro-osseous lesions, etc.) (Fig. 6.18) and malignant lesions [squamous cell carcinoma (SCCA), adenocarcinoma, adenoid cystic carcinoma, lymphoma, esthesioneuroblastoma, etc.] (Figs. 6.19 and 6.20).

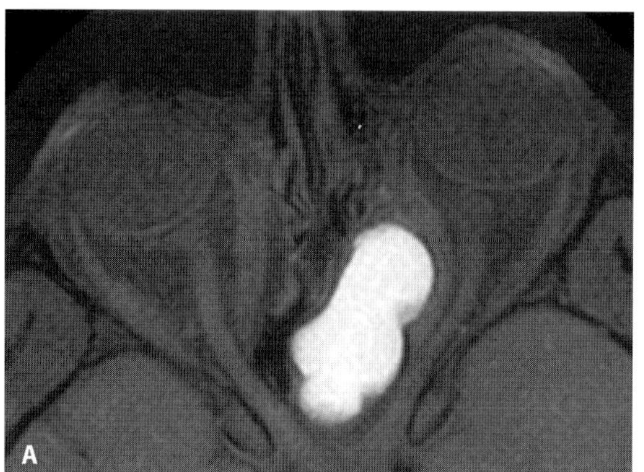

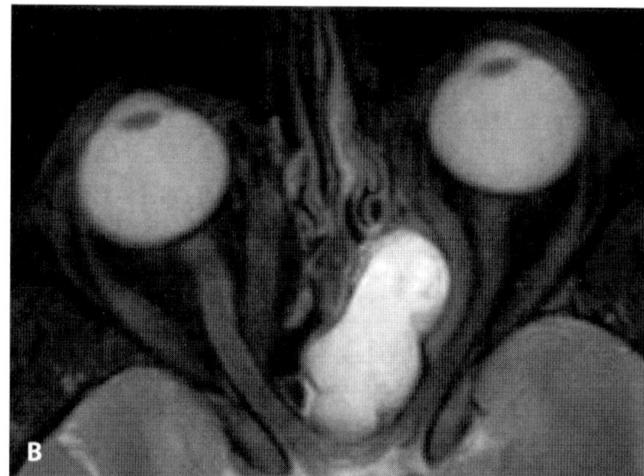

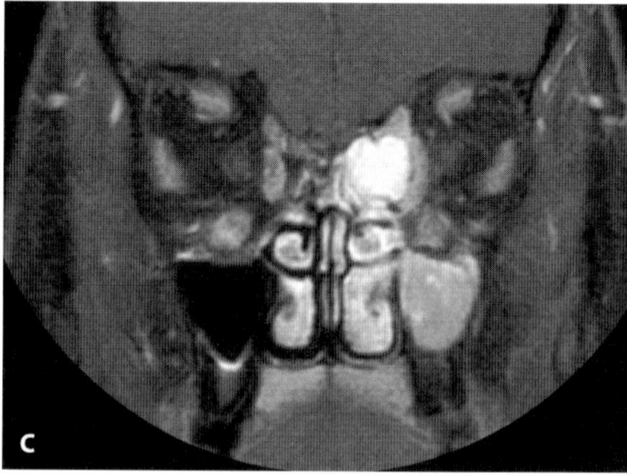

Fig. 6.21 A–C. Mucocoele. Transverse SE T1-WI (**A**) and transverse (**B**) and coronal WI (**C**) TSE T2-WI at the level of the sphenoid sinus in a patient who complained of progressive diplopia. Spectral fat saturation was applied in all sequences. An expansile lesion with high signal intensity is noticed at the sphenoid sinus. There is clear expansion of the sinus cavity with intraorbital extension of the mucocoele and displacement of the medial rectus muscle. The signal intensity of a mucocoele depends on the viscosity of the secretions

Table 6.7. Paranasal sinus masses

Mucocoele
Mucus retention cyst
Polyp
Antrochoanal polyp
Inverted papilloma
Sinusitis
Carcinoma

6.4 Skull Base

6.4.1 Introduction

The bony structures of the skull base are easier to recognize on CT. However, lesions of the skull base can also involve the extracranial and intracranial soft tissues, the nerves and vessels in the skull base foramina, and the bone marrow. Only MRI provides adequate contrast and spatial resolution to distinguish all these structures and has, therefore, become the method of choice to study skull-base lesions and cranial nerve involvement.

6.4.2 Coils and Patient Positioning

A standard, circularly polarized head coil provides the best images of the skull base. Patients are examined in the supine position, and their head is placed as high as possible in the head coil. The closer the skull base is to the centre of the head coil, the better the image quality. Images are made parallel and/or perpendicular to the part of the skull base to be examined.

6.4.3 Sequence Protocol

The MR technique will depend on the structures surrounding the region of interest.

1. Gd-enhanced, high-resolution SE T1-WI are used when cortical bone, soft tissues and nerves surrounded by bone or soft tissues must be visualized (Fig. 6.20).
2. In the central skull base and especially in the posterior skull base, nerves and vessels approach the skull base surrounded by cerebrospinal fluid (CSF). In these regions, normal nerves and tumour extension along nerves are best seen on transverse GRE T2-WI. On these images the tumour/nerves are seen as intermediate to low signal-intensity structures, outlined by high signal-intensity CSF (Fig. 6.22).
3. Within the skull-base foramina, the nerves, vessels and surrounding bone are best distinguished from one another when high-resolution (3DFT-FISP) time-of-flight MRA images are used. These images should be contrast enhanced so that the venous lakes become hyperintense and provide a different signal intensity from the nerves and surrounding bone (Fig. 6.23).
4. Lesion characterization and screening of the skull base can be performed using high-resolution transverse TSE T2-WI (Fig. 6.24). This sequence can also be used as the first screening sequence in severe pathology.

The parameters of these four routine skull-base sequences are shown in Table 6.8.

Contrast-enhanced, high-resolution T1-WI with fat suppression can be used to detect bone-marrow invasion, and they sometimes are better at distinguishing tumour from normal fat. Unenhanced SE T1-WI remain the most sensitive images to detect bone-marrow invasion.

6.4.4 Pathology

MRI is used in the skull base mainly to evaluate tumour extension (especially along nerves and vessels), detect bone invasion and achieve better tumour characterization. Tumours can originate intracranially in the marrow/cortical bone of the skull base or in the extracranial soft tissues. All possible extension routes through neuroforamina should be checked. Inflammatory lesions, congenital malformations, traumatic lesions and all types of cranial nerve pathology may also involve the skull base and be studied by MRI. However, congenital malformations and traumatic lesions are best studied with CT, with some exceptions. The anterior skull base is best studied in the coronal and sagittal planes. Unenhanced and Gd-enhanced high-resolution SE T1-WI are best suited to study the olfactory bulbs

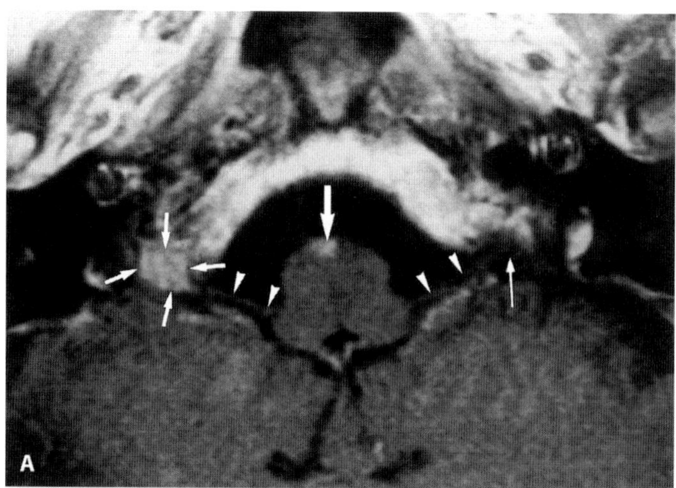

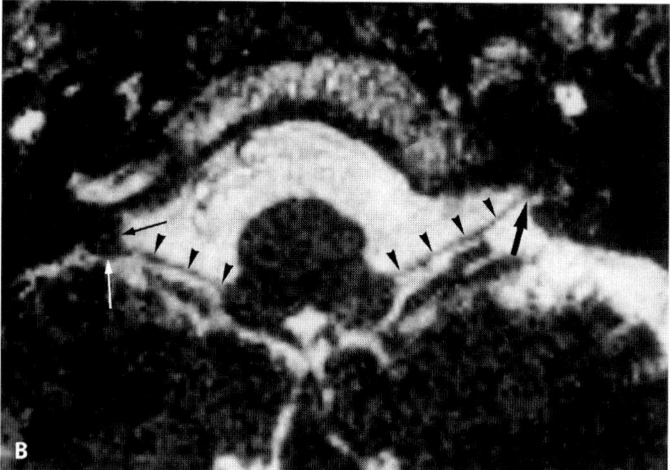

Fig. 6.22A,B. Skull-base metastasis near the right jugular foramen. Transverse Gd-enhanced SE T1-WI (**A**) and GRE T2-WI (**B**) at the level of the medulla oblongata in a patient with hoarseness and difficulty swallowing. A nodular enhancing structure (*small white arrows*) is observed near the entrance of the right jugular foramen, and it is unclear whether we are dealing with flow in a venous structure or with a mass (**A**). There is an enhancing metastasis that can be seen in the anterior part of the brain stem (*large white arrow*). Notice the normal appearance of the left jugular foramen (*long white arrow*). The glossopharyngeal nerve is seen bilaterally (*arrowheads*). On the thin GRE images (**B**), a low signal-intensity metastasis on the glossopharyngeal nerve replaces the CSF near the intracranial entrance of the jugular foramen (*long arrows*). Compare with the normal CSF, which can be followed until the jugular foramen is reached on the left side (*large black arrow*). Again, the glossopharyngeal nerves are seen even better (*arrowheads*)

Table 6.8. Magnetic resonance imaging protocol recommendations for examinations of the skull base

Pulse sequence	WI	Plane	No. of sections	TR (ms)	TE (ms)	Flip angle	Echo train length	Section thickness (mm)	Matrix	FOV	recFOV	BW	No. of acq.	Acq. time (min:s)
SE (T1+Gd)	T1	tra/cor/ sag	20	450	12	90	–	4	384×512	220	75	130	3	8:41
GRE 3DFT-CISS	T2	tra	46	12.25	5.9	70	–	0.7	192×256	95	–	195	1	7:14
GRE-MRA 3DFT-FISP	–	tra	64	39	7	25	–	1.15	192×512	240	75	81	1	8
TSE-T2	T2	tra	20	4000	99	180	11	4	242×512	300	50	130	2	3

Abbreviations: *WI* weighted image; *TR* repetition time (ms); *TI* inversion time (ms); *TE* echo time (ms); *TD* time delay (sec); *no part* number of partitions; *Matrix* (phase×frequency matrix); *FOV* field of view (mm); *recFOV* % rectangular field of view; *BW* bandwidth (Hz)

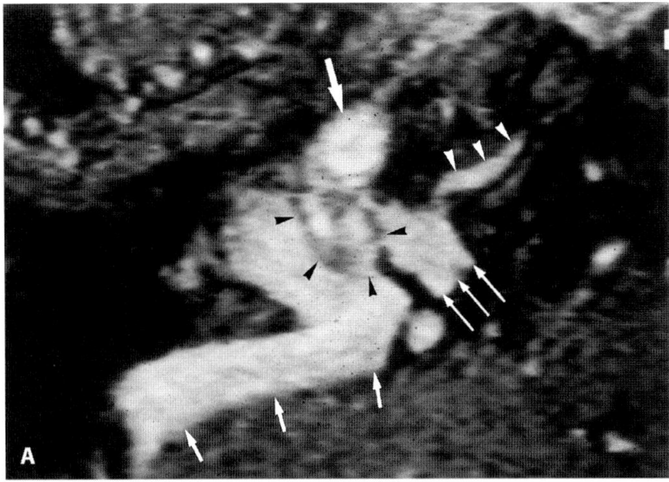

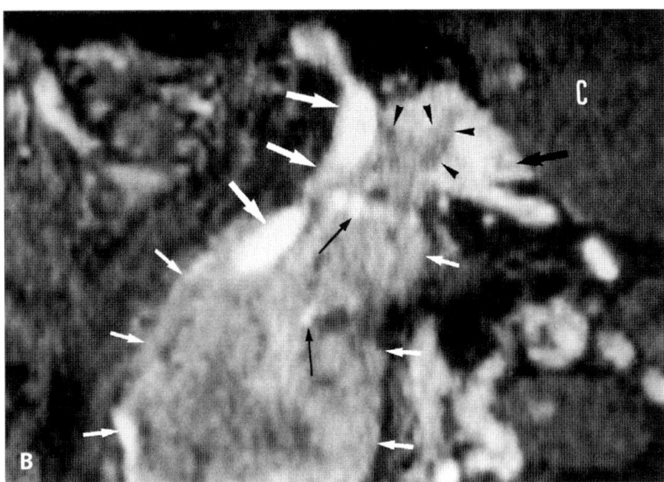

Fig. 6.23A,B. Glomus vagale. Transverse Gd-enhanced 1-mm-thick MRA image through the right jugular foramen (**A**) and parasagittal MRA reconstruction (**B**) in a patient with a glomus vagale tumour. A hypointense mass (*black arrowheads*) with central hyperintense signal intensities (flow) can be seen behind the internal carotid artery (*large white arrow*). The adjacent Gd-enhanced sigmoid sinus (*small white arrows*) and venous structures in the hypoglossal canal (*long white arrows*) make the hypointense mass visible (**A**). The inferior petrosal sinus is identified (*white arrowheads*). In the reconstructed image (**B**), the glomus vagale tumour has an intermediate inhomogeneous signal intensity (*small white arrows*), and high signal-intensity vessels are present inside the tumour (*long black arrows*), revealing the nature of the mass. The exact extension of the intermediate signal-intensity tumour (*black arrowheads*) inside the jugular foramen can be recognized, due to the high signal intensity of the surrounding Gd-enhanced venous blood (*large black arrow*) (**B**). *C*, cerebellum; carotid artery (*large white arrows*)

and tracts (trauma patients, congenital anosmia, etc.) and tumours originating in the sinuses or intracranially (meningiomas, esthesioneuroblastomas, etc.). Coronal, thin GRE T2-WI are only required when a CSF leak or meningo(encephalo)coele is suspected. The central skull base and especially the parasellar region and neuroforamina are best studied in the coronal and transverse planes with high-resolution SE T1-WI. Most of the tumoral lesions and cranial nerve lesions may be studied this way and, when necessary, be further characterized using TSE T2-WI. Transverse MRA images are only used when aneurysms or vascular pathology is suspected. Transverse GRE T2-WI are used when posterior extension into the prepontine cistern or CPA is present. In the posterior skull base, axial and coronal images perform best. The sagittal plane is only used to study midline lesions of the clivus and craniocervical junction. High-resolution T1-WI are used to study tumours and look for abnormal enhancements in tumoral and inflammatory lesions. Thin, transverse GRE T2-WI are often used to study the relationship of the lesions to the cranial nerves VI to XII in the cisterns surrounding the lower brainstem. Finally, transverse, high-resolution, Gd-enhanced MRA images are needed when a lesion involves or grows through the jugular foramen.

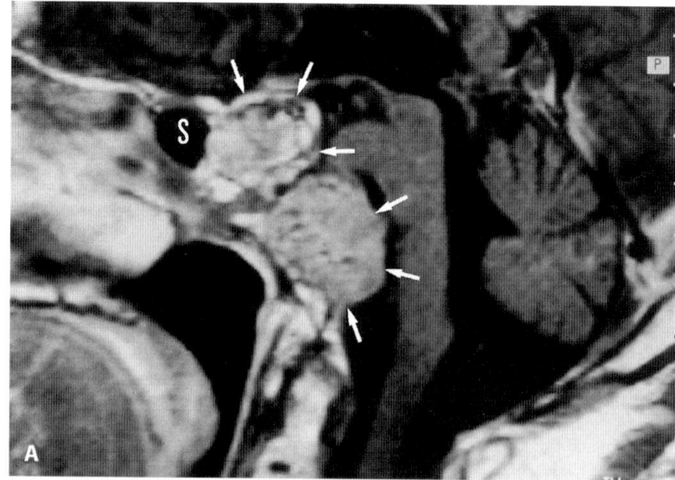

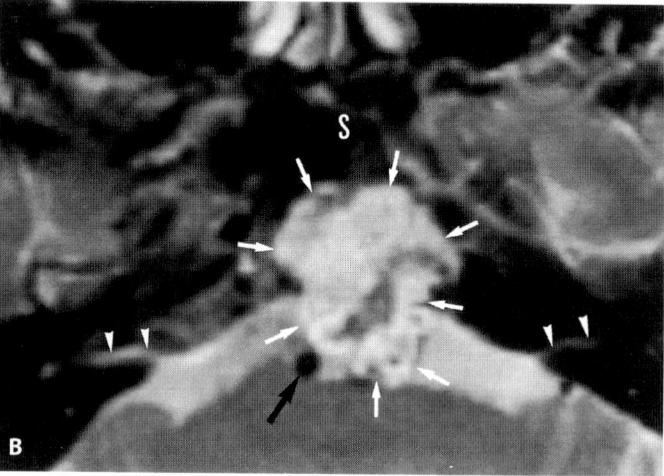

Fig. 6.24A,B. Clival chordoma. Sagittal Gd-enhanced T1-WI (**A**) and axial T2-WI (**B**) through the clivus in a patient with a chordoma. A bilobular enhancing mass can be seen behind the sphenoid sinus (*S*) and in the clivus (*white arrows*). The sagittal plane is best suited to image these midline lesions and also demonstrates the displacement of the brainstem. On the T2-WI (**B**) through the level of the IAC (*arrowheads*), the mixed signal intensities inside the tumour (*white arrows*), the multiple convex peripheral protrusions and the midline location further help to establish the diagnosis of a chordoma. The basilar artery (*black arrow*) is compressed between the chordoma and the brainstem

6.5 Nasopharynx and Surrounding Deep Spaces and Parotid Glands

6.5.1 Introduction

The nasopharynx is an anatomic area in the head and neck region, which is difficult to visualize clinically. Moreover, the surrounding deep spaces cannot be examined clinically, and lesions in these spaces only become visible when they become sufficiently large or start to involve surrounding structures, such as nerves, blood vessels, etc. Therefore, high-quality imaging is needed in these anatomical regions. Only MRI is able to consistently provide images with sufficient tissue-contrast resolution and spatial resolution in these regions and, therefore, is the imaging modality of choice.

6.5.2 Coils and Patient Positioning

A selective examination of the nasopharynx and surrounding spaces is best performed with a standard head coil. Patients are examined in the supine position with the head positioned as high as possible in the head coil. To obtain high-quality images, the patients should be instructed to avoid motion, swallowing and talking, because it degrades the images. Breathing through the nose with the mouth closed also reduces motion artefacts.

A dedicated neck coil is used when the complete oral cavity or complete oropharynx must also be included, or when a complete staging of the neck lymph nodes is required (see Sect. 6.6).

The parotid glands can be examined with surface coils. With these coils, higher spatial resolution can be achieved, but there is a drop in signal intensity from the superficial to the deep part of the gland, and this may result in insufficient visualization of the deep lobe. Another drawback is that only one gland is examined with a surface coil. Therefore, we prefer a head coil for imaging the parotid glands. In order to increase the spatial resolution, a 512×512 matrix is used. Another advantage is that the patient is better fixed in a head coil, and this will result in fewer motion artefacts than with a surface coil. Again, the patient must be positioned as high as possible in the head coil so that the inferior part of the parotid gland can be included in the imaging FOV (Fig. 6.25). The preferred slice orientation for the above-mentioned studies is the axial plane, parallel to the hard palate. A nasopharynx study should start at the superior border of the pituitary fossa in order to exclude intracranial extension. The inferior reference is the inferior border of the mandible; however, the signal is often already insufficient at this level when a head coil is used. A parotid-gland study starts at the superior border of the external auditory canal and ends at the inferior border of the mandible. When additional coronal slices are used, they are made in a plane perpendicular to the hard palate.

6.5.3 Sequence Protocol

The nasopharynx, surrounding deep spaces and parotid glands are best examined in the transverse plane; the MR imaging protocol for examinations of these regions is shown in Table 6.9.

1. Transverse high-resolution TSE T2-WI can be used as the first sequence. These images have a high contrast and spatial resolution, making them very sensitive for the detection of parotid lesions. Moreover, these images are needed when further tissue characterization is necessary (Fig. 6.25).
2. The MR examination continues with transverse unenhanced and Gd-enhanced high-resolution SE T1-WI. The unenhanced images are the most sensitive images in the detection of bone-marrow involvement and, therefore, can detect early skull-base or mandible invasion. Moreover, they prevent confusion of areas with high signal intensity on T1 images (blood, fat, proteinaceous fluid, etc.) with areas of enhancement. Gd-enhanced T1-WI have a better signal-to-noise ratio than the unenhanced images, and this results in better tumour delineation. The solid and cystic parts of a tumour are also better distinguished on the Gd-enhanced images (Figs. 6.25 and 6.26).
3. Additional coronal Gd-enhanced T1-WI of a nasopharynx lesion or a lesion of the surrounding spaces or the parotid gland often provide important information about the exact location and extension of the tumour. These are mandatory when the skull base is invaded.
4. Finally, the transverse and coronal Gd-enhanced images can be replaced by similar images with spec-

Table 6.9. Magnetic resonance imaging protocol recommendations for nasopharyns, surrounding deep spaces and parotid gland examinations

Pulse sequence	WI	Plane	No. of sections	TR (ms)	TE (ms)	Flip angle	Echo train length	Section thickness (mm)	Matrix	FOV	recFOV	BW	No. of acq.	Acq. time (min:s)
TSE-T2	T2	tra	20	4000	99	180	11	4	242×512	300	50	130	2	3
SE (T1±Gd)	T1	tra/cor	20	450	12	90	–	4	384×512	220	75	130	3	8:41

Abbreviations: *WI* weighted image; *TR* repetition time (ms); *TI* inversion time (ms); *TE* echo time (ms); *TD* time delay (sec); *no part* number of partitions; *Matrix* (phase×frequency matrix); *FOV* field of view (mm); *recFOV* % rectangular field of view; *BW* bandwidth (Hz)

tral fat suppression. On these images, tumour enhancement can be better distinguished from the surrounding fat. The drawback of fat suppression is that fewer slices are available when the same acquisition time is used. Therefore, the slice thickness should be increased if the complete region must be imaged, or the total acquisition time must be increased. Also, the signal-to-noise ratio is inferior on images with fat suppression.

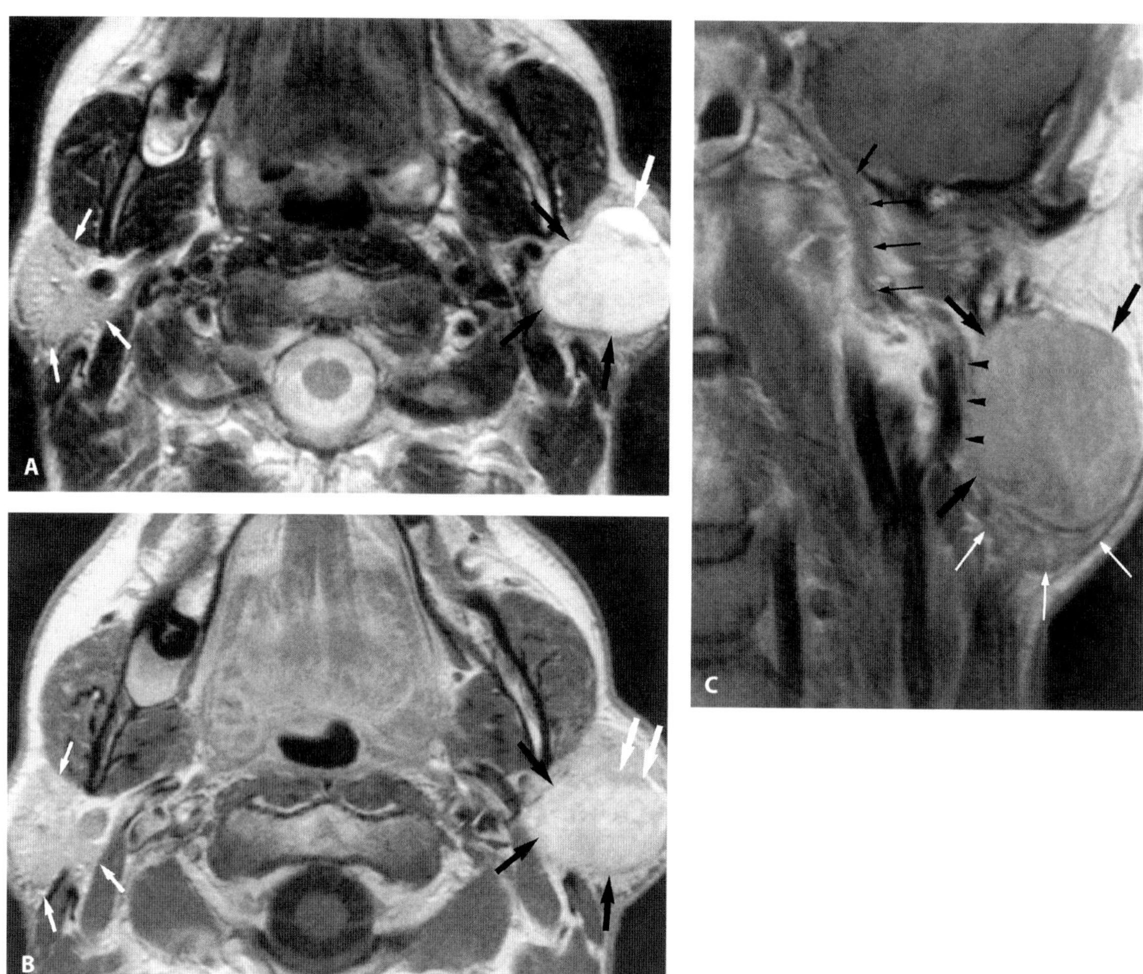

Fig. 6.25A–C. Pleomorphic adenoma. Transverse TSE T2-WI (**A**) and Gd-enhanced SE T1-WI in the transverse (**B**) and coronal planes (**C**) in a patient with a pleomorphic adenoma of the left parotid gland. Both the pleomorphic adenoma (*black arrows*) in the left parotid gland and the normal right parotid gland (*small white arrows*) can be studied in detail on high-resolution T2-WI when the head coil is used (**A**). The T2-weighting helps to distinguish the high-contrast lesion from the intermediate signal of the gland and also highlights the cystic component of the tumour (*large white arrow*). After Gd injection (**B**), both parotid glands can be studied in detail, but the solid part (*black arrows*) and cystic part (*large white arrows*) of the tumour are more difficult to distinguish from each other and from the surrounding normal parotid gland. The right parotid gland is normal (*small white arrows*). The coronal plane (**C**) often provides additional information about the position of the tumour (*large black arrows*) with regard to the remaining normal gland (*white arrows*), the adjacent blood vessels (*arrowheads*) and the skull base. The signal-to-noise ratio is still sufficient to allow evaluation of the inferior part of the parotid gland when the head coil is used. Notice the mandibular nerve in the oval foramen (*small black arrow*) and masticator space (*long black arrows*)

6.5.4 Pathology

6.5.4.1 Nasopharynx

About 70% of nasopharynx tumours are SCCAs, while lymphomas account for approximately 20% of lesions. Hence, the differential diagnosis is not the major problem. In these patients, the main role of MRI is to delineate the exact extent of the tumour, and this is only possible when 512×512 matrix images are used (Fig. 6.26).

6.5.4.2 Surrounding Spaces

These spaces (pre- and poststyloid parapharyngeal space, retropharyngeal space, prevertebral space, masticator space, etc.) contain different anatomical structures and can give rise to different kinds of tumours. The list of possible tumours is long but can be reduced considerably if one can recognize in which space the tumour originates. This is easier when high-resolution images are available because they show the anatomical landmarks of the different spaces better as well as the displacement of the fat of the prestyloid parapharyngeal space (Figs. 6.26, 6.27). Lesions originating in dif-

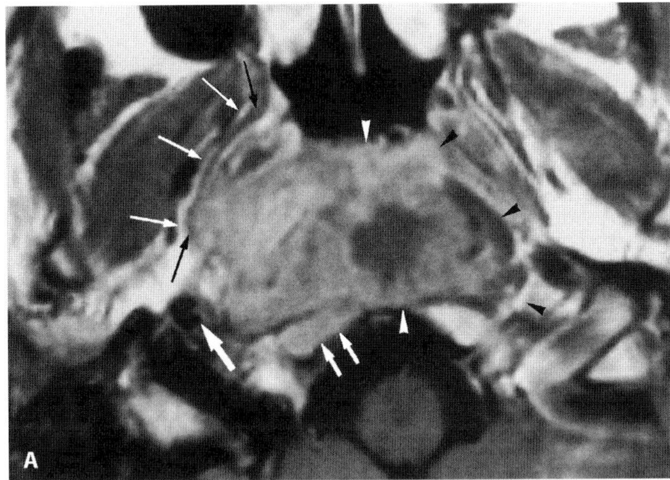

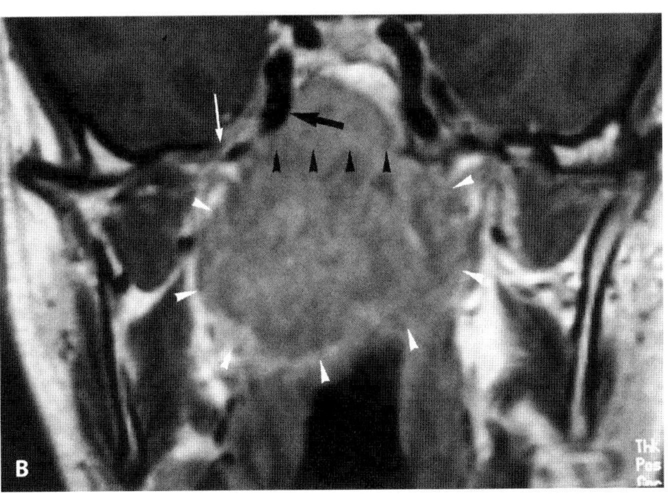

Fig. 6.26A,B. Nasopharyngeal squamous cell carcinoma (SCCA). Transverse (**A**) and coronal (**B**) Gd-enhanced SE T1-WI in a patient with SCCA of the nasopharynx. A large tumour (*arrowheads*) completely fills the nasopharynx lumen and pushes the right tensor veli palatini muscle (*long black arrows*) and prestyloid parapharyngeal space (*long white arrows*) laterally, but has not invaded these structures (**A**). The prevertebral muscles have been invaded, and signal loss is seen in the marrow of the skull base on the right side (*small white arrows*), indicating bone invasion. The closest and most frequently reached vital structure by nasopharynx tumours is the internal carotid artery; in this patient, the signal void of the internal carotid artery is only 1 mm away from the tumour (*large white arrow*). The destruction of the skull base (*black arrowheads*) by the large nasopharynx tumour (*white arrowheads*) is best seen in the coronal plane (**B**). The sphenoid sinus is completely filled with tumour, and the tumour reaches the medial wall of the internal carotid artery at this level (*black arrow*). The normal mandibular nerve inside the oval foramen (*white arrow*) has not been reached by the tumour

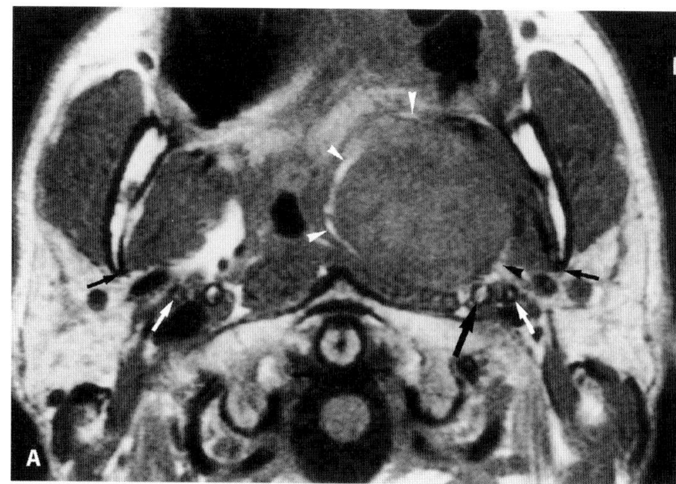

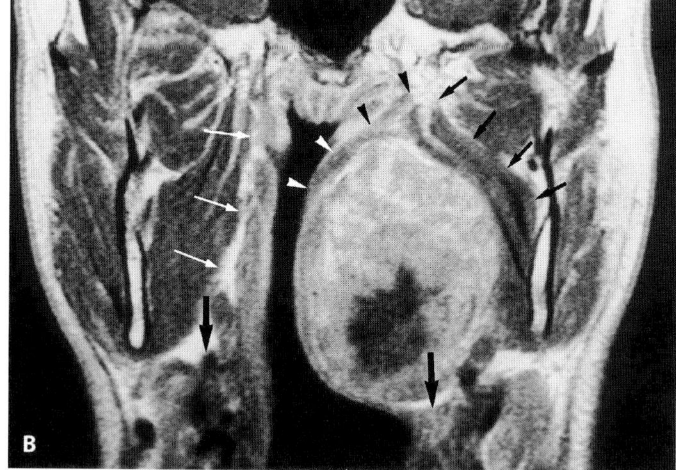

Fig. 6.27A,B. Minor salivary gland pleomorphic adenoma. Transverse unenhanced (**A**) and coronal Gd-enhanced SE T1-WI (**B**) in a patient with a pleomorphic adenoma arising from the minor salivary glands in the prestyloid parapharyngeal space. On the precontrast image (**A**), a round mass, slightly hyperintense in comparison with the muscles, is seen between the pharyngeal constrictor muscle and medial pterygoid muscle and is, therefore, situated in the prestyloid parapharyngeal space. The internal carotid artery is located posterior to the mass (*large black arrow*), and the fat of the space is displaced anteriorly (*white arrowheads*). The fat of the prestyloid space is also pushed backwards (*black arrowhead*) and indicates that we are not dealing with a lesion originating in the deep lobe of the parotid gland. The distance between the styloid process (*white arrows*) and the ramus of the mandible (*small black arrows*) is, therefore, not increased. After Gd injection (**B**), the solid part of the tumour enhances, and a less vascularized part of the tumour can now be seen. The tumour is stopped near the skull base by the medial pterygoid muscle (*small black arrows*) and tensor veli palatini muscle (*arrowheads*). The fasciae of these structures fuse near the skull base and attach medial to the oval foramen. In this way they prevent intracranial extension of prestyloid parapharyngeal space tumours. The left submandibular gland is pushed downward by the mass, compared with the position of the contralateral gland (*large black arrows*). Normal prestyloid parapharyngeal fat space on the right (*white arrows*)

ferent spaces medial, lateral, posterior to the prestyloid parapharyngeal space) displace the fat in different directions. The direction of fat displacement indicates the space in which the lesion originates.

6.5.4.3 Parotid Gland

Most parotid gland tumours are benign, and up to 80% of the benign tumours are pleomorphic adenomas (Fig. 6.25). The role of MRI is to demonstrate whether the deep lobe is involved and whether the tumour is located near the known (not visualized) course of the main branch of the facial nerve. Aggressive characteristics, suggesting malignant degeneration or the presence of a malignant tumour, can sometimes be seen but are not always present in the case of malignant tumours.

6.6 Oropharynx and Oral Cavity

6.6.1 Introduction

CT is frequently used in the staging of oropharynx and oral cavity tumours. Both the local and nodal staging can be performed easily with CT. MRI can also be used as the initial technique, but today MRI is most often performed when additional information concerning local tumour extension or tumour characterization is required.

6.6.2 Coils and Patient Positioning

Dedicated neck coils are necessary when the complete oropharynx and oral cavity must be covered. Images with sufficient signal-to-noise ratio at the level of the mandible and under the mandible can only be obtained when such dedicated coils are used (Fig. 6.28). Moreover, dedicated neck coils also allow imaging of the lower neck, which is mandatory if simultaneous MR assessment of the lymph nodes is required. On MR imaging, lymph node staging is much easier in the coronal plane; this is possible with a dedicated neck coil as these coils easily cover the region from the skull base to the upper mediastinum. Patients are examined in the supine position. They are instructed not to move, swallow or talk during the examination, and they are also asked to close their mouths and to breath quietly through their noses. Images are made parallel and/or perpendicular to the floor of the mouth or inferior border of the mandible. In the oropharynx, images are made in the axial plane; coronal images are optional. In the oral cavity, at least one sequence should be made in the coronal plane, preferably a fat-suppressed, high-resolution, Gd-enhanced SE T1-W sequence.

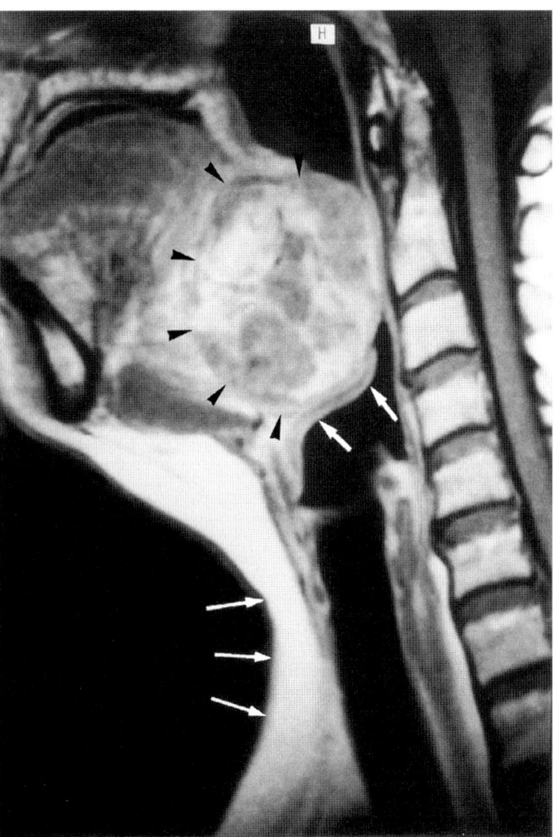

Fig. 6.28. Lingual thyroid. Sagittal Gd-enhanced T1-WI in a patient with a goitre in a lingual thyroid. The complete neck can be studied when a dedicated neck coil is used. Note the absence of a normal thyroid gland in the lower neck (*long white arrows*) and the presence of an inhomogeneous enhancing mass (*arrowheads*) in the base of the tongue, pushing the epiglottis backward (*small white arrows*)

6.6.3 Sequence Protocol

1. The examination starts with a transverse TSE T2-WI sequence, covering the complete region of interest. These images are very sensitive in the detection of lesions and, therefore, well suited as an initial sequence (Fig. 6.29).
2. Transverse high-resolution, unenhanced and Gd-enhanced SE T1-WI are then performed. The unenhanced images are needed as they are the most sensitive images to detect early bone marrow involvement (Fig. 6.30). Moreover, spontaneous hyperintensities (fat = dermoid cyst, blood = haemangioma or vascular malformations, etc.) can be detected on these images. Gd-enhanced T1-WI are used to evaluate the extent of the lesions. Solid lesions can sometimes become isointense with the surrounding soft tissues or fat on these images. Therefore, fat-suppressed images are often more sensitive, especially in the oral cavity.

The longest diameter of the oropharynx and oral cavity is anteroposterior; hence, when a rectangular FOV is used in the transverse plane, phase encoding should be chosen in the left-right direction. In the infrahyoid neck, the phase encoding should be chosen in the anteroposterior direction in order to avoid infolding of the shoulders.

For the MR imaging protocol for examinations of the oropharynx and oral cavity, see Table 6.10.

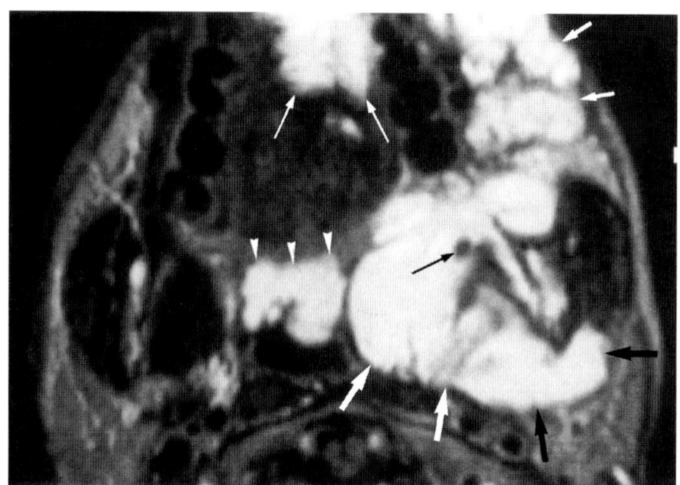

Fig. 6.29. Venous malformation. Transverse T2-WI in a patient with venous malformations (slow flow) in the soft tissues of the face, oral cavity and oropharynx. The high signal intensity of the lesions in the oropharynx (*arrowheads*), oral cavity (*large white arrows*), prestyloid parapharyngeal space (*large white arrows*), parotid space (*large black arrows*) and the buccomasseteric region (*small white arrows*) helps to visualize the exact extent of the lesion and also makes lesion characterization possible. The presence of a phlebolith further confirms the diagnosis (*long black arrow*)

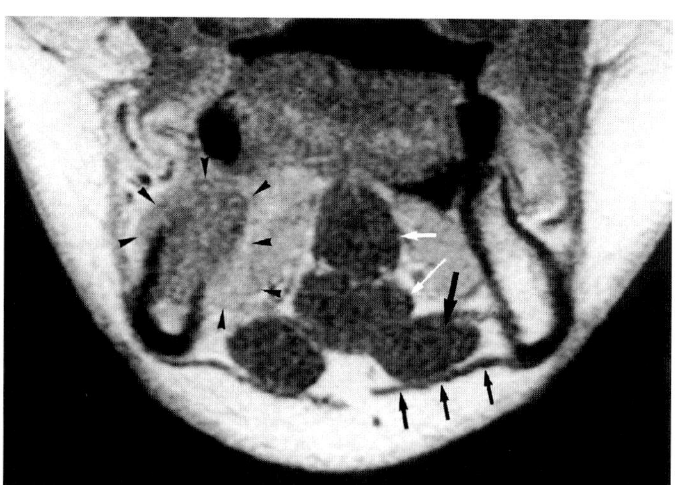

Fig. 6.30. Gingival squamous cell carcinoma (SCCA). Coronal T1-WI through the oral cavity in a patient with SCCA of the gingiva. The tumour can be seen covering the alveolar ridge of the right mandible (*arrowheads*). The cortical bone of the right mandible is destroyed, and the bone marrow is invaded; compare with the normal high signal-intensity bone marrow on the left side. Genioglossus muscle (*small white arrow*), geniohyoid muscle (*long white arrow*), anterior belly of the digastric muscle (*large black arrow*), platysma (*small black arrows*)

Table 6.10. Magnetic resonance imaging protocol recommendations for examinations of oropharynx and oral cavity

Pulse sequence	WI	Plane	No. of sections	TR (ms)	TE (ms)	Flip angle	Echo train length	Section thickness (mm)	Matrix	FOV	recFOV	BW	No. of acq.	Acq. time (min:s)
TSE-T2	T2	tra	20	4000	99	180	11	4	242×512	300	50	130	2	3
SE (T1–Gd)	T1	tra/cor	20	450	12	90	–	4	384×512	220	75	130	3	8:41
SE (T1+Gd, fat suppression)	T1	tra/cor	20	1180	12	90	–	4	384×512	220	75	130	1	10:57

Abbreviations: *WI* weighted image; *TR* repetition time (ms); *TI* inversion time (ms); *TE* echo time (ms); *TD* time delay (sec); *no part* number of partitions; *Matrix* (phase×frequency matrix); *FOV* field of view (mm); *recFOV* % rectangular field of view; *BW* bandwidth (Hz)

6.6.4
Pathology

The majority of tumours involving the oropharynx are SCCAs. Again, the cardinal role of MRI is the precise evaluation of tumour extent. The preferred imaging direction is the axial plane, because it allows comparison of both sides. Coronal images are only of benefit when the lateral walls of the oropharynx are involved.

In the oral cavity SCCA is, again, the most frequently encountered pathology. However, congenital malformations, inflammatory lesions and benign tumours also occur in this anatomical region. Therefore, unenhanced T1-WI should be used to detect the presence of fat, blood or proteinaceous fluid in these lesions, and TSE T2-WI can be used to further characterize the lesions.

Malignant tumours in the oropharynx are situated close to the mandible and maxilla and often invade these bony structures. Early involvement can be recognized as loss of the high signal-intensity bone marrow on the unenhanced T1-WI (Fig. 6.30). The loss of high-signal marrow is, however, not specific for tumoral invasion; it also occurs in cases of inflammation. At least one sequence in the coronal plane should be performed in order to avoid partial volume problems in the region between the floor of the mouth and the tongue, and at the superior and inferior borders of the mandible.

6.7
Larynx and Hypopharynx

6.7.1
Introduction

The major indication for MR imaging is to demonstrate the exact extent of the tumour in patients with laryngeal-hypopharyngeal cancer. The piriform sinus and retrocricoid hypopharynx are located so close to the laryngeal structures that a tumour arising in these regions necessitates total laryngectomy, as in patients with advanced laryngeal cancer. Today, however, partial (voice-sparing) laryngectomy can be performed successfully, depending on the depth extent of the tumour. Therefore, landmarks for conservative surgery should be carefully checked. Anterior commissure extension, spread in the pre-epiglottic fat space and the perilaryngeal fat, and cartilage invasion are important signs to look for in patients with laryngeal cancer. Both CT and MRI can detect tumoral spread beneath the mucosa. Moreover, submucosal lesions, tumours arising at the subglottic level or at the apex of the piriform sinus, can be visualized where endoscopic techniques fail (so-called blind mucosal areas). The advantage of MRI over CT is that this region can be better evaluated because of its high soft-tissue contrast, its high spatial resolution, and the multiplanar approach of this technique, without radiation. These factors contribute to the higher sensitivity and accuracy of MRI in detecting early cartilage invasion. The disadvantage of MRI is the longer

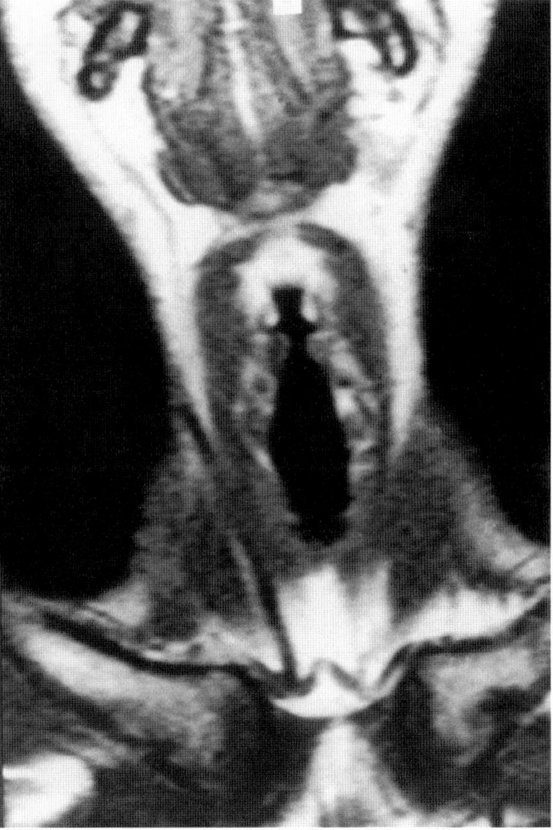

Fig. 6.31. Normal MR anatomy of the larynx. Coronal SE T1-WI through the ventricles of Morgagni in a normal volunteer. The false cords are displayed with high signal intensity (fat) indicating the level of the supraglottic region. Immediate below it, the air-filled ventricles are seen. The true vocal cords (posterior thyroarytenoid muscles) are displayed with a signal intensity comparable to muscle

examination time, resulting in more artefacts due to swallowing, respiration and blood flow.

6.7.2 Coils and Patient Positioning

The patient is placed in the standard supine position. It is important to explain to the patient the importance of the examination to achieve maximal cooperation (quiet breathing through the nose, avoiding swallowing and coughing). A special surface coil dedicated for imaging of the neck and cervical spine should be used to obtain the best results. The coil is centred at the level of the thyroid prominence (Fig. 6.31).

6.7.3 Sequence Protocol

1. The MR study starts with semiaxial high-resolution unenhanced SE T1-WI and TSE T2-WI, parallel to the true vocal cords.
2. After Gd injection, high-resolution SE T1-WI are obtained in the axial and coronal planes. To demonstrate tumoral extension in the base of the tongue, sagittal images are used instead of (or in addition to) coronal slices.
3. Fat-suppressed images after Gd injection can demonstrate enhancing tumour tissue in the paralaryngeal fat space even better.

For MR imaging protocol for examinations of the larynx and hypopharynx, see Table 6.11.

6.7.4 Pathology

Most frequently, MRI is performed to delineate the exact extent of the tumour in patients with SCCA (Fig. 6.32). Other tumours include adenoid cystic carcinoma (Fig. 6.33), lymphoma, plasmocytoma, chondrosarcoma and melanoma. Pseudotumoral lesions can also be encountered (laryngocoele, haematoma, etc.).

6.8 Temporomandibular Joint

6.8.1 Introduction

Clinically, it is almost impossible to differentiate patients with internal derangement of the temporomandibular joint (TMJ) from patients with myofascial pain dysfunction syndrome. The latter is a stress-related psychophysiological disorder, whereas the former is caused by an asynchrony of the various anatomic subunits of the joint. Today, MRI provides direct visualization of these different components, and therefore, it has surpassed techniques such as CT and arthrography. The most important structure within this joint is the articular disc, a biconcave dense fibrocartilaginous plate, which separates the mandibular condyle from the mandibular fossa. The role of MRI is to demonstrate the position and morphology of the disc and its relationship to the mandibular condyle during motion. The presence of bony abnormalities (mandibular condyle, glenoid fossa and articular prominence) should also be looked for.

Table 6.11. Magnetic resonance imaging protocol recommendations for examinations of the larynx hypopharynx

Pulse sequence	WI	Plane	No. of sections	TR (ms)	TE (ms)	Flip angle	TI (ms)	Echo train length	Section thickness (mm)	Matrix	FOV	recFOV	BW	No. of acq.	Acq. time (min:s)
SE	T1	tra/cor	19	570	15	90	–	–	3	196×512	230	75	130	2	3:44
TSE	T2	tra	19	4000	19–93	90	–	3	5	192×256	230	75	130	1	4:16
spectral	T1	tra/cor	11	650	15	90	–	–	3	192×256	230	75	130	2	4:10
fatsat	–	tra/cor	–	–	–	–	–	–	–	–	–	–	FS63		

Abbreviations: *WI* weighted image; *TR* repetition time (ms); *TI* inversion time (ms); *TE* echo time (ms); *TD* time delay (sec); *no part* number of partitions; *Matrix* (phase × frequency matrix); *FOV* field of view (mm); *recFOV* % rectangular field of view; *BW* bandwidth (Hz)

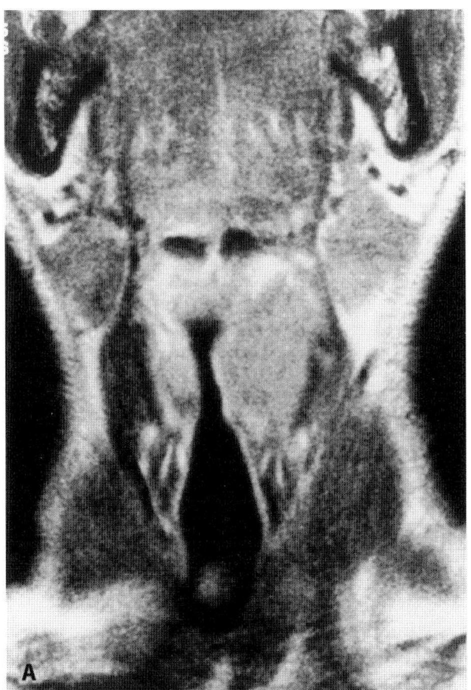

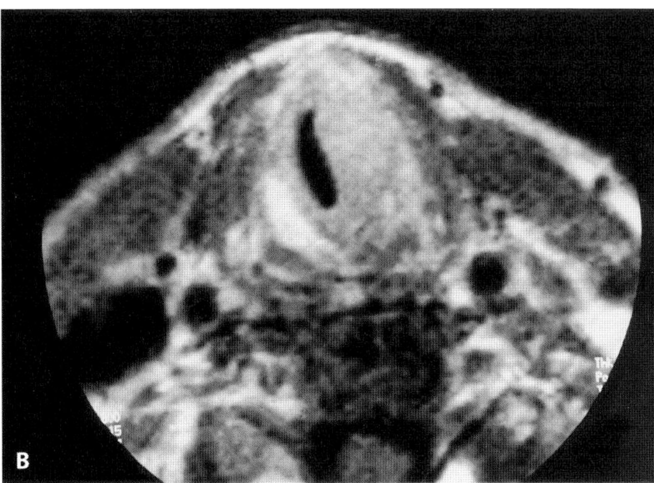

Fig. 6.32A,B. Laryngeal carcinoma. Gd-enhanced coronal (**A**) and transverse (**B**) SE T1-WI in a patient with T4 laryngeal squamous cell carcinoma. A bulky tumour is seen on the left side. The epicentre of the tumour is located in the paralaryngeal fat, indicating free access of the tumour to the supraglottic and subglottic regions. The normal architecture of the cricoid cartilage as seen on the right side has disappeared on the left side (**A**). Subglottic extension of the tumour is seen as a thickening of the soft tissues at the level of the cricoid ring (**B**). Invasion of the cricoid cartilage is also noticeable

6.8.2 Coils and Patient Positioning

As in most examinations, the patient is placed in a supine position. Examination of the TMJ can best be performed using a surface coil. A surface coil diameter between 8 cm and 12 cm provides an optimal signal-to-noise ratio. Bilateral dedicated surface coils (when available from the manufacturer of your MR system) that are placed symmetrically on both sides of the head and lateral to the joint are preferred, since both TMJs are simultaneously examined. This can be important, since bilateral abnormalities can be noticed in up to 60% of patients, and it allows comparison of both joints.

6.8.3 Sequence Protocol

Standard imaging of the TMJ should include oblique sagittal and coronal images obtained in both the closed- and open-mouth positions. Pseudodynamic imaging becomes possible when at least four images at different degrees of opening of the mouth are made (Fig. 6.34). The Burnett bidirectional TMJ device, which is made of plastic, can be used by the patient to control the degree of mouth opening. For the MR imaging protocol for examinations of the temporomandibular joint, see Table 6.12.

1. The basic MR examination, used for screening, consists only of oblique sagittal and coronal SE T1-WI. The direction of the oblique sagittal scans is parallel to the mandibular ramus.

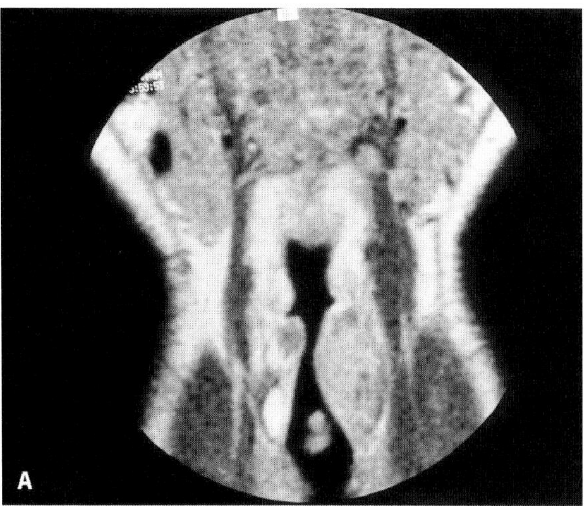

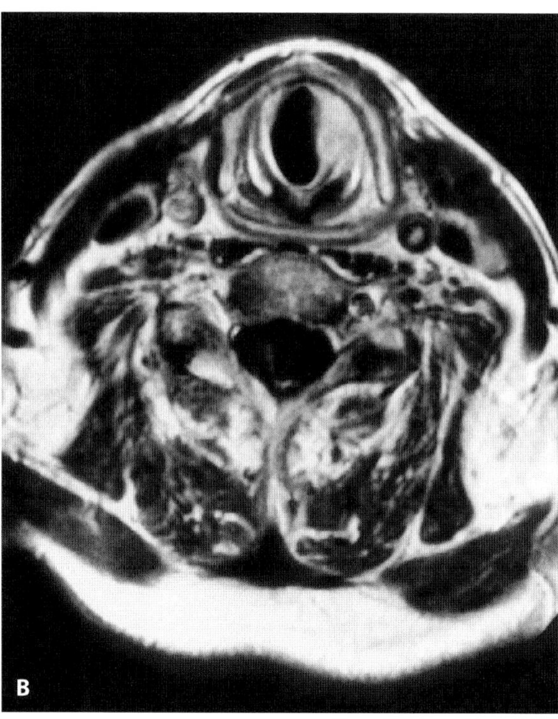

Fig. 6.33A,B. Adenoid cystic carcinoma. Gd-enhanced coronal (**A**) and transverse (**B**) SE T1-WI in a patient with adenoid cystic carcinoma of the larynx. There is submucosal spread of the tumour in the subglottic region on the left side (**A**). When a subglottic tumour is observed, the first differential diagnosis should be adenoid cystic carcinoma. Thickening of the soft tissues at the level of the cricoid ring with cricoid cartilage invasion is noticeable (**B**)

Table 6.12. Magnetic resonance imaging protocol recommendations or examinations of the temporomandibular joint

Pulse sequence	WI	Plane	No. of sections	TR (ms)	TE (ms)	Flip angle	Echo train length	Section thickness (mm)	Matrix	FOV	recFOV	BW	No. of acq.	Acq. time (min:s)
SE	T1	para-sag	9	500	20	90	–	3	210×256	180	63	78	3	5:15
SE	T1	cor	9	400	20	90	–	3	448×512	180	88	78	2	6
TSE	T2	sag	14	4500	91	90	8	3	128×256	180	50	130	3	3:36

Abbreviations: *WI* weighted image; *TR* repetition time (ms); *TI* inversion time (ms); *TE* echo time (ms); *TD* time delay (sec); *no part* number of partitions;*Matrix* (phase × frequency matrix); *FOV* field of view (mm); *recFOV* % rectangular field of view; *BW* bandwidth (Hz)

2. Additional TSE T2-WI in sagittal or coronal planes can be added to look for the presence of joint effusion and inflammatory changes in the joint capsule.
3. GRE T2-WI can also be applied, but these sequences are more vulnerable to artefacts arising from magnetic susceptibility, chemical shift and blood flow.

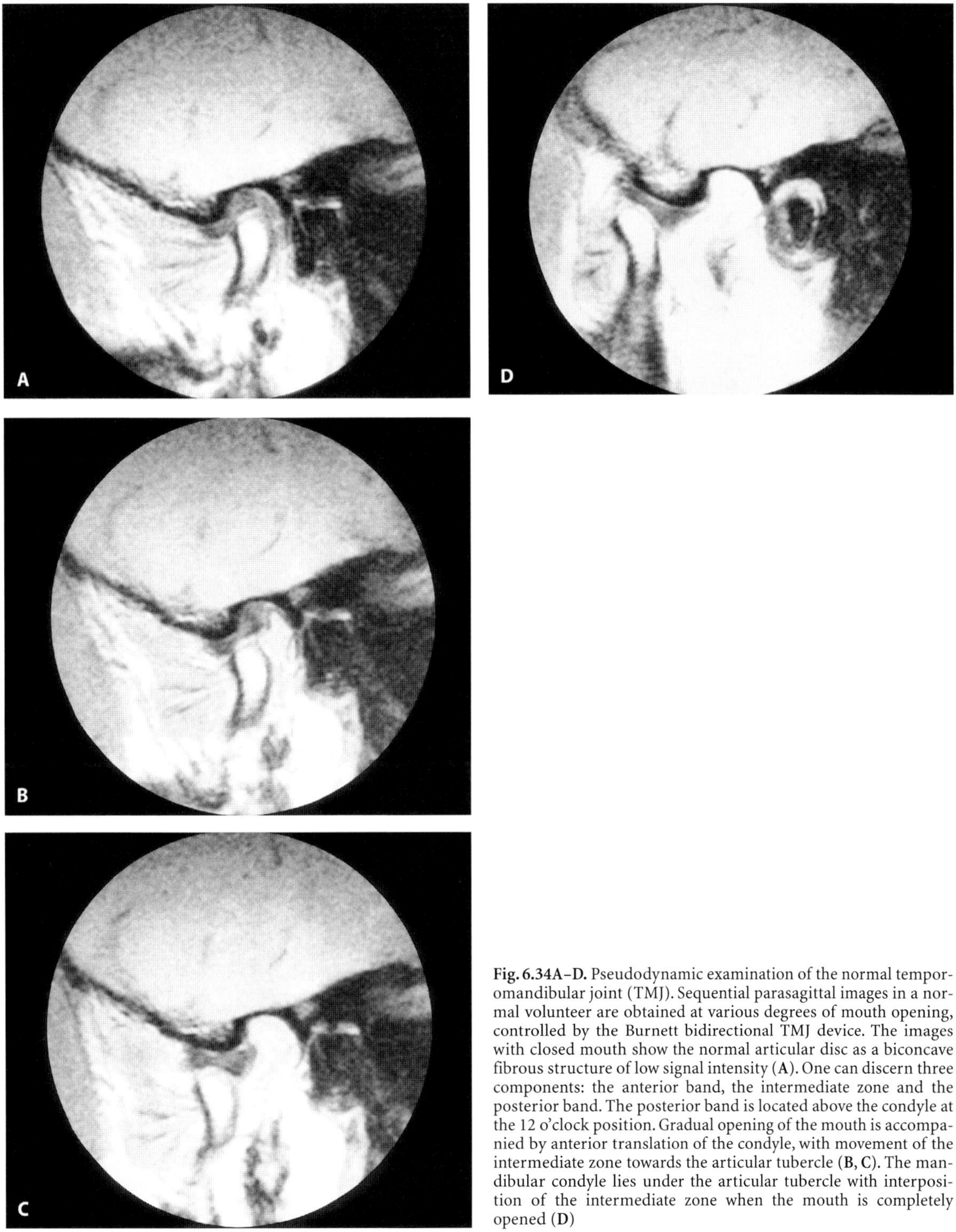

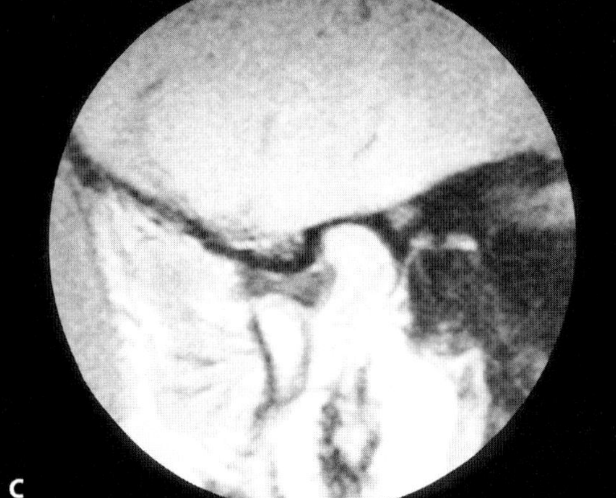

Fig. 6.34A–D. Pseudodynamic examination of the normal temporomandibular joint (TMJ). Sequential parasagittal images in a normal volunteer are obtained at various degrees of mouth opening, controlled by the Burnett bidirectional TMJ device. The images with closed mouth show the normal articular disc as a biconcave fibrous structure of low signal intensity (**A**). One can discern three components: the anterior band, the intermediate zone and the posterior band. The posterior band is located above the condyle at the 12 o'clock position. Gradual opening of the mouth is accompanied by anterior translation of the condyle, with movement of the intermediate zone towards the articular tubercle (**B, C**). The mandibular condyle lies under the articular tubercle with interposition of the intermediate zone when the mouth is completely opened (**D**)

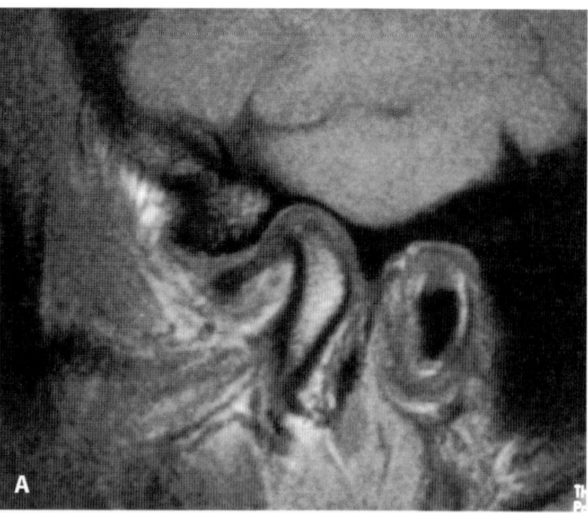

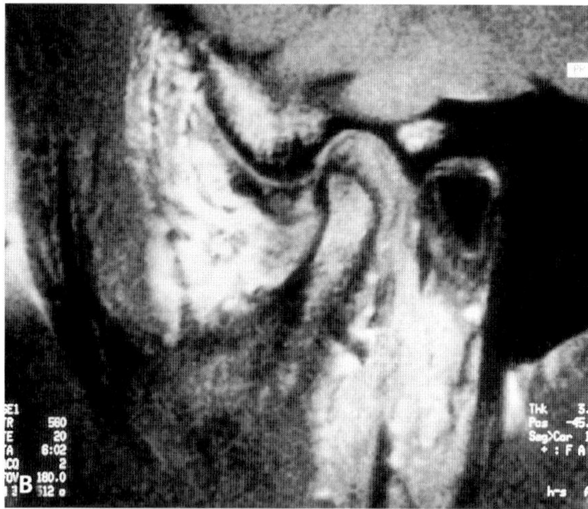

Fig. 6.35A,B. Disc dislocation. Anterior dislocation of the articular disc with the mouth closed (**A**) and mouth opened (**B**) in a patient with a click in the left temporomandibular joint (TMJ). The disc is positioned anteriorly of the condyle with the mouth closed (**A**). Note the disappearance of the biconcave morphology. There is no reduction of the disc on opening of the mouth (**B**)

6.8.4 Pathology

Internal derangement (mostly anterior disc displacement) and degenerative joint disease are the most common findings (Fig. 6.35). Other abnormalities include joint effusion (capsulitis), bone marrow oedema (avascular necrosis of the condyle) and tumours (synovial chondromatosis, osteoma, osteochondroma, etc.).

Further Reading

Armington WG, Bilaniuk LT, Zimmerman RA (1996) Visual pathways. In: Som PM, Curtin HD (eds) Head and neck imaging, 3rd edn. Mosby Year Book, St Louis, pp 1184–1232

Casselman JW (1996) Temporal bone imaging. Neuroimaging Clin North Am 6:265–289

Castelijns JA, van den Brekel MWM, Niekoop VA, Snow GB (1996) Imaging of the larynx. Neuroimaging Clin North Am 6:401–425

Curtin HD (1996) Larynx. In: Som PM, Curtin HD (eds) Head and neck imaging, 3rd edn. Mosby Year Book, St Louis, pp 612–710

Curtin HD (2002) The skull base. In: Atlas SW (ed) Magnetic resonance imaging of the brain and spine, 3rd edn. Lippincott/Williams and Wilkins, Philadelphia, pp 1243–1282

Curtin HD, Hasso AN, Swartz JD, Lo WWM (1996a) Temporal bone. In: Som PM, Curtin HD (eds) Head and neck imaging, 3rd edn. Mosby Year Book, St Louis, pp 1233–1535

De Potter P, Shields JA, Shields CL (1995) MRI of the eye and orbit. Lippincott, Philadelphia

Harnsberger R (1995) The normal and diseased orbit. In: Harnsberger R (ed) pp 300–338

Lustrin ES, Robertson RL, Tilak S (1994) Normal anatomy of the skull base. Neuroimaging Clin North Am 4:465–478

Mafee MF, Atlas SW, Galetta SL (2002) Eye, orbit, and visual system. In: Atlas SW (ed) Magnetic resonance imaging of the brain and spine, 3rd edn. Lippincott / Williams and Wilkins, Philadelphia, pp 1433–1526

Mark AS, Casselman JW (2002) Anatomy and disease of the temporal bone. In: Atlas SW(ed) Magnetic resonance imaging of the brain and spine, 3rd edn. Lippincott/Williams and Wilkins, Philadelphia, pp 1363–1432

Mukherji SK, Holliday RA (1996) Pharynx. In: Som PM, Curtin HD (eds) Head and neck imaging, 3rd edn. Mosby Year Book, St Louis, pp 437–487

Sigal R (1996) Oral cavity, oropharynx, and salivary glands. Neuroimaging Clin North Am 6:379–400

Smoker WRK (1996) Oral cavity. In: Som PM, Curtin HD (eds) Head and neck imaging, 3rd edn. Mosby Year Book, St Louis, pp 488–544

Som PM, Brandwein M (1996a) Salivary glands, tumors and tumor-like conditions. In: Som PM, Curtin HD (eds) Head and neck imaging, 3rd edn. Mosby Year Book, St Louis, pp 877–914

Som PM, Brandwein M (1996b) Sinonasal cavities: inflammatory diseases, tumours, fractures and postoperative findings. In: Som PM, Curtin HD (eds) Head and neck imaging, 3rd edn. Mosby Year Book, St Louis, pp 126–318

Som PM, Curtin HD (1995) Lesions of the parapharyngeal space. Role of MR imaging. Otolaryngol Clin North Am 28:515–542

Vogl TJ (1992a) Larynx and hypopharynx. In: Vogl TJ (ed) MRI of the head and neck. Springer, Berlin Heidelberg New York, pp 156–179

Vogl TJ (1992b) Temporomandibular joint. In: Vogl TJ (ed) MRI of the head and neck. Springer, Berlin Heidelberg New York, pp 207–223

Vogl TJ, Balzer JO (1996) Base of the skull, nasopharynx, and parapharyngeal space. Neuroimaging Clin North Am 6:357–378

Vogl TJ, Juergens M, Balzer JO, Mack MG, Bergman C, Grevers G, Lissner J, Felix R (1994) Glomus tumors of the skull base: combined use of MR angiography and spin-echo imaging. Radiology 192:103–110

Westesson PL, Katzberg RW (1996) Temporomandibular joints. In: Som PM, Curtin HD (eds) Head and neck imaging, 3rd edn. Mosby Year Book, St Louis, pp 375–436

Joints

7

H. Imhof, F. Kainberger, M. Breitenseher, S. Grampp, T. Rand, and S. Trattnig

Contents

Joints are examined in up to 40% of all MR examinations, which make them, after examinations of the brain and spine, the third most frequent site. Almost all of the different joint diseases are found (in different frequencies) in each joint. In this chapter, joint diseases are discussed only with reference to where they are found with the highest frequency. But the basic MR symptoms are similar in all joints!

7.1 Special Coils/Planes/Positioning

The following indicates the coil, plane, and positioning associated with various joints.

- Shoulder: circular surface coil (circular wrap-around coil)
  - Oblique parasagittal = angulated sagittal (parallel to M. supraspinatus = 'scapular' plane)
  - Axial
  - Oblique parasagittal (to M. supraspinatus)

  Positioning: supine, arm in supination or in abduction and external rotation (ABER) position, contralateral body supported by pillows
- Elbow: wrap-around coil, flexible rectangular surface coil
  - Coronal
  - Axial
  - Sagittal

  Positioning: supine, arm in supination and straightened, parallel to the body
- Hand: circular surface coil (wrap-around coil)
  - Coronal
  - Axial

  Positioning: prone and semi-oblique, arm above head in relaxed position, hand fixed with sandbags, fingers straightened.
- Sacro-iliacal: spine coil (or phased-array whole-body coil)
  - Paracoronal
  - Axial

  Positioning: supine, cushion under knees to reduce lumbar lordosis
- Hip: body (phased-array) coil
  - Coronal
  - Parasagittal
  - Axial

  Positioning: supine, feet inward rotated 15° and fixed; small pillow under knees
- Knee: knee quadrature coil
  - Sagittal
  - Coronal
  - Axial

  Positioning: supine, straightened leg, relaxed position; fixation with sand bags
- Ankle/foot: head quadrature coil or head and neck quadrature coil
  - Coronal
  - Axial

  Positioning: supine, optional fixation in plaster-cast, and sandbags

7.2 Sequence Protocols and Contrast Medium Application

In all joints, T1-W and T2-W FSE are standard sequence protocols. In addition, there are the T2-W FS sequences (STIR and SPIR), which are most sensitive to edema or effusion. For the evaluation of cartilage lesions, 3D-GRE sequences (with fat suppression) and FSE with FS are recommended. Intravenous (i.v.) application of contrast media is indicated in all cases of malignant blastomas, for staging and follow-up, and in cases of questionable inflammations.

Arthrography is a technique which is mainly used in the shoulder, ankle, knee and hip joints. There are two different techniques:

1. i.v. administration of contrast medium (indirect technique)
2. intraarticular administration of contrast medium (direct technique)

Both techniques may be used in questionable cases of cartilage, ligament or tendon lesions, or in the postoperative follow-up of cartilage lesions.

With the i.v. technique, no puncture of the joint is necessary, but the joint capsule is not expanded, and there are many overlying structures. Moreover extravasation of contrastmaterial in capsule-tears cannot be delinated. With direct arthrography, joint puncture is necessary (in many cases with fluoroscopic guidance), but the contrast within the joint is excellent. One additional drawback is that in many European countries, intraarticular injection of MR contrast media is not permitted (Table 7.1).

Table 7.1a. Pulse sequence recommendations for shoulder

Pulse sequence	WI	Plane	No. of sections	TR (ms)	TE (ms)	Flip angle	Echo train length	Section thickness (mm)	Matrix	FOV	recFOV	No. of acq.	Acq. time (min:s)
SE	T1	Paracoronal	19	530	14	–	–	3	512×256	180	90	3	5:28
FSE+SPIR	T2	Paracoronal	19	1400	130	–	12	3	512×256	200	60	6	4:12
3D-GRE	T2	Axial	70	50	19	20°	–	1	512×256	180	70	3	9:52
SE+SPIR +i.v. contrast	T1	Paracoronal	19	600	20	–	5	3	512×256	180	75	3	12:10
SE+SPIR direct arthrogr.	T1	Paracoronal/ sagittal/ axial	19	600	20	–	–	3	512×256	180	75		11:20
3D-GRE	T1	Axial	50	49	9	45°		1.5	512×256	180	75	1	4:05

Table 7.1b. Pulse sequence recommendations for elbow

Pulse sequence	WI	Plane	No. of sections	TR (ms)	TE (ms)	Flip angle	Echo train length	Section thickness (mm)	Matrix	FOV	recFOV	No. of acq.	Acq. time (min:s)
SE	T1	Coronal/ sagittal	19	555	14	–	–	3	256×512	150	95	2	4:32
FSE+SPIR	T2	Coronal	19	4090	95	–	5	3	256×512	250	100	3	7:51
SE+SPIR +i.v. contrast	T1	Axial/ coronal	19	575	14	–	5	3	256×512	150	95	2	9:24

Table 7.1c. Pulse sequence recommendations for wrist/hand

Pulse sequence	WI	Plane	No. of sections	TR (ms)	TE (ms)	Flip angle	Echo train length	Section thickness (mm)	Matrix	FOV	recFOV	No. of acq.	Acq. time (min:s)
FSE+STIR	WI	Coronal/axial	15	1200	16	–	5	2.4	256×512	140	100	4	6:75
SE	T1	Coronal	15	500	20	–	–	2.4	256×512	140	100	3	4:70
3D-GRE	T2	Coronal	30	60	17	20	–	1.0	256×512	140	90	1	9:11

Table 7.1d. Pulse sequence recommendations for SI joints

Pulse sequence	WI	Plane	No. of sections	TR (ms)	TE (ms)	Flip angle	Echo train length	Section thickness (mm)	Matrix	FOV	recFOV	No. of acq.	Acq. time (min:s)
FSE+STIR	T2	Paracoronal	21	2010	15	–	5	3	256×512	250	100	4	6:10
SE	T1	Paracoronal	21	450	14	–	–	3	256×512	250	100	3	4:70
3D-GRE	T2	Paracoronal	30	60	17	20	–	1.0	256×512	140	100	1	7:28
SE+SPIR +i.v. contrast	T1	Paracoronal	21	575	14			3		259	100	2	11:10

Table 7.1e. Pulse sequence recommendations for hip

Pulse sequence	WI	Plane	No. of sections	TR (ms)	TE (ms)	Flip angle	Echo train length	Section thickness (mm)	Matrix	FOV	recFOV	No. of acq.	Acq. time (min:s)
FSE+STIR	T2	Coronal/ sagittal	19	1200	13	–	5	4	256×256	450	100	2	4:12
SE	T1	Coronal/ sagittal	19	520	14	–	–	4	256×256	450	100	2	4:27
SE+SPIR +i.v. contrast	T1	Coronal	19	575	14	–	–	4	256×256	450	100	2	9:52
SE+SPIR direct arthrogr.	T1	Coronal	19	575	14	–	–	4	256×256	450	100	2	9:52
3D-GRE	T1	Coronal/ sagittal	60	49	9	45	–	1.0	256×256	450	90	1	6:51

Table 7.1f. Pulse sequence recommendations for knee

Pulse sequence	WI	Plane	No. of sections	TR (ms)	TE (ms)	Flip angle	Echo train length	Section thickness (mm)	Matrix	FOV	recFOV	No. of acq.	Acq. time (min:s)
SE	T1	Sagittal	23	555	14	–	–	3	256×512	150	95	3	6:32
FSE-DUAL	T2	Sagittal	23	2500	120/ 90	–	11	3	256×512	180	100	4	8:25
3D-GRE+SPIR	T2	Axial	70	575	14	–	–	1	256×512	180	90	1	12:04
FSE+STIR +i.v. contrast	T2	Coronal	19	1200	13	–	6	4	256×512	200	80	3	4:02
SE	T1	Sagittal	23	550	14	–	–	3	256×512	150	95	2	4:32
SE+SPIR	T1	Axial	19	575	14	–	–	3	256×512	150	95	2	9:24

Table 7.1g. Pulse sequence recommendations for knee

Pulse sequence	WI	Plane	No. of sections	TR (ms)	TE (ms)	Flip angle	Echo train length	Section thickness (mm)	Matrix	FOV	recFOV	No. of acq.	Acq. time (min:s)
SE	T1	Sagittal/ coronal	13	550	20	–	5	3	256×512	160	70	3	4:05
FSE+STIR	T2	Coronal	15	1500	13	–	10	3	256×512	180	80	3	5:10
SE	T2	Axial/ sagittal	13	3500	120	–	–	3	256×512	160	70	3	4:05
SE+SPIR +i.v. contrast	T1	Coronal/ axial	13	550	20	–	–	3	256×512	160	70	3	8:05
SE+SPIR direct arthrogr.	T1	Coronal/ sagittal	13	550	20	–	–	3	256×512	160	70	3	8:05
3D-GRE	T1	Coronal/ sagittal	60	49	9	45	–	1.0	256×512	160	90	2	8:50

- Indirect arthrography:
  a) i.v. injection of 0.1 mmol Gd-chelate/kg BW
  b) Joint motion (5′)
  c) Do imaging within 30 min
- Direct arthrography:
  a) Intraarticular injection of 2 mmol Gd-chelate (=0.2 ml of 0.1 mmol Gd-Chelate in 50 ml physiol. saline)
  b) Joint motion
  c) Do imaging within 30 min

Volume for intraarticular application: shoulder: 10–20 ml; wrist: 2–7 ml; hip: 10–20 ml; knee: 30–40 ml; ankle: 6–12 ml

7.3 Artifacts

Artifacts often occur from metallic implants or metallic remnants of previous surgery; depending on the iron content, they may produce areas with signal loss of varying size. A different form is the magic angle artifact, which is visible if the course of linearly directed anatomic structures form an angle of about 55° to the static magnetic field B_0. This artifact may be of importance in anatomic structures, such as the shoulder or ankle joint, which have curved courses, i.e., the rotator cuff.

7.4 Shoulder Joint

Slice orientation is demonstrated in Table 7.2.

Table 7.2. Slice orientation with anatomic and pathologic key elements

Slice orientation	Anatomic key structures	Pathologic key elements
Axial	Glenoid labrum Humeral head Joint space Biceps tendon	Defects of labrum Hill-Sachs lesion Capsulolabral lesion, effusion Tendinitis, effusion
Angulated coronal	Supraspinatus tendon and muscle Acromioclavicular joint Subacromial space Subacromial bursa	Tendinitis, rupture Degeneration, arthritis, other Narrowing Fluid collection
Angulated sagittal	Acromioclavicular arch Acromion Rotator cuff	Abnormal shape Abnormalities in form Tendinitis, rupture

7.4.1 Trauma

Rupture of the rotator cuff – as visible with MRI – occurs in the form of dehiscence of torn fibers. There may be partial or complete rupture. At times, differentiation between partial and complete ruture, as well as between rupture and degeneration, may be difficult. Effusion of the subdeltoidea bursa and thickening of muscle bellies due to retraction are indirect signs of rotator cuff ruptures (Fig. 7.1).

Instability of the glenohumeral joint leads to subluxation or luxation. In most cases, there is anterior dislocation of the humeral head, leading to varying degrees of defect in the anterior labrum (Bankart lesion) that occurs with or without bony defects (Fig. 7.2). Characteristic MR signs are interruption, deformity, or absence of labrum with effusion. The interrupted space should be filled with fluid or – in MR arthrography – with contrast medium. Diagnostic pitfalls may arise in cases, where there is – as variation in 10% of all cases – in parts of the glenoid rim no labrum at all or the labrum is dehiscent. Finally the completeness of the three gleno-humeral ligaments is mandatory.

Hill-Sachs lesion is a defect of the dorsolateral circumference of the humeral head that results from impression on the anteroinferior part of the capsular labrum. Both abnormalities are readily visible with MRI. Normal variants of the labrum shape include triangular and, less commonly, rounded, cleaved, notched, flat, or even absent labrum (Fig. 7.3). These variants should not be mistaken for defects due to instability. In all unclear cases, MR arthrography is absolutely indicated.

Defects in other parts of the articular labrum may rarely occur posteriorly, due to inverted luxation of the humeral head, or at the superior aspect, due to single or repetitive forces of the biceps tendon such as occur during sporting activities (SLAP lesion, i.e., superior labral tear with anterior and posterior extension). Old bone fractures of the humeral head, the scapula, or the clavicle present with fracture lines and appear hypointense

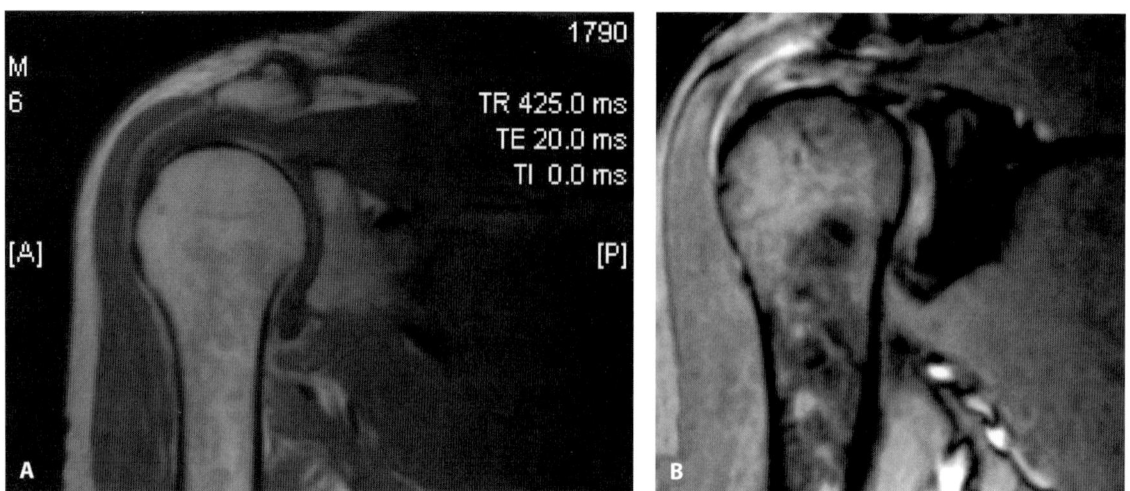

Fig. 7.1A,B. Rupture of the rotator cuff. **A** T1-W image with intermediate hyperintensity of the peripheral part of the supraspinatus tendon. **B** Hyperintense defect on T2-WI with hyperintense fluid in the joint space and the subdeltoid bursa indicating effusion

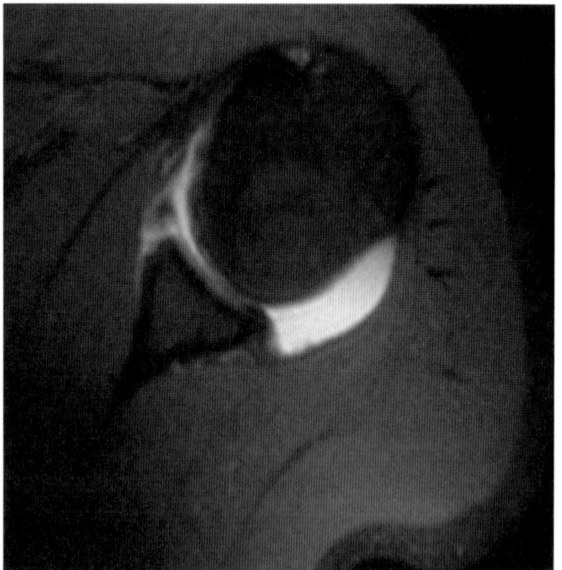

Fig. 7.2. Direct MR arthrography with basal defect of interior articular labrum due to luxation

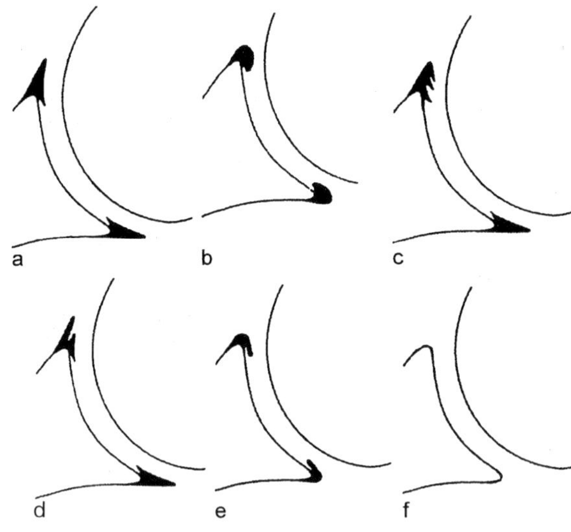

Fig. 7.3. Variation of shape of the labrum
a) triangular, b) round, c) stubby, d) cleaved, e) flat, f) absent

on all sequences, while acute fractures show T2-W hyperintense fracture-lines, dislocation of fracture segments, and bone-marrow edema. The latter, referred to as bone bruise, may be of significant importance in otherwise clinically occult fractures (Fig. 7.4).

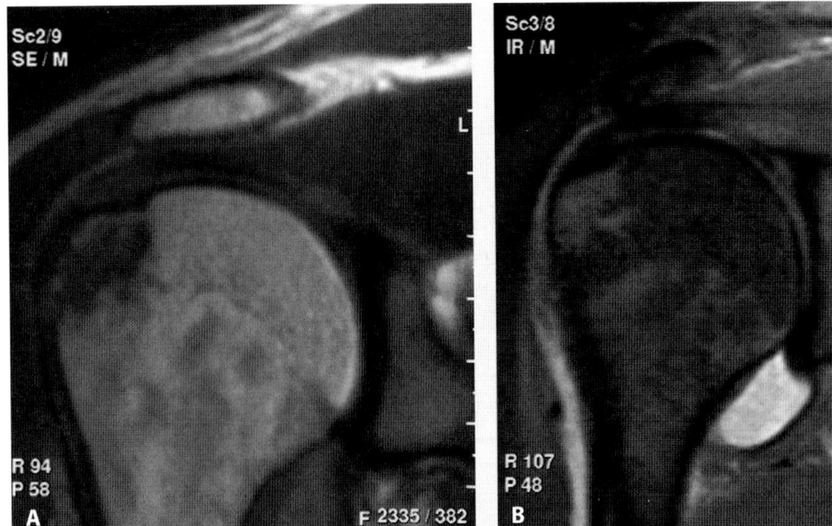

Fig. 7.4. **A** Bone bruise due to fracture of greater tubercle of humerus. T1-WI, angulated coronal, with hypointense signal changes in the bone marrow of the greater tubercle. Slight hypointense line as a sign of fracture without dislocation was hardly visible on plain films. **B** On T2-W fat-suppressed image (STIR), extensive hyperintensities are visible indicating bone-marrow edema

7.4.2 Degeneration

Due to narrowing of the subacromial space and mechanical overload, the components of the rotator cuff, i.e., the supraspinatus, the infraspinatus, the subscapularis muscle, and the teres minor muscle, are specifically prone to tendinitis and eventual rupture. Clinically, pain and impairment of motion are referred to as the impingement syndrome. Abnormalities of the rotator cuff strongly correlate with age. They are graded clinically and pathologically according to Neer. Grading with MRI was proposed by Tyson (Table 7.3).

Narrowing of the subacromial space may be due to an abnormal form and shape of the acromion, formation of a subacromial spur, osteoarthritis of the acromioclavicular joint, or hypertrophy of the supraspinatus muscle. The shape of the acromion may be classified as flat, curved, or hooked. Tendons, which are normally hypointense on all sequences, appear with intermediate or hyperintense signal intensity (Table 7.4) and with or without thinning and/or discontinuity of contours. These findings occur particularly in the lateral parts of the supraspinatus tendon.

Table 7.3. Grading of impingement of the shoulder. Morphologic grading proposed by Neer (1983). Findings with magnetic resonance imaging (MRI) modified after Tyson et al. (1993) and Kang et al. (1991) correlated with morphologic abnormalities of tendon or rotator cuff

Grade	Pathology	Typical age of disease	Course	Morphology	MRI signal intensity	
	Normal (no pathology)			T1 ⇓	T2 ⇓	
I	Edema, hemorrhage	<25 years	Reversible	Mild abnormality	T1 ⇑	T2 ⇓
II	Fibrosis, tendinitis	25–40 years	Recurrent pain	Severe abnormality	T1 ⇑⇑	T2 ⇑
III	Osteophytes, rupture	>40 years	Progressive	Tear	T1 ⇓	T2 ⇑⇑⇑

7.4.3 Inflammation

Arthritis is observed mainly in patients with rheumatoid arthritis; septic arthritis or inflammation due to other systemic rheumatic diseases are rare. On T2-W images, hyperintense joint effusions or effusions of the juxtaarticular bursae (either with or without bony erosions and synovial thickening) are the main MRI features. The contrast enhancement of synovium depends on the severity of inflammation. This feature can be used in therapeutic control. Tendinitis and/or ruptures of the rotator cuff may occur (see Sect. 7.4.2).

7.4.4 Tumors

The frequency-distribution of primary (malignant or benign) tumors in the shoulder joint is comparable to that in other locations. The only lesions that occur with the highest frequency in the shoulder are simple bone cysts and chondroblastomas. Only in unclear cases is MRI indicated for simple bone cysts. These cysts appear hyperintense on T2-W images and hypointense on T1-W images. Chondroblastomas are hypointense on T1-W images and moderately hyperintense on T2-W images.

7.4.5 Metabolic Diseases

Pyrophosphate arthropathy or periarthropathy due to hydroxyapatite crystal deposition is most often observed in the shoulder joint. In the latter, crystal deposits within the rotator cuff may calcify and, eventually, extend into the subdeltoid bursa. In the former, intraarticular crystal formation mainly occurs in the hyaline cartilage, either with or without calcification. It generally presents with signs of osteoarthritis of the humeroglenoidal joint.

With MRI, varying degrees of effusion, with or without osteophyte formation, are visible. Calcified crystal deposits within the rotator cuff are generally hypointense on all sequences, with hyperintense tendon abnormalities on T2-W images due to reactive inflammation with an increased water content.

7.5 Elbow Joint

7.5.1 Trauma

7.5.1.1 Ligaments

Physiologically, the collateral ligaments are visible as thin, hypointense bands in the coronal plane. After acute trauma (partial rupture, rupture) (Table 7.5), signal-intensity changes are visible; simplified, high signal intensity on T2-W images is due to edema and blood (Table 7.4). Furthermore, irregular borders and band laxity can be observed. In cases of chronic or repetitive trauma, secondary degenerative changes appear and are characterized by moderate to high signal-intensity changes on T1-W and T2-W SE images that occur without evidence of fluid or signs of rupture.

7.5.1.2 Injuries in Tendons (Biceps, Triceps)

General morphological features and signal characteristics of acute injuries are given in Table 7.5. The field of view (FOV) should include imaging of the complete tendon from the musculotendinous part to the insertion on the radius. A comparison with the contralateral joint is not necessary.

Additional MR signs for ligamentous or tendinous ruptures are: loss of visibility of the distal part of the tendon, fluid in the tendon sheath, a soft-tissue mass in the antecubital fossa, potential muscle edema, and/or atrophy in cases of an older rupture. Regarding recent

Table 7.4. Grading of tendolipament injuries

Grade	Pathology	MRI symptoms
1	Edema	Thickening, hyperintensity
2	Partial rupture	Thinning, spreading, hyperintensity, partial interruptlon
3	Complete rupture	Complete interruption, retraction of ends, hyperintensity, bleeding
4	Rupture and bone fracture	Grade 3 + bone-marrow edema, bone structures interrupted

ruptures, high signal intensity changes (T2-W images) are visible with in the ligament or tendon. Equivalent signs appear for ruptures of the triceps tendon; however, on T2-W images, signs of a bursitis olecrani and/ or bone-marrow edema in the area of the olecranon process might be visible. Chronic or repetitive injuries cause secondary degenerative changes (see Sect. 7.5.2)

7.5.1.3 Overuse Syndrome and Epicondylitis

Chronic stress is frequently induced by sports activities (golfers' elbow, tennis elbow). In complete ruptures of the collateral ligaments, a dissociation between the tendon and the adjacent bone is visible, with accumulation

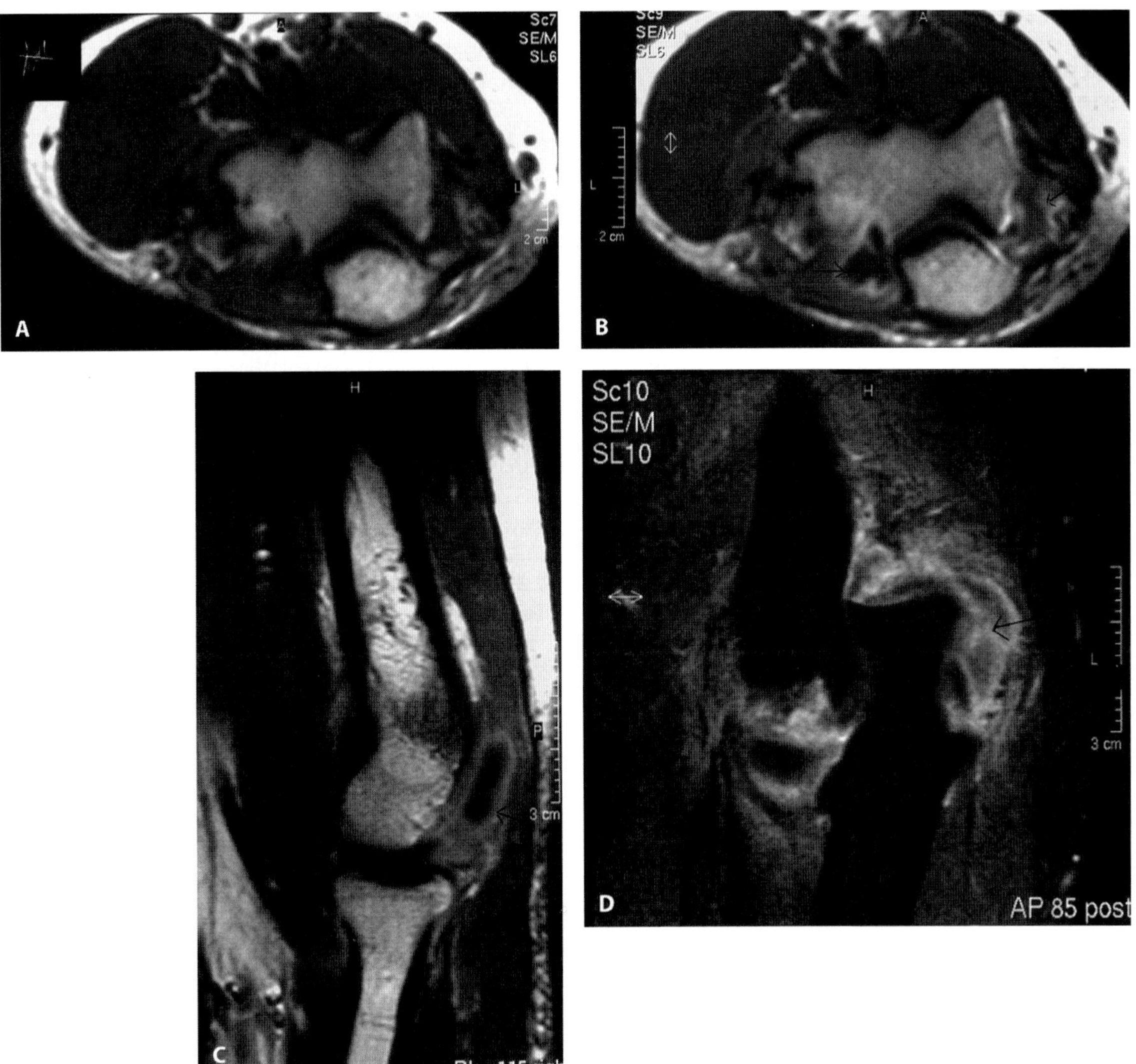

Fig. 7.5A–D. Synovitis of the elbow joint in a patient with rheumatoid arthritis. **A** Axial T1-W image precontrast, **B** axial postcontrast, and **C** sagittal postcontrast images, demonstrating synovial enhancement (*arrows*). **D** Coronal FS images demonstrating edema (*arrow*)

of fluid and high signal-intensity changes on T2-W images. Partial ruptures are characterized by a thinning of the ligament, with irregularity or discontinuation of individual fibers. Tendinosis and degenerative changes have an intermediate signal on T1-W sequences, without a significant increase in signal intensity on T2-W images. STIR images increase the signal alteration in complete or partial ruptures. Contrast application is not necessary but does potentially increase the signal intensity on T1-W postcontrast images.

7.5.1.4 Osteochondritis Dissecans

The most frequent location for osteochondritis dissecans (OD) is the area of the capitulum. MR imaging characteristics are similar to those other joints (see Sect. 7.9). Critical areas for the evaluation of loose bodies are the olecranon fossa, fossae radii, and coronoidea (Fig. 7.5).

7.5.2 Degeneration

Degenerative changes of the tendons are characterized by punctate lesions, bands, or areas of high signal intensity on T1 and T2-W images, without extension of the altered signal intensity to the surface of the tendon. Primary degenerative changes of the cartilage are rare; secondary changes are, in the majority of cases, due to previous trauma (see Sect. 7.9.2).

7.5.3 Inflammation

In cases of chronic polyarthritis (CP) and other inflammatory processes (Fig. 7.6), synovial proliferation is best demonstrated using T1-W contrast-enhanced images. Edematous changes and fluid are characterized by hypointense signal characteristics on T1-W and hyperintense signal characteristics on T2-W images. With gadolinium-enhanced T1-SE image, enhancement of the otherwise not visible synovium can be observed. The degree and activity of synovial proliferations may also be evaluated usin6 dynamic MR imaging.

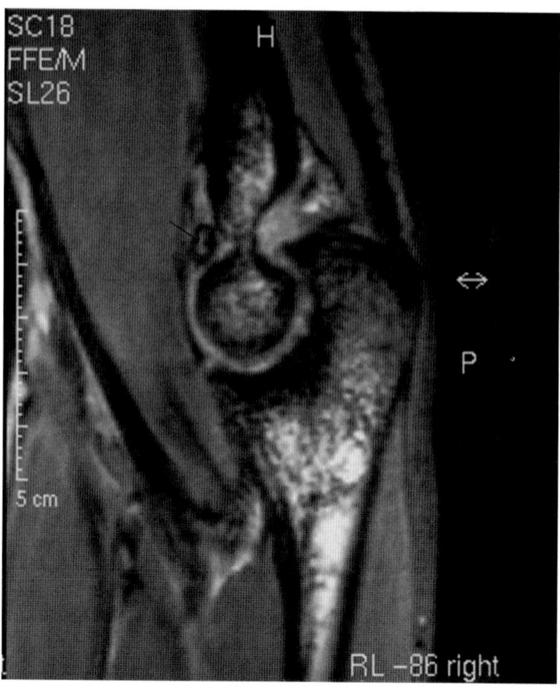

Fig. 7.6. Osteochondritis dissecans in the elbow joint; sagittal T2-W GRE images (*arrow*)

7.5.4 Tumors

Synovial chondromatosis is accompanied by synovial proliferation and the formation of intrasynovial nodules of cartilage. The nodules may calcify, ossify, or become free within the joint cavity and later embed in a distant synovial site. The appearance on MR images depends on the composition of the nodules and, specifically, on the degree of calcification and ossification. Calcification is typically hypointense on T1-W and T2-W images. Ossification must have bone marrow, which shows (in the case of fatty marrow) the characteristic MR signs of fat. Due to their high water content, mature chondroid lesions demonstrate hypointensity on T1-W images and hyperintensity on T2-W images. In the absence of calcification, the nodules have a signal intensity similar to that of fluid (hypointense on T1-SE images, hyperintense on T2-W images).

Chondromas are frequently seen in the elbow joint. Intracapsular chondromas are associated with masses of variable size that may calcify. Either inhomogeneous or homogeneous signal intensity may be noted on MR imaging, and there is a fluent continuation between benign chondromas and low-grade chondrosarcomas. The degree of high signal intensity on T2-W images gives some information about the biological characteristics. An exact differentiation of low-grade chondrosarcoma and chondroma is not possible in many cases.

7.6 Wrist Joint

7.6.1 Trauma and Degeneration

7.6.1.1 Tendinous and Ligamentous Injuries

Generally, degenerative changes are defined as small, intraligamentous, hyperintense signal alterations on T1 and T2-SE images. In the case of partial ruptures, more extensive signal alteration is visible, reaching the tendinous or ligamentous surface, albeit with evidence of intact residual fibers. Ruptures show high signal-intensity changes on T1 and T2-W images that comprise the total diameter and can be found with or without retraction.

Due to their size, intrinsic ligament indications are limited to the evaluation of the scapholunate (SL) and lunotriquetral (LT) ligaments. A perforation of the SL or LT ligament appears as a discontinuity in the normal signal intensity of the intact ligament; however, complete perforations do not always result in the physical dislocation of the two bones. With detachment, the remnants retract, making these portions of the ligament appear thicker. Otherwise, because about 30% of all cases with lesions do not have any clinical symptoms, the radiological diagnosis of a nonsymptomatic lesion remains questionable.

Regarding extrinsic ligaments, disruptions are combined with SL dissociation, midcarpal instability, and displaced scaphoid fractures. Because extrinsic ligaments are larger, MR imaging can discern mechanical disruption or significant degenerative lesion, and help stage and quantify ligamentous defects.

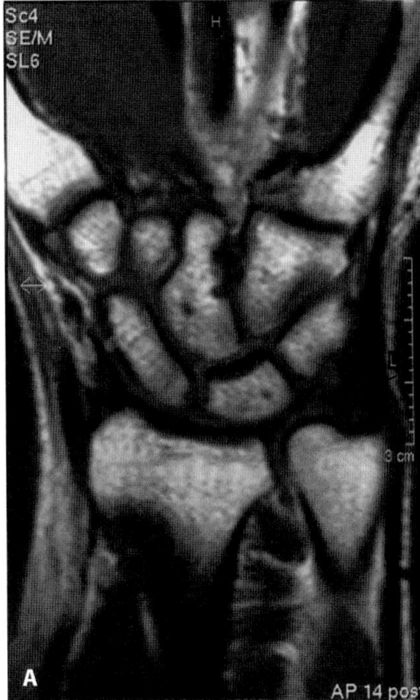

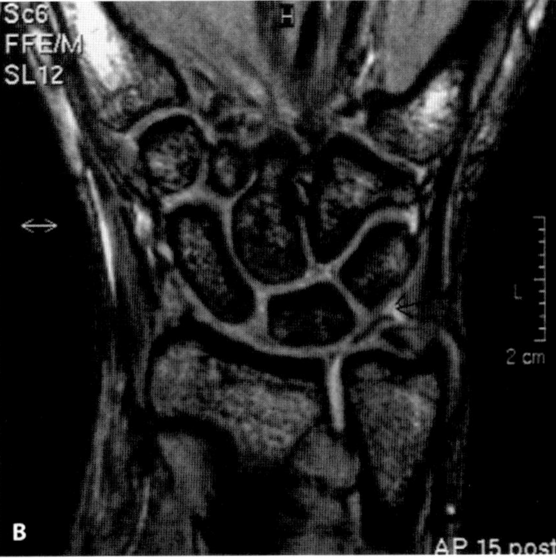

Fig. 7.7A,B. Rupture of the triangular fibrocartilage. **A** Coronal T1 and **B** coronal T2-W images (*arrow*)

7.6.1.2
Triangular Fibrocartilage

Triangular fibrocartilage (TFC) lesions may be either traumatic or degenerative. MRI can potentially localize defects within the TFC sufficiently to permit noninvasive staging and classification of the lesion. Perforations and disruptions appear as high signal-intensity areas on T1-W and T2-W images, interrupting the continuity of the low signal of the intact disc (Fig. 7.7).

Partial thickness perforations are recognized as irregular areas of higher signal intensity on T1-W and T2-W images that appear along the otherwise smooth proximal or distal surface of the TFC. Degenerative changes appear as hyperintense intradiscal irregularities on T1-W images, without an increase of signal intensity on T2-W images.

7.6.1.3
Dislocations and Instabilities

Although instabilities can be evaluated with plain film radiographs and conventional arthrography, use of MRI offers additional information concerning the TFC, ligaments, and tendons, by allowing for the evaluation of associated traumatic or degenerative changes. At the moment, it is thought that the use of intraarticular application of contrast agents does not have any specific indications in the wrist joint except in special cases.

7.6.2
Inflammation

MR imaging can be used to assess the extent of rheumatoid arthritis and other synovial inflammatory diseases. It allows assessment of cartilage and bone destruction, the extent of synovial inflammation, and the activity of the disease process. Marginal and central bone erosions and subchondral cystic lesions can be identified due to the high signal intensities of synovial fluid and inflammatory tissue on the T2-W SE and GRE images. For the differentiation of fluid and synovial pannus, the use of intravenous gadolinium is necessary. Signal enhancement within the inflamed synovial tissue allows for its differentiation from joint fluid, which does not enhance on T1-W SE MR images obtained immediately after injection. Due to the leakage of the contrast agent into the joint fluid, MR images that are delayed relative to i.v. administration of gadolinium are not useful for this differentiation. Postcontrast imaging can also be used to evaluate the extent of tendon sheath involvement in rheumatoid arthritis. Signal enhancement in synovial tissue on gadolinium-enhanced T1-W images generally implies active inflammation; the technique is beneficial in monitoring the therapeutic response.

7.6.3
Tumors

Lipomas are one of the most common tumors found and are revealed by signal characteristics of fat (high signal intensity on T1 and T2-W images). Ganglion cysts are seen as well-defined, smooth masses with signal-intensity characteristics of fluid (hyperintense on T2-W images, hypointense on T1 images). However, with increased protein concentration inside the ganglion, the signal intensity on T1-W images increases.

Hemangioma is the most common vascular tumor and has a typical MR appearance, with inhomogeneous intermediate signal intensity on T1 weighted and high signal intensity on T2 weighted and fat-suppression images. Moreover, it shows hypointense irregular septa (often serpentine).

7.7
Sacroiliac Joints

7.7.1
Trauma

Indications for MR imaging are insufficiency fractures (particularly with osteoporosis) and complex pelvis fractures with complications (unclear neural deficits, bleeding). Insufficiency fractures of the sacrum typically run parallel to the linear joint lesions, which are hypointense on T1-W and hyperintense on T2-W images (Fig. 7.8).

7.7.2
Degeneration

There are no indications for MRI in degenerative diseases of the SI joint.

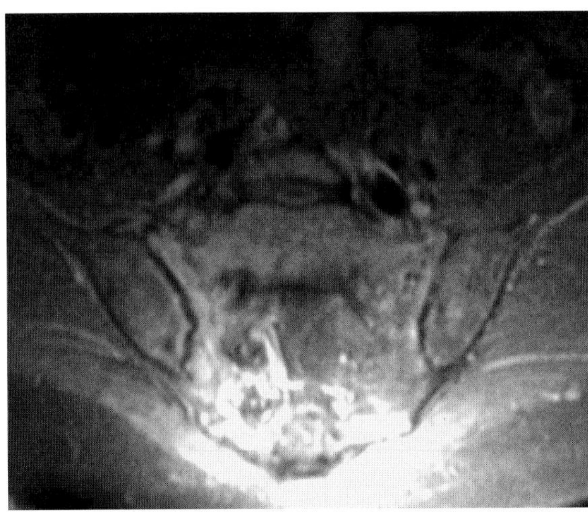

Fig. 7.8. Sacroiliacal joint (paracoronal, T2-W + STIR): insufficiency fracture. Hyperintense line parallel to the S1 joints, right more prominent than left

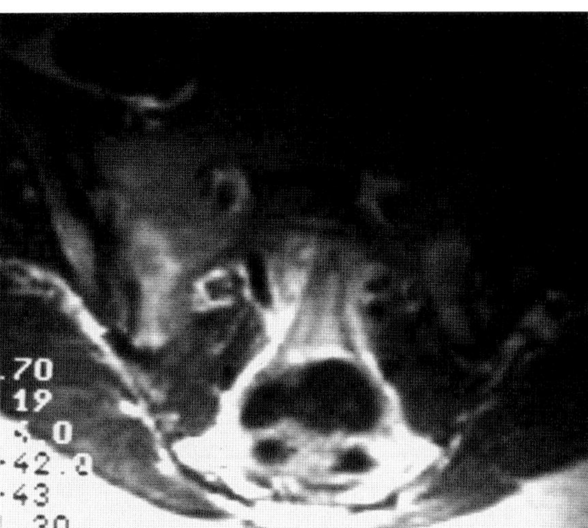

Fig. 7.9. Sacroiliacal joints (Daracoronal, T1-W + i.v. contrast). Ankylosing spondylitis bilateral enhanced hyperintensity in subchondral bone marrow (= active inflammation) and effusion

7.7.3 Inflammation

In cases of unclear inflammatory processes or for the grading and follow-up of inflammatory abnormalities, MR imaging is an add-on imaging modality. MR imaging allows for the exact differentiation of grades 2 and 4a inflammation (Table 7.5). The problem is that in all inflammatory processes, except septic sacroiliitis, there are different inflammatory grades present at the same time. With dynamic MR (time-intensity curves after i.v. injection of contrast medium), therapeutic control is possible. Symmetric or asymmetric distributions of lesions, the presence of erosions and/or sclerosis, ankylosis, and osteoporosis allow the differentiation of the forms of inflammation (rheumatoid arthritis, ankylosing spondylitis, enteropathic arthritis, psoriasis, Reiter's disease, degeneration; see Fig. 7.9, Table 7.6).

Table 7.5. Grading of inflammation of sacroiliac joints in rheumatoid disease

Grade	Pathology	MRI
0	Antigen to T-cells	0
1	Synovial hyperemia and edema Effusion Bone-marrow edema	T1, T2, i.v. contrast
2	Subchondral micro-edema, necrosis, porosis	MRI?
3	a) Bone erosions (active or nonactive) b) Cartilage: fibrillation, thinning, baldness calcification	T1, T2, i.v. contrast MRI? (3D-GRE)
4	Pannus (activity) New bone formation Cysts, sclerosis Ankylosis	T1, T2, i.v. contrast fatty conversion fibrosis

7.7.4 Tumors

Primary tumors of the SI joints are rare. The most common ones are osteochondroma, chordoma, aneurysmatic bone cysts, and chondrosarcomas. For malignant tumors, MR with i.v. contrast administration is required for the staging and follow-up. Secondary tumors in the SI region can be found in breast, prostate and renal cell cancer. Direct invasion may be seen in cancer of the rectum or uterus.

Table 7.6. Differential diagnosis of (inflammatory) sacroiliac joint lesions

	Rheumatoid arthritis	Inflammatory bowel disease, ankylosing spondylitis	Psoriasis, Reiter's syndrome	Septic arthritis	Hyperpara-thyroid	Degeneration
Distribution	Asymmetric	Bilateral and symmetric	Symmetric, asymmetric, unilateral, bilateral	Unilateral	Bilateral symmetric	Symmetric, asymmetric uni- and bilateral
Erosions	Superficial	Deep	Superficial	Deep	Superficial	0
Sclerosis	Mild	Moderate or severe	Severe	Mild	Moderate	Mild-moderate
Ankylosis	Rare	Common	Rare-common	0	0	Rare
Osteoporosis	Common	0	0	Common	0	o

7.8 Hip Joint

7.8.1 Trauma

Secondary traumatic lesions are more common than primary lesions. The most frequent imaging signs are bone-marrow edema, ischemic necrosis after hip neck fractures, and occult fractures, which are especially frequent in elderly, osteoporotic patients. All these lesions are recognized by localized hyperintensity on T2-W images, due to edema.

7.8.2 Degeneration

Degenerative changes of the hip joint are very common. Indications for MRI exist only in unclear cases to rule out nondegenerative lesions like blastoma and inflammation.

7.8.2.1 Labral Lesion

Tears of the acetabular labrum often develop as secondary degenerative changes in patients with congenital hip dysplasia or as sequelae of injury, especially after hip dislocation. In most cases, the anterior and superior parts of the labrum are involved. When the femoral head articulates with the torn part of the labrum, the cartilage at the head may be eroded. In this case, MR arthrography ensures excellent depiction of labral lesions as well as the cartilage of lesions. The superior diagnostic ability of MR arthrography compared with conventional MR imaging is due to the distention of the joint capsule by the intraarticular contrast agent, which fills defects in the labrum and, therefore, allows for superior contrast of tear and tissue. The typical horseshoe configuration of the normal acetabular cartilage is very well delineated. The normal continuation of the labrum in the caudal part is the lig. transversum. The configuration of the labrum varies from triangular (66–80%) to flat and round shaped. In 1–14% the labrum may be absent. A ganglion-cyst is an indirect sign for a labrum-pathology.

7.8.3 Inflammation

Imaging patterns similar to those present for ischemic lesions can be observed for infection and inflammation of the marrow cavity (i.e., osteomyelitis). Most of these changes may be well-depicted by MR imaging and manifest in focal or disseminated edema and hyperemia (T1 hypointense/T2 hyperintense). Effusion of the joint capsule (T2 hyperintense) can be adjacent to an osteomyelitis; however, this sign is not pathognomic because it can also be present in seronegative, HLA-B27-positive spondyloarthropathies (rheumatoid variants). A bacterial infection does have a propensity to be isolated to one side, usually shows a more widespread affection of bone marrow, and may spread into the surrounding tissues.

7.8.4
Tumors

Primary (malignant or benign) blastoma or tumor-like lesions are very rarely found in the hip joint. In these rare cases, osteoid osteoma, chondroblastoma, synovial chondromatosis, and fibrous dysplasia are most common. An indication for a MR examination exists only in unclear cases.

7.8.5
Edema and Ischemia

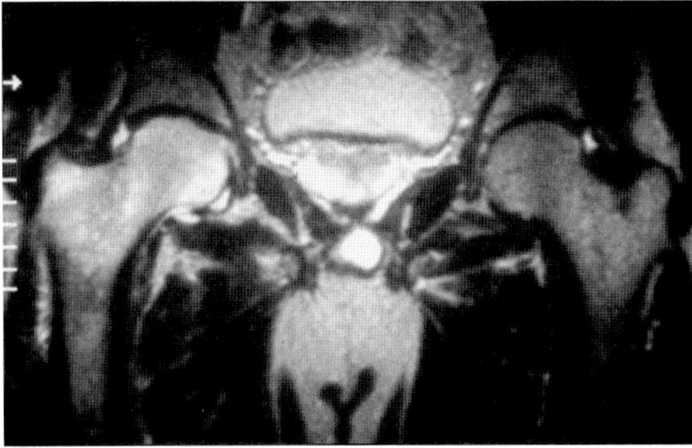

Fig. 7.10. Hip joint (T2-W STIR). Bone-marrow edema syndrome: large hyperintensity in the head of the hip-joint, synovial effusion

Marrow edema is characterized by increased intramedullary signal intensity on T2-W images and decreased signal intensity on T1-W images. Bone-marrow edema is caused by a variety of conditions, such as avascular necrosis, fractures, bone bruises, bone-marrow edema syndrome, osteomyelitis and infection, primary tumors and metastases. Most of those conditions can be distinguished by their clinical symptoms, as well as by their characteristic MR appearance.

The term bone-marrow edema syndrome (BMES) is used for a condition in which in the absence of specific signs for avascular necrosis, the characteristic bone-marrow edema pattern in MR imaging occurs in combination with nonspecific hip pain. BMES is, in most cases, a self-limiting condition, which should be distinguished from avascular necrosis. In BMES, most of the femoral head is usually affected, and the edema may also be visible in parts of the femoral neck and in the intertrochanteric region (Fig. 7.10).

Ischemic lesions involving bone and bone marrow usually show focal changes and may demonstrate a characteristic imaging pattern with subarticular osteonecrosis and intramedullary bone infarction, which appears hyperintense on T1-W images and T2-W images with a reactive margin. In intramedullary infarction, reactive T2-W hyperintensity may involve the whole infarcted region in an early phase. In this case, it shows a high contrast enhancement, too. Aseptic necrosis of the adult is called idiopathic if no trauma or other predisposing conditions (e.g., steroid therapy) are present. It is most commonly found in the hip joint (up to 50% bilateral), femoral condylus, distal tibia, proximal humerus, elbow and lunate. In the femur, changes appear mostly in the cranial weight-bearing portion of the head. In most cases, the area of necrosis is oval-shaped. Appreciation of its size may be of prognostic value. The imaging pattern of the necrosis depends on the ratio of different internal tissues (fat, subacute bleeding, edema, fibrosis). In early stages, one may find a small subcortical edema (T2-W hyperintense). Later, T1-W and T2-W hypointensities (necrosis) are found. In the majority of cases, there is an area of low intensity (on T1-W images) between the area of necrosis and the area of normal bone marrow, which is called the interface. On T2-W images, the border of the interface to the necrosis shows a hyperintense line, and the border of the interface to the regular marrow shows a hypointense line. This pattern is called the double-line sign

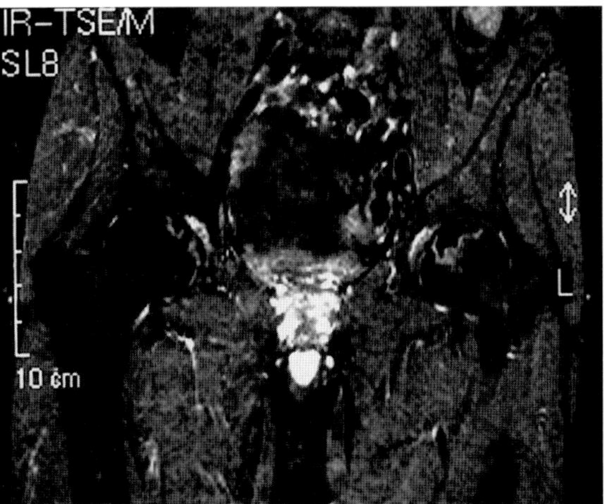

Fig. 7.11. Hip joint (T2-W STIR). Bilateral aseptic femoral head necrosis on the left side more pronounced than on the right with double-line sign (ARCO-Stage 2)

Table 7.7. ARCO staging of avascular necrsis (Association Recherche de Circulation Osseusse)

Stage	Pathology	MRI
0	Micronecrosis and edema	0
1	Subcortical edema	T1 hypointense T2 hyperintense
2	Demarcation of necrosis (fibrov. tiss.)	Double-line sign, necrosis = hypointense
3	Cortical impression	X-ray, CT
4	Deformation, see degeneration	X-ray, CT

(Fig. 7.11, Table 7.7). When i.v. contrast material is given, the inner border shows a strong enhancement. MRI plays a very important role in the early detection of avascular necrosis (stage 1) and in treatment decisions (e.g., conservative, drilling).

Morbus Perthes occurs in children between the ages of 6–8 years and probably represents a manifestation of idiopathic bone necrosis (due to discrepant vascular supply) and presents with imaging signs similar to aseptic femoral head necrosis of the adult. The epiphysis shows low signal intensities on T1-W and T2-W sequences which, in the early stages, may have a patchy appearance. With the course of the disorder, the entire epiphysis and parts of the metaphysis can be affected. The role of MRI, again, is in the early detection and follow-up of treatments that delineate containment of the hip joint.

7.9 Knee Joint

7.9.1 Trauma

7.9.1.1 Menisci

The posterior third of the medial meniscus is considerably larger than the anterior third. The anterior and posterior thirds of the lateral meniscus are equal in size and height. Accuracy rates of MRI for meniscal derangement are reported to be between 85% and 95%. Several observations help to differentiate between tear and degeneration. Degeneration:

1. Tends to be located in the body and horn of the medial meniscus.
2. Shows a horizontal and not a vertical orientation.
3. Does not involve the inner third of the meniscus.
4. Has only a low signal-intensity increase.

On the other hand, the majority of tears are identified by fluid equivalent signals (linear hyperintensity) extending to an articular surface. These can be divided into horizontal, vertical, or complex tears. Occasionally, tears present as a combination of horizontal and vertical components. These complex tears are usually unstable.

Two important tear patterns that do not demonstrate this characteristic appearance are radial and evulsion (bucket-handle) tears (Fig. 7.12). Radial tears are identified as fluid-filled gaps in the meniscal body that are significantly smaller than bucket-handle tears. Once again, the margins are generally well-demarcated, and the tear often completely traverses the body, in which case they are frequently associated with meniscal cysts.

Bucket-handle tears may present as:

1. Large fluid-filled defects in the meniscal body ('meniscal ghost').
2. The occurrence of the avulsed fragment centrally within the notch, where it can mimic the cruciate ligaments (ACL and PCL).
3. Occasional displacement of the meniscal fragment anteriorly and adjacent to the anterior horn (flipped meniscus sign or the pseudo-hypertrophied anterior horn sign).

7.9.1.2 Anterior Cruciate Ligament

MR imaging is highly sensitive and specific in diagnosing ACL tears. A normal ACL is seen as a single fiber or as several fibers running parallel to the roof of the intercondylar notch. In acute and complete ACL tears, direct MR findings are (Fig. 7.13):

1. Complete disruption of the fibers.
2. The occurrence of disruption (usually) in the proximal or mid-portions of the ligament.
3. A mass of high or heterogeneous signal intensity on T2-W images.

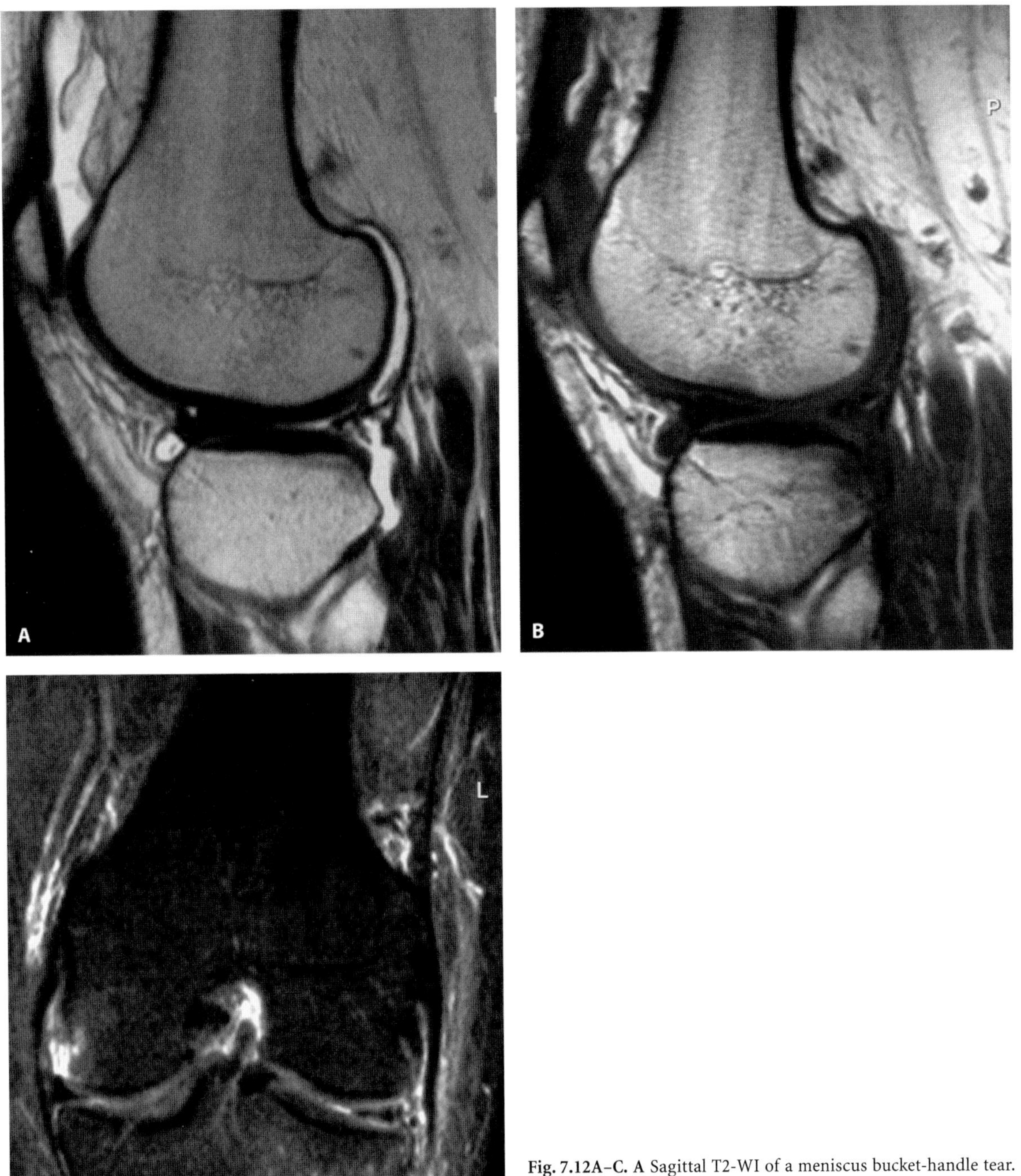

Fig. 7.12A–C. **A** Sagittal T2-WI of a meniscus bucket-handle tear. Fluid-filled defect in the posterior meniscal horn ('meniscal ghost') and the displaced meniscal fragment lying anterior adjacent to the anterior horn (flipped meniscus sign). **B** Corresponding sagittal T1-WI of a meniscus bucket-handle tear. **C** Coronal STIR MR image of a meniscus bucket-handle tear. The avulsed fragment lies centrally within the notch, where it can mimic the ACL or PCL

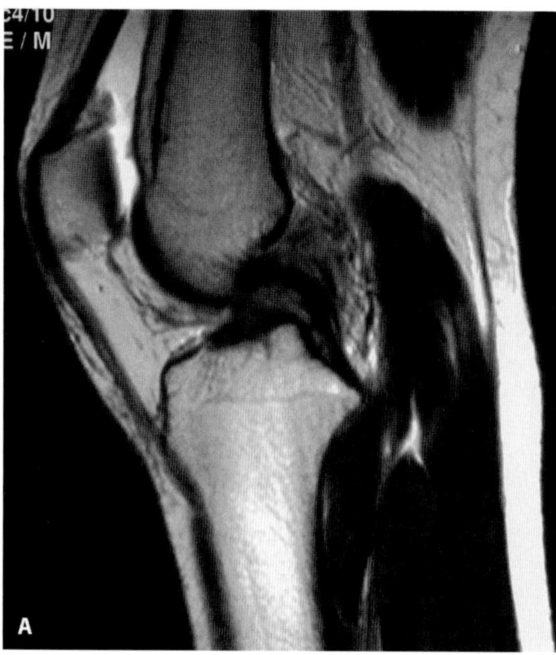

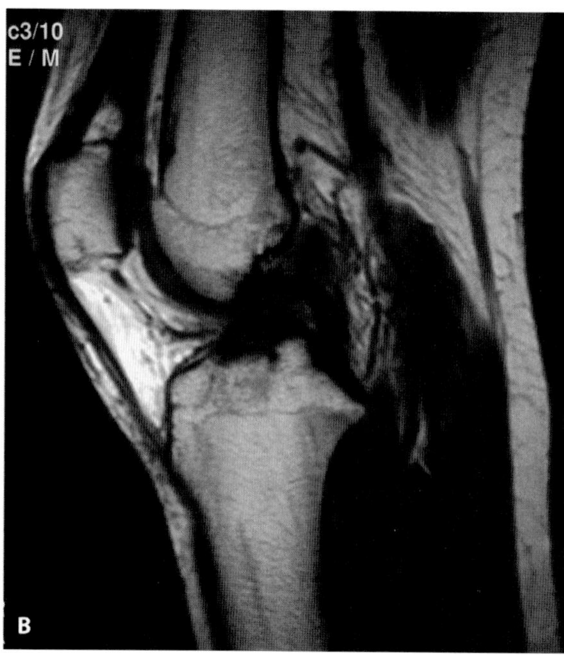

Fig. 7.13. A Sagittal T2-WI of an acute and complete ACL tear with complete disruption of the fibers in the mid-portions of the ligament appearing like a mass of high or heterogeneous signal intensity. **B** Corresponding sagittal T1-WI of a complete ACL tear can also be delineated

In old or chronic tears, the ACL ligament is either not visualized or is seen to be lying in an abnormally horizontal plane.

Several secondary MR signs of ACL disruption include:

1. An abnormal signal within the posterior aspect of the lateral tibial plateau (impaction).
2. A corresponding lesion in the lateral femoral condyle (impaction).
3. An increased depth of the normal lateral condylar sulcus (small impaction fracture).
4. Anterior translation of the tibia.
5. Buckling of the PCL due to anterior subluxation of the tibia.

Secondary signs do not significantly improve the diagnostic accuracy when compared with direct signs alone. They may help to distinguish partial from complete tears. MRI signs of partial tear of the ACL are:

1. Thickening or thinning of the ligament.
2. High signal within the ligament.
3. Laxity of the ligament.

7.9.1.3 Posterior Cruciate Ligament

The PCL is a strong structure that rarely ruptures. Injuries occur usually as a result of posterior displacement of the tibia in a flexed knee or as a hyperextension injury. The normal PCL is easily identified on MRI. MR signs of a partial or complete tear resemble the ACL findings. MRI is also highly sensitive and specific for PCL rupture (sensitivity and specificity: 90%–95%).

7.9.1.4 Medial Collateral Ligament

The medial collateral ligament (MCL) has a superficial component that runs from the medial epicondyle to the medial aspect of the tibial metaphysis and a deep component that attaches to the joint margin and is closely applied to the medial meniscus. The MCL is best visualized on coronal images.

Tears of the superficial ligament:
1. Are usually partial.
2. Occur close to either the tibial or femoral insertions.
3. Show an increase in signal intensity on T1-W and T2-W images and thickening.

Tears of the deep fibers alone:
1. Occur with the knee in the flexed position and in a valgus injury.
2. Show high signal intensity on T1-W and T2-W images between the superficial layer and the medial meniscus.

MR imaging has only a limited role in the assessment of MCL tears, given that X-rays and clinical examination are sufficient for diagnosis and that treatment is invariably conservative.

7.9.1.5 Lateral Collateral Ligament

The lateral collateral ligament is a strong cord-like structure which runs in a posterior oblique fashion from the lateral femoral epicondyle to the head of the fibula. It is:
1. Usually torn as a result of a major trauma such as a dislocation.
2. Rare as an isolated injury – it is usually associated with injuries of the popliteus tendon, iliotibial band, or arcuate ligament.
3. Torn at the fibular attachment or in its mid portion.

Tears may be treated conservatively or repaired surgically.

7.9.1.6 Meniscofemoral Ligament

The meniscofemoral ligament runs from the posterior aspect of the posterior third of the lateral meniscus to the lateral surface of the medial femoral condyle. There are two components, one lying anterior (ligament of Humphrey) and one posterior (ligament of Wrisberg) to the PCL. It is important to be aware of the meniscofemoral ligament, because its attachment to the posterior portion of the lateral meniscus may mimic a meniscal tear on sagittal images.

7.9.1.7 Postoperative Imaging of Cartilage Repair

With recent advances in the treatment of acute cartilage trauma (e.g., fracture with cartilage defects) in young patients, including autologous osteochondral defects and autologous chondrocyte implantation, noninvasive MRI has gained additional importance. Cartilage transplants should be evaluated with respect to their morphology and signal intensity. For morphology, the degree of defect repair (filling of the defect), the integration with the border zone, the surface of the transplant, the subchondral lamina, and the subchondral bone should be evaluated.

7.9.2 Degeneration

Degeneration is a cartilage and subchondral disease. For visualization of these abnormalities, high-resolution cartilage sequences (3D-GRE + fat suppression, dual FSE) must be used. Chondromalacia is the forerunner of degeneration. It can be graded with MRI into four types, depending on the degree of cartilage involvement:
1. Grade 1: surface softening or blistering.
2. Grade 2: fissuring of the surface (fibrillation).
3. Grade 3: cartilage defect extending to the bone.
4. Grade 4: baldness.

Grade 4 lesions are readily identified on MRI. The majority of grade 3 lesions can be also detected with MRI. Grade 2 will generally only be seen with high-resolution sequences or, more readily, with direct arthrography. Grade 1 lesions can only identified in 40%–50% with MR arthrography.

7.9.2.1 Patellar Tendinitis (Jumper's Knee)

Patellar tendinitis is particularly associated with jumping sports. When suspected, the lesion is detected on ultrasound and is also easily seen on MRI. MR signs of a jumper's knee are:
1. Focus of high signal.
2. A swollen tendon.
3. Lesion close to the patellar tendon origin.
4. Fluid may be seen in the adjacent soft tissue.

7.9.3 Inflammation

7.9.3.1 MRI in Rheumatoid Conditions of the Knee

MRI is able to give precise morphological information about the synovial, cartilage, and bone-marrow components and the effusions or pannus tissue in rheumatoid knee joint diseases. MR signs synovitis are:

1. Increase in joint fluid.
2. Thickening of the synovium.
3. Synovial enhancement following intravenous contrast medium.
4. Correlation of the rate of contrast medium enhancement with the degree of inflammation.
5. Rapid transfer of synovial contrast medium into joint fluid (10 min).

As synovitis becomes invasive, destructive pannus may be formed (Fig. 7.14). The synovium itself may be thickened and lobulated, with areas of intermediate or low signal reflecting mixed active or fibrous pannus tissue. Extremely low signal may occur in a number of conditions, including 'burnt out' synovitis (fibrosis), bleeding disorders, synovial chondromatosis, and amyloidosis.

Nowadays, MRI is not used routinely in the assessment of rheumatoid diseases. However, there are important indications:

1. When there is monarthropathy and the diagnosis is in doubt.
2. To evaluate periarticular involvement, including tendinitis and tendon rupture.
3. To evaluate distant complications of rheumatoid diseases, such as craniocervical instability, spondylodiscitis, and endplate changes.

The disease occurs intermittently. It leads to cartilage destruction, starting at the surface and subchondral region. At the moment, MRI is not included in the Larsen grading of rheumatoid disease. But it is well accepted that MRI is the best imaging method for visualizing synovitis and active erosions. Differential diagnosis of rheumatoid arthritis and other diseases with synovial thickening includes:

1. Synovial tumors including pigmented villonodular synovitis (PVNS): in this condition, a combination of thick synovium with low signal iron deposits is found (this can also be seen in hemophilia).

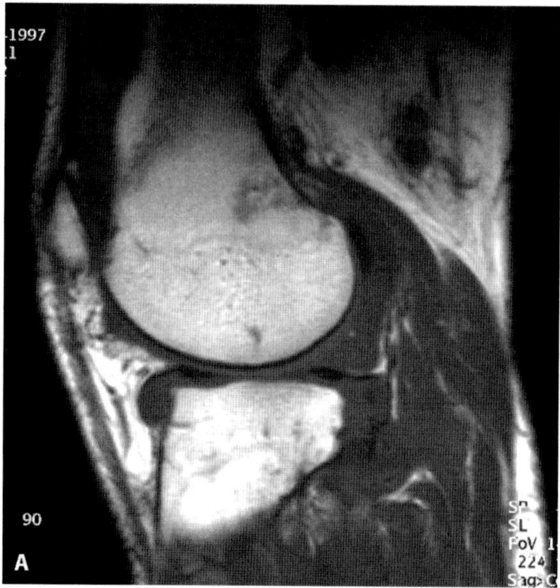

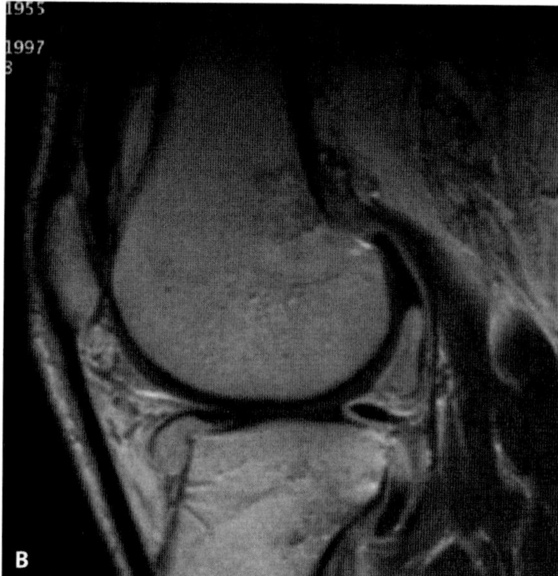

Fig. 7.14. A Sagittal T1-WI of a rheumatological arthritis demonstrates a pannus-like thickening of the synovial tissue. **B** Corresponding sagittal contrast-enhanced T1-W MR image shows a high signal increase of the synovitis

2. Synovial chondromatosis: thickened synovium with areas of low signal due to the calcified chondroid masses can be detected.
3. Lipoma arborescens: the fat content of the tumor is characteristic.

7.9.4 Blastoma

7.9.4.1 Diagnosis and Differential Diagnosis

In a limited number of tumors, MR characteristics allow a specific diagnosis: hemangioma, intraosseous lipoma (fatty tissue characteristica), fibromatosis, giant-cell tumor of the tendon sheath, and pigmented villonodular synovitis. In cases of aneurysmal bone cyst, solitary bone cyst, chondromatous tumors, and chondromas, MRI can contribute a tissue-specific diagnosis together with other imaging modalities.

7.9.4.1.1 Synovial Hemangioma

Synovial hemangioma is a soft-tissue mass within the joint that typically exhibits an intermediate signal intensity on T1-W images and a very high signal intensity on T2-W images (brighter than subcutaneous fat tissue). Moreover, it shows thin, often serpentive low-intensity septa within it. After i.v. injection of gadolinium, enhancement of the hemangioma may be seen.

7.9.4.1.2 Pigmented Villonodular Synovitis and Giant-Cell Tumor of Tendon Sheath

Pigmented villonodular synovitis (PVNS) is an uncommon benign and monoarticular condition. MR signs of PVNS are:

1. Joint fluid
2. Synovial mass
3. Low-signal intensity of the mass
4. Erosions

The low signal intensity at the synovial mass on all sequences is from repeated intraarticular bleeding (hemosiderin). The mass may be focal or generalized within the joint and often extends away from the joint. The giant-cell tumor of the tendon sheath shows the same typical MR imaging features, but outside of the joint.

7.9.4.1.3 Synovial Sarcoma

Only 10% of synovial sarcomas are actually in joints. The remainder arise in the periarticular tissues, such as tendon sheaths or bursae. Synovial sarcomas are prevalent in young adults (20–40 years) and men (3:2). It is highly malignant. The knee joint is the most frequently affected site. MR signs are:

1. Knee joint mass.
2. Two forms: localized sessile and diffuse infiltrative form.
3. Heterogenous, multilocular mass with internal septations.
4. Possible multiple fluid-fluid levels.
5. High signal on T2-W images.

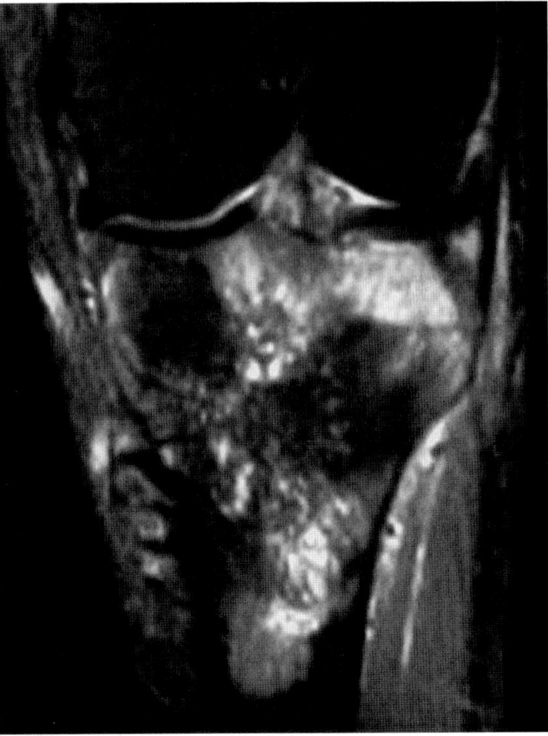

Fig. 7.15. Cor. STIR sequence of an osteosarcoma demonstrates the infiltration of the ACL. Such an infiltration can only be seen with MRI

Tumor-free margins are the goal of surgical intervention. In local tumor staging, MRI is superior to all other imaging modalities (Fig. 7.15) and identifies:

1. Bone marrow involvement (MR > CT)
2. Cortical bone involvement (MR = CT)
3. Muscular compartment involvement (MR > CT)
4. Neurovascular involvement (MR>angiography; MR > CT)
5. Joint involvement (MR tends to overstage), joint effusion is nonspecific

MR recurrence signs during follow-up after tumor surgery, chemotherapy, and/or radiation therapy (relative to a baseline study 3–6 months after surgery) include:

1. Growing mass
2. High signal T2-W
3. Gadolinium enhancement with a steep early phase

7.1 0 Ankle and Foot Joints

7.10.1 Trauma

7.10.1.2 Osteochondritis Dissecans

Osteochondritis dissecans (OCD) is a common disorder that may affect the talus, knee joint, and elbow joint. It is more common in adolescents and young adults and usually affects men. Most authors believe that repetitive chronic trauma is the usual cause of this disorder, with resulting necrosis. The cause of this injury is typically a shear or compressive force. When the injury occurs early in life, the cartilage is resilient in transmitting the vector to the underlying bone. Because the bone is less elastic than cartilage, the bone fractures without a chondral fracture. Healing of this lesion is dependent on both the osseous stability of the fragment and the degree to which the overlying cartilage remains intact. The imaging stage of the lesion is therefore the main determinant of the prognosis. Medial OCD is more common and also more commonly posterior than lateral. The stages of OCD are stable, partially loose, loose in situ, and intraarticular bodies. Loose fragments are surrounded by high signal interface on T2-W or STIR images. Any lesion with an underlying cyst is also invariably loose (Fig. 7.16). Incompletely circumferential

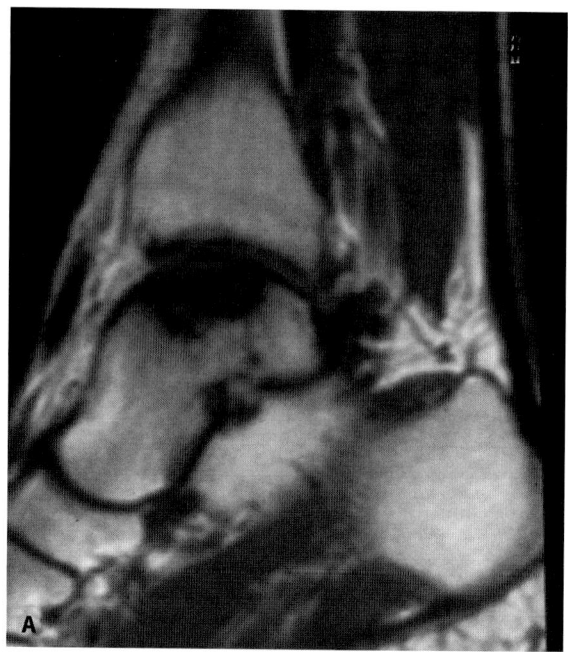

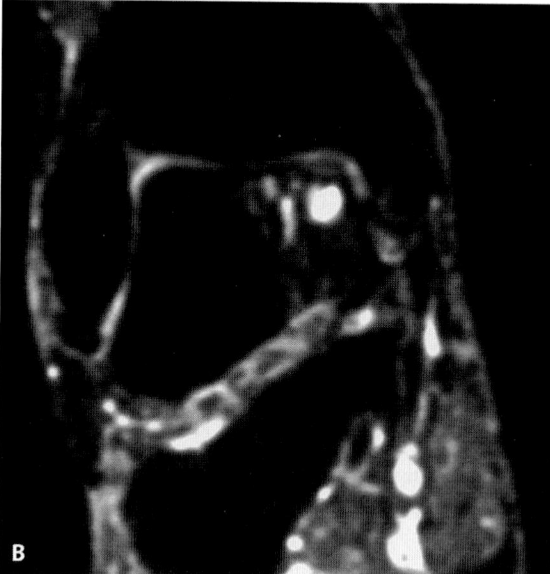

Fig. 7.16. A Sagittal T1-W SE. A lenticular-shaped subchondral lesion of the talus can be seen with marked hypointense demarcation to the normal bone marrow and flattening of the corresponding articular surface which represents a mechanical insufficiency of osteochondritis dissecans. **B** Osteochondritis dissecans of the medial border of the talus with cystic components on this coronal fat-suppressed STIR sequence indicating instability of the lesion

high signal is consistent with a partially loose fragment. Irregular peripheral high signal is usually seen in more stable fragments. Signal intensity at the fragment itself is of no clinical relevance. MRI can also assess the intactness of the overlying cartilage using high resolution and cartilage-sensitive techniques such as fat-suppressed 3D GRE or T2-W FSE with fat suppression. With i.v. injection of contrast media, the healing process can be monitored.

7.10.1.3 Ligament Injuries

Inversion injuries are the most common ankle injuries and among the most common musculoskeletal complaints presented to the emergency room. Because the medial (deltoid) ligament is so strong, avulsion fractures occur medially. The lateral ligamentous complex is where ankle ligament tears occur. The laterally supporting ligamentous structures can be divided into ankle and hindfoot ligaments. The lateral ankle collateral ligaments consist of the anterior talofibular ligament and the calcaneal fibular ligament. The posterior talofibular ligament is also part of the lateral collateral ligaments, although it is only rarely injured. Supporting the hind foot are fibers of the inferior extensor retinaculum, the cervical ligament, and the interosseous talocalcaneal ligament.

Acute ankle-ligament injuries typically affect the anterior talofibular ligament, but frequently will also affect the calcaneal fibular ligament. Acute injuries can be classified according to the grade of strain. Grade I is stretching and microscopic injury to the ligament, grade II is a partial tear, and grade III is a complete tear. However, 10%–20% of lateral ankle-ligament injuries lead to chronic symptoms and require surgical intervention. The anterior and posterior talofibular ligaments are best seen on axial MR images in 10°–20° dorsiflexion. The anterior ligament does not normally demonstrate internal signals and is usually half the thickness of the posterior ligament (Fig. 7.17a). The calcaneal-fibular ligament is best seen on semiaxial images with the foot in 45° plantar flexion. The tibiofibular membrane is infrequently torn, but may be avulsed off the tibia. Injury to the anterior talofibular ligament may be demonstrated by thickening, wavy appearance, hyperintensity, discontinuity, and joint fluid violation of its anterior border (Fig. 7.17b). With chronic instability, the ligament may scar and thicken, demonstrate an unusually low signal on T2-W images, or become wavy.

The sinus tarsi is a cone-shaped space between the talus and calcaneus; it has a lateral opening and consists of fatty tissue, ligaments, and vessels. The inferior extensor retinaculum inserts into the most lateral aspect of sinus tarsi, where it is best seen on lateral sag-

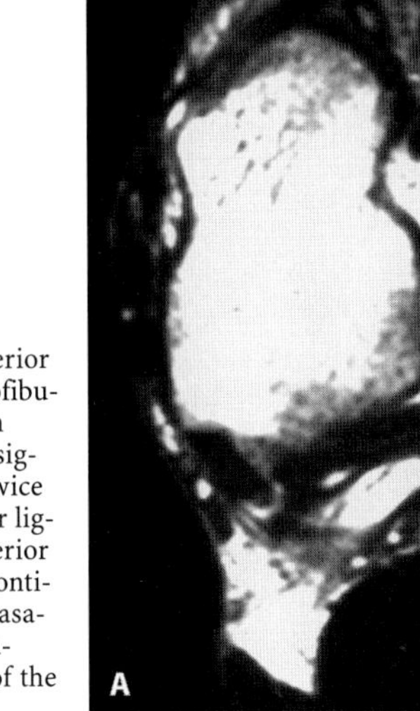

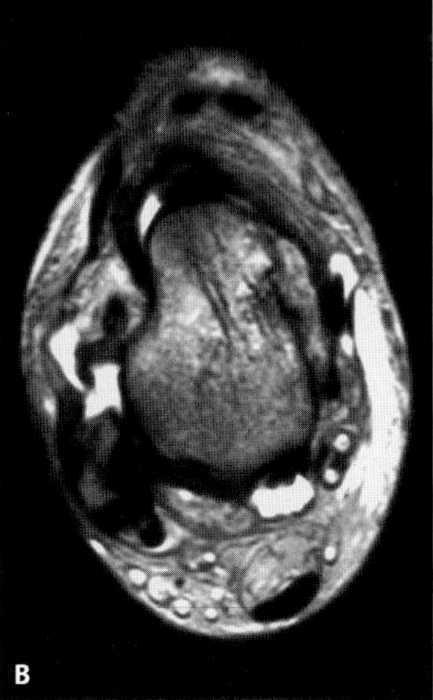

Fig. 7.17. A Normal appearance of anterior talofibular ligament and posterior talofibular ligament on axial T2-W TSE, which shows both ligaments, of marked low signal intensity and posterior ligament twice the diameter of the anterior talofibular ligament. **B** Complete rupture of the anterior talofibular ligament which shows discontinuity, increase in diameter, and extravasation of joint fluid anteriorly to the ligament, which represents an acute tear of the anterior talofibular ligament

ittal images. The cervical ligament lies in the anterior sinus tarsi. It may be seen on coronal or sagittal MR images. The interosseous talocalcaneal ligament is seen just posterior to the cervical ligament and is a thicker band within the sinus tarsi fat. Injuries to this ligament may therefore cause abnormally high signal intensity within the sinus tarsi on STIR sequence and replacement of fatty tissue on T1-W images. The MR differential diagnosis of this appearance is idiopathic or rheumatoid sinus tarsi syndrome, which may cause a similar appearance of edema. In sinus tarsi syndrome, however, the ligaments are intact.

7.10.1.4 Tendons

There are 13 tendons that cross the ankle. Of these, 12 have sheaths; the exception is the Achilles' tendon. In a large percentage of asymptomatic patients, small amounts of fluid are observed in most of these sheaths. The extensor tendons and the distal posteroir tibial tendon are the exceptions, in that normal patients rarely have fluid in these areas. Fluid seen in these locations is always abnormal.

The Achilles' tendon is the largest and strongest tendon in the body. All normal tendons are strong, and if a stress is applied, they rarely tear. Therefore, for a tendon to tear, regardless of the force, it must be degenerated. Similar to the supraspinatus tendon, the Achilles' tendon has a watershed area 2–4 cm above the insertion; this leads to degeneration and is where most Achilles disorders occur. The first stage of injury is tendinitis, which represents degeneration. Without treatment and continued activity, these patients may develop chronic tendinitis, hypertrophy, and scarring. Finally, partial tears or complete tears may occur.

The normal tendon has no internal signal on any sequence (Fig. 7.18). The tendon with tendinitis may or may not develop an internal signal. When present, it is most likely to be seen on T1-W and STIR images. Differentiation between an abnormal signal caused by tendinitis versus that caused by a partial tear is often difficult unless a hyperintense or fluid-like signal can be seen on T2-W sequences and appears linearly on longitudinal images (Fig. 7.19). On axial MR imaging, the normal Achilles' tendon is typically lenticular (kidney)-shaped. In chronic Achilles' tendinitis, the tendon enlarges, with enlargement on sagittal images seen at up to 2–4 cm above the insertion. On cross-sectional images, the tendon loses its normal lenticular shape and becomes ovoid and, finally, rounded. In a degenerated tendon, complete Achilles' tears usually occur 2–4 cm from the insertion. Frequently, a tendon gap is visible. This gap will be minimized or absent with plantar flexion.

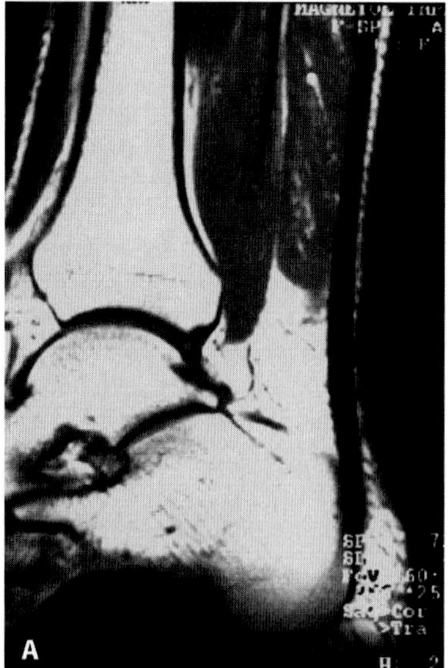

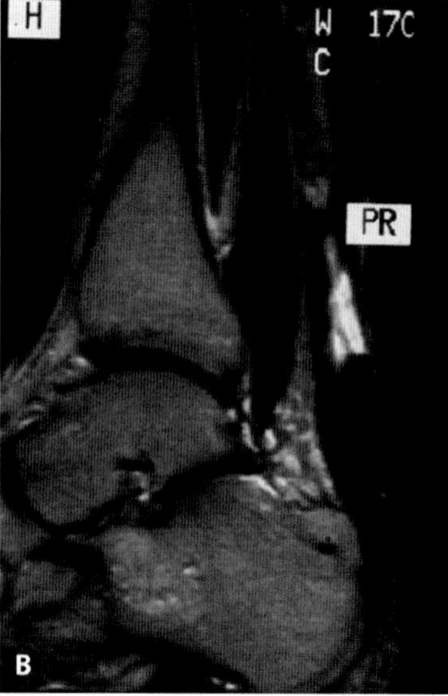

Fig. 7.18. A Normal appearance of Achilles' tendon on sagittal T1-W SE which shows a band without internal signal and of the same diameter over its entire course. **B** In complete tear of the Achilles' tendon on T2-W TSE in sagittal plane shows a fluid-like signal alteration about 4 cm proximal to the insertion with marked thickening of the tendon in this area

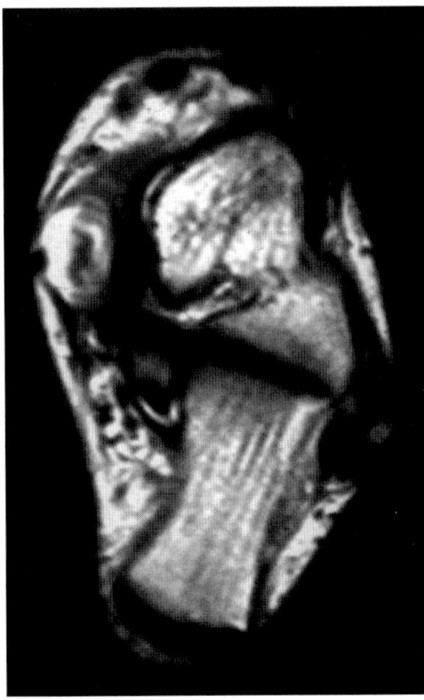

Fig. 7.19. Complete tear of the posterior tibialis tendon on axial T2-W TSE, which shows a large amount of fluid and hematoma within the tendon sheath and some of hypointense residual fibers centrally

7.10.1.4.1
Posterior Tibial Muscle Tendon

The posterior tibial muscle tendon (PTT) is the most anterior of the medial ankle tendons, passing just behind the medial malleolus. This tendon is enclosed in a synovial sheath. The PTT inverts the hindfoot, maintains the plantar arc and everts in plantar flexion. PTT disorders are more common in women, usually middle-aged to elderly. Because of a zone of relative hypovascularity as well as friction against the medial malleolus, the typical location for injury is at or just below the medial malleolus. Type I tears are partially ruptured, with longitudinal split and tendon hypertrophy. Type II tears are partial tears, with tendon attrition. Type III injuries are complete tears. The PTT typically is twice the diameter of the flexor digitorum longus tendon. When this ratio is disturbed, the tendon is also either atrophic from partial tears or hypertrophic from chronic injury and inflammation. When completely torn, a fluid-filled gap may be seen or the tendon may be retracted (Fig. 7.6). The presence of either a hypertrophied medial tubercle or accessory navicular is associated with PTT disorders.

7. 10.1.4.2
Peroneal Tendons

The peroneus longus (PL) and brevis (PB) act as pronators and evert the foot. PB and PL share a common synovial sheath up to the region of Chopart's joint. The PL tendon lies lateral and posterior to the PB tendon. Tenosynovitis may be seen in patients with osteoarthritis and osteophyte formation or as a result of calcaneal fractures. Internal signals, which are uncommon in these tendons, represent tendinitis or interstitial tears and are always abnormal. Subluxation or dislocation of the peroneal tendons may occur. On MR images, the tendon is seen lateral to the lateral aspect of the fibula. Subluxations and dislocations may demonstrate absent or torn peroneal retinacula and a hypoplastic, absent, or convex peroneal groove in the distal fibula. Ruptures of the peroneal tendons are rare, more often affecting the PB, and usually occur at the level of the calcaneal cuboid joint. Tendon split is a final entity affecting PB. These splits result from mechanical attrition within the fibular groove as a result of trauma.

7.10.2 Degeneration

Primary degenerative changes in the ankle joint are very uncommon. Secondary degenerative changes are in the majority of cases due to repetitive chronic trauma (see Sect. 7.9.1).

7.10.3 Inflammation

Primary inflammations of the ankle joint are rare. As in other joints, the basic signs are effusion, synovial thickening, and reactive edema in the neighboring bone marrow. All of these abnormalities are best visualized with fat-suppressed images (STIR and SPIR), followed by i.v. contrast medium administration.

Secondary inflammation of the ankle and foot joints may be due to soft-tissue cellulitis or osteomyelitis (e.g., diabetic foot). Systemic (metabolic) diseases (e.g., gout, Reiter's, rheumatoid) very often involve the ankle and foot joints. At the moment, there is no real MRI indication in these diseases.

7.10.4 Tumors

Primary neoplasms of the ankle and foot joints are rare. The most common are PVNS and synovial sarcoma. The typical features are described in Sect. 7.9.8.

Further Reading

Beltran I, Campanni DS, Knight C et al (1990) The diabetic foot: magnetic resonance imaging evaluation. Skeletal Radiology 19:37–41

Bigliani LU, Morisson DS (1986) The morphology of the acromion and its relationship to rotator cuff tears. Orthop Trans 10:228–231

Bohndorf K, Imhof H, Pope TL (2001) Musculoskeletal imaging. Thieme, Stuttgart

Bollow M, Loreck D, Braun J, Hamm B (1997) Die Sakroliitis: Das Schlüsselsymptom der Spondyloarthropathien. Röfo 166:95–100, 275–289

Bollow M, Braun J, Hamm B, Eggens U, Schilling A, König H, Wolf KJ (1995) Early sacroiliitis in patients with spondyloarthropathy: evaluation with dynamic gadolinium-enhanced MR-imaging. Radiology 194:529–536

Deutsch AL, Mink JH, Kerr R (1992) MRI of the foot and ankle. Raven, New York

De Smet AA, Fisher DR, Burnstein MI, Graf B, Lang RH (1990) Value of MR imaging in saging osteochondral lesions of the talus (osteochondritisdissecans). Am J Roentgenol 154:555–558

Erickson SJ, Cox ICH, Hyde JS, Carrera GF, Strandt JA, Estkowski LD (1991) Effect of tendon orientation on MR imaging signal intensity: a manifestation of the 'magic angle' phenomenon. Radiology 181:389–392

Fitzgerald SW (1994) Magnetic resonance imaging clinics of North America: the knee. Saunders, Philadelphia

Gilula AL, Yin Y (1996) Imaging of the wrist and hand. Saunders, Philadelphia, pp 441–479

Greenspan A, Remagen W (1998) Differential diagnosis of tumor-like lesions of bones and joints. Lippincott-Raven, Philadelphia

Gross MS, Nasser S, Finerman GAM (1994) Hip and pelvis. In: DeLee JC, Drez D (eds) Saunders, Philadelphia, pp 1063–1085

Kang HS, Kindynis P, Brahme SK (1991) Triangular fibrocartilage and intercarpal ligaments of the wrist: MR imaging – cadaveric study with gross pathologic and histologic correlation. Radiology 181:401–404

Kerr R (1997) MR imaging of sports injuries of the hip and pelvis. Semin Musculoskeletal Radiol 1:65–82

Lang P, Genant HK, Majumdar S (1994) Bone marrow disorders. In: Chan W, Lang PH, Genant HK (eds) MRI of the musculoskeletal system. Saunders, Philadelphia, pp 445–486

Marcus DS, Reider MA, Kellerhouse LF (1989) Achilles' tendon injuries: the role of MR imaging. J Comput Assist Tomogr 13:480–486

Mitchell DM, Kundel HL, Steinberg ME, Kressel HY, Alavi A, Axel L (1986) Avascular necrosis of the hip: comparison of MR, CT and Scintigraphy. Am J Roentgenol 147:67–71

Murphy BJ (1992) MR imaging of the elbow. Radiology 184:525–529

Neer CS (1983) Imingement lesions. Clin Orthop 173:70–77

Plenk H, Hofmann S, Eschberger J, Gstettner M, Kramer J, Schneider W, Engel A (1977) Histomorphology and bone morphometry of the bone marrow edema syndrome of the hip. Clin Orthop 334:73–84

Reiser MF, Bongartz GM, Erlemann R (1989) Gadolinium-DTPA in rheumatoid arthritis and related diseases: first results with dynamic magnetic resonance imaging. Skeletal Radiol 18:591–597

Reiser M, Heuck A (1997) Hüftgelenk und Becken. In: Vahlensieck M, Reiser M (eds) MRT des Bewegungsapparats. Thieme, Stuttgart, pp 143–168

Resnick D (1995) Diagnosis of bone and joint disorders, 3rd edn. Saunders, Philadelphia

Resnick D (1997) Internal derangements of joints: emphasis on MR Imaging. Saunders, Philadelphia

Resnick D, Kang HS (1997) Internal derangements of joints. WB Saunders, Philadelphia

Schneck CD, Mesgarzadeh M, Bonakdarpour A, Ross GJ (1992) MR imaging of the most common ankle ligaments, part II, ligaments injuries. Radiology 184:507–512

Steinbach LS, Tirman PFJ, Peterfy CG, Feller JF (1998) Shoulder magnetic resonance imaging. Lippincott-Raven, Philadelphia

Tyson LL, Crues JV (1993) Pathogenesis of rotator cuff disorders. Magnetic resonance imaging characteristics MRI. Clin North Am 1:37–46

Vahlensieck M (1997) Schulter. In: Vahlensieck M, Reiser M (eds) MRT des Bewegungsapparates. Thieme, Stuttgart, pp 53–82

Vahlensieck M, Reiser M (1997) MRT des Bewegungsapparates. Thieme, Stuttgart

Van de Berg B, Malghem JJ, Labaisse MA (1993) MR imaging of avascular necrosis and transient marrow edema of the femoral head. Radiographics 13:501–520

Bone and Soft Tissues

8

J. van Gielen, A. Van der Stappen, A. M. De Schepper

Contents

8.1 Introduction and General Remarks

The introduction of magnetic resonance (MR) imaging has dramatically changed imaging of the musculoskeletal system. The clinical relevance of this new imaging technique equals the importance of the introduction of X-rays to examine the skeleton, which occurred more than one hundred years ago.

The excellent spatial and contrast resolution of MRI allows recognition of abnormalities in bone and joints, hyaline and fibrous cartilage, tendons, ligaments (Fig. 8.1), muscles, and vessels. MRI improves the characterization of soft-tissue abnormalities and, due to its multiplanar imaging capacity, has the greatest potential for staging inflammatory and neoplastic processes. Finally, this method offers unique possibilities for studying normal and replaced bone marrow.

MRI provides the evaluation of an entire anatomical area – bone structures included – but is only good for the study of a limited part of the skeleton. This is in contrast to scintigraphy, with which the whole skeleton can be evaluated at once. Otherwise, MRI helps to elucidate the true nature of highly nonspecific hot spots on scintigraphy.

The diagnostic duo of conventional radiology and MRI guarantees the best accuracy in bone studies, while ultrasonography and MRI are complementary in soft-tissue examination. Although the high-field strength setting of the MR equipment results in a better signal-to-noise ratio, low-field MRI of the musculoskeletal system also yields useful diagnostic information.

The musculoskeletal system, especially in the extremities, is not influenced by motion, and as a consequence, motion artifacts are rare. Infolding artifacts can be avoided by selecting an appropriate imaging matrix, saturating anatomical areas outside the region of interest, and off-center imaging. Artifacts due to dis-

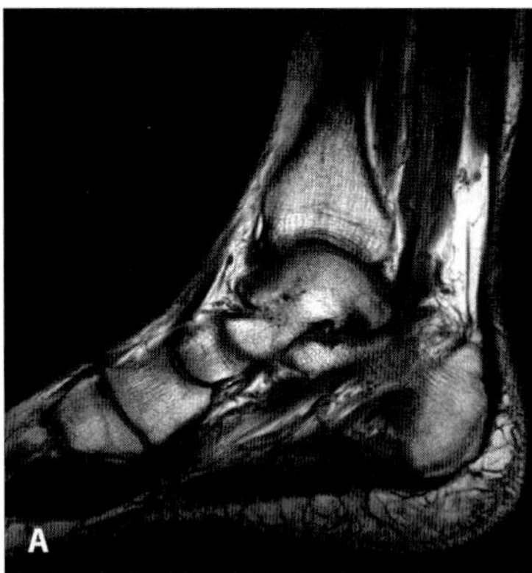

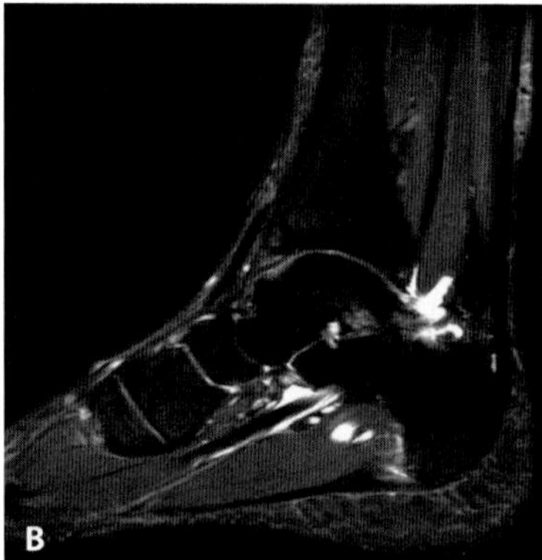

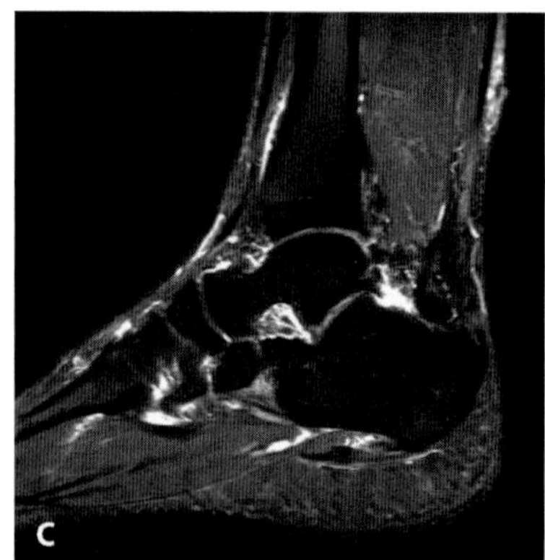

Fig. 8.1 A–C. Late findings after inversion trauma in a 52-year-old man with chronic, diffuse ankle pain: sinus tarsus syndrome with tear of the interosseous and cervical ligament, posterior impingement with edema of the posterior process of the talar bone and osteochondral lesion stage III at the posterior subtalar joint. Concomitant effusion in the ankle joint and posterior subtalar joint with distention into the tendon sheath of the flexor hallucis longus tendon. Sagittal spin-echo (SE) T1-weighted image (WI) shows an undetached, undisplaced, hypointense fragment in the posteroinferior part of the talus adjacent to the posterior subtalar joint (**A**). Sagittal turbo SE (TSE) T2-WI with fat suppression demonstrates hyperintense bone edema in the subtalar region due to an osteochondral fracture stage III. Concomitant effusion in the ankle joint and posterior subtalar joint with extension towards the tendon sheath of the flexor hallucis longus tendon. Hyperintense posterior talar process. There is also an enthesophyte at the calcaneum with concomitant fasciitis plantaris (**B**). A more lateral sagittal TSE T2-WI with fat suppression shows effusion in the sinus tarsi without delineation of the interosseous and cervical ligament in a sinus tarsi syndrome (**C**)

tortions of the local magnetic fields are attributable to ferromagnetic and, to a lesser degree, nonferromagnetic orthopedic devices. The use of surface coils will improve the signal-to-noise ratio; indeed, smaller slice thickness and larger matrices are essential for soft-tissue imaging. The choice of small 'field-of-view' without changing the matrix size will increase the spatial resolution. Sometimes, imaging of the contralateral side is necessary, requiring a larger field-of-view and the use of a body coil. Imaging in two orthogonal planes is recommended, but the choice of imaging plane, slice thickness, and slice spacing are related to the anatomical region and the pathology that is being sought. The choice of pulse sequences in musculoskeletal MRI

Table 8.1. Pulse recommendations for soft-tissue and bone scanning

Location	Sequence	WI	No. of slices	TR	TE	Flip angle (°)	Slice interval (mm)	Slice thickness (mm)	Matrix	FOV	Rectangular FOV	No. of acq.	Acq. time (min:s)	Fat saturation
Knee	TSE	PD	19	3000	21		10	4	512	180	80%	1	3:29	No
Knee	SE	T1	19	500	14		10	3	512	180	75%	2	3:16	No
Knee	SE	T1												Yes
Knee	TSE	PD	19	3000	30		10	4	512	180	100%	2	4:11	Yes
Knee	Dess 3D		1/28	20	5.7	25°	20		256	150	100%	1	3:33	Yes
Hip	TSE	PD	19	3000	36		25	4	512	350	100%	1	3:47	No
Hip	TSE	PD	19	3270	37		10	3	256	250	100%	1	2:19	Yes
Hip	SE	T1	19	938	13		10	3	512	350	100%	2	3:16	No
Spine	GE	Out of phase	16	500	14.3		20	4	512	380	100%	1	5:09	No

WI weighting of images, *Acq.* acquisition(s)

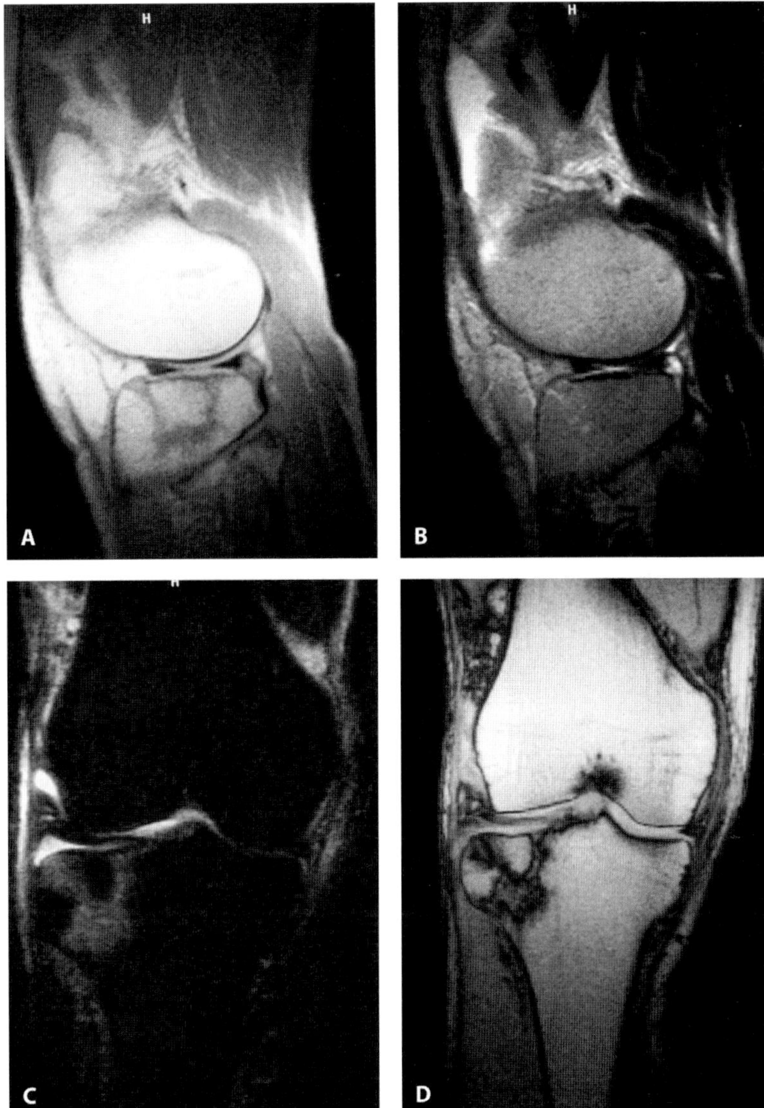

Fig. 8.2A–D. Impaction fracture of the lateral tibial plateau in a 42-year-old man after a soccer trauma. Sagittal SE T1-WI shows a square of decreased signal intensity (SI) in the tibial epiphysis (**A**). Conventional radiographic findings were normal. Sagittal fast SE (FSE) T2-WI demonstrates a faint hypointense line in the lateral tibial plateau without alteration of the tibial cortex. No apparent bone edema (**B**). Coronal STIR image demonstrates the surrounding bone edema well, but the fracture lines are not accurately shown (**C**). On coronal GRE, out-of-phase image, the impaction fracture is seen as a very sharp hypointense line with mild displacement of the fracture components which is not obvious on other imaging sequences. This sequence, however, underestimates the bone edema (**D**)

depends on the suspected disease and the MR system available (Fig. 8.2) (Table 8.1). The most frequently used pulse sequences and their respective advantages and disadvantages are listed in Table 8.2.

Because of the multidirectional capacity of the method and the lack of ionizing radiation, computed tomography (CT) guidance of bone biopsies will probably be replaced by MR guidance. Moreover, more open gantries will provide easier patient access. The use of gadolinium (Gd) contrast material aids in quantifying extracellular spaces in inflammatory and neoplastic diseases (neovascularization) and in demonstrating the presence of intralesional necrosis (which is a major parameter of malignancy).

Because separate chapters will deal with MR imaging of the joints and spine, topics to be highlighted in this chapter are: (1) normal and pathological bone marrow, (2) disorders of tendons, (3) disorders of muscles, (4) tumors of bone, and (5) tumors of soft tissues. Infectious lesions (abscesses, cellulitis, fasciitis, poly-

Table 8.2. Frequently used pulse sequences and their respective advantages and disadvantages

Pulse sequencea	Advantages	Disadvantages
SE T1-WI	Best anatomic detail Superior contrast between pathology and fat Detection of methemoglobin	No differentiation between muscles and non-fatty structures
SE T1-WI after Gd injection	Detection of vascularization Detection of necrosis	
Subtraction images	Detection of subtle areas of Gd-contrast enhancement	
FS SE T1-WI	Better demonstration of Gd-contrast enhancement Differentiation of fat and methemoglobin	
SE T2-WI	Detection of fluid	Long acquisition time
Turbo (fast) SE T2-WI	Superior contrast between pathology and fat/muscle Detection of fluid	Fat remains bright
FS TSE T2-WI	Excellent detection of fluid Best fat suppression	Necessitates high field equipment
FS TSE Intermediate WI	Good detection of fluid with preservation of anatomical detail Good differentiation between hyaline cartilage and joint effusion	
STIR TURBO STIR	Best detection of fluid Excellent fat suppression T1- and T2-weighting	Must not be used in combination with Gd injection Limited slice number
GRE T2* WI (low grade flip angle)	Short acquisition time allows dynamic Gd-studies	Susceptibility artifacts Limited soft-tissue contrast (not commonly used)
GE out-of-phase	SI is the result of the difference between fat and water signal in each proton High sensitivity	Low specificity

[a] Echo planar imaging (EPI) is not discussed because this application in musculoskeletal imaging is rarely described

myositis, bursitis), inflammatory conditions (myopathies, bursitis), and granulomatous lesions (foreign bodies, granulomatous myopathies) will not be discussed in this chapter.

8.2 MR of Bone Marrow

8.2.1 Introduction

Conventional radiography, CT, and bone scintigraphy have a low sensitivity for the detection of bone-marrow disorders. In contrast, MRI provides information about bone and about soft tissues that either surround the bones or fill in their medullary cavity. As such, MRI is a highly sensitive method for imaging normal and abnormal bone and can thereby differentiate between fatty, cellular, fibrotic, and hemosiderotic marrow.

8.2.2 Imaging Technique

Spin-echo (SE) T1-weighted image (WI), short tau inversion recovery images (STIR or turbo STIR), fat-presaturated turbo SE (TSE) T2-WI, and chemical-shift imaging (in phase, out of phase) are used routinely in the axial skeleton, whereas SE T2-WI and gradient-echo (GE) T2*-WI are less suitable for marrow examination. A standard protocol includes a coronal T1-WI and a STIR (or fat-presaturated TSE T2-WI) of the pelvis.

8.2.3 Normal Bone-Marrow Imaging

Yellow marrow contains aliphatic protons in fat cells (80%), whereas red marrow contains an overwhelming amount (60%) of water protons in hematopoietic cells.

Because they have different physicochemical properties, MRI is able to demonstrate the proportion and distribution of yellow versus red marrow under normal and pathological conditions. Otherwise, mineralized substances of bone (trabecular and cortical) lack mobile protons and yield little or no detectable signal; nevertheless, they may cause susceptibility artifacts on GE images.

In an adult, red marrow is located between the bony trabeculae and predominates in the axial skeleton, ribs, and proximal metaphyses of long bones (femur and humerus). Through aging and under normal conditions, red marrow will progressively be replaced by yellow marrow in the peripheral bones and, to a lesser degree, in the axial skeleton. This phenomenon is called marrow conversion. This process proceeds centripetally, i.e., from the peripheral to the axial skeleton; centrifugally, i.e., from the mid-diaphyses to the epimetaphyses; and symmetrically.

In SE T1-WI, conversion from red to yellow marrow results in an increasing signal intensity (SI) – from SI of muscle in the newborn to SI of fat in the adult. SI changes from high to intermediate on SE T2-WI and from high to low (the fat signal is nulled) on FS TSE T2-WI or intermediary (TE30–40) WI or STIR images. Fatty marrow has a low SI on fat presaturated SE T2-WI and GE out-of-phase images. Gd enhancement of normal bone marrow is subtle and only visible on subtracted images or FS SE T1-WI. With aging, increasing signal is found on SE T1-WI in the long bones and vertebrae, reflecting both the reduction of cellular components and the loss of cortical and trabecular bone (replaced by fat).

Hematopoietic marrow hyperplasia is a paranormal presentation in healthy individuals and is characterized by patchy, low-SI marrow in adults. It is more frequently seen in pregnant women, obese persons, and heavy smokers. Isolated islands of cellular marrow may be present in the fatty marrow and vice versa. This pattern is observed in the menstruating age group and under physical stress, i.e., in marathon runners.

8.2.4 MR Imaging of Marrow Disorders

Vogler and Murphy discerned four patterns of bone-marrow alteration: (1) red-marrow reconversion is the reversal of red-marrow conversion and is due to an increased demand for hematopoiesis (in hemolysis), (2) marrow infiltration or replacement, in which normal marrow is replaced by tumoral or inflammatory cellular

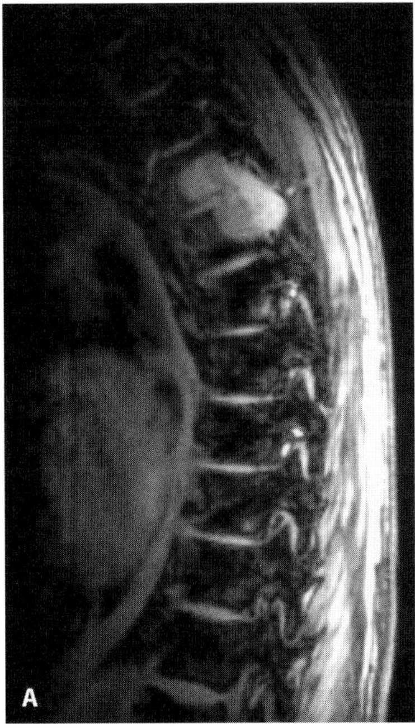

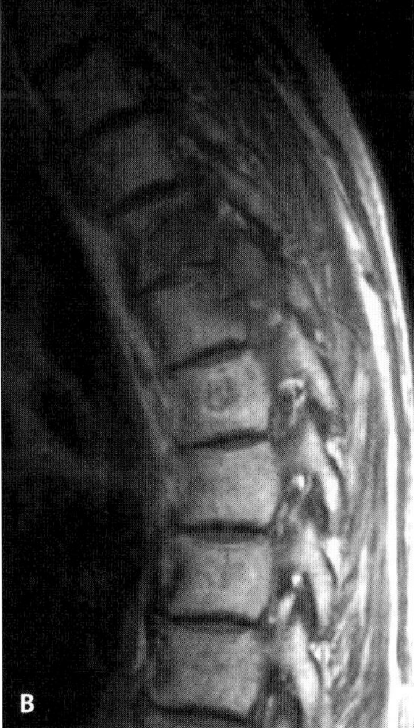

Fig. 8.3A,B. A 73-year-old woman with known multiple myeloma after chemotherapy. SE T1-WI (**B**) and GE T2-WI in opposed phase (**A**) reveal a well-defined lesion in two adjacent vertebral bodies (T4–5) with destruction of the dorsal wall and protrusion into the neural canal. The lesion has a high SI on T2-WI and a low SI on T1-WI

infiltrates, (3) myeloid depletion, which is characterized by a decrease in hematopoietic cells (aplastic anemia) and an increase in fat content; these conditions include metastatic cancer and leukemia, infection, damage by chemical agents and ionizing radiation, and (4) marrow edema, which is due to an increased amount of interstitial water.

Vande Berg proposed a more logical approach to the understanding of MR imaging of bone marrow changes that is based on SI changes on T1-WI.

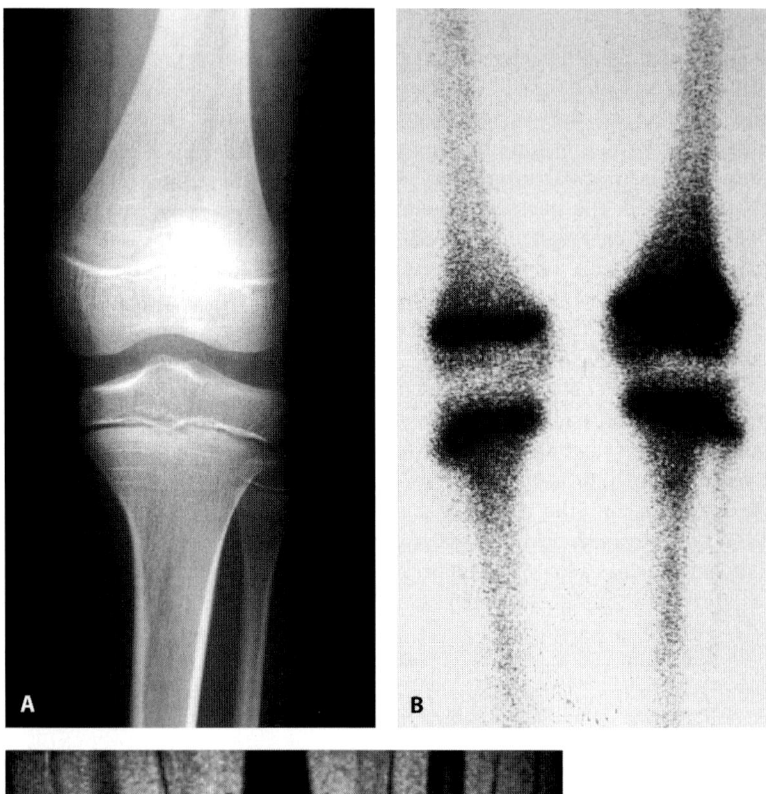

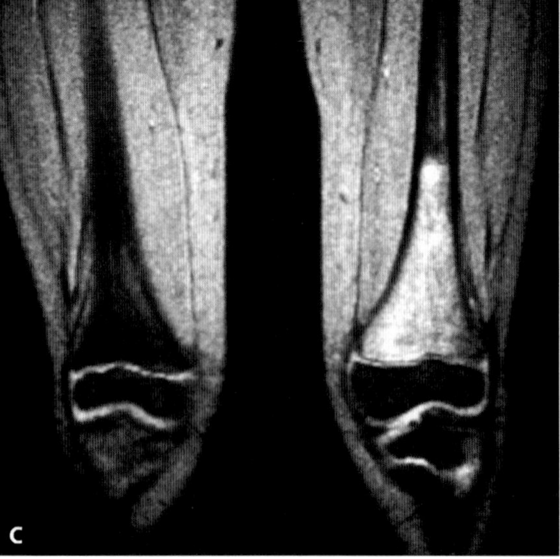

Fig. 8.4A–C. Thirteen-year-old boy presenting with fever, increased inflammatory parameters, and knee pain. Normal findings on plain film of the left knee (**A**). Hyperfixation at the distal metaphysis of the left femur on bone scintigraphy (**B**). Fat-suppressed T2-WI shows a well-demarcated area of high SI at the distal metadiaphysis of the left femur, without involvement of the distal epiphysis (**C**)

1. Red marrow depletion (increased SI on T1-WI). An increase in fat content can be seen as a consequence of radiation therapy, in aplastic anemia, in vertebral hemangiomas, and adjacent to degenerative bone changes.
2. Marrow infiltration (subtle or moderate decrease in SI on T1-WI and inhomogeneity of SI). This condition may be seen in marrow edema, transient osteoporosis, avascular necrosis, and reflex sympathetic dystrophy, and also in response to anemia, cyanotic heart disease, chronic infection, neoplastic infiltration, and storage disorders.
3. Marrow replacement (marked decrease in SI on T1-WI). This condition is mostly seen in primary marrow changes, such as neoplasms and infections (Fig. 8.3).
4. Marrow signal void (dramatic decrease in SI on T1-WI). This condition is seen in compact bone islands and marrow hemosiderosis.

On T2-WI, the SI depends on the type of tissue that replaces fat. Fibrosis and osteoblastic metastases have low SI, cellular infiltration produces intermediate or high SI, and hemorrhagic material generates high SI on both SE sequences. Although MRI is a very sensitive method for detecting marrow disorders, it has a rather low specificity because there is a substantial overlap between various conditions. Therefore, factors such as clinical history, location of the abnormality, lesion multiplicity, and morphological features must be considered when marrow abnormality is assessed.

MRI can provide additional information in scaphoid fracture healing, it can confirm bony union in a high proportion of patients deemed clinically nonunited.

8.2.5 Osteomyelitis

In osteomyelitis, inflammatory cells replace bone marrow, and cellular material and fluid produce decreased SI on T1-WI and increased SI on T2-WI and STIR-images (Fig. 8.4). In cases of osteomyelitis, parosseal edema is best demonstrated on STIR images. Enhancement of a thick, ill-defined abscess rim is best appreciated on T1-WI, following injection of Gd contrast.

In the case of Brodie's abscess, chronic recurrent multifocal osteomyelitis (CRMO), or SAPHO (synovitis, acne, pustulosis, hyperostosis, osteitis), a sterile form of osteitis associated with pustulosis plantopalmaris and enthesitis and posttraumatic or exogenous osteomyelitis, MRI will be of additional value in demonstrating the presence or absence of marrow and soft-tissue involvement. Especially with children, MRI makes a significant additional contribution in the evaluation of the extent of epiphyseal involvement. As a consequence, plain SE T1-WI, FS SE T2-WI, and STIR images are the most suitable pulse sequences, whereas Gd contrast application with subtraction of pre- and postcontrast SE T1-WI or in combination with fat-presaturated SE T1-WI is mandatory to differentiate abscesses from edema and to demonstrate intralesional necrosis.

MRI is also valuable in differentiating between osteomyelitis and neuropathic bone pathology of the foot (Charcot), two conditions which are hardly differentiated on conventional radiography, not even on bone scintigraphy in combination with nanocolloid scan. In neuropathic foot disorders, there is an absence of extraosseous edema (which is often present in acute osteomyelitis).

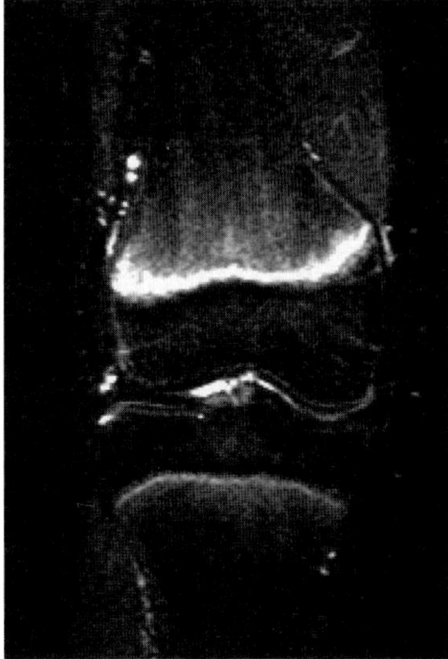

Fig. 8.5. Pain at rest and night in the right knee after trauma in a 15-year-old boy. Coronal STIR image shows an increased SI over the growth plate with widening of the physis in case of a Salter Harris type I lesion. Also increased SI in the adjacent metaphyseal bone due to bone edema

8.2.6 Bone-Marrow Edema

Bone-marrow edema is characterized by increased fluid in the extravascular, interstitial compartment of the bone marrow. Increased capillary permeability is seen under variable conditions, such as inflammation, overuse, trauma (Figs. 8.5 and 8.6), ischemia, and also around tumoral processes. The pattern of bone contusion after trauma is like a footprint; by studying the distribution of bone marrow edema on MR images, one can frequently determine the type of injury that occurred. Armed with the knowledge of the mechanism of injury, one can search more diligently for the commonly associated but sometimes less conspicuous MR imaging signs of soft-tissue injuries.

8.2.7 Transient Marrow Edema or Transient Osteoporosis

This disorder occurs mostly at the femoral neck, head, and intertrochanteric region, preferentially in young and middle-aged men and pregnant women (Fig. 8.7), and in the absence of risk factors for osteonecrosis (steroid abuse, chronic alcohol abuse). Conventional radiography shows profound osteopenia 3–6 weeks after the onset of clinical symptoms. Laboratory findings are normal. On MRI, there are signs of diffuse bone-marrow edema with decreased SI on T1-WI and increased SI on (FS) T2-WI or STIR images. A subtle accompanying joint effusion may be seen. The disease is self-limiting, and clinical improvement occurs within 2–6 months. MRI will show complete resolution at that time. Possible causes of transient osteoporosis include

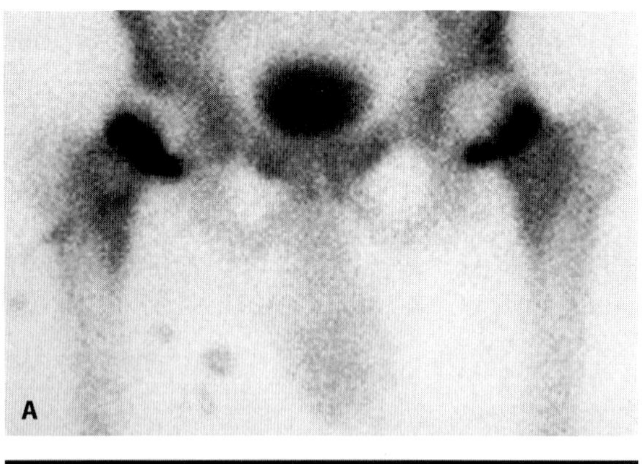

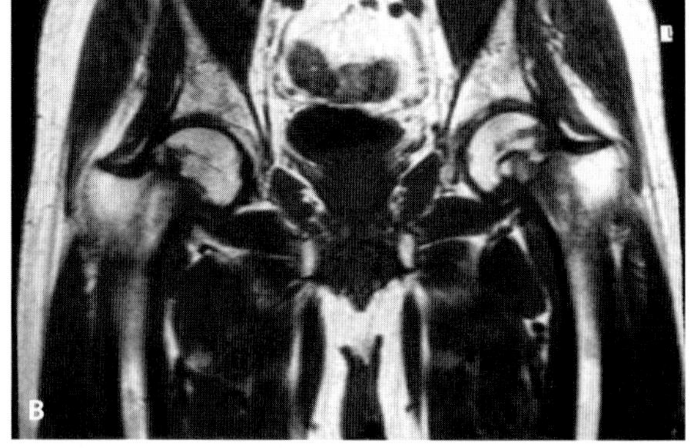

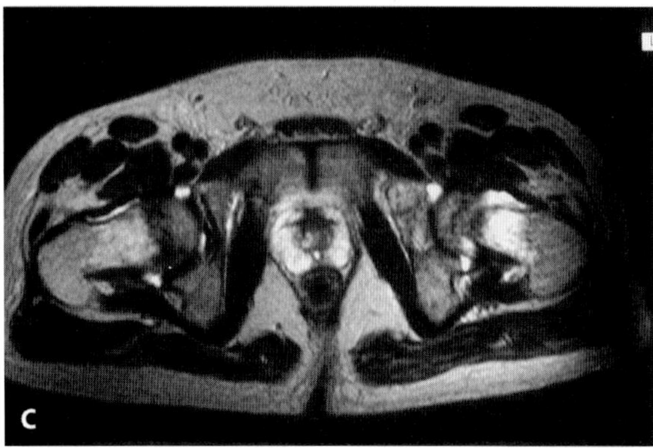

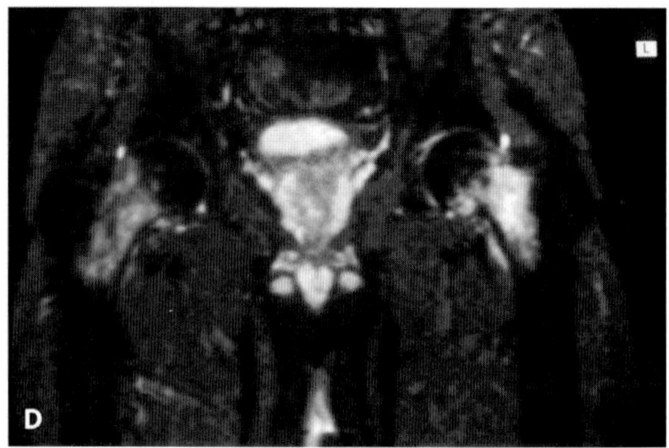

Fig. 8.6A–D. Bilateral femoral stress fracture in a 54-year-old man with 3 months of chronic hip pain after occult trauma. Bone scintigraphy shows bilateral increased uptake at the femoral neck (**A**). Coronal SE T1-WI shows a subcapital band of hypo-intensity with decreased SI of the surrounding bone marrow (**B**). Axial FSE T2-WI demonstrates massive edema at the level of both femoral necks (**C**). Coronal STIR-image confirms the impacted fracture lines with the diffuse surrounding edema (**D**)

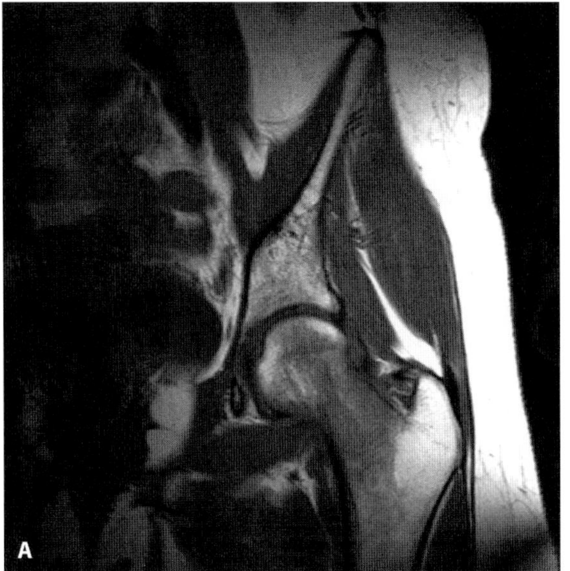

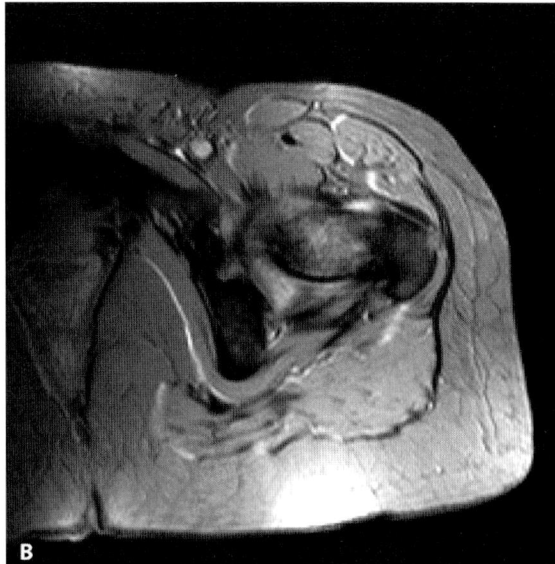

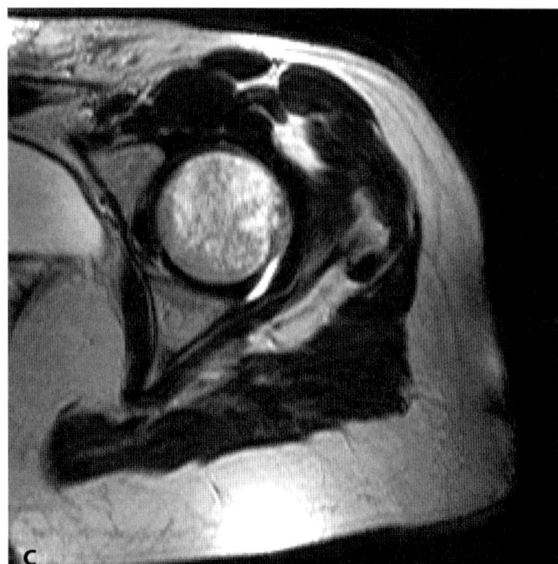

Fig. 8.7A–C. Postpartum MRI in a 29-year-old woman with right hip pain since delivery. Coronal SE T1-WI demonstrates decreased SI in the subchondral area and femoral neck without a demarcation line. Intact subchondral bone layer (**A**). Axial GE T2*-WI with fat suppression gives a better illustration of the bone marrow edema as a high SI region (**B**) compared with axial TSE T2-WI (**C**). This case is illustrative for a transient osteoporosis (bone marrow edema)

trauma, synovitis, reflex sympathetic dystrophy, and transient ischemia or early reversible osteonecrosis. Subchondral fractures as a consequence of the osteoporotic nature of transient osteoporosis of the hip were recently described.

In Table 8.3, marrow pathology is listed according to SI on T1-WI and T2-WI.

8.3 Diseases of the Musculotendinous Unit

The region of lowest resistance at the musculotendinous unit (MTU) is age and activity dependent. In children, the region of lowest resistance in acute trauma and chronic overuse is found at the apophyseal growth

Table 8.3. Marrow pathology according to signal intensities on T1- and T2-weighted images

T1WI	STIR/FS T2-WI	Bone-marrow disorder
Very low SI	Low SI	Hemosiderosis (iron storage)
Low SI	High SI	Bone-marrow edema (trauma, infection) Acute leukemia (homogeneous, diffuse, symmetric)
Low SI	Variable SI	Myeloma (diffuse or patchy) Metastases
Low SI	Intermediate SI	Marrow reconversion (patchy) Sickle cell anemia (+ marrow infarction) Polycythemia vera
Low SI	Low SI	Gaucher's disease (patchy, coarse, diffuse) (+ marrow infarction) Sclerotic metastasis (nodular) Myelofibrosis
Intermediate SI	High SI	Chronic leukemia Lymphoma (nodular or diffuse)
High SI	Intermediate SI	Irradiation (regional) Aplastic anemia (diffuse) Hemangioma (local) Denegerative bone changes (local)

plate. In adults, the region of lowest resistance in acute trauma is found at the musculotendinous junction, in chronic overuse syndrome, the worst vascularised mid-tendinous region is at risk.

8.3.1 Lesions of the Tendons and Tendo-osseous Junctions

Because of their high collagen content, normal tendons demonstrate low SI on all MR pulse sequences. MRI of tendons and tendo-osseous junctions is performed in at least two orthogonal planes. Routinely used pulse sequences are SE T1-WI and FS T2-WI or STIR and GRE T2* images (low-grade flip-angle; see also imaging protocol for muscular diseases).

Tenovaginitis and paratenonitis are easily visualized on axial and longitudinal FS T2-WI. Tenovaginitis is an associated finding in impingement syndromes and stenosing tenovaginitis; it is found in De Quervain stenosing tenovaginitis of the wrist, flexor hallucis longus tenovaginitis in posterior ankle impingement syndrome, and iliotibial band friction syndrome.

Tendon derangement may be a consequence of acute injury (partial or complete tear) or the result of recurrent mechanical attrition or overuse syndromes. Infection of the Achilles tendon is a known complication of diabetic foot pathology. Amyloid deposition may present with tendon thickening with low SI on all pulse sequences; it is found in long-term dialysis patients. Partial or complete tendon rupture is frequently seen after repetitive injections of corticosteroids for tendinosis or bursitis. Pathological findings on MRI consist of morphological changes and intratendinous SI changes – mainly due to increased water content in the tendons and tendon sheaths. Bone marrow edema due to overlying tendon friction or hyperemia of the overlying tendon sheath is described in dysfunction of tendons around the ankle. Subtendinous bone marrow edema has a high association with location of symptoms and overlying tendon abnormality; it may be a reliable indicator of true disease.

Morphological changes of tendon disease are tendon (sub)luxation; longitudinal tendon split, resulting in a multipartite appearance of the tendon on axial images; increased diameter and ill-defined or feathery borders on cross-section in cases of partial rupture; and tendon discontinuity with fluid-filled gap in cases of complete rupture (Fig. 8.8). SI changes are high SI fluid in the tendon sheath (tenosynovitis or tenovaginitis), high SI fluid around tendons without synovial sheath (paratenonitis), increased linear or heterogeneous intrasubstance signals, geographical intratendinous areas of intermediate SI on T1-WI and high SI on T2- or T2* images, and areas of hyperintensity at the osteotendinous junction. SI changes in complete rupture are due mainly to intratendinous fluid collections and hematoma.

Acute tendon avulsions are rare and are usually seen in the lower extremities. Acute lesions of the MTU are typical in muscles that work across two joints, a flexion in one and extension in the other joint confuses the muscle and predisposes it to tearing. They occur at the anterior inferior iliac spine (rectus femoris muscle), the anterior superior iliac spine (sartorius muscle and fascia lata), the ischial tuberosity (hamstrings), and the trochanter major (gluteus medius and obturator muscle). Luxation or subluxation of tendons is seen in acute injuries or as a result of chronic tendinosis. Common sites of luxation are the tendon of the long head of the biceps muscle and the peroneal tendons.

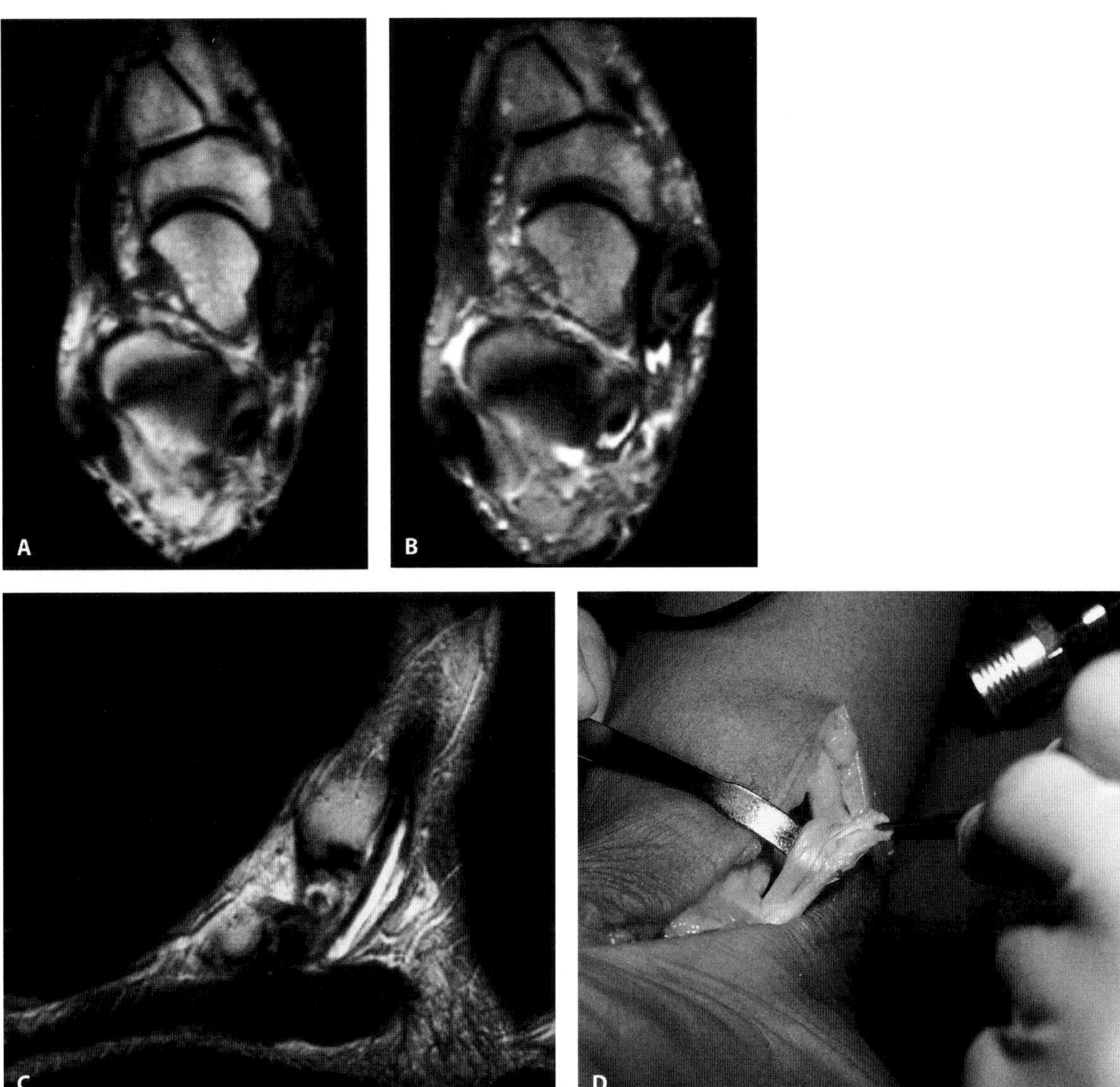

Fig. 8.8A–D. Posterior tibial tendon (PTT) tear in a 24-year-old patient with a symptomatic flat foot. Axial SE T1-WI at the level of the talar head shows ruptured distal tendon fibers with intratendinous increased SI (**A**). Axial FSE T2-WI depicts disruption of the normal tendon structure and intrasynovial effusion and presence of reparative tissue with increased intratendinous SI compared with the low SI of normal tendon (**B**). Sagittal FSE T2-WI illustrates an intact flexor digitorum tendon (FDT) adjacent to the empty synovial sheet of the retracted PTT (**C**). Peroperatively, the torn PTT is shown with an intact FDT (**D**)

All tendons may be affected by tendinosis at their tendo-osseous junction. More common sites of tendinosis are the gluteus medius and obturator tendon, adductor, rectus femoris, biceps femoris (Fig. 8.9), sartorius and fascia lata, patellar (jumper's knee), Achilles, and peroneal and posterior tibial tendons, extensor tendons of the forearm (tennis elbow), and rotator cuff with the long head of the biceps muscle. Tendinosis may be accompanied by chronic bursitis (tendinobursitis), frequently seen in the trochanteric region (three largest bursae in the human body) and in the iliotibial band friction syndrome (de novo bursitis). At the end stage of

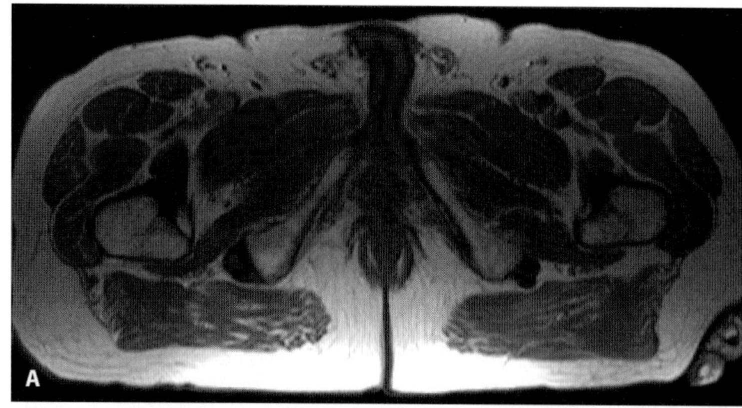

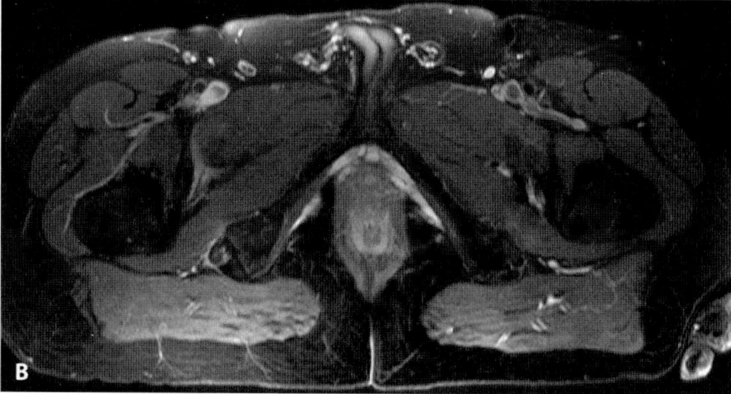

Fig. 8.9A,B. A 50-year-old patient with longstanding pain on the right tuber ischiadicum during forward bending with extended knee. Axial SE T1-WI demonstrates a slightly increased volume of the lateral part of the tendon insertion on the right tuber ischiadicum (**A**). Axial TSE T2-WI with fat suppression shows increased SI in the insertion region (**B**). Typical example of insertion tendinosis of the biceps femoris muscle on the right tuber ischiadicum

tendinosis fibrosis, mucoid degeneration and/or fibrovascular repair known as angiofibrous dysplasia (neovascularization) is found. Fibrosis is seen as areas of intermediate SI on all pulse sequences, and fibrovascular repair is seen as areas of intermediate SI on T1-WI and T2-WI and high SI on GE T2* images. Neovascularization is easily seen on Doppler sonographic examination, which is an advantage of sonography over MRI. Insertion tendinosis (tendo-osseous junction) on the other hand is better detected with MRI than with sonography.

False-positive results consisting of intrasubstantial hyperintensity can be a consequence of the so-called 'magic angle phenomenon' that results from changes in the direction of the collagen fibers and the orientation of the peroneal, tibial, and supraspinatus tendons. The 'magic angle phenomenon' may cause a false-positive intratendinous SI increase on pulse sequences with short TE (T1-WI and Pd-WI) which disappears on pulse sequences with long TE (T2-WI).

Morphological changes and changes in SI in different tendinous diseases are listed in Table 8.4.

8.3.2 Diseases of the Muscle and Musculotendinous Junction

Like tendon injuries, muscle injuries may be the result of a single acute traumatic event or of a more chronic, muscle-overuse syndrome occurring in both recreational and occupational activities, e.g., tennis leg. Increased intra- and extracellular water in muscle injuries correlates well with an increase in both T1- and T2-relaxation times.

Because muscles have a relatively short T2-relaxation time, even subtle changes in their composition will result in changes of SI on T2-WI. The STIR sequence reveals any prolongation of T1- and T2-relaxation times. With both sequences, muscle injuries appear

Table 8.4. Morphological and signal intensity changes in different tendinous diseases

Disease	Morphological changes	Changes in signal intensity
Early tendinosis	Increased diameter	Intermediate intrasubstance SI (T2-WI/STIR)
Early tendinosis with paratenonitis or tenovaginitis	Fluid accumulation	High SI (T2-WI/STIR) around the tendon or within the tendon sheath
Late tendinosis	Fibrosis/mucoid degeneration	Intermediate intrasubstance SI (T1-WI), intermediate intrasubstance SI (T2-WI)
	Fibrovascular repair	High SI (GE T2*)
	Decreased or increased diameter	Enhancing intrasubstance areas
Partial tear (incomplete rupture)	Increased or decreased diameter	Intermediate and heterogeneous intrasubstance SI (T1-WI)
	Ill-defined-feathery borders	Foci of high SI (T2-WI/STIR)
	Longitudinal splitting	
Acute complete rupture	Discontinuity	High SI (T2-WI/STIR) around the tendon or within the tendon sheath
	Retraction of ends	SI of hematoma within the tendon gap
Luxation/subluxation	Abnormal location	Normal

hyperintense. To overcome some drawbacks of the STIR sequence, a fast STIR technique was introduced. Comparable results are obtained with spectral fat presaturation T2-WI. Use of this sequence necessitates a higher field strength, whereas STIR images can be obtained with both high- and low-field equipment. GE sequences with a low flip-angle generate a T2* effect and may be useful in demonstrating susceptibility effects.

The response of muscle to denervation deserves some attention. The subacute stage of the denervation process reveals prolonged T1 and T2 values due to increased extracellular water with hyperintensity on T2-WI with or without fat suppression and STIR sequences (Fig. 8.10). In chronic denervation, muscles will atrophy with fatty infiltration (Fig. 8.11).

Proposed protocols for MRI of the muscular system include: (1) axial STIR sequence or fat-presaturated T2 or intermediate WI with 10-mm sections and a 2.5-mm interslice gap; this sectioning allows simultaneous visualization of the muscles; (2) coronal or sagittal STIR sequence (or fat-presaturated T2-WI); the alignment of the image is parallel to the long axis of the involved muscles; (3) axial or longitudinal SE T1-WI in case of acute or subacute hematoma. Surface coils are used for small sizes, providing excellent SNR, whereas body coils afford a large field-of-view, allowing comparative examination of the contralateral side.

MRI will give objective information about muscle imaging by demonstrating the integrity of strained muscles, the musculotendinous unit, the tendon and the tendo-osseous junction. As such, it allows for improved classification of the various types of muscle injuries. MRI will also aid in appropriate legal judgements and decisions about worker compensation.

8.3.2.1 Muscle Contusion

This disorder results in a combination of hemorrhage and edema and is due to a direct trauma. Hematoma pushing aside muscle fibers is frequently associated with muscle contusion and results in a volume increase of the muscle. MR image appearance is a direct reflection of superficial capillary rupture, interstitial hemorrhage, edema, and inflammatory reaction. SI of hematomas depends on the field strength used and on the age of the lesion itself. Variable signal intensities on different pulse sequences result from the variable influence of blood degradation products on relaxation times. Different SI of hematomas are listed in Table 8.5.

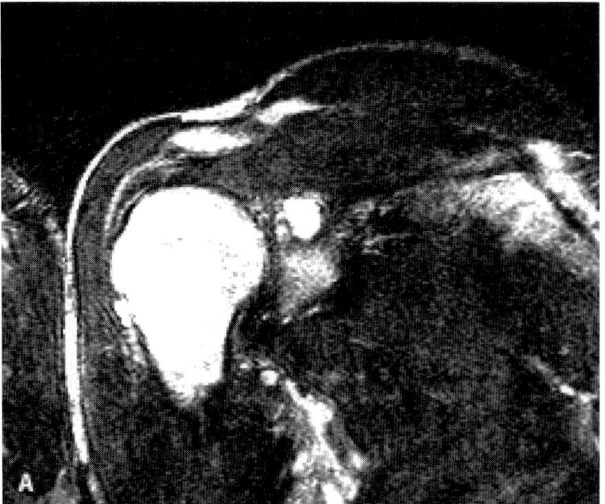

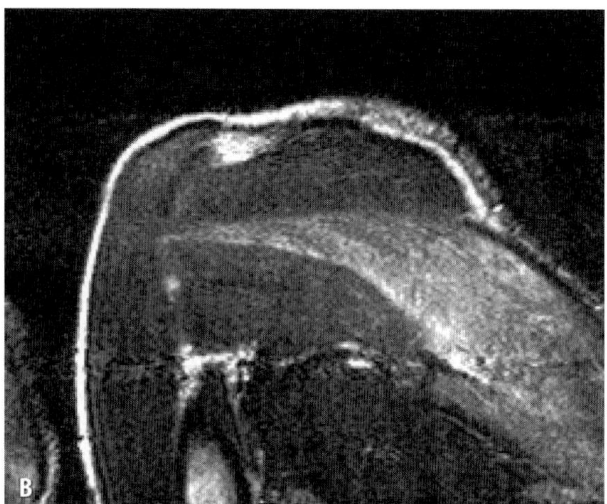

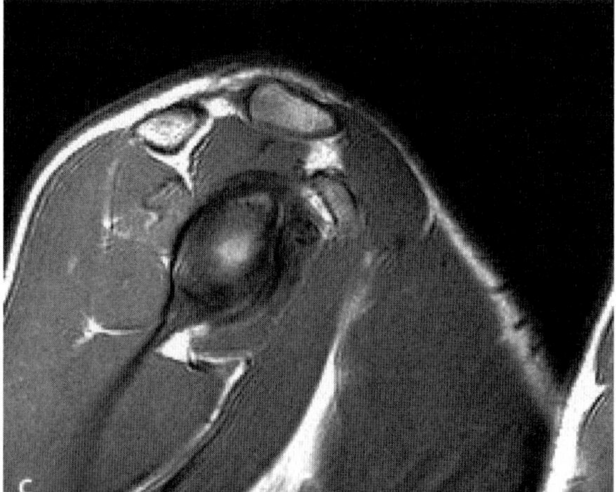

Fig. 8.10A–C. Increasing soreness and power loss in the right shoulder in a 28-year-old man. TSE T2-WI (**A**) and proton-density-WI (**B**) with fat suppression show an overall increase of signal in the infraspinatus muscle due to edema. No muscle atrophy is seen. SE T1-WI with fat suppression reveals an additional structure with intermediate SI in the supraglenoidal notch (**C**). This lesion has a high SI on T2-WI (**A**) with fat suppression. Acute denervation with diffuse muscle edema in the infraspinatus due to paralabral cyst with compression on the subscapular nerve

Table 8.5. Different SI of hematomas

	T1-WI	T2-WI (STIR)	Pathophysiology
Fresh hematoma (<24 h)	SI of muscle	Increased SI	Effect of oxyhemoglobin
Acute hematoma (1–7 days)	SI of muscle	Strongly decreased SI	Effect of desoxyhemoglobin
Subacute hematoma (1–4 weeks)	Increasing SI	Intermediate SI	Decreasing water content – increasing protein content – Effect of intracellular methemoglobin
Chronic hematoma (>4 weeks)	High SI	High SI Peripheral rim of low SI (hemosiderin)	Lysis of erythrocytes-effect of hemosiderin

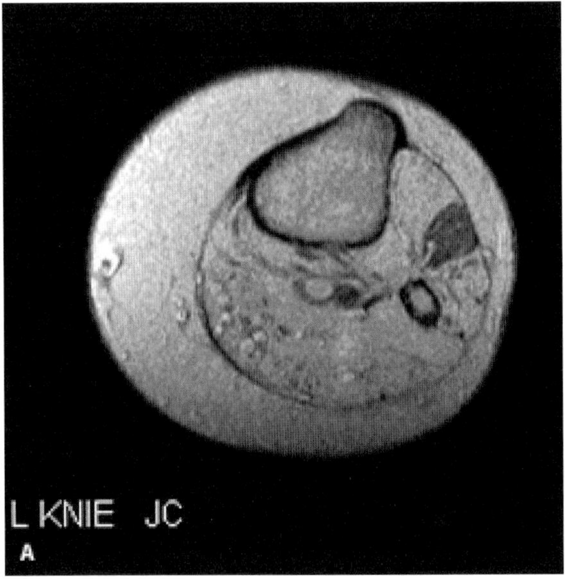

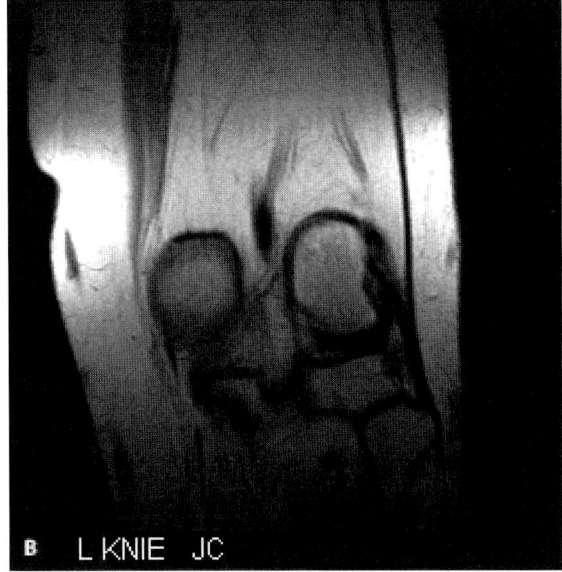

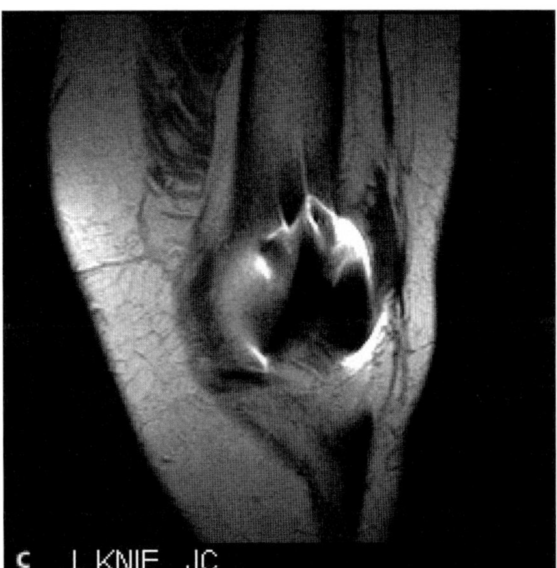

Fig. 8.11A–C. Chronic pain/soreness in the left knee after neurolysis in a 67-year-old woman. Axial TSE T2-WI (**A**) shows a diffuse high SI of all muscles; SI is comparable with that of normal subcutaneous fat. On coronal SE T1-WI (**B**), fatty infiltration-involution of all muscles is demonstrated. Sagittal TSE proton-density-WI also demonstrates the higher SI in the muscles because of fatty involution due to chronic denervation (**C**)

8.3.2.2 Muscle or Musculotendinous Junction Strain

Muscle strain is an indirect traumatic event caused by excessive stretching of the myotendinous unit. Certain muscles are more vulnerable to muscle strain, including those with the highest proportion of fast-twitch, type-II muscle fibers and those that span more than one joint, i.e., the hamstrings, rectus femoris, gastrocnemius (tennis leg; Fig. 8.12), adductor, and soleus muscles. The most frequent site of muscle strain is the musculotendinous junction of the lower extremity muscles. Multiple muscles may be involved concomitantly. On MRI, muscle strain is characterized by a hyperintense signal on

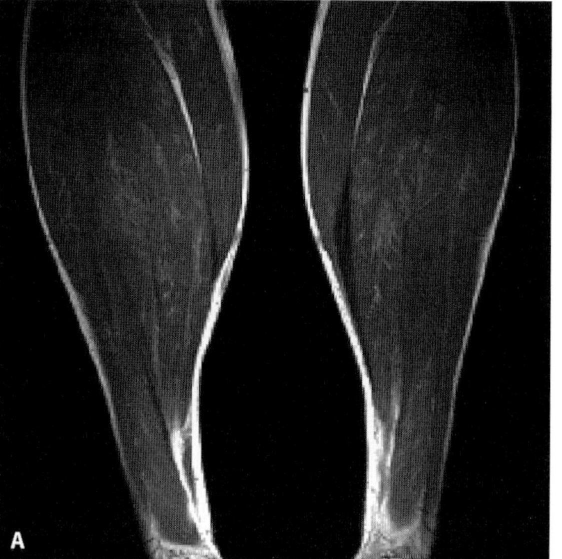

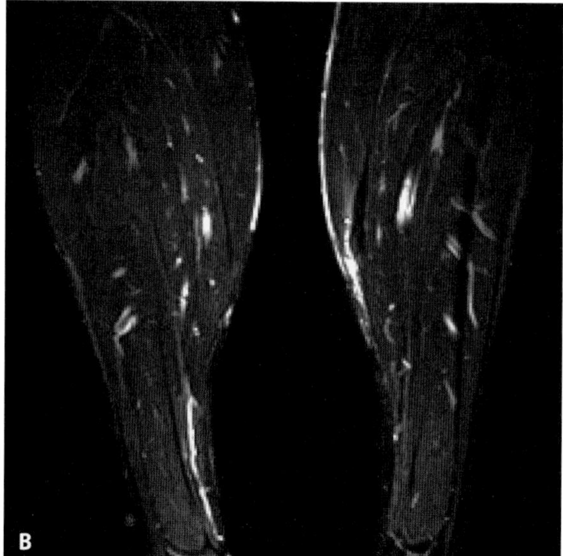

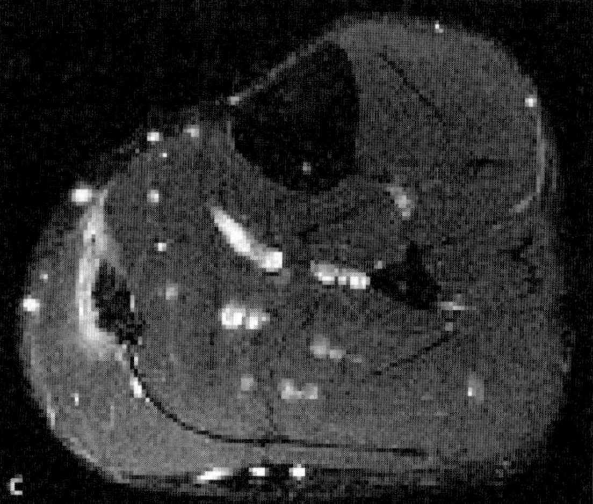

Fig. 8.12A–C. Sustained and repetitive soreness in left lower leg in a 47-year-old man after an acute pain attack in the calf region. Coronal SE T1-WI demonstrates a hypointense, band-like lesion at the musculotendinous junction of the left medial gastrocnemius (**A**). On STIR-WI (**B**) there is a long, high SI area adjacent and medial to the hypointense bandlike lesion. Axial TSE T2-WI with fat suppression shows an area of increased, slightly inhomogeneous SI at the musculotendinous junction of the medial gastrocnemius muscle around a hypointense fusiform mass (**C**). Tennis leg with chronic scar tissue and acute muscle strain with edema

STIR or fat-presaturated T2-WI, with the degree of hyperintensity being related to the severity of the injury.

Muscles strains are graded as follows:

1. Grade I strain: low-grade inflammation without myofascial disruption. There is mild hyperintensity of the affected muscle.
2. Grade II strain: muscle fiber tearing. There are multiple foci of hyperintensity on a background of mildly elevated SI, with or without perifascial blood collection.
3. Grade III strain: complete disruption of the muscle or muscle-tendon unit. There is separation of muscle fibers or the muscle-tendon unit, hyperintense fluid within the area, and perimuscular hematoma. In the severest form of this type of complete rupture and injury, retraction of muscle ends surrounded by hematoma may be seen on longitudinal (coronal or sagittal) images. This pathological image is known as the bell-clapper sign. Grade II and grade III strain are responsible for muscle volume loss.

8.3.2.3
Delayed-Onset Muscle Soreness

This condition is mostly the result of eccentric muscle lengthening. In this type of muscle injury, related symptoms develop following a delay of 24 h. Associated findings are increased intramuscular fluid pressure, elevation of plasma enzymes, and myoglobinemia. Rhabdomyolysis is the extreme form of delayed-onset muscle soreness (DOMS).

8.3.2.4
Compartment Syndrome

In case of muscle injury, edema and hemorrhage may raise the intracompartmental pressure (40–60 mmHg) within intact fascial boundaries. Common locations affected by compartment syndrome are calf, arm, and thigh. Untreated compartment syndrome may result in myonecrosis and invalidating outcome. MRI is the only imaging modality to visualize the early, prenecrotic stages of compartment syndrome which sonography cannot.

8.3.2.5
Chronic Overuse Syndromes

These conditions consist of pain and stiffness as a result of repetitive movements used in certain occupations and recreational activities. There is a combined pathology of tendons, muscles, and bony structures (see Sect. 8.3). For example: shin splints refer to a periostitis, myositis, or tendinosis, or a combination of these in case of chronic overuse of the anterior tibial muscle (Fig. 8.13).

Chronic-overuse syndrome may cause stress fractures. These are also called fatigue fractures and are defined as an interruption of the cortical bone caused by repetitive and cyclic loads (Fig. 8.5). Insufficiency fractures are fatigue fractures in osteopenic bone (osteoporotic or osteomalacic). Risk factors are professional sports and previous irradiation. Preferential locations are the metatarsals, the symphyseal and parasymphyseal area of the pubis, the lateral part of the sacral wings, the posteromedial part of the tibia, the tibial plateau, and the pars interarticularis (isthmus) of the vertebrae. Frequently, there is an associated reaction of the periosteum, the subperiosteal bone, and the fasciae. Well-known aspects include traction-induced stresses of the soleus muscle, rectus abdominis muscle, obturator muscle, and adductor muscles.

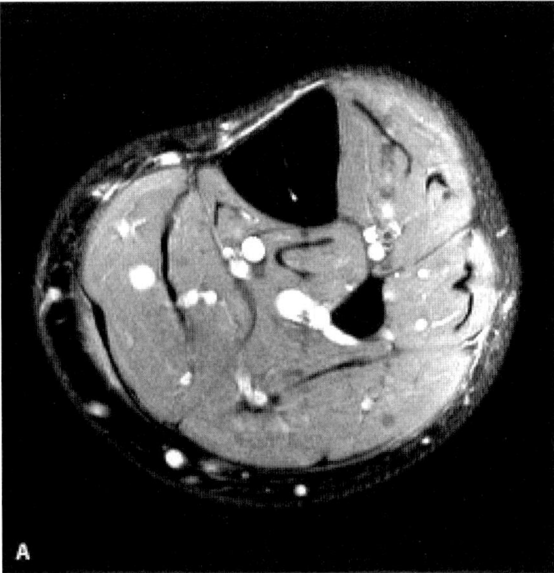

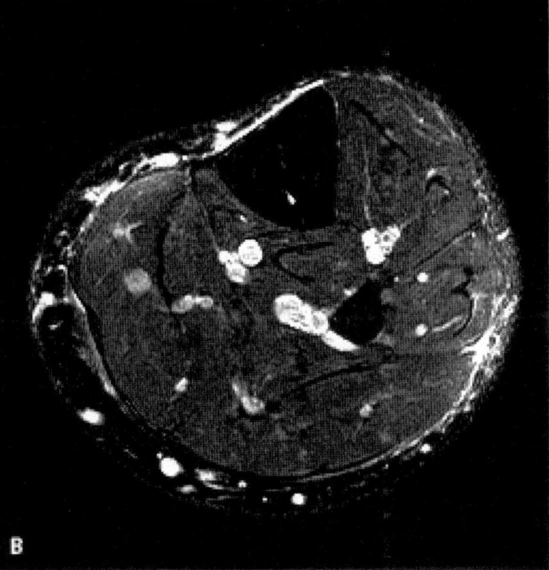

Fig. 8.13A,B. Pain anteriorly in the left lower leg in a 46-year-old long distance runner. Axial TSE proton-density (**A**) and T2-WI (**B**) with fat suppression reveal a high SI periosteum and adjacent subcutaneous tissue anteromedially of the tibia. Normal aspect of the muscles. Characteristic pattern of periostitis in shin splint

On MRI, the fracture itself is seen as a low SI line or zone in the medullary bone, surrounded by a zone of intermediate SI on T1-WI. On T2-WI (fat-presaturated or STIR), a zone of high SI is seen, containing the fracture line itself and the surrounding edema. Conventional radiographs are normal in 72% of stress fractures in the initial phase.

Soft-tissue lesions in overuse syndromes consist of irritation at the muscle-tendon junction, tendinosis, impingement syndromes, and chronic inflammation. Well-known examples are: (1) iliotibial band-friction syndrome, caused by repetitive friction between the iliotibial band and the lateral condyle of the femur, (2) jumper's knee, which is an overuse syndrome of the tendo-osseous junction of the quadriceps and patellar tendon, (3) waitress or tennis elbow, which is an overuse syndrome of the tendo-osseous junction of extensor muscles of the forearm (especially the extensor carpi radialis brevis and extensor digitorum longus at their common insertion), and (4) Achilles tendinosis, which may also be the result of chronic overuse.

8.3.2.6 Muscle Fibrosis

Muscle fibrosis is a sequel of third-degree muscle strain or muscle contusion and is related to the severity of the muscle injury. Fibrotic areas present with hypointense signal on all MR sequences. Fibrosis occurs in close proximity to the musculo-tendinous junction. Distinguishing between hypointense tendon and fibrosis is sometimes difficult and requires comparative axial and coronal images. MRI is useful in differentiating chronic scar and recurrent acute muscle tear Fig. 8.12.

8.3.2.7 Myositis Ossificans

Myositis ossificans is generally a solitary, benign, self-limiting ossifying process occurring in the musculature of the extremities in young men and is related to direct trauma in about half of the cases. Infection and coagulopathy have been mentioned as other causative factors. Furthermore, the disease may also occur in association with burns, paraplegia, and quadriplegia or with other neuromuscular disorders such as tetanus.

Pain and tenderness are the first symptoms, followed by a diffuse swelling of the soft tissues. This swelling typically becomes more circumscribed and indurated after 2–3 weeks. Thereafter, it changes progressively into a firm, hard mass – approximately 3–6 cm in diameter – that is well outlined on palpation. Principal sites of involvement are the limbs, which are affected in more than 80% of cases. The quadriceps muscle and brachialis muscle are favored sites in the lower and upper extremity, respectively. Areas prone to trauma are more commonly afflicted.

Three different appearances of myositis ossificans are noted on MRI, corresponding to the stage of maturation. Early stages of myositis ossificans, the so-called acute form, present on MRI as a mass that is isointense or even slightly hyperintense to muscle on T1-WI, but hyperintense on T2-WI. The lesion is surrounded by variable amounts of edema, appearing hyperintense on T2-WI. Following administration of Gd, a well-defined rim of enhancement is observed. The MR appearance of the lesions during the intermediate or subacute stage is characterized by isointensity with muscle on T1-WI and by a mild increase in SI on T2-WI. These findings are explained by a central fibrous transformation. Mature lesions (i.e., the 'chronic stage') show more extensive signal voids on all sequences, corresponding to a considerable degree of peripheral calcification and ossification. In this stage, lesions demonstrate increased SI in an 'onion-skin pattern' on T2-WI.

8.4 MR of Primary Bone Tumors

8.4.1 Introduction

MR imaging has been recognized as a powerful diagnostic tool in the work-up of bone tumors. Plain films, however, remain of utmost importance in the analysis of bone tumors and tumor-like lesions, i.e., in detecting the lesion, differentiating between benign and malignant tumors, and predicting a correct histological diagnosis. When the lesion is not visible on radiography in a symptomatic patient, other imaging modalities should be applied, such as scintigraphy or MRI since they are more sensitive in detecting bony abnormalities than radiography. MRI, however, became the cornerstone in locoregional staging of primary bone tumors. Because of its high spatial resolution, high soft-tissue contrast, and multiplanar imaging capabilities, MR imaging provides precise information about the intramedullary extent of the tumor and its relationship to adjacent extraosseous structures.

In the future, diffusion-weighted imaging (DWI) may allow for improved differentiation of acute benign and neoplastic vertebral compression fractures. DWI may aid in therapy control, in the distinction between necrotic and viable tumor tissue, and in the differentiation between post-therapeutic soft-tissue changes and tumor recurrence. DWI may also be useful in the differential diagnosis of bone neoplasms and soft-tissue tumors.

8.4.2 Imaging Technique

To avoid diagnostic errors and misinterpretations, plain films should be the first step in a diagnostic work-up of bone tumors. If possible, MR imaging should be performed with a dedicated surface coil to improve the signal-to-noise ratio and spatial resolution. Imaging should be performed in at least two orthogonal planes. After scout views in three orthogonal planes, we perform mostly SE T1-WI in a sagittal or coronal plane, depending on the localization of the tumor in the bone. This sequence is necessary for accurate determination of any intraosseous extension. Afterwards, axial SE or fast SE T2-WI is performed, covering the whole tumor volume. T2-WI are mandatory for adequate depiction of extension into the adjacent soft tissues.

The main drawback of fast SE T2-WI is the high SI of fat. Therefore, fat-presaturated T2-WI or STIR sequences should be performed. Thus, the inability of fast SE T2-WI sequences in detecting bone-marrow edema is resolved. On STIR images, lesion conspicuity is high, but delineation of the intra- and extraosseous extent is hampered since the tumor, peritumoral edema, and fracture all have high SI. Fat-saturated T2-WI may be reliable for determining the extension into the soft tissues, encasement of the neurovascular bundle, and visualizing intratumoral necrosis in osteosarcomas and Ewing's sarcomas. This sequence is a valuable alternative to T2-WI.

In most cases, SE T1-WI after i.v. injection of Gd-chelates is performed in the same imaging plane as that of the precontrast series and in the axial plane. Gd-enhanced T1-WI affords an excellent demonstration of intratumoral necrosis, differentiation of bone-marrow edema versus tumor, depiction of extraosseous extension, and differentiation of recurrent tumor versus postoperative fibrosis. Subtraction of post- from pre-Gd-enhanced images may be of use to demonstrate subtle enhancement and to delineate the tumor from fatty surrounding tissues.

8.4.3 Tissue Characterization

MRI has only a limited role in offering a tissue-related diagnosis. Plain films, indeed, are indispensable for characterization. They accurately depict calcification/ossification of the tumor matrix, cortical permeation or disruption, and faint periosteal reaction, less clearly visualized by MR imaging. Furthermore, most tumors have low SI on T1-WI and high SI on T2-WI.

In certain cases, however, a combination of distinctive findings (e.g., SI, enhancement patterns) allows for an accurate diagnosis or else narrows the differential diagnosis. Intratumoral fluid-fluid levels are often seen in aneurysmal bone cyst, but also in fibrous dysplasia, chondroblastoma, (telangiectatic) osteosarcoma, and giant cell tumor. Ring-and-arc ('septal') enhancement is seen in immature enchondromas and low-grade chondrosarcoma, whereas high-grade chondrosarcomas show strong inhomogeneous contrast enhancement (Fig. 8.14). Intraosseous lipomas are easily recognized by their high SI on T1-WI. Giant-cell tumor is characterized by its low SI on T1-WI and T2-WI (Fig. 8.15). Eosinophilic granuloma manifests as an expansile, lytic lesion with rather high SI on T1-WI, abundant intramedullary and soft-tissue edema, and often firm periosteal reaction. Fibrous cortical defects are sharply circumscribed metaphyseal lesions with characteristic low SI on T1-WI, T2-WI, and STIR images. In general, MRI provides additional value in the diagnosis of bone tumors. In a study performed at our institution, lipoma, chondrosarcoma, and osteomyelitis were the three most common pathologies with the strongest gain concerning diagnosis. A diagnostic gain of MRI was seen in 50% of cases.

8.4.4 Grading

The role of MR imaging in grading bone tumors is limited, because plain films are highly accurate in differentiating benign from malignant tumors. In a study performed at our institution on 79 bone tumors in chil-

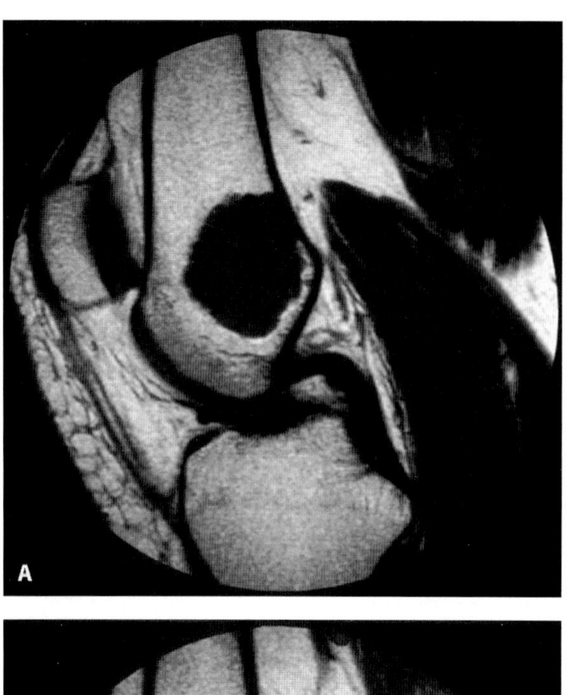

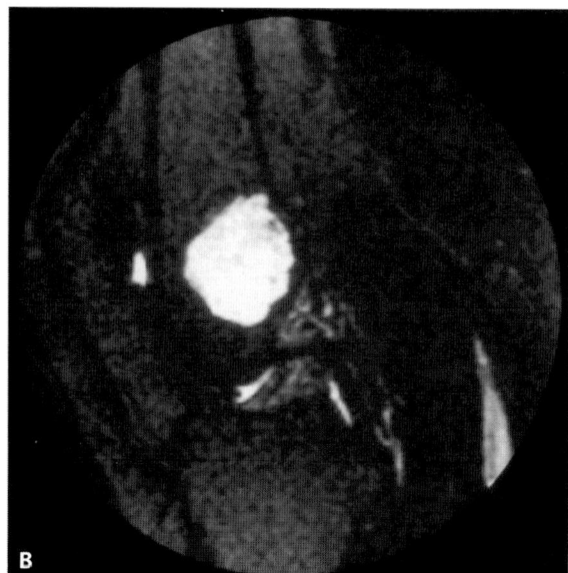

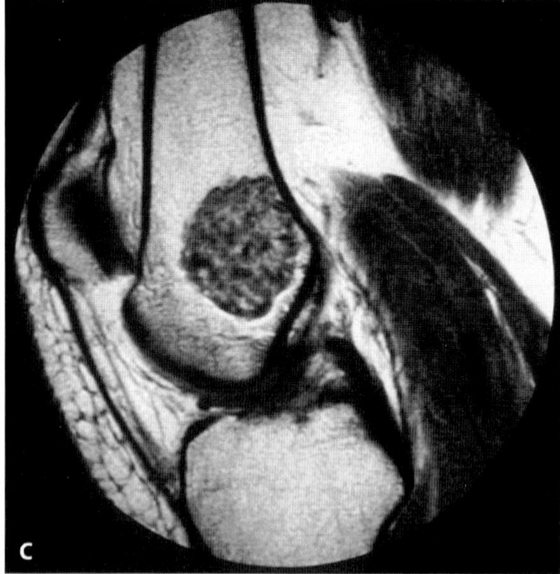

Fig. 8.14A–C. Enchondroma of the right distal femur in a 40-year-old woman. Sagittal SE T1-WI (**A**) shows a sharply circumscribed mass with intermediate SI. On STIR images (**B**), the lesion has high SI with some small intralesional septations of low SI. No peritumoral edema is seen. Sagittal SE T1-WI after i.v. injection of Gd (**C**) shows a 'ring-and-arc' enhancement pattern. The combined findings of a high SI mass with low SI septations on T2-WI, without perilesional marrow edema, together with 'ring-and-arc' enhancement are characteristic for an enchondroma

dren, correct grading on plain films occurred in 89% of cases. One may never solely rely on MR images to distinguish benign from malignant tumors. In a study by Ma et al., only 55% of masses could be assessed correctly with MR imaging.

STIR and FS T2-WI images differentiate between benign and malignant intramedullary cartilaginous tumors because peritumoral and soft-tissue changes are seen in chondrosarcomas, whereas this phenomenon is not seen in enchondromas (Fig. 8.14). One should be aware not to misdiagnose an enchondroma with associated pathologic fracture that shows peritumoral high-SI areas (as with chondrosarcoma).

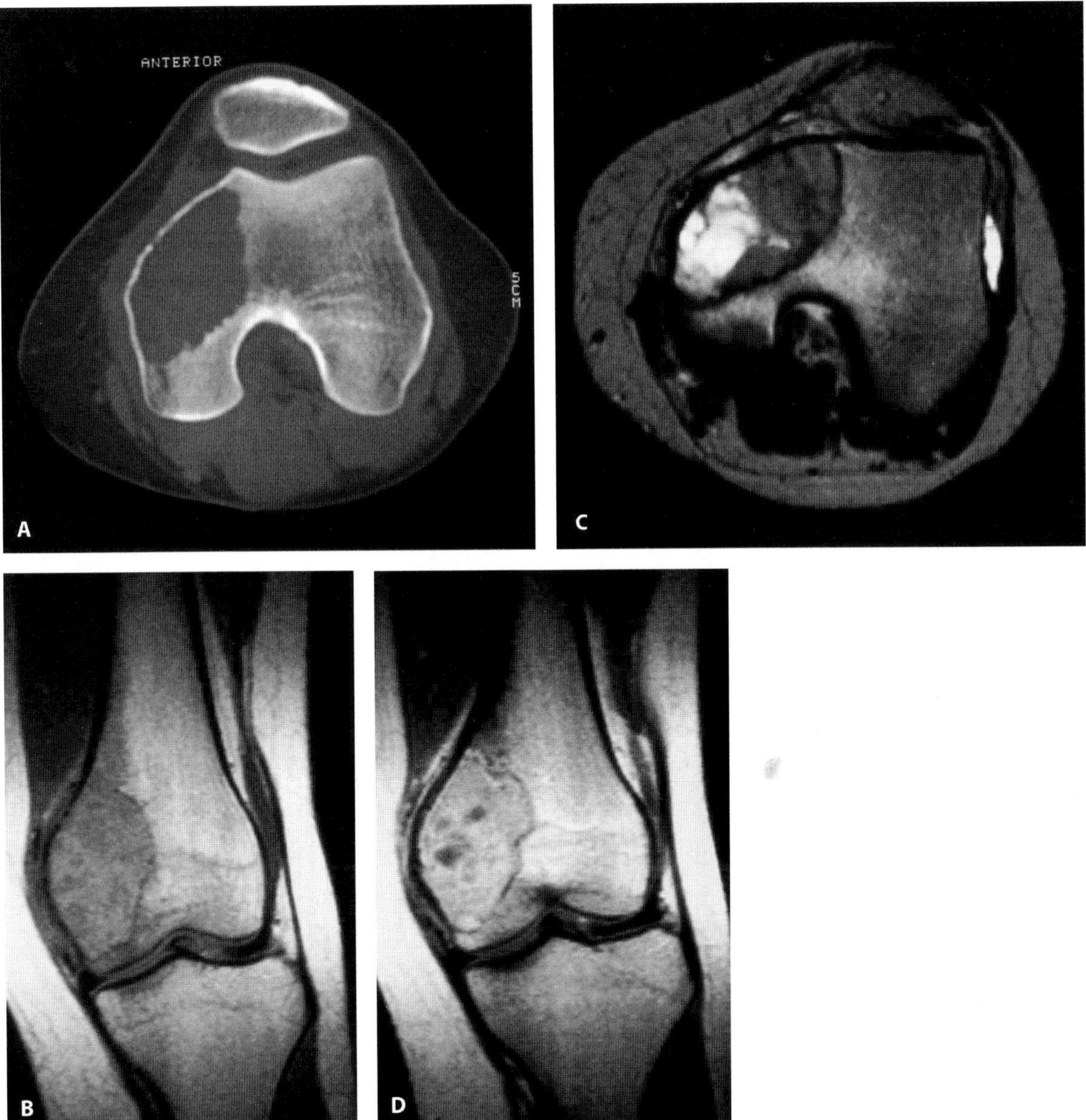

Fig. 8.15A–D. Giant-cell tumor of the left distal femur in a 27-year-old woman. On axial CT scan, an osteolytic area is seen at the medial condyle. The cortex is disrupted, and a small soft-tissue mass is seen (**A**). On coronal SE T1-WI, a well-circumscribed mass is noted (**B**). Presence of perilesional bone-marrow edema, which is better demonstrated on T2-WI (**C**). There is marked enhancement after i.v. injection of Gd (**D**). The low SI of the lesion on this sequence, together with the epiphyseal location and the age of the patient, prompts the diagnosis of giant-cell tumor

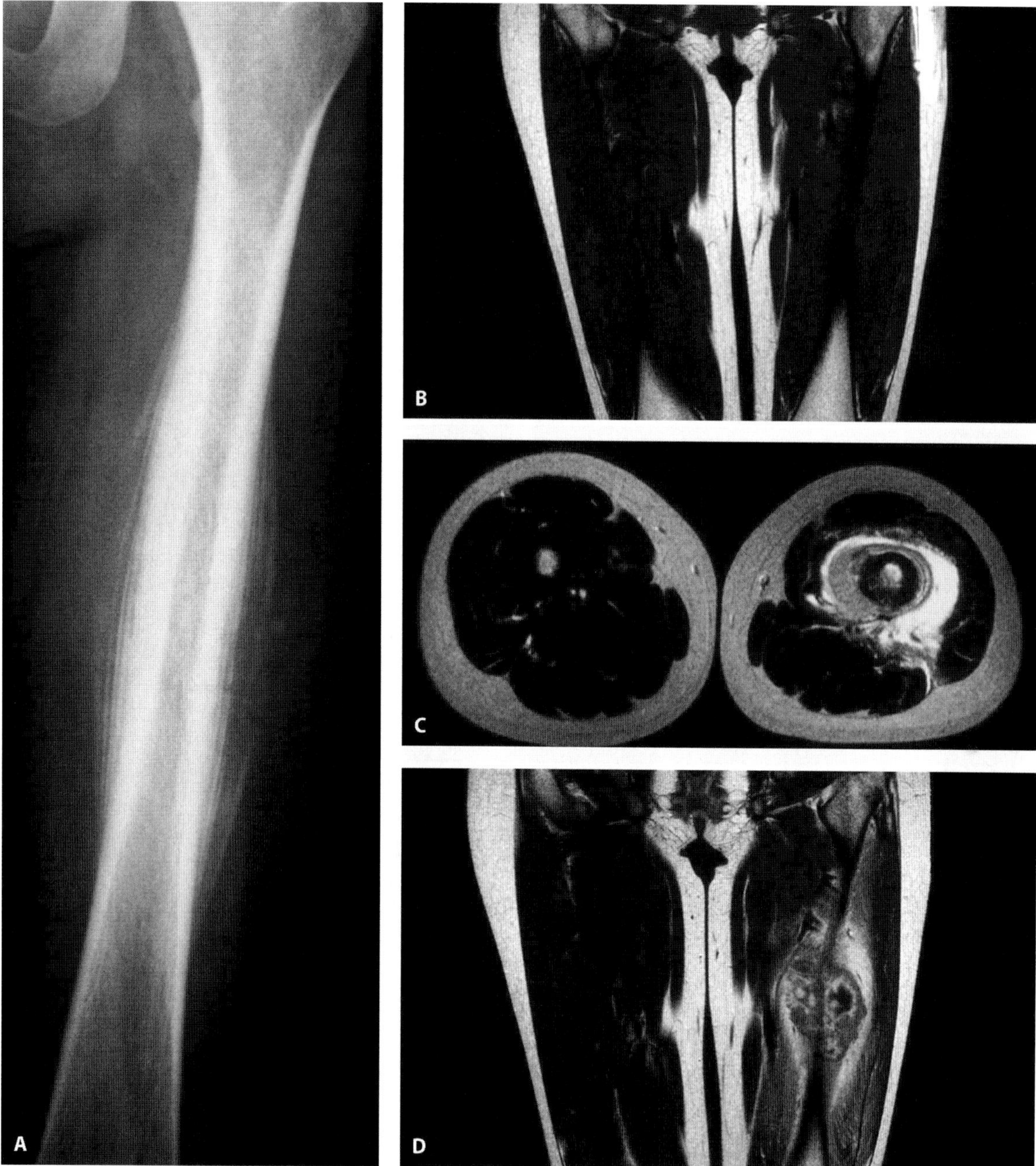

Fig. 8.16A–D. Ewing's sarcoma of the left femur in a 13-year-old girl. A plain film shows thickened cortical bone at the midportion of the left femur, surrounded by an 'onion-peel' periosteal reaction. The radiographic image affords to make a reliable diagnosis, since it is almost pathognomonic for Ewing's sarcoma (**A**). However, MR imaging much better demonstrates the extent of the lesion. Coronal T1-WI shows a huge medullary mass (**B**). The cortical disruption, periosteal reaction, and surrounding soft-tissue edema are better seen on axial TSE T2-WI (**C**) and on Gd-enhanced SE T1-WI (**D**). Large field-of-view images allow the orthopedic surgeon to measure the required length of the allogreffe accurately

8.4.5 Locoregional Staging

Because of its unequaled soft-tissue contrast and spatial resolution, MR imaging is the cornerstone of locoregional staging. This means defining intra- and extraosseous extent and the relationship to adjacent soft tissues and neurovascular elements. Exact tumor extent can be determined most accurately by a combination of T1-WI, T2-WI, and Gd-enhanced T1-WI (Fig. 8.16). On these Gd-enhanced images, intramedullary edema will enhance differently and can be differentiated from primary tumor. Some authors have reported the value of MR angiography in demonstrating tumor neovascularity. The promising initial results need to be confirmed in larger prospective series.

Correlative MR imaging histopathology contradicts the misconception of the ability of the growth plate to limit tumor spread. Indeed, transphyseal spread occurs in 50%–88% of osteosarcomas in patients with an apparently normal growth plate. While plain radiography and even axial CT scan do not allow accurate visualization of the relationship between the tumor, physeal plate, and epiphysis, MRI is highly accurate in this regard. In contrast to transphyseal spread, involvement of an adjacent joint by a bone tumor is rarely seen, given that cartilage is an effective barrier against tumoral spread. When transarticular spread occurs, MR imaging can easily show it.

In the diagnostic work-up of malignant bone tumors, it is important to detect skip metastases (small intraosseous metastatic deposits beyond the reactive zone, but within the same compartment as the primary tumor). Therefore, a large field-of-view, T1-weighted sequence may be added to the imaging protocol to visualize the largest possible peritumoral area (Fig. 8.16).

8.4.6 Dynamic MR Imaging

Gd-chelates, currently used for musculoskeletal imaging, have a small molecular size and are distributed in the intravascular and interstitial space. This allows them to diffuse in necrotic tissue, leading to enhancement and, thus, underestimation of the presence and amount of intratumoral necrosis. Therefore, static Gd-enhanced MR imaging does not accurately show the amount of intratumoral necrosis.

Dynamic MR imaging after i.v. injection of Gd is a useful diagnostic tool that overcomes this problem. Different techniques have been developed, but the first-pass and subtraction techniques are used most frequently. Fast or ultrafast sequences with a temporal resolution of 2–3 s per image or a set of parallel images are available and mandatory for the measurement of tissue enhancement during the first pass of the contrast agent. Various parameters, such as time of onset of enhancement, wash-out, maximal enhancement, and slope values can be measured. Because a large overlap exists in slope values of benign and malignant bone tumors, the role of dynamic imaging in grading and tissue characterization is limited. Recently, Ma et al. reported that rim-to-center enhancement (RTC) ratios, based on the difference in vascularity pattern between benign and malignant masses, might be useful in differentiating them more accurately. These results need to be confirmed in larger series.

8.4.7 Post-treatment Follow-up and Detection of Recurrences

Dynamic Gd-enhanced MR imaging is well established in the detection of residual or recurrent tumors. In the postoperative follow-up of a patient with a malignant bone tumor, regular MR studies are mandatory when searching for evidence of residual or recurrent tumor. On plain films or CT, a large recurrent tumor can present as an osteolytic area that may be accompanied by a soft-tissue mass and periosteal reaction. When performing MRI, small recurrences can be detected, enabling early therapeutic actions.

First, MR examination after surgical intervention should be performed within 9–15 weeks. When imaging is done within the first 6 weeks after surgery, any residual mass cannot be differentiated from postoperative changes, such as edema, subacute hematoma, and inflammatory granulation tissue. The imaging protocol starts with a T2-weighted sequence. When no areas of high SI are seen, no tumor recurrence is present. When high SI areas are present, one must evaluate whether such areas are mass-like or not. An inhomogeneous high-SI area without mass lesion may correspond to postoperative inflammatory changes. When a mass lesion is encountered, intravenous administration of Gd-contrast is necessary to differentiate between postoperative seroma/lymphocele and recurrence. Cystic space-occupying lesions, such as seroma or lymphocele, will show either no or only rim enhancement, whereas recurrences enhance more homogeneously.

A major problem arises when postoperative MR imaging must be performed in patients who have undergone reconstructive surgery with ferromagnetic osteosynthetic devices, such as nails, plates, and screws. Susceptibility artifacts will disturb the image quality. However, most recurrences will be detected by the meticulous comparison of pre- and post-contrast series. Nowadays, most prosthetic devices consist of titanium, causing fewer artifacts. Further options available to minimize susceptibility artifacts are: (1) performing the examination with a magnet at low field strength, (2) accurately choosing and optimizing the sequence type and parameters (susceptibility artifacts are negligible on SE images, and less-pronounced on FSE sequences than on GE sequences), (3) shortening the TE value, and (4) decreasing the voxel size.

Soft-tissue edema poses another problem for the radiologist viewing MR follow-up studies of patients who have undergone radiation therapy for bone or soft-tissue sarcomas. Postirradiation edema of the soft tissues complicates the postoperative picture characterized by myositis, peritumoral edema, hemorrhage, fibrosis, and even toxic edema (due to chemotherapeutic agents). These changes will subside within 1 year post-treatment, whereas postirradiation edema persists for more than 2–4 years in 20%–50% of the patients treated with photon or neutron radiation therapy. On T2-WI and STIR images, diffuse bone-marrow edema is seen very early and lasts for weeks to months, until fatty replacement occurs.

Different authors have reported on the role of dynamic Gd-enhanced MR imaging in the evaluation of preoperative chemotherapy of bone sarcomas. The ultimate goal is to reveal the presence and amount of intratumoral necrosis, in order to differentiate responders from non-responders. This enables the prediction of definitive outcomes in individual cases. Accuracy levels of 86%–100% in differentiating these two groups have been achieved using dynamic Gd-enhanced MR to depict tissue vascularization and nests of remaining viable tumor. By this means, the best biopsy site can be determined.

Further applications of this technique are on the way, for example, the use of dynamic MR imaging in distinguishing tumor and peritumoral edema, slope values for differentiating regions of microscopic intramedullary invasion from tumor-free bone marrow in patients with osteosarcoma after chemotherapy, and – more recently – diffusion-weighted MR images to refine the assessment of intratumoral necrosis (differences in molecular diffusion and, thus, in membrane integrity between viable and necrotic tissue are easily detected).

8.5 MR of Soft-Tissue Tumors

8.5.1 Introduction

Staging means defining the local and distal extent of pathological processes and their relationship to adja-

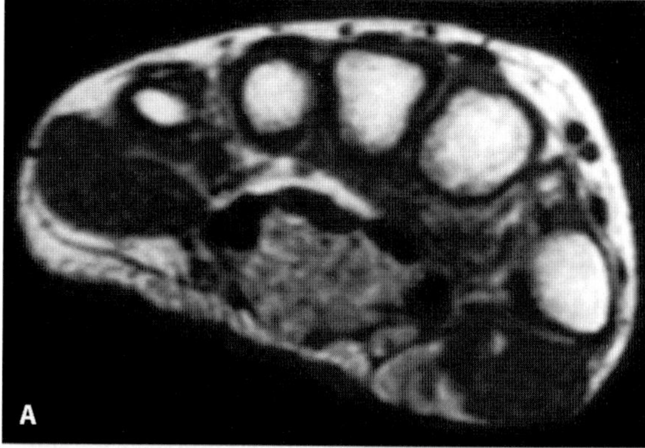

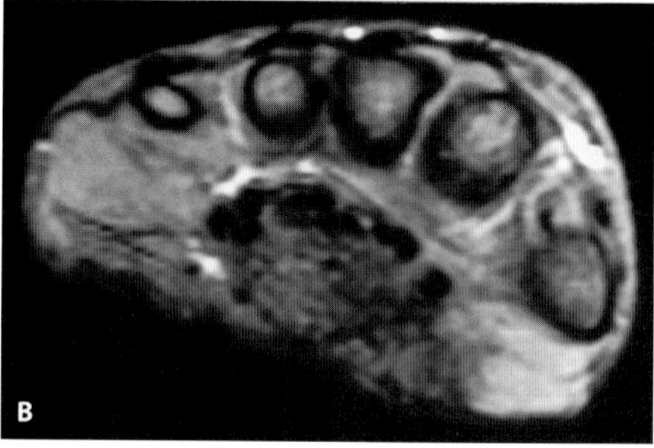

Fig. 8.17A,B. Fibrolipohamartoma of the median nerve in a 40-year-old man. Axial SE T1-WI (**A**) and GRE T2-WI (**B**) show a heterogeneous mass with mixed SI, corresponding to lipomatous tissue, fibrous tissue, and intervening enlarged neural fascicles. This lesion has a characteristic location and SI. (Reprinted with permission from De Schepper et al. 1997)

cent structures, such as bone, muscles, tendons, and neurovascular bundles. Characterization consists of both grading and a tissue-specific diagnosis. While a tissue-specific diagnosis implies pathological typing, grading implies differentiating benign and malignant processes and defining the malignancy grade.

Although pathology will always remain the gold standard in the diagnosis of soft-tissue tumors, the prediction of a specific histological diagnosis remains one of the ultimate goals of each new imaging technique (Fig. 8.17). Moreover, decisions regarding biopsy and treatment could be simplified if a specific diagnosis or a limited differential diagnosis could be provided on the basis of imaging. Because the tumor grade is also a major staging parameter, there is a close relationship between staging, grading, and characterization of soft-tissue tumors (Fig. 8.18).

8.5.2 Staging

A useful staging system should incorporate prognostic factors (higher stages mean higher risks), allow the planning of surgical margins needed for local tumor control (narrow margins mean less favorable outcome), and provide guidelines for the use of adjunctive therapies. Moreover, it should facilitate the communication of data.

There are different staging systems. The most useful is the Musculoskeletal Tumor Society (MTS) system, which is based on the interrelationship of the grade (benign G_0, low-grade malignant G_1, high-grade malignant G_2), the site, and the presence or absence of metastases (M_0 vs M_1). The site or local extent is defined as intra- (T1) or extra-compartmental (T2), if the outer-

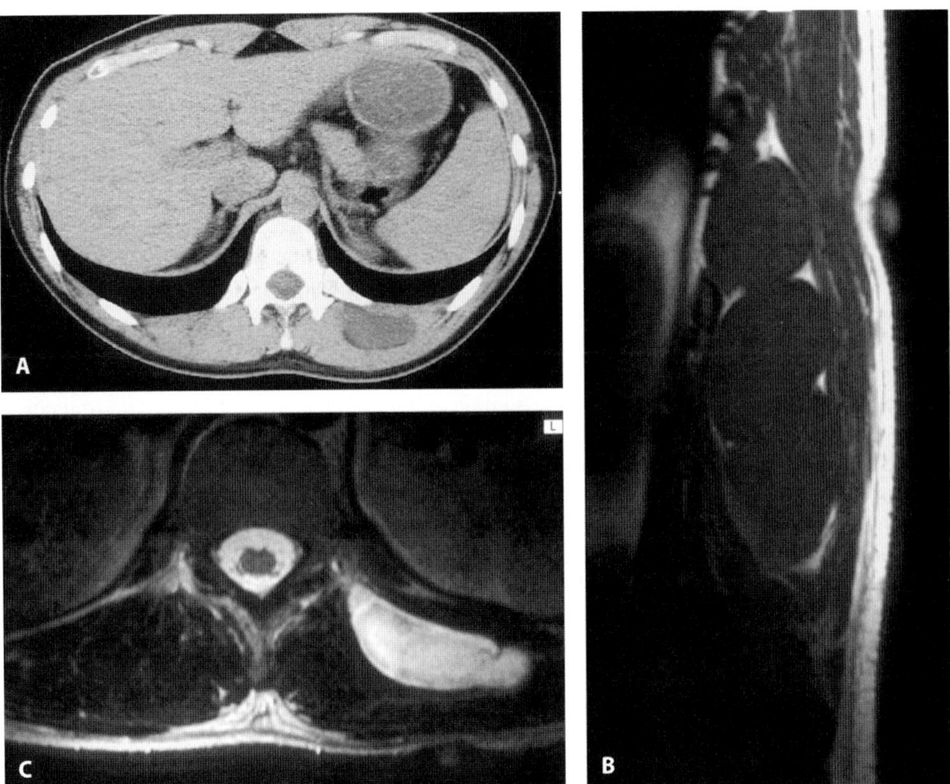

Fig. 8.18A–C. Collagenous neurofibroma in the paravertebral region in an 18-year-old man. The exact delineation and shape of the tumor, leading to a correct preoperative diagnosis, are better appreciated on sagittal SE T1-WI (**B**) than on axial CT scan (**A**). Furthermore, the extension to an adjacent neuroforamen is excellently depicted on axial TSE T2-WI (**C**), since contrast resolution is better than on CT scan

most margin is bounded by natural anatomic barriers (bone, cartilage, fascial septa, tendons, and ligaments). Local staging must be completed before a biopsy is performed. There is no doubt that MRI is by far the best imaging modality for local staging of soft-tissue tumors.

8.5.3 Grading

The prognosis for soft-tissue tumors is determined by the tumor stage and grade. Well-known histologic grading parameters, such as cellularity, mitotic rate, matrix, and presence of necrosis, all influence SI on MR imaging. As a consequence, the grading capacity of MR imaging seemed promising. Nevertheless, there is still much controversy regarding the value of MR imaging in the differentiation of benign and malignant soft-tissue tumors.

Table 8.6 lists soft-tissue tumor grading parameters described in the literature. The value of these signs, both alone and in combination, has been discussed by several authors. With a few exceptions, the grading of soft-tissue tumors on the basis of individual parameters is not useful. Combinations of different parameters guarantee higher sensitivity and specificity.

Table 8.6. Soft-tissue tumor (STT) grading parameters

Origin (subcutaneous, fascial, intramuscular, mixed)
Size
Shape
Margins
Signal homogeneity
Changing pattern of homogeneity (T1–T2)
Contrast enhancement
Static studies (type, intensity)
Dynamic studies (ratio, slope)
Low signal intensity septations
Hemorrhage
Peritumoral edema
Distribution
Intracompartmental
Extracompartmental
Neurovascular bundle displacement/encasement
Bone involvement
Growth rate

8.5.3.1 Individual Parameters

Examples of commonly used individual parameters for predicting malignancy are intensity and homogeneity of the MR signal on different pulse sequences. With the exception of fibrosarcoma, malignant soft-tissue tumors exhibit high SI on T2-WI. Although SI is highly sensitive for predicting malignancy, its specificity is very low. Evaluation of the homogeneity of the SI pattern has been reported by several authors. The sensitivity of the inhomogeneous SI pattern on T1-W images is between 70% and 88%, the specificity between 25% and 76%. Recently, a sensitivity of 72% and a specificity of 87% in predicting malignancy was reported for changing homogeneity (from homogeneous on T1-WI to heterogeneous on T2-WI), and a sensitivity of 80% with a specificity of 91% was reported for low-signal intratumoral septations (Table 8.6).

Concerning the size of the lesions, combined data from three investigations show that a lesion of less than 3 cm diameter is a reasonable indicator of benignity, as this threshold is associated with a predictive value of 88%. Conversely, a diameter threshold of 5 cm predicts a malignant soft-tissue mass with a sensitivity of 74%, specificity of 59%, and an accuracy of 66%.

The parameter 'shape' is unlikely to contribute significantly to tumor grading. Although benign tumors tend to be well delineated and, conversely, malignant tumors have rather ill-defined margins, several studies concluded that the margin of a soft-tissue mass on MR imaging is of no statistical relevance in predicting malignancy.

Peritumoral edema, shown on T2-WI as an ill-defined area of high SI, can indicate infiltrative tumor, edema, or both. As a consequence, it is not helpful as a grading parameter. The involvement of adjacent bone, extracompartmental distribution, or encasement of the neurovascular bundle are relatively uncommon findings which are specific but insensitive signs of malignancy. They are also seen in aggressive benign soft-tissue lesions, including desmoids, hemangiomas, and pigmented villonodular synovitis. The same holds true for 'growth rate', which is related to the aggressiveness of a soft-tissue tumor rather than its malignancy grade. Although malignant tumors show increased vascularity and have large extracellular spaces, depending on tumoral activity or aggressiveness, we found no correlation between the degree and pattern of enhancement and malignancy grade.

Dynamic contrast-enhanced studies are valuable in distinguishing benign from malignant lesions. On time-intensity plots, increases in SI were always lower than 100% for benign and between 80% and 280% for malignant tumors. Slopes with greater than a 30% per minute increase in SI were seen in 84% of malignant tumors, and slopes with lower than a 30% per minute increase in SI were seen in 72% of benign tumors. Some overlap was, however, observed. Largely necrotic malignant tumors showed slopes of less than 30%, whereas aggressive benign lesions, such as myositis ossificans, showed slopes similar to those of malignant tumors.

Although a statistically significant difference was found between the 'first-pass' slope values of benign and malignant lesions, pathologic and angiographic findings indicated that 'first-pass' images reflect tissue vascularization and perfusion, rather than benignity or malignancy. In 25% of the cases, the images provide new information for diagnosis, choice of biopsy site, and follow-up of chemotherapy.

Intratumoral hemorrhage is a rare finding, which can be observed in benign as well as in malignant lesions, and is difficult to differentiate from non-tumoral soft-tissue hematoma. In a recent study, intratumoral hemorrhage was observed in 23 benign and 5 malignant tumors among a total number of 225 masses. Hemorrhage was diagnosed on the basis of high signal on T1-WI, coupled with low or high signal on T2-WI, provided that the tissue was not isointense to fat on all sequences. A low signal hemosiderin rim was interpreted as evidence of prior hemorrhage (see also Table 8.10, fluid-fluid levels).

8.5.3.2 Combined Parameters

Although most investigators failed to establish reliable criteria for distinguishing benign from malignant lesions, a combination of individual parameters yields higher sensitivity and specificity. Reported important criteria, such as size, margins, and homogeneity of SI, predict malignancy with a specificity of 82%–96%, a negative predictive value of 92%–96%, and a positive predictive value of 88%–90%. These figures have never been confirmed. Moreover, the accuracy of MR imaging declines when typically benign tumors are excluded from the analysis. A significant percentage of malignant lesions may appear deceptively 'benign' with the criteria that are used currently.

We performed multivariate statistical analyses to determine the accuracy of ten parameters, individually and in combination, for predicting malignancy. When the following signs were observed, malignancy was portended with a sensitivity of 81% and a specificity of 81%: absence of low SI on T2-WI, signal inhomogeneity on T1-WI, and mean diameter of the lesion greater than 33 mm (Fig. 8.19). Malignancy was predicted with the highest sensitivity when a lesion had high SI on T2-WI, was larger than 33 mm in diameter, and had an inhomogeneous SI on T1-WI.

Signs that had the greatest specificity for malignancy included the presence of tumor necrosis, bone or neurovascular involvement, and a mean diameter of more than 66 mm. A poorly circumscribed area of low SI on T1-WI and high SI on T2-WI, showing no contrast enhancement, was considered an area of necrosis. Of the malignant lesions, 80% had irregular or partially irregular margins, while a similar percentage of benign masses had well-defined or partially irregular margins. The majority of both benign and malignant lesions showed moderate or strong enhancement; no predominant enhancement pattern emerged for either type of mass. In contrast to previous studies, margin, SI on T2-WI, SI on T1-WI, shape, and enhancement pattern were statistically nondiscriminatory.

It is likely that the divergence in results is a consequence of differences in the specific population studied, of the varying experience of the interpreters, and of variability in the parameters used. Prospective studies with a statistically relevant number of patients and well-defined diagnostic parameters are needed to overcome these drawbacks.

8.5.4 Characterization

Because of its high intrinsic contrast resolution, it was expected that MR imaging had great potential for the histological classification of soft-tissue tumors. Unfortunately, the basis for the initial enthusiasm has not been confirmed.

There are two reasons for this. First, by showing SI related to some physicochemical properties of tumor components (e.g., fat, blood, water, collagen) and, consequently, reflecting gross morphology of the lesion rather than underlying histology, MR images provide only indirect information about tumor histology. Soft-tissue tumors belonging to the same histologic group may have a different composition or different propor-

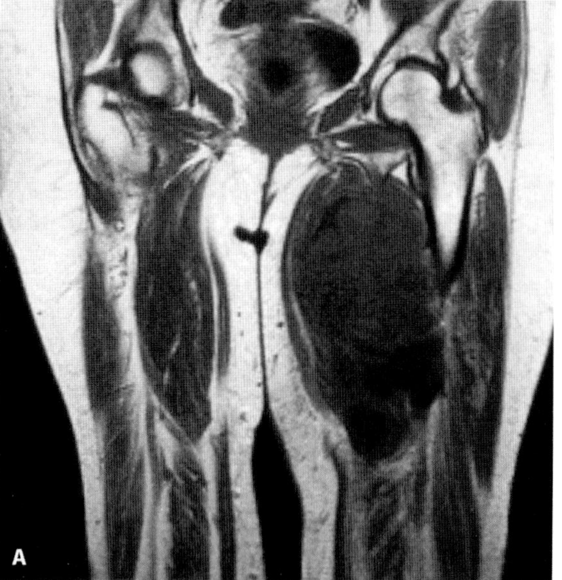

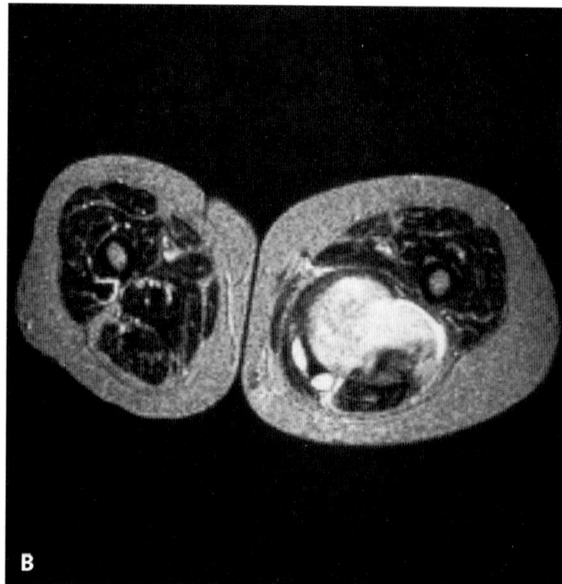

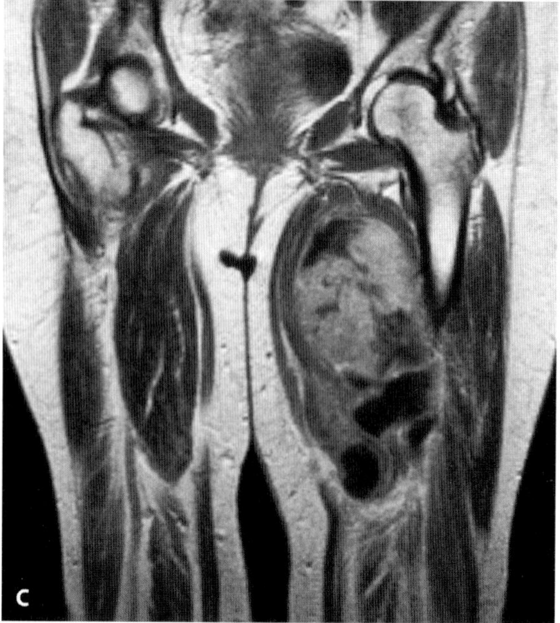

Fig. 8.19A–C. Liposarcoma of the left thigh in a 71-year-old man. Coronal SE T1-WI shows a huge inhomogeneous mass within the adductor region (**A**). On Axial TSE T2-WI, the mass has low, intermediate, and high SI components (**B**). Coronal SE T1-WI after i.v. injection of Gd shows inhomogeneous enhancement (**C**). The combination of inhomogeneous SI on T1-WI, diameter greater than 33 mm, and absence of low SI on T2-WI suggests the diagnosis of malignancy

tions of tumor components, resulting in different MR signals. This feature is well exemplified by the group of liposarcomas that may be well-differentiated (lipomatous), myxoid, round cell, or pleiomorphic, or contain different proportions of these components. Only well-differentiated liposarcomas are predominantly fatty, whereas the other histologic subtypes have less than 25% fat or no fat at all. As a consequence, there are no specific MR characteristics for liposarcomas as a group.

The second reason for the poor performance of MRI in characterizing tumors histologically involves time-dependent changes during natural evolution or as a consequence of therapy. Young desmoid tumors are highly cellular with a high water content; this results in high SI on T2-WI. With aging, they become more collagenous and less cellular, which results in a decreasing SI. The same transformation has been described for many tumors of fibrous tissue and also for malignant fibrous histiocytomas. Furthermore, the SI of large malignant tumors undergoes changes as a consequence of intratumoral necrosis and/or bleeding.

These limitations have prompted M. Kransdorf to state 'a correct histological diagnosis reached on the basis of imaging studies is possible in only approximately one quarter of cases'. We would like to be somewhat more optimistic. The highest confidence in characterization is reached when the majority of the cases are benign lesions, such as lipomas, hemangiomas and arteriovenous malformations, benign neural tumors, periarticular cysts, hematomas, pigmented villonodular synovitis, giant-cell tumors of tendon sheath, and abscesses. The use of intravenously injected paramagnetic contrast agents is valuable in the detection and staging of soft-tissue tumors, but neither the intensity nor the pattern of enhancement contributes to further histological characterization of these lesions. Dynamic contrast studies are useful for assessing the response of soft-tissue tumors to chemotherapy and for differentiating postoperative edema from recurrent tumor. 'First-pass' imaging may aid in differentiating hemangioma from arteriovenous malformation.

As a guideline for the reader, we have summarized the value of different parameters, such as preferential location (Table 8.7), shape (Table 8.8), presence of signal voids (Table 8.9), fluid-fluid levels (Table 8.10), signal intensities on different pulse sequences (Table 8.11), multiplicity (Table 8.12), and concomitant diseases (Table 8.13) in concise tables.

Table 8.7. Preferential location of soft-tissue tumors

Location		Tumor
Neck	Infants	Cystic hygroma – lymphangioma capillary hemangioma
	Dorsal neck	Nuchal fibroma
	Sternocleidomastoid muscle (children)	Fibromatosis colli
	Carotid bifurcation	Glomus tumor
Trunk	Axilla	Cystic hygroma – lymphangioma
	Subscapular	Elastofibroma
	Paraspinal gutter	Neurogenic tumor
Abdomen	Rectus abdominis muscle (postpuerperal women)	Abdominal desmoid
	Paraspinal gutter	Neurogenic tumor
	Psoas muscle, parapsoatic	Plexiform neurofibroma
Pelvis	Presacral	Plexiform neurofibroma
	Buttock, lateral aspect	Desmoid
		Injection granuloma
	Coccyx	Extraspinal ependymoma
Upper limb	Deltoid, subcutaneous	Desmoid
		Injection granuloma
	Wrist	Ganglion cyst
	Wrist, volar aspect	Fibrolipohamartoma of median nerve
	Hand	(Gouty tophi)
	Hand, volar aspect	Palmar fibromatosis
		Fibrolipohamartoma of median nerve
	Finger, volar aspect	Giant cell tumor of tendon sheath
	Finger, dorsal aspect (children)	Digital fibroma
	Finger, tip	Epidermoid cyst
		Glomus tumor

Table 8.7. (continued)

Location		Tumor
Lower limb	Flexor aspect, along major nerves	Schwannoma
	Thigh (older men)	Sarcoma (liposarcoma)
	Thigh (adults)	Alveolar soft part sarcoma
	Thigh (infants)	Fibrohamartoma of infancy
	Knee	Synovial hemangioma
	Knee (young, middle aged men)	Pigmented villonodular synovitis
	Knee (older men)	Lipoma arborescens
	Knee, popliteal fosa	Pigmented villonodular synovitis
		Baker's cyst
		Synovial cyst
		Ganglion cyst
		Meniscal cyst
		Nerve sheath tumors
		(Aneurysm of popliteal artery)
	Knee, tibio-fibular joint	Ganglion cyst
	Ankle	Ganglion cyst
	Foot, extensor aspect	Ganglion cyst
	Sole (young adults)	Synoviosarcoma
		Plantar fibromatosis
	Heel	Clear cell sarcoma
	Metatarsals (women)	Morton's neuroma
	Toes	Giant cell tumor of tendon sheath
Lower limb	Flexor aspect, along major nerves	Schwannoma
	Thigh (older men)	Sarcoma (liposarcoma)
	Thigh (adults)	Alveolar soft part sarcoma
	Thigh (infants)	Fibrohamartoma of infancy
	Knee	Synovial hemangioma
	Knee (young, middle aged men)	Pigmented villonodular synovitis
	Knee (older men)	Lipoma arborescens
	Knee, popliteal fosa	Pigmented villonodular synovitis
		Baker's cyst
		Synovial cyst
		Ganglion cyst
		Meniscal cyst
		Nerve sheath tumors
		(Aneurysm of popliteal artery)
	Knee, tibio-fibular joint	Ganglion cyst
	Ankle	Ganglion cyst
	Foot, extensor aspect	Ganglion cyst
	Sole (young adults)	Synoviosarcoma
		Plantar fibromatosis
	Heel	Clear cell sarcoma
	Metatarsals (women)	Morton's neuroma
	Toes	Giant cell tumor of tendon sheath
Upper and lower limbs		Fibrous histiocytoma
		Malignant fibrous histiocytoma
		(Myositis ossificans)
	Extensor aspect (young adults)	Leiomyoma
Tendons	(Achilles tendon. bilateral)	Xanthoma
		Giant cell tumor of tendon sheath
		Clear cell sarcoma
Joints, periarticular		Synovial hemangioma
		Pigmented villonodular synovitis
		Synoviosarcoma
Cutis, subcutis		Desmoid
		Neurofibroma
		Nodular fasciitis
		Dermatofibrosarcoma protuberans

Table 8.8. Distinguishing shapes of soft tissue tumors

Fusiform (ovoid)	Neurofibroma Lipoma
Dumbbell	Neurofibroma Desmoid
Moniliform	Neurofibroma
Round	Cyst Schwannoma
Serpiginous	Hemangioma
Soap bubbles	Lipoma arborescens
Nodular	Fibromatosis (plantaris, palmaris)
Branching (bilateral) finger-like, bag of worms	Plexiform neurofibroma

Table 8.9. Intratumoral signal void

Flow	Hemangioma (capillary) Arteriovenous malformation
Calcification	Hemangioma (phlebolith) Lipoma (well-differentiated and dedifferentiated) Desmoid Cartilaginous tumors Osteosarcoma of soft tissue Synoviosarcoma (poorly defined, amorphous) Chordoma Alveolar soft part sarcoma Myosilis ossificans (marginal)

Table 8.10. Fluid-fluid levels

Hemangioma
Hematoma
Cystic lymphangioma
Synoviosarcoma
Myxoma
Myositis
Metastasis

Table 8.11. Signal intensities on spin-echo sequences

High SI on T1-WI + intermediate SI on T2-WI	Lipoma Liposarcoma Lipoblastoma Hibernoma Elastofibroma Fibrolipohamartoma Metastasis of melanoma (melanin) Clear cell sarcoma (melanin)
High SI on T1-WI + high SI on T2-WI	Hemangioma Lymphangioma Subacute hematoma Myxoma Small arteriovenous malformation
Low SI on T1-WI + high SI on T2-WI	Cyst Myxoma Myxoid liposarcoma Sarcoma
Low to intermediate SI on T1-WI + low SI on T2-Wl	Desmoid and other fibromatoses Pigmented villonodular synovitis Morton's neuroma Fibrolipohamartoma Giant cell tumor of tendon sheath Acute hematoma (few days) Old hematoma Xanthoma High flow arteriovenous malformation Mineralized mass Scar tissue Amyloidosis
Intermediate SI on T1-WI + high SI on T2-WI	Neurogenic tumor Desmoid

Table 8.12. Multiplicity

Venous malformation
Lipoma (5%–8%)
Lipoma of tendon sheath (50%)
Desmoid
Neurofibroma
Myxoma
Metastasis
Dermatofibrosarcoma protuberans
Kaposi's sarcoma

Table 8.13. Concomitant diseases

Concomitant osseous involvement	Pigmented villonodular synovitis Lymphoma Desmoid Angiomatosis Parosteal lipoma
Concomitant osseous involvement + nodular soft-tissue tumors	Infantile myofibromatosis
	Infantile fibromatosis Fibrosarcoma multiforme
Concomitant osseous involvement + nodular soft-tissue tumors + hypertrophic gingiva + flexion contractures + acroosteolysis	Juvenile hyalin fibromatosis
Maffucci's disease	Cavernous hemangioma(s)
Fibrous dysplasia (Mazabraud)	Myxoma(s)
Neurofibromatosis	Schwannoma(s) Neurofibroma(s)
Gardner's syndrome	Fibromatosis
Dupuytren's disease (flexion contractures)	Palmar fibromatosis
Macrodystrophia lipomatosa of the digits –	Fibrolipohamartoma of the median nerve
Familial hypercholesterolemia	Xanthoma
Normolipidemia + lymphoma or granuloma	Cutaneous xanthoma
Turner's syndrome	Lymphangioma
Noonan's syndrome	
Fetal alcohol syndrome	
Down's syndrome	
Familial pterygium colli	
Diabetes + degenerative joint disease + trauma	Lipoma arborescens
Multiple myeloma	Amyloidosis

Further Reading

Aström M, Gentz CF, Nilsson P et al (1996) Imaging in chronic achilles tendinopathy. Skeletal Radiol 25:615–620

Baur A, Reiser M.F. (2000) Diffusion-weighted imaging of the musculoskeletal system in humans. Skeletal Radiol 29: 555–562

Berquist T, Ehman R, King B, Hodgman C, Ilstrup D (1990) Value of MR imaging in differentiating benign from malignant soft-tissue masses: study of 95 lesions. Am J Roentgenol 155: 251–1255

Bloem JL, van der Woude HJ, Geirnaerdt M et al (1997) Does magnetic resonance imaging make a difference for patients with musculoskeletal sarcoma? Br J Radiol 70:327–337

Bohndorf K (1997/1998) Differential diagnosis of bone marrow edema. In: Musculoskeletal MRI, Erasmus Course on MRI. Birmingham, pp 13–16

Bohndorf K, Imhof H, Pope TL (2001) Musculoskeletal imaging. Thieme, Stuttgart, pp 230–231

Cerofolini E, Landi A, Desantis G, Maiorana A, Canossi G, Romagnoli R (1991) MR of benign peripheral nerve sheath tumors. J Comput Assist Tomogr 15:593–597

De Beuckeleer LH, De Schepper AM, Ramon F, Somville J (1995) Magnetic resonance imaging of cartilaginous tumors: a retrospective study of 79 patients. Eur J Radiol 21:34–40

De Schepper AM, Parizel PM, De Beuckeleer L, Vanhoenacker F (eds) (2001) Imaging of soft-tissue tumors. Springer, Berlin Heidelberg New York

Erlemann R, Sciuk J, Bosse A et al (1990) Response of osteosarcoma and Ewing sarcoma to preoperative chemotherapy: assessment with dynamic and static MR imaging and skeletal scintigraphy. Radiology 175:791–796

Fletcher B, Hanna S, Fairclough D, Gronemeyer S (1992) Pediatric musculoskeletal tumors: use of dynamic contrast-enhanced MR imaging to monitor response to chemotherapy. Radiology 184:243–248

Gielen JL, Vanholsbeeck MT (1990) Growing bone cysts in long-term hemodialysis. Skeletal Radiol 19:43–49

Golfieri R, Baddeley H, Pringle JS, Souhami R (1990) The role of the STIR sequence in magnetic resonance examination of bone tumours. Br J Radiol 63:251–256

Gronemeyer SA, Kauffman WM, Rocha MS et al (1997) Fat-saturated contrast-enhanced T1-weighted MRI in evaluation of osteosarcoma and Ewing sarcoma. J Magn Reson Imaging 7:585–589

Hermann G, Abdelwahab I, Miller T, Klein M, Lewis M (1992) Tumour and tumour-like conditions of the soft tissue: magnetic resonance imaging features differentiating benign form malignant masses. Br J Radiol 65:14–20

Imhof H, Breitenseher M, Haller J, Kainberger F, Tratting S (1998) Tendinous diseases. In: Masciocchi C (ed) Radiological imaging of sports injuries. Springer, Berlin Heidelberg New York, pp 49–63

Janzen L, Logan PM, O'Connell JX et al (1997) Intramedullary chondroid tumors of bone: correlation of abnormal peritumoral marrow and soft-tissue MRI signal with tumor type. Skeletal Radiol 26:100–106

Khoury NJ, El-Khoury GY, Saltzman CL et al (1996) MR Imaging of posterior tibial tendon dysfunction. Am J Roentgenol 167:675–682

Kransdorf M (1995) Benign soft tissue tumors in a large referral population: distribution of specific diagnoses by age, sex and location. Am J Roentgenol 164:395–402

Kransdorf M (1995) Malignant soft tissue tumors in a large referral population: distribution of specific diagnoses by age, sex and location. Am J Roentgenol 164:129–134

Kransdorf M, Jelinek J, Moser R (1993) Imaging of soft tissue tumors. Radiol Clin North Am 31:359–372

Lang P, Grampp S, Vahlensieck M et al (1995) Primary bone tumors: value of MR angiography for preoperative planning and monitoring response to chemotherapy. Am J Roentgenol 165:135–142

Lang P, Wendland MF, Saeed M et al (1998) Osteogenic sarcoma: noninvasive in vivo assessment of tumor necrosis with diffusion-weighted MR imaging. Radiology 206:227–235

Ma LD, Frassica FJ, Scott WW Jr et al (1995) Differentiation of benign and malignant musculoskeletal tumors: potential pitfalls with MR imaging. Radiographics 15:349–366

Ma LD, Frassica FJ, McCarthy EF et al (1997) Benign and malignant musculoskeletal masses: MR imaging differentiation with rim-to-center differential enhancement ratios. Radiology 202:739–744

Major NM, Helms CA (1997) Pelvic stress injuries: the relationship between osteitis pubis and sacroiliac abnormalities in athletes. Skeletal Radiol 26:711–717

McLoughlin RF, Raber EL, Vellet AD et al (1995) Patellar tendinitis: MR imaging features, with suggested pathogenesis and proposed classification. Radiology 197:843–848

McNally EG, Goodman R (2000) The role of MRI in the assessment of scaphoid fracture healing: a pilot study Eur Radiol 10: 1926–1928

McNamara MT, Greco A (1998) The role of MR imaging in sports injuries of the muscles. In: Masciocchi C (ed) Radiological imaging of sports injuries. Springer, Berlin Heidelberg New York, pp 31–47

Miller T, Potter H, McCormack R (1994) Benign soft tissue masses of the wrist and hand: MRI appearances. Skeletal Radiol 23:327–332

Miyanishi K, Yamamoto T (2001) Subchondral changes in transient osteoporosis of the hip. Skeletal Radiol 30:255–261

Morrison W B, Carrino JA (2001) Subtendinous bone marrow edema patterns on MR images of the ankle: association with symptoms and tendinopathy. AJR 176:1149–1154

Moulton J, Blebea J, Dunco D, Braley S, Bisset G, Emery K (1995) MR imaging of soft tissue masses: diagnostic efficacy and value of distinguishing between benign and malignant lesions. Am J Roentgenol 164:1191–1199

Panuel M, Gentet JC, Scheiner C et al (1993) Physeal and epiphyseal extent of primary malignant bone tumors in childhood. Correlation of preoperative MRI and the pathologic examination. Pediatr Radiol 23:421–424

Parizel PM, Wilmink JT (1998) Imaging of the spine: techniques and indications. In: Algra PR, Valk J, Heimans JJ (eds) Diagnosis and therapy of spinal tumors. (Medical radiology. Diagnostic imaging and radiation oncology.) Springer, Berlin Heidelberg New York, pp 15–48

Peterfy CG, Linares R, Steinbach L (1994) Recent advances in magnetic resonance imaging of the musculoskeletal system. Radiol Clin North Am 32:291–311

Pöyhiä T, Azouz EM (2000) MR imaging evaluation of subacute and chronic bone abcesses in children. Pediatr Radiol 30:763–768

Potter HG, Hannafin JA, Morwesse RM et al (1995) Lateral epicondylitis: correlation of MR imaging, surgical and histopathological findings. Radiology 196:43–46

Richardson ML, Zink-Brody GC, Patten RM et al (1996) MR characterization of post-irradiation soft tissue edema. Skeletal Radiol 25:537–543

Sanders TG, Medynski MA (2000) Bone contusion patterns of the knee at MR imaging: footprint of the mechanism of injury. Radiographics 20:135–151

Seiderer M (1995) Musculoskeletal applications: soft tissue. In: Rinck P (ed) The rational use of magnetic resonance imaging. Blackwell Science, Oxford, pp 201–216

Seo GS, Aoki J, Kazakida O, Sone S, Ishii K (1997) Ischiopubic insufficiency fractures: MRI appearances. Skeletal Radiol 26:705–710

Slavotinek JP, Coates PT (2000) Shoulder appearances at MR imaging in long-term dialysis recipients. Radiology 217:539–543

Stevens SK, Moore SG, Kaplan ID (1990) Early and late bone-marrow changes after irradiation: MR evaluation. Am J Roentgenol 154:745–750

Stoller DW (1997) Magnetic resonance imaging in orthopaedics and sports medicine. Lippincott-Raven, Philadelphia

Sundaram M, McLeod R (1990) MR imaging of tumor and tumor-like lesions of bone and soft tissue. Am J Roentgenol 155:817–824

Swan JS, Grist TM, Sproat IA et al (1995) Musculoskeletal neoplasms: preoperative evaluation with MR angiography. Radiology 194:519–524

Vanel D, Lacombe MJ, Couanet D et al (1987) Musculoskeletal tumors: follow-up with MR imaging after treatment with surgery and radiation therapy. Radiology 164:243–245

Vanel D, Verstraete KL, Shapeero LG (1997) Primary tumors of the musculoskeletal system. Radiol Clin North Am 35:213–237

Wang X (2001) Additional value of Magnetic Resonance Imaging (MRI) in the diagnosis of bone tumors: a comparative study between radiography and MRI. Thesis presented to obtain Master degree in Medical Sciences at the 'Universitaire Instelling Antwerpen'. Promoter: Prof Dr A De Schepper

Wolf RE, Enneking WF (1996) The staging and surgery of musculoskeletal neoplasms. Pediatr Orthoped Oncol 27:473–481

Upper Abdomen: Liver, Pancreas, Biliary System, and Spleen

9

P. Reimer, B. Tombach

Contents

9.1 General Clinical Indications

Magnetic resonance (MR) imaging is a widely used modality for the evaluation of diffuse liver disease and the detection as well as further characterization of focal liver disease. Compared with spiral-computed tomography (CT), multislice CT, and ultrasound, MRI was considered more of a problem-solving tool for the pancreas and spleen. However, recent developments have changed this view, with MRI presenting a comprehensive but also more complex approach compared with other imaging modalities. In particular, the biliary system requires clinical attention because of its noninvasive and unenhanced visualization of the biliary tree and pancreatic ducts compared with invasive endoscopic retrograde cholangiopancreatography (ERCP).

9.2 Coils

Patients are scanned in the supine position (feet or headfirst) with either the body coil, which is implemented in every system inside the magnet bore, or preferably a phased-array coil. Phased-array coils combine a number of small coils, typically positioned anterior and posterior to the patient and wrapped together (wrap-around coil), providing a higher signal-to-noise ratio and a better image quality. These coils increase the hardware costs, depending on the vendor and the amount of data acquired, which increases the demand for better data processing and storage capacity. Since the anteroposterior diameter of patients varies considerably, scanning technicians need to adjust the signal amplification of the middle third of the body specifically to the individual's anteroposterior diameter to avoid a layering effect with a higher signal towards the coil and a lower signal towards the middle of the body. The inhomogeneous signal within phased-array coils makes signal measurements for signal quantification more difficult than within the body coil.

9.3 Pulse Sequences

The minimum protocol for the parenchymal organs of the upper abdomen consists of two-dimensional (2D) or 3D T1-weighted (T1-W) and 2D or 3D T2-W sequences obtained in the axial plane. The section thickness varies from 4 mm to 8 mm for the liver and spleen, 2 mm to 4 mm for the pancreas, and 1 mm to 4 mm for vessels and cholangiopancreatography. Breathing-related movements are the major source of artifacts of the upper abdomen, and a variety of compensatory techniques have been developed, such as respiratory compensation, cranial, caudal, and anterior saturation pulses, multiple averaging, fat suppression, and navigator echoes. An effective technique is to use breathhold sequences with acquisition times of 25 s or less, combined with cranial and caudal saturation pulses to further minimize pulsation artifacts. Typically, an expiratory breathhold is performed to ensure reproducible slice positioning. If the patients cannot suspend respiration for around 20 s, a non-breathhold sequence with multiple averaging and saturation pulses is preferable. Fat suppression may be applied with both T1-W and T2-W pulse sequences, using the available technology for fat suppression on each scanner; this provides more advantages for the pancreas and biliary system than for the liver and spleen.

Breathhold spoiled gradient-echo (GRE) sequences, such as fast low-angle shot imaging (FLASH), are preferable for T1-W imaging (T1-WI) and are referred to within the text. The echo time (TE) of spoiled GRE sequences should be chosen close to in-phase (1.0 T: 6.9 ms and 1.5 T: 4.6 ms) and out-of-phase (1.0 T: 3.45 ms and 1.5 T: 2.3 ms) to characterize fatty tissue. TE close to optimal in-phase echo-times may be used, depending on specific pulse-sequence optimization strategies. Current sequences allow for coverage of the entire liver during a single breathhold at the cost of some artifacts, because the increase in the number of sections is typically achieved by applying the spoiler pulses just before acquisition of the data set and not before each phase-encoding step (see also Chapter 1). More recently, 3D T1-W spoiled GRE sequences with fat saturation have been developed, allowing the acquisition of even thinner sections of the order of 3–4 mm at the cost of some artifacts (see Chapter 1). T1-W sequences are combined with extracellular gadolinium-chelates (Magnevist®, Dotarem®, Omniscan®, ProHance®, or Gadovist®), paramagnetic hepatobiliary agents (Teslascan® or MultiHance®), and superparamagnetic iron oxides (Endorem® or Resovist®). In this chapter, the use of clinically approved agents will be referred to (see also Chapter 2).

Table 9.1. Pulse sequence recommendations for the upper abdomen

Pulse sequence	WI	Plane	No. of sections	TR (ms)	TE (ms)	Time delay (ms)	Flip angle	Echo train length	Section thickness (mm)	Matrix	FOV	No. of acq.	Acq. time
MR imaging:													
FLASH breath-hold	T1	Axial	10–20	100–200	4.1 (1.5 T)		60–90°		3–10	128×256	300–450	1	<25 s
In-phase FLASH breath-hold	T1	Axial	10–20	100–200	4.6 (1.5 T) 6.9 (1 T)		60–90°		3–10	128×256	300–450	1	<25 s
Out-of-phase FLASH breath-hold	T1	Axial	10–20	100–200	2.3 (1.5 T) 3.45 (1 T)		60–90°		3–10	128×256	300–450	1	<25 s
3D out-of-phase FS-breath-hold FLASH	T1	Axial	20–40	<10	2–3 (1.5 T)		10–20°		2–6	128×256	300–450	1	<25 s
SE/TSE non-breath-hold	T2	Axial	15–20	>2500	1:40–100 2:150–200		<180°	<12	3–10	128×256	300–450	2–6	>4 min
TSE breath-hold	T2	Axial	5–15	<4000	75–150		<180°	>20	5–10	100×256	300–450	1	<20 s
HASTE breath-hold	T2	Axial	15–20	<10	50–100	800–1000	<180°	>128	5–10	128×256	300–450	1	<25 s
True-FISP breath-hold	T2	Axial or coronal	10–20	<10	2 –5 (1.5 T)		60–90°	>128	5–30	256×256	300–450	1	<25 s
MR angiography:													
3D CE-MRA	T1	Coronal	=40	=5	=2		20–50°		=2	>128×256	300–450	1	<25 s
2D TOF	T1	Axial or coronal	1–3	5–10	2–10		20–50°		=5	>128×256	300–450	1	<5 s
MR cholangiopancreatography													
2D HASTE	T2	Coronal	<20	<20	>50		<180°	>128	=5	128×256	300–450	1	<30 s
3D TSE (respiratory triggered)	T2	Axial or coronal	10–20	>3000	>500		<180°	>128	1–10	128×256	300–450	1	>5 min
3D TSE (thick slab)	T2	Coronal	1 slab	>3000	>500		<180°	>128	50–100	128×256	300–450	1	<20 s

The FOV is individually adjusted to the patient using rectangular FOV, and the section thickness depends on the organ or pathology imaged. *WI* weighting of images, *Matrix* phase × frequency matrix, *Acq.* acquisition(s)

A variety of sequences are available for T2-WI. Turbo spin-echo imaging (TSE) is widely preferred over SE with different options for breathhold and non-breathhold sequences. However, conventional SE still represents a diagnostic standard for T2-WI of the liver and can be used with a 128×256 matrix, cranial and caudal saturation pulses, two acquisitions, and fat saturation. Breathhold TSE sequences use increasing numbers of echoes per TR (echo train length 'ETL') to decrease the acquisition time at the same anatomical resolution or increase the anatomical resolution at the same temporal resolution. However, the use of sequences with increasing ETL with numerous 180° refocussing pulses also decreases the susceptibility weighting, which is an important contributor to lesion contrast within parenchymal organs. Therefore, TSE sequences may provide lower lesion contrast for solid lesions than conventional SE sequences, but this disadvantage may be compensated by an increased image quality. Thus, non-breathhold sequences with a limited number of echoes but stronger susceptibility weighting are still relevant for clinical MR imaging and provide stable image quality. Breathhold, multishot, rapid-acquisition relation enhancement imaging (RARE) sequences have been recently improved by using fast read-outs, half-Fourier acquisitions, and single-shot half-Fourier TSE (HASTE) techniques and are becoming clinically useful. T2-W sequences with susceptibility weighting are combined with superparamagnetic iron oxides and will be referred to in this chapter.

MR angiography of the portal-venous system, supplying the visceral arteries and visceral veins, is increasingly performed with contrast-enhanced MR angiography (CE-MRA) techniques that utilize a combination of gadolinium-chelates and breathhold, coronal, 3D, nonspoiled GRE sequences as described in Chapters 1 and 13. Clinically approved low-molecular-weight gadolinium-chelates are intravenously injected by means of power injectors following calculation or automatic measurement of the individual bolus transit time. This technique requires fast gradients and is available mainly on high-field systems (≧1 T). Alternatively, plain breathhold axial or coronal 2D TOF sequences, which may also be combined with superparamagnetic iron oxides, are suited for imaging of the intrahepatic vasculature and vasculature of the upper abdomen. Individual angiographic sections should always be viewed together with postprocessed maximum intensity projection (MIP) angiograms. More recently, balanced nonspoiled GRE sequences have gained particular importance (true-FISP [Siemens] or balanced FFE [Philips]). Typically acquired as 2D sequences, this technique provides bright vessels almost irrespective of the flow direction and velocity as well as bright fluid-filled structures. Therefore, these sequences are useful in demonstrating the patency of a vessel without the use of contrast agents. This technique also requires fast gradients and is available mainly on newer high-field systems (≧1 T).

MR cholangiopancreatography (MRCP) has been improved with the refinement of TSE/FSE/HASTE pulse sequences. Current approaches differ according to scanner technology and use predominantly either breathhold 2D sequences or non-breathhold and often respiratory-triggered 3D sequences. Intraductal fluid is visualized bright, based on long TE compared with background tissues, which have already lost their signal. Individual sections should always be viewed together with postprocessed MIP cholangiograms and pancreaticograms.

Table 9.1 provides general guidelines for sequence parameters which are discussed further in the text (see also Chapter 1).

9.4 Liver

9.4.1 Liver Anatomy

The liver demonstrates higher SI (SI) on T1-W sequences and lower SI on T2-W sequences than the spleen. SI from normal parenchyma is homogeneous on both sequences (Fig. 9.1).

9.4.2 Contrast Agents for Liver MRI

Nonspecific, low-molecular-weight, extracellular gadolinium-chelates are currently most frequently used for contrast-enhanced liver MR imaging and are useful in characterizing liver disease. These compounds behave pharmacologically similarly to iodinated X-ray contrast agents and can be bolus injected to perform dynamic studies using multisection spoiled GRE techniques with approximately 20–25 sections in a single breathhold.

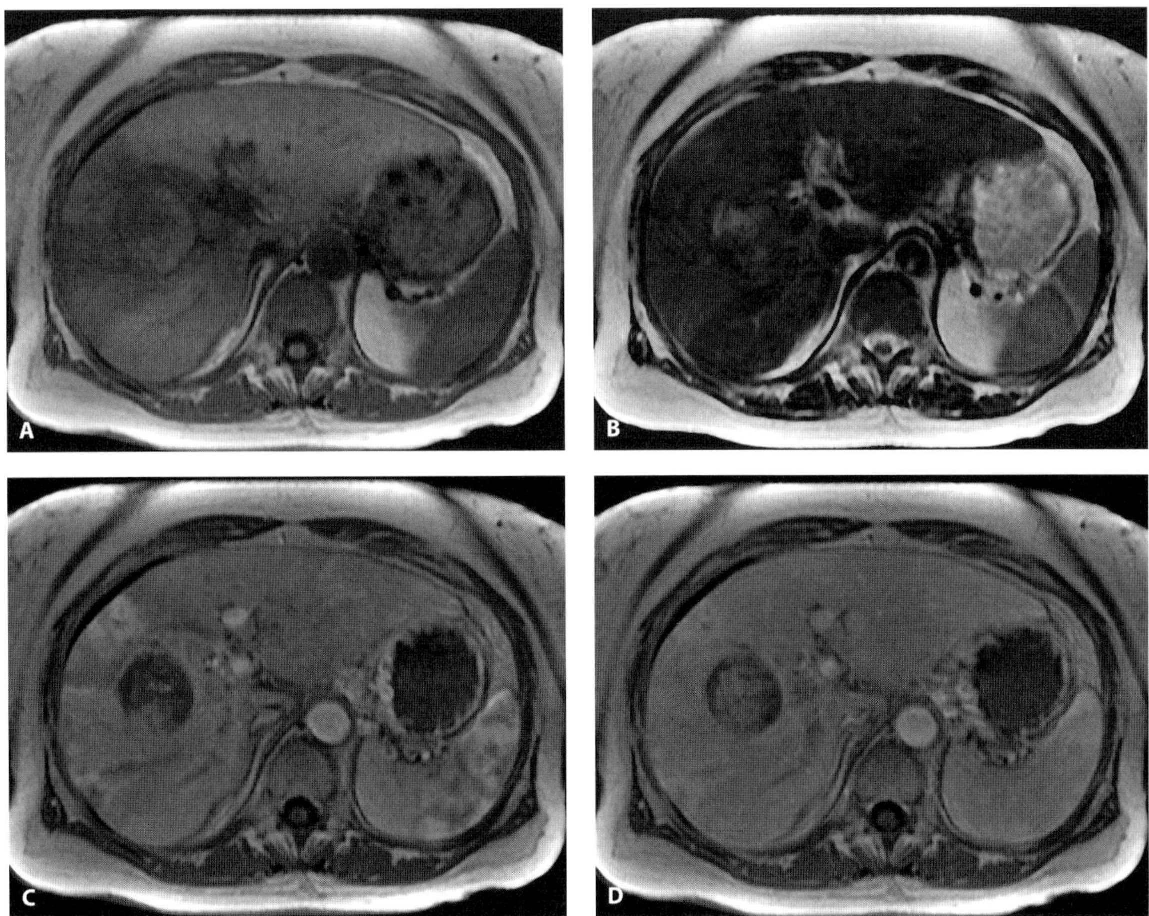

Fig. 9.1A–D. Perfusion defect in the right liver lobe. Plain T1-W spoiled GRE (**A**), T2-W TSE (TE 138 ms) (**B**), arterial phase, gadolinium-enhanced, T1-W spoiled GRE (**C**), and portal venous phase, gadolinium-enhanced, T1-W spoiled GRE (**D**) show a large mass in the right liver lobe with a perfusion defect. The biopsy-proven intrahepatic cholangiocarcinoma demonstrates low SI on T1-WI (**A**), slightly high SI on T2-WI (**B**), and peripheral contrast enhancement (**C**,**D**). The mass compresses the right portal vein, which causes a wedge-shaped portal perfusion defect. The liver parenchyma within the perfusion defect enhances more strongly during the capillary phase due to a relative increase in the arterial supply compared with liver parenchyma that has normal portal perfusion (**C**). The difference in parenchymal enhancement fades away on portal venous phase images (**D**)

Gadolinium-enhanced images can be interpreted very similarly to contrast-enhanced CT images, because gadolinium shortens the T1-relaxation time, resulting in tissue signal enhancement on T1-WI (Fig. 9.1). Contrast timing requires the acquisition of arterial phase (20–30 s following injection) images to detect and characterize hypervascular lesions [focal nodular hyperplasia (FNH), adenoma, hepatocellular carcinoma (HCC), hypervascular metastases: renal cell cancer, islet-cell tumors, carcinoid, pheochromocytoma, etc.]. In the arterial phase, contrast material is present in the visceral arteries, with strong enhancement of the pancreas and renal cortex without opacification of the hepatic veins. The normal spleen should show an arciform or serpiginous enhancement pattern (see Sect. 9.9). Portal phase images (50–90 s following injection) demonstrate strong parenchymal enhancement to detect hypovascular lesions with best conspicuity during this phase (Fig. 9.2). Equilibrium phase images acquired more than 2 min following injection (up to 10 min) result in a diffuse enhancement that can be useful to allow hemangiomas to fill in and inflammatory changes to enhance.

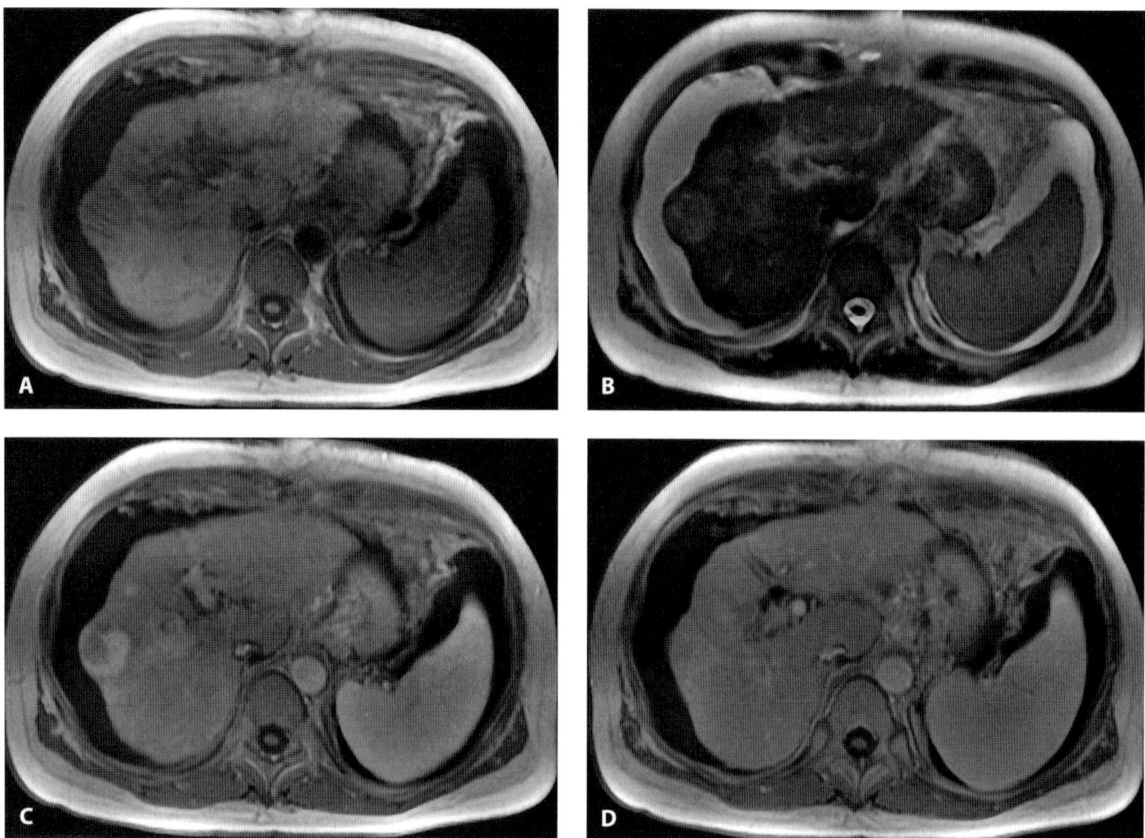

Fig. 9.2A–D. Hepatocellular carcinoma (HCC) in chronic hepatitis C with liver cirrhosis. Plain T1-W spoiled GRE (**A**), T2-W HASTE (TE 64 ms) (**B**), arterial phase, gadolinium-enhanced, T1-W spoiled GRE (**C**), and portal venous phase, gadolinium-enhanced, T1-W spoiled GRE (**D**) of a patient with HCC following chronic hepatitis C with liver cirrhosis, portal hypertension, and ascites. A mildly hypointense lesion on T1-W spoiled GRE (**A**) and mildly hyperintense lesion on T2-W HASTE (**B**) are depicted in the lateral right liver lobe. The liver demonstrates higher SI than the spleen on T1-W sequences and lower SI than the spleen on T2-W sequences. Liver cirrhosis with hypertrophy of the left lobe, splenomegaly, and ascites is present. Arterial phase images demonstrate the hypervascularity of the lesion already visible on plain images and two additional enhancing smaller lesions anterior to the larger lesion (**C**) with decreasing contrast on portal venous phase images (**D**). Imaging findings were confirmed following liver transplantation

Liver-specific intracellular contrast agents have been developed to further improve liver imaging, and some of them are already clinically available. The first clinically approved paramagnetic hepatobiliary agent Teslascan® (mangofodipir trisodium, formerly known as Mn-DPDP) is partially excreted into the bile following uptake into hepatocytes and causes an increase of SI on T1-WI. In Europe, Teslascan® is drip-infused, and therefore, dynamic scanning cannot be performed. The compound enhances the liver parenchyma and was advocated to differentiate tumors of hepatocellular origin from nonhepatocellular origin. However, the specificity for differentiation of hepatocellular tumors is lower than expected. Since tumors of nonhepatocellular origin show nonspecific intratumoral enhancement, a second MR study with a time delay of several hours (typically 1 day) is required to allow for diffusion of the contrast agent out of the intratumoral interstitium. A perilesional rim may be visible, and small metastases may be detected only on these images. A second compound with comparable enhancement characteristics on T1-WI, MultiHance® (gadobenate dimeglumine), is clinically available for liver imaging but has gained more attention for vascular imaging as off-label use. The compound can be bolus injected, and imaging studies may be designed as described for nonspecific gadolinium compounds combined with delayed scans some hours later for tumor detection because of nonspecific uptake in focal liver lesions (see Chapter 2). A third compound, Gd-EOB-DTPA, should become available in the near future. This compound is associated with a strong biliary excretion and can be bolus injected with imaging studies as described for nonspecific gadolinium compounds combined with delayed scans as early as 20 min postinjection (see Chapter 2).

Superparamagnetic iron-oxide particles (SPIO) accumulate efficiently within minutes of administration within phagocytic cells in the liver (approximately 80%) and in the spleen (5%–10% of the injected dose). Malignant tumors are typically devoid of a substantial number of phagocytic cells appearing as hyperintense/bright lesions in a hypointense/black liver on T2-W sequences. Tumors with a substantial number of phagocytic cells, such as focal nodular hyperplasia, hepatocellular adenoma, well-differentiated hepatocellular carcinoma, hypervascular metastases, and/or a significant blood pool (hemangiomas) may show sufficient uptake of SPIO and, thus, decrease in SI on T2-W sequences. The signal decrease is related to the Kupffer cell activity and tumor vascularity. Clinically approved Endorem® is currently administered by drip infusion in glucose or saline at a dose of 10–15 µmol Fe/kg body weight over 30 min with a flow rate of approximately 3 ml/min, since side-effects (facial flush, dyspnea, rash, lumbar pain) occur at higher injection rates. The patient is then brought back into the magnet, typically on the same day, with a large time-window of several hours to acquire postcontrast images. Resovist® is bolus-injectable and has been clinically available for liver MR imaging in Europe since 2001. Patients may either be scanned within one session or up to 1–4 days postcontrast (see also Chapter 2).

Ultrasmall SPIO particles (USPIO; Sinerem®) have a longer blood half-life and accumulate primarily in the liver, spleen, bone marrow, and lymph nodes. Since USPIO have a stronger T1 effect than SPIO and a longer blood half-life, they can also be used as T1 (brightening) blood-pool agents for MR angiography or liver lesion characterization. Well-perfused lesions increase in SI on T1-W images and decrease in SI on T2-W images. Thus, USPIO yields information regarding the vascular nature of liver lesions during accumulation phase images. This compound is under phase-3 clinical investigation and may become available within the near future (see also Chapter 2).

9.5 Liver Pathology – Diffuse Liver Disease

9.5.1 Fatty Liver

Fatty liver may cause severe problems with ultrasound (US) and CT by obscuring focal lesions; however, MRI is very effective in fatty liver since fat contributes to the SI, and a signal from fat can be eliminated selectively (fat suppression). The follow-up of patients with chemotherapy-induced fatty liver suspicious of metastases is therefore best evaluated by MRI. High signal on T1-WI and decreasing signal with fat-suppression techniques prove the presence of fat. Out-of-phase GRE techniques are clinically useful to differentiate focal fatty infiltration and focal sparing in diffuse fatty infiltration from mass lesions. Some lesions have to be considered for differential diagnoses. Well-differentiated HCC is typically better delineated and often encapsulated with spotted areas of fat. Hepatic adenoma can be differentiated by strong early enhancement following gadolinium injection, by late enhancement following infusion of hepatobiliary agents such as Teslascan®, or by late enhancement on delayed images following infusion or injection of SPIO (Fig. 9.3). Hemorrhage, melanin, protein, and copper may also cause increased signal on T1-WI (see Chapter 3).

9.5.2 Cirrhosis

Liver cirrhosis is characterized by irreversible fibrosis with destruction of the hepatic architecture. Atrophy of the right liver lobe and the medial segment of the left liver lobe with consecutive hypertrophy of the lateral segment of the left lobe and caudate lobe is frequently present. An irregular parenchymal pattern is often also present (Fig. 9.2). Regenerative nodules develop from heterogeneous regeneration and dysplasia. MR imaging is superior to CT and US in depicting regenerative nodules, which present with lower SI compared to the cirrhotic liver on T2-WI. SPIO-enhanced and gadolinium-

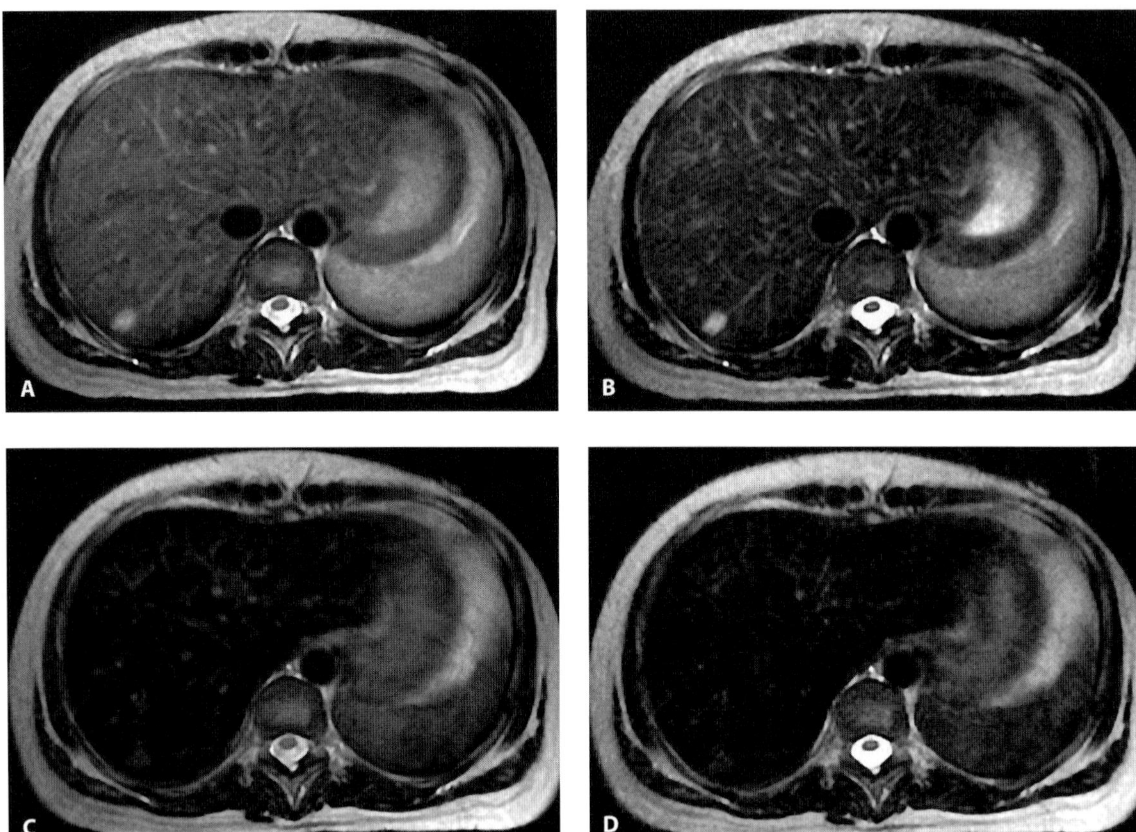

Fig. 9.3A–D. Liver adenoma. T2-W TSE images before (**A**: TE 83 ms and **B**: TE 165 ms) and 10 min following intravenous injection of 10 µmol Fe/kg body weight (Resovist) (**C**: TE 83 ms and **D**: TE 165 ms). The focal lesion in the dorsal part of the right liver lobe decreases slightly in signal at the longer echo-time on precontrast T2-W images (**A,B**). The lesion significantly decreases in SI on postcontrast T2-W images (**C,D**). Imaging was performed for tumor staging in a young woman with breast cancer and subsequent biopsy to rule out a hypervascular metastasis which revealed a liver adenoma

enhanced MR imaging can be used to differentiate regenerative nodules with higher SI on T2-WI compared to HCC. Regenerative nodules appear hypointense on early gadolinium-enhanced T1-WI and reveal a substantial uptake of SPIO, resulting in a signal decrease, which is rarely observed in well-differentiated HCC.

Liver cirrhosis is the most common cause of portal hypertension due to a sinusoidal obstruction with subsequent complications, such as variceal bleed, ascites, and splenomegaly (Fig. 9.2). The normal hepatopetal flow may reverse in severe cirrhosis and become hepatofugal, which can be easily demonstrated by MR flow measurements. Portal varices and shunts (splenorenal, splenocaval, etc.) are demonstrated by true-FISP, PC-MR, TOF-MR, and gadolinium-enhanced MR angiography.

9.5.3 Iron Overload

The signal appearance of iron overload is similar to postcontrast SPIO-enhanced images with low SI on T2/T2*-WI. Severe iron overload may also lead to low SI on T1-WI (Fig. 9.4). MR imaging is the most sensitive imaging technique to demonstrate iron overload, with muscle and fat serving as inherent reference tissues. Hepatic iron overload is caused either by idiopathic

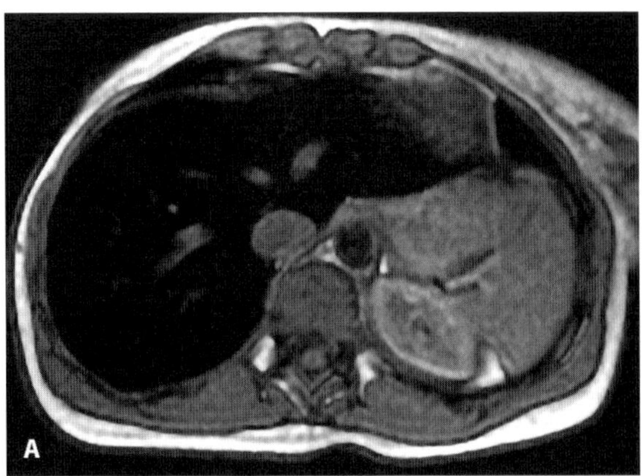

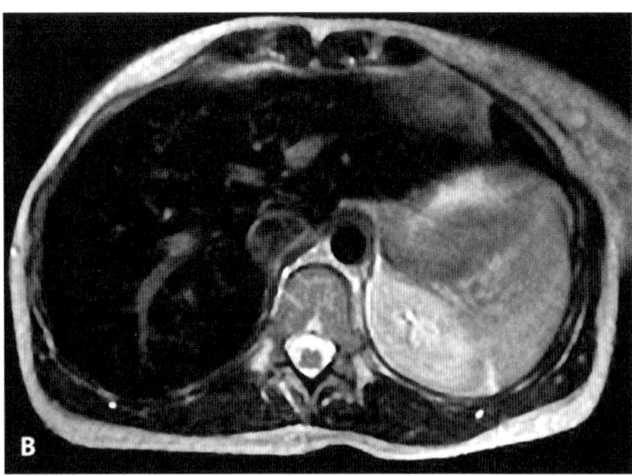

Fig. 9.4A,B. Idiopathic hemochromatosis. Plain T1-W spoiled GRE (TE 5 ms) (**A**) and T2-W TSE (TE 90 ms) (**B**) in a 23-year-old patient. The liver demonstrates low SI on T1-W and T2-W sequences without a signal decrease within the pancreas, heart, or spleen. No signs of liver cirrhosis are present

(primary) hemochromatosis, transfusional iron overload, hemolytic anemia, or associated with liver cirrhosis.

Idiopathic hemochromatosis results from increased absorption and accumulation of dietary iron, affecting primarily the liver, pancreas, and heart. Iron accumulation can be fatal due to the development of liver cirrhosis, HCC, diabetes mellitus, and cardiomyopathy. Iron accumulation starts in the liver; it should be diagnosed early, since therapy before accumulation in the pancreas and heart may result in a normal life expectancy. The spleen is typically spared, and involvement of the pancreas typically presents when liver cirrhosis has already developed. Patients with liver cirrhosis are at risk of HCC, and nonsiderotic nodules in patients with hemochromatosis should be considered as malignant until proven otherwise. Regenerative nodules contain iron and have a lower SI than HCC, which also serves as a test by means of SPIO-enhanced MR imaging to differentiate regenerative nodules from HCC in patients with liver cirrhosis but without iron overload. However, hepatocellular iron may also be mildly increased in patients with liver cirrhosis. Dysplastic nodules or adenomatous hyperplasia may show variable iron uptake and thus, may also appear as relatively bright lesions within the hypointense liver as a differential diagnosis to HCC.

Transfusional iron overload with iron deposition in the reticuloendothelial system (RES) of the liver, spleen, and bone marrow spares hepatocytes, pancreas, heart, and other parenchyma. Unless severe iron overload is present at later stages of the disease, involvement of the spleen (transfusional iron overload) versus the pancreas (idiopathic hemochromatosis) helps to differentiate RES iron from hepatocellular iron overload.

Hemolytic anemias frequently require blood transfusions, and, therefore, a coexisting transfusional iron overload may develop. Patients with thalassemia vera without transfusions but with increased absorption of dietary iron may develop erythrogenic hemochromatosis, primarily affecting the liver. Filtration and tubular absorption of free hemoglobin in sickle cell anemia explain the decreased signal of the renal cortex. Paroxysmal nocturnal hemoglobinuria often leads to iron overload in the liver and renal cortex.

9.5.4 Vascular Liver Disease

Portal thrombosis may occur in malignant liver tumors (HCC), coagulopathies (cirrhosis), inflammation (pancreatitis), or extrinsic compression (CCC, metastases, lymphomas, etc.) of portal veins and may lead to a cavernous transformation of the portal vein (Fig. 9.5). Higher signal on T2-WI and enhancement on T1-W gadolinium images typically characterize tumor thrombus. Bland thrombus (see Chapter 3) shows a lower signal on T2-WI and no gadolinium enhancement. Areas with decreased portal perfusion are usually wedge-

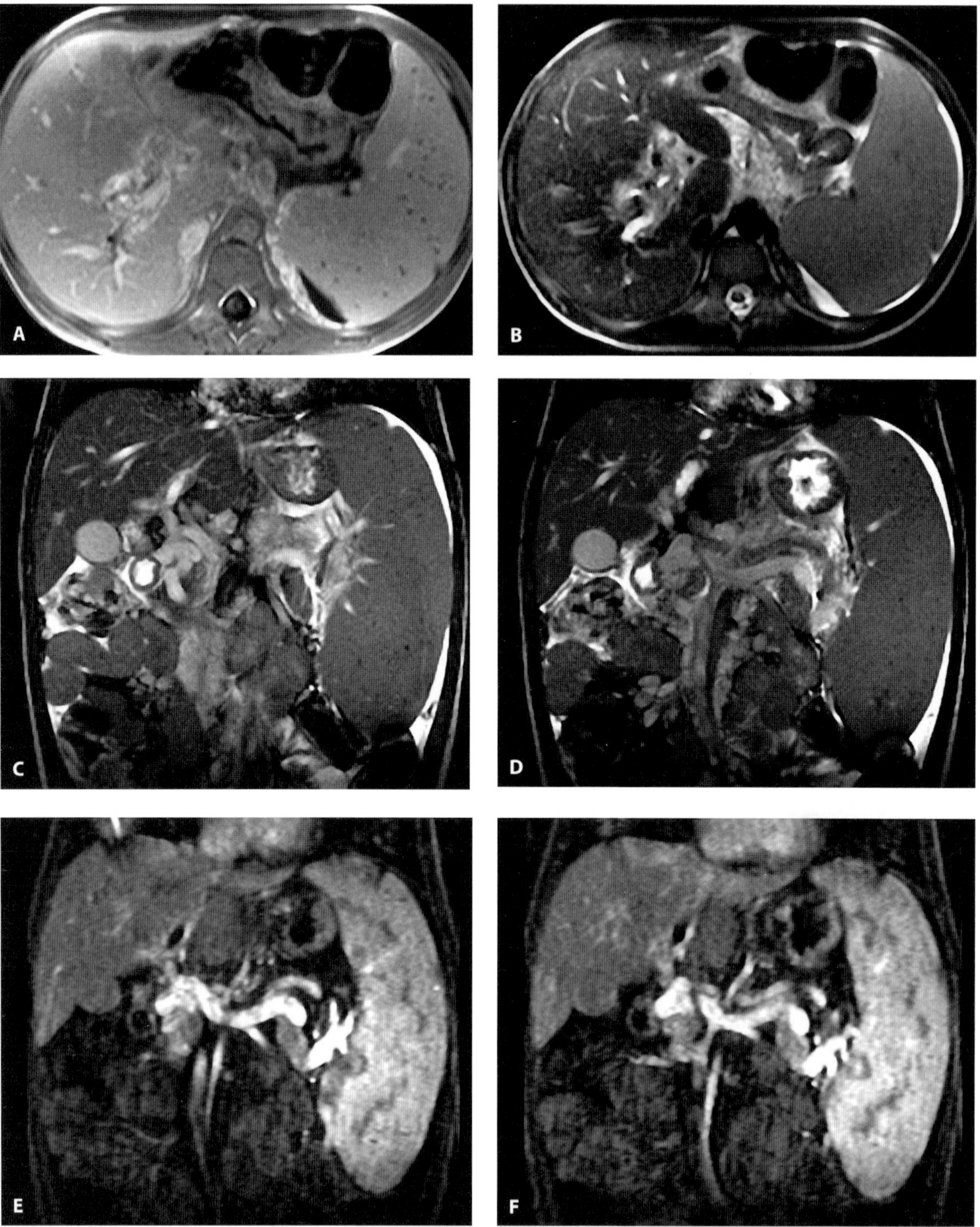

Fig. 9.5A–F.

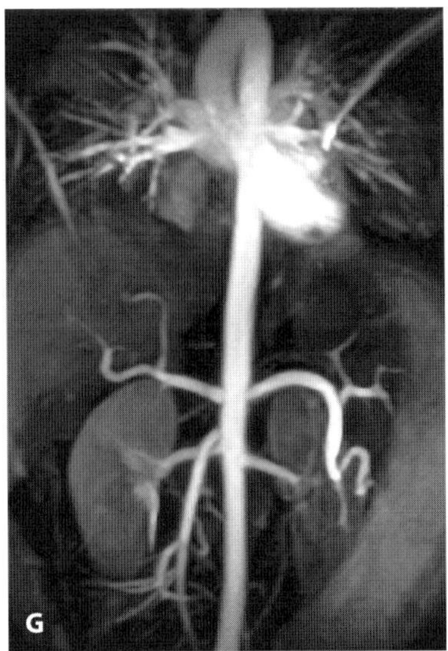

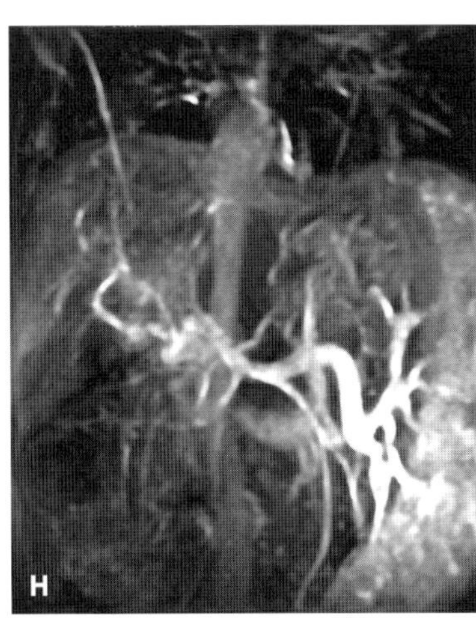

Fig. 9.5A–H. Cavernous portal vein transformation in a child. Portal venous phase, gadolinium-enhanced, T1-W spoiled GRE (**A**), T2-W HASTE (TE 90 ms) (**B**), coronal true-FISP (**C,D**), single sections from contrast-enhanced, time-resolved MRA during the portal phase (**E,F**), and MIPs of the arterial phase (**G**) and portal venous phase (**H**). The portal vein is absent, and large collateral vessels are visible within the hepatoduodenal ligament. The spleen is markedly enlarged, with small siderotic nodules within the parenchyma, and ascites is present. Displayed arteries are completely normal. The most likely reason is an umbilical vein catheter during the first weeks of life

shaped and may demonstrate an earlier and stronger enhancement during the capillary phase due to a relative increase in their arterial supply compared with liver regions with normal portal perfusion. The difference in parenchymal enhancement fades away on delayed contrast-enhanced images (Fig. 9.1). Liver infarcts may occur following surgery, chemoembolization, trauma, and portal thrombosis, resulting in hypoperfused wedge-shaped defects (Fig. 9.6). Extrahepatic and intrahepatic liver vessels are well demonstrated on gadolinium-enhanced 3D MR angiography (Fig. 9.7). Intrahepatic vessels are also visualized on iron-oxide-enhanced 2D TOF images, contrasting the portal venous system in the dark liver parenchyma (Fig. 9.8).

9.5.5 Budd-Chiari Syndrome

Venous outflow in Budd-Chiari syndrome is often not completely eliminated due to accessory hepatic veins, segmental obstruction, or small veins (Fig. 9.9). Shunting into the portal vein may cause reversed portal flow in patients with portal hypertension. Typically, the caudate lobe and central parts are spared, and the right lobe is atrophic. Portosystemic shunts, intrahepatic collaterals, and capsular collaterals are often present. Gadolinium enhancement varies from acute disease with more decreased enhancement to chronic disease with increased enhancement relative to normal or hypertrophied segments. Central parts may therefore appear as low SI mass-like lesions. Nodular regenerative hyperplasia may develop in chronic disease, demonstrating a similar signal pattern to adenomatous hyperplastic nodules with high SI on T1-WI, intermediate to low SI on T2-WI, and early enhancement on gadolinium-enhanced images. The differential diagnosis of HCC within individual patients may become quite difficult. Hepatobiliary agents cause an increased signal enhancement and SPIO a decreased signal enhancement.

9.5.6 Infectious Disease

Pyogenic abscesses typically show low SI on T1-WI, moderate to high SI on T2-WI (hyperintense necrotic center), and a thick rim of perilesional enhancement on gadolinium-enhanced T1-WI with an indistinct or irregular outer margin. Amebic abscesses basically reveal a similar pattern, although they are more encapsulated with enhancement of the capsule (Fig. 9.8).

Echinococcal disease presents as an encapsulated multicystic lesion with potential satellite cysts (<20% of patients). The signal behavior can be complex, with mixed signal (debris, protein) on T1-WI and T2-WI and

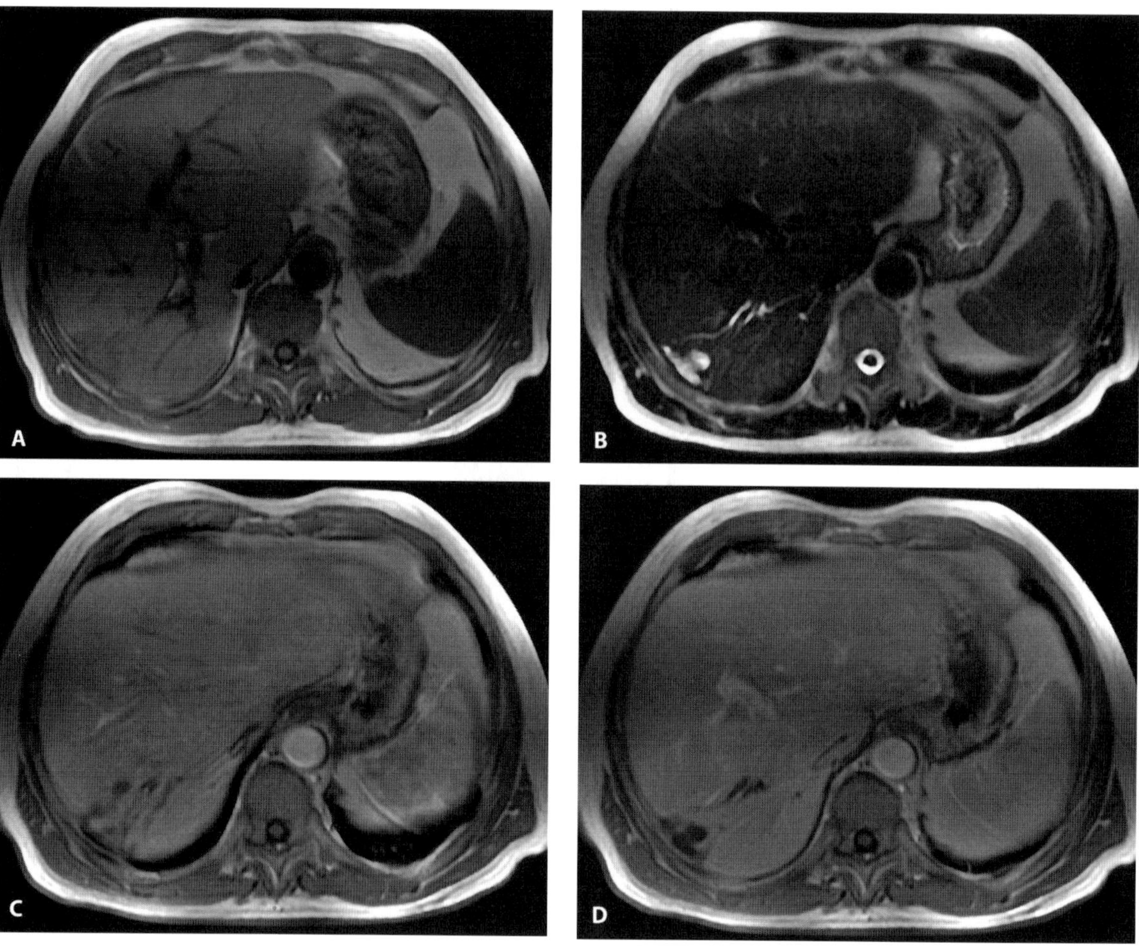

Fig. 9.6A–D. Liver infarct following chemoembolization. Plain T1-W spoiled GRE (**A**), T2-W HASTE (TE 90 ms) (**B**), arterial phase, gadolinium-enhanced, T1-W spoiled GRE (**C**), and portal venous phase, gadolinium-enhanced, T1-W spoiled GRE (**D**). The liver demonstrates a wedge-shaped perfusion in segment 5/6 with no enhancement following gadolinium injection and high signal on T2-W HASTE due to liquefactive necrosis

calcifications, which are often present within the cyst wall. MR imaging cannot reliably distinguish the fibrous tissue of the capsule from calcifications. The fibrous capsule and the internal septations are well shown on gadolinium-enhanced MR imaging.

Fungal infections, typically *Candida albicans*, present as microabscesses with small lesions in size (<2 cm) and low signal on T1-WI and T2-WI. *C. albicans* predominantly involves the liver and spleen (hepatosplenic candidiasis) and occasionally the kidney. FS T2-WI and gadolinium-enhanced, dynamic T1-WI is most useful in depicting the lesions. Acute lesions may show an almost cystic signal pattern (low SI on T1-WI and high SI on T2-WI) without peripheral enhancement. Granulomatous reactions as a treatment response demonstrate central high SI on plain T1-WI and T2-WI and gadolinium-enhancement on T1-WI with a dark peripheral ring. Chronic lesions with scarring show low SI on T1-WI and are typically invisible on T2-WI. Irregular lesions without gadolinium enhancement are best visualized on early gadolinium-enhanced T1-WI. Liver-specific agents do not provide additional clinically relevant information.

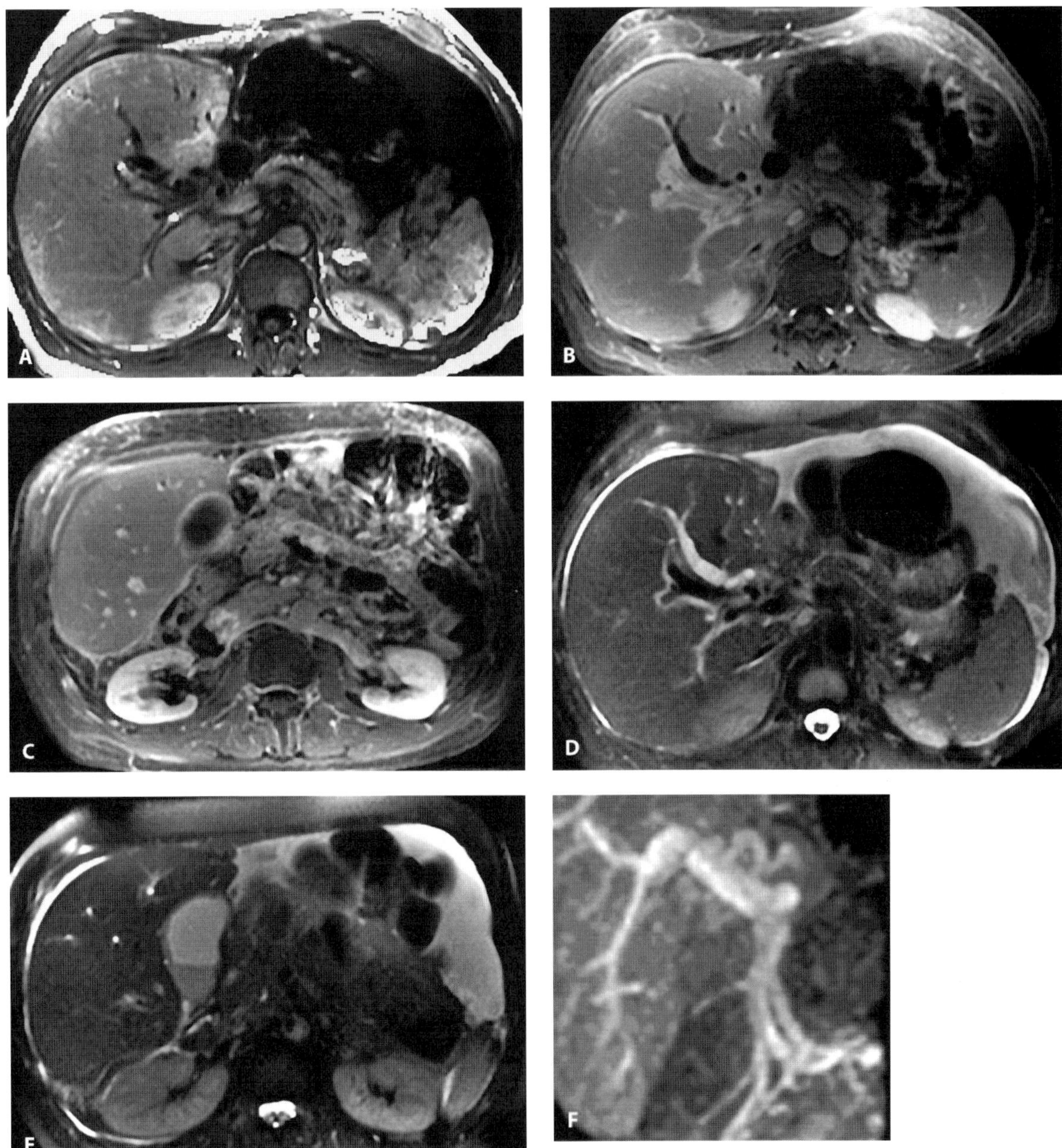

Fig. 9.7A–F. Klatskin tumor. Arterial phase, gadolinium-enhanced, T1-W spoiled GRE (**A**) and gadolinium-enhanced, FS T1-W spoiled GRE at the level of the tumor (**B**) reveal dilated intrahepatic biliary ducts (*dark*) and a relatively hypointense infiltrative mass lesion in the hilus surrounding the portal vein (*bright*). The second gadolinium-enhanced, FS T1-W spoiled GRE section (**C**) at the level of the papilla of Vater shows contrast enhancement of the tissue adjacent to the papilla due to inflammatory changes following ERCP. The two HASTE (TE 90 ms) images at the level of the tumor (**D**) and the gallbladder (**E**) portray the dilated intrahepatic ducts as bright and the portal vein as dark. The gallbladder shows a fluid-fluid level due to sludge (lower SI) below the bile (higher SI). Bright ascites is also present. CE-MRA displaying the portal venous phase (**F**) was obtained with 0.2 mmol gadolinium/kg body weight. The distal part of the main portal vein shows direct tumor infiltration with significant narrowing of the lumen. Explorative laparotomy confirmed tumor infiltration into the main portal vein with peritoneal carcinomatosis

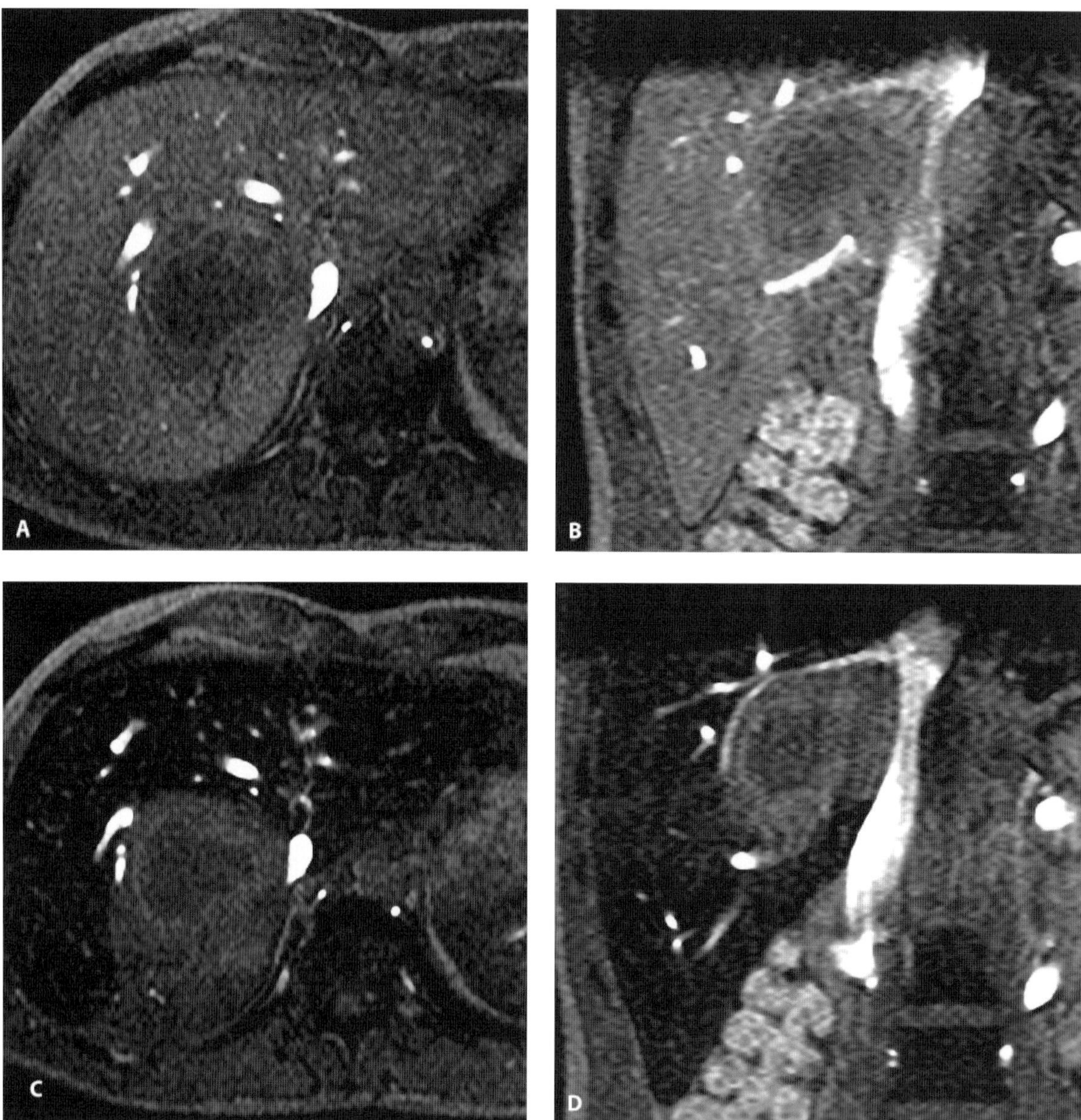

Fig. 9.8A–D. Amebic liver abscess. Axial and coronal 2D-TOF images before (**A**,**B**) and 10 min following i.v. injection (Resovist) of 10 µmol Fe/kg body weight (**C**,**D**) of a patient with an amebic liver abscess in the right liver lobe. A thick wall and a necrotic center characterize the abscess. Liver-vessel contrast is increased on SPIO-enhanced images due to a decrease in liver SI with improved visualization of the portal venous vessels

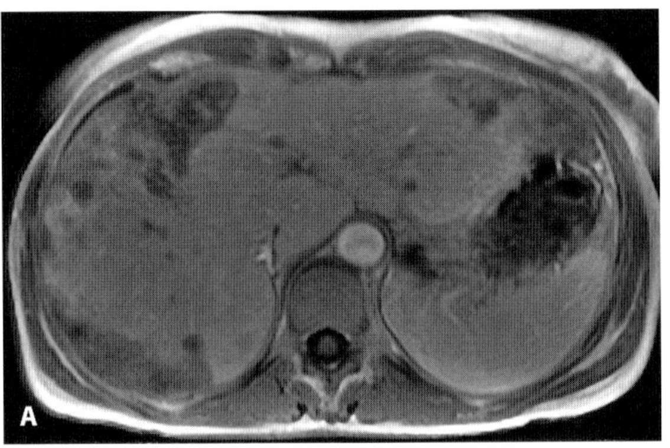

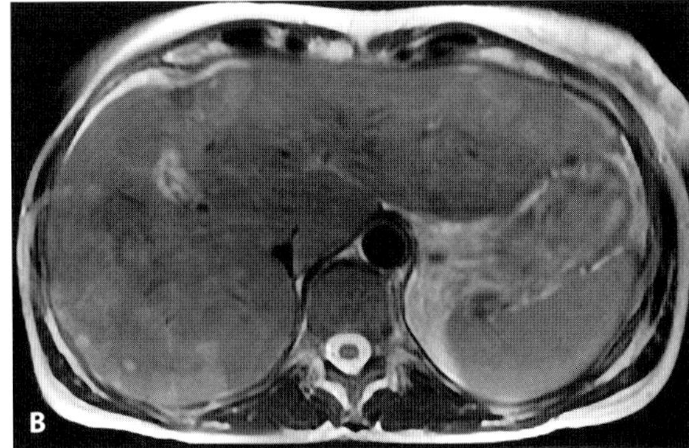

Fig. 9.9A,B. Budd-Chiari. Portal venous phase, gadolinium-enhanced, T1-W spoiled GRE (**A**) and T2-W HASTE (**B**) The liver demonstrates inhomogeneous SI on T1-WI and T2-WI with multiple peripheral infarcts and absent hepatic veins

9.5.7 Granulomatous and Lymphomatous Disease

Sarcoidosis typically presents as multifocal small lesions (1 cm) in the liver and spleen. Granulomas are hypointense on T1-WI and T2-WI and show delayed gadolinium enhancement. Focal lymphomatous disease demonstrates low signal on T1-WI and a slightly high signal on T2-WI. Gadolinium-enhanced T1-WI shows no significant increase in lesion SI, but occasionally perilesional enhancement. Liver-specific agents offer a better delineation of lesions on accumulation phase images.

9.6 Liver Pathology – Focal Liver Disease

Plain and contrast-enhanced MR imaging is useful for the detection and characterization of focal liver lesions. Hepatic MR imaging is best performed with breathhold T1-W GRE techniques, breathhold T2-W TSE or HASTE techniques, or non-breathhold T2-W TSE or SE techniques.

Metastases are the most common liver tumors in Western countries and HCC in Africa and Asia. Contrast-enhanced MR imaging exceeds the diagnostic ability of contrast-enhanced spiral CT and portal-enhanced spiral CT to detect and subsequently characterize malignant focal liver lesions. Lesion characterization is of particular importance in patients with primary malignancies, because even in this selected population up to 50% of small lesions (<10–15 mm) may be benign. Imaging protocols include transverse plain and contrast-enhanced T1-W and/or T2-W pulse sequences, depending on the contrast agents administered. The acquisition of an additional T1-W or T2-W sagittal or coronal plane may be useful to depict lesions on the upper surface of the liver.

Contrast enhancement with extracellular low-molecular gadolinium-chelates requires rapid T1-W spoiled GRE imaging before, during the arterial phase (hypervascular lesions), during the portal-venous phase (hypovascular lesions), and plain T2-W images with moderate (detection) and long (characterization) TE. Fat saturation of T2-W TSE sequences may be advantageous to facilitate the detection of superficial lesions. Delayed T1-WI are recommended to observe slow fill-in patterns.

Contrast enhancement with hepatobiliary agents is best performed with T1-WI before and at different time points following rapid contrast injection (MultiHance® and Gd-EOB-DTPA) or infusion (Teslascan®). T2-WI with moderate (detection) and long (characterization) TE is typically performed before contrast administration. Dynamic T1-WI is helpful to study the perfusion phase of lesions comparable to extracellular low-molecular gadolinium-chelates, and delayed imaging (>2 h for Teslascan® and MultiHance® and >20 min for Gd-EOB-DTPA) has to be performed because of nonspecific enhancement of lesions during the perfusion phase. Following an initial wash-out, malignant nonhepatocellular lesions exhibit a constant signal on T1-W delayed images. However, the presence of hepatocytes in the early stages of HCC may cause enhancement comparable with liver tissue (see adenoma and FNH).

It is recommended to acquire T1-WI in a second plane as part of the protocol for delayed scanning to look for small lesions close to the liver capsule beneath the diaphragm.

Contrast enhancement with iron oxides is best performed with T1-WI and T2-WI before and after 15–30 min following rapid contrast injection (Resovist®) or infusion (Endorem® and Sinerem®). Dynamic imaging is helpful to study the perfusion phase of lesions comparable with extracellular low-molecular gadolinium-chelates. Delayed imaging has to be performed to utilize the best lesion-liver contrast for the detection of lesions and provides features for lesion characterization. Malignant lesions without phagocytic cells exhibit constant signal on T2-W accumulation phase images with all three available or tested iron oxides. However, the presence of phagocytic cells in the early stages of HCC may cause enhancement comparable to adenomatous hyperplasia.

9.6.1 Cysts

Liver cysts appear as well-defined and frequently multiple focal lesions with a typical signal pattern demonstrating low signal intensity on T1-WI, homogeneous high SI on T2-WI, and no contrast enhancement with either extracellular or liver-specific contrast agents (Fig. 9.10). MR imaging is superior to CT and US in

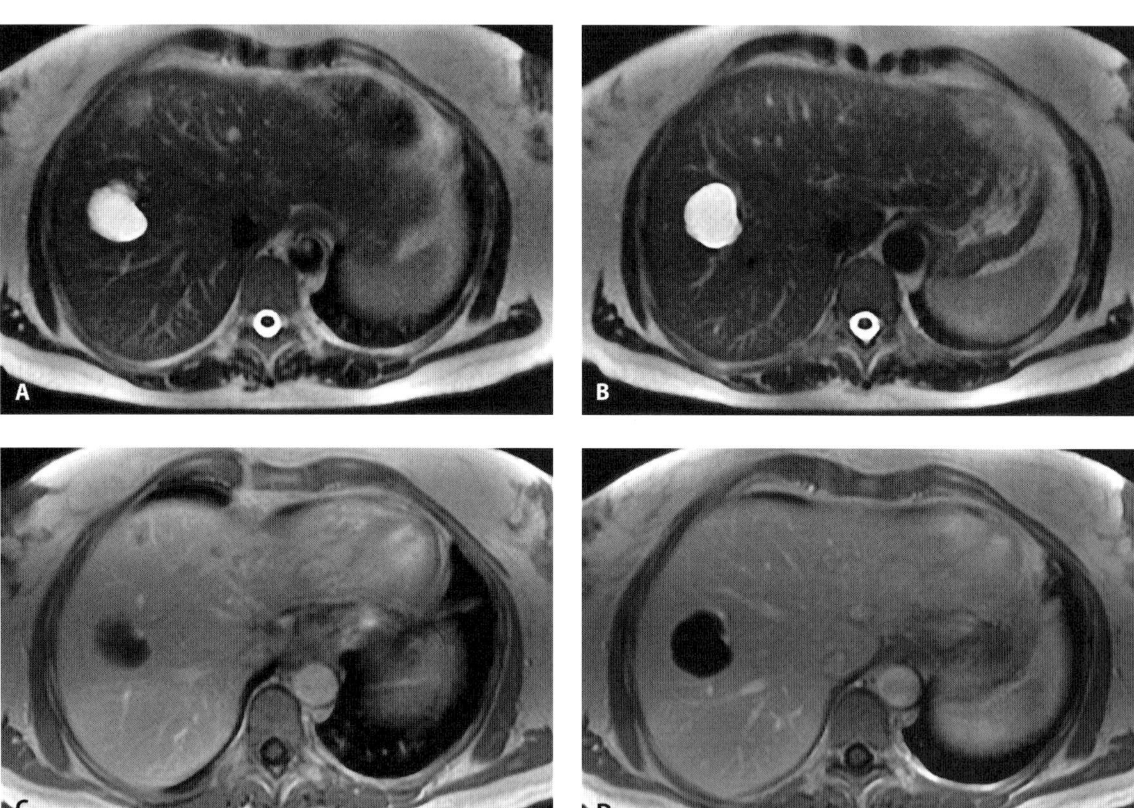

Fig. 9.10A–D. Liver cyst and liver metastases. Adjacent sections of T2-W HASTE (TE 90 ms) (**A**,**B**) and portal venous phase, gadolinium-enhanced, T1-W spoiled GRE (**C**,**D**) of a patient with colon carcinoma prior to liver surgery. A cyst with high SI on T2-WI (**B**) and absent gadolinium enhancement on portal venous phase, gadolinium-enhanced, T1-W spoiled GRE (**D**) is located in the right liver lobe. At least three ring-enhancing lesions are visible on portal venous phase, gadolinium-enhanced, T1-W spoiled GRE (**C**) in the left liver lobe, which appear only slightly hyperintense on T2-WI (**A**). Findings were confirmed at surgery

depicting and characterizing small cysts. Rarely, cysts may appear with higher signal on T1-WI due to a hemorrhagic or proteinaceous content.

9.6.2 Hemangioma

Hemangioma is the most common benign focal liver lesion and is typically detected incidentally. Cavernous liver hemangiomas are by far more common than capillary hemangiomas. The major clinical implication is the misclassification on CT, ultrasound, or scintigraphy, complicating patient management. MRI is the best modality to detect and characterize liver hemangioma and should be recommended widely for this clinical question. Hemangiomas appear as well defined and lobulated focal lesions. The signal pattern on unenhanced MR imaging is very similar to cysts with low signal intensity on T1-WI and high SI on T2-WI due to long T1- and T2-relaxation times (>120 ms), which are however shorter than for cysts. Dynamic and serial gadolinium-enhanced T1-WI are effective in distinguishing hemangiomas from malignant lesions, because hemangiomas typically enhance in a peripheral nodular fashion with subsequent complete or almost com-

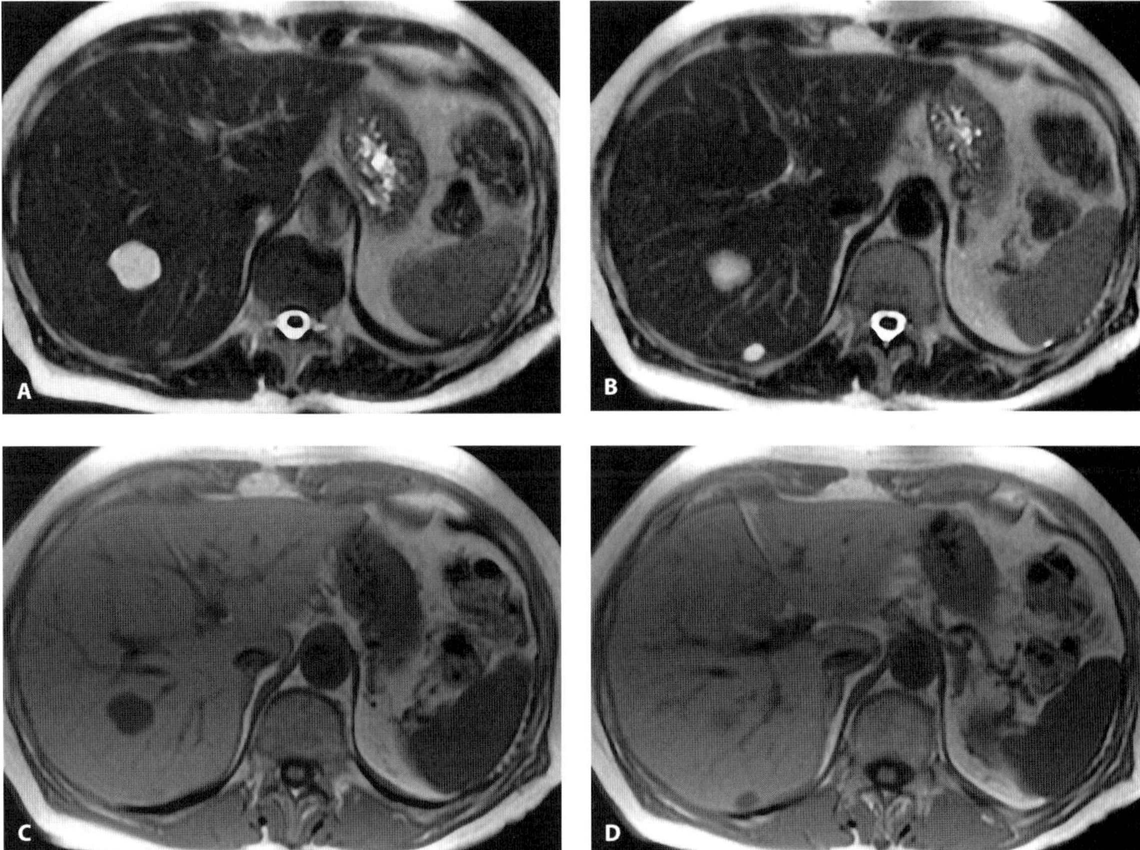

Fig. 9.11A–H. Liver hemangiomas. T2-W HASTE (TE 90 ms) (**A**,**B**), plain T1-W spoiled GRE (**C**,**D**), arterial phase, gadolinium-enhanced, T1-W spoiled GRE (**E**,**F**), and portal venous phase T1-W spoiled GRE (**G**,**H**). The liver demonstrates a larger hemangioma within the right liver lobe and a smaller subcapsular hemangioma showing high SI on T2-WI and low signal on T1-WI. The larger hemangioma demonstrates a type-3 enhancement pattern with peripheral nodular gadolinium enhancement, followed by a centripetal progression on delayed gadolinium-enhanced T1-WI without complete uniform signal enhancement. The smaller hemangioma reveals a type-1 enhancement pattern with early uniform high signal enhancement and homogeneous SI on delayed T1-WI

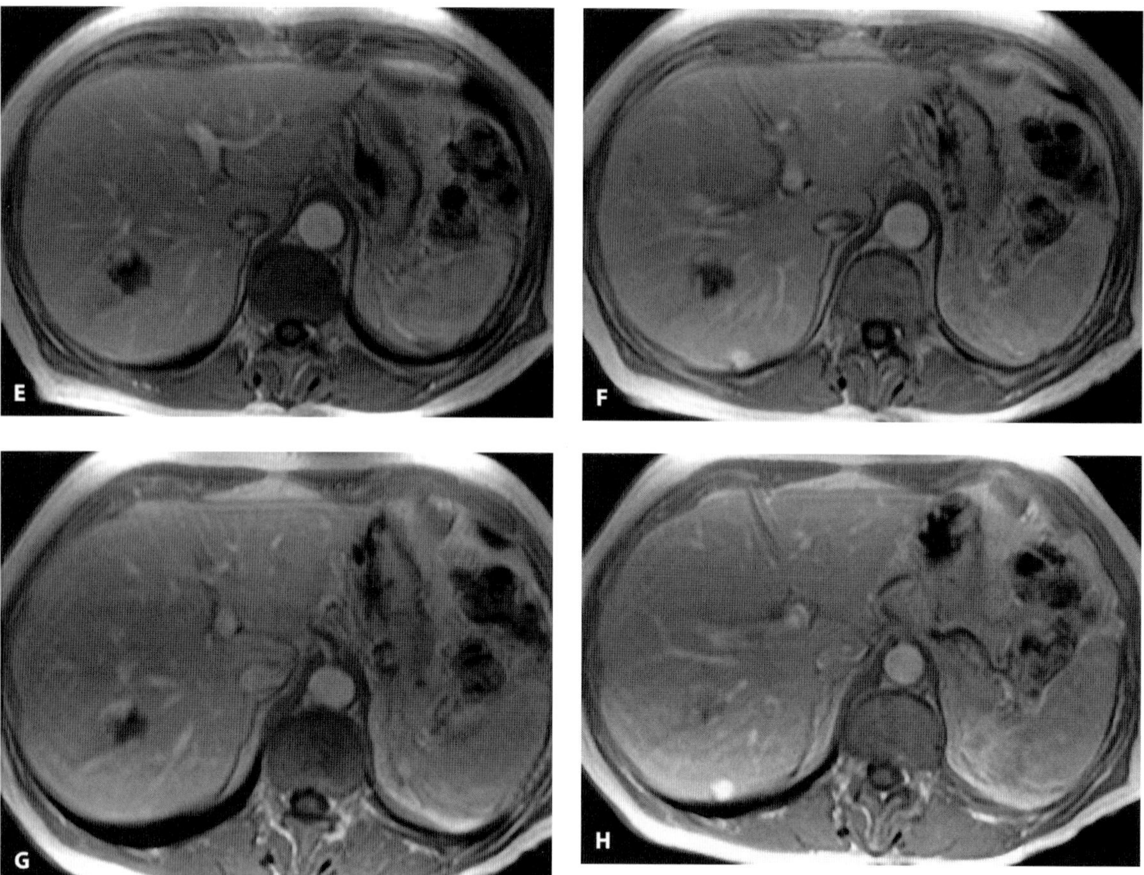

Fig. 9.11E–H

plete fill-in of the entire lesion over 5–10 min (Fig. 9.11). Three types of enhancement patterns for dynamic T1-WI have been described:

- Type 1 Uniform high signal enhancement during the early phase, without wash-out (metastases)
- Type 2 Peripheral nodular signal enhancement during the early phase, followed by a centripetal progression to uniform high signal enhancement
- Type 3 Peripheral nodular signal enhancement during the early phase, followed by a centripetal progression with a persistent central scar

Type-1 enhancement is present in small hemangiomas (15 mm), type-3 enhancement typically in large hemangiomas (>5 cm) or giant hemangiomas (Fig. 9.12), and type-2 enhancement in hemangiomas of each size. The dynamic pattern of enhancement provides additional criteria to establish the diagnosis of a hemangioma. Nodular enhancement is demonstrated immediately following gadolinium enhancement, which is also frequently eccentric. Enhancement fades away over time without a peripheral or heterogeneous wash-out (see metastases). Some hemangiomas may also enhance fairly rapidly, within less than 2 min (Fig. 9.11). Hypervascular malignant liver lesions (HCC, leiomyosarcoma, angiosarcoma, islet-cell tumors) may be indistinguishable from small hemangiomas, and consideration of the clinical history is a subjective criteria that may have to be applied. The absence of a central scar in an otherwise mass lesion appearing like a giant heman-

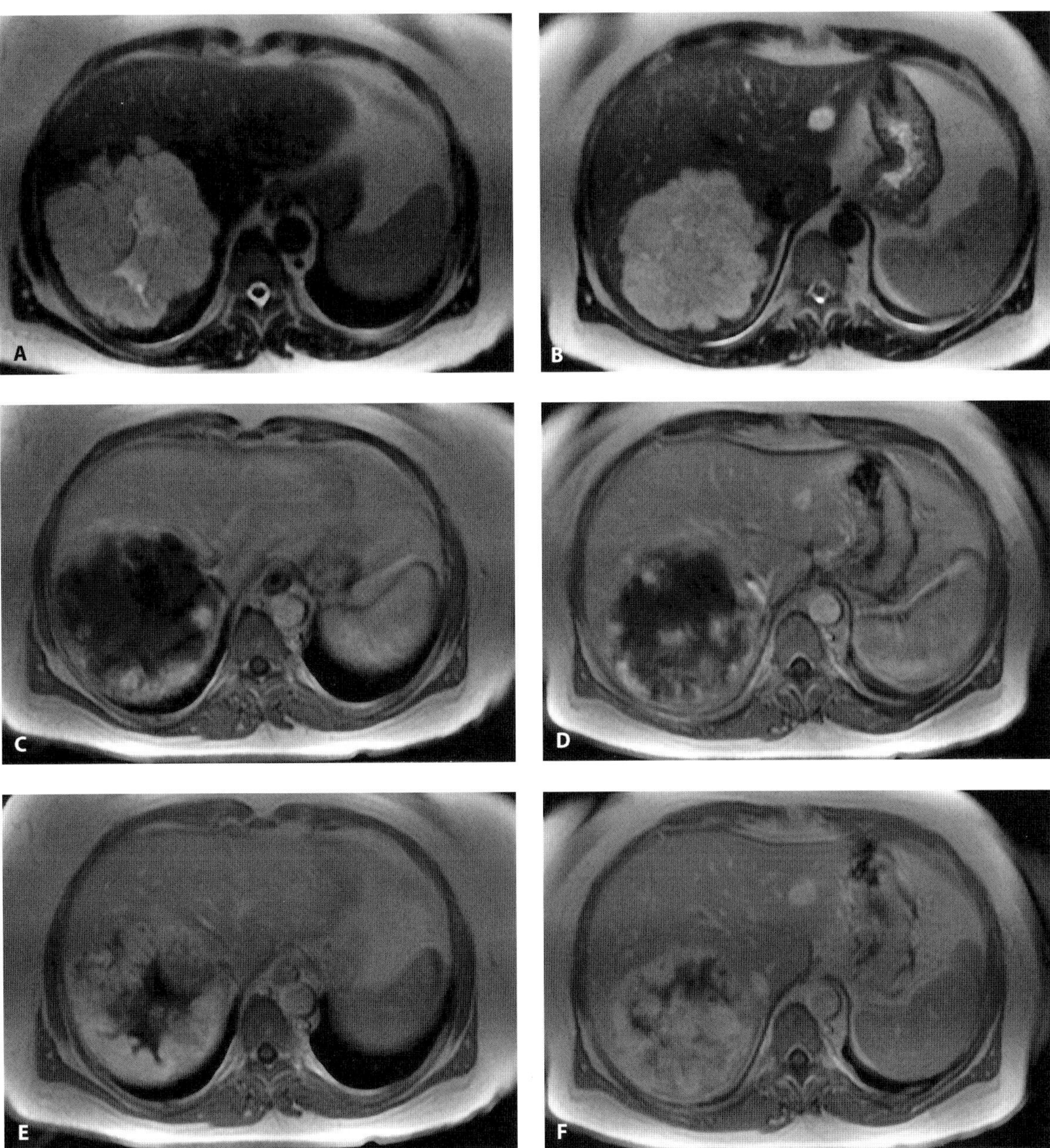

Fig. 9.12A–F. Giant liver hemangioma. T2-W HASTE (TE 90 ms) (**A,B**), arterial phase, gadolinium-enhanced, T1-W spoiled GRE (**C,D**), and delayed (5 min) gadolinium-enhanced T1-W spoiled GRE (**E,F**). The liver demonstrates a giant hemangioma in the right liver lobe with a central scar showing high SI on T2-WI and absent gadolinium enhancement (type 3). The giant hemangioma demonstrates peripheral nodular gadolinium enhancement (**C,D**), followed by a centripetal progression on delayed gadolinium-enhanced T1-W images (**E,F**). The smaller hemangioma in the left lobe reveals a type-1 enhancement pattern with early uniform high signal enhancement (**D**) and homogeneous filling on delayed T1-WI (**F**)

gioma should raise concern, and a biopsy may be required (Fig. 9.12). Large hemangiomas may rarely hemorrhage or compress the adjacent portal vein, resulting in transient increased enhancement on immediate post-gadolinium images secondary to an autoregulatory increased hepatic arterial blood supply.

Hepatobiliary contrast agents demonstrate similar patterns of signal enhancement following bolus injection, as is feasible with MultiHance or Gd-EOB-DTPA. Iron oxides show a decrease in SI on heavily T2-WI (Fig. 9.34), and dynamic imaging with Resovist again shows similar signal patterns as described for T1-W gadolinium-enhanced images (signal increase) and a reversed pattern (signal decrease) on T2 or T2*-WI. The blood-pool agent Sinerem also results in a signal increase on T1-WI and a signal decrease on early T2-WI.

9.6.3 Focal Nodular Hyperplasia

Focal nodular hyperplasia (FNH) is more frequently diagnosed in women (80%–90%) than in men (10%–20%). The tumor contains hepatocytes, bile-duct elements, Kupffer cells, fibrous stroma, and frequently possesses a central scar. Hemorrhage is very rare, and the lesion has no malignant potential. The typical signal pattern on plain MR imaging is either slightly lower SI on T1-WI and a slightly higher SI or isointensity on T2-

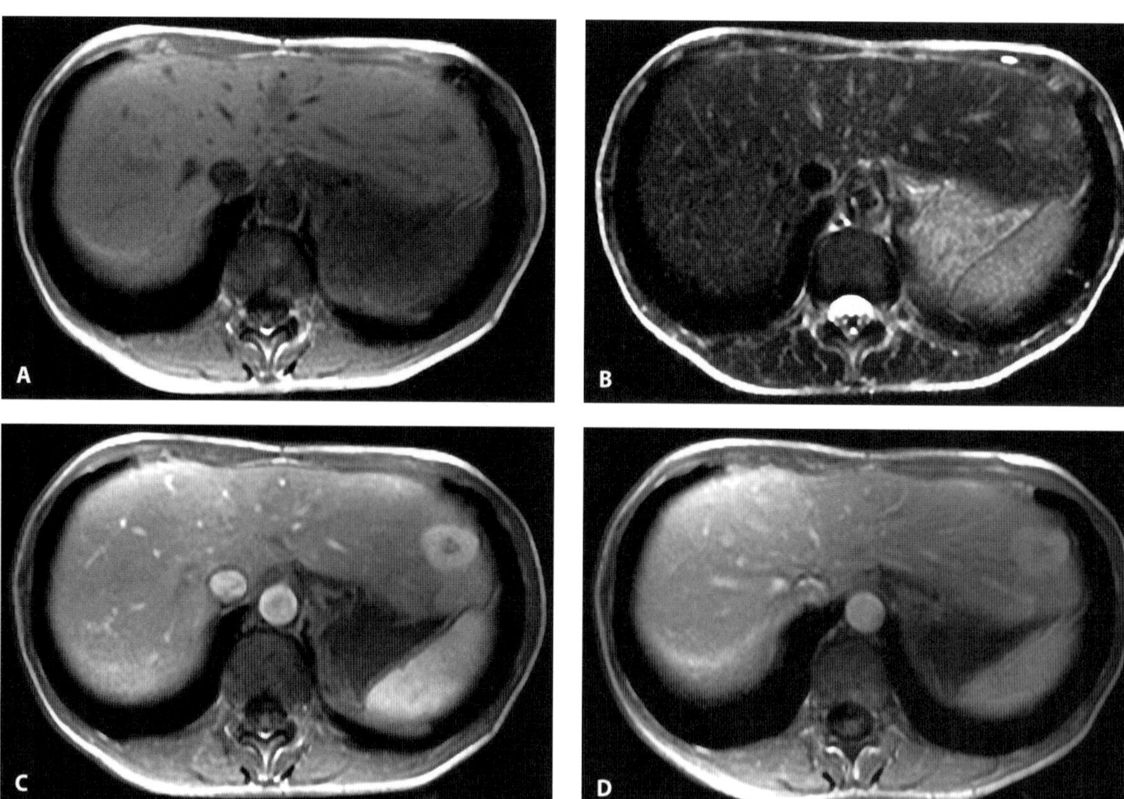

Fig. 9.13A–D. Focal nodular hyperplasia with central scar. Plain T1-W spoiled GRE (**A**), T2-W TSE (TE 165 ms) (**B**), arterial phase, gadolinium-enhanced, T1-W spoiled GRE (**C**), and portal venous phase, gadolinium-enhanced, T1-W spoiled GRE (**D**). The liver demonstrates an isointense lesion in the left liver lobe compared with liver on T1-W spoiled GRE and hypointense compared with liver on T2-W TSE. A central scar is visible (hypointense on T1-W spoiled GRE and hyperintense on T2-W TSE). The lesion strongly enhances on arterial phase, gadolinium-enhanced, T1-W spoiled GRE with persistent enhancement on portal venous phase, gadolinium-enhanced, T1-W spoiled GRE

WI than normal liver parenchyma (Fig. 9.13). The central scar is a relatively characteristic feature with high SI on T2-WI, but is only present in one-third of patients (Fig. 9.14).

Gadolinium-enhanced MR imaging is useful for the detection and characterization of FNH with a strong uniform blush on arterial phase, gadolinium-enhanced, T1-W spoiled GRE images, also with rapid fading of enhancement within less than 60 s (Figs. 9.13 and 9.14). A low SI central scar may enhance over time. Hepatobiliary agents enhance FNH, similar to adenomas, reflecting the presence of well-differentiated hepatocytes with well-differentiated HCC or early dedifferentiation as a differential diagnosis (Fig. 9.15).

All iron oxides are effective for the characterization of FNH on T2-W accumulation-phase images because of phagocytic cells within the tumor, resulting in a signal decrease. Therefore, lesions are less visible on SPIO-enhanced accumulation phase images than on plain images. Additional information for lesion characterization may be obtained by dynamic imaging with bolus injectable Resovist mimicking dynamic gadolinium-enhanced MR on T1-WI.

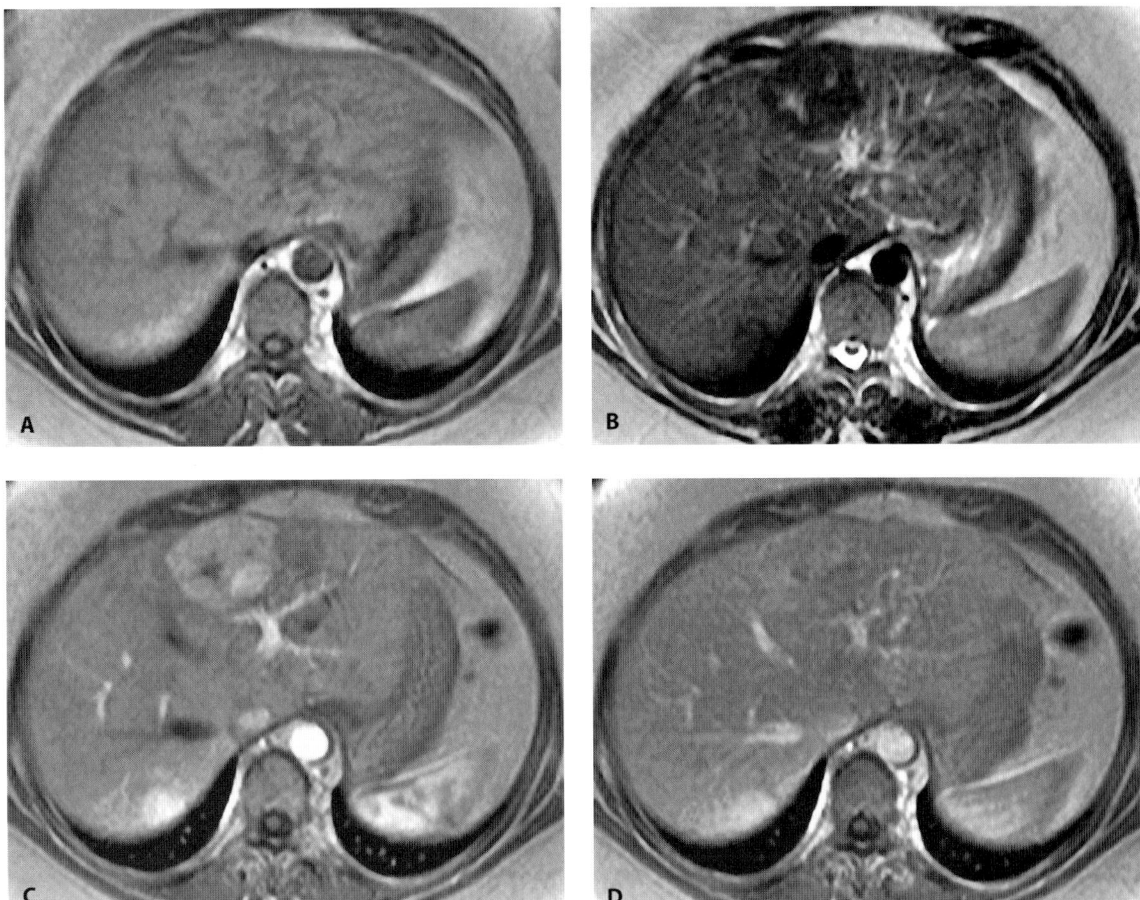

Fig. 9.14A–D. Focal nodular hyperplasia. Plain T1-W spoiled GRE (**A**), T2-W TSE (TE 165 ms) (**B**), arterial-phase gadolinium-enhanced T1-W spoiled GRE (**C**), and portal venous-phase gadolinium-enhanced T1-W spoiled GRE (**D**). The liver demonstrates two lesions in the left liver lobe (*ventral*) and right liver lobe (*dorsal*), which are isointense compared with liver on T1-W spoiled GRE and hypointense compared with on T2-W TSE. Only the larger lesions demonstrate a central hyper-intense scar on T2-W TSE. Both lesions strongly enhance on arterial-phase gadolinium-enhanced T1-W spoiled GRE with isointensity on portal venous phase gadolinium-enhanced T1-W spoiled GRE

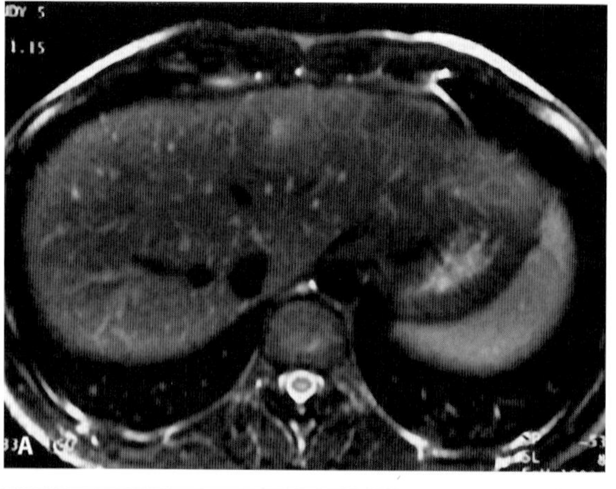

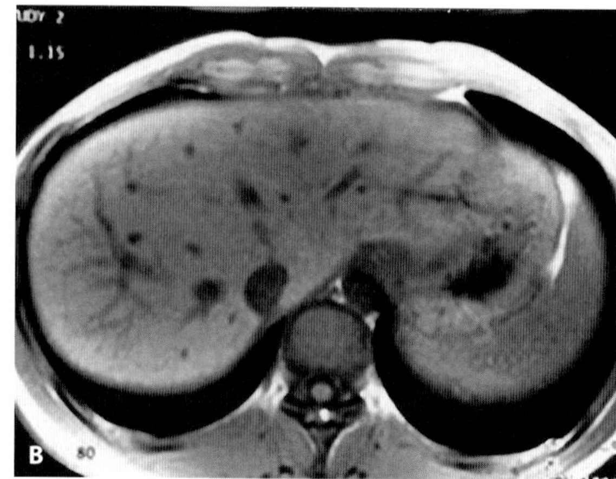

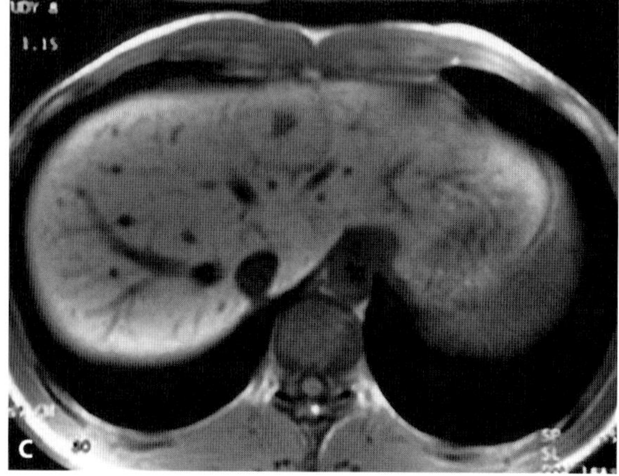

Fig. 9.15A–C. Focal nodular hyperplasia with Teslascan. T2-W TSE (**A**), plain T1-W spoiled GRE (**B**), and delayed manganese-enhanced T1-W spoiled GRE (**C**). The lesions demonstrate a typical signal pattern on unenhanced images (**A,B**) and persistent enhancement on delayed T1-WI due to hepatocellular uptake of manganese. (Courtesy of W. Schima, Vienna, Austria)

9.6.4 Adenoma

Liver adenomas have a strong association with oral contraception, and more than 90% are found in young women. Necrosis and hemorrhage, which may be life threatening, are common causes of pain. Adenomas may contain fat, intracellular glycogen, may present with a thin pseudocapsule, and show a loose architecture. They are primarily derived from hepatocytes. This explains why adenomas vary in signal from hypointense to hyperintense (fat content) on T1-WI and are typically slightly hyperintense on T2-WI. Some adenomas are almost isointense to normal liver. Fat-containing adenomas demonstrate a signal decrease on out-of-phase images, and hemorrhage causes mixed signal patterns. Gadolinium-enhanced MR imaging shows a strong transient blush on arterial phase, gadolinium-enhanced, T1-W spoiled GRE images, also with rapid vanishing of enhancement within less than 60 s. Hepatobiliary agents enhance adenomas, similar to FNH, reflecting the presence of well-differentiated hepatocytes within the tumors, again with well-differentiated HCC or early dedifferentiation as a differential diagnosis.

Iron oxides again show a similar pattern as described for FNH and observed for regenerating nodules and adenomatous hyperplasia with a signal decrease on T2-W accumulation phase images (Fig. 9.3). Additional information for lesion characterization may be obtained by dynamic imaging with bolus injectable Resovist mimicking dynamic gadolinium-enhanced MR on T1-WI.

9.6.5 Metastases

Metastases are typically hypointense on T1-WI and moderately hyperintense on T2-WI. The lesion border may be either irregular or sharp, and the lesion shape can be irregular, oval, or round. Hemorrhage may result in hyperintense lesions on T1-WI and hypointense lesions on T2-WI. Coagulative necrosis (colorectal metastases) results in a hypointense lesion center and hyperintense periphery (viable tumor) on T2-WI. Mucin-producing tumors demonstrate high SI on T2.

Hypovascular metastases (Fig. 9.10) represent the vast majority (colorectal) of metastases, and the perfusion pattern is based on a diminished blood supply. Thus, similar to CT, lesions are typically best detected on the portal-venous gadolinium-enhanced T1-WI (Fig. 9.16). Plain images typically show low SI on T1-WI and slightly higher SI or almost isointensity on T2-WI. Metastases with large amounts of liquefactive necrosis may appear as cystic lesions with a signal void on immediate gadolinium-enhanced T1-WI. A peripheral enhancement is common on portal venous phase and delayed T1-WI. Typically, peripheral ring enhancement begins on immediate contrast-enhanced images with potential enhancement towards the center of the lesion and peripheral wash-out on delayed T1-WI (Fig. 9.16). It has been demonstrated that the perilesional enhance-

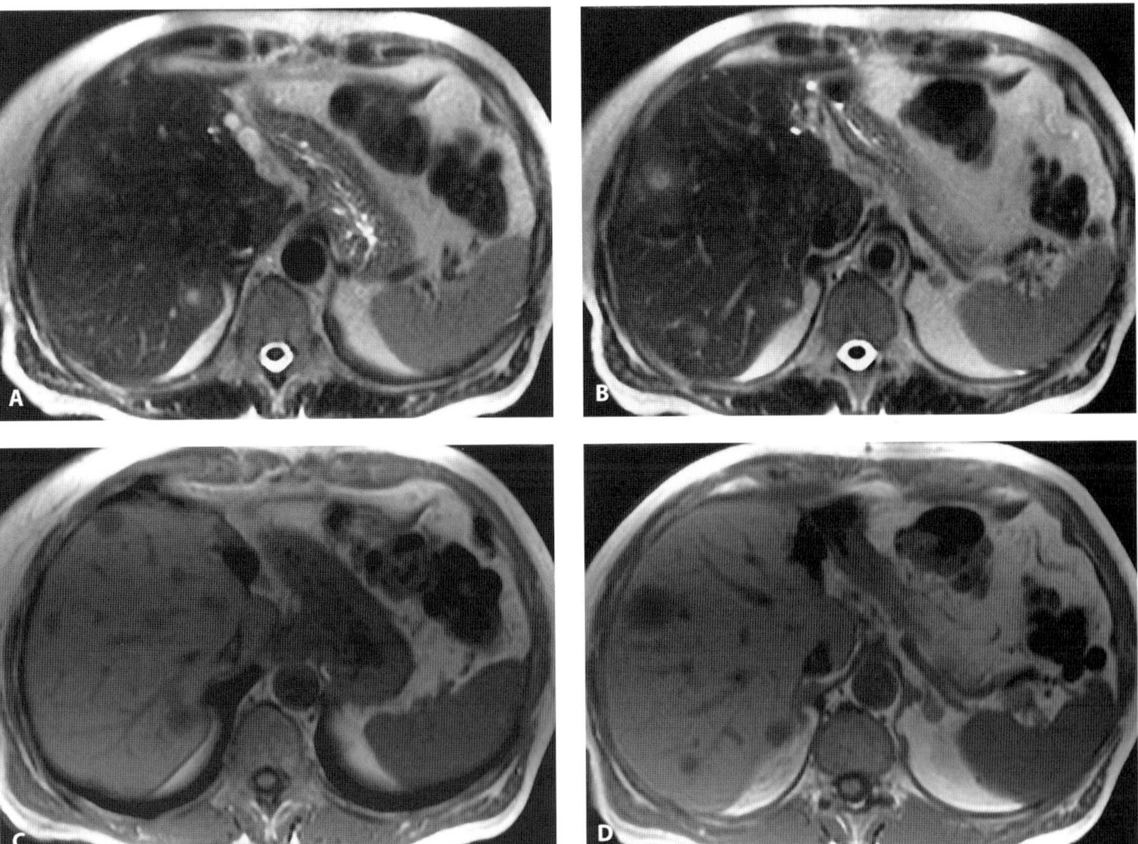

Fig. 9.16A–H. Hypovascular metastases. Two sections of each T2-W HASTE (TE 64 ms) (**A,B**), plain T1-W spoiled GRE (**C,D**), arterial phase, gadolinium-enhanced, T1-W spoiled GRE (**E,F**), and portal venous phase, gadolinium-enhanced, T1-W spoiled GRE (**G,H**) of a patient with a colorectal carcinoma and a probable lesion diagnosed within the right liver lobe at ultrasound. The sections demonstrate multiple metastases with a necrosis visible on T2-WI. Contrast enhancement clearly improves lesion conspicuity, and more lesions are detected than on T2-WI. Most metastases show peripheral ring enhancement with a wash-out on portal venous phase images, suggestive of malignancy. Some metastases demonstrate wedge-shaped perfusion phenomena

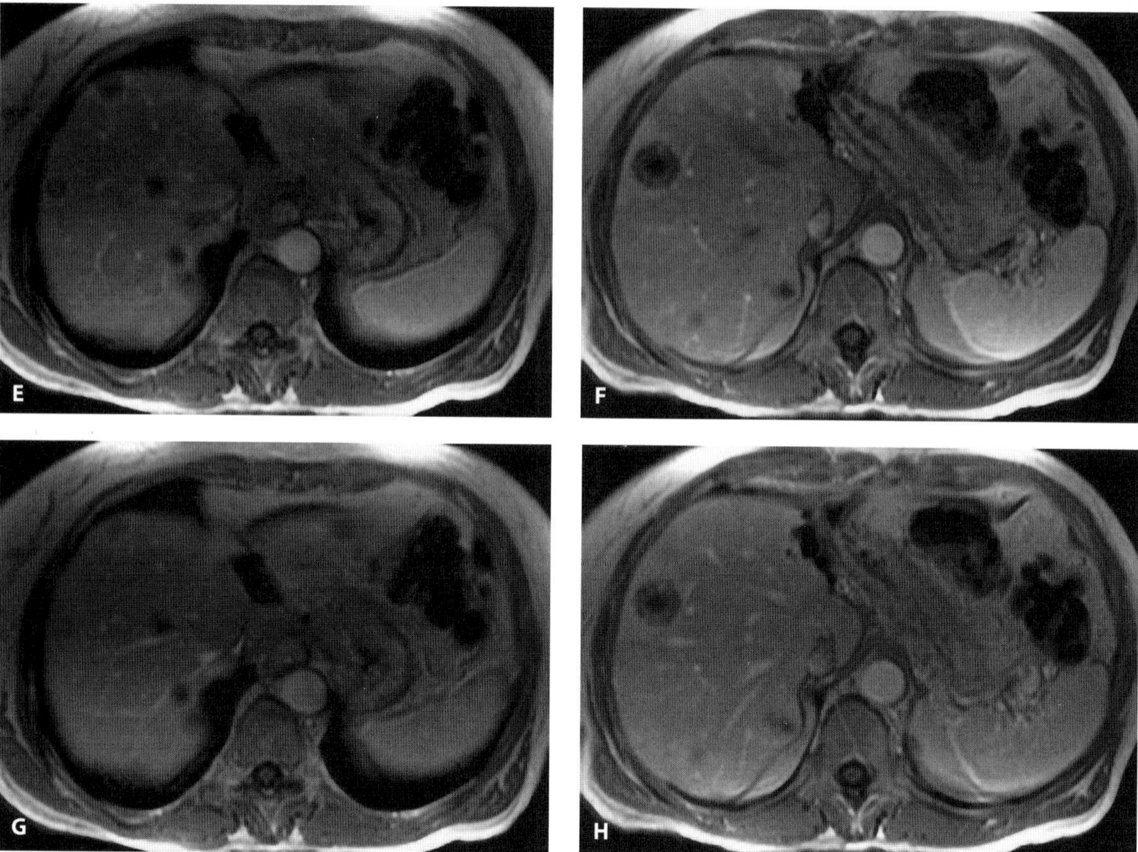

Fig. 9.16E–H.

ment of metastases on early gadolinium-enhanced MR images correlates with histopathologic hepatic parenchymal changes, which include peritumoral desmoplastic reaction, inflammatory cell infiltration, and vascular proliferation. Large colorectal metastases (Fig. 9.19) may show an additional inhomogeneous 'cauliflower enhancement'. These enhancement features are also observed with dynamically scanned, liver-specific contrast agents.

A variety of primary malignancies frequently cause hypervascular metastases (pheochromocytoma, renal cell, islet cell, carcinoid, leiomyosarcoma, thyroid, or melanoma). Hypervascular metastases (Fig. 9.17) may appear with high signal on T2-WI, comparable to hemangiomas, and show an intense peripheral ring enhancement with a potentially progressing centripetal enhancement. Small hypervascular metastases vary in contrast enhancement with immediate and often complete lesion enhancement. The different melanin content of melanoma metastases causes different hyperintense/hypointense patterns on T1-WI and T2-WI, because the paramagnetic property of melanin presents hyperintense on T1-WI (Fig. 9.18). Dynamic gadolinium-enhanced MR imaging is particularly useful for the detection and characterization of hypervascular liver lesions with immediate ring type, uniform, or irregular enhancement and subsequent wash-out effects. The absence of nodular enhancement within the enhancing ring type periphery, the uniform thickness of the enhancing ring, and the peripheral wash-out help to differentiate malignant lesions from hemangiomas, which also show enhancement over a longer period of time.

One of the major advantages of liver-specific contrast agents is the improved detection of hypovascular liver metastases as compared with gadolinium-enhanced

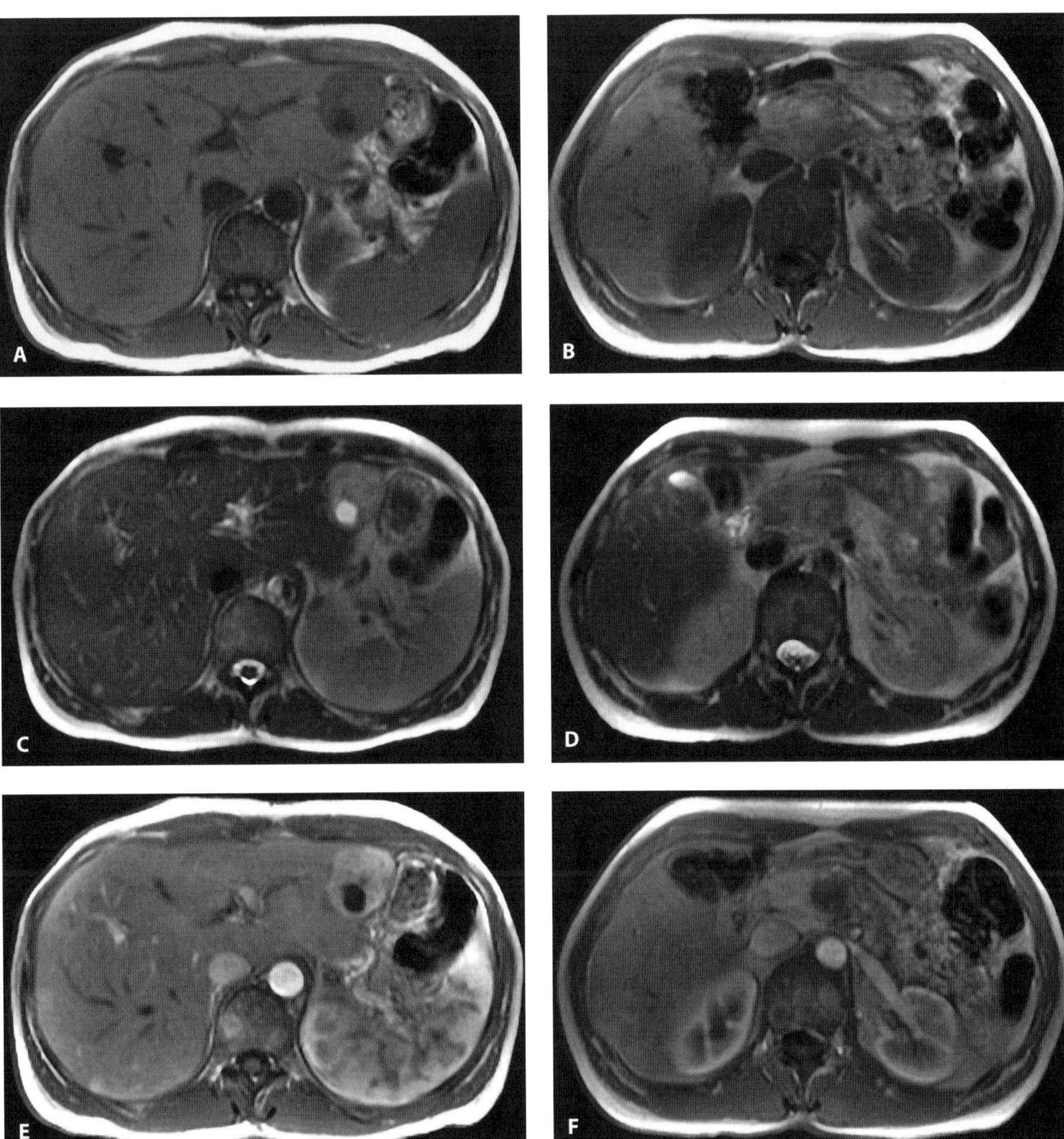

Fig. 9.17A–H. Hypervascular islet-cell tumor metastases and pancreatic tumor. Two sections of each plain T1-W spoiled GRE (**A**,**B**), T2-W HASTE (TE 64 ms) (**C**,**D**), arterial phase, gadolinium-enhanced, T1-W spoiled GRE (**E**,**F**), and portal venous phase, gadolinium-enhanced, T1-W spoiled GRE (**G**,**H**) of a patient with an islet-cell tumor of the pancreas and multiple hypervascular liver metastases. The sections in the *left column* demonstrate a large hypervascular metastasis in the lateral segment of the left liver lobe with a necrotic area. A small metastasis is visible in the laterodorsal right liver lobe. Both lesions show a strong arterial phase gadolinium enhancement and high SI on T2-W images. The pancreatic tumor is shown in the *right column* with central high SI on T2-WI (**D**) and good conspicuity on gadolinium-enhanced images (**F**,**H**)

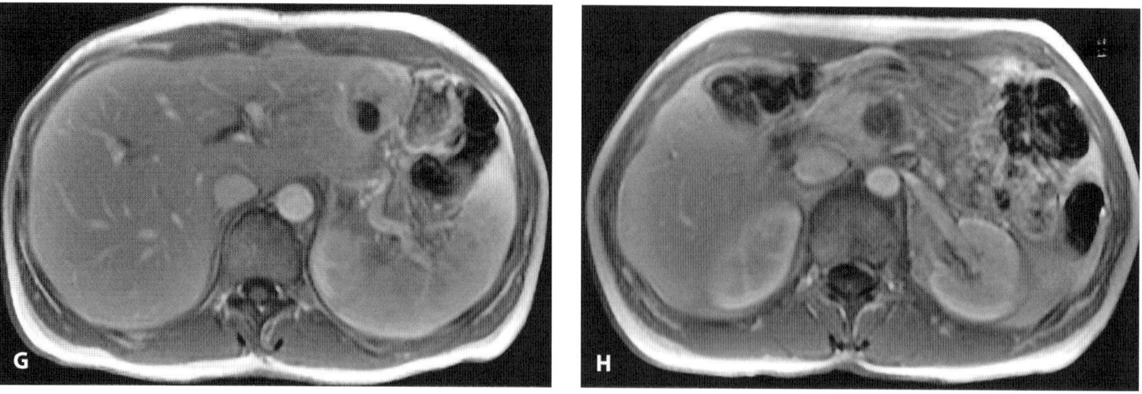

Fig. 9.17G, H.

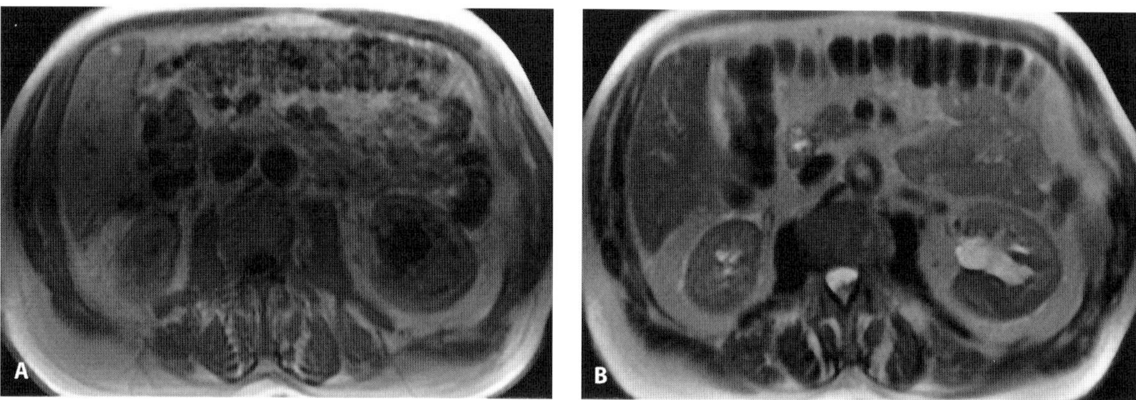

Fig. 9.18A,B. Melanoma metastasis. T1-W spoiled GRE (**A**) and T2-W HASTE (TE 90 ms) (**B**) images reveal a small hyperintense lesion in segment 5 of the right liver lobe in a patient with malignant melanoma

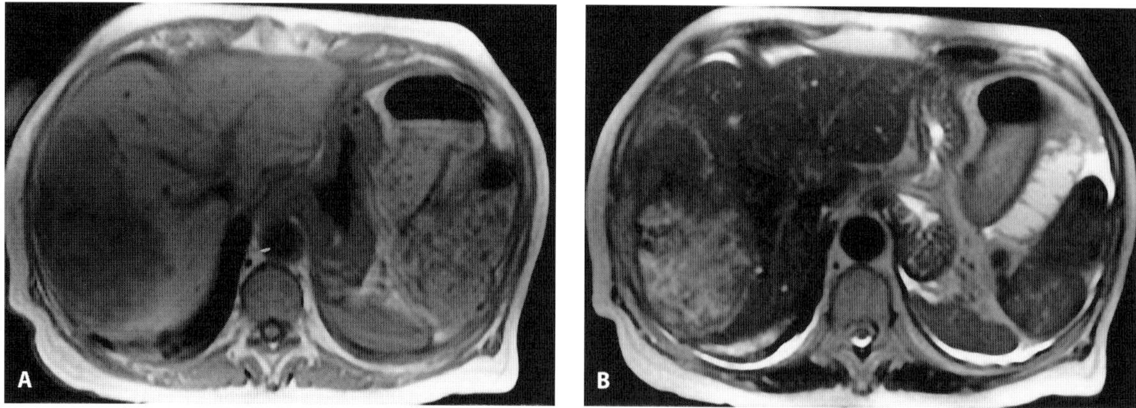

Fig. 9.19A–B.

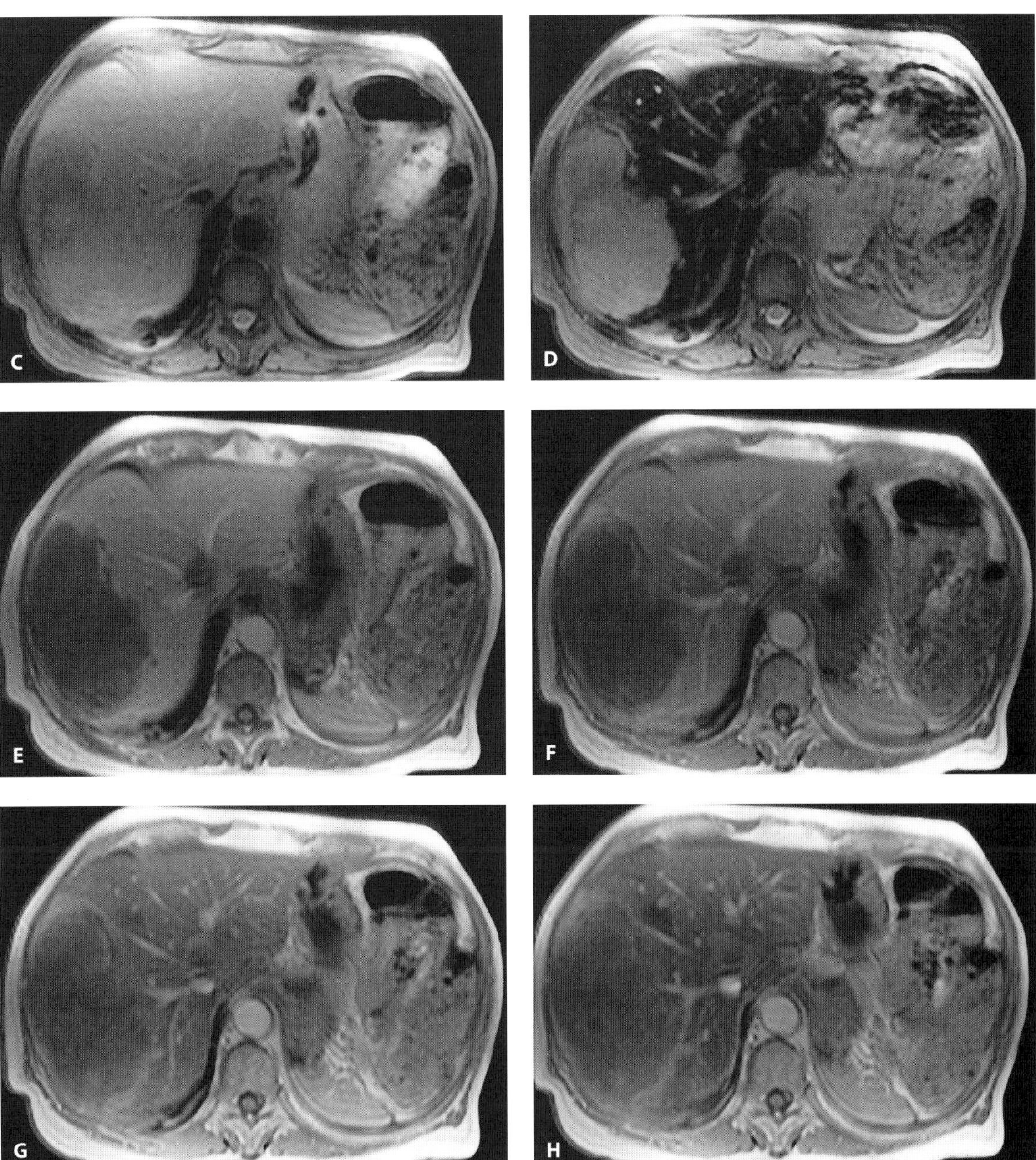

Fig. 9.19A–H. Liver metastases with SPIO. Plain T1-W spoiled GRE (**A**), plain T2-W HASTE (TE 90 ms) (**B**), plain PDW spoiled GRE before (**C**) and 10 min following (**D**) i.v. injection of 1.4 ml Resovist, and dynamic T1-weighted spoiled GRE images at multiple time points following injection (**E** 30 s, **F** 70 s, **G** 2 min, and **H** 5 min) in a patient with colorectal cancer and a large liver metastasis within the right liver lobe as diagnosed by ultrasound. Tumor-liver contrast and lesion conspicuity significantly increase on Resovist-enhanced PDW-GRE (**D**), and an additional lesion is now clearly visible near the confluence of the hepatic veins into the inferior vena cava. Dynamic T1-WI show increased and persistent signal enhancement within vessel demarcating lesions as known from contrast-enhanced CT or gadolinium-enhanced MRI. Lesion contrast decreases over time with decreasing liver signal (**G,H**)

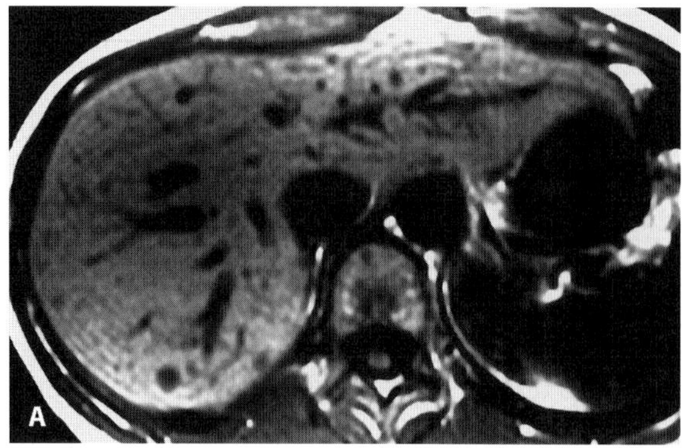

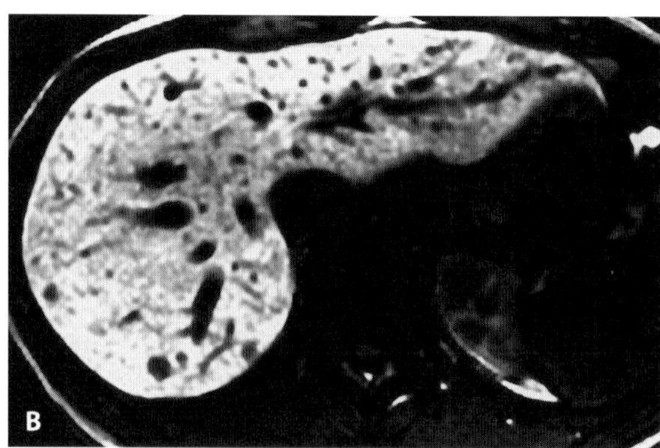

Fig. 9.20A,B. Liver metastases with Teslascan. T1-W spoiled GRE before (**A**) and 2 h following (**B**) Teslascan show an increase in lesion conspicuity on contrast-enhanced T1-WI. Lesions are more clearly visible, and additional lesions are detected. (Courtesy of W. Schima, Vienna, Austria)

MRI or contrast-enhanced CT techniques (Figs. 9.19 and 9.20). Results for lesion detection are equivalent to the most invasive CT technique (CTAP: CT arterial-portal) and superior for lesion characterization.

9.6.6 Hepatocellular Carcinoma (HCC)

Worldwide, HCC is the most common primary malignancy, because of its high prevalence in Asia and Africa. HCC in Europe and North America predominantly arises as a result of chronic liver disease, such as chronic active forms of hepatitis, alcoholic cirrhosis, and hemochromatosis. Japanese researchers have described a de novo development with progressive cellular atypias within adenomatous hyperplasia with progression to early differentiated HCC and with advanced dedifferentiated HCC as the final stage. Well-differentiated HCC typically shows a pseudocapsule appearing hypointense on T1-WI, potentially hyperintense on T2-WI, hypointense on early gadolinium-enhanced T1-WI, and with enhancement on delayed T1-WI. Advanced dedifferentiated HCC tends to infiltrate into the portal or hepatic veins. HCC grows predominantly as a solitary tumor in 50% of patients or multifocal in 40% of patients, but is rarely diffuse (in less than 10% of patients).

HCC show a variable signal pattern on plain MR images. As a rule of thumb, one-third appear hypointense, one-third isointense, and one-third hyperintense (fat, copper, or proteins) compared with liver SI on T1-WI. SI on T2-WI varies from almost isointensity to slight hyperintensity relative to liver parenchyma (Figs. 9.2 and 9.21).

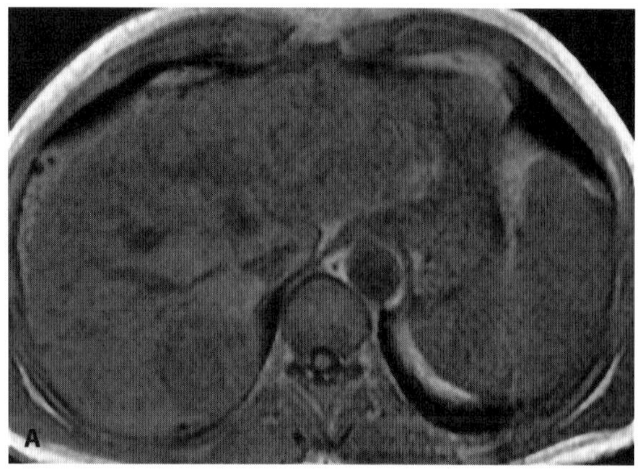

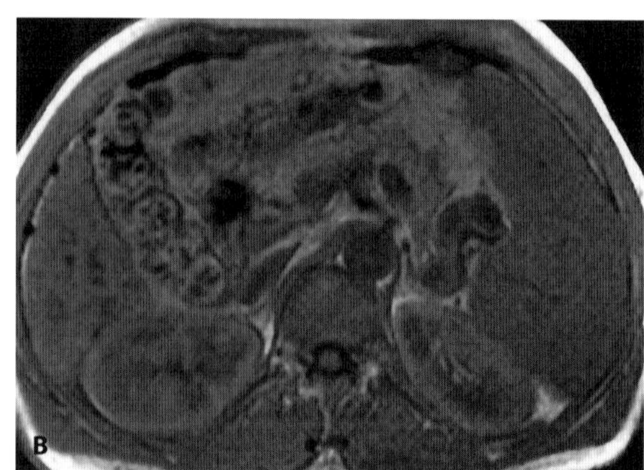

Fig. 9.21A, B.

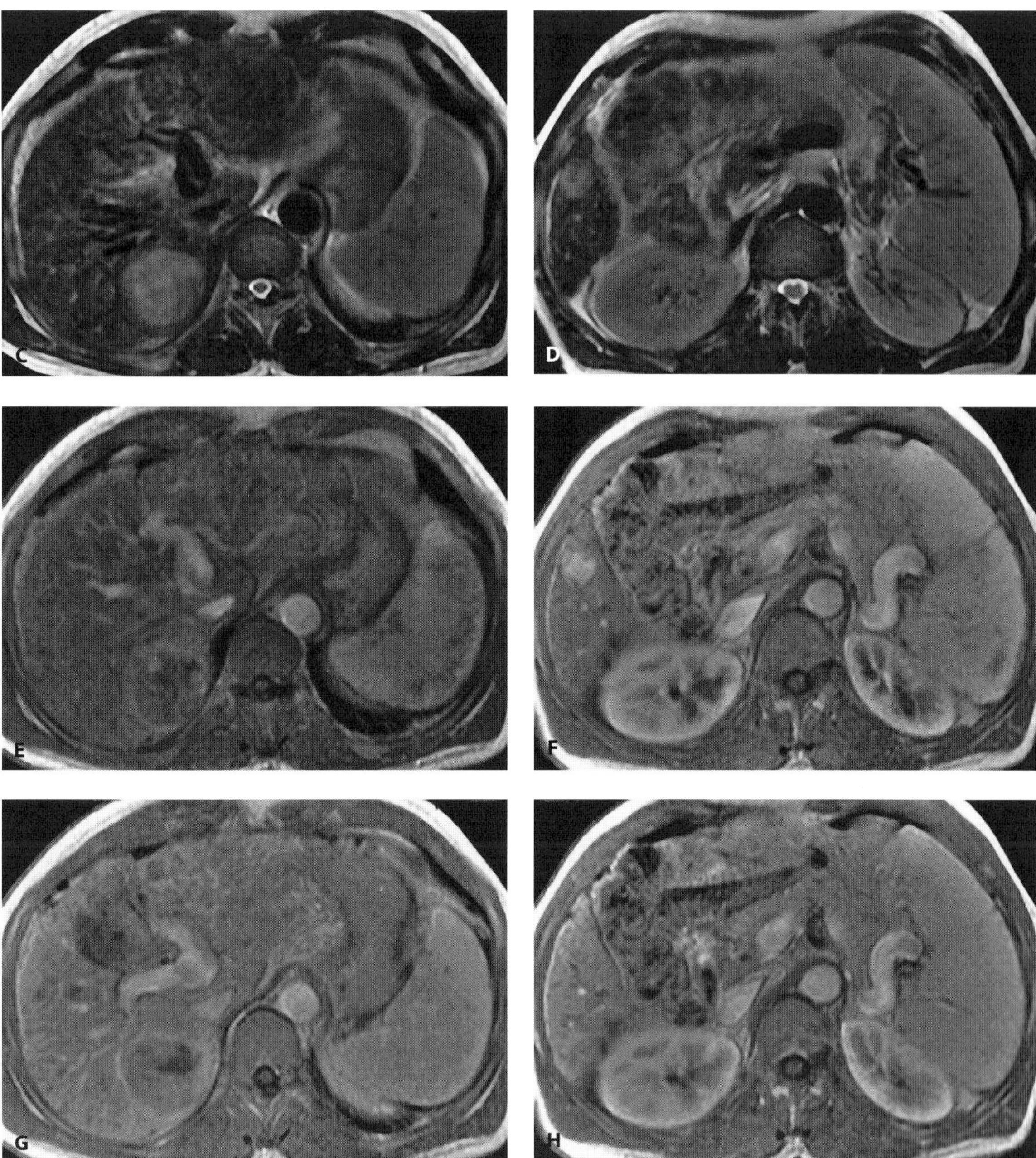

Fig. 9.21A–F. Multifocal HCC in hepatitis C with liver cirrhosis, iron overload, portal hypertension, and splenomegaly. Plain T1-W spoiled GRE (**A**,**B**), T2-W HASTE (TE 64 ms) (**C**,**D**), arterial phase, gadolinium-enhanced, T1-W spoiled GRE (**E**,**F**), and portal venous phase, gadolinium-enhanced, T1-W spoiled GRE (**G**,**H**) of a patient with HCC following chronic hepatitis C with liver cirrhosis, portal hypertension, and splenomegaly. The larger lesion is hypointense on plain T1-WI, while the smaller lesion is isointense. T2-WI demonstrates both lesions as relatively hyperintense (**C**,**D**). Both show strong contrast enhancement on arterial-phase images (**E**,**F**) which rapidly decreases on portal venous phase images (**G**,**H**). Imaging findings were confirmed following liver resection

Dynamic gadolinium-enhanced MR imaging demonstrates the hypervascular nature of tumors with often diffuse and intense enhancement, which typically involves the entire tumor stroma, while metastases predominantly reveal peripheral enhancement. The intensity of enhancement appears to correlate with tumor grading, and well-differentiated lesions may be completely hypovascular (Fig. 9.21).

Patients with pre-existing cirrhosis require careful image analysis, and any mass lesion with either hyperintensity on T2-WI or diffuse enhancement on gadolinium-enhanced images should be considered as potential HCC (Figs. 9.2 and 9.21).

Liver-specific contrast agents are helpful in the detection and characterization of HCC. The presence of hepatocellular cells in the early stages of HCC causes enhancement with hepatobiliary agents (Teslascan, MultiHance, and Gd-EOB-DTPA) on delayed images. Well-differentiated HCC may even show increased enhancement tissue because of persistent hepatocellular function combined with a decreased biliary clearance. Dynamic studies are also feasible with bolus-injectable MultiHance and Gd-EOB-DTPA, comparable with extracellular low-molecular-weight gadolinium-chelates. Iron oxides are suited to improve the detection of HCC in cirrhosis because both, regenerating nodules

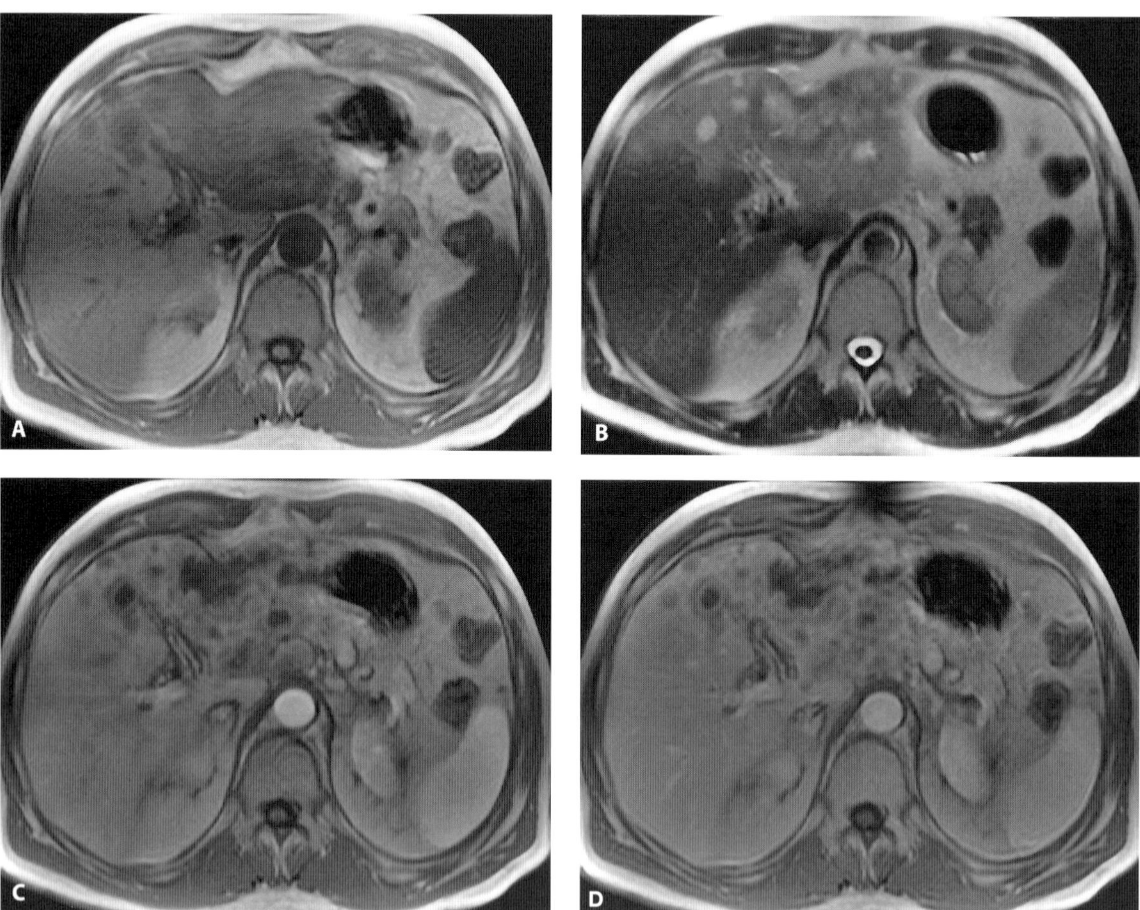

Fig. 9.22A–D. Multifocal cholangiocarcinoma. Plain T1-W spoiled GRE (**A**), T2-W TSE (TE 165 ms) (**B**), arterial phase, gadolinium-enhanced, T1-W spoiled GRE (**C**), and portal venous phase, gadolinium-enhanced, T1-W spoiled GRE (**D**) show a large mass in the left liver lobe with multiple satellite lesions. The biopsy-proven cholangiocarcinoma demonstrates low SI on T1-WI (**A**), slightly high SI on T2-WI with multiple hyperintense nodules (**B**), and peripheral contrast enhancement of multiple satellite lesions (**C**,**D**). Contrast-enhancement images clearly show the extent of disease much better than plain images

and adenomatous hyperplasia, contain RES cells and therefore show uptake of particles. Phagocytic cells may be present in the early stages of HCC, which may also show some enhancement. Dynamic imaging with bolus-injectable iron oxides is also suited to study the vascularity of HCC.

Fibrolamellar HCC represents a slow-growing subtype with a good prognosis that occurs predominantly in young women without underlying liver disease as a large and solitary lesion. A central scar with radiating appearance is common. Lesions demonstrate heterogeneous hypointensity on T1-WI and heterogeneous hyperintensity on T2-WI. Gadolinium enhancement is diffuse, without enhancement of the scar, which also appears hypointense on T2-WI (see also FNH).

9.6.7 Cholangiocarcinoma (CCC)

Intrahepatic cholangiocarcinoma (CCC) is not as common as HCC and typically presents as a large mass lesion in elderly patients with low SI on T1-WI and moderate SI on T2-WI. CCC causes compression of the portal veins and biliary system. Gadolinium-enhanced T1-WI typically demonstrates a hypovascular tumor with minimal to diffuse heterogeneous enhancement which then persists on delayed images (Figs. 9.1 and 9.22).

9.7 Biliary System

9.7.1 Biliary Anatomy

MR imaging of the intrahepatic and extrahepatic biliary system is tailored to visualize either the biliary fluid or the duct walls and adjacent soft-tissue structures. MRCP demonstrates bile within the ducts and gallbladder by using heavily T2-W sequences with TE longer than the T2-relaxation times of soft tissue, which then does not contribute to the signal on images (Figs. 9.23). This technique allows the visualization of fluid (bright) and may be considered as a fluid-W technique. T1-WI and T2-WI without or with fat suppression and gadolinium enhancement demonstrate the duct wall and adjacent soft-tissue structures (Fig. 9.7). Hepatobiliary agents show a bright ductal system on T1-WI based upon the biliary excretion of contrast agents into the bile. However, at the disadvantage of increased cost, the use of hepatobiliary agents has not been proven to be clinically advantageous compared with heavily T2-WI in visualizing the ductal system.

9.7.2 Technique

A variety of MRCP techniques is available with different approaches depending on scanner hardware and software, including 2D, 3D, breath-holding, or respiratory triggering (Table 9.1). One simple breathhold approach with a RARE sequence uses a thick slab with long TE and an oblique coronal image that requires no further postprocessing. The commonly used multisection techniques use a HASTE sequence with thin sections and postprocessing to generate maximum-intensity projections (MIP). However, consideration of the source images together with the postprocessed images is mandatory for clinical analysis. 3D techniques are typically based upon TSE sequences acquired with respiratory triggering using navigator techniques and thin overlapping reconstructions. The performance of these different approaches is somewhat vendor-specific and depends on the equipment available. When administered for other indications, hepatobiliary contrast agents also exhibit high SI within the bile and, thus, directly visualize the duct lumen. Gadolinium-enhanced T1-WI shows ducts with intraluminal low SI and can be used as a 'dark-fluid' technique. Gadolinium-enhanced FS T1-WI, preferably with breathhold techniques, is ideal to image the ducts and adjacent soft tissues.

9.7.3 Benign Biliary Disease

Acute and chronic cholecystitis are imaged with axial plain T1-WI, T2-WI, and gadolinium-enhanced T1-WI, using fat-suppression techniques. FS gadolinium-enhanced T1-WI demonstrates a strong enhancement of the gallbladder wall and pericholecystic tissues in acute cholecystitis. Chronic cholecystitis presents as a crumpled, irregularly shaped gallbladder with a thick-

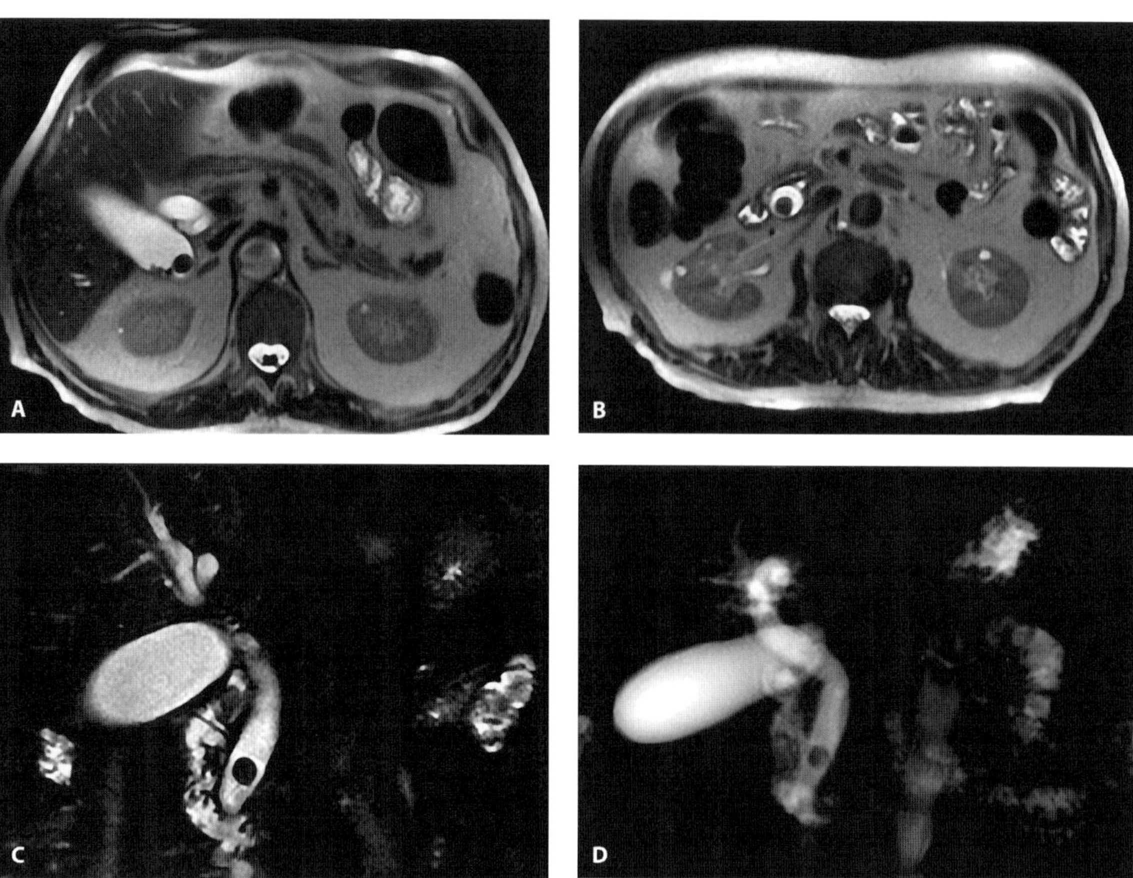

Fig. 9.23A–D. Gallbladder and common bile duct stones. Axial T2-HASTE (TE90 ms) (**A**,**B**), thin coronal MRCP section (**C**), and MIP of MRCP images (**D**) demonstrate multiple stones in the gallbladder and a distal common bile duct stone. The hypointense stones are well demarcated in the otherwise hyperintense bile (**A**–**C**). The common bile duct stone is better visualized with the single-section technique (**B**,**C**), and the gallbladder stones are completely missed on the MIP (**D**)

ened but only mildly enhancing wall. The degree of mural enhancement and enhancement of pericholecystic tissue reflect the activity and the degree of the inflammatory process.

Cholangitis occurs as infectious or sclerosing cholangitis. Infective cholangitis, by ascending infections, presents with ductal wall thickening which enhances on gadolinium-enhanced T1-WI. Ductal dilatation is best appreciated with MRCP techniques. A potential complication is the development of biliary abscesses, which are best visualized on FS T2-WI and FS gadolinium-enhanced T1-WI. Sclerosing cholangitis is characterized by a segmental dilatation of the biliary tree with interleaved narrowed segments resulting in a beaded and stenotic appearance that is best appreciated on MRCP. A second feature is mild ductal wall thickening, which is demonstrated best on FS gadolinium-enhanced T1-WI obtained during the portal venous phase. Enhancement correlates with the degree of inflammation. Cholangiocarcinoma is the most important pitfall. Its differential diagnosis should be considered when the ductal wall thickening tends to be greater than 5 mm and the degree of enhancement tends to be lesser than in infective cholangitis.

Calculous disease within the gallbladder and biliary ducts is best depicted with heavily T2-WI (e.g.,MRCP), rendering the bile bright and stones dark. The bile is typically dark on T1-WI and bright on T2-WI (Fig. 9.23). SI of the gallbladder content on T1-WI may vary from dark (water) to bright (fat, proteins), with fluid-fluid levels if sludge is present. Biliary obstruction is also best demonstrated using MRCP techniques, which are also helpful in the planning of endoscopic or percutaneous interventions. The specificity, sensitivity, and accuracy for the detection of choledocholithiasis has been reported to be 90% or better. ERCP is still the gold standard, combining diagnosis and treatment. However, MRCP is valuable in patients prior to laparoscopic cholecystectomy to rule out choledocholithiasis, with surgical bypass procedures such as hepatojejunostomy or gastrectomy, and in patients with acute pancreatitis. Pitfalls in diagnosing calculous disease are biliary prostheses, clips, aerobilia, hematobilia, and incrustations.

MRCP studies should be performed prior to the placement of biliary plastic prostheses or metal stents. Plastic prostheses are diamagnetic and provide no signal on MR images isointense to stones or sludge. Metal stents show susceptibility artifacts depending on their structure and composition. The assessment of the duct over the length of the stent is subsequently at least significantly reduced and in most stents impossible. Patients with surgical complications following laparoscopic cholecystectomy may be scanned without any harm since surgical clips are MR compatible, and the area of interest may be assessed without any restrictions. The major advantage of MRI is the comprehensive assessment of parenchymal structures, ductal structures, vessels, extrahepatic tissues, and fluid collections.

Cystic diseases, such as pancreatic cysts, choledochal cyst, choledochocele, or Caroli's syndrome (Fig. 9.24), are best visualized on coronal and axial MRCP images.

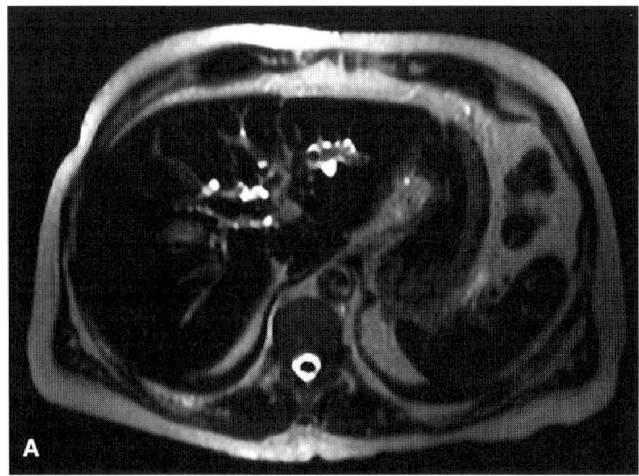

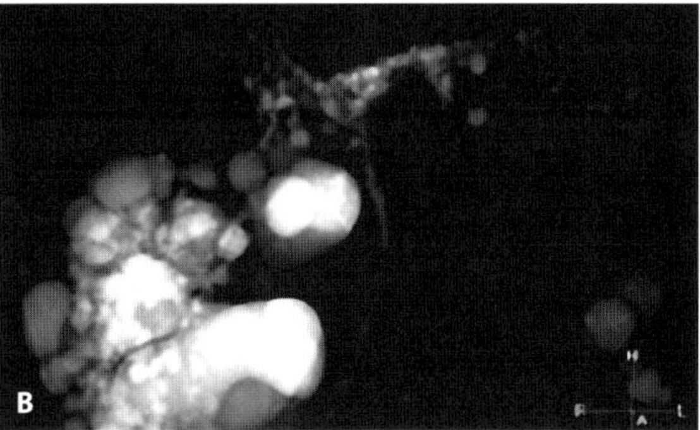

Fig. 9.24A–D. Caroli's syndrome. Axial navigator-echo-triggered T2-TSE (**A**) and coronal MRCP projection (**B**) demonstrate multiple intrahepatic bile-duct-associated cysts and extrahepatic cysts. The hyperintense cysts are well demarcated against the otherwise hypointense structures

9.7.4 Malignant Biliary Disease

Gallbladder cancer has a strong association with calculous disease, typically presenting as a defect within the gallbladder or a mass replacing the gallbladder. Focal or diffuse thickening (10 mm) of the gallbladder wall is suspicious. Invasion into the adjacent liver, duodenum, and pancreas occurs frequently. T2-WI and gadolinium-enhanced T1-WI are useful in depicting liver invasion. FS gadolinium-enhanced T1-WI better visualizes the extension into pancreas and adjacent tissue.

Extrahepatic cholangiocarcinoma typically occurs in older patients presenting with jaundice and weight loss. The tumor represents a primary malignancy of the bile ducts and is classified as central or peripheral. Central tumors refer to lesions arising from the main hepatic ducts (common bile duct: CBD) and peripheral tumors arise from intrahepatic branches. The most frequent location is the junction of the right and left hepatic ducts, where they are called Klatskin tumors. Tumors of the common bile duct are more frequent than tumors of the intrahepatic branches. The role of imaging is to determine the proximal extent of Klatskin tumors for planning resectability (Fig. 9.7). Biliary obstruction with intrahepatic ductal dilatation and ductal wall thickening of 4 mm or more are suggestive of cholangiocarcinoma. A combination of MRCP and gadolinium-enhanced T1-WI is useful to depict lesions that enhance moderately. Tumors within the pancreatic head present as hypointense lesions within the otherwise hyperintense pancreatic head. MRCP is particularly helpful in guiding palliative treatment and produces a 3D view of the intrahepatic and extrahepatic biliary tree, which is more difficult to obtain by ERCP. Gadolinium-enhanced T1-WI are useful to show superficial tumor spread by demonstrating thickened (2 mm) duct wall tissue with increased enhancement. It is mandatory to obtain axial and coronal/oblique contrast-enhanced images in order to assess the presence or absence of infiltration of the Klatskin tumor into the hepatic parenchyma, which is important for tumor staging. Inflammatory changes and susceptibility artifacts following stenting may complicate this diagnosis. The complete evaluation of Klatskin tumors includes imaging of the liver, biliary ducts, adjacent soft tissues, lymph nodes, and vessels, with focus on the portal vein. A comprehensive MR imaging and MR angiography protocol with conventional imaging, MRCP, and MR angiography (Figs. 9.7 and 9.30) is mandatory.

Periampullary and ampullary disease includes carcinomas, adenomas, and inflammatory changes. Patients with tumors present with a dilatation of the pancreatic duct and common bile duct (dual duct sign). Tumors are best depicted using a combination of MRCP and T1-WI. Tumors typically present as hypointense lesions contrasted against the hyperintense pancreas on FS T1-WI and show mild contrast enhancement. Inflammatory changes, such as those observed following ERCP, demonstrate stronger contrast enhancement, which is also best demonstrated on FS T1-WI (Fig. 9.30). The role of dedicated oral contrast agents as compared with water or studies without any additional oral contrast has not been clearly evaluated.

9.8 Pancreas

9.8.1 Pancreas Anatomy

The pancreas is best depicted on T1-W sequences with thin sections (<6 mm) which provide good contrast of pancreatic tissue with intermediate to slightly high SI against the high SI of surrounding adipose tissue. Pancreatic SI may be decreased by atrophy, pancreatitis, neoplasm, and iron overload. Fat suppression improves the conspicuity of pancreatic parenchyma and focal pancreatic lesions, which is of particular importance in small nonobstructing lesions. SI on T2-W sequences varies even more than on T1-W sequences, but T2-WI is useful to demonstrate fluid-filled structures. MR angiography scans are preferably obtained as breathhold 3D CE-MR angiography sequences. MRCP visualizes ductal structures by means of intraluminal fluid and is performed with heavily T2-W 2D or 3D sequences (see Table 9.1).

9.8.2 Technique

Two different intravenous contrast techniques are available to improve pancreatic MR, especially for the depiction of small focal lesions and vascular invasion. Gadolinium-enhanced T1-W MR shows a stronger and earlier capillary enhancement of the well-vascularized pancreas compared with the liver. The detection of hypovascular tumors relies on the visualization of a low-SI lesion contrasted against the well-vascularized pancreas before the arterial bolus diminishes. Contrast is also helpful to depict necrotic or less-perfused areas of the pancreatic tissues and inflammatory tissue.

Alternatively, Teslascan may be used to enhance the normal pancreatic parenchyma on T1-WI over a longer period of time. Originally developed as a hepatobiliary agent with intracellular uptake into hepatocytes, Teslascan has subsequently been tested for CE-MRI of the pancreas and is clinically approved for this indication in Europe (see Chapter 2); the compound has been noted to enhance the pancreas, probably due to the uptake of free manganese. The exact clinical role of Teslascan-enhanced pancreatic MRI compared with gadolinium-enhanced pancreatic MRI still has to be defined by controlled clinical studies.

Delineation of the pancreas from bowel can be improved by the administration of oral contrast media. The most inexpensive, well tolerated, and safe contrast agent is water with low SI on T1-WI and high SI on T2-WI. The effects of commercially available paramagnetic or superparamagnetic oral contrast agents on the intraluminal SI depend on the pulse sequences used. Paramagnetic oral contrast media show a predominantly high intraluminal SI on T1-W, and superparamagnetic oral contrast media show predominantly low intraluminal SI on T2-WI (see Chapters 1 and 2).

9.8.3 Congenital Anomalies and Diseases

9.8.3.1 Pancreas Divisum

Pancreas divisum is the most clinically important anatomic variant, with a lack of fusion of the dorsal and ventral main pancreatic ducts (Fig. 9.25). The common bile duct drains separately from the main pancreatic duct into the major papilla, and the dorsal part of the main pancreatic duct (Wirsung) drains into the minor papilla. The higher incidence of acute pancreatitis in patients with pancreas divisum is believed to be due to congestion in the duct from partial obstruction at the orifice of the minor papilla. MRCP is a tool to detect this anomaly in patients with acute pancreatitis, obviating the need for diagnostic ERCP.

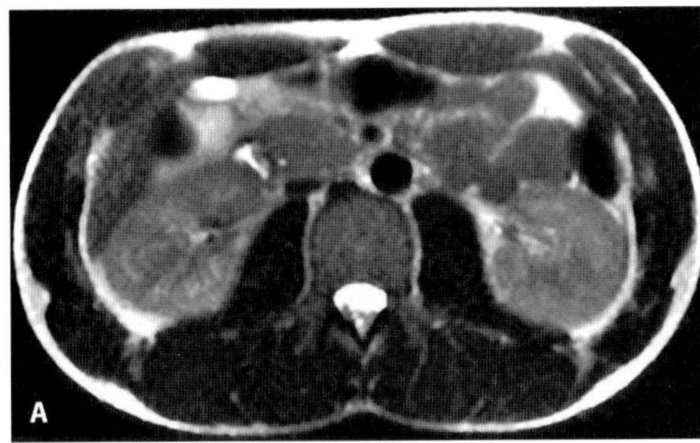

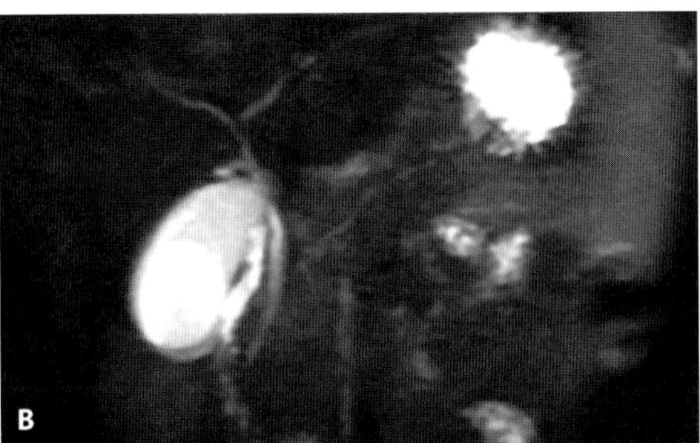

Fig. 9.25A,B. Pancreas divisum. Axial T2-W HASTE (TE 64 ms) (**A**) and MIP of a stack of coronal HASTE images (**B**) demonstrate a lack of fusion of the dorsal and the ventral main pancreatic ducts in a 20-year-old patient with two episodes of acute pancreatitis. The common bile duct drains separately from the main pancreatic duct into the major papilla, and the dorsal part of the main pancreatic duct (Wirsung) drains into the minor papilla

9.8.3.2 Hemochromatosis

Primary or idiopathic hemochromatosis may show low SI on T2/T2*-WI due to iron deposition within exocrine and b-islet cells, causing diabetes mellitus. The liver is involved earlier and more substantially, with the formation of liver cirrhosis. Deposition of iron in the pancreas and heart tends to occur during late stages of disease. Secondary hemochromatosis due to blood transfusion or hemolysis does not involve the pancreas.

9.8.3.3 Cystic Fibrosis

Cystic fibrosis is the major congenital disease that causes variable degrees of fatty replacement and atrophy. The fat content can be nicely demonstrated by T1-W sequences with and without fat suppression.

9.8.3.4 Lipomatosis

Severe lipomatous depositions within the pancreas may be observed in adult patients with excessive weight, senile atrophy, or cystic fibrosis. The parenchyma appears lobulated, with preserved margins and a reduced volume. T1-W techniques without and with fat saturation are mostly used to demonstrate and identify these lipomatous depositions.

9.8.4 Pancreatitis

Acute and chronic forms of pancreatitis may be grouped according to their clinical course and severity (edematous, exudative, infectious, hemorraghic, or necrotizing).

9.8.4.1 Acute Pancreatitis

Patients with suspected or known acute pancreatitis are usually imaged by US or CT complementary to clinical and laboratory findings. These imaging modalities can be performed in intensive care units and are therefore more easily arranged in clinical practice.

Uncomplicated acute pancreatitis resembles the normal pancreas with intermediate to slightly high SI on T1-WI and uniform gadolinium enhancement. Edematous pancreatitis and exudative pancreatitis are the most common presentations (Fig. 9.26). Severe pancreatitis may demonstrate abscess, superinfection, bleeding, necrosis, and vascular complications such as thrombosis or aneurysm. The assessment of pancreatitis requires a comprehensive MR protocol with MR imaging and MRCP and is more difficult to perform than CT with severely ill patients. MRI is more sensitive than CT and US in detecting the subtle changes of complicated acute pancreatitis, such as peripancreatic fluids, inflammatory changes, hemorrhage, pseudocyst

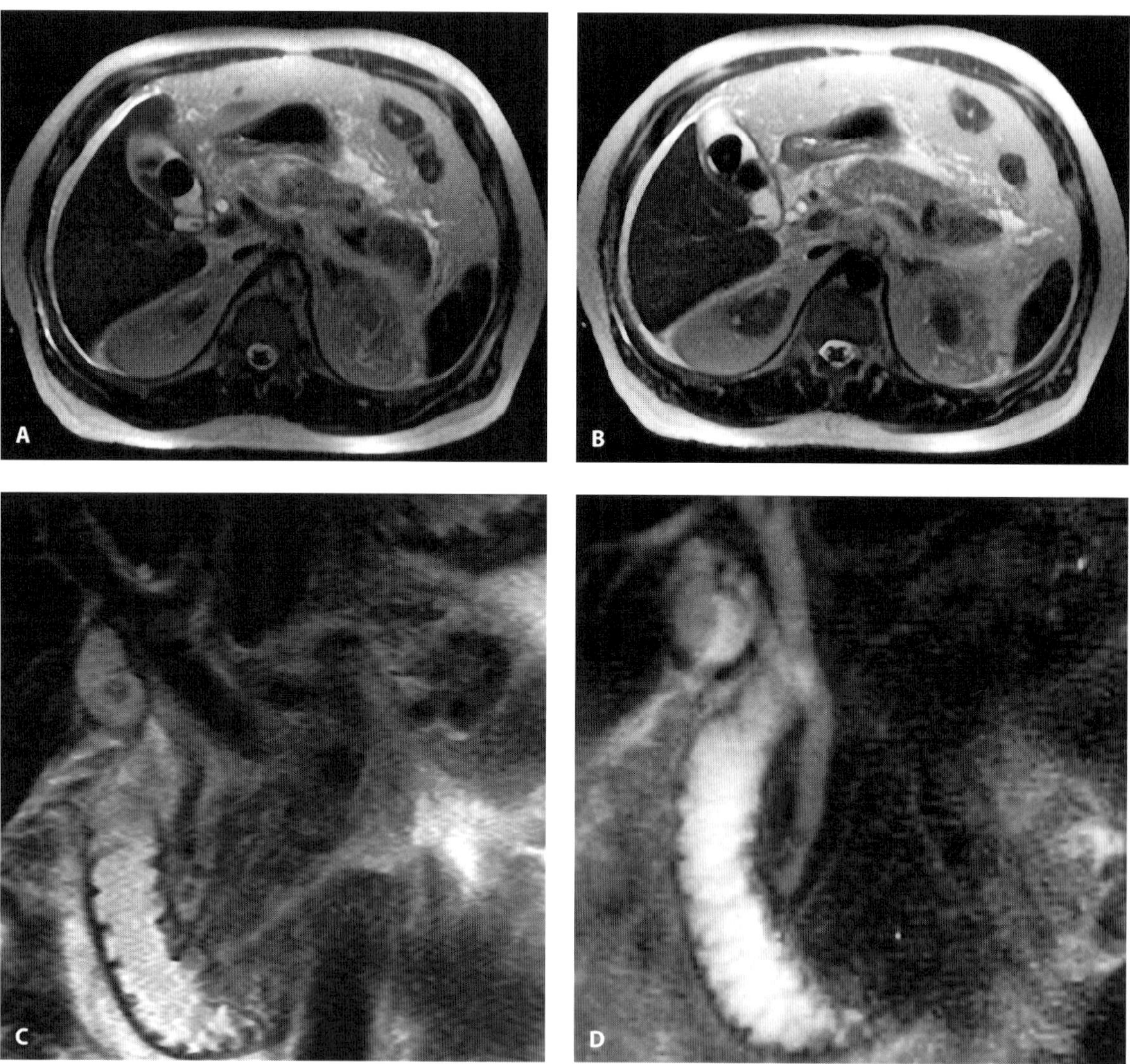

Fig. 9.26A–D. Common bile duct stones with acute pancreatitis. Axial T2-HASTE (TE90 ms) (**A,B**), thin true-FISP section (**C**), and MIP of MRCP images (**D**) demonstrate multiple stones in the gallbladder, two distal common bile duct stones, and an enlarged pancreas with surrounding fluid. The hypointense stones are well demarcated in the otherwise hyperintense bile (**A–D**). Pancreatitis was caused by an obstruction of the main pancreatic duct by the common bile duct stones, which were subsequently removed

formation, and necrosis. MR angiography can be useful to demonstrate vascular complications, obviating the need for invasive catheter angiography. The patient should be able to sustain breathhold acquisitions up to 20 s. RARE or HASTE type sequences are more robust to breathing artifacts due to their contiguous acquisition scheme than sequences with a multislice acquisition scheme (SE, TSE, or GRE).

9.8.4.2 Chronic Pancreatitis

End-stage chronic pancreatitis is characterized by irreversible damage of the endocrine and exocrine pancreatic function. Dilatation of the main pancreatic duct, parenchymal atrophy, calcification, pseudocyst, focal gland enlargement, and biliary ductal dilatation (Fig. 9.27) characterize chronic pancreatitis.

The most difficult diagnosis is the differentiation of adenocarcinoma and focal pancreatitis, which has similar features (low perfused areas with hypointense appearance on T1-WI). Unsuspected adenocarcinoma is pathologically detected in approximately 15% of patients following surgery for chronic pancreatitis. MRI shows decreased SI on T1-WI with decreased and more inhomogeneous gadolinium enhancement. Ductal dilatations and strictures can be well visualized with MRCP. Calcifications cannot be directly demonstrated.

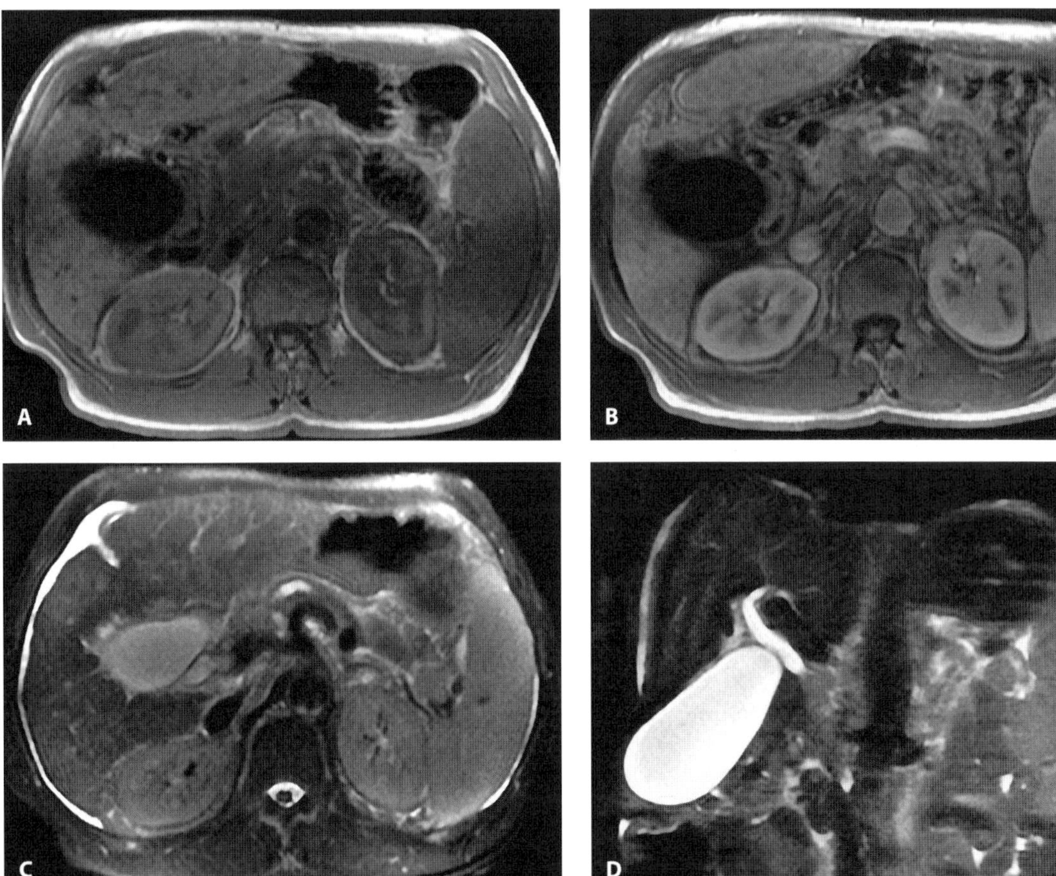

Fig. 9.27A–D. Chronic pancreatitis. Plain T1-W spoiled GRE (**A**), gadolinium-enhanced, T1-W spoiled GRE (**B**), T2-W HASTE (**C**), and a coronal T2-W HASTE (**D**) from a MRCP study in a patient with a long history of chronic pancreatitis. SI of the gland is decreased on plain T1-W spoiled GRE (**A**), and the contrast-enhanced study (**B**) reveals a decreased and more inhomogeneous gadolinium enhancement than the normal pancreatic parenchyma. T2-W HASTE demonstrates dilatation of the common bile duct (**D**) and main pancreatic duct (**C**) with parenchymal atrophy and focal enlargement of the pancreatic head

CE-MRI with gadolinium chelates and Teslascan exhibit similar contrast effects with a lower enhancement within chronic pancreatitis than in the normal pancreas and a sometimes even lower enhancement within areas of focal tumor. It appears that CE-MRI is more sensitive than CT or US in the detection of adenocarcinoma in patients with chronic pancreatitis, but focal chronic pancreatitis remains a diagnostic challenge.

9.8.5 Tumors

9.8.5.1 Cystic Tumors

9.8.5.1.1 Dysontogenic Pancreatic Cysts

Dysontogenic pancreatic cysts with an epithelial cell lining are very rare and incidentally detected. They are more frequently associated with cystic kidney disease, cystic liver disease, and von Hippel-Lindau disease. MR features of these well-circumscribed, round or oval cysts include low SI on T1-WI, high SI on T2-WI, and no contrast enhancement.

9.8.5.1.2 Pseudocysts

Pseudocysts may develop during the course of pancreatitis within areas of necrosis or exudation with a surrounding wall of granulation tissue and without an epithelial cell lining. The contents consist of pancreatic debris, pancreatic excretion, or old blood. A spontaneous and typically early regression (<6–8 weeks) is possible. Imaging of a pancreatic pseudocyst is not a strong indication for MRI, and pseudocysts are most often coincidentally detected when areas of focal chronic pancreatitis are imaged to rule out pancreatic cancer. The imaging appearance varies considerably according to the potentially different components. The center typically shows low SI on T1-WI and high SI on T2-WI. Sludge and hemorrhagic components cause a lower signal on T2-WI. The cystic wall may reach several millimeters thick and may demonstrate gadolinium enhancement due to the well-perfused granulation tissue. The wall shows low SI on T1-WI and T2-WI. Calcifications occur frequently and are best depicted on CT.

9.8.5.1.3 Cystic Neoplasm

MRI can be useful to differentiate benign microcystic adenoma (serous cystadenoma) and potentially malignant mucinous cystic neoplasms (cystadenoma or cystadenocarcinoma) along with clinical parameters such as age, location, and size. MRI evaluates the cystic components of these tumors better than CT or US.

Microcystic adenoma is a benign tumor characterized by multiple, small cysts occurring in older patients (Fig. 9.28). The tumor may contain an often calcified scar, has an average diameter of approximately 5 cm without invasion of surrounding structures, and is well defined on MR with hypointense cystic components on T1-WI and hyperintense cystic components on T2-WI. The cystic wall may show contrast enhancement.

Mucinous adenoma or adenocarcinoma is a macrocystic, potentially malignant, mucin-containing tumor (Fig. 9.29). These tumors are larger, with an average diameter of approximately 10 cm, multiloculated, usually located in the pancreatic body and tail, and occur more frequently in women. The rare subtype of a duct ectatic mucinous adenoma is predominantly located in the uncinate process. Single cysts are typically larger than 20 mm in diameter. Smaller daughter cysts may occur within larger cysts. Small tumors appear partially solid with smaller cysts and may, therefore, be difficult to differentiate from microcystic adenomas. T1-W FS gadolinium-enhanced images demonstrate irregular, hypointense, cystic spaces and thick septa. The mucin content tends to appear hyperintense on T1-WI and T2-WI, and the cystic components are more readily visible compared to CT. Aqueous cysts demonstrate water-equivalent contrast features. It appears almost impossible to safely rule out a malignant transformation or focus since only small areas with a lesser degree of contrast enhancement may be involved. Therefore, surgical resection of the tumor is recommended.

The differential diagnosis of macrocystic adenoma includes the rare entity of a solid and papillary epithelial neoplasm. This low-grade tumor with a low risk of metastasis is typically observed in young women during their third decade of life. The diagnosis of a solid and papillary epithelial neoplasm should be considered when a large (>10 cm) mass is present within the

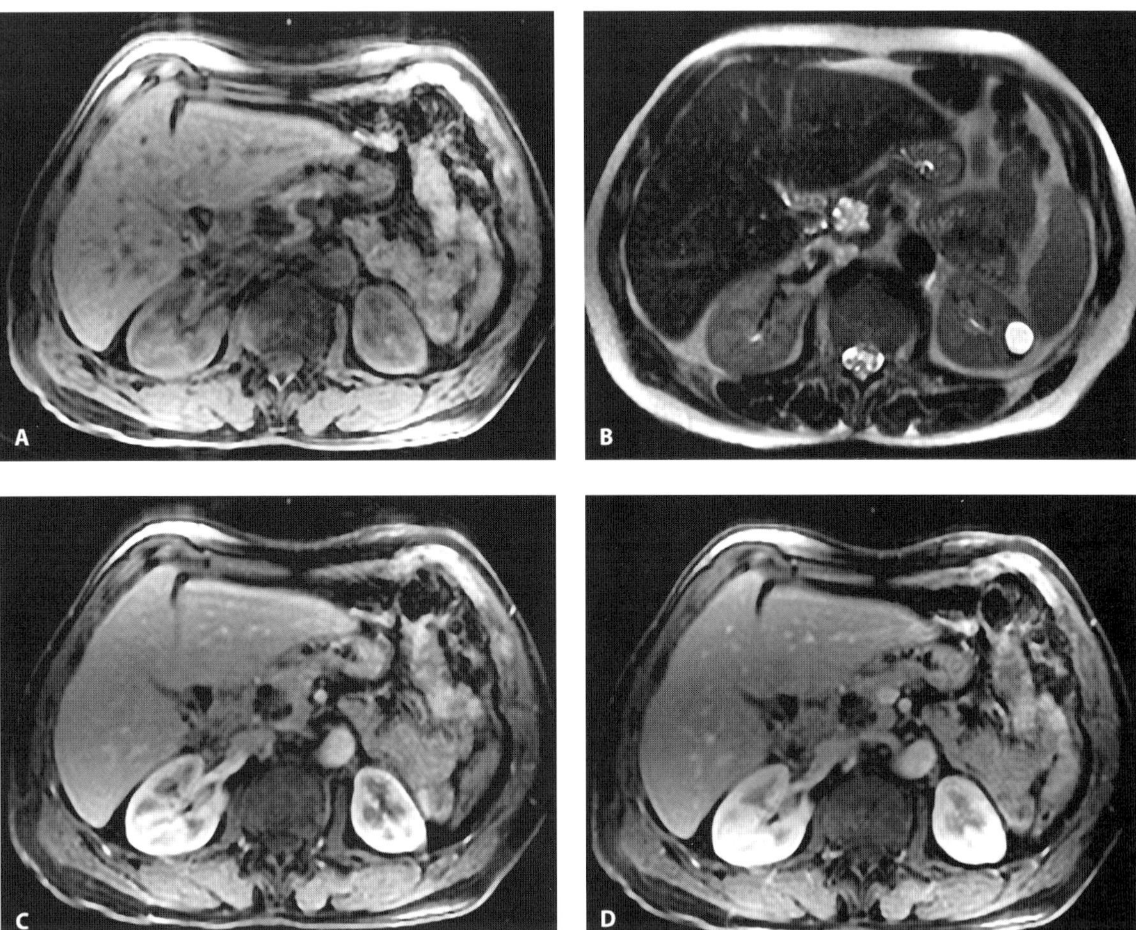

Fig. 9.28A–D. Microcystic adenoma. Plain T1-W spoiled GRE (**A**), axial HASTE (**B**), arterial phase, gadolinium-enhanced, T1-W spoiled GRE (**C**), and portal venous phase, gadolinium-enhanced, T1-W spoiled GRE (**D**) in a patient with a mass lesion in the pancreatic head. The mass is lobulated (**A**–**D**) and consists of small cysts [T1-hypointense (**A**) and T2-hyperintense (**B**)] without noticeable wall enhancement (**C**,**D**)

pancreatic tail mimicking features of a macrocystic adenoma.

9.8.5.2
Solid Tumors – Pancreatic Adenocarcinoma

The most common pancreatic tumor is ductal adenocarcinoma, accounting for 95% of all malignant tumors of the pancreas and known for its dismal prognosis. Staging of the disease is still the main role of imaging modalities, while the incidental detection of a ductal adenocarcinoma is rare. Focal disease is present in 80% and diffuse involvement in 20%. Location of focal disease is predominantly confined to the pancreatic head in 60%, followed by the body in 15%, and tail in 5%. Since pancreatic carcinomas of the pancreatic head tend to obstruct the CBD and produce jaundice, these tumors are typically smaller than tumors of the body and tail at the time of onset of clinical symptoms and imaging tests. However, in less than 15%, the tumor is still confined to the pancreas when detected, without the presence of lymph node or distant metastases.

MRI is the only imaging modality offering a comprehensive evaluation of the tumor, parenchymal organs,

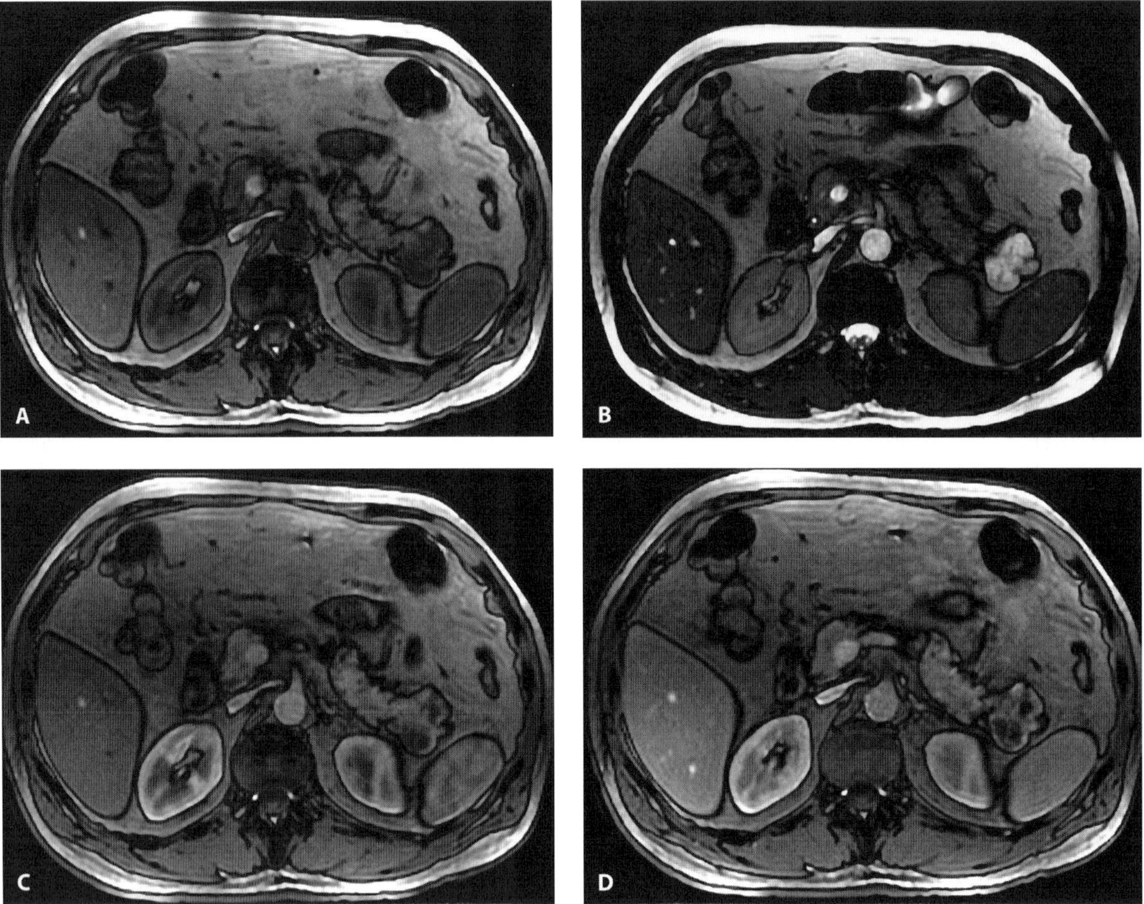

Fig. 9.29A–D. Macrocystic carcinoma. Plain T1-W spoiled GRE (**A**), axial true-FISP (**B**), arterial phase, gadolinium-enhanced, T1-W spoiled GRE (**C**), and portal venous phase, gadolinium-enhanced, T1-W spoiled GRE (**D**) in a patient with a mass lesion in the pancreatic tail. The mass is lobulated (**A–D**) and consists of large confluent cysts [T1-hypointense (**A**) and T2-hyperintense (**B**)] with thick enhancing walls (**C**,**D**)

surrounding soft tissue, vessels, and ductal structures. Pancreatic adenocarcinoma is hypointense on T1-WI, and fat suppression potentially improves the conspicuity. Rapid scanning following gadolinium injection during the capillary phase (<30–60 s postinjection) should demonstrate tumors as hypointense (hypovascular) lesions, and some enhancement of viable tumor may be visible on later scans (Fig. 9.30). Consecutive pancreatic atrophy, causing low SI of the normal pancreas, may reduce the contrast relative to focal tumors, and as a rule of thumb, the pancreas should only be considered normal if the SI is equal to or higher than the liver or renal cortex. Ductal obstruction is best visualized with MRCP techniques (Fig. 9.30). However, the depiction and differentiation of a pancreatic adenocarcinoma close to the ampulla of Vater, ampullary tumors, periampullary tumors, and distal bile duct calculi may still be difficult and require ERCP also for histopathologic proof and palliative intervention. T2-WI may help to rule out stones, which appear with low SI, while tumors appear with intermediate SI; however, the detection of a stone does not rule out cancer.

Imaging analysis has to include all relevant structures. A dilatation of the pancreatic duct may already be suggestive for a tumor. Irregular ductal dilatations following the course of chronic pancreatitis and stone-related dilatations have to be considered. A pronounced tumor necrosis may mimic a pseudocyst but will not contain calcifications and will show an irregularly thickened wall. Some tumors are associated with an inflammatory reaction, and thus the tumor may appear larger. Regional lymph node metastases are observed in up to two-thirds of patients. End-stage disease is characterized by peritoneal carcinomatosis with ascites, tumor infiltration into surrounding organs or soft-tissue structures, and liver metastases (Fig. 9.30). The

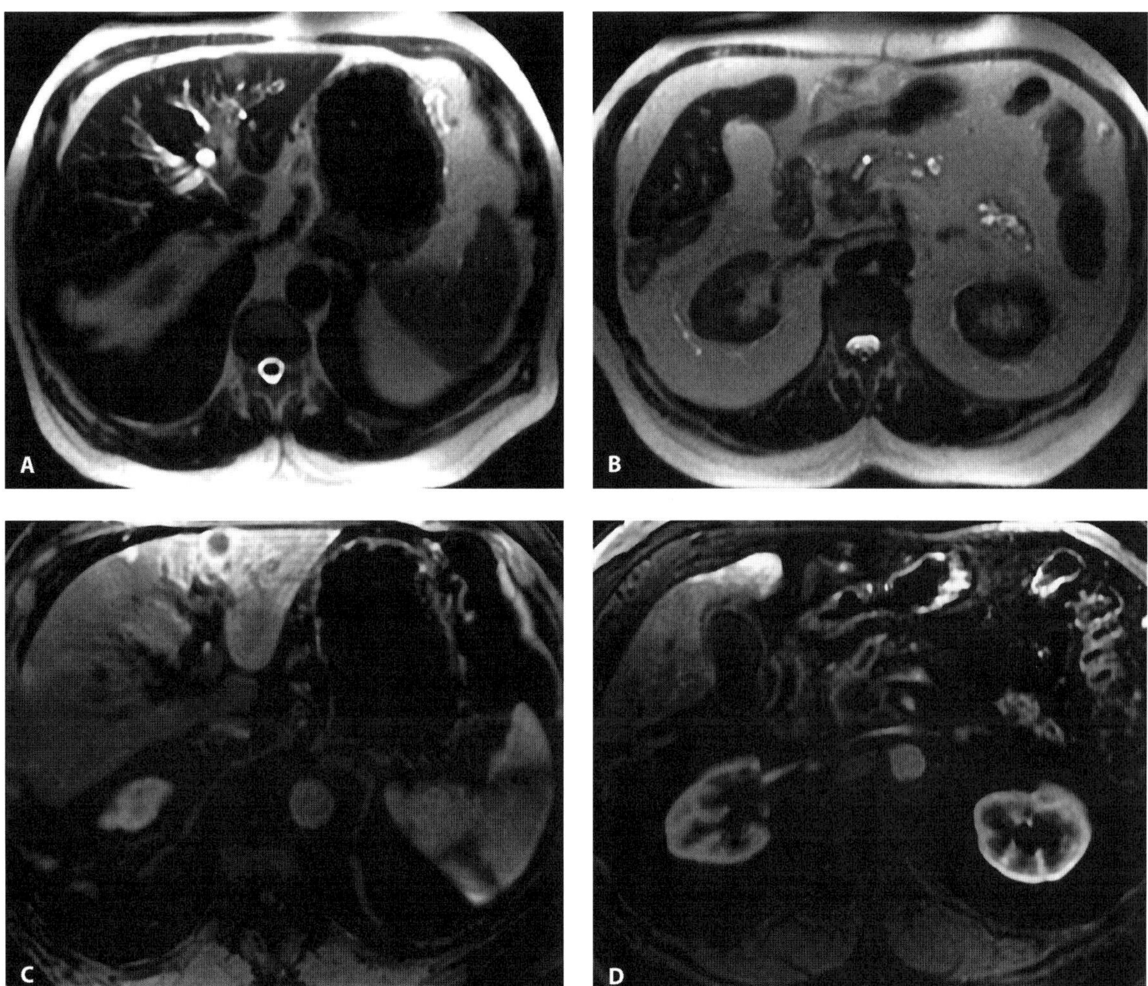

Fig. 9.30A–H. Pancreatic adenocarcinoma. Axial HASTE (**A**,**B**), axial, arterial phase, gadolinium-enhanced, FS-3D T1-W spoiled GRE (**C**,**D**), portal venous phase, gadolinium-enhanced, FS-3D T1-W spoiled GRE (**E**,**F**), thick-slab MRCP (**G**), and MIP of the portal venous phase of CE-MRA (**H**). Sections through the liver (**A**,**C**,**E**) demonstrate intrahepatic ductal dilatation and a subcapsular metastasis with ring enhancement. The common bile duct and the main pancreatic duct are obstructed at the level of the pancreatic head. The tumor is best seen as a hypoperfused, hypointense mass on contrast-enhanced FS-3D spoiled GRE images (**D**,**F**) and is barely visible as a hyperintense mass on T2-W HASTE (**B**). MRCP-MIP (**G**) from a stack of thin coronal HASTE images demonstrates the obstruction at the level of the pancreatic head close to the papilla of Vater. Arterial phase (**D**) and portal venous phase (**F**), gadolinium-enhanced, FS-3D T1-W spoiled GRE images show extension of the tumor to the confluence of the splenic vein and the SMV into the proximal portal vein (**D**,**F**). CE-MRA during the portal venous phase (**H**) displays findings from axial images with a visualized obstruction of the venous confluence. The tumor growth was confirmed at surgery, and a palliative gastroenterostomy was performed

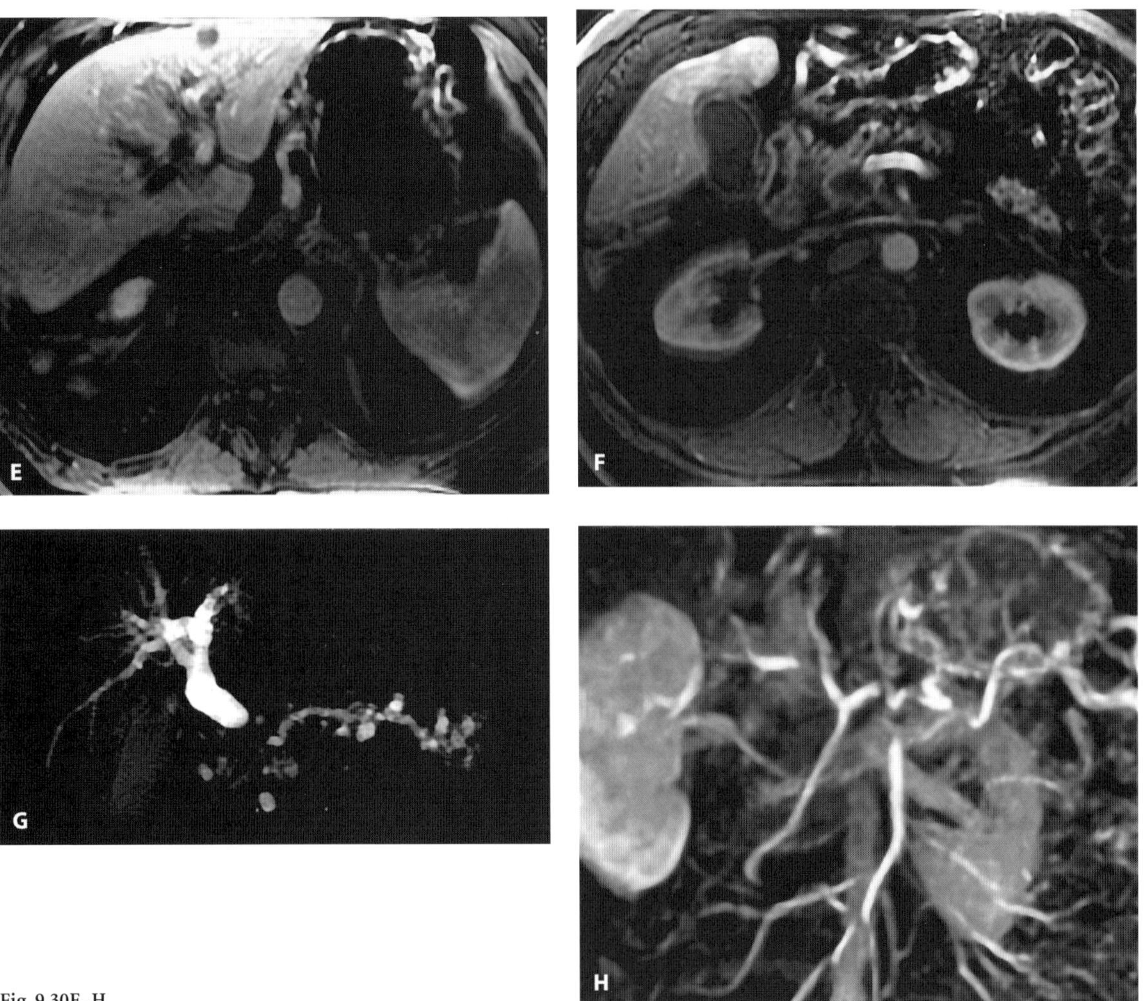

Fig. 9.30E–H.

most difficult indication is to rule out or depict carcinoma within chronic pancreatitis (see Chronic pancreatitis).

Signs of inoperability (infiltrative growth, vascular involvement, lymph node metastases, and distant metastases) are best identified by a comprehensive protocol including plain T1-WI, T2-WI, gadolinium-enhanced MRI, MRCP, and CE-MRA (Figs. 9.30 and 9.31). A capsule does not surround the pancreas, and thus, pancreatic carcinoma tends to invade along perivascular, lymphatic, and perineural structures. Therefore, the celiac axis, SMA, SMV, portal vein, and hepatoduodenal ligament are often encased or infiltrated at an early stage (Fig. 9.30). Obliteration of fat planes and direct tumor growth into canalicular structures are useful signs of inoperability. The detection of lymph nodes is comparable to that with CT; however, nodes along the celiac axis and porta hepatis may be more readily visible with MRI. Liver metastases are hypointense on T1-WI, slightly hyperintense on T2-WI, show rim enhancement on immediate gadolinium-enhanced T1-WI, and demonstrate no enhancement on delayed SPIO-enhanced T2-WI or delayed hepatobiliary-enhanced T1-WI (Figs. 9.19 and 9.20). MR offers the potential of a comprehensive test for the detection and staging of pancreatic adenocarcinoma; however, this requires that the study be specifically tailored to individual patients.

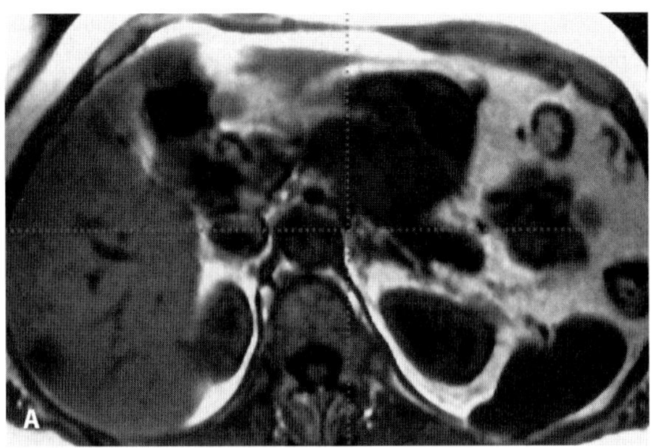

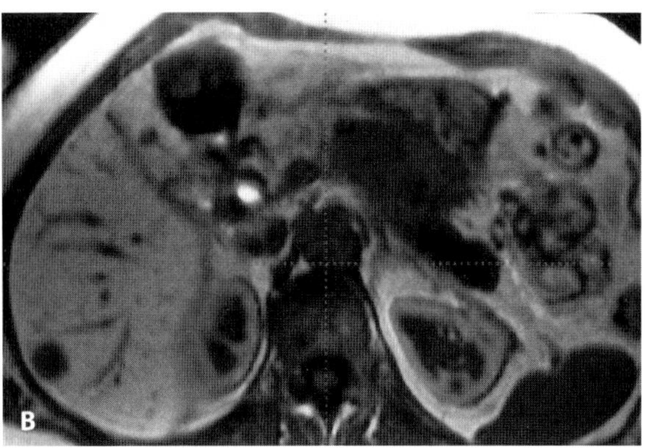

Fig. 9.31A,B. Teslascan-enhanced pancreatic adenocarcinoma. Plain T1-W spoiled GRE (**A**) and Teslascan-enhanced T1-W spoiled GRE (**B**) demonstrate a mass lesion within the pancreatic body and a lesion within the right liver lobe. Paramagnetic Teslascan (5 µmol/kg body weight) enhances the normal pancreas (signal increase), while the lesion shows no contrast enhancement. The pancreatic cancer has already infiltrated into surrounding tissue structures, and a liver metastasis is present. Imaging with Teslascan can be performed during a broader time window than with extracellular contrast agents, with a higher anatomic resolution than is possible for dynamic gadolinium-enhanced images where the lesion has to be preferably depicted during the arterial phase. However, areas of chronic pancreatitis also show no enhancement comparable to tumors, and Teslascan is therefore not able to solve this clinical problem. (Courtesy of W. Schima, Vienna, Austria)

9.8.5.3 Islet-Cell Tumors

The majority of islet-cell tumors, which are of neuroendocrine origin, arise from the pancreas. Islet-cell tumors are classified either as functional (80%) or nonfunctional (20%) and appear histologically as insulinoma, gastrinoma, glucagonoma, VIPoma, somatostatinoma, and carcinoid. The majority of islet-cell tumors are benign. Functional tumors are typically detected when smaller in size (typically <2 cm) than nonfunctional tumors because of symptoms related to the hormone secretion. Functional tumors may be part of multiple endocrine neoplasm (MEN I). Malignant islet-cell tumors (insulinoma 10% and glucagonoma 60%) are typically nonfunctional. T1-W FS gadolinium-enhanced sequences during the arterial phase and T2-W FS sequences are the most sensitive methods. Tumors are well defined and hypointense on T1-WI, demonstrate strong ring (larger tumors) or complete (smaller tumors) gadolinium enhancement, and are mostly hyperintense on T2-WI. This also differentiates islet-cell tumors from pancreatic adenocarcinoma, and liver metastases show similar features. Vessels are typically not encased, no ductal dilatation is present, and central necrosis is rare compared with pancreatic adenocarcinoma. Insulinomas are usually more hypervascular than the other islet-cell tumors (Fig. 9.17). Calcifications are frequent and best depicted on CT.

9.8.5.4 Lymphoma

Non-Hodgkin's lymphoma may directly involve the pancreas or peripancreatic lymph nodes, appearing with lower SI than the pancreas on T1-WI. Lymphomas are not very hyperintense on T2-WI and show only mild contrast enhancement. Pancreatic lymphomas are typically large and often present with a ventral displacement of the pancreas. Patients typically do not complain about pain and do not suffer from jaundice.

9.8.5.5 Metastases

Primary malignancies metastasizing to the pancreas or peripancreatic lymph nodes include melanoma, lung, kidney, breast, and gastrointestinal cancers. Direct infiltration into the pancreas from tumors either originating in surrounding organs (hypernephroma) or following the development of metastases within these organs may occur as well. The signal increase on gadolinium-enhanced T1-WI reflects the vascularity of metastases and primary malignancies.

9.8.6 Trauma and Surgical Complications

9.8.6.1 Trauma

Since MRI with MRCP and CE-MRA is a comprehensive tool to assess all pancreatic components, it is also a valid tool in acute trauma (Fig. 9.32). Lacerations show a broad range from contusions to complete transections of the parenchyma with vessels or ducts typically within the pancreatic body with possible early pancreatitis. Ductal injuries, typically evaluated by ERCP, may also be demonstrated by MRCP. Further complications are pseudocysts, strictures, aneurysms, or fistulas.

9.8.6.2 Pancreatic Resection

Detailed information on surgical procedures performed in individual patients is helpful to interpret MR studies following pancreatic surgery. Surgical materials like vascular clips or clips from stapled intestinal anastomoses are no contraindication but may cause a signal void or susceptibility artifact. Ultrasound and CT are the imaging methods of choice for the imaging of most surgical complications. MRI is useful to rule out or detect recurrent pancreatic tumor. Problems located in the biliary ducts or pancreatic duct are a good indication since some surgical techniques do not always allow a postoperative ERCP.

9.8.6.3 Transplantation

MRI is typically performed to evaluate severe surgical complications such as transplant rejection or necrosis. The most common surgical technique connects afferent and efferent pancreatic vessels with the iliac vessel and implants the pancreatic duct into the urinary bladder. Acute rejections are characterized by an edematous swelling of the organ and fluid collections. Dynamic perfusion studies with gadolinium-chelates are useful to evaluate organ vascularization in chronic rejection. CE-MRA is useful for the assessment of vascular complications.

9.9 Spleen

9.9.1 Spleen Anatomy

The spleen is hypointense on T1-WI and hyperintense on T2-WI (Fig. 9.1). This signal behavior is similar to that of many splenic lesions, limiting the value of plain MRI for detecting focal or diffuse splenic disease. An accessory spleen occurs in up to 40% of patients and has to be differentiated from other mass lesions.

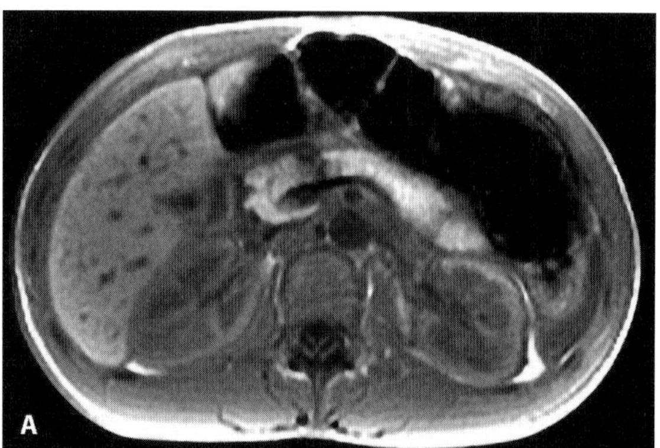

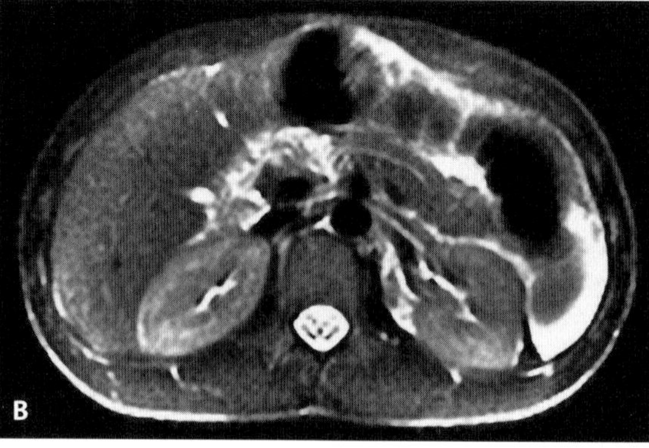

Fig. 9.32A,B. Pancreatic trauma with transection. Plain T1-W spoiled GRE (**A**) and FS-T2-W HASTE (TE 64 ms) (**B**) in a child with abdominal pain following a bicycle accident. The pancreas shows a complete transection [T1-hypointense (**A**) and T2-hyperintense (**B**)] anterior to the spinal column between the pancreatic head and the pancreatic body. Free intra-abdominal fluid (hemorrhage) is present (**B**). Imaging findings were confirmed at surgery

9.9.2 Technique

Two different contrast techniques are available to further differentiate splenic lesions. Gadolinium-enhanced early-phase T1-WI shows an arciform pattern turning homogeneous within 1 min of contrast injection and uses the perfusion difference of spleen versus lesions. Alternatively, delayed SPIO-enhanced T2-WI demonstrates a signal decease in normal spleen based on the RES content without a signal change within lesions such as metastases or lymphoma. A similar contrast pattern may be present in hemochromatosis due to hemosiderin deposition. We also recommend postcontrast scanning in the coronal plane in addition to precontrast and regular postcontrast images in the axial plane to improve the visualization of the spleen.

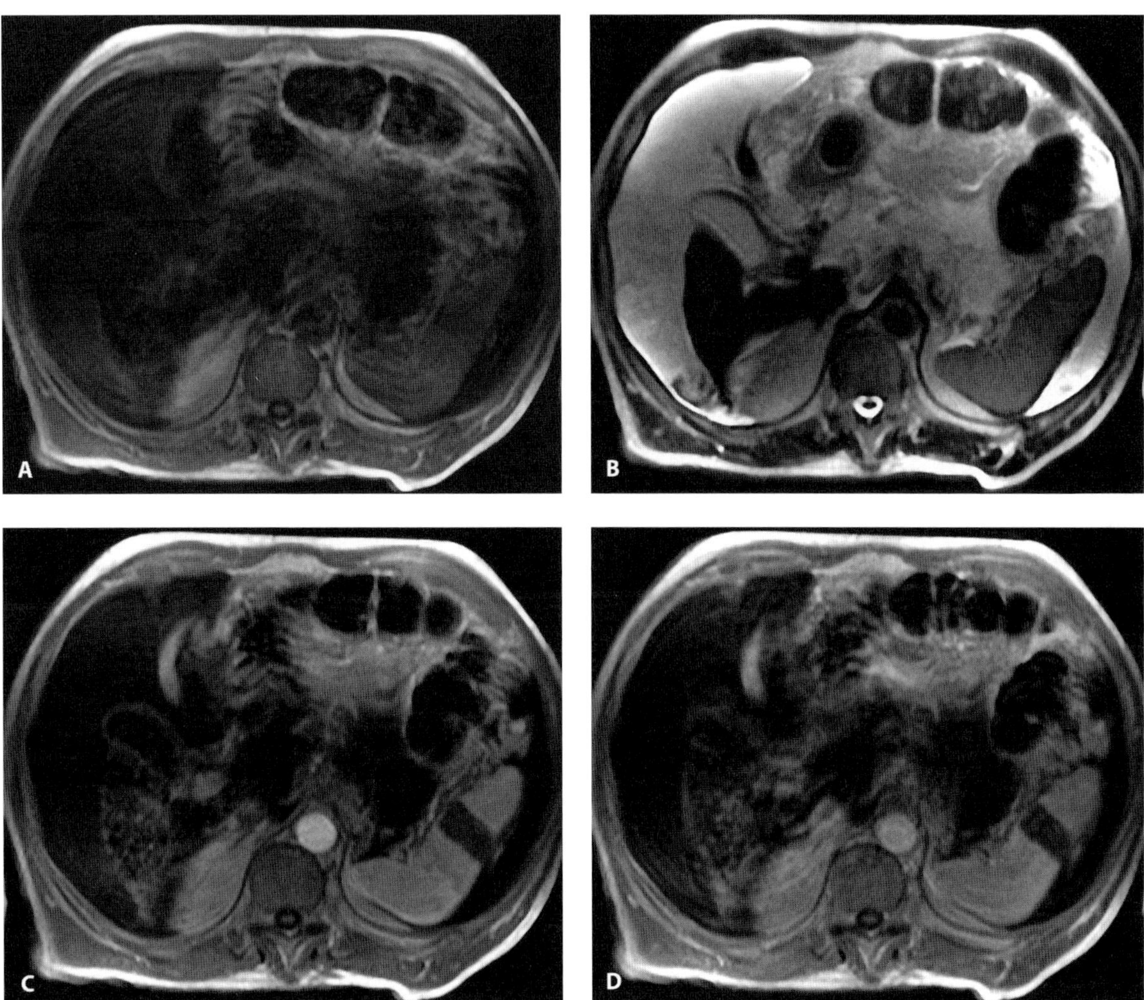

Fig. 9.33A–D. Splenic infarct and liver cirrhosis. Plain T1-W spoiled GRE (**A**), T2-W HASTE (TE 90 ms) (**B**), arterial phase, gadolinium-enhanced, T1-W spoiled GRE (**C**), and portal venous phase, gadolinium-enhanced, T1-W spoiled GRE (**D**). Contrast-enhanced T1-W images (**C**,**D**) reveal a wedge-shaped perfusion defect in the spleen that is almost isointense to the normal spleen parenchyma on plain T1-WI and T2-WI (**A**,**B**). The cirrhotic liver demonstrates an irregular parenchymal perfusion pattern and a signal decrease on T2-W HASTE (**B**) due to iron overload. Severe ascites is present with low SI on T1-WI and high SI on T2-WI

9.9.3 Diffuse Diseases

The spleen is the most commonly involved organ in trauma, with the formation of hematoma, contusion, laceration, and infarcts, which may also develop based on thromboembolic disease (Fig. 9.33).

Patients with cirrhosis or portal hypertension may develop small (<1 cm) foci of iron deposition appearing particularly hypointense on T2-WI which are called Gamna-Gandy bodies (Fig. 9.5).

Granulomatous lesions, such as sarcoid, are small (<1 cm) and typically hypovascular, explaining their low SI on T2-WI and almost no enhancement on gadolinium-enhanced T1-WI.

Patients with sickle cell anemia may present with a hypointense spleen, mainly due to iron deposition following multiple blood transfusions. In this case, hyperintense lesions on T1-WI most likely represent secondary infarcts.

9.9.4 Infection

Viral and bacterial infections may cause splenomegaly. Fungal infection with *Candida albicans* is common in immunocompromised patients. Fungal microabscesses are typically scattered throughout the spleen, appear hyperintense on T2-WI and hypointense on gadolin-

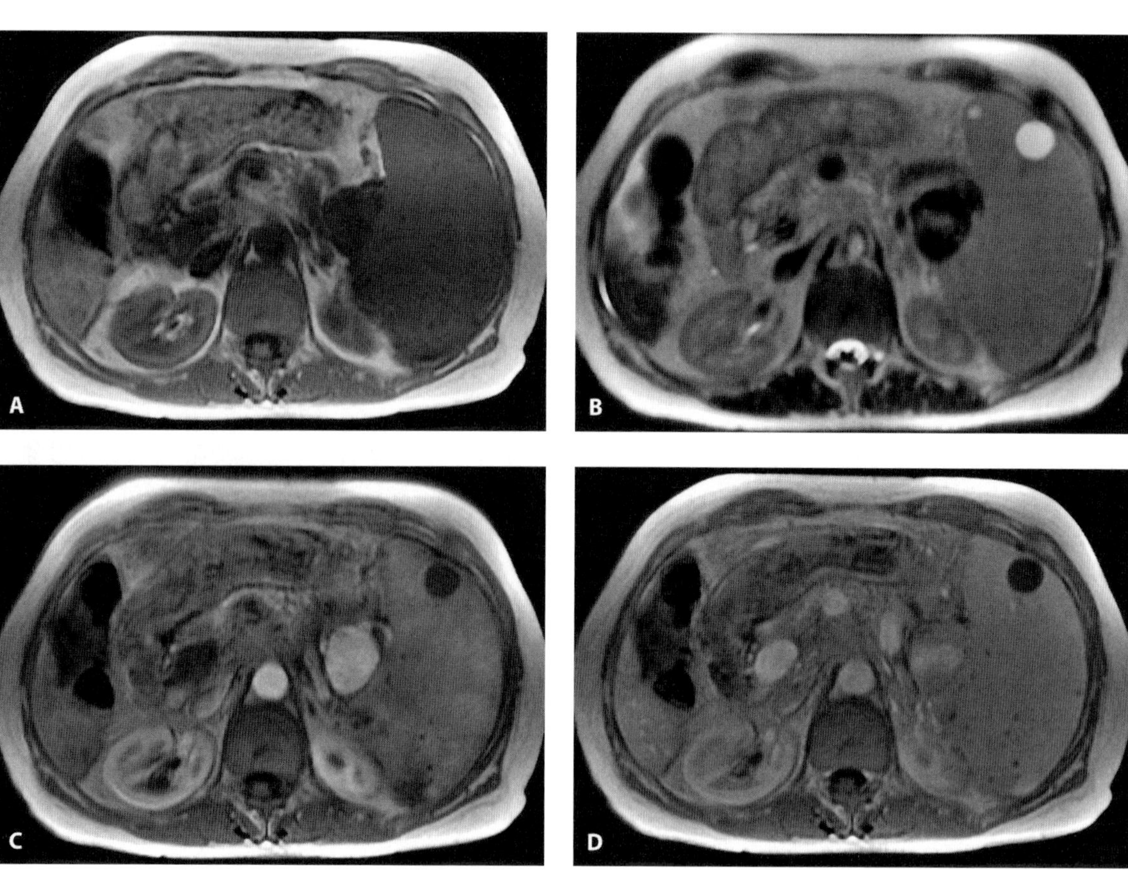

Fig. 9.34A–D. Splenic cysts and splenic artery aneurysm. Plain T1-W spoiled GRE (**A**), T2-W HASTE (TE 90 ms) (**B**), arterial phase, gadolinium-enhanced, T1-W spoiled GRE (**C**), and portal venous phase, gadolinium-enhanced, T1-W spoiled GRE (**D**). Plain and contrast-enhanced T1-W images (**A,C,D**) reveal splenic cysts without contrast enhancement and homogeneous high SI on T2-WI (**B**). Arterial-phase images (**C**) demonstrate an enhancing mass lesion in the splenic hilus with the normal-sized splenic artery visible on both sides of the aneurysm

ium-enhanced T1-WI without significant enhancement. Fat suppression may improve lesion conspicuity, and MRI is superior to CT for the detection and follow-up of fungal microabscesses. Splenic abscesses may develop following infected thromboembolism, as in patients with endocarditis. These larger bacterial abscesses are typically hyperintense on T2-WI and hypointense on gadolinium-enhanced T1-WI with significant enhancement of the abscess wall.

9.9.5 Benign Lesions

Cystic lesions are the most common, are differentiated benign, focal splenic lesions and three benign types: pseudocysts, epidermoid cysts, and hydatid cysts. Most cystic lesions in industrialized countries are posttraumatic pseudocysts without an epithelial cell lining. Epidermoid cysts are true cysts with an epithelial cell lining and are usually discovered incidentally in young patients. Hydatid cysts or echinococcal cysts are more frequent in southern Europe and may show extensive wall calcification. All cysts are well demarcated, hypointense on T1-WI, hyperintense on T2-WI, and show no contrast enhancement (Fig. 9.34).

Hemangiomas are the most common, benign, solid, focal splenic lesions. Splenic hemangiomas are typically cavernous hemangiomas and are smaller in size than liver hemangiomas. Hemangiomas are generally hypointense on T1-WI, hyperintense on T2-WI, and show contrast enhancement (Fig. 9.35). Gadolinium enhancement on T1-WI may be early and homogeneous or nodular with a filling-in pattern; however, these features are not as pronounced as those known for liver hemangiomas. Iron oxides show a decrease in T2-WI due to pooling of particles within hemangiomas (Fig. 9.35).

Cystic lymphangiomas and hamartomas are rare benign focal lesions. Cystic lymphangiomas appear as well-defined multiloculated masses with high SI on T2-WI. Hamartomas are predominantly solid, show intermediate SI on T1-WI, high SI on T2-WI, and a relatively strong gadolinium enhancement.

9.9.6 Malignant Lesions

Secondary focal malignant lesions are much more frequent than primary malignant splenic lesions. Splenic metastases are mostly seen in advanced stages of cancer disease, typically originating from breast carcinoma, lung carcinoma, or malignant melanoma. Plain MRI often fails to detect lesions because of a similar contrast behavior of the normal spleen. Malignant melanoma represents an exception since the melanin content may

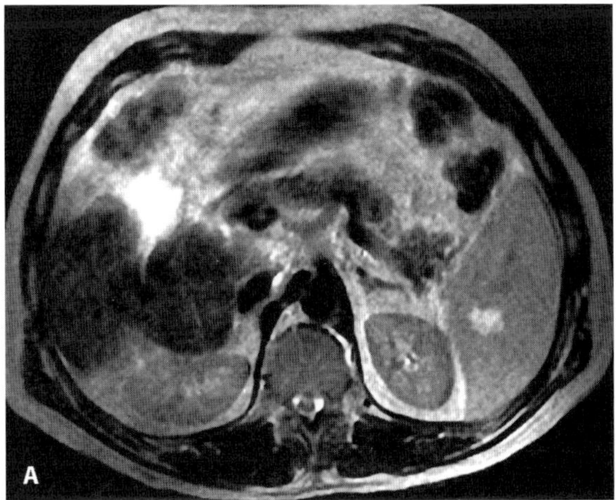

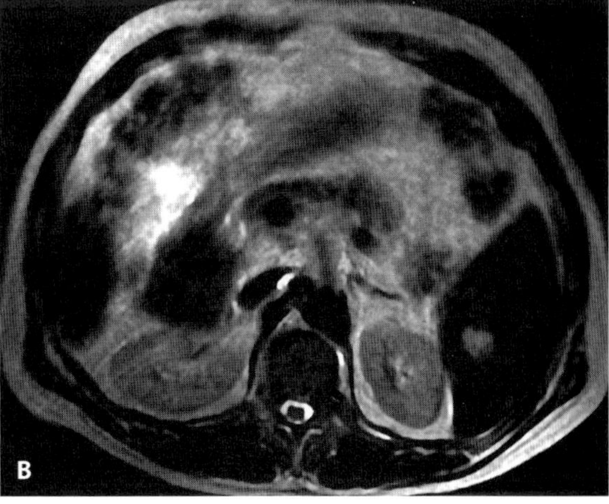

Fig. 9.35A,B. Splenic hemangioma. T2-W TSE (TE 165 ms) images before (**A**) and 10 min following (**B**) i.v. injection of 10 µmol Resovist/kg body weight. Liver and spleen SI decrease on postcontrast images due to the uptake of iron oxide particles in the RES. The hemangioma in the spleen also decreases in SI on postcontrast images due to pooling of blood in the lesions. The same pattern applies to liver hemangiomas

cause high SI on T1-WI. Contrast-enhanced techniques help to improve lesion conspicuity by means of hypointense lesions on early (30 s) gadolinium-enhanced T1-WI or hyperintense lesions on iron-oxide-enhanced T2-WI with a broader time window (3 days).

Lymphomatous disease (Hodgkin's and non-Hodgkin's lymphoma) often involves the spleen, and again, plain MRI often fails to detect focal or diffuse splenic involvement because of the similar contrast behavior of normal spleen and lesions. Visible lymphomas are typically hypointense on T2-WI and enhance on early (30 s) gadolinium-enhanced T1-WI. Diffuse involvement may demonstrate a disturbance of the regular arciform perfusion pattern, and diffusely scattered focal lesions appear as multiple hypointense lesions on early gadolinium-enhanced T1-WI. Iron oxides improve the conspicuity of splenic lymphoma, presenting as hyperintense lesions compared with the hypointense spleen due to the uptake of particles in the RES present in the normal spleen. The dose of SPIO required to effectively decrease the SI of normal splenic tissue is somewhat higher than currently approved for the liver, but a mild signal decrease is observed at the current approved doses as well.

Acknowledgements. We are indebted to Wolfgang Schima for many helpful comments.

Further Reading

Buck JL, Elsayed AM (1993) Ampullary tumors: radiologic-pathologic correlation. RadioGraphics 13:193–212

Edelman RR, Hesselink JR, Zlatkin MB (1996) Clinical magnetic resonance imaging, 2nd edn. WB Saunders, Philadelphia

Fulcher AS, Turner MA, Franklin KJ, et al (2000) Primary sclerosing cholangitis: evaluation with MR cholangiography – a case-control study. Radiology 215:71–80

Higgins CB, Hricak H, Helms CA (1997) Magnetic resonance imaging of the body, 3rd edn. Lippincott-Raven, New York

Holzknecht N, Gauger J, Sackmann M, et al (1998) MR cholangiography with snapshot techniques: prospective comparison with endoscopic retrograde. Radiology 206:657–664

Lavelle MT, Lee VS, Rofsky NM, Krinsky GA, Weinreb JC (2001) Dynamic contrast-enhanced three-dimensional MR imaging of liver parenchyma: source images and angiographic reconstructions to define hepatic arterial anatomy. Radiology 218:389–394

Lim JH, Choi D, Cho SK, et al (2001) Conspicuity of hepatocellular nodular lesions in cirrhotic livers at ferum oxides-enhanced MR imaging: importance of Kupffer cell number. Radiology 220:669–676

Kanematsu M, Shiratori Y, Hoshi H, Kondo H, Matsuo M, Moriwaki H (2000) Pancreas and peripancreatic vessels: effect of imaging delay on gadolinium enhancement at dynamic gradient-recalled-echo MR imaging. Radiology 215:95–102

Krinsky GA, Lee VS, Theise ND, et al (2001) Hepatocellular carcinoma and dysplastic nodules in patients with cirrhosis: prospective diagnosis with MR imaging and explantation correlation. Radiology 219:445–454

Mirowitz S (1996) Pitfalls, variants and artifacts in body MRI. Thieme, Stuttgart

Park MS, Yu JS, Kim KW, et al (2001) Recurrent pyogenic cholangitis: comparison between MR cholangiography and direct cholangiography. Radiology 220:677–682

Petersein J, Spinazzi A, Giovagnoni A, et al (2000) Focal liver lesions: evaluation of the efficacy of gadobenate dimeglumine in MR imaging – a multicenter phase III clinical study. Radiology 215:727–736

Semelka RC, Hussain SM, Marcos HB, Woosley JT (2000) Perilesional enhancement of hepatic metastases: correlation between MR imaging and histopathologic findings – initial observations. Radiology 215:89–94

Stark DD, Bradley WG (1998) Magnetic resonance imaging, 3rd edn. Mosby, St. Louis

Van Hoe L, Vanbeckevoort D, Van Steenbergen W (1999) Atlas of cross-sectional and projective MR cholangiopancreatography. Springer, Berlin Heidelberg New York

Ward J, Guthrie JA, Scott DJ, et al (2000) Hepatocellular carcinoma in the cirrhotic liver: double-contrast MR imaging for diagnosis. Radiology 216:154–162

Yu JS, Kim KW, Jeong MG, Lee JT, Yoo HS (2000) Nontumorous hepatic arterial-portal venous shunts: MR imaging findings. Radiology 217:750–756

Kidneys and Adrenal Glands

10

C. Catalano, G. Cardone, A. Laghi, A. Napoli, F. Fraioli, F. Pediconi

Contents

10.1 MR Imaging of the Kidneys

The role of magnetic resonance (MR) imaging in the evaluation of renal pathologies is becoming increasingly important. MR imaging is now considered a modality complementary to computed tomography (CT) and ultrasound (US). Using up-to-date equipment, it is possible to obtain high-quality images of the kidneys and perirenal spaces; MR imaging provides information particularly useful for the staging of renal neoplasms. The use of fast imaging techniques may also provide information regarding renal function and allow for selective direct imaging of the entire urinary tract.

MR imaging is used mainly for staging renal neoplasms and has become more than a mere alternative to intravenous (i.v.) urography and CT in those patients for whom the use of iodinated contrast agents is contraindicated. MR imaging is also a valuable technique for characterizing renal masses – in particular, for differentiating between cystic and solid lesions. By providing direct imaging of the dilated urinary tract, MR urography may also substitute for invasive procedures.

10.1.1 Coils and Patient Positioning

MR imaging of the kidneys is performed with a phased-array coil that increases the signal-to-noise ratio by factor of 2 to 3, allowing the use of smaller fields-of-view (FOV) to obtain high-resolution images. The patient is positioned supine in the gantry. It is preferable to ask the patient to fast from solid and liquid foods to avoid filling the intestinal loops. This is particularly important when performing MR urography, given that the gastrointestinal tract could be superimposed over the upper urinary tract during three-dimensional reconstruction, and thereby impair the final image quality. To reduce motion artifacts due to excursion of the abdominal wall during respiration, it may be helpful to use a compression band. Breath-hold sequences or respiratory compensation should be used to avoid misregistration artifacts due to respiration. A further reduction of motion artifacts due to peristalsis of the gastrointestinal tract can be achieved by using either glucagon or scopolamine hydrobromide. Intramuscular and/or intravenous injection of one of these drugs immediately prior to MR examination reduces peristalsis.

10.1.2 Sequence Protocol

Both in-phase and opposed-phase T1-weighted gradient-echo (T1-GRE) and axial, fat-suppressed Turbo-Spin-Echo (TSE) T2-weighted images are acquired from the dome of the diaphragm to the lower pole of the kidneys (Table 10.1). These T1-weighted GRE images are acquired with both a TE of 4.2 ms (in-phase) and a TE of 2.1 ms (out of phase) to detect lipid in renal or adrenal lesions. Breath-hold fat-saturated T1-GRE images are acquired before and during the dynamic intravenous administration of gadolinium; the same GRE sequence is repeated over time, e.g., after 30 s, 60 s, 90 s, 120 s, and 180 s. The contrast-enhanced portion of the examination may be performed either as two-dimensional (2D) or three-dimensional (3D) sequences. The plane of 2D imaging should be chosen to allow dynamic evaluation of both kidneys and is generally the coronal plane. The coronal plane is often advantageous for imaging of renal neoplasms, because it allows evaluation of both kidneys, the renal vessels, the inferior vena cava, and the spine in a small number of slices. The imaging FOV generally varies between 30 cm and 40 cm, according to the size of the patient. The matrix size is 192–256 (phase) × 256–512 (frequency), depending on the characteristics of the MR equipment.

If the upper urinary tract has to be studied, MR urography can be performed. If a hydroureteronephrosis is present, either a respiratory-compensated 3D heavily T2-W TSE sequence or a breath-hold half-Fourier acquisition single-shot turbo spin-echo (HASTE) sequence can be acquired in the coronal plane (Table 10.1). To reduce the fat signal and increase the contrast resolution, a technique for fat suppression should be used when performing TSE MR urography. Contrast-enhanced MR urography is not routinely performed as part of the evaluation of renal masses, although it is included as part of the evaluation of suspected transitional cell carcinoma. For this examination, 10 mg of furosemide is injected along with the gadolinium, dynamic-enhanced 2D or 3D images of the kidney are acquired as described previously, and then the kidneys, ureters, and urinary bladder are imaged with a coronal, fat-suppressed 3D GRE sequence with or without respiratory triggering.

Table 10.1. Pulse sequence recommendations for the kidneys

Sequence	WI	Plane	No. of slices	TR (ms)	TE (ms)	Flip angle	Slice thicknes (mm)	Matrix	FOV	No. of acq.	Acq. time (min)
GRE (in-phase and opposed-phase) breath-hold	T1	Axial	10–20	50–300	4.2, 2.1	90	6	196×256	300–400	1	<0.30
TSE (fat-suppressed) breath-hold	T2	Axial	10–20	4000–6000	100–150	60–90	6	256×256	300–400	2	<0.30
GRE (fat-suppressed) breath-hold	T1	Axial or coronal	10–20	50–300	Min	90	6	128–192	300–400	1	<0.30
MR urography 2D or 3D TSE/HASTE	T2	Coronal	15–20	>3000	>500	<180	2–4	128×256	300–400	2–4	<5
3D GRE (fat-suppressed) breath-hold		Coronal	10–20	Min	Min	20	2	512×192	300–400	2	<30

WI weighting of images, *Matrix* phase × frequency matrix, *Acq.* acquisition(s)

Single TSE, HASTE MR urography and contrast-enhanced MR urography images have to be reconstructed to obtain a 3D display; this is typically done using a maximum intensity projection (MIP) algorithm. For the assessment of pathologies in MR urography, it is important also to evaluate the raw data, which allows identification of small obstructing pathologies that are often not visible on the 3D display.

10.1.3 Normal Anatomy and MR Imaging Patterns of the Kidney

T1-GRE images allow for differentiation between the hyperintense peripheral cortex of the kidneys and the hypointense central medulla. Although evident in all planes, the septa of Bertin and the medullary pyramids are particularly noticeable in coronal images. Differentiation between the cortex and medulla can be improved using FS T1-W sequences. The cortex is highly vascularized by the arterial network; therefore, dynamic studies following i.v. injection of contrast agent allow for better differentiation between the renal zones and enable the collection of functional information about the kidneys. On T2-WI, both the renal cortex and medulla are hyperintense. Therefore, T2-WI do not provide good anatomical information for differentiating between the two renal zones.

10.1.4 Clinical Applications

10.1.4.1 Congenital Anomalies

The kidneys may present with abnormalities in number, position, rotation, and fusion. Bilateral renal agenesis is not compatible with life, whereas unilateral agenesis is not so rare (0.01%–0.02%). The kidneys may also be located in an anomalous position (in any possible location from the thorax to the pelvis) or may be fused. Several fusion abnormalities exist, but the more common ones are the horseshoe and pancake kidneys. The multiplanar capabilities of MR imaging in combination with breath-hold sequencing greatly facilitate the identification of renal anomalies.

10.1.4.2 Medical Renal Diseases

MR imaging is not currently used for the assessment of medical renal pathologies, either infectious or noninfectious. In fact, US or CT are typically employed for this purpose. If CT is needed but the patient is intolerant to iodinated contrast agents, MR imaging may be requested. Diffuse bilateral enlargement of the kidneys may be seen in a variety of renal parenchymal diseases, including acute glomerulonephritis, interstitial nephritis, postactinic nephritis, and nephrotic syndrome. In all of these pathologies, edema and loss of the corticomedullary junction are evident in T1-WI. MR imaging may also be useful for demonstrating parenchymal atrophy in small kidneys that have reduced corticomedullary differentiation and sinus lipomatosis.

10.1.4.3 Obstructive Nephropathy

Dilatation of the renal collecting structures, pelvis, and ureters can be seen well in both T1-WI and T2-WI. The degree of obstruction can be determined by analyzing sequential axial images, heavily T2-W MR urography, and contrast-enhanced MR urography images. The cause of obstruction can also be determined by evaluating either axial images or coronal MR urograms (Fig. 10.1). The appearance of the renal parenchyma varies depending on the duration of the obstruction. In the case of chronic obstruction, a marked reduction of the corticomedullary junction is evident, whereas in the case of acute obstruction, it remains normal. Renal function can be evaluated using i.v. contrast agents, which normally do not become concentrated in obstructed kidneys.

10.1.4.4 Renal Cystic Disease

Simple renal cysts are the most common benign renal masses. They typically appear as well-defined round masses, with a homogeneously low signal intensity on T1-WI, a homogeneously high signal intensity on T2-WI, and no contrast enhancement (Fig. 10.2). Infected cysts may present with an inhomogeneous signal intensity on both T1-WI and T2-WI.

MR is particularly useful to differentiate typical simple cysts (Fig. 10.2) from complicated cysts, abscesses,

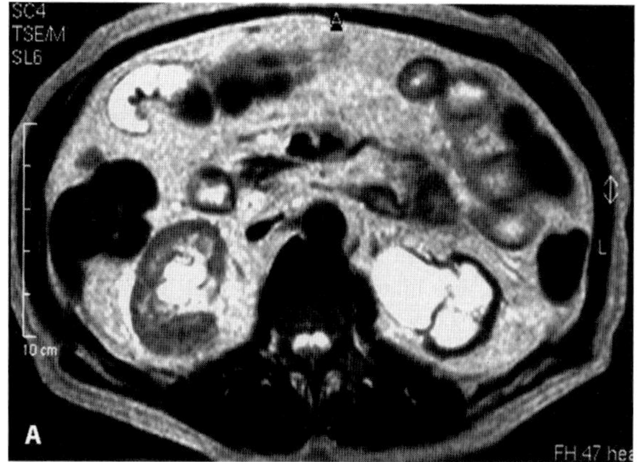

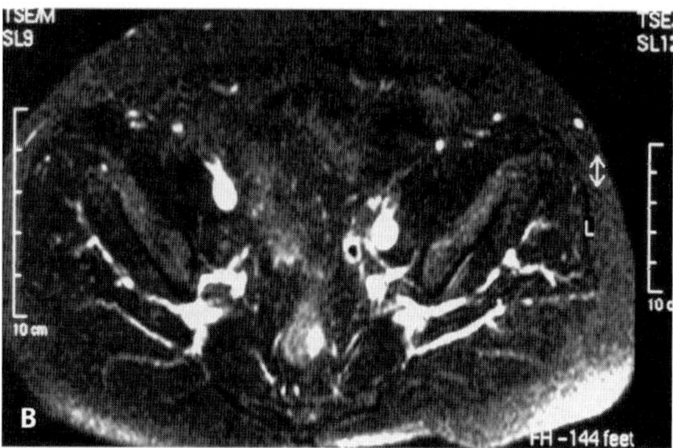

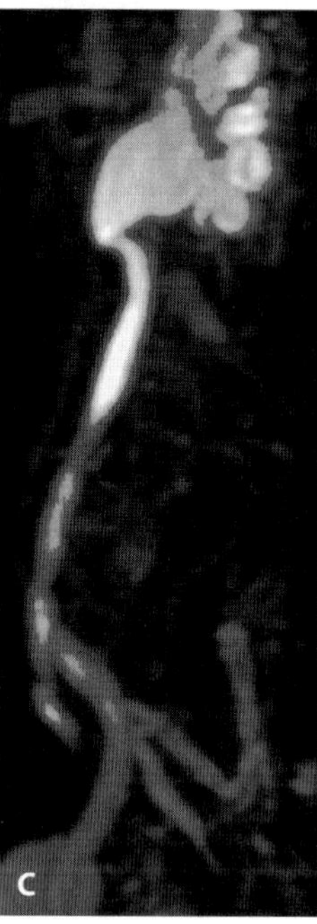

Fig. 10.1A–C. Hydroureteronephrosis. Axial T2-weighted (T2-W) turbo spin-echo (TSE) (**A**) and T2-W FS-TSE (**B**) show a filling defect within the dilated left ureter. MR urography (**C**) clearly demonstrates the dilated ureter and the level of obstruction

and cystic or hypovascular renal carcinomas. A good measure for this purpose is Bosniak's classification where cystic lesions are described into four categories.

Category 1: simple benign cyst (T1-hypointense, T2-hyperintense, T1+Gd-no enhancement) with a thin wall, protein content may cause high SI on T1-WI.

Category 2: probably benign cyst with some additional features like thin septa which may show some contrast enhancement, small calcifications, signs of hemorrhage or protein (T1-hypointense – hyperintense, T2-hyperintense – hypointense, T1+Gd-no enhancement), but homogeneous, a smooth wall, and no contrast enhancement.

Category 3: indeterminate cyst and potentially malignant with inhomogeneous signal, irregular walls, thick and irregular calcifications (CT), and thickened contrast enhancing septa.

Category 4: probably malignant cyst with an irregular and thickened wall, areas of contrast enhancement are typically present, solid components on T2-WI.

10.1.4.5 Benign Renal Neoplasms

Benign renal neoplasms are quite uncommon. The most frequent benign lesion that can be accurately diagnosed with MR imaging is angiomyolipoma, due to the presence of fat within the lesion. The use of fat-suppressed sequences, either T1-W or T2-W, allows for the detection of fat within the lesion and for making the diagnosis of an angiomyolipoma (Fig. 10.3).

Further clinically presenting benign renal neoplasm's are lipoma, oncocytoma, and adenoma. Lipomas are diagnosed applying the same criteria as explained for angiomyolipomas. Oncocytomas (Fig. 10.4) are typically small in size (<3 cm), may exhibit a central scar, a capsule, are hypointense on T1-WI, hyperintense on T2-WI, are well perfused, and may show a wheel-type perfusion pattern (20–80%). Adenomas do not present with typical imaging patterns.

10.1.4.6 Malignant Renal Neoplasms

Renal cell carcinoma is the most frequent malignant renal neoplasm. In many cases, it is quite advanced at the time of diagnosis, given that the neoplasm is asymptomatic when small. In the preoperative assessment, MR

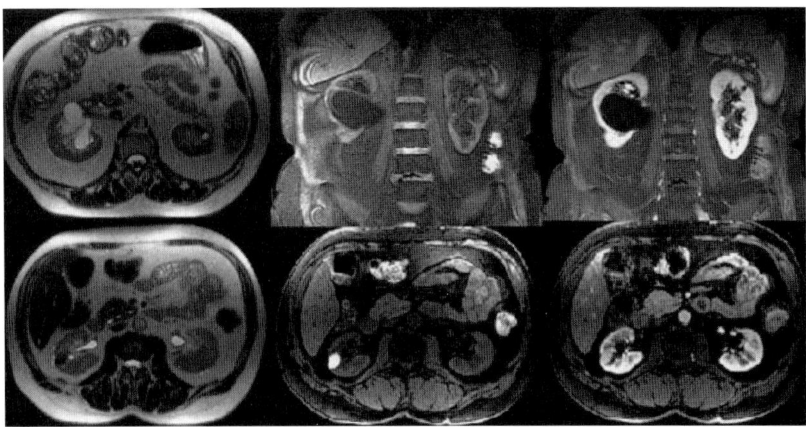

Fig. 10.2. Renal cyst. Category 1 renal cysts (upper row) and category 2 renal cyst (lower row) in two different patients. The simple bilateral benign cysts show typical high SI on T2-W HASTE (left), low SI on plain FS-2D GRE-coronal T1 (middle), and no enhancement on Gd-enhanced FS-2D GRE-coronal T1 (right). The category 2 cyst (right kidney) shows signal characteristics consistent with hemorrhage. T2-W HASTE (left) demonstrates the cyst homogeneously hypointense, FS-3D GRE-axial T1 (middle) with homogeneous high SI, and with constant high SI on Gd-enhanced FS-3D GRE-axial T1 (right) without further enhancement

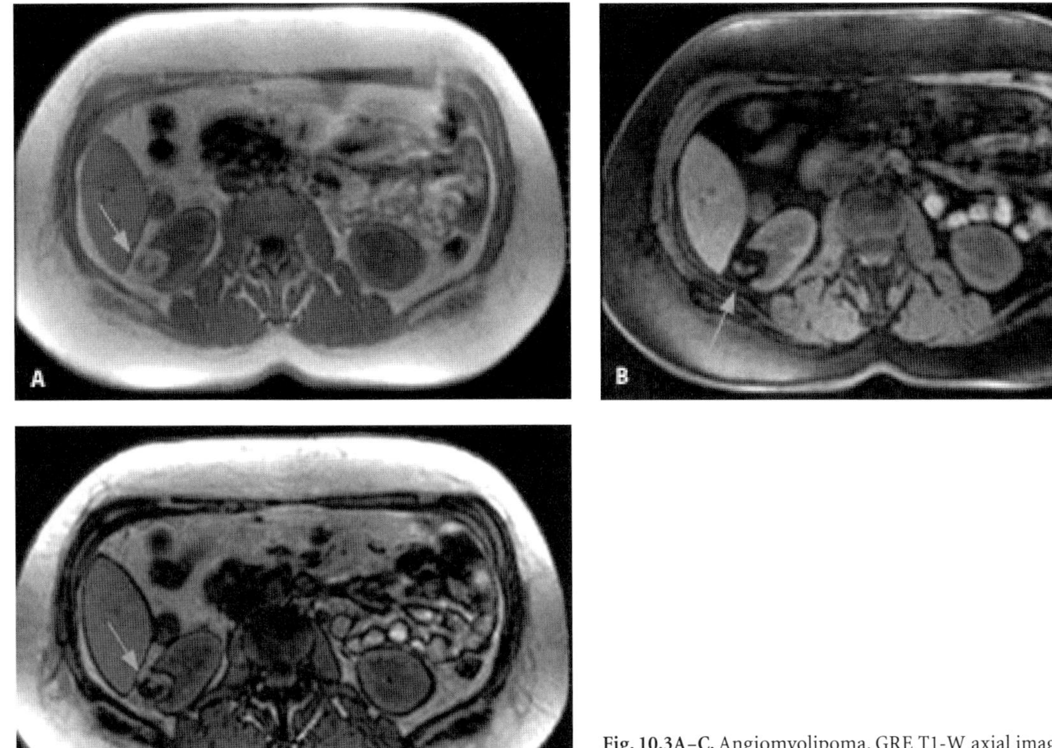

Fig. 10.3A–C. Angiomyolipoma. GRE T1-W axial image (**A**) shows the presence of angiomyolipoma in the right kidney. The presence of fat is well demonstrated by GRE FS T1-weighted image in-phase (**B**) and T1-weighted image opposed-phase (**C**)

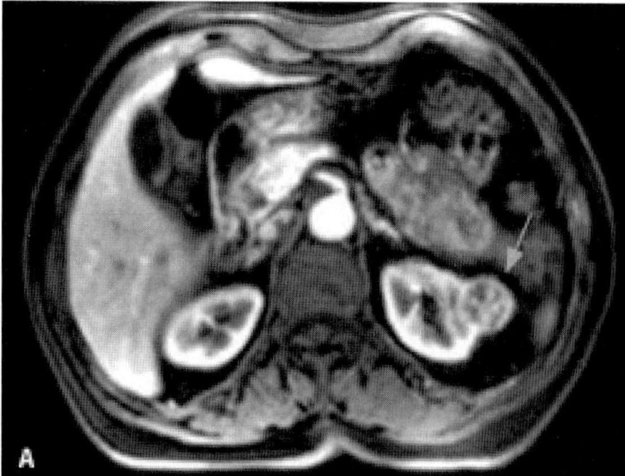

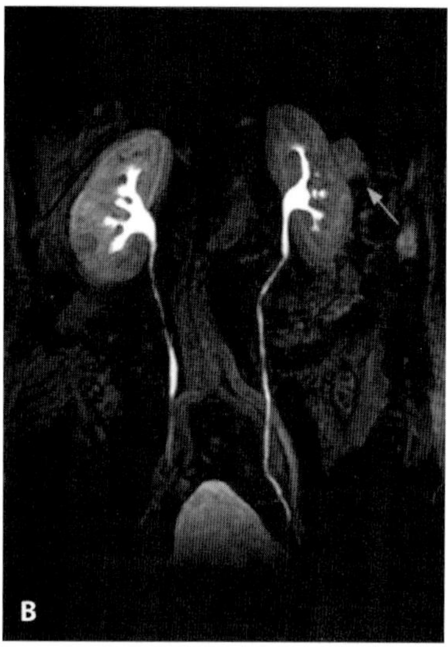

Fig. 10.4A, B. Oncocytoma. Axial GRE T1-W post-contrast image shows an oncocytoma in the left kidney (**A**), well demonstrated also in the coronal urogram (**B**)

imaging may be useful in identifying the lesion and determining the degree of infiltration into the perinephric space and/or adjacent organs, the presence of enlarged lymph nodes, and venous tumoral thrombosis. Renal cell carcinoma has a variable appearance in MR images; in most instances, it is isointense in both T1-WI and T2-WI, although it is generally more obvious in T1-WI, especially if small. Postcontrast images may be helpful in identifying small renal cell carcinomas. Renal cell carcinoma is typically hypervascular and thus appears hyperintense in the early phase following i.v. administration of paramagnetic contrast agents. Rapid contrast-enhanced MR imaging has a greater sensitivity for the detection of small (<3 cm) renal cell carcinomas than conventional sequences (Fig. 10.5).

MR imaging has also proved accurate for staging renal cell carcinomas. Although the most accurate technique in all stages, MRI is particularly useful in stage III, in which there is infiltration of the renal vein and/or inferior vena cava, and in stage IV, in which there is infiltration of adjacent organs. The neoplastic thrombus generally has the same signal intensity as the tumor. MR imaging is more accurate for demonstrating tumor extension into the vena cava than CT or US; however, the accuracy of MR imaging for demonstrating renal vein thrombosis is somewhat lower. The infiltration of adjacent organs can be demonstrated by exploit-

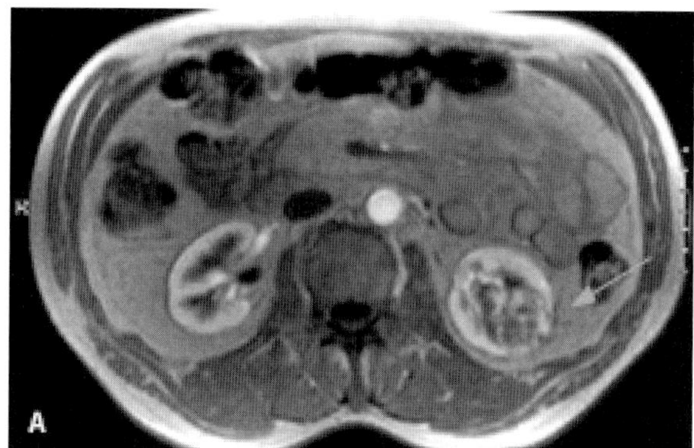

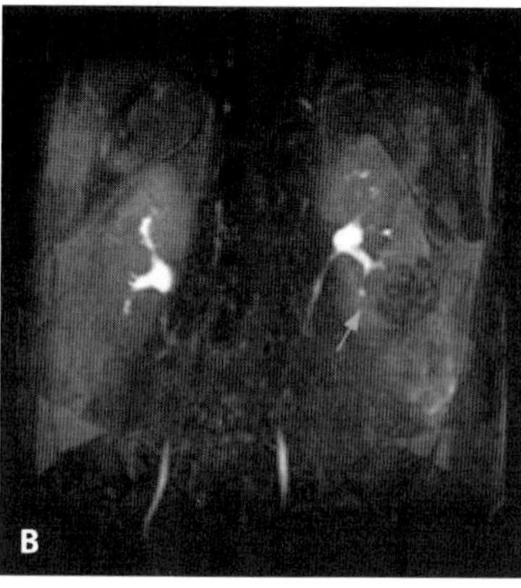

Fig. 10.5A, B. Renal cell carcinoma. Axial GRE T1-W post-contrast image shows a renal cell carcinoma at the inferior pole of the left kidney (**A**) invading the pelvis, as demonstrated in the coronal urogram (**B**)

ing the multiplanarity of MR imaging – particularly using coronal and sagittal images – and the alteration of signal intensity that can be observed in an infiltrated organ. The accuracy of MR imaging in stage IV ranges between 80% and 95%. MR imaging is at least comparable to CT in the assessment of recurrent renal cell carcinomas (Fig. 10.6).

10.1.4.7 Uroepithelial Neoplasms

Uroepithelial neoplasms are much less common than renal cell carcinoma; uroepithelial carcinomas are generally localized in the ureter or in the bladder and rarely occur in the kidney. In most cases, they result in dilatation of the calices and/or the pelvis, depending on where the neoplasm is located. Conventional MR images do not have great sensitivity for the identification of uroepithelial carcinomas; these are better identified by means of MR urography, which can substitute for i.v. urography and more invasive exams, such as ascending pyelography (Fig. 10.7). Transitional-cell carcinomas appear as a filling defect within the collecting system, similar to that seen using conventional methods. The most common renal neoplasm in children is Wilms' tumor or nephroblastoma. It is a large solid mass, which generally appears isointense on T1-WI and hyperintense on T2-WI.

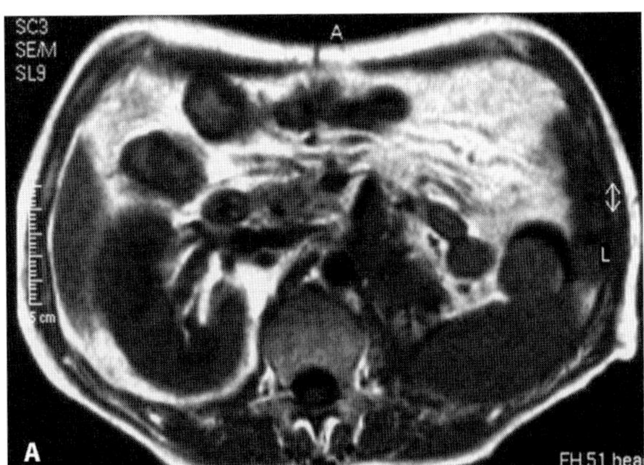

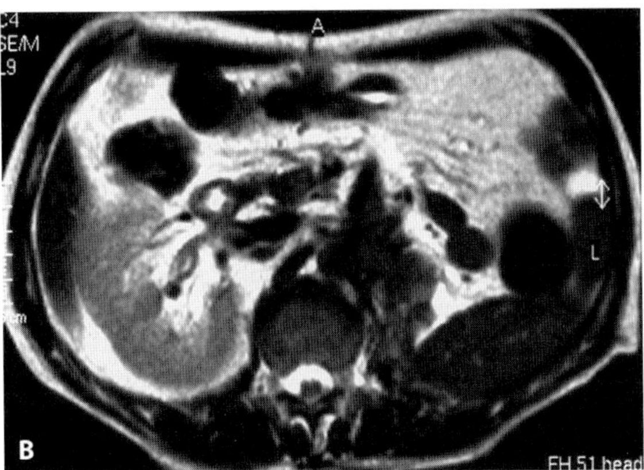

Fig. 10.6A, B. Recurrent renal cell carcinoma. Axial T1-W SE (**A**) and T2-W TSE (**B**) demonstrate a large left retroperitoneal mass following nephrectomy. The recurrent tumor demonstrates low signal intensity on T1-W SE (**A**) and T2-W TSE (**B**)

10.1.4.8 Metastatic Disease

Several primary neoplasms, including those of the lung, breast, colon, and stomach, and those associated with melanoma, leukemia, and lymphoma may metastasize to the kidneys. Focal renal metastasis is rare, usually small, and cannot be easily differentiated from renal cell carcinoma. Metastasis from lymphoma and leukemia generally determine an unilateral or bilateral parenchymal enlargement with loss of corticomedullary differentiation on T1-WI. Lymphoma may also produce focal metastasis to the kidneys, which is not different from other cases of focal metastasis.

10.1.4.9 Evaluation of Renal Allografts

Transplanted kidneys must often be evaluated using several imaging modalities. For this purpose, sonography is generally utilized, although MR imaging may also provide important information about renal function and for identifying the presence of lymphoproliferative disorders. For this purpose, pre- and postcontrast images should be acquired. Precontrast T1-WI and T2-WI provide information about the morphology of the kidneys and the presence of surgical complications (fluid collections). Dynamic postcontrast images can be useful to determine renal function and, in particular, to demonstrate the presence of lymphoproliferation (with poor differentiation between the renal cortex and medulla).

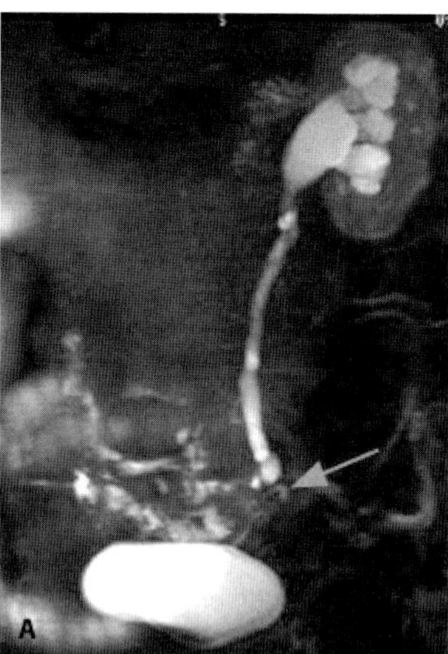

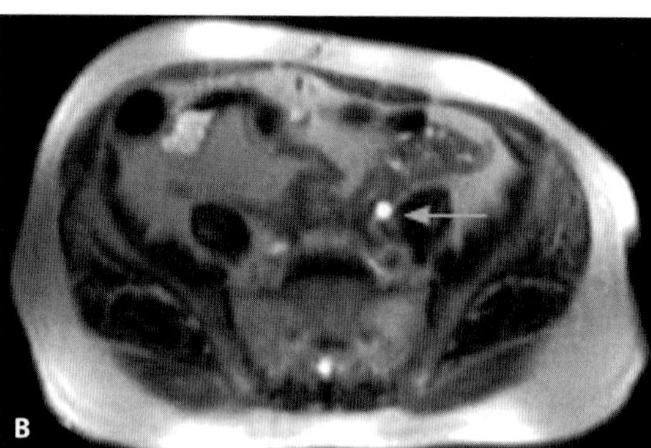

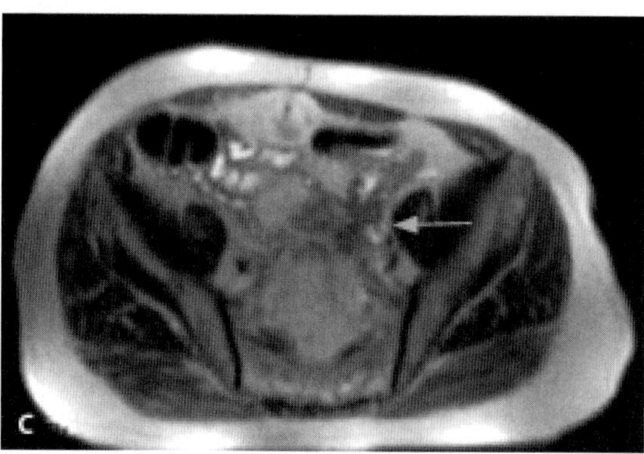

Fig. 10.7A–C. Uroepithelial neoplasm. HASTE T2-WI, in coronal (A) and axial (B) view, show a dilatation of the left uretheres due to a mass in a distal portion (**C**)

10.2 MR Imaging of the Adrenal Glands

The retroperitoneally located, paired adrenal glands are comprised of two separate functional units: the cortex, developing from the mesoderm, and the medulla, developing from ectodermal cells of the neural crest. The adrenal cortex comprises three distinct histological areas: (1) the zona glomerulosa, (2) zona fasciculata, and (3) zona reticularis. The mineralocorticoids, the main representative of which is aldosterone, are synthesized and secreted in the zona glomerulosa, whereas the glucocorticoid steroids and androgens are synthesized and secreted in the zona fasciculata and reticularis. In the adrenal medulla, the chromaffin cells synthesize, store, and secrete the catecholamines adrenaline and noradrenaline. The excellent soft-tissue contrast of MRI allows for good morphological delineation of adrenal masses. In addition to morphological evaluation, MRI is useful for differentiating between benign and malignant etiologies. MRI is frequently employed to further characterize adrenal masses incidentally identified on CT or US.

10.2.1 Coil and Patient Positioning

The patient should be positioned so that the adrenal glands are at or near the plane of the isocenter of the magnet. Adrenal MRI is typically performed with a body phased-array coil.

10.2.2 Sequence Protocol

The image quality can be further improved using flow compensation, spatial presaturation pulses above and below the imaging volume, and respiratory compensation (phase-encoding artifact reduction for T1-WI and respiratory triggering for T2-WI). The phase-encoding direction must, however, be chosen carefully in the different planes so as not to obscure the region of interest with ghost artifacts. In addition, axial FS T2-W TSE sequences and coronal T1-W GRE sequences may be helpful (Table 10.2). Fat suppression also reduces respiratory-motion-induced artifacts and noise, thus giving a sharper depiction of the adrenals. The dynamic range of the abdominal signal intensity is reduced and the gray scale expanded, accentuating small differences in tissue contrast. Although screening examinations generally require imaging in only the transverse plane, coronal T1-WI are useful for defining the relationships between the adrenal glands and the surrounding organs.

If an adrenal mass lesion is detected, in-phase and opposed-phase breath-hold GRE sequences are performed (Table 10.2). This approach reveals fat within adenomas, which is typically not present within metastases. The signal of an in-phase image is derived from the signal of water plus fat protons, whereas the signal of an opposed-phase image is derived from the difference between the signal of water and fat protons. A fat-containing lesion will therefore show significantly less signal in opposed-phase images than in in-phase images. Clinically, a 50% decrease in signal is accepted as a cut-off value for diagnosing an adenoma. No further imaging tests or biopsies are required to establish the diagnosis of an adenoma and to rule out a metastasis. If no signal decrease can be measured, further imaging is required. This includes T2-W and dynamic gadolinium-enhanced T1-W MR imaging. Postcontrast T1-WI are useful for determining the enhancement characteristics of adrenal masses. Angiographic studies are useful for identifying vascular structures or assessing vascular invasion of adrenal malignancy. Phase-contrast sequences and breath-hold CE 3D MR angiography (MRA) sequences are both useful.

10.2.3 Normal Anatomy and MR Imaging Patterns of Adrenal Glands

The adrenal glands are located at the level of the eleventh or twelfth rib, lateral to the vertebrae, bound by the superior portion of Gerota's fascia in the anterosuperior aspect of the perinephric space, and surrounded by fatty areolar tissue. The right adrenal gland is superior to the upper renal pole, immediately posterior to the inferior vena cava, medial to the posterior segment of the right hepatic lobe, and lateral to the crus of the diaphragm. The left adrenal gland is slightly lower in relation to the left kidney and lies anteromedial to its upper pole, lateral to the crus, posterolateral to the aorta, and posteromedial to the splenic vessels and pancreatic tail. Morphologically, the adrenal gland is separated into an anteromedially located body and two posterior or posterolateral limbs. The configuration of the adrenals is quite varied, with inverted *V* or *Y* shapes being the most common (Fig. 10.8). The normal adrenal gland appears dark on both MR T1-WIs and T2-WIs, relative to most other tissues. The gland is of similar or lower signal intensity when compared with liver and muscle. MR cannot differentiate the cortex from the medulla.

Table 10.2. Pulse sequence recommendations for the adrenal glands

Sequence	WI	Plane	No. of slices	TR (ms)	TE (ms)	Flip angle	Slice thicknes (mm)	Matrix	FOV	No. of acq.	Acq. time (min)
GRE (in-phase and opposed-phase) breath-hold	T1	Axial	10–20	50–300	4.2, 2.1	90	6	196×256	300–400	1	<0.30
TSE (fat-suppressed) breath-hold	T2	Axial	10–20	4000–6000	100–150	60–90	6	256×256	300–400	2	>2
GRE (fat-suppressed) breath-hold	T1	Axial or coronal	10–20	50–300	Min	90	6	128–192	300–400	1	<0.30
TSE breath-hold	T2	Axial	10–20	4000–6000	100–150	60–90	6	256×256	300–400	1	<0.30

WI weighting of images, *Matrix* phase × frequency matrix, *Acq.* acquisition(s)

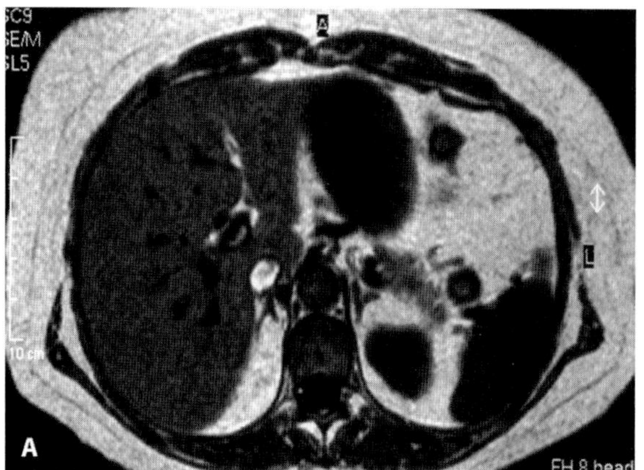

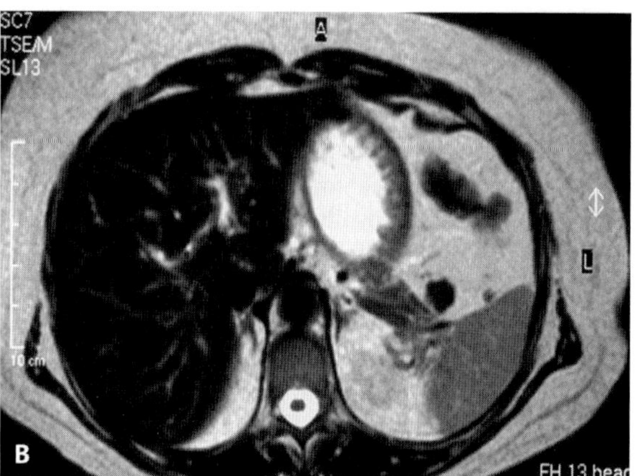

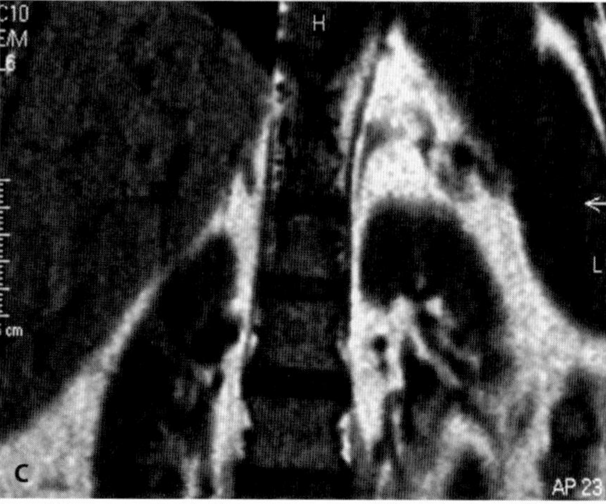

Fig. 10.8A–C. Normal adrenal glands. Axial T1-W SE (**A**), T2-W TSE (**B**), and coronal T1-W SE (**C**) demonstrate normal Y-shaped adrenal glands. The normal adrenal gland appears dark on both T1-W and T2-W MR images. The gland is of similar or lower signal intensity than liver and muscle. MRI cannot be used to differentiate the cortex from the medulla

10.2.4 Clinical Applications of Adrenocortical Mass Lesions

10.2.4.1 Adrenal Hyperplasia

Hyperplasia of the adrenal cortex may develop in response to a variety of physiological and pathological stresses and may be associated with normal, elevated, or diminished production of adrenocortical hormones. Enlargement of the adrenal gland is usually more obvious in patients with Cushing's syndrome than in those with Conn's syndrome. Diffuse adrenocortical hyperplasia is characterized by bilateral homogeneous enlargement with preservation of normal glandular configuration and signal intensities on T1-WI and T2-WI. Macronodular hyperplasia, seen less commonly than diffuse hyperplasia, produces diffuse adrenal enlargement with one or more macroscopic cortical nodules, and it is more common in long-standing pituitary adrenocorticotropic hormone (ACTH) secretion. MRI demonstrates glandular enlargement and nodules based on contour distortion in patients with macronodular hyperplasia.

10.2.4.2 Adenoma

Adrenal adenomas consist of cords of clear cells separated by fibrovascular trabeculae. Macroscopically, the adrenal adenoma is a well-defined, rounded, homogeneous mass, typically less than 3 cm in diameter. Calcification, central necrosis, and hemorrhage are uncommon. Nonfunctioning adenomas are common, with a prevalence in the general population of approximately 3% and on abdominal CT examination of 0.6%–1.5%. Adrenal adenomas are imaged as homogeneous, localized masses of variable size, with a signal decrease on opposed-phase images relative to in-phase images (Table 10.2). The signal characteristics of nonhyperfunctioning adenomas are similar to those of the normal adrenal gland. They are typically hypointense on T1-WI and isointense or slightly hyperintense on T2-WI. On FS T2-WI, adenomas show a hyperintense rim that corresponds to a tumor capsule or peripherally compressed normal adrenal tissue, with a lower signal intensity core (Fig. 10.9). Relative to nonfunctioning adenomas, hyperfunctioning adenomas, especially aldosteronomas, exhibit increased signal intensities on T2-WI (Fig. 10.10). However, atypical nonfunctioning

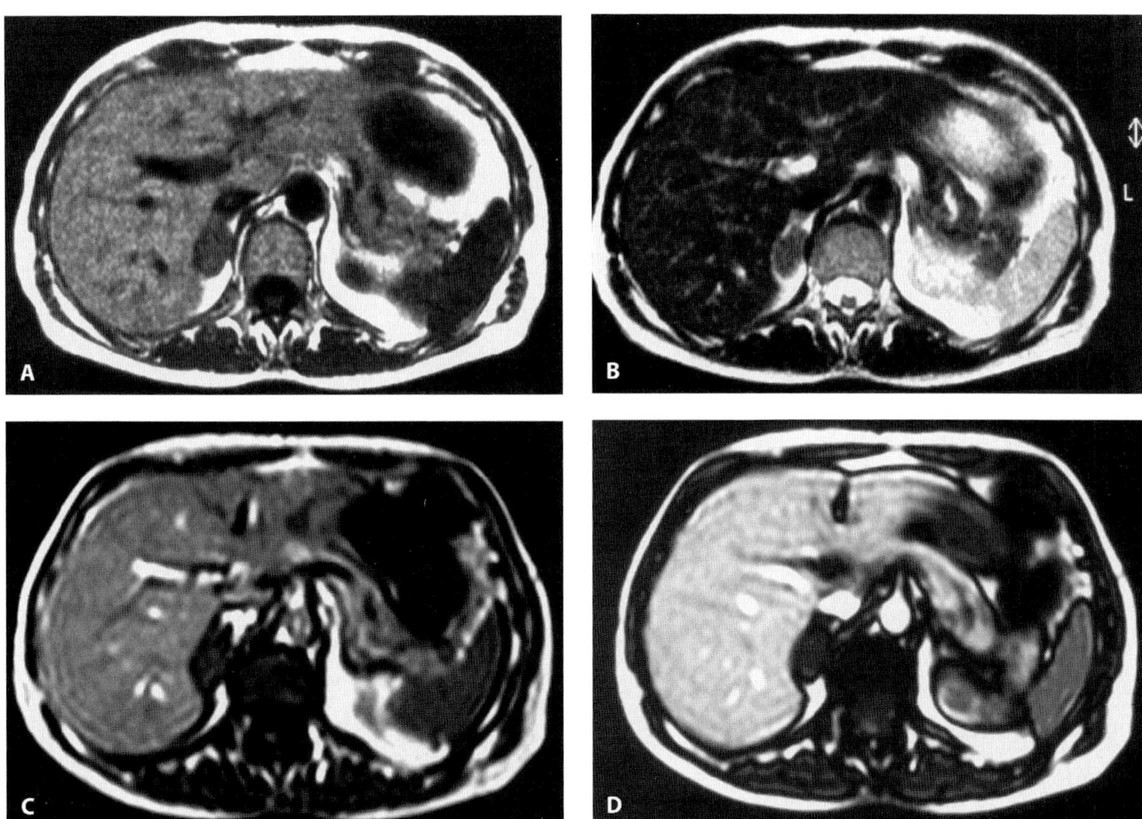

Fig. 10.9A–D. Nonfunctioning adrenal adenoma. Axial T1-W SE (**A**), T2-W TSE (**B**), in-phase (**C**), and opposed-phase GRE images (**D**) of a patient with a nonfunctioning adenoma within the right adrenal gland. The nonhyperfunctioning adenoma demonstrates similar signal characteristics to the normal adrenal gland with low signal intensity on T1-W image (**A**), moderate to slightly high signal intensity on T2-W image (**B**), and a signal decrease on the opposed-phase image (**D**) compared with the in-phase image (**C**)

adenomas exist that can be considerably hyperintense relative to liver on T2-WI, due to hemorrhage and necrosis. Thus, although a higher proportion of functional adenomas are hyperintense relative to the liver on T2-WI when compared with nonfunctioning adenomas, no consistent relationship between the MR characteristics and the adrenocortical function exists (Fig. 10.11).

10.2.4.3 Carcinoma

Adrenal cortical carcinoma is a rare, highly malignant tumor, accounting for less than 0.2% of all cancer deaths. It occurs more commonly on the left than on the right, and approximately 10% are bilateral. Approximately 50% of these tumors are functional, with hypercorticalism, virilization, and mixed syndromes predominating. Relative to liver, adrenal carcinomas typically show lower signal intensity in T1-WI and higher signal intensity in T2-WI (Fig. 10.12). Tumor heterogeneity, best demonstrated by the use of T2-WI, demonstrates areas of necrosis, hemorrhage, and dystrophic calcifications. Following the administration of paramagnetic contrast agents, large signal-intensity increases in the first minute, with delayed washout, are characteristic of adrenal carcinoma. Local invasion of adjacent organs is common, and extension through the adrenal vein, renal vein, or inferior vena cava may be seen. Lack of signal void in the morphological T1-WI and T2-WI indicates the presence of thrombus. Vascular involvement can be further evaluated using GRE imaging or CE 3D-MRA.

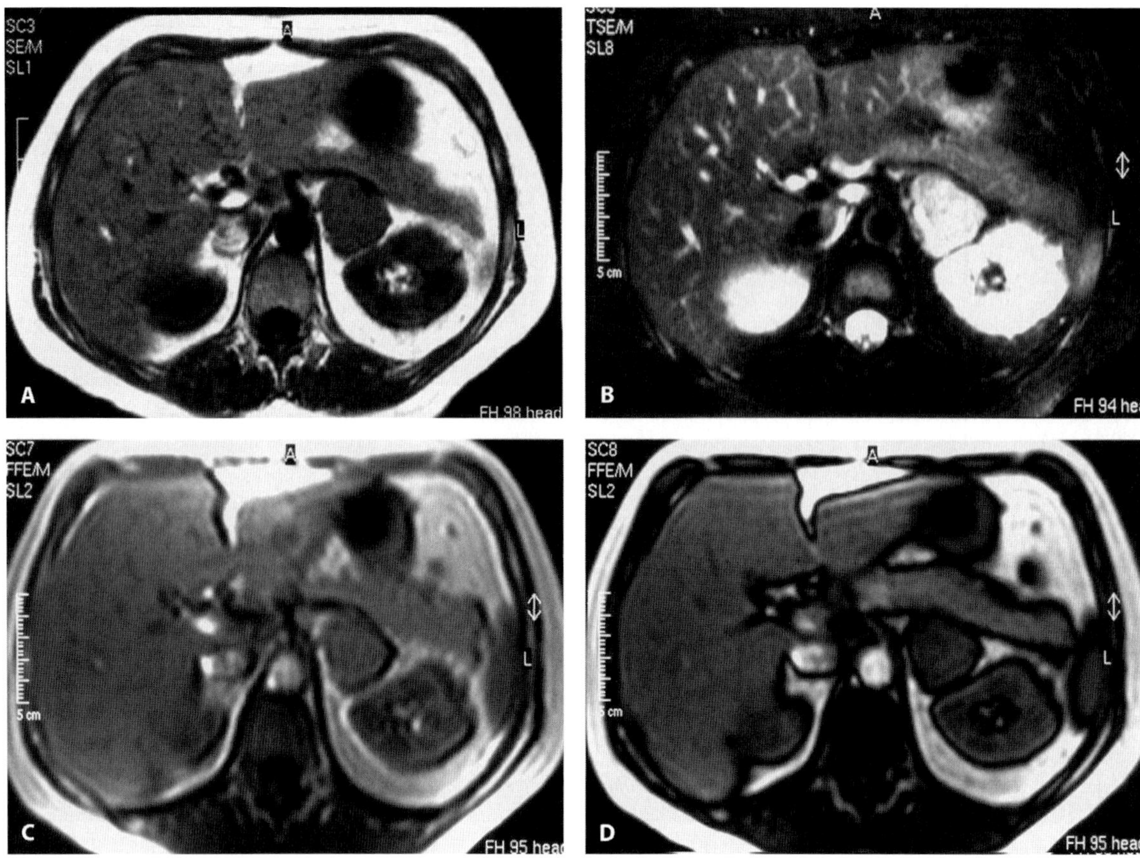

Fig. 10.10A–D. Functioning adenoma. Axial T1-W SE (**A**), FS-T2-W TSE (**B**), in-phase (**C**) and opposed-phase (**D**) GRE images. The functioning aldosteronoma within the left adrenal gland shows higher signal intensity on T2-W MR imaging (**B**) than the non-functioning adenoma (see Fig. 10.9). Opposed-phase GRE (**D**) demonstrates a significant signal decrease compared with in-phase GRE (**C**)

10.2.4.4 Myelolipoma

Myelolipomas are benign tumors of the adrenal cortex, composed of mature adipose cells and hematopoietic tissue. Although associated endocrine disorders have been reported (Cushing's syndrome, Conn's syndrome, hermaphroditism, and intersex), those tumors are not hormonally active and are usually detected incidentally. On MR images, myelolipoma is hyperintense on all pulse sequences, and its intensity is similar to that of subcutaneous or retroperitoneal fat, with a significant signal decrease on FS T1-WI and FS T2-WI.

10.2.5 Clinical Applications of Medullary Mass Lesions

10.2.5.1 Pheochromocytoma

Pheochromocytomas are the most common tumors of the adrenal medulla. They arise from chromaffin cells and secrete catecholamines. Patients may present with a variety of symptoms, including episodic hypertension, flushing, and palpitations. The diagnosis of pheochromocytoma is made by the biochemical assay of catecholamines and their metabolites in blood or urine.

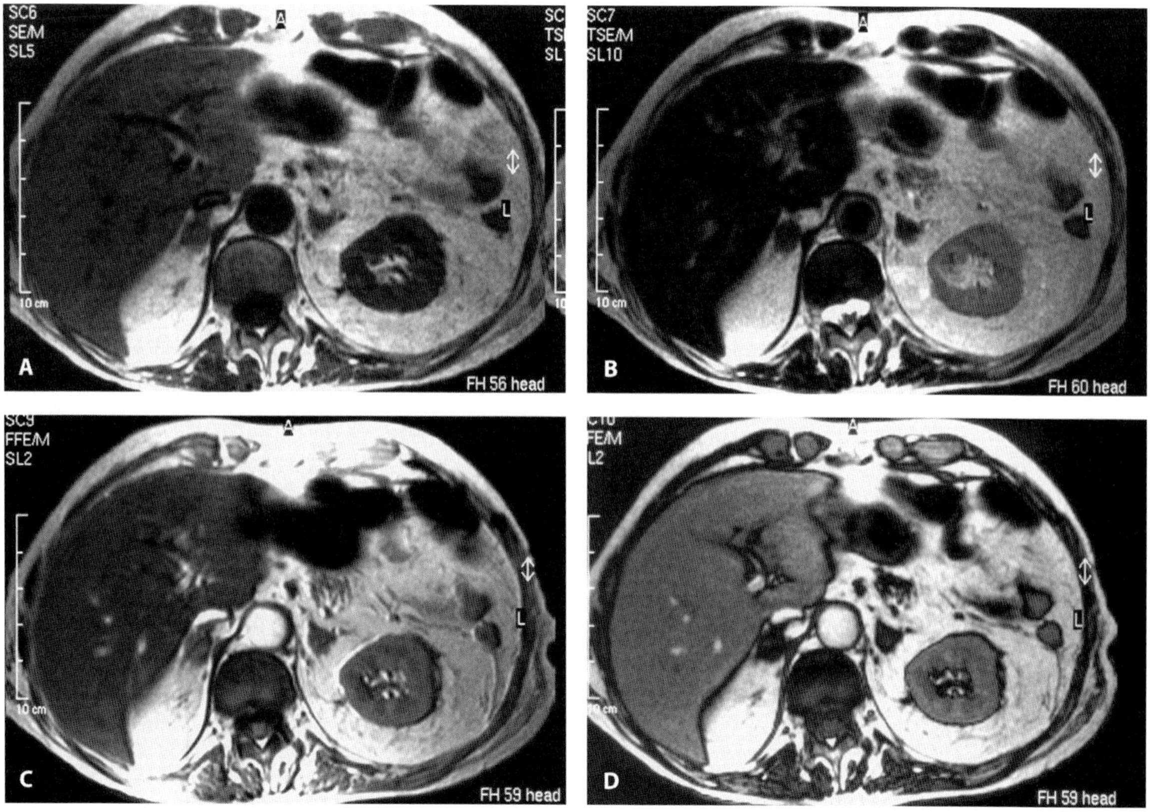

Fig. 10.11A–D. Bilateral adrenal adenomas. Axial T1-W SE (**A**), T2-W TSE (**B**), in-phase (**C**) and opposed-phase (**D**) GRE images of a patient with bilateral adenomas. The signal behavior on T1-W (**A**) and T2-W (**B**) images does not allow bilateral metastases in patients with malignant disease to be ruled out. However, the typical signal decrease on the opposed-phase image (**D**) compared with the in-phase image (**C**) clearly demonstrates the benign nature of the masses

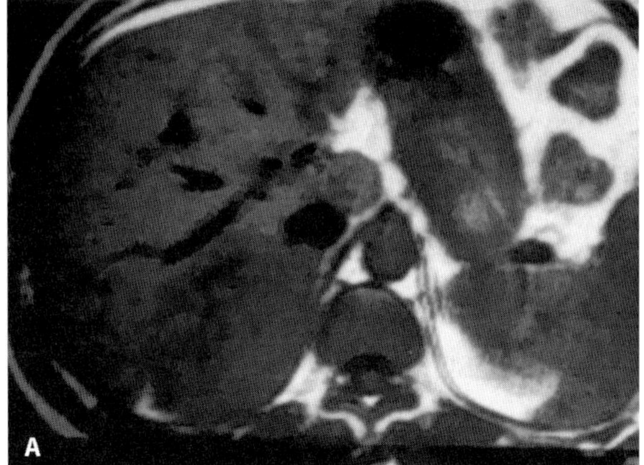

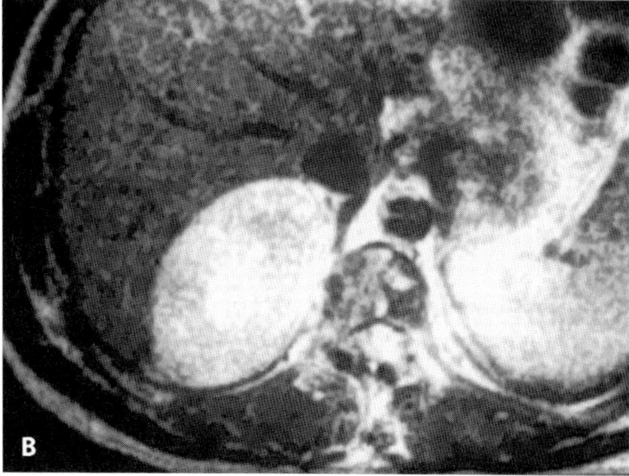

Fig. 10.12A,B. Adrenal carcinoma. Axial T1-W SE (**A**) and T2-W TSE (**B**) images of a large adrenal carcinoma within the right adrenal gland demonstrate low signal intensity on T1-W MR and high signal intensity on T2-W MR images

Imaging tests are used primarily to localize the tumor. Pheochromocytomas can arise anywhere in the autonomic nervous system. However, 98% originate in the abdomen, predominantly (90%) in the adrenal medulla. Some 90% are sporadic, and 10% are part of a systemic disease, such as multiple endocrine neoplasia syndrome (MEN IIa or IIb), neurofibromatosis, or von Hippel-Lindau disease. Approximately 10% of pheochromocytomas are malignant, but the incidence is higher in extra-adrenal masses and in tumors greater than 6 cm in diameter. Malignancy can often be identified only by the presence of metastases and not by the microscopic appearance. Hormonal activity is detected in 90% of pheochromocytomas. Most pheochromocytomas are hypointense on T1-WI and markedly hyperintense on T2-WI. Although typical, these appearances on T2-WI are not specific, as there is some overlap with necrotic adrenal metastases, and 35% of pheochromocytomas may not have a long T2. Although the use of paramagnetic contrast agents is rarely necessary, as with CT, pheochromocytomas enhance markedly following injection (Fig. 10.13).

10.2.5.2 Hemorrhage

Adrenal hemorrhage is usually found in the adrenal medulla and invades the surrounding cortex. Adrenal hemorrhage may be spontaneous, traumatic, or related to anticoagulation. Most adrenal hematomas are resorbed, but sometimes they liquefy and persist as adrenal pseudocysts. The MR appearance of adrenal hemorrhage varies as it evolves from acute to chronic stages (see Chapter 3). High signal intensity on T1-WI and T2-WI in the acute and subacute stages of adrenal hemorrhage reflect the presence of hemoglobin oxidation products (methemoglobin) that are paramagnetic (Fig. 10.14).

10.2.5.3 Neuroblastoma

Neuroblastoma is the most common tumor in children younger than 5 years of age. The tumor originates from undifferentiated cells of the neural crest ectoderm of the sympathetic ganglia. Frequently, neuroblastomas are hormonally active, producing catecholamines or less-active precursors that may be detected in urine. Neuroblastomas are iso- to hyperintense in T1-WI and hyperintense in T2-WI, relative to muscle or liver. Calcifications, seen in 40%–50% of neuroblastomas, are not well imaged with MRI. This disadvantage is offset by the ability to use MRI to image the orthogonal planes, which may be of help in staging.

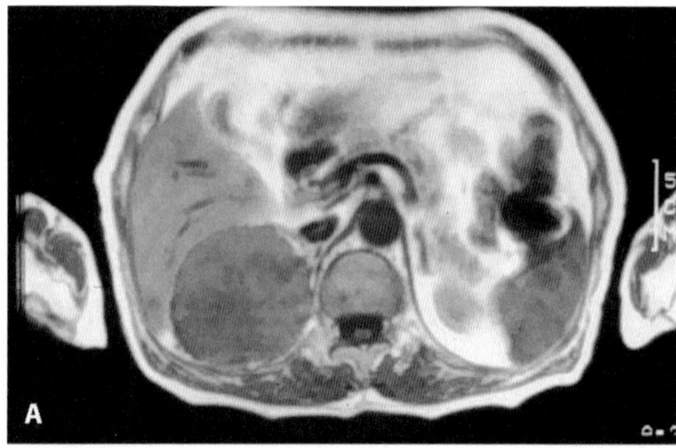

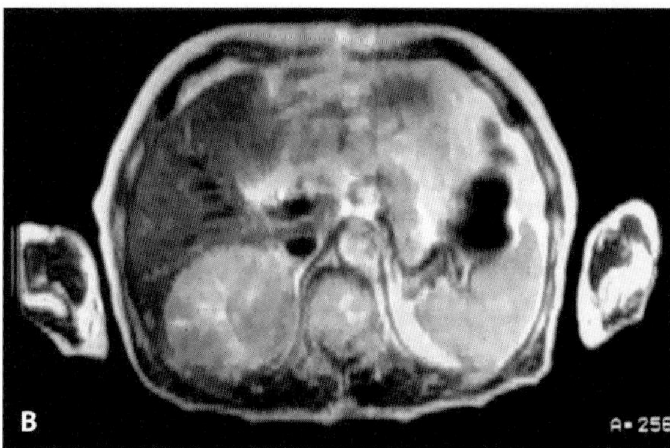

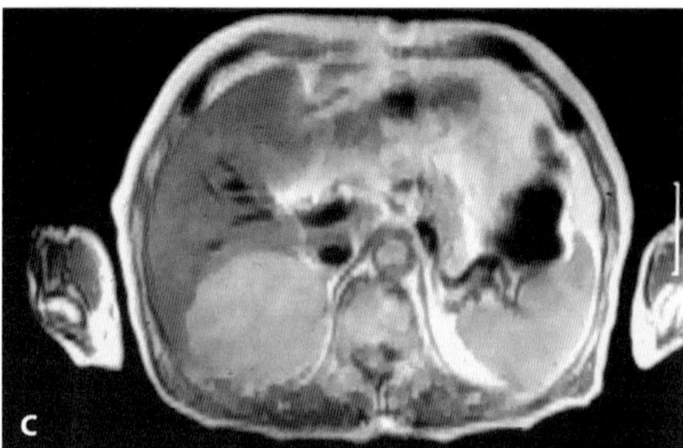

Fig. 10.13A–C. Pheochromocytoma. Axial plain T1-W SE (**A**), contrast-enhanced T1-W SE (**B**), and T2-W TSE (**C**) images demonstrate a large mass within the right adrenal gland. The mass is hypointense on T1-W MR (**A**) with strong contrast enhancement (**B**) and high signal intensity on T2-W MR (**C**), reflecting the hypervascular nature of this tumor

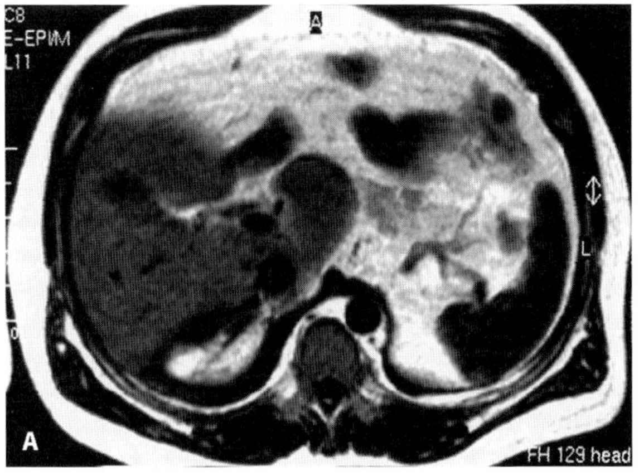

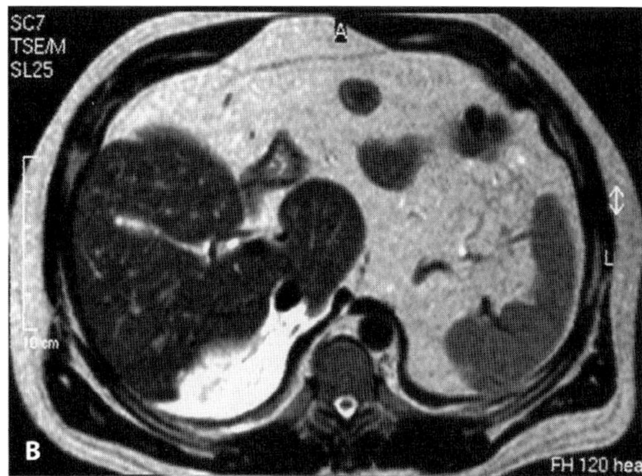

Fig. 10.14A,B. Adrenal hemorrhage. Axial T1-W SE (**A**) and T2-W TSE (**B**) images of right-sided adrenal hemorrhage demonstrate high signal intensity on T1-W and T2-W images, suggesting an acute to subacute stage of hemorrhage

10.2.6 Lesions Affecting Both Cortex and Medulla

10.2.6.1 Cysts

Adrenal cysts are uncommon lesions that may occur at any age. Based on their pathological origin, adrenal cysts have been classified into four types: (1) endothelial cysts (45%), (2) pseudocysts (39%), (3) epithelial cysts (9%), and (4) parasitic cysts (7%). Simple adrenal cysts are hypointense on T1-WI, hyperintense on T2-WI, and demonstrate no contrast enhancement.

10.2.6.2 Metastases

Virtually any malignancy may spread hematogenously to the adrenals. Lung and breast carcinomas are the most common source of adrenal metastasis, followed by gastric, thyroid, and pancreatic carcinomas. During autopsy, adrenal metastases have been detected in up to 27% of cancer patients. Adrenal metastases are pleomorphic; the majority are relatively small, although they may attain almost any size. As with other adrenal neoplasms, the small lesions are generally homogeneous; the larger ones are commonly heterogeneous as a result of hemorrhage and necrosis. Adrenal metastases are bilateral in approximately 40% of cases. In MR imaging, metastases are generally hypointense to liver on T1-WI but significantly hyperintense to liver on T2-WI obtained with or without fat-suppression techniques. Metastases show no significant signal decrease on opposed-phase images (Fig. 10.15).

10.2.7 Incidental Masses

Unknown adrenal masses are detected incidentally in up to 1% of abdominal CT examinations. Characterization is necessary in those patients with extra-adrenal primary malignancy, because curative surgery or radiation therapy for the primary tumor is usually contraindicated if the adrenal mass is depicted as a metastatic lesion. Different therapeutic approaches are usually undertaken for primary malignant lesions if the adrenal mass can be shown to be benign. On SE imaging, most adenomas appear hypointense to isointense in both T1-WI and T2-WI relative to liver; most nonadenomas, including metastasis, appear hyperintense in T2-WI. Quantitatively, when calculating signal-intensity ratios, a 20%–30% overlap between adenomas and nonadenomas exists. Gadolinium-enhanced images show mild enhancement of adenomas with a quick washout, whereas malignant tumors and pheochromocytomas show strong enhancement and slower washout. However, considerable overlap of benign and malignant masses also exists for gadolinium-enhanced MRI. The in-phase/opposed-phase approach provides a better discrimination of adenomas and nonadenomas, because adenomas generally contain large lipid-laden

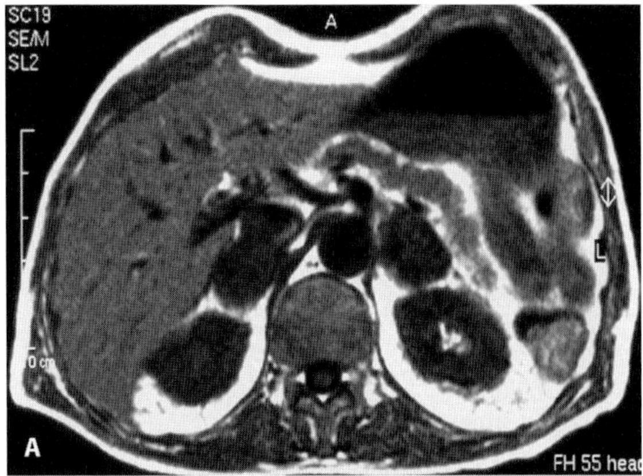
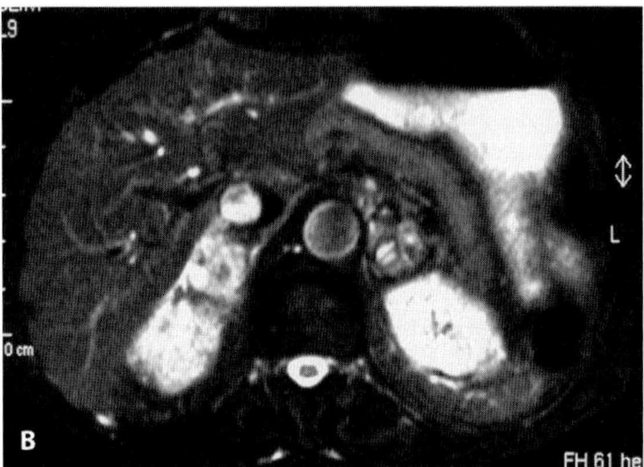
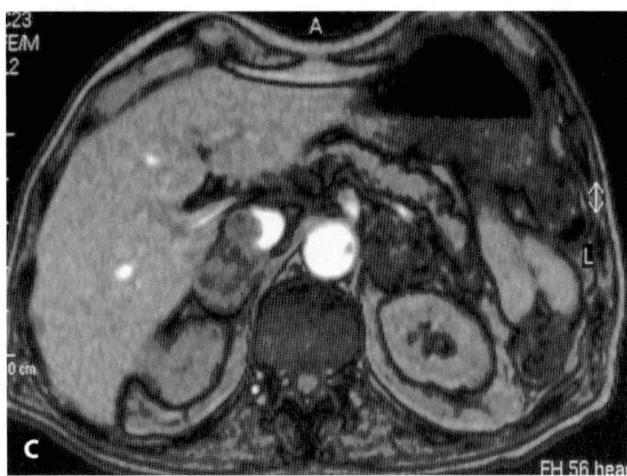

Fig. 10.15A–C. Bilateral adrenal metastases. Axial T1-W SE (**A**), T2-W FS TSE (**B**), and opposed-phase (**C**) GRE images of a patient with bilateral metastases from lung cancer. The signal behavior on T1-W MR (**A**) does not allow the diagnosis of bilateral metastases to be made. However, the irregular high signal intensity on T2-W FS TSE (**B**) and the absent signal decrease on opposed-phase GRE (**C**) demonstrate the malignant nature of the masses

cells, whereas malignant lesions contain little or no fat. Therefore, adenomas homogeneously lose signal intensity on opposed-phase images when compared with in-phase images, whereas metastases remain unchanged (Figs. 10.9, 10.11, 10.15). Differential diagnoses to be considered when a heterogeneous signal decrease is present include fat-containing metastases, HCC, and liposarcoma. Rarely, functioning adenomas may contain such a low lipid content that a significant loss of signal on opposed-phase images cannot be observed.

Further Reading

Bilal MM, Brown JJ (1997) MR imaging of renal and adrenal masses in children. Magn Reson Imaging Clin North Am 511:179–197

Cryer PE (1985) Phaeochromocytoma. Clin Endocrinol Metab 14:203–220

Dawson P (2002) Contrast agents in patients on dialysis. Semin Dial 15:232–236

Dunnick NR, Korobkin M (2002) Imaging of adrenal incidentalomas: current status. AJR Am J Roentgenol 179:559–568

Hussain S, O'Malley M, Jara H, Sadeghi-Nejad H, Yucel EK (1997) MR urography. Magn Reson Imaging Clin North Am 511:95–106

Katzberg RW, Buonocore MH, Ivanovic M, et al (2001) Functional, dynamic, and anatomic MR urography: feasibility and preliminary findings. Acad Radiol 8:1083–1099

Kocak M, Sudakoff GS, Erickson S, Begun F, Datta M (2001) Using MR angiography for surgical planning in pelvic kidney renal cell carcinoma. AJR Am J Roentgenol 177:659–660

Lockhart ME, Smith JK, Kenney PJ (2002) Imaging of adrenal masses. Eur J Radiol 41:95–112

Mitchell DG, Nascimento AB, Alam F, Grasel RP, Holland G, O'Hara BJ (2002) Normal adrenal gland: in vivo observations, and high-resolution in vitro chemical shift MR imaging-histologic correlation. Acad Radiol 9:430–436

Namimoto T, Yamashita Y, Mitsuzaki K, et al (2001) Adrenal masses: quantification of fat content with double-echo chemical shift in-phase and opposed phase FLASH MR images for differentiation of adrenal adenomas. Radiology 218:642–646

Nascimento AB, Mitchell DG, Zhang XM, Kamishima T, Parker L, Holland GA (2001) Rapid MR imaging detection of renal cysts: age-based standards. Radiology 221:628–632

Outwater EK, Siegelman ES, Huang AB, et al (1996) Adrenal masses: correlation between CT attenuation value and chemical shift ratio at MR imaging with in-phase and opposed-phase sequences. Radiology 200:749–752

Peppercorn PD, Reznek RH (1997) State of the art CT and MRI of the adrenal gland. Eur Radiol 7:822–836

Pretorius ES, Wickstrom ML, Siegelman ES (2000) MR imaging of renal neoplasms. Magn Reson Imaging Clin N Am 8:813–836

Scialpi M, Di Maggio A, Midiri M, Loperfido A, Angelelli G, Rotondo A (2000) Small renal masses: assessment of lesion characterization and vascularity on dynamic contrast-enhanced MR imaging with fat suppression. AJR Am J Roentgenol 175:751–757

Siegelman ES (2000) MR imaging of the adrenal neoplasms. Magn Reson Imaging Clin N Am 8:769–786

Slywotzky CM, Bosniak M A (2001) Localized cystic disease of the kidney. AJR Am J Roentgenol 176:843–849

Tello R, Davison BD, O'Malley M, et al (2000) MR imaging of renal masses interpreted on CT to be suspicious. AJR Am J Roentgenol 174:1017–1022

Pelvis

11

D. MacVicar, P. Revell

Contents

11.1 Patient Preparation, Positioning, and Coil Selection

Magnetic resonance (MR) imaging is established as the investigation of choice for most neurological and musculoskeletal imaging. Its role in body imaging is less well established, but up-to-date machinery allows good quality, and reproducible images can be obtained from most parts of the body. In general, MR imaging of the pelvis is well-researched, presents few technical problems, and is rapidly gaining acceptance as the technique of choice in many clinical situations, particularly in urological and gynecological oncology. The pelvis is sufficiently distant from the diaphragm that respiration artifacts are minimal. Bowel peristalsis may be modified pharmacologically, and positioning maneuvers and bladder filling can help remove the small bowel from the field-of-view. The major vessels in the pelvis rarely cause clinically distracting artifacts. Demonstration of disease within the pelvis depends on good quality images using sequences that are reliable and reproducible. Therefore, up-to-date instruments operating at high field strength (1.0–1.5 T) are ideally suited to pelvic imaging. Nevertheless, clinically adequate images can often be obtained with low-field systems, usually by extending the imaging times. With a cooperative patient, clinically useful images may be obtained with machines operating at a field strength as low as 0.2 T.

Patient selection for pelvic MR imaging rarely causes problems, as few patients are confused or agitated. Some patients with severe pelvic pain may require shortening of the protocol, but some images are obtainable in virtually all patients. Whether the images are clinically useful depends on the degree of cooperation between the radiologist and the referring physician, and protocols may vary with the clinical question. Details of surgical procedures, e.g., cystectomy and gut resection, are particularly important and may alter the way in which the patient is prepared for the investigation. Unless they are particularly anxious or claustrophobic, patients for pelvic MR imaging need no sedation. The urinary bladder should not be emptied prior to the investigation, as it is a useful and immediately recognizable anatomical landmark. Ideally, the patient should be instructed, at the time of scheduling, to empty the bladder 2–3 h before the investigation and, subsequently, drink normally. Overfilling of the bladder is also to be avoided, as this can generate patient discomfort, particularly if imaging times are protracted. The usefulness of bowel-marking contrast agents is less clear for pelvic MR imaging than it is for upper abdominal studies. We do not use oral or rectal gut-marking agents on a routine basis. However, if the patient is thin and, therefore, considered unlikely to have adequate natural contrast within the pelvis and lower abdomen to identify bowel loops clearly, oral contrast is sometimes given. Likewise, if the upper-pelvic and retroperitoneal nodal groups are of paramount clinical importance, as is frequently the case in the investigation of gynecological malignancy, contrast agents may be given. The agents used may be positive contrast agents, which are designed to increase the signal return from the bowel on T1-W sequences, or negative contrast agents, which reduce the signal from the bowel. An example of a positive contrast agent is gadolinium-diethylene triamine penta-acetic acid (Gd-DTPA; Oral Magnevist, Schering). This preparation is largely water based and contains mannitol. The advantages of this preparation are ease and speed of administration, as well as the production of a fairly reliable contrast column, which reaches the pelvis within 30 min under normal circumstances. However, it may induce brisk peristalsis, necessitating administration of a gut-relaxing agent. Several other gadolinium-based preparations are available. An alternative approach is to coat polymer balls of suitable size with a super-paramagnetic iron-oxide preparation, which reduces signal from the bowel, particularly on T2-weighted imaging (T2-WI). An example of this is Abdoscan® (Nycomed). This preparation has a 2-h administration time, but produces a well-distributed contrast column. It is tolerable but unpleasant to drink, and care is needed in sequence selection, as some gradient-echo sequences may be associated with susceptibility artifacts around the contrast.

Antiperistaltic gut-relaxing agents are given routinely in our department for all pelvic studies that involve structures above the prostate, including those that involve a nodal survey of the pelvis. The only studies exempt from gut-relaxing agents are those directed to the external genitalia, perineum, or anal canal. Hyoscine butylbromide (Buscopan, Boehringer Ingelheim) is a quaternary ammonium compound with antimuscarinic action causing smooth-muscle relaxation. Parenteral injection of 20 mg by the intravenous or intramuscular route will reduce peristalsis for 30–40 min. Reflex hyperperistalsis may then ensue, and further doses may be necessary if imaging times are prolonged. Side effects such as dry mouth, impairment of visual accommodation, and hesitant micturition are common. The drug should be avoided in patients with a history of glaucoma. The drug is extremely inexpensive.

An alternative muscle relaxant is glucagon, which may be given by subcutaneous, intramuscular, or intravenous injection in a dose of 1 mg (1 mg/ml). The antiperistaltic action lasts longer than hyoscine (usually over 1 h). Nausea and vomiting occur rarely, and hypersensitivity reactions have been described, although these are also rare. In the UK, the dose costs approximately 30 times as much as hyoscine, but remains inexpensive when the cost of the total examination is considered.

Positioning of the patient is influenced by individual preference. In our unit, patients are routinely scanned lying supine. With the bladder adequately filled, the small bowel is displaced from the pelvis, allowing visualization of the pelvic organs. Respiratory artifacts are rarely distracting. Some investigators prefer to use the prone position on the basis that the anterior abdominal wall movement during respiration is reduced. In addition, the gut is squashed upward away from the pelvis. The disadvantage of the prone position is that many patients are less comfortable, and thus patient movement is more likely.

A variety of coils can be used for imaging the pelvis. In most up-to-date high-field systems, the body coil gives adequate images and is used for surveying the pelvis and retroperitoneum for nodal enlargement in cases of pelvic malignancy. More detailed pelvic anatomy and pathology can be demonstrated by a variety of surface coil designs. Most manufacturers use a system that involves anterior and posterior surface coils. Phased-array electronics are available on many, and the signal-to-noise ratio, spatial resolution, and contrast resolution are excellent. The quest for increased signal-to-noise ratio and the convenient placement of pelvic orifices has led to the development of a number of intracavitary coils, including endorectal coils, endoanal coils, and endovaginal coils. Of these, only the endorectal coil, most frequently used for prostate imaging, is widely used. Some manufacturers offer integrated endorectal and pelvic phased-array coils. The practical utility of increasingly sophisticated coil design will be discussed individually, with reference to the clinical setting, later in the chapter.

11.2 Sequence Protocols

11.2.1 General Considerations

As a general rule, sequence selection in the pelvis involves a compromise between maximizing the signal-to-noise ratio, contrast resolution, and spatial resolution while keeping imaging times to a minimum. The anatomy of the pelvis lends itself to MR imaging, as there are easily recognizable anatomical landmarks separated in most individuals by some fat. Spin-echo (SE) sequences and spoiled gradient recalled echo (GRE) sequences form the basis of most protocols. T1-W SE sequences and T2-W turbo spin-echo (TSE) sequences can be completed on high-power machines with acquisition times of 1–5 min. Since motion artifacts are less problematic than in the upper abdomen, the reliance on very fast scanning techniques is reduced. A wide range of pathologies is found in the pelvis, but malignant tumors and inflammatory conditions, including infection, form the majority of the case load. These conditions generate edema and excess free water within the pathological tissues, and the resulting prolonged relaxation times alter the signal characteristics, increasing disease conspicuity, especially on T2-W sequences. In cases where doubt exists as to whether pathology is present, very high contrast techniques, such as short tau inversion recovery (STIR), will also function satisfactorily in the pelvis. The STIR sequence has the added advantage of suppressing signal from fat. Other sequences suppressing fat signal include chemical-shift fat-saturation techniques. These are usually performed with T1-W and can be repeated following intravenous gadolinium administration to increase the sensitivity for pathological tissue.

Some pelvic organs, notably the cervix and body of the uterus and the prostate gland, have a zonal anatomy that is clearly demonstrable on T2-W sequences. SE/TSE sequences also demonstrate urine and other pelvic fluid collections as areas of high signal. As a result, they are frequently the most important single sequence, and if imaging time is limited, for example, by patient claustrophobia, the T2-W sequence is carried out first. The suggested sequence protocols for individual organs within the pelvis may be varied according to the pathology under investigation. Some general advice is given in this section regarding basic imaging techniques, and in the following clinical section, some refinements for specific pathologies are suggested.

In all the sequences where a field-of-view of less than 200 mm is used, a reduced bandwidth is used to maintain an adequate signal-to-noise ratio. The effect of this produces a chemical-shift misregistration of one pixel between the water and the lipid image. This must be considered in the interpretation of the resultant images. If the bandwidth is increased to 210 Hz/pixel or greater (at 1.5 T), the water and lipid signals will fall within the same pixel, but the signal-to-noise ratio will be reduced.

The use of spatial presaturation produces significant improvements in the quality of the images obtained in the pelvic region. This is especially true if a phased-array surface coil is being used. In these cases, correct adjustment of the normalization filter (if available) is also necessary.

Imaging sequences in the transverse plane require spatial presaturation of tissue, both proximal and distal to the imaging volume, to saturate the spins of inflowing blood and to prevent a variation in the signal returned from blood vessels passing through the image stack. If the sequences are acquired within a breath-hold, this is sufficient; if not, the image quality can be improved by the use of spatial presaturation of the anterior and posterior abdominal-wall subcutaneous fat. In sequences using a small field-of-view, these areas of presaturation should extend from the edge of the imaging volume to beyond the skin surface.

In sagittal acquisitions, the use of anterior and posterior spatial presaturation produces improvement in image quality. As in the transverse plane, the areas should be prescribed up to the limit of the imaging volume or, if necessary, slightly beyond it.

In the coronal plane, spatial presaturation is only necessary if large blood vessels are flowing into the imaging volume. Signal normalization should not be used in the coronal plane.

11.2.2 Nodal Survey

A common indication for pelvic MR imaging is staging urological or gynecological malignancy. An integral part of this investigation is surveying the pelvis and retroperitoneum for enlarged nodes (Table 11.1). It is wise to complete this part of the investigation first, as gut relaxation is maximized early in the procedure, and if oral contrast agents have been used, the contrast column is less likely to have broken up. Images of the pelvis are obtained using T2-W and T1-W spoiled GRE (breath-hold) sequences, in the axial plane, from the aortic bifurcation to the inguinal region just below the femoral canal. Slice thickness should be 8–10 mm using a 0-mm to 4-mm gap. This may be varied to accommodate patients of varying heights. Subsequently, a survey of the retroperitoneum should be carried out. If the pelvis is clear of enlarged nodes, the incidence of metastasis to the retroperitoneal nodes from the low pelvic tumors (cervix, bladder, prostate, and rectum) is very low, but metastatic lymph node spread from the body of the uterus or ovaries may occur directly to the retroperitoneum. If the pelvis is clear, a single sequence through the retroperitoneum using T1-W in the coronal plane will usually suffice. This should be included routinely in the protocol if there are no suitably trained personnel available to review the pelvis at the time of imaging. Following this node survey, the local staging of the malignancy should be pursued using the appropriate protocol for the primary site.

11.2.3 Uterus and Cervix

Initially, a localizing sequence should be obtained in the axial plane, using a rapid-acquisition technique that is able to identify the uterus. If a node survey has been completed, one of the axial images of the pelvis may be used as a localizer. Following this, T2-W SE/TSE sequences form the basis of imaging of the cervix and body of the uterus, as the sequences demonstrate the zonal anatomy, sometimes in exquisite detail (Table 11.2). The zonal anatomy is difficult to appreciate on T1-W sequences. A sagittal sequence should be acquired first, from which the orientation of the uterus can be ascertained. Subsequent T2-W images should be obtained in a plane perpendicular to the long axis of the uterus. This will usually be paraxial, but in patients with

Table 11.1. Pulse sequence recommendations for pelvic nodal survey. (Breath-held sequences, each of two interleaved acquisitions)

Sequence	WI	Plane	No. of slices	TR (ms)	TI (ms)	TE (ms)	Flip angle	Echo train length	Slice thickness (mm)	Matrix	FOV	recFOV (%)	Band-width	No. of acq.	Acq. time (min:s)
GE	T1	ax	16	163	–	4.1	75	1	5	256×128	300	62.5	260	1	0:13
TSE	T2	ax	16	5000	–	120	–	65	5	256×128	300	62.5	557	1	0:21
Turbo-IR	T2	cor	15	4800	150	60	–	11	6	256×176	230	100	130	2	4:38

Table 11.2. Pulse sequence recommendations for uterus and cervix

Sequence	WI	Plane	No. of slices	TR (ms)	TI (ms)	TE (ms)	Flip angle	Echo train length	Slice thickness (mm)	Matrix	FOV	recFOV (%)	Band-width	No. of acq.	Acq. time (min:s)
TSE	T2	sag	13	3500	–	120	–	15	5	256×192	180	100	130	2	3
TSE	T2	ax	15	4000	–	120	–	15	4	256×192	160	100	130	2	3:46
TSE	T1	ax	15	700	–	12	–	3	4	256×192	160	100	195	3	5:02

Imaging plan will vary with orientation of the anatomical structures
Abbreviations: *WI* weighted image; *TR* repetition time; *TI* inversion time; *TE* echo time; *Matrix* matrix (phase × frequency matrix); *FOV* field of view (mm); *recFov* % rectangular field of view; *Acq* number of acquisitions

extreme anteversion of the uterus, this may be closer to a true coronal plane. Occasionally, the uterus may be anteflexed, i.e., there is a considerable angle between the cervix and body of the uterus. In these circumstances, the main clinical question should be addressed, and if the procedure is being carried out, for example, for the staging of a cervical carcinoma, then the imaging plane should be perpendicular to the long axis of the cervix.

If parametrial spread of cancer is suspected, a T1-W sequence perpendicular to the long axis of the uterus can demonstrate tumor spread. If this is equivocal, a fat-suppression sequence, such as STIR, may be helpful; alternatively, fat suppressed (FS) T1-W images may be acquired before and after gadolinium enhancement. Coronal plane imaging is occasionally helpful, particularly if disease spread to the vagina is suspected on the initial imaging sequences. Investigation of benign conditions of the uterus, such as leiomyoma and adenomyosis, will usually require a shorter protocol than a preoperative staging procedure for malignancy.

The best quality images of the uterus and cervix are obtained using TSE sequences in a machine operating at 1.0–1.5 T. SE sequences generally perform better than GRE sequences, giving greater clarity of anatomy. Older and lower power machines using standard SE sequences can still give reasonable image quality, but at a cost of relatively long imaging times.

11.2.4 Ovary

The ovary and adnexal structures are relatively difficult to image with any technology. Ultrasound is frequently the first technique used, but MR is capable of imaging masses and cysts in the adnexa. Once again, T2-W and T1-W sequences will usually demonstrate the pathology adequately (Table 11.3). The axial plane is of paramount importance, and coronal imaging is often helpful in clarifying the relationship of masses to the uterus and vessels. The sagittal plane is of limited use.

11.2.5 Vagina

T2-W SE/TSE images once again form the mainstay of the imaging technique (Table 11.4). Small field-of-view

Table 11.3. Pulse sequence recommendations for ovary

Sequence	WI	Plane	No. of slices	TR (ms)	TI (ms)	TE (ms)	Flip angle	Echo train length	Slice thickness (mm)	Matrix	FOV	recFOV (%)	Band-width	No. of acq.	Acq. time (min:s)
TSE	T2	ax	15	4000	–	120	–	15	5	256×128	239	75	220	2	3:46
TSE	T1	ax	15	700	–	14	–	3	5	256×192	230	75	220	3	5:02
Turbo-IR	T2	ax	15	4800	150	60	–	11	6	256×176	230	75	130	1	5:24
TSE	T2	cor	11	4000	–	120	–	15	5	256×192	230	100	130	2	3:01

Table 11.4. Pulse sequence recommendations for vagina

Sequence	WI	Plane	No. of slices	TR (ms)	TI (ms)	TE (ms)	Flip angle	Echo train length	Slice thickness (mm)	Matrix	FOV	recFOV (%)	Band-width	No. of acq.	Acq. time (min:s)
TSE	T2	sag	13	3000	–	120	–	15	4	256×192	200	100	130	2	3
TSE	T2	cor	13	3000	–	120	–	15	4	256×192	200	100	130	2	5:24
TSE	T2	ax	13	3000	–	120	–	15	6	256×192	180	100	130	2	3:46
TSE	T1	sag	13	600	–	12	–	3	4	256×192	200	100	195	2	3:54
TSE	T1	cor	13	600	–	12	–	3	4	256×192	200	100	195	2	3:54
TSE	T1	ax	13	600	–	12	–	3	6	256×192	180	100	195	4	5:02

Abbreviations: *WI* weighted image; *TR* repetition time; *TI* inversion time; *TE* echo time; *Matrix* matrix (phase × frequency matrix); *FOV* field of view (mm); *recFov* % rectangular field of view; *Acq* number of acquisitions

high-resolution images can sometimes differentiate layers of the vaginal wall. Axial, coronal, and sagittal planes are all of use in demonstrating the relationship of the vagina to the adjacent organs. Coronal images demonstrate the relationship to the levator ani muscle to its best advantage, while axial and coronal images demonstrate the relationship to the rectum and bladder. Tampons should preferably be removed, particularly if soiled, as hemorrhagic debris may obscure diagnostic detail.

11.2.6 Prostate

The zonal anatomy of the prostate is well-demonstrated by T2-W SE/TSE sequences (Table 11.5). Good contrast can be demonstrated between the inner gland, which is predominantly transition zone, and the outer gland, which is predominantly peripheral zone. The zonal contrast is lost on T1-W sequences, but pathological entities can be seen to enhance to a greater degree than normal tissue with gadolinium on T1-W sequences. T2-W SE/TSE sequences should be obtained in the axial plane initially. Coronal and sagittal images are useful in staging malignancy. Best results are obtained using a local surface coil, such as a pelvic phased-array coil. We use a small field-of-view high-resolution technique for imaging the prostate and seminal vesicles (Table 11.6). The impact of endorectal coil imaging on patient management remains under investigation.

11.2.7 Urinary Bladder

A variety of techniques have been employed to study the bladder. T2-W SE/TSE sequences are particularly

Table 11.5. Pulse sequence recommendations for prostate

Sequence	WI	Plane	No. of slices	TR (ms)	TI (ms)	TE (ms)	Flip angle	Echo train length	Slice thickness (mm)	Matrix	FOV	recFOV (%)	Band-width	No. of acq.	Acq. time (min:s)
TSE	T2	ax	13	4000	–	120	–	15	4	256×162	182	75	130	4	4:20
TSE	T2	cor	13	3600	–	120	–	15	4	256×162	160	100	130	4	4:07

Table 11.6. Pulse sequence recommendations for prostate (endorectal receiver coil)

Sequence	WI	Plane	No. of slices	TR (ms)	TI (ms)	TE (ms)	Flip angle	Echo train length	Slice thickness (mm)	Matrix	FOV	recFOV (%)	Band-width	No. of acq.	Acq. time (min:s)
TSE	T2	ax	15	6000	–	112	–	15	3	256×240	120	100	130	3	4:49
SE	T1	ax	15	600	–	17	–	–	3	256×256	120	100	130	2	5:10
TSE	T2	cor	15	6000	–	112	–	15	3	256×240	120	100	130	3	3:41

Table 11.7. Pulse sequence recommendations for bladder

Sequence	WI	Plane	No. of slices	TR (ms)	TI (ms)	TE (ms)	Flip angle	Echo train length	TD (s)	Slice thickness (mm)	Matrix	FOV	recFOV (%)	Band-width	No. of acq.	Acq. time (min:s)
TSE	T2	sag	15	4000	–	120	–	15	–	5	256×192	180	100	130	2	3:01
TSE	T1	sag	15	800	–	14	–	3	–	5	256×192	180	100	195	2	3:54

The imaging plane for investigations of the bladder is dependent on the position of the lesion within the bladder. Sagittal or coronal planes are most commonly used

Abbreviations: *WI* weighted image; *TR* repetition time; *TI* inversion time; *TE* echo time; *TD* time delay; *Matrix* matrix (phase × frequency matrix); *FOV* field of view (mm); *recFov* % rectangular field of view; *Acq* number of acquisitions

useful for demonstrating the extent of malignant disease within the bladder wall (Table 11.7). T1-W SE/TSE sequences are often critical in demonstrating perivesical spread of tumors when treatment options are being contemplated. The most useful imaging plane can often only be established once the site of disease within the bladder has been identified. We commence imaging with an axial T2-W sequence, unless there is cystoscopic evidence that there is a small tumor lying at the bladder base or at the dome, where it is unlikely to be adequately visualized by axial imaging. Fat-suppression sequences can be extremely useful for demonstrating perivesical spread. It should be noted that the bladder is particularly susceptible to chemical-shift artifacts, because of the markedly different signal characteristics of urine, bladder wall, and perivesical fat, and sequence selection should reflect this fact.

11.2.8 Anorectal Region

Two main indications for MR imaging of the anorectal region have developed in recent years (Tables 11.8, 11.9). The first is imaging of inflammatory disease and fistula formation. Axial and coronal images can be used to demonstrate the muscles of the pelvic floor, and the coronal plane is particularly important in demonstrating the extent of inflammatory conditions such as fistulae. Penetration of the pelvic floor by a fistula is most reliably detected by MRI. A variety of inversion recovery sequences have been tried, and STIR images are the most widely used, supplemented by T1-W SE sequences. Some authors recommend the use of gadolinium to demonstrate fistula extent.

The second major indication is in the preoperative staging of rectal carcinoma. Initial imaging is in the sagittal plane, from the perineum to the sacral promontory. Most rectal tumors will be visible, and once local-

Table 11.8. Pulse sequence recommendations for anorectal region

Sequence	WI	Plane	No. of slices	TR (ms)	TI (ms)	TE (ms)	Flip angle	Echo train length	Slice thickness (mm)	Matrix	FOV	recFOV (%)	Band-width	No. of acq.	Acq. time (min:s)
TSE	T2	sag	13	4000	–	120	–	15	4	256×162	160	100	130	3	3:01
TSE	T2	cor	13	4000	–	120	–	15	4	256×162	160	100	130	4	5:24
TSE	T2	ax	13	4000	–	120	–	15	5	256×162	160	100	130	4	4:20
TSE	T1	ax	13	750	–	14	–	3	5	256×192	160	100	195	3	4:01
Turbo-IR	T2	cor	13	4000	150	60	–	11	4	256×162	160	100	130	2	3:40
Turbo-IR	T2	ax	13	4000	150	60	–	11	5	256×162	160	100	130	2	3:40

Abbreviations: *WI* weighted image; *TR* repetition time; *TI* inversion time; *TE* echo time; *Matrix* matrix (phase × frequency matrix); *FOV* field of view (mm); *recFov* % rectangular field of view; *Acq* number of acquisitions

Table 11.9. Pulse sequence recommendations for the rectum

Sequence	Plane	WI	No. of slices	TR (ms)	TE (ms)	Flip angle	TI	Echo train length	Slice thickness	Matrix	FOV	recFOV (%)	Band-width
TSE	Trans.	T1	25	600	11	–	–	3	8	512×384	380	75	130
TSE	Trans.	T2	25	5000	130	–	–	15	8	512×400	380	75	220
TSE	Sagittalsag	T2	19	5000	130	–	–	15	3	512×358	300	60	130
TSE	Trans.	T2	26	6600	130	–	–	15	3	256×192	140	100	130

Abbreviations: *WI* weighting of images; *TR* repetition time; *TI* inversion time; *TE* echo time; *Matrix* phase × frequency matrix; *FOV* field of view (mm); *recFOV* rectangular field of view
For high-resolution demonstration of local spread of rectal tumors, the transverse scans should be oriented perpendicular to the long axis of the tumor, and may therefore be paraxial or even paracoronal

ized should be imaged using a T2-W sequence. Thin slice (3–4 mm), small field-of-view, high image matrix scans should be obtained in a plane perpendicular to the long axis of the tumor. The exact imaging plane will depend on the orientation of the rectum at the site of the tumor. For example, if the tumor is close to the rectosigmoid junction, a plane perpendicular to the axis of the tumor may be closer to coronal than true axial. Using this technique, it should be possible to resolve the tumor within the wall, and nodules in the perirectal fat. It is also possible to see the mesorectal fascia and predict the likelihood of successful removal by modern surgical procedures such as total mesorectal excision (TME). Sagittal and coronal imaging planes are useful in demonstrating the proximity of the tumor to the anal sphincter complex, and give an indication of whether the sphincter can be preserved and reanastomosis effected.

Satisfactory imaging is usually achievable using the body coil, but high quality, small field-of-view images are best obtained using pelvic phased-array coils. Tumor staging has been performed using endorectal coils. As with prostate cancer, its place in clinical practice is not yet established. Endoanal coils are being developed that are capable of identifying the individual muscle groups of the anal sphincter, and these are likely to take on a role in the assessment of incontinence (for example following obstetric trauma) and perianal fistulae.

11.2.9 External Genitalia

The male external genitalia are very suitable for MR imaging (Table 11.10). The corpus spongiosum and corpora cavernosa are separated by layers of fascia, and the urethra runs through the corpus spongiosum in the ventral compartment of the penis. Tumors of the penile urethra and a variety of inflammatory and traumatic conditions can be demonstrated. T2-W images yield excellent contrast, and T1-W images following gadolinium administration are useful in demonstrating tumors. A pelvic phased-array coil is ideal, and attention to detail when positioning the male organ can result in greater ease of interpretation of images. A small local surface coil can be used that will yield a good signal and reduce the need to oversample, in controlling aliasing artifacts.

The scrotal contents may be imaged using T2-W and T1-W images. The axial plane is useful to orientate the testes and epididymis, and coronal images are also useful. A wide variety of pathologies, including tumors and trauma, are demonstrable by MRI, but the technique has not replaced ultrasound for most clinical indications.

The female external genitalia may also be imaged using a pelvic coil. Indications are limited, but it is useful for the staging of vulval carcinoma, and tumors of the urethra may be demonstrated.

Table 11.10. Pulse sequence recommendations for external genitalia

Sequence	WI	Plane	No. of slices	TR (ms)	TI (ms)	TE (ms)	Flip angle	Echo train length	Slice thickness (mm)	Matrix	FOV	recFOV (%)	Band-width	No. of acq.	Acq. time (min:s)
TSE	T2	sag	13	4000	–	120	–	15	3	256×192	160	100	130	3	3:01
TSE	T1	sag	13	750	–	14	–	3	3	256×192	160	100	195	2	3:54
TSE	T2	ax	15	4500	–	120	–	15	5	256×192	160	100	130	2	3:46
TSE	T1	ax	15	800	–	14	–	3	5	256×192	160	100	195	4	5:02

Abbreviations: *WI* weighted image; *TR* repetition time; *TI* inversion time; *TE* echo time; *Matrix* matrix (phase × frequency matrix); *FOV* field of view (mm); *recFov* % rectangular field of view; *Acq* number of acquisitions

11.3 Clinical Applications of Pelvic MR Imaging

11.3.1 Uterus and Cervix

11.3.1.1 Anatomy

The uterus is divided into three segments: the fundus lies above the cornua, the body or corpus uteri lies between the fundus and the most caudal part of the uterus, which is the cervix (Fig. 11.1). Histologically, the uterine corpus has three tissue layers: the serosa, which is a covering of peritoneum draped over the uterus; the myometrium, which consists of smooth muscle, and the endometrium. The inner third of the myometrium is composed of smooth-muscle bundles, which are densely packed and orientated mostly along the long axis of the uterus. The outer myometrium contains more loosely packed and randomly orientated smooth-muscle fibers. The MR imaging anatomy of the uterine body and fundus is well-demonstrated by sagittal T2-W SE/TSE sequences. A high signal-intensity stripe represents normal endometrium and secretions within the cavity. The width of the endometrial stripe varies with the menstrual cycle, and the average thickness has been reported to be 3–6 mm in the follicular phase and 5–13 mm during the secretory phase. Below the endometrial stripe, there is band of low signal referred to as the junctional zone. Beyond this is an outer layer of myometrium, which returns intermediate signal intensity on T2-W images. There is some controversy about the histological basis for the low signal intensity of the junctional zone. The hypothesis that it represents the densely packed muscle bundles of the inner layer of the myometrium is attractive; however, some in vitro studies have demonstrated that the thickness of the inner layer of myometrium does not correspond exactly to the junctional zone on either MRI or ultrasound. Some authors have attributed the low signal from the junctional zone to a lower water content, while others have drawn attention to an increase in the percentage of nuclear area within the cells of the junctional zone compared with that of the outer myometrium.

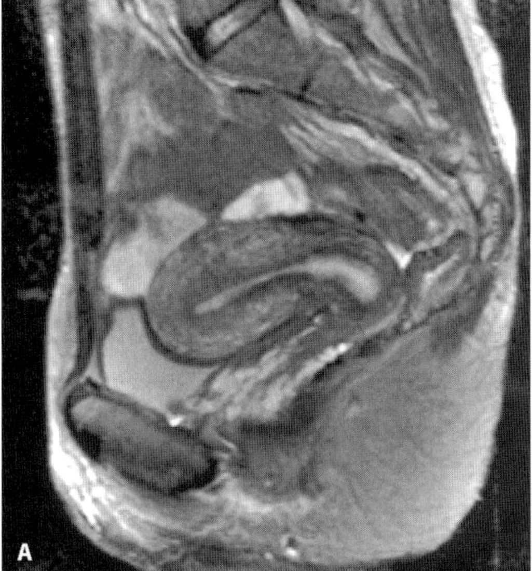

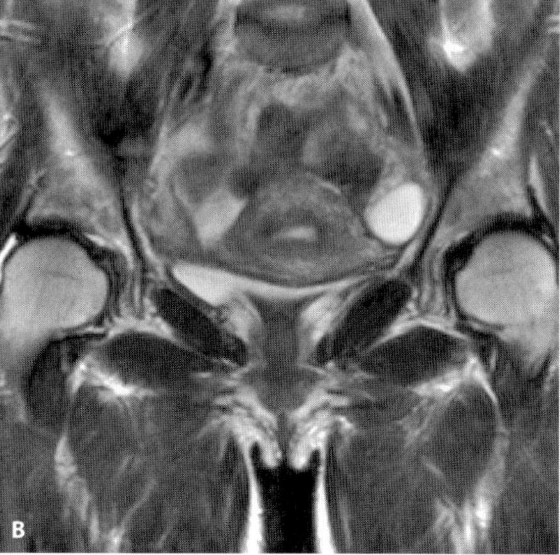

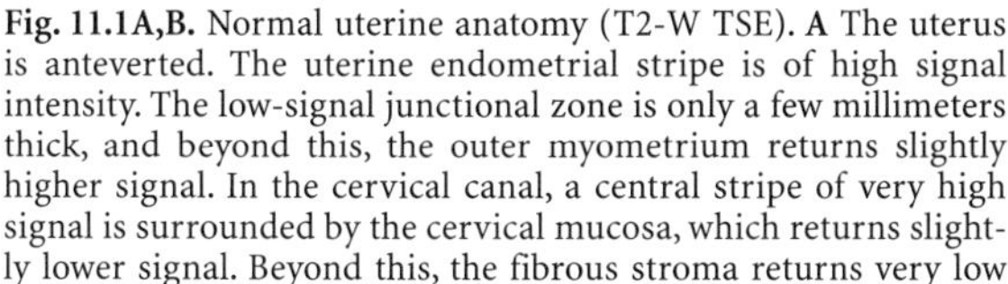
Fig. 11.1A,B. Normal uterine anatomy (T2-W TSE). **A** The uterus is anteverted. The uterine endometrial stripe is of high signal intensity. The low-signal junctional zone is only a few millimeters thick, and beyond this, the outer myometrium returns slightly higher signal. In the cervical canal, a central stripe of very high signal is surrounded by the cervical mucosa, which returns slightly lower signal. Beyond this, the fibrous stroma returns very low signal, and the outermost layer of the cervix is of intermediate signal, representing muscle in continuity with the outer myometrium. **B** An image has been obtained in a plane perpendicular to the long axis of the uterus. Because of the degree of anteversion of the uterus, this is close to a true coronal image. It demonstrates the high signal returned by the endometrium and luminal secretions, surrounded by the junctional zone and outer myometrium

The cervix is separated from the uterine corpus by the internal os, which corresponds to a slight constriction, marked by the entrance of the uterine vessels. The cervical canal is lined by the columnar epithelium of the endocervix. Small folds can sometimes be seen (plicae palmatae). Surrounding the cervical endothelium is a dense, fibrous stroma. The outermost layer of the cervix is composed of muscle, which becomes increasingly thin in the lower cervix toward the external os and is marked histologically by the squamocolumnar mucosal junction. On T2-W images, the secretions in the canal form a zone of very high signal. The cervical mucosa itself returns slightly lower signal, and the plicae palmatae may be seen. The fibrous stroma is of very low signal, and the muscular outer cervix is of intermediate signal. This muscular layer is continuous with the outer myometrium of the uterine corpus. The MR appearance of the cervix varies little with the menstrual cycle.

The parametrium and suspensory ligaments of the uterus may serve as pathways for local spread of disease. The parametrium lies between layers of the broad ligament, which is a folded double sheet of peritoneum that reflects from the ventral and dorsal surface of the uterus and extends to the pelvic side wall. The lower border of the broad ligament is thickened by a condensation of connective tissue and muscle, forming the cardinal ligaments. The paired uterosacral ligaments are fused anteriorly with the cardinal ligaments and extend posteriorly to the sacrum. The uterovesical ligaments extend from the cervix to the base of the urinary bladder. These are the main suspensory ligaments of the uterus. The round ligaments run from the posterolateral aspect of the uterine fundus through the inguinal canal to the labia majora. The ligaments are of low signal intensity on T1-WI and of variable intensity on T2-WI. The parametrium contains multiple venous plexuses and some loosely packed connective tissue, which is of intermediate signal intensity on T1-W sequences and isointense with fat on T2-W sequences.

11.3.1.2
Congenital Anomalies

The fallopian tubes, uterus, and upper two-thirds of the vagina are derived from the paired Müllerian ducts. Agenesis or hypoplasia may affect any part of the female genital tract. A variety of partial and complete duplications may also result from embryological aberrations. Simple anomalies can usually be identified on transvaginal ultrasound. MR imaging should be reserved for patients with technically difficult or indeterminate ultrasound examinations, which may occur in patients with vaginal malformations and multiple complex anomalies. The coronal plane using T2-W sequences is frequently the most informative sequence.

11.3.1.3
Benign Pathology

Endometrial polyps and hyperplasia can usually be detected using transvaginal ultrasound, at which time endometrial sampling may be undertaken. MRI currently has no established role in the initial investigation of endometrial pathology, although thickening of the endometrial stripe can be clearly demonstrated. In cases where there is difficulty in assessing the endometrium, for example, in cervical stenosis, MRI may provide useful information. Thickening of the endometrial stripe is of pathological significance, particularly in postmenopausal women, but the normal ranges are not clearly defined. It has been suggested that the postmenopausal endometrial thickness should not exceed 3 mm in women not receiving hormone-replacement therapy and should not exceed 6 mm in women on hormone-replacement treatment. On T2-W images, endometrial polyps return a slightly lower signal than normal endometrium. When they are large, endometrial polyps may be markedly heterogeneous with areas of high and low signal. They show variable degrees of enhancement on T1-W sequences following the administration of gadolinium. Typically, they enhance less than endometrium but more than adjacent myometrium.

Leiomyoma is the most common type of uterine tumor and is estimated to be present in 20%–30% of premenopausal women over the age of 35 years. Following menopause, they may regress, as they are estrogen dependent. Most leiomyomas exhibit some form of degeneration pathologically, particularly if they are large. Degeneration may be hyaline, myxomatous, cystic, fatty, or hemorrhagic. In addition, they may calcify, and these diverse degenerative features account for the variable signal changes seen on MR imaging. T2-W sequences provide optimal contrast between leiomyomas and adjacent myometrium or endometrium. T1-W sequences may be useful in depicting hemorrhagic degeneration and may be helpful in demonstrating clear fat planes between the uterus and adnexal structures in cases where difficulty is encountered in dis-

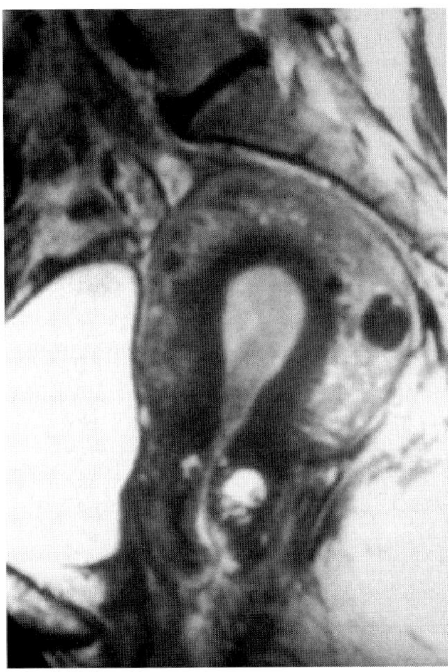

Fig. 11.2. Uterine fibroid (T2-W TSE, sagittal plane). The endometrial stripe is wide in this premenstrual patient. The junctional zone is within normal limits. There are low-signal lesions in the outer myometrium, none of which exceed 1 cm in maximum dimension. These are uterine fibroids

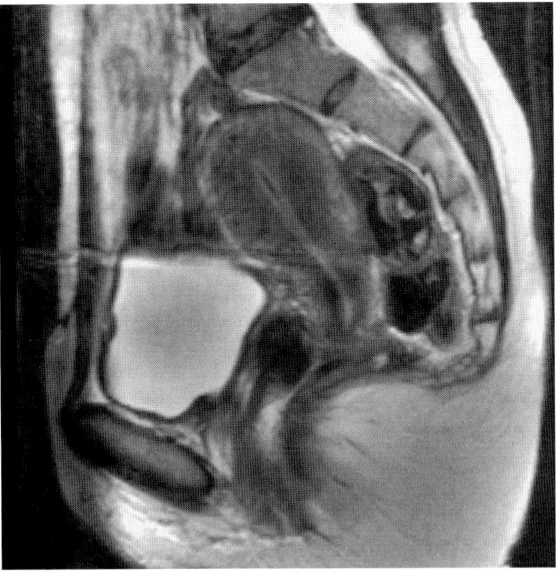

Fig. 11.3. Adenomyosis (T2-W TSE). The endometrial stripe is within normal limits, but the junctional zone is diffusely thickened. The outer myometrium returns normal signal

criminating a uterine leiomyoma from an ovarian mass. Leiomyomas typically appear as well-marginated masses of low signal intensity relative to myometrium on T2-W sequences (Fig. 11.2). Very small lesions are frequently identified, and MRI is more sensitive than transvaginal ultrasound. The detail available on MR imaging may help demonstrate the myometrial origin of a submucosal leiomyoma protruding into the endometrial cavity, thus assisting in discrimination from an endometrial polyp.

The cellular subtype of leiomyoma and those with significant degeneration are the most likely tumors to cause confusion, as they may return high signal on T2-W sequences. The appearance of leiomyomas following the administration of gadolinium is variable. The majority enhance to a lesser degree than the surrounding myometrium on both early and delayed contrast-enhanced images. However, early intense enhancement may be seen with the cellular subtype. Bizarre signal change in large leiomyomas should raise the possibility of sarcomatous degeneration, which is rare and cannot be reliably diagnosed by MRI alone.

The greatest utility of MR imaging in the diagnosis of uterine leiomyoma is in unequivocally demonstrating the myometrial origin of a lesion, where other investigations such as transvaginal ultrasound are indeterminate.

Uterine adenomyosis is a common condition caused by heterotopic endometrial gland and stroma in the myometrium. This ectopic tissue appears to be independent of hormonal stimuli, and the clinical presentation usually involves irregular or excessive bleeding, pelvic pain, and sometimes uterine enlargement. Adenomyosis may be focal, diffuse, or microscopic and is frequently found incidentally following hysterectomy for other indications.

Because the presenting symptoms are nonspecific, imaging is of value if the diagnosis is to be made preoperatively. In this clinical setting, MRI has some advantages over transvaginal ultrasound, primarily its reproducibility and relative lack of operator dependency. T2-W sequences are ideal for diagnosing adenomyosis. The heterotopic endometrium generates adjacent myometrial hyperplasia, and this is represented as diffuse or focal thickening of the junctional zone (Fig. 11.3). On T1-W sequences, small hyperintense foci may be seen, which are thought to represent hemorrhage.

Gadolinium enhancement does not assist in the diagnosis. Various values for the maximum thickness of the junctional zone have been proposed, but the consensus view is that it should be no thicker than 12 mm. A value in excess of this is highly predictive of the presence of adenomyosis. If the junctional zone is less than 8 mm, adenomyosis is very unlikely. Between 8 mm and 12 mm, the diagnosis relies on other features, such as the presence of localized hemorrhagic areas, poor definition of the junctional zone, and focal thickening of the junctional zone. The main differential diagnosis, clinically and radiologically, is from leiomyoma. MRI, despite some overlap of features, is the most reliable method of preoperative diagnosis. This is an important point, since uterine leiomyoma may be treated conservatively, whereas the treatment for clinically debilitating adenomyosis is hysterectomy.

Benign conditions of the cervix include nabothian cysts, cervical stenosis, and cervical incompetence. Nabothian cysts result from distension of the endocervical glands, and these very common lesions return high signal on T2-WI and are usually asymptomatic. Cervical stenosis may be congenital, inflammatory, iatrogenic, or neoplastic. MR imaging can identify the location of cervical stenosis and demonstrate neoplasms. It can also demonstrate the degree of distension of the proximal uterus by retained secretions.

11.3.1.4 Malignant Disease

Endometrial carcinoma is a common malignancy of the female genital tract in the developed world. Its peak incidence occurs between the ages of 55 and 65 years. Most patients present with postmenopausal bleeding or irregular bleeding, usually early in the course of the disease. Patients are referred for dilatation and curettage if no obvious cause is found on clinical grounds. This allows for prompt diagnosis and treatment. Approximately 85% of endometrial carcinomas are adenocarcinomas, although papillary serous and clear-cell carcinomas, which carry a worse prognosis, may also be found. Endometrial carcinoma may spread locally. Lymphatic spread may be directly to para-aortic nodes. Most clinicians use the staging system of the Federation Internationale de Gynaecologie et d'Obstetrique (FIGO) (Table 11.11).

Tumor grade, stage of disease, and depth of myometrial invasion are the most important prognostic factors. MR imaging is well-suited to staging endometrial carcinoma, and T2-W sequences in the sagittal and transverse planes are extremely helpful for assessing the depth of myometrial invasion. The MR appearance of noninvasive endometrial carcinoma (stage IA) is nonspecific, and MR imaging, therefore, has no role as a screening technique. Histological sampling is required for the diagnosis, and discrimination from hyperplasia is not possible by MRI. The signal intensity of endometrial carcinoma is variable. It may be isointense with normal endometrium or slightly hypointense on T2-W sequences. Alternatively, a heterogeneous mass of mixed high and low signal intensity may be seen. Thickening of the endometrial stripe in postmenopausal women is a suspicious sign.

In patients with myometrial invasion (stage IB and IC), segmental or complete disruption of the junctional zone by a mass of intermediate signal intensity on T2-W sequence should be seen (Fig. 11.4). Disruption of the junctional zone should be seen on two imaging planes. There is overlap with the MR findings in adenomyosis, but once a histological diagnosis of carcinoma has been made, the MR signs can be interpreted with reasonable confidence. The percentage of myometrial invasion is estimated, separating patients into stage IB (less than 50% wall invasion) or stage IC (greater than 50% wall invasion). Superficial extension of endometrial carcinoma into the cervical mucosa (stage

Table 11.11. Federation Internationale de Gynaecologie et d'Obstetrique (FIGO) staging of endometrial carcinoma

Stage 0	Carcinoma in situ
Stage I	Tumor confined to corpus
IA	Tumor limited to endometrium
IB	Invasion <50 % of myometrium
IC	Invasion >50 % of myometrium
Stage II	Tumor invades cervix but does not extend beyond uterus
IIA	Invasion of endocervix
IIB	Cervical stromal invasion
Stage III	Tumor extends beyond uterus but not outside true pelvis
IIIA	Invasion of serosa, adnexa, or positive peritoneal cytology
IIIB	Invasion of vagina
IIIC	Pelvic and/or para-aortic lymphadenopathy
Stage IV	Tumor extends outside of true pelvis or invades bladder or rectal mucosa
IVA	Invasion of bladder or rectal mucosa
IVB	Distant metastases (includes intra-abdominal or inguinal lymphadenopathy)

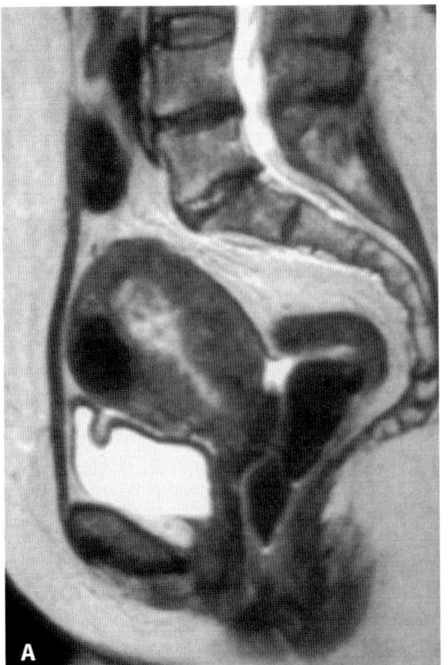

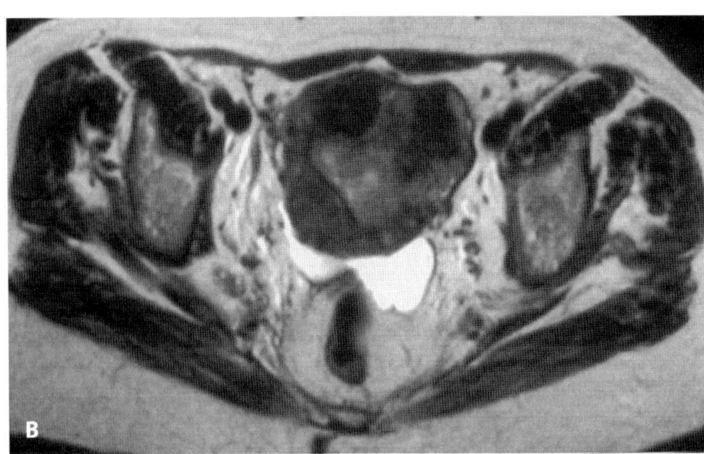

Fig. 11.4A,B. Endometrial carcinoma (T2-W TSE). **A** Sagittal sequence demonstrates some mixed signal within the endometrial stripe. The junctional zone is not clearly identified. Anteriorly, a uterine fibroid is noted. **B** Paraxial plane (perpendicular to long axis of uterus). The endometrial signal is mixed. The junctional zone and anatomy of the outer myometrium are disrupted by endometrial carcinoma spreading to the left of midline and anteriorly. Low-signal areas within the myometrium are uterine fibroids. Hysterectomy demonstrated no parametrial spread of the tumor

IIA) can be demonstrated on T2-WI by widening of the endocervical canal and internal os. If the low signal-intensity fibrous stroma of the cervix is invaded, stage IIB disease is diagnosed. MR imaging has been demonstrated to be an accurate technique for staging of early endometrial carcinoma. Few data are available in the literature regarding stage III and stage IV endometrial carcinoma, but MRI is certainly capable of demonstrating bulky tumors with parametrial invasion, invasion of the vagina, and regional lymphadenopathy. It is less reliable in demonstrating peritoneal spread. In practice, many centers do not employ MR staging of endometrial carcinoma since surgeons proceed to hysterectomy in early-stage disease, and surgical/histological staging is, therefore, available.

Cervical carcinoma is the third most common malignancy of the female genital tract in the developed world, but it is also extremely common in Africa. Screening by cytology picks up cervical intraepithelial neoplasia, which is considered to be a precursor of cervical carcinoma. The disease may, therefore, be picked up when asymptomatic. It is estimated that 80%–90% of cervical carcinomas are squamous-cell carcinomas, but adenocarcinoma is undoubtedly becoming more common and carries a worse prognosis. In women under 35 years of age, most cervical carcinomas arise from the squamocolumnar junction, which lies on the vaginal surface of the cervix. These tumors grow in a polypoid fashion (Fig. 11.5). In older women, most tumors occur within the endocervical canal, resulting in a barrel-shaped cervix. Tumors located within the cervical canal are more difficult to evaluate clinically and have a high incidence of parametrial invasion (Fig. 11.6). Cervical carcinoma is usually staged clinically, using the FIGO system (Table 11.12), despite its well-known limitations.

T2-W sequences provide optimal contrast between tumors and the normal cervical structures. Sagittal and transverse imaging planes will normally evaluate local tumor extension accurately. Coronal sections may be useful in providing additional information regarding the parametrium and the lateral vaginal fornices. Carcinoma in situ or microinvasive tumors (stage IA)

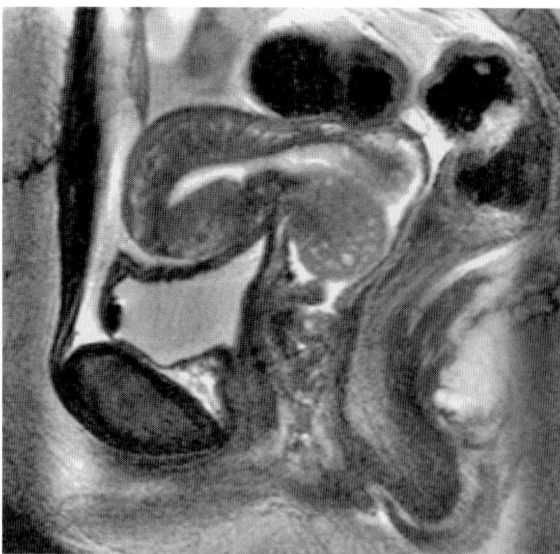

Fig. 11.5. Carcinoma of cervix (T2-W TSE, sagittal plane). There is a mass protruding from the anterior lip of the cervix. The canal appears intact, but the fibrous stroma has been disrupted. A mixed-signal mass is projecting into the vagina. The appearance is of carcinoma of the cervix. The uterus is slightly enlarged and the junctional zone indistinct, as this patient presented postpartum

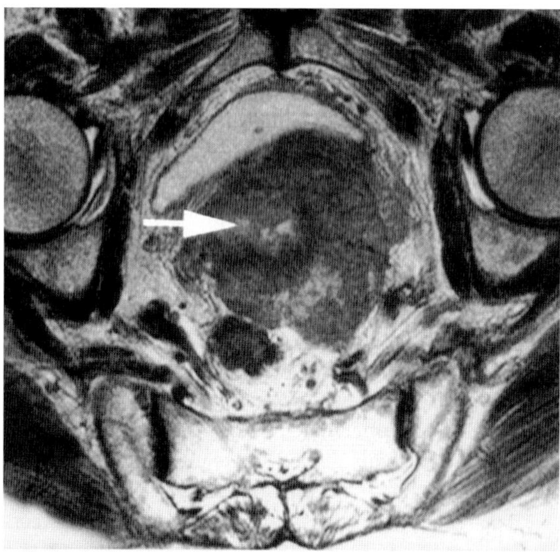

Fig. 11.6. Bulky, locally advanced carcinoma of the cervix (T2-W TSE, axial plane). This axial image through the cervix shows an outline of the cervical anatomy (*arrow*). The low-signal ring of the fibrous stroma is irregular and disrupted. Beyond this, there is extensive parametrial invasion, almost to the pelvic side wall on the left. The posterior wall of the bladder is involved by the tumor

Table 11.12. Federation Internationale de Gynaecologie et d'Obstetrique (FIGO) staging of cervical carcinoma

Stage 0	Carcinoma in situ
Stage I	Tumor confined to cervix (extension of corpus should be disregarded)
IA	Microinvasion
IB	Clinically invasive. Invasive component >5 mm in depth and >7 mm in horizontal spread
Stage II	Tumor extends beyond cervix, but not to pelvic side wall or lower third of vagina
IIA	Vaginal invasion (no parametrial invasion)
IIB	Parametrial invasion
Stage III	Tumor extends to lower third of vagina or pelvic side wall; ureter obstruction
IIIA	Invasion of lower third of vagina (no pelvic side wall extension) peritoneal cytology
IIIB	Pelvic side wall extension or ureteral obstruction
Stage IV	Tumor extends outside true pelvis or invades bladder or rectal mucosa
IVA	Invasion of bladder or rectal mucosa
IVB	Distant metastases

The presence of metastatic lymph nodes is not included in the FIGO classification

are not normally identified by MR imaging. However, MRI will identify tumors that invade the fibrous stroma, despite relatively normal-appearing epithelium. Macroinvasive cervical carcinoma (stage IB) is defined as an invasive component greater than 5 mm in depth and 7 mm in horizontal spread; these appear on T2-WI as masses of intermediate signal intensity that deform the canal or disrupt the very low signal-intensity fibrous band. The lateral margins of the cervix, which are formed by muscle incontinuity with the outer myometrium, should remain smooth in stage-IB disease. On T1-WI, cervical tumors are usually isointense with normal cervix, and the zonal anatomy is difficult to appreciate. Small tumors are, therefore, not visible on T1-W sequences unless gadolinium is given. Cervical carcinoma will demonstrate increased enhancement relative to cervical stroma, which is most marked on images acquired within 60 s of administration, using a dynamic sequencing technique.

Cervical carcinoma is classified as stage IIA when it invades the upper two-thirds of the vagina. On T2-W images, disruption of the vaginal wall or diffuse thickening with high signal intensity are signs of tumor invasion. One of the crucial clinical decisions takes place in the diagnosis of stage-IIB disease, in which parametrial invasion is present. Under most circumstances, surgery is not considered for these patients, and radiotherapy is the treatment of choice. It has been shown that a completely intact ring of cervical stroma accurately excludes parametrial extension. However, full-thickness disruption of the fibrous stroma with abnormal signal intensity in the parametrium has a significant false-positive rate in stage I tumors, and it seems that overstaging results from peritumoral inflammatory change.

Locally advanced (stage III or stage IV) disease is usually diagnosed clinically and can easily be confirmed with MR imaging. There is relatively little histologically correlated data in the literature, as these tumors are rarely removed. Large masses frequently invade the pelvic sidewall, bladder, and rectum. When large, cervical carcinomas return mixed signal on T2-WI and low signal on T1-WI. The T2-W image is useful in demonstrating tumor invading muscles, such as levator ani, obturator internus or piriformis, as the muscles are usually of lower intensity than the invading tumor. T1-W sequences maximize contrast if there is sufficient fat in the pelvis. Fat-suppression techniques may also be helpful in clarifying the anatomy.

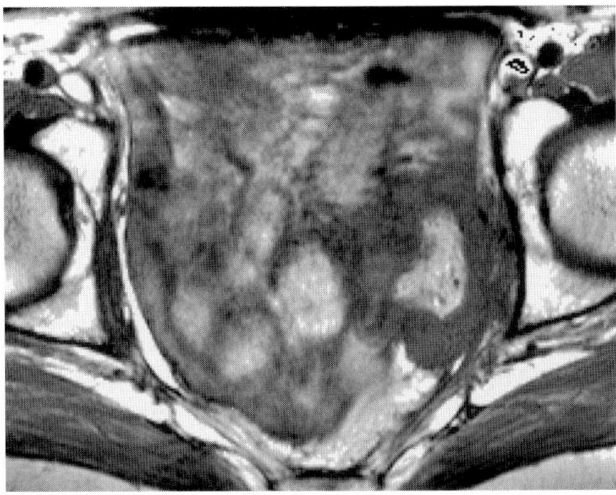

Fig. 11.7. Recurrent cervical carcinoma (T2-W TSE, axial plane). This patient presented with pelvic pain following hysterectomy and radiotherapy for carcinoma of the cervix. On the left side of the pelvis, there is a mass returning predominantly low signal peripherally with an area of high signal centrally. The central area represents necrotic and hemorrhagic debris. The outer layer was biopsy proven to represent recurrent carcinoma. The diagnosis may be made on the morphology of the mass, which is clearly invasive, rather than the signal characteristics per se. The mass is penetrating fat planes laterally and disrupting the cortical bone of the acetabulum

Following radiotherapy for cervical carcinoma, diagnosis of suspected recurrent disease is a frequent and difficult clinical problem. By 12 months after completion of the radiation treatment, the uterus and cervix should return low signal. However, during the initial 6–12 months after treatment, developing radiation changes may return high signal, due to inflammation and increased vascularity. Enhancement with gadolinium is not normally seen later than 12 months after radiation treatment. However, the rate of development of the typical hypointense signal from radiation fibrosis is extremely variable from patient to patient, and an abnormal signal may persist for years. Recurrent tumor should, therefore, be diagnosed on the basis of a demonstrable mass, rather than on signal change alone (Fig. 11.7).

11.3.2 Parametrium and Ovaries

MR imaging is capable of diagnosing adnexal masses as cystic or solid, and can characterize the components as fluid, fatty, or hemorrhagic. Up-to-date machinery using pelvic phased-array coils can usually demonstrate the ovaries and parametrial structures on T2-W SE sequences. The axial and coronal planes are most useful. T1-W SE sequences following gadolinium may be helpful, as may FS images. Transvaginal ultrasound remains the investigation most commonly performed first for investigation of the ovaries. However, in selected cases, MR imaging can yield additional information.

In women of reproductive age, the normal ovaries may demonstrate zonal anatomy on T2-W images. The medulla has a slightly higher signal intensity than the cortex. Cysts are frequently seen, returning high signal on T2-W sequences. On T1-W sequences, follicular cysts have thin walls, which enhance variably. Thick enhancing rims are typical of the corpus luteum, which is also prone to hemorrhage. Bizarre and complex cystic structures with irregular thickening and enhancement should raise a suspicion of malignant disease (Fig. 11.8). Solid tumors are also frequently malignant, although benign teratoma masses may demonstrate areas of signal intensity consistent with fat.

Pelvic inflammatory disease is fundamentally a clinical diagnosis. Tubo-ovarian abscess, a well-recognized complication of pelvic inflammatory disease, can be

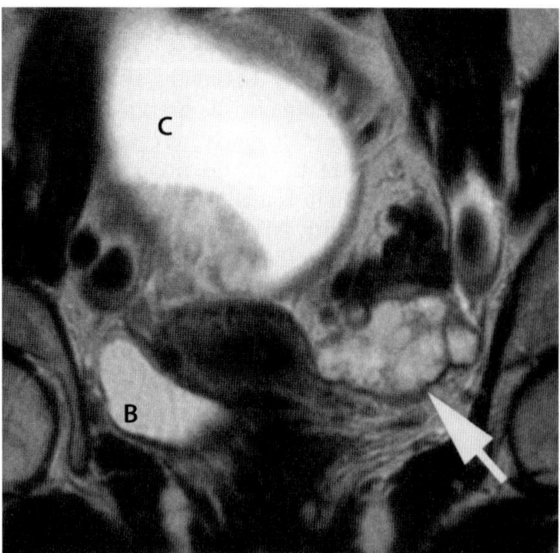

Fig. 11.8. Bilateral ovarian carcinoma (T2-W TSE, coronal plane). The anteverted uterus is seen centrally, showing the myometrium and junctional zone in cross-section. The bladder (*B*) contains high-signal urine. Fluid is also present in a right adnexal cyst (*C*), which has a thick wall and a nodular mass lying inferiorly. An intermediate- to high-signal solid mass is present in the left adnexum (*arrow*). These features are characteristic of malignant ovarian masses (ovarian adenocarcinoma)

demonstrated by MRI, although transvaginal ultrasound remains the imaging investigation of first choice.

11.3.3 Urinary Bladder

11.3.3.1 Anatomy

The urinary bladder lies in a subperitoneal position. It has an outer adventitial layer of connective tissue, and the dome of the bladder is covered by peritoneum. Below the adventitia, there is a layer of smooth muscle (the bladder detrusor). The outer part of the muscle layer consists of more loosely packed muscle fibers, while the inner layer is more compact. The muscle layer appears on MR imaging as a structure of low signal intensity on T2-W sequences, and low to intermediate signal on T1-W sequences. It is sometimes possible to discern a slight difference in signal between the two muscle layers, the compact inner layer being slightly lower in signal intensity than the outer. The mucosa and submucosa of the bladder return a higher signal intensity than the muscle on T2-W sequences, and the normal mucosa will enhance on T1-W sequences following the administration of gadolinium. The total bladder-wall thickness is approximately 5 mm, although this is significantly influenced by bladder filling. The degree of distension of the bladder is of considerable importance for a number of reasons; the overfilled bladder will induce involuntary motion artifacts, but some degree of filling is helpful to push the bowel out of the way to reduce bowel-related motion artifact. Overfilling may also stretch the muscle layer and obscure early-stage, flat bladder tumors. Underfilling thickens the detrusor, which would also obscure small tumors. Blood in the urine from hemorrhagic tumors can result in distracting artifacts. Following gadolinium administration, increasing urinary concentration of contrast can also cause problems.

T2-W and T1-W SE/TSE sequences will demonstrate most pathology. Imaging planes are best selected with knowledge of the site of pathology. This is frequently known, since most imaging techniques have a limited role in the initial diagnosis of bladder lesions. Presenting symptoms, such as hematuria and dysuria, are usually investigated by bacteriological and cytological examination, and if the cause remains uncertain, cystoscopy is performed. The nature and site of pathology are therefore frequently known at the time of imaging. The multiplanar imaging capability of MRI makes it the best available technique for imaging all forms of bladder pathology. Imaging acquisition in different planes will minimize the partial volume effect. Sagittal images are utilized for investigating lesions of the anterior and posterior wall and dome of bladder, while the coronal imaging plane is ideal for lesions of the lateral walls and dome.

Chemical-shift artifacts occur at the interfaces between urine, bladder wall, and surrounding fat. This can result in a dark or bright band along the lateral wall on either side of the bladder. Rotation of the frequency-encoding gradient or chemically selective fat suppression can be used to minimize this artifact. Alternatively, suitable selection of bandwidth can reduce the artifact, but at the cost of reducing the signal-to-noise ratio.

11.3.3.2
Benign Bladder Pathology

A variety of fascinating but rare disease entities may affect the bladder. Leiomyoma is the most common of these lesions. They have a predilection for the region around the trigone, and may cause bladder-outflow obstruction. They are of intermediate signal intensity on T1-W images and of high signal intensity relative to the normal muscle of the bladder on T2-W images. Intramural extent of the tumor can, therefore, be assessed. They may degenerate, resulting in mixed signal intensities. Neurofibromas, hamartomas, and pheochromocytomas are also reported. Endometriosis may involve the bladder, classically presenting as cyclical hematuria, although persistent hematuria may occur. Evidence of hemorrhage may be present on MRI, and extravesical manifestations of the disease are usually seen (Fig. 11.9). Granulomatous disease of the bladder is common in the setting of genitourinary tuberculosis, but the lesions on MRI have no specific features and may simulate malignant lesions. Transitional-cell papillomas are important, although they account for only 2%–3% of all primary bladder tumors. They are superficial, may be multiple, and have a tendency to recurrence and malignant transformation. They are best demonstrated on gadolinium-enhanced images, where the degree of enhancement is normally in excess of the adjacent normal bladder wall.

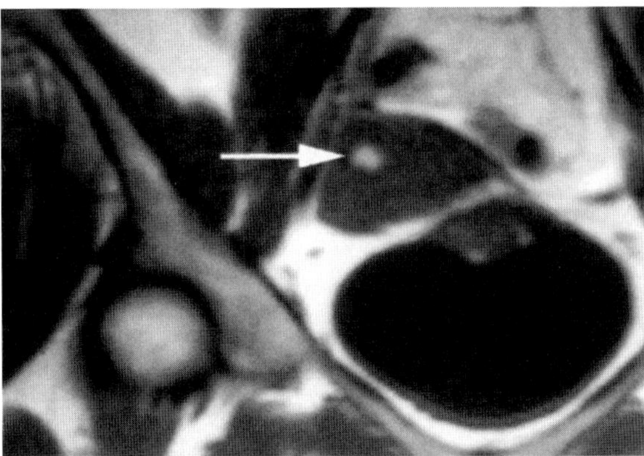

Fig. 11.9. Endometriosis of bladder (T1-W TSE, coronal plane). At the dome of the bladder, there is a mass thickening the bladder wall with an intraluminal polypoid component. Some high signal is present on this unenhanced scan, indicating a hemorrhagic component. There is also a hemorrhagic focus (*arrow*) in the uterus. Biopsy is usually necessary to confirm the diagnosis, although in some clinical circumstances, typical MRI features of endometriosis can establish the diagnosis with reasonable certainty. On this occasion, transurethral resection of the bladder lesion confirmed the diagnosis of endometriosis

11.3.3.3
Bladder Carcinoma

Malignant epithelial neoplasms of the bladder are common, particularly in the elderly, and carry a poor prognosis. They are classified according to cell type, pattern of growth, and histological grade. Transitional-cell carcinoma (TCC) accounts for almost 90% of all bladder malignancies. Squamous cell carcinoma, adenocarcinoma, and carcinosarcoma account for the rest, although squamous cell carcinomas are more prevalent in regions where schistosomiasis is common. The growth pattern may be papillary or sessile, and infiltrating or noninfiltrating. Histological grading runs from I through III, with grade-III tumors more likely to be sessile and infiltrating. MRI is the best way of staging malignant bladder neoplasms and should form a crucial part of the evaluation of treatment options. The tumor node metastasis (TNM) system is used for staging bladder cancer (Table 11.13). Bladder carcinoma returns low to intermediate signal on T1-WI. The tumor will be of higher signal intensity than urine within the bladder lumen on unenhanced scans, although the signal may be similar to the muscle layer of the bladder wall. Bladder carcinoma returns higher signal than the muscular layer on T2-W images. If the appropriate plane is used, the extent of tumor within the wall may be assessed. The depth of invasion of the bladder wall is of considerable importance to the prognosis. If the deep layer of muscle is involved, the incidence of nodal involvement is increased, and the 5-year survival is

Table 11.13. TNM staging classification of bladder cancer

TX	Primary tumor cannot be assessed
T0	No evidence of primary tumor
T1	Tumor invades subepithelial connective tissue
T2	Tumor invades muscle
T2a	Tumor invades superficial muscle (inner half)
T2b	Tumor invades deep muscle (outer half)
T3	Tumor invades perivesical tissue:
T3a	Microscopically
T3b	Macroscopically (extravesical mass)
T4	Tumor invades any of the following: prostate, uterus, vagina, pelvic wall, abdominal wall
T4a	Tumor invades prostate or uterus or vagina
T4b	Tumor invades pelvic wall or abdominal wall

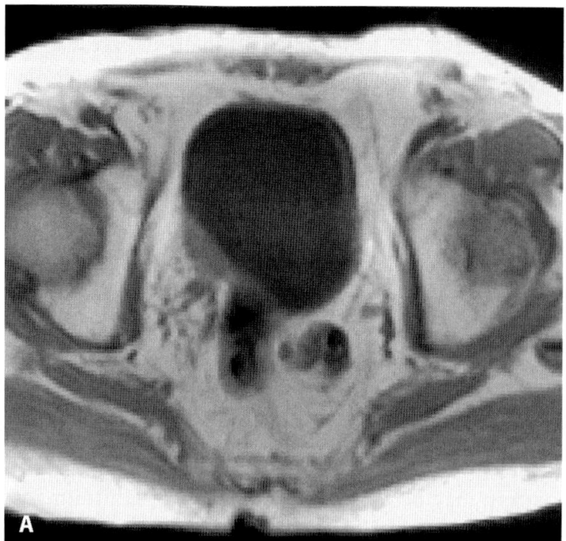

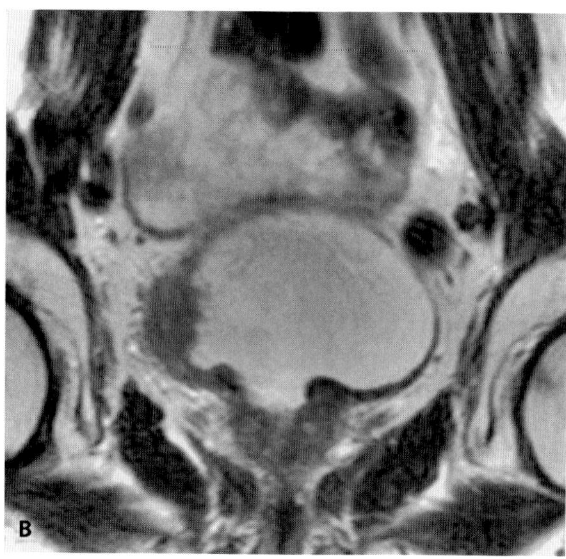

Fig. 11.10A,B. Carcinoma of bladder. **A** T1-W spoiled GRE images (breath-hold) in axial plane. Along the right bladder wall, there is a mass lesion of intermediate signal. This is projecting into the perivesical fat, although the mucosa of the bladder on this image looks flat. Urine returns low signal, and good contrast is obtained between the tumor, urine, and perivesical fat. **B** T2-W TSE, coronal plane. In this plane, there is obvious extravesical spread of the tumor and also projection into the bladder lumen. Abnormal signal within the bladder wall is seen to extend superiorly to the tumor mass. Normal bladder wall, seen *inferolaterally* on the left, returns a low signal from the muscular layer. (Local staging of bladder tumor is T3b)

reduced. The latest revision of the TNM staging classification acknowledges the fact that a genuine extravesical mass forms a contraindication to an attempt at radical cystectomy, but the prognosis for patients whose disease shows microscopic extravesical spread following cystectomy is not significantly worse than patients with invasion of the deep muscle layers without extravesical spread. Staging with MRI should, therefore, attempt to discriminate visible, macroscopic, extravesical spread (Fig. 11.10). Estimation of the depth of invasion within the wall is somewhat subjective, but as a rule of thumb, abnormal signal in more than 50% of the thickness of the bladder wall indicates spread to the deep muscle layer.

The natural history of TCC is characterized by evolution from a relatively low grade histology and polypoid growth pattern to a more malignant tumor of sessile morphology, which is frequently found at multiple sites (Fig. 11.11).

In the context of diffuse but potentially resectable bladder tumors, intravenous gadolinium is extremely useful. Bladder tumors are enhanced early on dynamic images. These tumors are usually vascular, and gadolin-

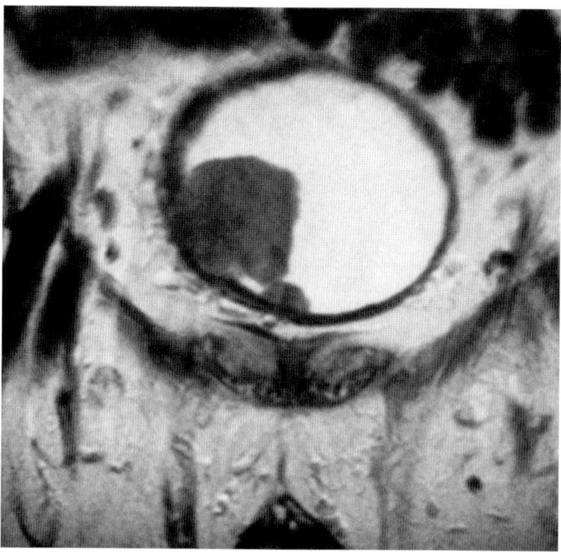

Fig. 11.11. Multifocal bladder carcinoma (T2-W TSE, coronal plane). There is a large mass arising from the right side of the bladder with evidence of invasion of the muscularis. A further small focus of sessile tumor is present inferiorly. The remainder of the scan showed two further areas of sessile tumor formation similar to the smaller nodule

ium leaks into the extracellular space. Images acquired within 30–60 s of gadolinium administration will demonstrate brisk enhancement before excreted gadolinium reaches the urinary bladder, and give excellent depiction of tumor spread within the bladder walls (Fig. 11.12). Delayed images may also outline the intraluminal portion of the bladder tumor against high-signal urine, but layering artifacts are common, and small tumors may be obscured. Unfortunately, in our experience, many bladder tumors present late (Fig. 11.13). Once an extravesical mass or nodal spread has been demonstrated, there is little to be gained by giving gadolinium.

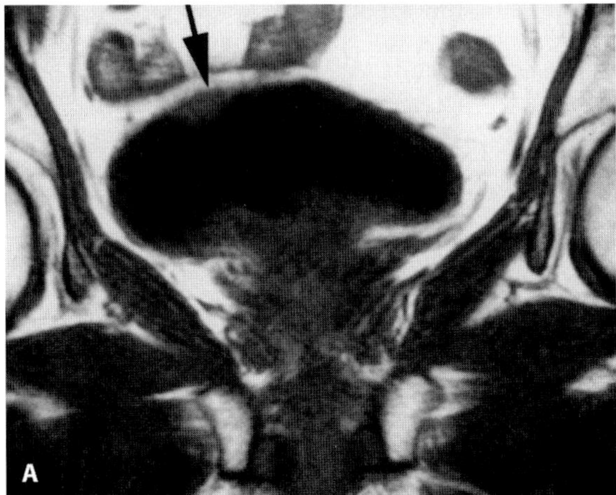

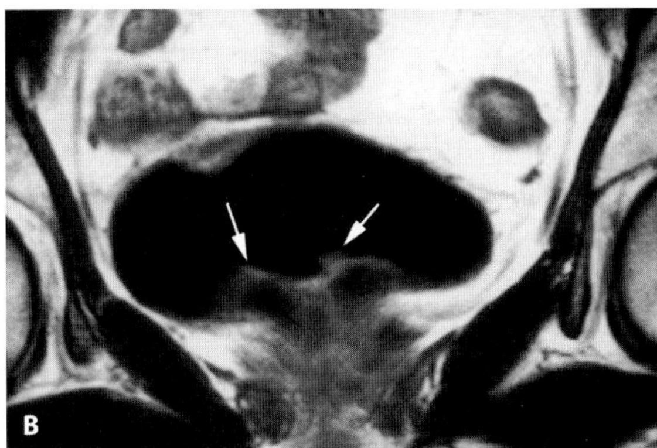

Fig. 11.12A,B. Diffuse superficial bladder tumor. **A** T1-W TSE, coronal plane. Cytoscopy had demonstrated a small tumor at the dome of the bladder (*arrow*). **B** T1-W TSE, coronal plane following gadolinium administration. The images were obtained within 60 s of a bolus dose of intravenous gadolinium, prior to the arrival of contrast within the bladder. The small mass at the dome of the bladder enhances. There is also focal abnormal enhancement of the bladder epithelium at the trigone (*arrows*), extending into the bladder outlet and proximal prostatic urethra. Transitional-cell carcinoma frequently develops a diffuse or multifocal growth pattern

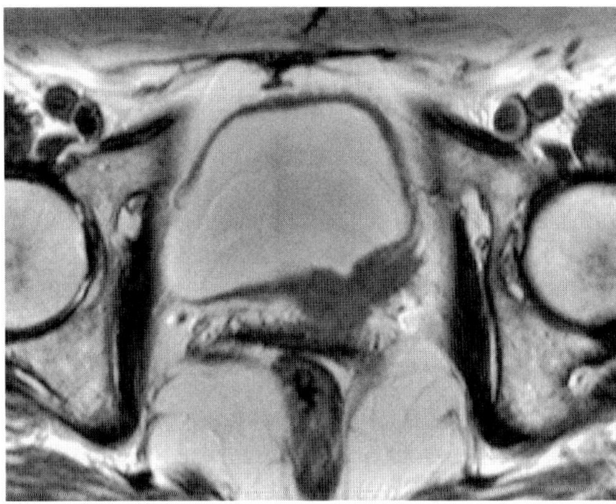

Fig. 11.13. Carcinoma of the bladder. T2-W TSE, axial plane. There is an irregular mass in the left posterolateral aspect of the bladder. This returns intermediate signal, higher than normal bladder muscle but lower than urine and the surrounding perivesical fat. There is evidence of direct spread into the left lateral vaginal fornix

11.3.3.4 Diffuse Disease of the Bladder

Hypertrophic change is common, particularly in the presence of benign prostatic disease. The absence of areas of abnormal signal within the thickened bladder wall should allow discrimination from tumor.

Signal changes occur in the bladder wall following therapeutic radiation. The bladder mucosa and bladder wall return abnormally high signal on T2-W images, and the changes are thought to be due to edema of the bladder mucosa. These may occur in the asymptomatic patient. Severe radiation change may cause bladder-wall thickening and fistula formation.

Hemorrhagic cystitis may result from infection by bacteria such as *E. coli*, and may also occur following radiation treatment and some forms of chemotherapy (particularly involving cyclophosphamide). A variety of interesting signal changes may occur within the bladder wall and in the urine. These may be confusing if a telltale history of hematuria is concealed from the investigating radiologist.

11.3.4 Prostate

11.3.4.1 Anatomy

The lobar concept of prostatic anatomy, first described by Lowsley in 1929, has now been replaced, for the purpose of cross-sectional imaging, by the zonal concept of prostatic anatomy, first described by McNeal in 1966. The zonal anatomy is well-demonstrated on T2-W SE/TSE sequences. The prostate is a cone-shaped glandular organ, with the apex of the cone lying caudally and the base lying cranially, abutting the bladder where the urethra starts. The prostatic urethra runs through the gland to the apex, where it becomes the membranous urethra. The muscular wall of the membranous urethra forms the external sphincter. At mid-gland level, the transition zone surrounds the urethra. The transition zone contains a relatively high proportion of stromal elements compared with glandular tissue and, therefore, has an intermediate signal intensity on T2-WI. When the transition zone enlarges with age, benign prostatic hypertrophy develops, which is common enough to be considered virtually normal in patients over the age of 45 years. As prostatic hypertrophy increases, cystic spaces and discrete nodules may develop, but the zonal anatomy of the prostate should remain recognizable. Around the transition zone lies the peripheral zone. This area has a high glandular content, is relatively lacking in stromal elements, and returns a high signal on T2-WI. At the apex of the gland, below the transition zone, it accounts for virtually the entire gland. However, if there is a significant degree of benign prostatic hypertrophy at mid-gland level, the peripheral zone is compressed into a horseshoe shape (Fig. 11.14). The central zone is an area of gland lying in the midline, cranial to the transition zone. The ejaculatory ducts run through the central zone to the verumontanum, a small ovoid structure, which returns high signal. The central zone is frequently indistinguishable as a separate structure and accounts for only a small percentage of the prostatic volume. The anterior border of the prostate is marked by a band of thickened fibromuscular tissue, which thins laterally to form the capsule of the prostate. This is frequently only a few cells thick and, in places, is completely deficient, glandular tissue merging directly with periprostatic fat. The neurovascular bundles are located posterolaterally. The seminal vesicles lie immediately superior to the base of the gland.

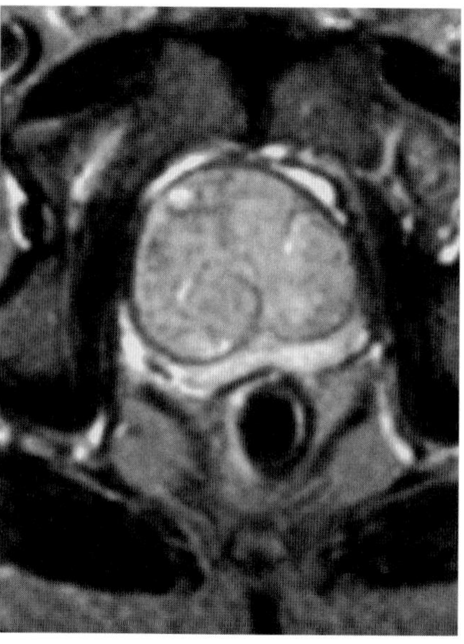

Fig. 11.14. Benign prostatic hypertrophy (T2-W SE, axial plane). The prostate is grossly enlarged. The transition zone accounts for most of the bulk of the gland. The peripheral zone is compressed posterolaterally into a band of high signal. The fibromuscular septum is thinned and stretched anteriorly. However, the zonal anatomy of the gland is preserved, no masses are present in the peripheral zone, and the mixed glandular and stromal elements of the transition zone are characteristic of a nodule of benign prostatic hypertrophy

T2-W sequences are crucial to the demonstration of zonal anatomy. TSE sequences function extremely well, although the degree of contrast between transition and peripheral zone is slightly reduced, compared with standard SE sequences. T2-W GRE sequences and STIR have been found to be less useful. T1-W sequences demonstrate good contrast between the prostate and surrounding periprostatic fat, but the zonal anatomy is obliterated by lack of contrast.

11.3.4.2 Benign Disease

Severe congenital anomalies, such as agenesis and hypoplasia, are rare and are usually associated with other congenital abnormalities of the genital or urinary tract. However, developmental cysts, such as utricular and Müllerian-duct cysts, may be seen. They return high signal on T2-W images and low signal on T1-W images. Benign prostatic hypertrophy results from enlargement of the transition zone. Signal characteristics may be variable on T2-WI, depending on the relative preponderance of glandular hyperplasia, compared with interstitial or stromal hyperplasia. Cystic ectasia, resulting from dilatation of glandular elements, shows up as small areas of high signal intensity. Areas of infarction may cause low signal intensity. The appearance of benign prostatic hypertrophy is usually characteristic (Fig. 11.14). Infiltration of the peripheral zone by benign prostatic hypertrophy has been described, but it is extremely rare, and for practical purposes, an abnormality visible on MR imaging in the peripheral zone is not benign prostatic hypertrophy.

11.3.4.3 Malignant Disease

Adenocarcinoma of the prostate accounts for over 95% of malignant prostatic tumors. It is frequently latent, and its clinical behavior depends on histological grade, disease stage, and tumor bulk. Of all prostate carcinomas, 70% arise in the peripheral zone, 10% in the central zone, and 20% in the transition zone. Tumors are frequently small or diffusely infiltrative. Benign prostatic hypertrophy is common enough that the diseases may coexist, and therefore, the typical appearance of benign prostatic hypertrophy does not exclude coexistent carcinoma.

Prostatic carcinoma typically shows a low signal, relative to the glandular tissue of the peripheral zone (Fig. 11.15). Rarely, these tumors are isointense or hyperintense, and they usually have mucinous elements. There is some overlap between the appearance of prostatic carcinoma and chronic inflammatory conditions of the prostate, e.g., chronic granulomatous prostatitis, and the diagnosis must always be confirmed by biopsy. Patients may be referred for MRI following biopsy. Ideally, 6 weeks should be allowed for artifacts to resolve, but this is often impractical, and biopsy artifacts may cause confusion (Fig. 11.16). Once the diagnosis is confirmed, MRI is the most accurate method of staging prostate cancer. Staging accuracy reported in the literature exceeds that of transrectal ultrasound and computed tomography (CT), and nodal staging can be accomplished at the same investigation. The TNM system is used for staging prostatic carcinoma (Table 11.14). This is similar to the American Joint Committee on Cancer Staging system, but differs mark-

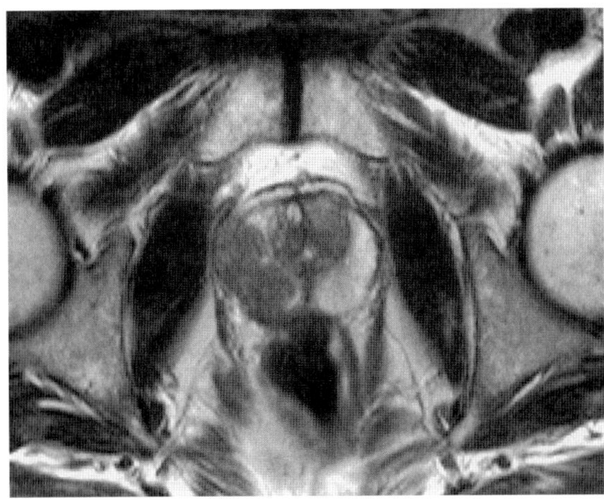

Fig. 11.15. Carcinoma of the prostate (T2-W TSE axial images using small field-of-view).There are nodules of low signal in the peripheral zone on the right. There is also a nodule of low signal in the transition zone anteriorly on the left. The transition zone is not enlarged but is surrounded by tumor tissue. The peripheral zone on the left is normal. Although this is not a large tumor, there is evidence of bulging of the prostatic capsule to the right, and some abnormal signal projects into the periprostatic fat. These signs correlate closely with the presence of extracapsular tumor spread. Locally advanced disease discourages attempts at radical prostatectomy, and this patient went on to radiation therapy

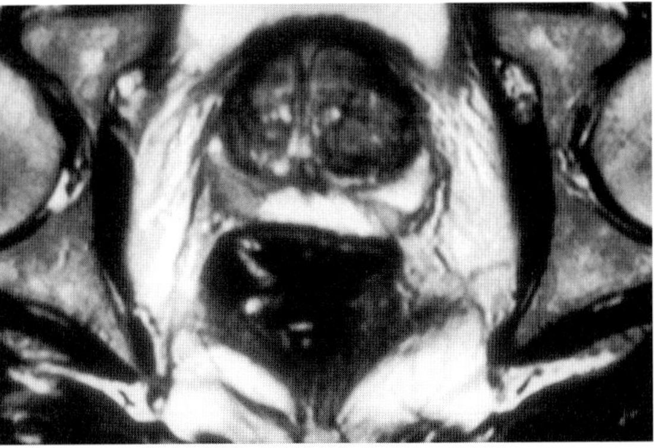

Fig. 11.16. Biopsy artifacts in prostate (T2-W TSE, axial plane). A nodule of benign prostatic hypertrophy is present. Two weeks previously, TRUS-guided cores from the transition zone had revealed adenocarcinoma of the prostate. Wedge-shaped low-signal areas are present in the peripheral zone. These are typical of biopsy artifacts and do not necessarily imply the presence of tumor. There is no evidence of extracapsular spread of tumor, and indeed the areas of carcinoma diagnosed histologically are difficult to identify on MRI with any confidence

Table 11.14. TNM staging classification of prostate cancer

TX	Primary tumor cannot be assessed
T0	No evidence of primary tumor
T1	Clinically unapparent tumor not palpable or visible by imaging
T1a	Tumor incidental histological finding in 5% or less of tissue resected
T1b	Tumor incidental histological finding in more than 5% of tissue resected
T1c	Tumor identified by needle biopsy (e.g., because of elevated PSA)
T2	Tumor confined within the prostate
T2a	Tumor involves one lobe
T2b	Tumor involves both lobes
T3	Tumor extends through the prostatic capsule
T3a	Extracapsular extension (unilateral or bilateral)
T3b	Tumor invades semional vesicle(s)
T4	Tumor is fixed or invades adjacent structures other than seminal vesicles: bladder neck, external sphincter, rectum, levator muscle, and/or pelvic wall

edly from the American Urological Association system. Tumor spread initially penetrates the capsule, and the first route of spread is frequently to the neurovascular bundles or seminal vesicles. Locally advanced disease (Fig. 11.17) is common at presentation, although if routine screening of asymptomatic men becomes prevalent, early-stage disease may be picked up. The tell-tale signs of extracapsular spread are the bulging of the prostatic outline (Fig. 11.15) and 'beaks' pointing out toward the neurovascular bundle. These signs correlate well with the discovery of extracapsular spread in pathological specimens following radical prostatectomy. In general, the unequivocal detection of an extracapsular tumor mass is considered a contraindication to radical prostatectomy. Infiltration of the seminal vesicles (Fig. 11.18) and extracapsular spread near the apex of the gland can be difficult to diagnose, and for this reason, coronal images may be used to supplement the routine axial images. In some centers, sagittal images are recommended for evaluation of the spread to the seminal vesicles.

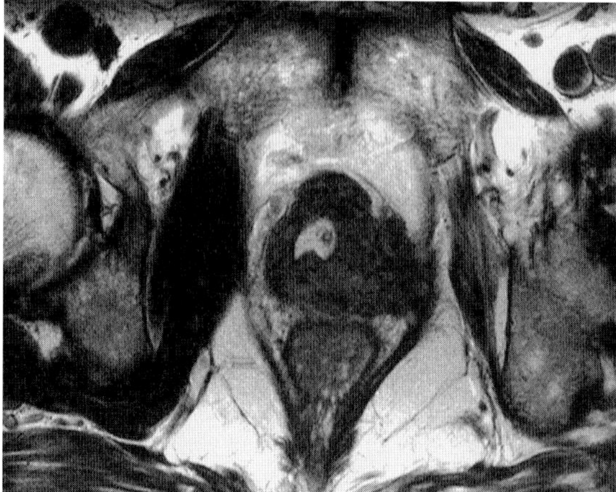

Fig. 11.17. Carcinoma of the prostate (T2-W SE, axial plane). This patient presented to us with locally advanced carcinoma of the prostate following transurethral resection. The transurethral resection of prostate (TURP) defect is seen centrally as an area of high signal. The zonal anatomy of the prostate is completely unrecognizable, as it has been obliterated by very extensive tumor. Extracapsular spread is penetrating the muscles of the pelvic sling to the left. Local disease stage is T4b. Unfortunately, a large percentage of patients present with this type of disease

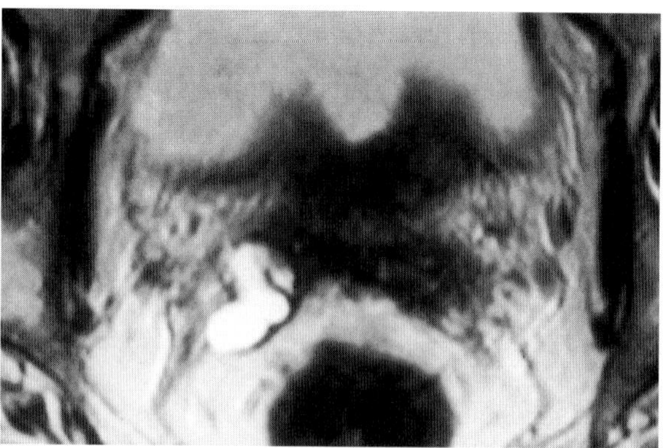

Fig. 11.18. Prostatic carcinoma with seminal vesicle invasion (T2-W TSE, axial plane). Low-signal tumor extends from the base of the gland through the central zone into the seminal vesicles. The right seminal vesicle is seen to contain high-signal fluid. The leaf-like anatomy of the seminal vesicle is well demonstrated on the *right*, whereas on the *left* it is replaced by low signal, irregular tumor. The diagnosis of seminal vesicle invasion is frequently more difficult than on this occasion, particularly at the insertion of the vasa deferentia and in the presence of nodules of benign prostatic hypertrophy extending cranially

Endorectal coil imaging (Fig. 11.19) in the evaluation of the disease stage is controversial. Some authors have reported that the staging accuracy is improved by the use of endorectal coils, while others have reported quite the opposite. There is no doubt that some artifacts are generated, particularly near the high field signal, which may obscure subtle signs of extracapsular spread toward the neurovascular bundle. Good quality pelvic phased-array coil images obtained on a high field system can be excellent, and endorectal coils can now be electronically integrated. The use of the endorectal coil is time-consuming; however, patient tolerance is

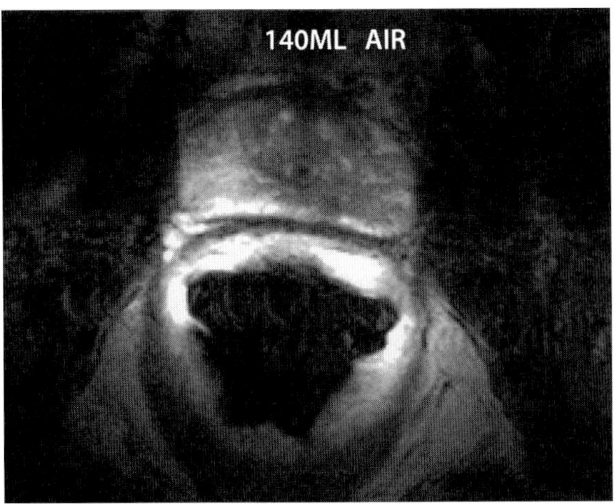

Fig. 11.19. Carcinoma of the prostate, endorectal coil imaging (T2-W TSE, axial plane. Coil inflated with 140 ml air). Diffuse low signal is infiltrating the transition zone and peripheral zone on the left. The zonal anatomy of the prostate is recognizable. There is no bulging or penetration of the capsule. Local disease stage is T2, and the patient is a suitable candidate for radical prostatectomy

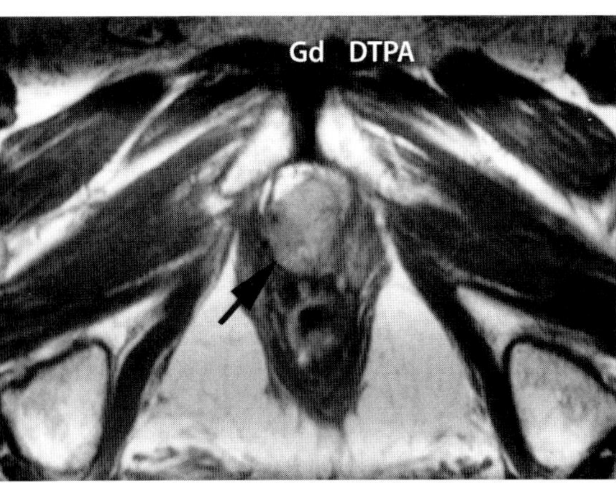

Fig. 11.20. Recurrent prostatic carcinoma (T1-W TSE, following gadolinium administration). Following radical prostatectomy, the area of the prostatic bed immediately posterior to the pubic symphysis should return low signal on all pulse sequences as a result of mature fibrosis following surgery. On this occasion, there is a nodule of enhancing tissue as a result of recurrent prostatic carcinoma (*arrow*). Early recurrence may not be detectable on MRI, and in the presence of a rising PSA following prostatectomy, blind or ultrasound-guided biopsy of the surgical site is frequently necessary to confirm the diagnosis

surprisingly good, although this depends on age, attitude, and educational background. Currently, a consensus on its clinical utility has not been reached.

Gadolinium enhancement is not used routinely in our center for prostate imaging. However, it is frequently helpful in confirming disease spread to the seminal vesicles. Prostatic carcinoma enhances early and to a greater extent than the surrounding normal gland. A dynamic run using fast acquisitions of sequential T1-W images over 2–3 min following bolus injection of gadolinium may clarify the extent of tumor spread. There is considerable research interest in the field of tumor vascularity and extracellular leakage of contrast in prostate cancer, but its clinical relevance has not yet been established.

MRI following hormonal or radiation therapy for prostate cancer usually demonstrates a reduction in size and loss of contrast within the gland. Following radical prostatectomy, recurrence can be difficult to detect. The postsurgical prostatic bed returns low signal, and a local recurrence produces an enhancing mass (Fig. 11.20). Most local recurrences following surgery need TRUS-guided biopsy confirmation.

11.3.5 Anorectal Region

11.3.5.1 Anatomy

The rectum is an extraperitoneal structure, although the anterior part of the lateral surface of the rectum is covered by peritoneum, which is reflected anteriorly. Above the rectosigmoid junction, the sigmoid colon becomes intraperitoneal. The rectum consists of four layers: the mucosa, submucosa, muscularis, and adventitia. The muscularis consists of an inner-circular and outer-longitudinal layer. Inferiorly, the rectum traverses the levator ani. The circular layer of muscle continues into the anal canal. The longitudinal muscle layer is joined by fibers from the levator ani to form the conjoined muscle. Outside this, the powerful anal sphincter consists of deep, superficial, and subcutaneous layers. Using body-coil images, the individual layers and components of the sphincter cannot be identified. However, recently developed endoanal coil imaging can clearly identify the individual muscles of the anal-sphincter complex.

11.3.5.2
Benign Conditions

Congenital anomalies, such as anorectal atresia, can be demonstrated by MRI. Imaging in multiple planes can be extremely helpful in demonstrating the presence or absence of fibrous bands and residual muscle running through to the perineum, which may be helpful in planning reconstructive techniques.

MRI is established as the investigation of choice in imaging of perianal fistulae. MRI is able to demonstrate the anatomy of the anorectal canal, the ischioanal and ischiorectal fossae, and the structures on either side of the pelvic floor in multiple directly imaged planes; in addition, MR imaging can contrast pus and granulation tissue with normal structures. Experience suggests the use of T1-W SE/TSE sequences for anatomical detail and STIR images for contrasting pathology against normal tissue. The literature confirms that MRI is a more accurate method of assessment of complex perianal fistulae than examination under anesthetic, even by experienced surgeons.

Fecal incontinence may be investigated using endoanal MR imaging, and atrophy of muscles may be seen following trauma (usually obstetric or postoperative).

11.3.5.3
Malignant Disease of the Anorectal Region

Colorectal carcinoma is common and increasing in frequency in the developed world. Rectal adenocarcinoma can be regarded as a separate pathological entity when considering large-bowel tumors, because of the location of these tumors within the bony pelvis, which renders adequate removal of the primary tumor technically difficult. One of the major problems following rectal cancer surgery is local recurrence, which occurs in up to 40% of patients. Clinical results following treatment for such recurrences are uniformly poor. In recent years, there have been major developments that promise to improve disappointing survival figures. These are focused on reducing the incidence of local recurrence. Many centers now use preoperative chemotherapy and radiotherapy to downstage local tumor when necessary. This is followed by total mesorectal excision surgery (TME). Standardized pathology assessment of rectal cancer specimens should now include scrutiny of the circumferential resection margin. Initial staging of rectal cancer has become much more important with the increasing sophistication of the therapeutic approach, and staging with imaging should form an integral part of the presurgical planning.

Widespread acceptance of TME surgery as the gold standard operative procedure for patients promises to reduce local recurrence. The technique was first described by Heald and Ryall in 1986 and is associated with a local recurrence rate of 6%. The principles behind the surgical approach include total removal of the rectum and its draining lymph nodes en bloc, anal sphincter preservation, and autonomic nerve preservation. TME surgery involves division of the peritoneum at the level of the inferior mesenteric artery, and a posterior dissection takes place that follows the visceral peritoneum over the surface of the mesorectum. Inferiorly, the plane between the mesorectal fascia and presacral fascia is developed down to the levator ani. The dissection plane is then developed laterally between the mesorectal fascia and the hypogastric nerves, which lie just lateral to the mesorectal fascia. Preservation of the neural plexus is necessary to maintain sexual and bladder function. The tumor, rectum, and mesorectum are removed as a single package. A breach of the mesorectum and tears of the fascia may result in incomplete removal of the tumor and mesorectum. As with all surgical procedures, suitable patient selection improves the success rate. Accurate preoperative staging is integral to patient selection, and certain issues must be addressed. The tumor should be clear of adjacent structures, namely prostate, seminal vesicles, bladder, and pelvic sidewalls. The tumor should also be clear of the mesorectal fascia, which is well demonstrated by MR imaging (Fig. 11.21). Tumor extending to the mesorectal fascia or breaching the fascia will result in cutting through the tumor during TME surgery. A further issue is to establish whether the tumor is invading through the levator ani or extending into the anal sphincter complex. Sphincter preservation will not be feasible in these patients. Patients in whom the tumor is close to the sphincter complex may require a technically difficult low stapled anastomosis. Tumor deposits elsewhere in the pelvis, for example lateral to the mesorectal fascia, should also be identified at staging MRI. Failure to resolve these important issues preoperatively may result in unnecessary 'open and close' laparotomies. Accurate staging will allow a rational choice of treatment which may involve chemoradiation to downstage the tumor.

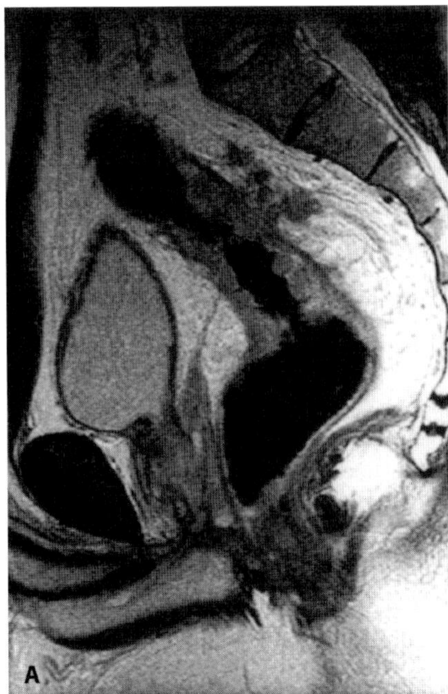

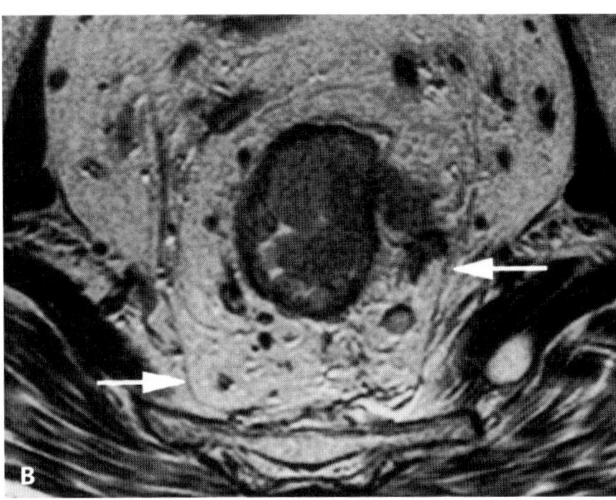

Fig. 11.21A,B. Carcinoma of the rectum. **A** T2-W TSE, sagittal plane. Extensive, irregular mural thickening is present in the upper third of the rectum extending into the lower sigmoid. There is transmural spread anteriorly and posteriorly. **B** T2-W TSE, high-resolution, fine-cut technique. The plane of orientation of the scan cuts perpendicularly through the tumor demonstrated in A, and is therefore paraxial rather than true axial. The tumor is demonstrated penetrating the wall to the left. The mesorectal fascia is seen as a fine layer of low-signal tissue (*arrows*) which surrounds the rectum. This is the fascial plane which is dissected by the surgeon at TME surgery. On this occasion, an irregular nodule is present close to the mesorectum, and the patient may benefit from downstaging by chemotherapy and radiotherapy prior to surgery. Well-circumscribed nodules within the mesorectum sometimes represent reactive lymph nodes, but irregular extramural masses should be interpreted as tumor deposits. The caudal limit of the tumor is seen to be clear of the anal sphincter

Thin-slice, high-resolution MRI has recently been described by Brown et al. (see Table 11.9). Using this scanning technique with a surface pelvic phased-array coil, an in-plane resolution can be achieved similar to that obtained with an endorectal coil. One of the advantages of the technique is the ability to image all patients, even those with stenosing lesions which prevent insertion of an endorectal coil. The layers of the rectal wall can frequently be depicted. The outer muscle layer has an irregular corrugated appearance, and there may be interruptions in this layer where vessels penetrate the rectal wall. The perirectal fat returns high signal on the T2-weighted sequence, surrounding the muscularis propria. The mesorectal fascia is seen as a fine low-signal layer enveloping the perirectal fat and rectum; it is this layer that defines the surgical excision plane for TME surgery (Fig. 11.21). Sagittal images identify the peritoneal reflection which lies on the surface of the bladder and then attaches to the anterior aspect of the rectal wall, and from this the relationship of the tumor to the peritoneal reflection may be determined. The sagittal plane imaging also demonstrates the proximity of the tumor to the anal sphincter (Fig. 11.22).

Tumor morphology is of paramount importance for image interpretation (Table 11.15). The returned signal may be mixed. It is important to stress that MR diagnosis of T3 (locally advanced) lesions is based on the presence of a tumor mass extending into the perirectal fat with a broad-based configuration. The mass should be in continuity with an intramural tumor. Irregularity and disruption of the outer longitudinal muscle do not necessarily signify locally advanced tumor. Masses with extensive pushing margins are frequently associated with extensive nodal involvement and vascular invasion. The MR features of mucinous tumors are distinctive, as they may have high signal intensity on the T2-

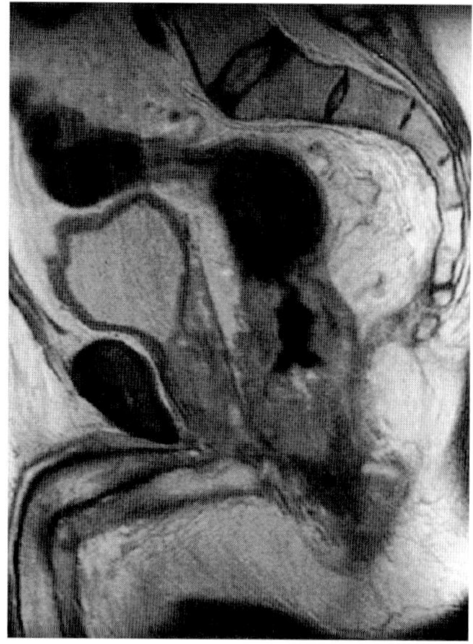

Fig. 11.22. Carcinoma of the rectum (T2-W TSE, sagittal plane). These images demonstrate a bulky circumferential tumor of the low rectum. In contrast to Fig. 11.21A, there is no normal mucosa between the tumor and the anal sphincter which appears to be involved. It is unlikely that reanastomosis will be possible at surgery

Table 11.15. MRI reporting criteria for T and N staging of rectal carcinoma

T1 lesion	A low-signal mass demonstrated within the bright mucosal/submucosal layer but with preservation of the muscularis propria layer
T2 lesion	A low-signal mass demonstrated within the submucosal layer causing loss of the interface between the submucosa and muscularis propria
T3 lesion	Tumor is of higher signal intensity than muscle. Breach of the outer rectal longitudinal muscle layer with broad based/nodular extension of the tumor signal into the perirectal fat
T4 lesion	Extension of the tumor signal intensity into adjacent structures or extension through peritoneal reflection in high anterior rectal tumors
Nodal involvement	Presence of involved perirectal lymph nodes; tumor signal/irregular contour

weighted sequence as opposed to the intermediate signal seen with most rectal tumors. Spiculation has often been defined as a manifestation of extramural spread, particularly on CT. However, pathological specimens frequently show intense desmoplastic response and fibrosis, and spiculation does not always indicate tumor extension.

Lymph nodes and tumor nodules are frequently identified within the mesorectum (Fig. 11.21). However, pathological examination reveals that some enlarged nodes contain only reactive hyperplasia. Lymph nodes within the mesorectum are usually classified as normal if they have smooth, sharply demarcated borders, and irregular, small masses are usually classified as malignant. However, if they are within the mesorectal sleeve, they should be removed. None of the current staging investigations is able to detect microscopic or partial nodal involvement by tumor, but micrometastases within the mesorectum do not appear to be prognostically significant.

MRI is a more adaptable staging procedure than endoluminal ultrasound, and the usefulness of CT in the staging of rectal carcinoma has been disappointing. Digital rectal examination remains widely used as a preoperative assessment, relying on the ability of the examining finger to detect fixity of a low rectal tumor; the accuracy of this approach is limited.

Anal carcinoma can be imaged using a technique which relies more on axial and coronal imaging planes (Fig. 11.23). Clinical examination of anal carcinoma is more reliable than for rectal carcinoma, and the treatment of choice is usually radiotherapy. The precise definition of the tumor suitable for surgery is still appropriate when planning radiation fields, but currently the role of MR imaging in planning the treatment of anal carcinoma is developing.

Following radiation to the anorectal region or other pelvic organs, abnormality of signal and enhancement characteristics can persist for up to 2 years before the typical appearance of fibrosis appears. Unfortunately, the time course of these changes is unpredictable, and therefore considerable caution needs to be exercised in interpreting MR images of the anorectal region following radiation therapy, usually in the clinical context of suspected recurrence.

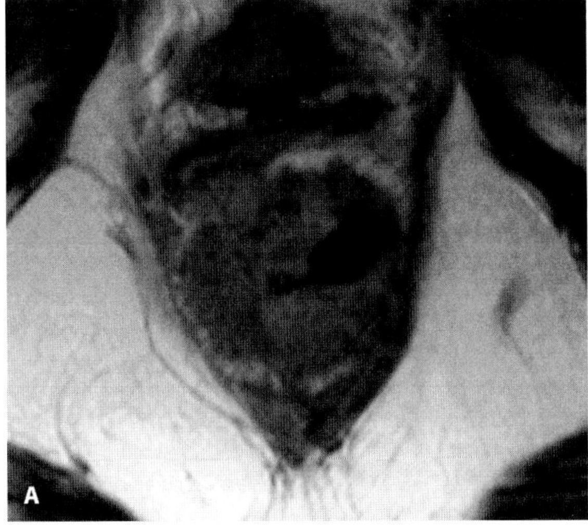

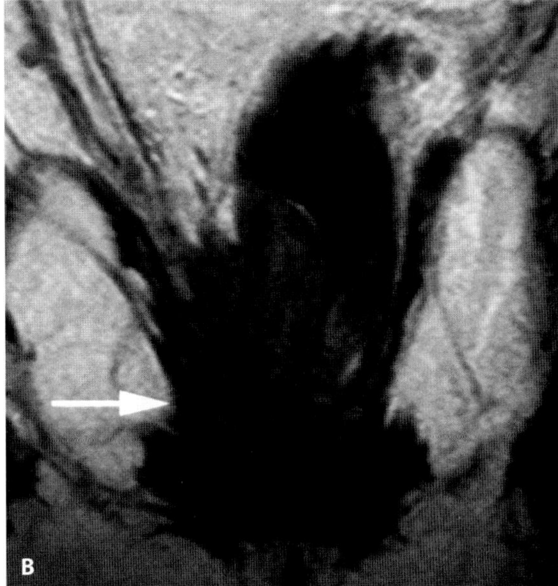

Fig. 11.23A,B. Carcinoma of the anus. **A** T2-W TSE, axial plane. The anatomy of the anal sphincter is disrupted by a circumferential mass which is predominantly to the right of the midline. The levator ani on the left is largely normal, but on the right has been infiltrated by tumor. The posterior wall of the vagina, seen anteriorly, is also involved. **B** T2-W TSE, coronal plane. These confirm a bulky tumor mass involving almost the entire length of the anal sphincter, and extending into the lower rectum. Tumor crosses the lower part of the levator ani muscle (*arrow*)

11.3.6 Male External Genitalia

11.3.6.1 Penis and Scrotum

The anatomy of the male external genitalia is considered by some to be at its most beautiful when demonstrated by MR imaging using T2-W SE/TSE sequences. Following careful positioning to orientate the penis in a craniocaudal direction, thin sagittal slices (3 mm) should be obtained, supplemented by images perpendicular to the long axis of the penile shaft.

The anterior urethra runs through the corpus spongiosum, which is enveloped by a thin layer of tunica albuginea. These structures comprise the ventral compartment of the penis. The dorsal compartment contains the paired corpora cavernosa. The two compartments are separated by Buck's fascia, which also surrounds both compartments and their tunica albuginea. The posterior portion of the corpus spongiosum expands to form the bulb, and the anterior part expands to form the glans.

The testes lie within the scrotum, a sac comprised of internal cremasteric and external fascial layers, the dartos muscle, and skin. The testes are encased by the tunica albuginea, which invaginates the testis posteriorly to form the mediastinum. The seminiferous tubules, coiled within each testis, converge to form the rete testis and the efferent ductules. These ductules form the epididymis, which lies posterior to the testis. The tail of the epididymis leads into the vas deferens. The supplying vessels pass into the mediastinum. When MR imaging is performed, the scrotal contents should be supported by a towel placed between the thighs. Axial and coronal T2-W and T1-W SE/TSE sequences will demonstrate the anatomy. Under normal circumstances, the glandular tissue of the testis returns high signal on T2-W sequences and intermediate to low signal on T1-W sequences. Following gadolinium enhancement, the epididymis will be enhanced to a greater extent than the normal testis.

11.3.6.2 Benign Conditions

Congenital abnormalities of the penis are usually clinically apparent. The characteristic signal returned by the testis makes MR a useful technique for hunting the testis in cases of cryptorchidism. Fat-suppression techniques such as STIR can be very helpful in this clinical setting. Most benign conditions of the penis can be evaluated clinically. The rare but fascinating Peyronie's disease (induratio penis plastica) is caused by focal inflammation of the tunica albuginea and corpora cavernosa. The condition is painful and eventually leads to fibrosis, which, if unilateral, leads to deviated erections and, if bilateral, leads to shortening of the penis. On T2-W images, low-signal-intensity fibrotic plaques are visualized within the corpora cavernosa. These plaques will be enhanced following gadolinium, particularly where there is an element of active inflammation.

A number of prostheses are available for the treatment of impotence. Some of these contain silicone and some are inflated with fluid. Care should be taken to ensure that no metallic prosthetic structures are present.

Hydrocele, varicocele, torsion, and epididymo-orchitis may all be identified, but clinical examination and ultrasound are sufficient for establishing the diagnosis in the vast majority of cases.

11.3.6.3 Malignant Conditions

MR imaging is extremely useful in the evaluation of tumors of the penile urethra. The majority of penile urethral carcinomas are squamous (approximately 80%), with transitional-cell carcinomas and adenocarcinomas accounting for the rest. Squamous-cell carcinomas are, to some extent, radiosensitive, and the extent of disease can be well demonstrated by MR imaging (Fig. 11.24). Tumor masses are usually of a signal intensity slightly lower than the adjacent corpus spongiosum and corpora cavernosa on T2-WI. T1-WI following gadolinium application is useful. Tumors show moderate enhancement, and there is often a flare of adjacent enhancement in the corpus spongiosum due to increased vascularity and extracellular diffusion locally. Extension of prostatic carcinoma down the urethra may also be demonstrated.

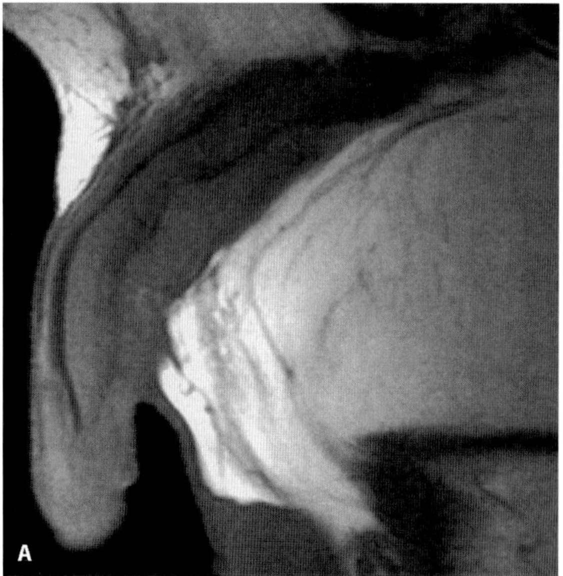

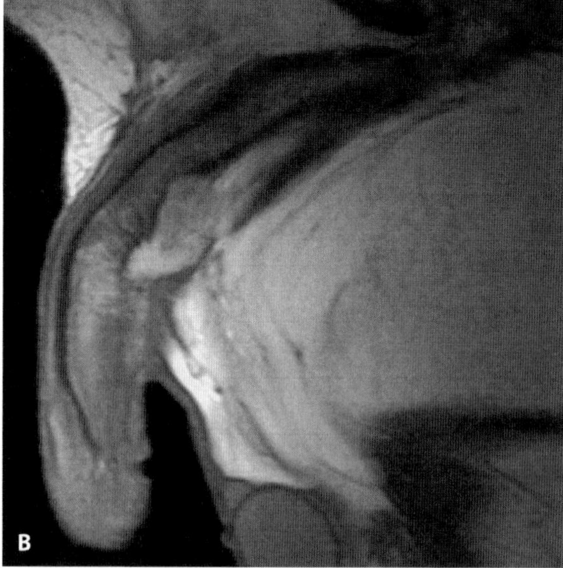

Fig. 11.24A,B. Carcinoma of the penile urethra. **A** T1-W SE sagittal images. The low signal bands of Buck's fascia separate the dorsal and ventral compartments of the penis. There is some upward displacement of the posterior part of the intercavernous septum of Buck's fascia. **B** Following gadolinium enhancement, at the site of upward displacement, there is a clear nodular tumor mass. Surrounding this, in the corpus spongiosum, there is intense enhancement, which is a result of local inflammation and capillary leakage into the extracellular space, and this enhancement does not represent tumor spread

Squamous-cell carcinoma of the glans can usually be evaluated clinically, but the depth of infiltration can be assessed using MRI.

Malignant tumors of the testes are well demonstrated by MR imaging. When small, they return a slightly lower signal than normal testes on T2-W images. However, frequently they are large, and teratoma may be hemorrhagic. Often, little normal testicular anatomy can be identified. Once again, most cases are evaluated clinically and, if necessary, with ultrasound.

11.3.7 Female External Genitalia

The lower third of the vagina and the vulva are demonstrable on MR imaging using axial images initially, and sagittal or coronal images according to the clinical problem. Most pathology of the female external genitalia is demonstrable by clinical examination, but the extent of some vaginal tumors can be demonstrated in detail by MR imaging. Staging of vulval carcinoma is of importance, but currently, clinical examination and ultrasound are used in most instances.

11.4 Pediatric Pelvic MR Imaging

The general principles described above can be extrapolated to the pediatric population. Using general anesthetic or sedation with suitable monitoring equipment, patients of all ages can be imaged. Complex congenital anomalies of the urogenital tract can be assessed using MRI. In addition, pelvic rhabdomyosarcoma is the third most common solid tumor of childhood, and MRI is an extremely useful imaging technique to assess the organ of origin, usually the vagina in girls and the prostate in boys (although it may be difficult to identify the exact organ of origin, owing to the extreme bulk of some of these tumors). MRI is also excellent for demonstrating the response to chemotherapy and the site of residual mass lesions prior to surgical clearance of the tumor bed. Other tumors that may occur in the pelvis include neuroblastoma, sacrococcygeal teratoma, and recurrent Wilm's tumor, which may sometimes be found in the pouch of Douglas (see also Chapter 16).

Acknowledgements. We are very grateful to Janet Macdonald and Maureen Watts for their assistance in the preparation of this text. Thanks are also due to our colleagues, Professor Janet Husband, Dr. Aslam Sohaib, and Dr. Gina Brown, for some of the images used. Figure 11.9 is reproduced by kind permission of Dr. Julie Olliff and the Editor of the BJR.

Further Reading

Allen KS, Kressel HY, Arger PH, Pollack HM (1989) Age-related changes of the prostate. Am J Roentgenol 152:77–81

Appleton C, Krn J, Abeler VM (1991) Cancer of the endometrium: value of MR imaging in determining depth of invasion into the myometrium. Am J Roentgenol 157:1221–1223

Ascher SM, Arnold LL, Patt RH et al (1994) Adenomyosis: prospective comparison of MR imaging and transvaginal sonography. Radiology 190:803–806

Balfe D, Semin M (1998) Colorectal cancer. In: Husband JE, Reznek RH (eds) Imaging in oncology. ISIS Medical Media, Oxford, pp 129–150

Barentsz JO, Ruijs SHJ, Strijk SP (1993) The role of MR imaging in carcinoma of the urinary bladder. Am J Roentgenol 160: 937–947

Barker PG, Lunniss PJ, Armstrong P et al (1994) Magnetic resonance imaging of fistula-in-ano: technique, interpretation and accuracy. Clin Radiol 49:7–13

Brown G, MacVicar D, Ayton V, Husband J (1995) The role of intravenous contrast enhancement in magnetic resonance imaging of prostatic carcinoma. Clin Radiol 50:601–606

Brown G, Richards C, Dallimore NS et al (1999) Rectal carcinoma: thin section MR imaging for staging in 28 patients. Radiology 211:215–222

Chang YCF, Hricak H, Thurnher S, Lacey C (1988) Vagina: evaluation with MR imaging, part II. Neoplasms. Radiology 169: 175–179

deSouza NM, Scoones D, Krausz T, Gilderdale DJ, Soutter WP (1996) High-resolution MR imaging of stage I cervical neoplasia with a dedicated transvaginal coil: MR features and correlation of imaging and pathologic findings. Am J Roentgenol 166:553–559

Hall TB, MacVicar AD (2001) Imaging bladder cancer. Imaging 13:1–10

Halligan S (1998) Imaging fistula-in-ano. Clin Radiol 53:85–95

Halligan S, Healy JC, Bartram CI (1998) Magnetic resonance imaging of fistula-in-ano: STIR or SPIR? Br J Radiol 71:141–145

Hawnaur J Uterine and cervical tumours. In: Husband JE, Reznek RH (eds) Imaging in oncology. ISIS Medical Media, Oxford, pp 309–328

Heald RJ, Ryall RD (1986) Recurrence and survival after total mesorectal excision for rectal cancer. Lancet 1:1479–1482

Hricak H, Chang YCF, Thurnher S (1988a) Vagina: evaluation with MR imaging, part I. Normal anatomy and congenital anomalies. Radiology 169:169–174

Hricak H, Lacey CG, Sandles LG, Chang YC, Winkler ML, Stern JL (1988b) Invasive cervical carcinoma: comparison of MR imaging and surgical findings. Radiology 166:623–631

Hricak H, Carrington BM (eds) (1991) MRI of the pelvis.

Husband JE (1998) Bladder cancer. In: Husband JE, Reznek RH (eds) Imaging in oncology. ISIS Medical Media, Oxford, pp 215–238

Jager G, Barentsz J (1998) Prostate cancer. In: Husband JE, Reznek RH (eds) Imaging in oncology. ISIS Medical Media, Oxford, pp 239–257

MacVicar D, Husband J (1993) Imaging in the management of prostatic cancer. Imaging 5:29–37

McDermott VG, Meakem TJ III, Stolpen AH, Schnall MD (1995) Prostatic and periprostatic cysts: findings on MR imaging. Am J Roentgenol 164:123–127

Padhani AR, MacVicar AD, Gapinski CJ, Dearnaley DP, Parker GJM, Suckling J, Leach MO, Husband JE (2001) Effects of androgen deprivation on prostatic morphology and vascular permeability evaluated with MR imaging. Radiology 218: 365–374

Quinn S, Franzini D, Demlow T, Rosencrantz D, Kim J, Hanna RA, Szumowski J (1994) MR imaging of prostate cancer with an endorectal surface coil technique: correlation with whole mount-specimens. Radiology 190:323–327

Reinhold C, McCarthy S, Bret PM et al (1996) Diffuse adenomyosis: comparison of endovaginal US and MR imaging with histopathologic correlation. Radiology 199:151–158

Scoutt LM, McCauley TR, Flynn SD, Luthringer DJ, McCarthy SM (1993) Zonal anatomy of the cervix: correlation of MR imaging and histologic examination of hysterectomy specimens. Radiology 186:159–162

Scoutt LM, McCarthy SM, Flynn SD et al (1995) Clinical stage I endometrial carcinoma: pitfalls in preoperative assessment with MR imaging. Radiology 194:567–572

Semelka RC, Ascher SM, Reinhold C (eds) (1997) MRI of the abdomen and pelvis. A text atlas. Wiley-Liss, New York

Sohaib S, Reznek R, Husband JE Ovarian cancer. In: Husband JE, Reznek RH (eds) Imaging in oncology. ISIS Medical Media, Oxford, pp 277–308

Spencer JA, Ward J, Ambrose NS (1998) Dynamic contrast-enhanced MR imaging of perianal fistulae. Clin Radiol 53: 96–104

Subak LL, Hricak H, Powell CB, Azizi L, Stern JL (1995) Cervical carcinoma: computed tomography and magnetic resonance imaging for preoperative staging. Obstet Gynecol 86:43–50

Tempany CM (1996) MR staging of prostate cancer: How we can improve our accuracy with decision aids and optimal techniques. In MRI Clin North Am 4(3):519–532

Tempany CMC, Fielding JR (1996) Female pelvis. In: Edelman RR, Hesselink JR, Zlatkin MB (eds) Clinical magnetic resonance imaging. Saunders, Philadelphia, pp 1432–1465

Umaria N, Olliff JF (2001) Imaging features of pelvic endometriosis. Br J Radiol 74:556–562

Heart

12

M. G. Lentschig

Contents

12.1 Patient Preparation, Positioning, and Coil Selection

12.1.1 Introduction

In the evaluation and investigation of heart disease, reaching a specific diagnosis may require the use of various noninvasive and invasive diagnostic tests. Often, several of these diagnostic techniques are utilized, and a final diagnosis is achieved by interpreting the combined results. Over the past 10 years, magnetic resonance (MR) imaging has been evolving as a method for investigating the heart. It is a noninvasive or minimally invasive method, with high tissue-contrast resolution that provides excellent anatomical information in any imaging plane. In addition, it may provide temporal resolution high enough to evaluate cardiovascular dynamics.

Prior to the development of electrocardiogram (ECG) gating, MR imaging of the heart was of little value because of the disturbing motion artifacts caused by the complex contractile motion. The application of ECG gating to trigger the acquisition of pulse sequences helps suppress these motion artifacts and makes the technique different from MR imaging of other organs. Another advance in cardiac MR imaging was the development of breath-hold sequences to further minimize motion artifacts.

Today, electrocardiographically gated cardiac MR imaging is useful for evaluating congenital and acquired heart disease.

MR imaging is absolutely contraindicated in patients with an active pacemaker or other electrical stimulators, which are implanted. Mediastinal clips, coronary stents, and most cardiac prostheses stents may produce artifacts and may limit diagnostic sensitivity, but do not contraindicate the examination.

12.1.2 Preparation

Communication between the referring physician and the radiologist is essential, and before a cardiac MR examination is done, a specific clinical question has to be identified to tailor the study to the specific problem. This is essential, because the available pulse sequences provide different as well as overlapping information about the anatomical section being viewed; the choice of pulse sequence is determined by the question being asked. For most patients, there is also an important role for physician supervision of the cardiac MR examination. Diagnosis- or problem-specific examination protocols speed individual studies and enhance examinations by allowing for the selection of specific parameters for image acquisition, manipulation, and display.

Most patients know about MR but are unaware of its use in cardiac imaging. Therefore, the radiologist should explain the general nature of the examination to the patient (e.g., that the technique provides important morphological and functional information; it is a minimally or noninvasive technique; it requires no catheterization of the heart), indicate the duration of the examination (up to 1 h), and explain that it might be uncomfortable to lie still for this time, that some sequences need breath-holding for up to 20 s, and that there is a constant contact to the patient (via microphone and by monitoring their heartbeat). Some anxious patients need mild sedation, e.g., diazepam 5–10 mg, given by mouth or intravenously. It is very helpful if the patients void their bladders immediately before the examination.

In cardiac-triggered techniques, respiration induces changes in the heart rate. By performing these studies using a breath-hold technique, respiratory modulation is avoided, and more consistent cardiac synchronization can be assured. For these breath-hold sequences, the patient should be instructed carefully prior to initiating scanning; patient cooperation is required to guarantee high image quality. Normal end-expiration should be used for consistent breath-hold positions.

12.1.3 ECG Gating

The contraction of the heart muscle has devastating effects on the MR image quality. This major determining factor can be significantly reduced by different methods for coupling the data acquisition to the contraction and motion.

Using ECG gating, each successive phase-encoded line is acquired at the same part of the cardiac cycle. Multislice imaging is possible, although each slice is acquired at a different phase of the cardiac cycle. The ECG gating signal may be obtained by placing three monitoring electrodes on the anterior or posterior chest wall close to the position of the heart. We prefer to place the ECG leads on the anterior chest wall. The leads should pass directly over the patient's body without forming loops. The obtained ECG signal is useless for diagnostic electrocardiographic purposes; it may only be used to calculate the heart rate and discern arrhythmias.

During MR scanning, a temporally variable magnetic flux is generated mainly as a result of changes in the magnetic field that occur when imaging gradients are applied. The changes in the electromagnetic field are superimposed (as artifacts) on the ECG signal, which is observed outside of the magnetic field. In addition, magneto-hydrodynamic effects further degrade the ECG signal.

It is very important to assure good contact between the electrodes and the patient's skin. Therefore, disposable electrodes, which are coated with electrode jelly, are recommended. The patient's skin should be cleaned with alcohol or another cleansing agent.

In patients with severe ventricular ectopia, tachyarrhythmia, very low voltage ECGs (e.g., pericardial effusion), or after acute myocardial infarction, an adequate gating may not be obtained. In these patients, peripheral pulse gating may be helpful.

12.1.4 Coil Selection

In high-field MR systems, the body is the predominant source of noise. Careful selection of radiofrequency (RF) coils that are optimized for imaging specific anatomical structures allow the detector to be as near as possible to the region of interest and have, therefore, proven very beneficial for image quality. Today, there is no special cardiac surface coil available, although numerous suboptimal local coils have been used (e.g., a spine coil placed across the chest). We prefer the body phased-array coil, with its high image quality. Its signal-to-noise ratio, spatial resolution, and contrast resolution are excellent. These coils combine a number of individual elements that are positioned anterior and posterior to the patient and wrapped together. Each element receives a signal from only a small part of the body, and this results in a larger signal-to-noise ratio. Individual coil elements can be activated, and all activated elements are combined automatically to generate one image. Images acquired with a phased-array coil are not uniform in signal intensity, due to surface characteristics. Objects closer to the coil appear brighter than objects further away. The effect is more predominant in T1-weighted images (WI), given that fat is closest to the coil. A normalization filter can be incorporated to create a more uniform signal intensity distribution. Optimal results are achieved with the heart positioned in the center of the magnet (±10 cm).

Infants and small children may be examined from within a head-imaging coil. This has the advantage of allowing thinner slices and a smaller field-of-view for greater spatial resolution.

12.1.5 Image Plane Construction

Because the cardiac axes are not parallel to the body axes, a great advantage of MR imaging is the ability to select and image in any plane, parallel or orthogonal to the cardiac axes. Standard image plane acquisition allows for comparison of the MR images with information obtained using other cross-sectional techniques, such as echocardiography, and projection techniques, such as angiocardiography. The most commonly used cardiac axes are the short axis (two-chamber view) and long axis (four-chamber view). To obtain these axes, a series of low-resolution, ungated, gradient-echo (GRE) scout images (localizers) have to be acquired:

1. Coronal (one to three images), through the middle third of the chest to provide cranial and caudal landmarks (Fig. 12.1).
2. Axial (six images), planned in the coronal scout, through the heart (Fig. 12.2).
3. Oblique (six images), planned in the axial scout, parallel to the ventricular septum (Fig. 12.3).

In the parasagittal images obtained, the short and long axes of the heart can be planned, as shown in Fig. 12.4.

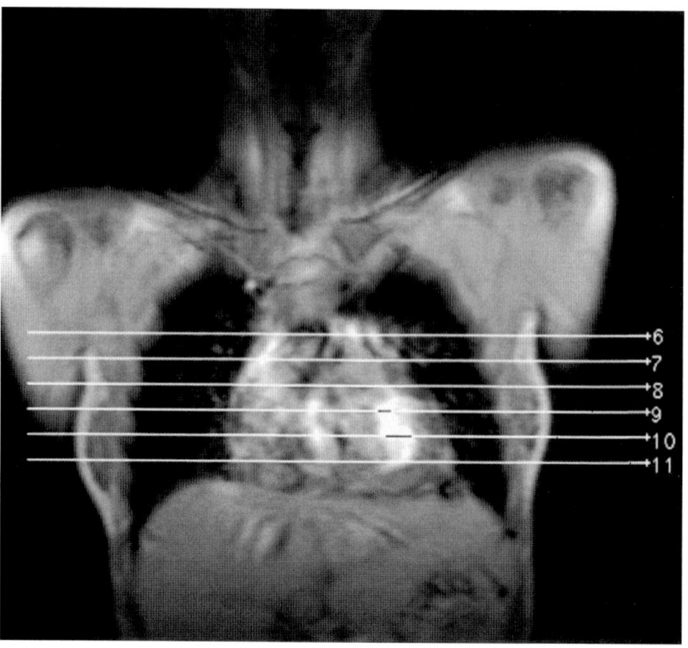

Fig. 12.1. Coronal scout [fast imaging into steady precession sequence (FISP 2D)] through the middle third of the chest to provide cranial and caudal landmarks

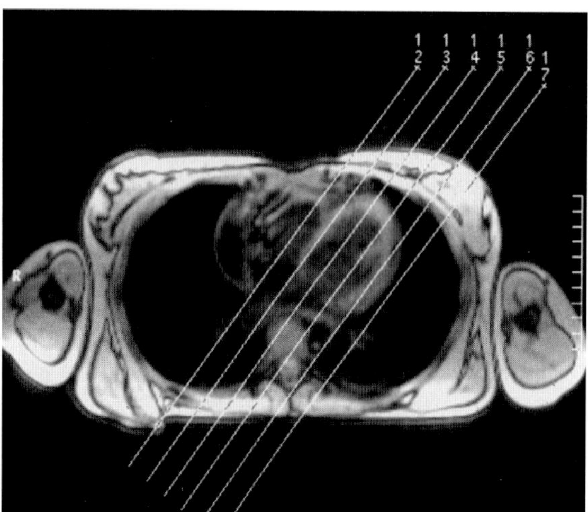

Fig. 12.2. Axial scout [turbo fast low-angle shot sequence (FLASH)] through the heart, planned in the coronal scout

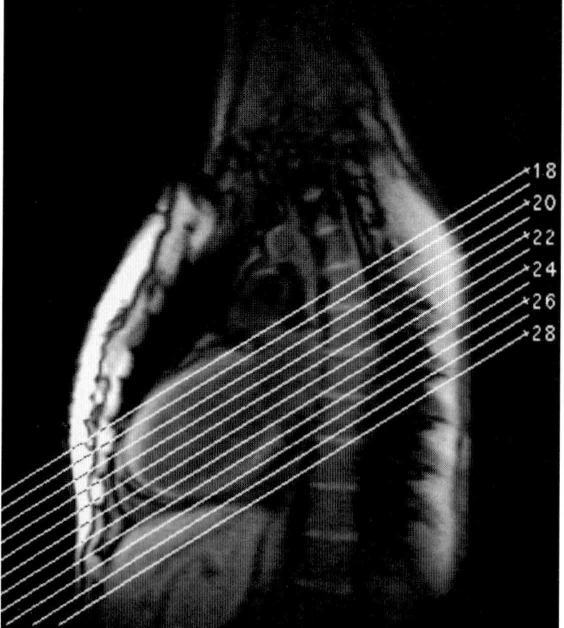

Fig. 12.3. Oblique scout (turbo FLASH) parallel to the ventricular septum, planned in the axial scout

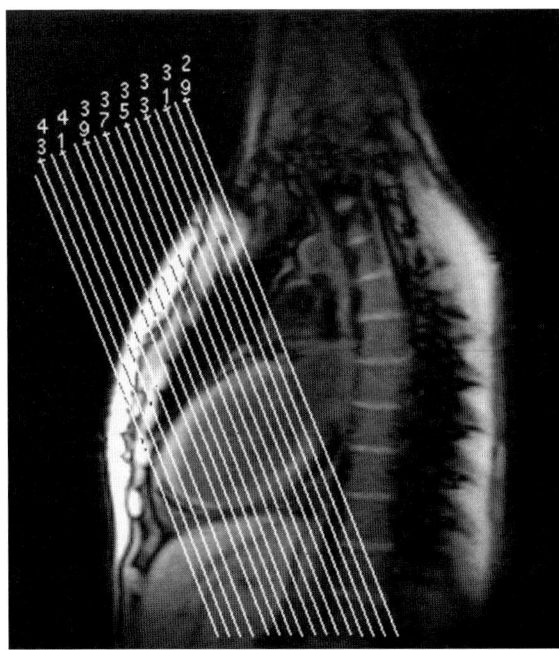

Fig. 12.4. Parasagittal images obtained (turbo FLASH). Short axis and long axis of the heart can be planned

12.2 Sequence Protocols

12.2.1 Localizer/Scout

The fast imaging into steady precession (FISP), two-dimensional (2D) sequence is a standard scout protocol used with non-breath-hold imaging techniques. Multiple acquisitions may be used to reduce respiratory and cardiac motion artifacts. The turbo fast low-angle shot sequence (FLASH) combines a dark-blood single-shot sequence which freezes respiratory motion. It is triggered on every second cardiac cycle to allow sufficient signal recovery between image acquisitions (Table 12.1).

12.2.2 Morphology

Spin-echo (SE) sequences are very sensitive to respiratory motion, particularly when used in combination with the body array coil. Increasing the number of acquisitions that are averaged together reduces motion artifacts at the cost of longer scan times. Turbo spin-echo (TSE) sequences reduce the scan time considerably, allowing for an increased number of acquisitions (to reduce respiratory motion artifacts).

The breath-hold turbo FLASH technique allows for the acquisition of bright-blood, high-resolution, 2D anatomical images. A trigger delay should be incorporated so that scanning occurs during a relatively quiet period of the cardiac cycle, mid- to late-diastole.

Dark-blood-prepared TSE is used with breath-hold TSE-sequences. T1-W breath-hold TSE shows a higher signal-to-noise ratio than T2-W TSE, but is not as sensitive to pathology that is associated with an increased water content.

Single-shot half-Fourier acquired single-shot TSE (HASTE) sequences with dark-blood preparation show no respiratory motion artifacts because of the short acquisition window. STIR techniques (short tau inversion time inversion recovery TSE) with dark-blood preparation have a lower signal-to-noise ratio than breath-hold T2-W TSE sequences, but are highly sensitive to edema and inflammation (Table 12.2).

Table 12.1. Short sequences used to construct the cardiac axes, which are not parallel to the body axes

Sequence	WI	Plane	No. of slices	TR (ms)	TE (ms)	Flip angle	TI (ms)	Echo train length	Slice thickness (mm)	Matrix	FOV	recFOV (%)	No. of acq.	Acq. time (min:s)
FISP2 D	T1	ax	6	90	7	40			8	128×256	450		1	>0:06
TFLA SH	T1	ax	6	1100	2.3	10			8	128×256	4000		1	>0:06

Abbreviations: *WI* weighting of images; *TR* repetition time; *TI* inversion time; *TE* echo time; *Matrix* phase × frequency matrix; *FOV* field of view (mm); *recFOV* % rectangular field of view, *Acq.* acquisition(s)

Table 12.2. Morphological imaging of the heart. The techniques proposed here are sensitive to pathologic changes in T1 and T2 relaxation times of the myocardium

Sequence	WI	Plane	No. of slices	TR (ms)	TE (ms)	Flip angle	TI (ms)	Echo train length	Slice thickness (mm)	Matrix	FOV	recFOV (%)	No. of acq.	Acq. time (min:s)
SE	T1	Long	19	600	14	90			6	128×256	350	75	1	>3:53
TSE	T1	Long	11	600	12	180		3	6	156×256	350	75	5	>2:39
FL2D[a]	T1	Long	1	167	6.2	30			6	154×256	280	100	1	>0:10
TSE[a]	T1	Short	1	700	32	160		9	6	126×256	350	75	1	>0:10
TSE[a]	T2	Short	1	800	57	160		15	6	120×256	350	75	1	>0:11
STIR[a]	T2	Short	1	800	57	160	170	15	8	120×256	350	75	1	>0:11
HASTE	T2	Short	21	800	43	150			6	128×256	350	75	1	>0:31
HASTEIRM	T2	Short	21	800	43	150	170		8	128×256	350	75	1	>0:31

[a] Breath-hold

Abbreviations: *WI* weighting of images; *TR* repetition time; *TI* inversion time; *TE* echo time; *Matrix* phase × frequency matrix; *FOV* field of view (mm); *recFOV* % rectangular field of view; *Acq.* acquisition(s)

12.2.3
Function

We prefer the breath-hold cine FLASH 2D sequence. One has to adjust the number of phases so that the product of the repetition time (TR) and number of phases is about 10% less than the duration of the cardiac cycle (R–R interval). The short axis orientation results in the best blood/myocardium contrast, whereas the long axis orientation is compromised because of spin saturation effects. The untriggered ultrafast FLASH 2D technique is fast enough to freeze cardiac and respiratory motion, at the cost of relatively low spatial and temporal resolution. It may be useful for rapid functional assessment in critically ill patients (Table 12.3).

Another means of visualization of myocardial motion is tagging (grid and stripe tagging). Myocardial tagging is a MR imaging method that uses a sequence of RF pulses to presaturate thin planes of the myocardium prior to the examination. These grid or stripe tags persist in the myocardium throughout the cardiac cycle and can be used to track the motion of the heart. If postprocessing software is available, it can be used to obtain accurate estimates of tag displacement for visualizing segmental dyskinesias or hypokinesias.

MR dobutamine stress testing has been employed for the evaluation of coronary artery disease by means

Table 12.3. Sequences are used for dynamic cine visualization of cardiac function with prospective or retrospective triggering. Another means for visualization of myocardial motion is tagging (grid and stripe tagging)

Sequence	WI	Plane	No. of slices	TR (ms)	TE (ms)	Flip angle	TI (ms)	Echo train length	Slice thickness (mm)	Matrix	FOV	recFOV (%)	No. of acq.	Acq. time (min:s)
FL2D[a]	T1	Short	2	40	4.8	30	–	–	8	128×256	320	75	3	>4:07
FL2D[b]	T1	Short	2	40	4.8	30	–	–	8	128×256	320	75	1	>3:26
FL2D[c]	T1	Short	5	30	4.8	30	–	–	8	132×256	320	75	3	>5:19
FL2D[d]	T1	Short	1	60	4.8	20	–	–	8	128×256	320	75	1	>0:19
FL2D[e]	T1	Short	1	2.4	1.2	8	–	–	10	50×256	320	75	60	>0:07

[a] Prospective triggering; [b] Retrospective gating; [c] Segmented sequential; [d] Breath hold; [e] Untriggered

Abbreviations: *WI* weighting of images; *TR* repetition time; *TI* inversion time; *TE* echo time; *Matrix* phase × frequency matrix; *FOV* field of view (mm); *recFOV* % rectangular field of view; *Acq.* acquisition(s)

of the detection of wall motion abnormalities under pharmacological stress. Dobutamine increases contractility, heart rate, and myocardial oxygen consumption. Drug administration is discontinued if wall motion abnormalities develop, if there is a new onset of symptoms, e.g., dyspnea or chest pain, or if the target heart rate has been reached (0.85×[220-age]).

12.2.4 Angiography

Two-dimensional techniques can be used to visualize the coronary arteries when using a breath-hold technique. Three-dimensional navigator techniques allow for visualization of the coronary arteries, with respiratory motion compensation. Contrast-enhanced 3D angiography techniques are used to evaluate the abdominal and thoracic vasculature following contrast injection (Table 12.4).

12.2.5 Flow Quantification

Phase-difference techniques are used with prospective or retrospective triggering to assess blood-flow velocities. Through-plane and in-plane flow measurement is available with a set of predefined velocity-encoding (VENC) values. Segmented techniques allow for breath-hold measurement of flow velocities. The number of phases have to be adjusted to scan over the complete cardiac cycle. The selected VENC must be larger than the maximum expected flow velocity to avoid aliasing (Table 12.5).

12.2.6 Perfusion

Single-slice techniques with a TI of 200 ms result in the best overall image quality. Sixty acquisitions should be performed. The patient should be asked to breath-hold for as long as possible. Contrast injection should be started at the same time as the measurement. Multiple slices are possible with longer TRs. The protocol may be applied along the short or the long axis of the heart. Typically, a first-pass experiment is comprised of 60acquisitions of up to 5 sections (Table 12.6).

A power injector is useful for controlling the contrast media injection. Low doses (0.02–0.06 mmol/kg bodyweight) of the MR contrast agent should be injected at a rate of 5 ml/s. Repeated measurement with 0.02 mmol/kg bodyweight are possible.

Table 12.4. MR two- and three-dimensional coronary angiography techniques

Sequence	WI	Plane	No. of slices	TR (ms)	TE (ms)	Flip angle	TI (ms)	Echo train length	Slice thickness (mm)	Matrix	FOV	recFOV (%)	No. of acq.	Acq. time (min:s)
FL2D[a]	T1	Var	1	167	6.2	30			4	160×256	280	75	1	>0:10
FISP3D[b]	T1	Var	Slab	5.0	2.0	25			Var	160×256	320	100	1	>0:26
FL3D[c]	T1	ax	Slab	600	2.7	30			2	160×256	300	100	5	>6:26

[a] Breath-hold, with fat suppression; [b] Breath-hold, gadolinium enhanced; [c] Navigator technique

Table 12.5. Phase difference techniques to assess blood flow velocities

Sequence	WI	Plane	No. of slices	TR (ms)	TE (ms)	Flip angle	TI (ms)	Echo train length	Slice thickness (mm)	Matrix	FOV	recFOV (%)	No. of acq.	Acq. time (min:s)
FL2D[a]	T1	Var	1	24	5	30			6	160×256	300	75	1	>1:56
FL2D[b]	T1	Var	1	25	6	30			6	160×256	300	75	1	>3:00

[a] Through plane; [b] In plane

Abbreviations: *WI* weighting of images; *TR* repetition time; *TI* inversion time; *TE* echo time; *Matrix* phase × frequency matrix; *FOV* field of view (mm); *recFOV* % rectangular field of view; *Acq.* acquisition(s)

Table 12.6. Ultrafast single-shot imaging techniques to assess myocardial perfusion, based on dynamic enhancement of myocardial signal intensity following contrast injection

Sequence	WI	Plane	No. of slices	TR (ms)	TE (ms)	Flip angle	TI (ms)	Echo train length	Slice thickness (mm)	Matrix	FOV	recFOV (%)	No. of acq.	Acq. time (min:s)
TFLASH	T1	Var	1	416	1.2	8	200		10	90×128	380	75	–60	>0:30
TFLASH	T1	Var	3	664	1.2	16[b]	10		10	90×128	380	75	–60	>0:40
TFLASH	T1	Var	5	844	1.2	18[b]	10		10	90×128	380	75	–60	>0:50

[a] Set TR to RR –50 ms to image every heart beat; [b] Lager FA can cause image artifacts
Abbreviations: *WI* weighting of images; *TR* repetition time; *TI* inversion time; *TE* echo time; *Matrix* phase × frequency matrix; *FOV* field of view (mm); *recFOV* % rectangular field of view; *Acq.* acquisition(s)

12.2.7 Contrast Agents

Clinical contrast agents are paramagnetic gadolinium chelates. In the normal myocardium, water is homogeneously distributed and relatively free to pass through the capillary wall and cellular membrane. Low-molecular gadolinium chelates are free to equilibrate throughout the interstitium, but they do not enter the intracellular space. The distribution of low-molecular contrast media is approximately 30% of the myocardial volume. Macromolecular contrast agents are classified as intravascular or blood-pool agents. Contrast agents should be used for perfusion studies in cases of acute coronary occlusion, occlusive or reperfused myocardial infarctions, and the work-up of cardiac tumors. However, contrast agents are not mandatory for all examinations.

12.3 Clinical Applications of Cardiac MR Imaging

12.3.1 Ischemic Heart Disease

12.3.1.1 Introduction

Ischemic heart disease remains a leading cause of morbidity and mortality in industrial nations. MR imaging offers a comprehensive, noninvasive evaluation of cardiac morphology, function, and perfusion and can be used for coronary angiography, providing high spatial resolution and 3D imaging. The application of MR imaging techniques to patients with ischemic heart disease is advancing rapidly. Ultrafast pulse sequences combined with high-performance gradient hardware in high-field-strength magnet systems are rapidly realizing the comprehensive 'one-stop-shop' cardiac MR imaging.

Determining the presence, size, and location of acute myocardial infarctions and differentiating between acute and chronic myocardial infarctions is possible. MR imaging may reveal complications associated with myocardial infarctions and may allow for the assessment of global and regional myocardial function, cardiac morphology, and blood flow through native coronary arteries and bypass grafts. Moreover, the application of contrast agents may allow for the evaluation of regional myocardial perfusion at different stages of ischemic heart disease, including characterizing occlusive and reperfused myocardial infarctions and determining the presence of stunned and hibernating myocardium in regions being considered for revascularization. Cardiac MR imaging is effective in the management of coronary artery disease by means of assessment of the coronary microvasculature with myocardial perfusion imaging, evaluation of wall motion with pharmacological stress testing, and direct visualization of the coronary arteries.

12.3.1.2 MR Imaging Protocol

For MR studies in patients with ischemic heart disease, we recommend a combined protocol with morphological and functional studies, MR coronary angiography, and perfusion studies referring to the clinical question (Table 12.7).

Table 12.7. MR imaging protocol recommended for ischemic heart disease

Sequence	WI	Plane	No. of slices	TR (ms)	TE (ms)	Flip angle	TI (ms)	Echo train length	Slice thickness (mm)	Matrix	FOV	recFOV (%)	No. of acq.	Acq. time (min:s)
TSE	T1	Long	11	600	12	180		3	6	160×256	320	75	5	>2:39
TSE[d]	T1	Short	1	700	32	160		9	6	160×256	320	75	1	>0:10
HASTE	T2	Short	21	800	43	150			6	160×256	320	75	1	>0:31
STIR[d]	T2	Short	1	800	57	160	170	15	6	160×256	320	75	1	>0:11
or														
HASTEIRM	T2	Short	21	800	43	150	170		6	160×256	320	75	1	>0:31
FL2D[a,d]	T1	Var	1	167	6.2	30			4	160×256	280	75	1	>0:10
or														
FL3D[b] Perfusion	T1	ax	Slab	230	2.7	30			2	128×256	300	100	5	>6:26
TSE[c]	T1	Long	11	600	12	180		3	6	156×256	320	75	5	>2:39
TSE[c]	T1	Short	1	700	32	160		9	6	126×256	320	75	1	>0:10

[a] With fat suppression; [b] Navigator technique; [c] Post gadolinium; [d] Breath-hold
Abbreviations: *WI* weighting of images; *TR* repetition time; *TI* inversion time; *TE* echo time; *Matrix* phase × frequency matrix; *FOV* field of view (mm); *recFOV* % rectangular field of view; *Acq.* acquisition(s)

12.3.1.3 MR Findings

12.3.1.3.1 Morphology

In regions affected by acute myocardial infarction, ECG-gated MR images show a high signal intensity on T2-WI. This is consistent with myocardial edema and the pattern of contrast change that occurs with increasing echo time (TE). Animal studies have revealed a significant prolongation of the T2-relaxation time as early as 4 h after myocardial ischemia is induced by coronary occlusion. Initial hypoperfusion, followed by evolving edema in the infarct and the surrounding region, plays a role in producing transient changes in T1- and T2-relaxation times. The size of the infarcted region can be determined very accurately with MR imaging (Figs. 12.5–12.7).

Even though changes in T1 and T2 due to infarction and edema provide excellent MR contrast, infarcted regions can be better distinguished from normal myocardium using contrast-enhanced MR imaging. Chronic myocardial infarctions do not show enhancement by gadolinium, because the ischemic myocardium is replaced by scar tissue. Regional wall thinning also occurs in patients with chronic myocardial infarction (Figs. 12.8 and 12.9).

Myocardial infarctions involving the left ventricle often produce aneurysms and mural thrombi. Aneurysms are frequently located in the apex or the anterolateral region and are recognized as severe wall thinning and diastolic bulging of the left ventricular wall (Fig. 12.10). Mural thrombi are recognized as a

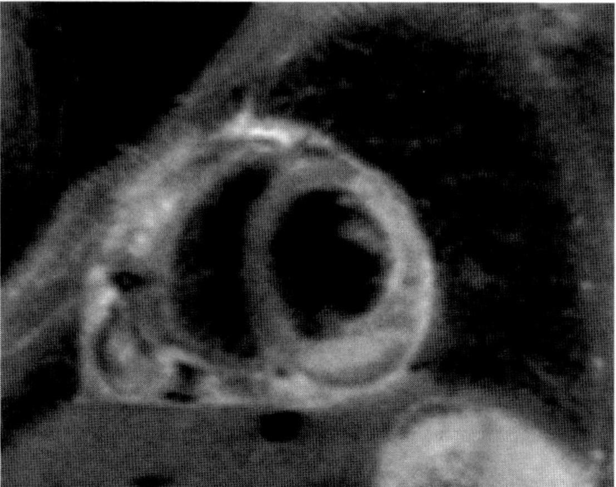

Fig. 12.5. Acute myocardial infarction. Short-axis view. Half-Fourier acquired single-shot turbo spin-echo (HASTE) sequence (repetition time 800 ms, echo time 43 ms) with dark-blood preparation. Acute myocardial infarction of the inferior and lateral region. High signal intensity of the ischemic myocardium

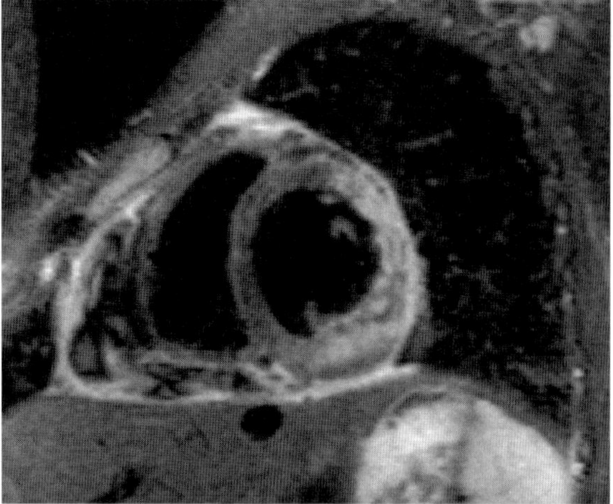

Fig. 12.6. Acute myocardial infarction. Short-axis view. Short tau inversion recovery (STIR) sequence (repetition time 1936 ms, echo time 76 ms) with dark-blood preparation, breath-hold, single-slice acquisition. Acute myocardial infarction of the inferior and lateral region of the left ventricular wall. High signal intensity of the ischemic myocardium, best visualization because of the high sensitivity to edema

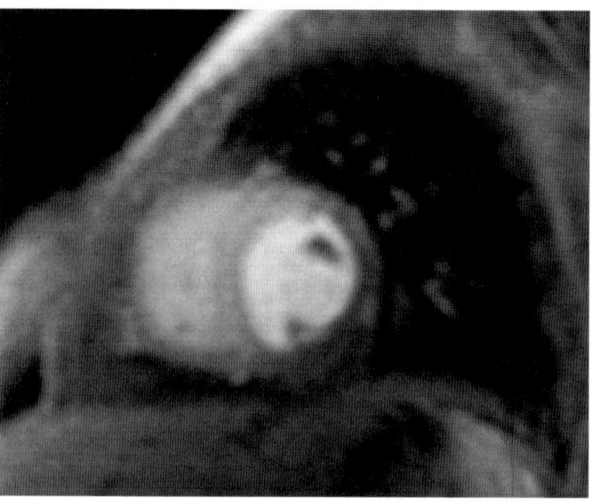

Fig. 12.7. Acute myocardial infarction. Short-axis view. Perfusion study, turbo Fourier acquisition in steady-state (FLASH) sequence (repetition time 416 ms, echo time 1.2 ms) after application of gadolinium chelate, 0.02 mmol/ kg body weight. Acute myocardial infarction of the inferior and lateral region of the left ventricle. Normal perfusion of the septal and anterior parts of the left ventricle, hypoperfusion of the infarcted regions

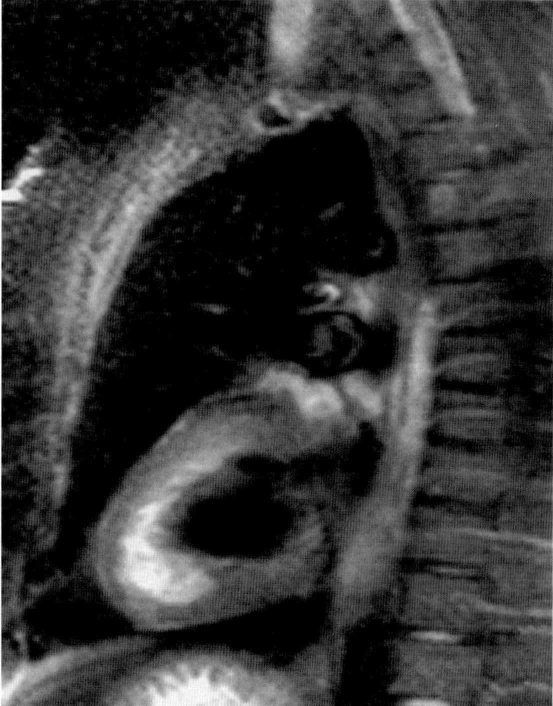

Fig. 12.8. Acute myocardial infarction. Parasagittal view. HASTE sequence (repetition time 800 ms, echo time 43 ms). Non-transmural acute myocardial infarction of the left ventricular apex. High signal intensity of the ischemic myocardium

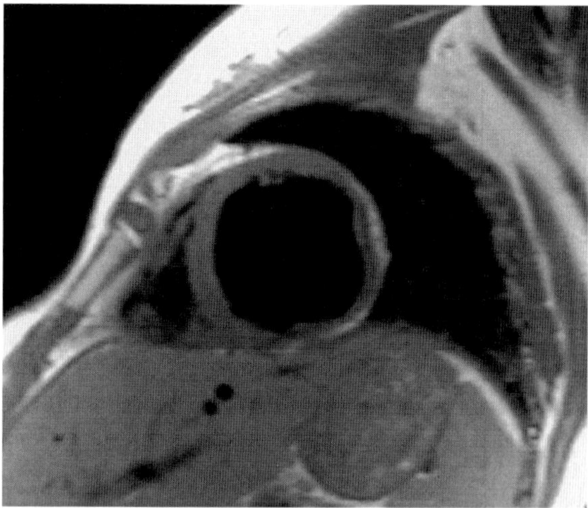

Fig. 12.9. Chronic myocardial infarction. Short-axis view. T1-weighted TSE sequence (repetition time 842 ms, echo time 32 ms) with dark-blood preparation. Chronic myocardial infarction of the left ventricular lateral wall. Regional wall-thinning, the ischemic myocardium is replaced by scar and shows an isointense signal to the normal left ventricular myocardium

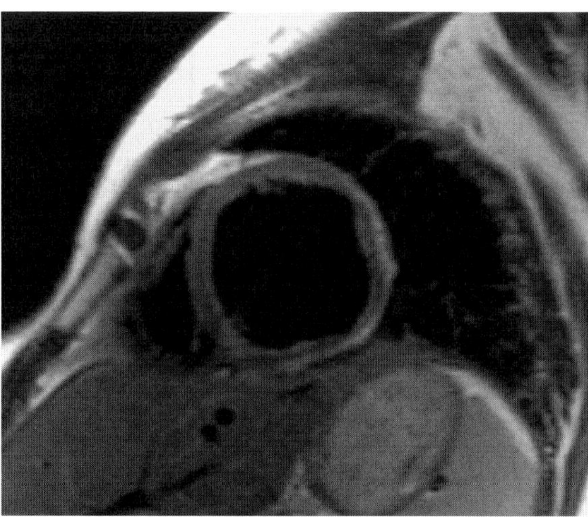

Fig. 12.10. Chronic myocardial infarction. Short-axis view. T2-weighted TSE sequence (repetition time 1743 ms, echo time 76 ms) with dark-blood preparation of the left ventricular lateral wall. Regional wall-thinning, the ischemic myocardium is replaced by scar and shows an isointense signal to the normal left ventricular myocardium, no edema

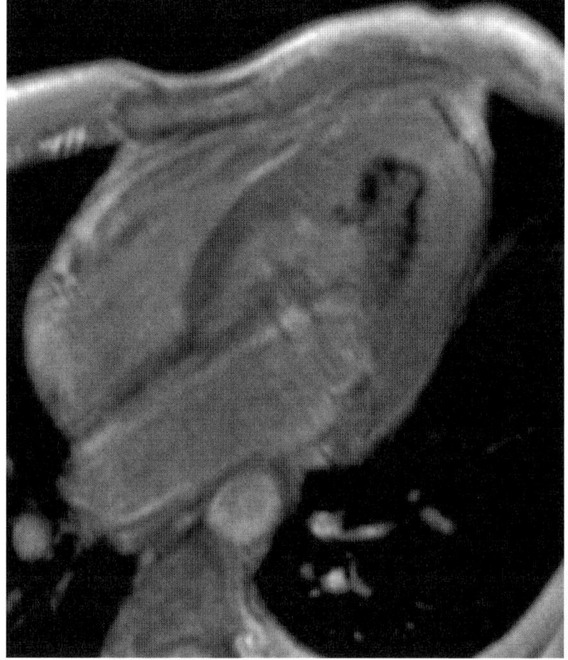

Fig. 12.11. Thrombus of the left ventricle. Long-axis view. T1-weighted FLASH 2D sequence (repetition time 1419 ms, echo time 6.2 ms). Thrombus in the left ventricular apex, partially calcified. Hypointense signal. Perfusion studies do not show any enhancement, no blood flow in this region

mass adhering to the myocardium or filling an aneurysm (Fig. 12.11). The signal intensity of mural thrombi varies, depending on their age. In subacute cases, the thrombus shows an intermediate or high signal intensity on T1-WI and a high signal intensity on T2-WI. The signal decreases with increasing age, and an organized thrombus has a low signal intensity in both weighted images. It is difficult to differentiate a thrombus from slow-flowing blood on SE images (non-breath-holding) in some cases. However, on the cine-mode images, the thrombus produces low signal intensity and is visualized within the high signal of the left ventricular blood pool.

12.3.1.3.2
Function

Cine MR imaging is useful for defining focal areas of decreased or absent myocardial wall thickening during the cardiac cycle. Normal thickening is about 60% and absolute wall thickening is greater than 2 mm in normal myocardium. At sites of prior myocardial infarction, the relative and absolute wall thickening decreases. Comparative studies of fluorodeoxyglucose (FDG) positron emission tomography (PET) and cine MR imaging have concluded that wall thickness and systolic wall thickening provide reliable evidence that regions with a moderate reduction in FDG activity represent viable myocardium. Absence of systolic wall thickening may be present both in hibernating and nonviable myocardium; however, the combination of severely reduced or absent FDG activity associated with significant wall thinning and no systolic wall thickening indicates nonviable myocardium. Using MR imaging, regional wall thinning in ischemic cardiomyopathy can be distinguished from uniform wall thinning in patients with idiopathic congestive dilated cardiomyopathy.

12.3.1.3.3
Perfusion

With the development of ultrafast imaging techniques, such as fast GRE or echo-planar imaging (EPI), it has become possible to visualize regional myocardial perfusion by monitoring first-pass kinetics of contrast media, such as low-molecular-weight gadolinium chelates. Image signal intensities are a measure of the regional concentration of the contrast media, resulting from a change in relaxation time. A normally perfused

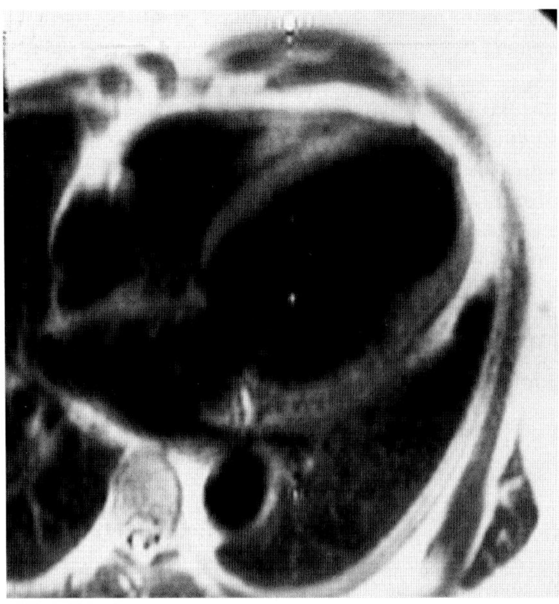

Fig. 12.12. Aneurysm of the left ventricle. Long-axis view. T1-weighted TSE sequence (repetition time 1000 ms, echo time 32 ms) with dark-blood preparation. Aneurysm of the left ventricular apex as complication of myocardial infarction, severe wall thinning, diastolic bulging in functional studics

myocardial region demonstrates a T1-shortening effect, with an increase in signal intensity, followed by washout from the tissue after intravenous bolus administration of contrast agent. Hypoperfused myocardial regions with subsequently reduced concentrations of the contrast media exhibit a lesser decrease in signal intensity compared with normal myocardium (Fig. 12.12). Advances in hardware and pulse sequence technology allow the acquisition of multiple imaging planes during every heartbeat while tracking a contrast agent bolus. The perfusion in the entire ventricle can be evaluated following a single bolus injection of gadolinium chelates. The spatial and temporal resolution cannot be matched by any other modality, and information on myocardial perfusion can be obtained in a totally non-invasive manner without the application of radioactive tracers. Interpretation of the large number of images will be simplified by the availability of automated pixel-based programs and the creation of perfusion maps.

12.3.1.3.4 Dobutamine Stress MR Imaging

In addition to the MR studies performed at rest, cine GRE imaging provides the choice of pharmacological stress testing following the administration of dipyridamole or dobutamine. MR imaging during dynamic exercise, as in an ECG laboratory, is currently not feasible within conventional magnets. Studies have visualized stress-induced wall motion or wall-thickening abnormalities of ischemic myocardium in patients with coronary artery disease but who have normal left ventricular function. Dipyridamole stress MR studies are safe; however, they provide limited sensitivity and specificity for detecting coronary artery disease. The sensitivity of dipyridamole MR imaging for localizing hemodynamically significant stenoses associated with major coronary arteries is up to 85%; the specificity reaches 90%. Dobutamine stress MR imaging, using the analysis of ventricular wall segment thickening, showed an overall sensitivity up to 100% for three-vessel disease. With dobutamine stress MR imaging, first wall motion abnormalities can be induced in myocardial areas fed by coronary arteries with hemodynamically significant and subcritical stenoses (insufficient coronary reserve) which are secondly directly related to the assessment of myocardial viability. Cine MR imaging with dobutamine stress testing correlates with results of myocardial stress scintigraphy and has demonstrated higher sensitivity and specificity than dobutamine stress echocardiography, because cardiac MR imaging has a consistently superior image quality and the possibility of tissue tagging to allow the detection of subtle wall motion abnormalities.

12.3.1.3.5 Coronaries

Direct visualization of coronary atherosclerotic plaques and stenoses is essential for the diagnosis and treatment of coronary artery disease. Physiological motion and the small size of coronary vessels present a challenge for conventional MR techniques. Several new ultrafast techniques have been applied to evaluate the coronary arteries.

Two-dimensional MR angiography (MRA) uses a single breath-hold, which requires excellent patient cooperation. Consistency in breath-holding is also needed to follow the course of coronary vessels; this

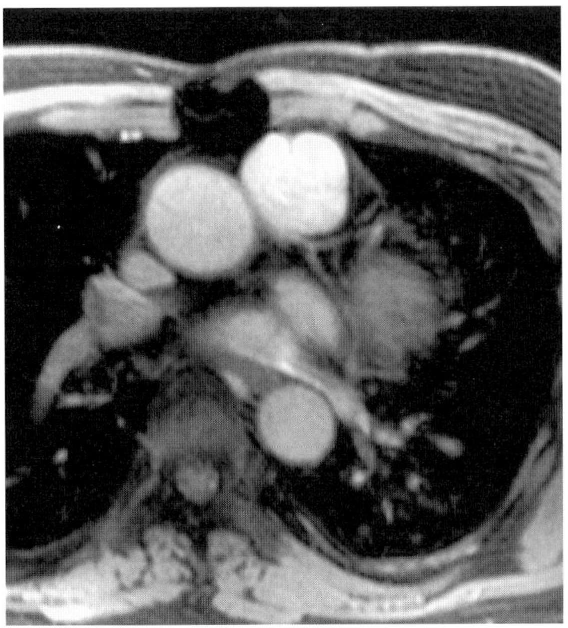

Fig. 12.13. Left coronary artery. FLASH 2D sequence with single breath-hold and fat suppression (repetition time 1450 ms, echo time 6.2 ms), single-slice technique. Good visualization of the left main artery, the left anterior descending, and the left circumflex artery

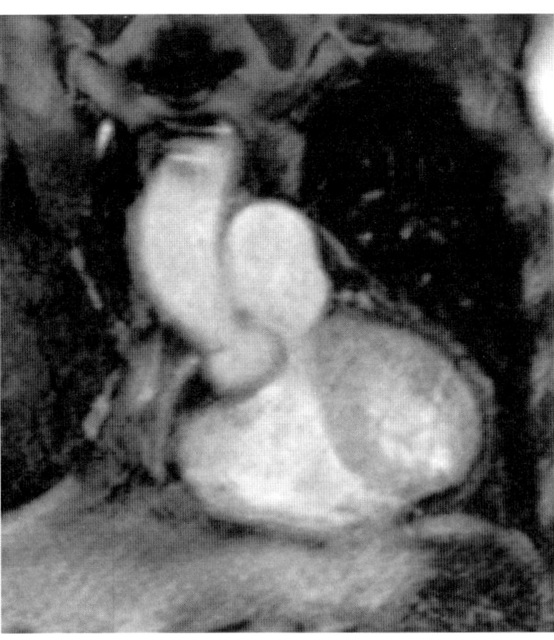

Fig. 12.14. Right coronary artery. FLASH 2D sequence with single breath-hold and fat suppression (repetition time 1425 ms, echo time 6.2 ms), single-slice technique. Excellent visualization of the right coronary artery, proximal and middle segments

requires significant physician time and interaction to select the imaging planes properly (Figs. 12.13 and 12.14). Breath-hold 2D coronary MRA can depict up to 76% of hemodynamically significant stenoses in the proximal coronary arterial tree. The best image quality is found for the right coronary artery (RCA) and the left anterior descending (LAD) coronary artery, whereas the left circumflex branch (LCX) of the coronary arteries had the worst quality. The image quality is disturbed by insufficient breath-holding, ghost artifacts, and incomplete fat suppression. Diagnostic problems include incomplete differentiation of the coronary arteries from cardiac veins and from the pericardial sac.

The navigator echo technique is a 3D approach that reduces respiratory effects by decreasing the range of signal intensities of the diaphragm position during data acquisition. Navigator echo signals can be acquired to sample the diaphragm position before and after the image data readout. The use of navigator echo-based real-time respiratory gating can effectively reduce motion blur and ghost artifacts in coronary imaging (Fig. 12.15). Because of the much longer acquisition

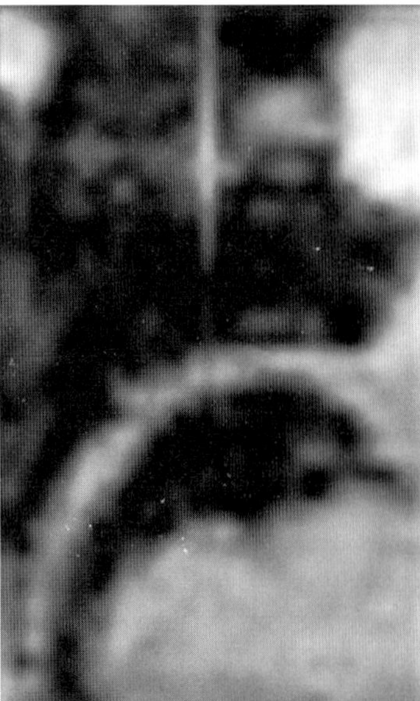

Fig. 12.15. Right coronary artery. FLASH 3D sequence with navigator echo technique and fat suppression (repetition time 1342 ms, echo time 2.7 ms). Multiplanar reconstruction of the right coronary artery, proximal and middle segments

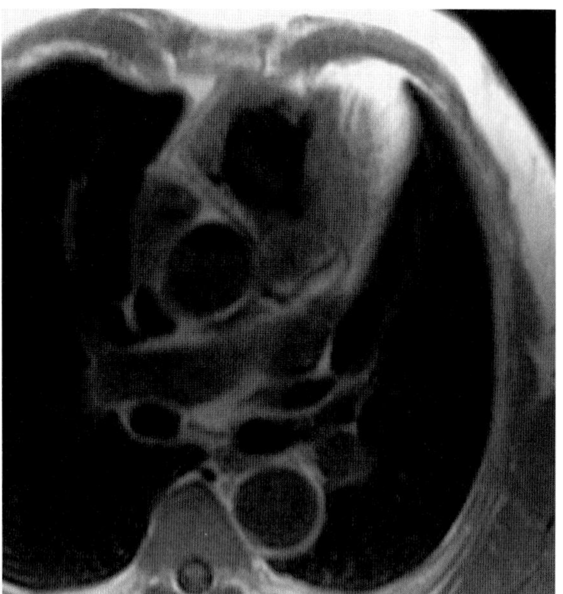

Fig. 12.16. Abnormal origin of the right coronary artery out of the left coronary sinus. FLASH 2D sequence with single breath-hold and fat suppression (repetition time 1425 ms, echo time 6.2 ms), single-slice technique

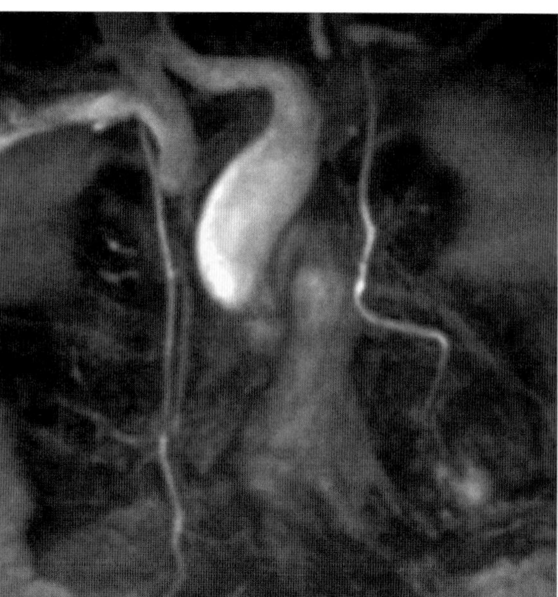

Fig. 12.17. Bypass graft. Fast imaging into steady precession (FISP) 3D sequence (repetition time 5.0 ms, echo time 2.0 ms) after application of gadolinium chelate, 0.1 mmol/kg body weight. Postoperative evaluation of the bypass graft. Excellent visualization of the left internal mammary artery. The anastomosis to the left anterior descending (LAD) coronary artery and the bypass graft patency are clearly visualized

time of the 3D navigator technique (up to 14 min), the image quality is often disturbed by motion artifacts and inconsistent breathing.

Contrast-enhanced 3D MR angiography techniques are used to evaluate the abdominal and thoracic vasculature following contrast injection. They can sufficiently depict the left internal mammary artery and are a very useful noninvasive technique for the preoperative work-up of patients with coronary disease of the LAD who are scheduled for minimally invasive coronary artery bypass grafting, and could also be useful in conventional bypass surgery (Fig. 12.17).

The clinical role of coronary MRA still needs to be defined. The in-plane image resolution of current coronary MRA techniques is about 1 mm. This is sufficient for the detection of abnormalities (Fig. 12.16) and stenoses in large coronary arteries but insufficient for the exact detection of stenoses in smaller branches. The future role of coronary MRA will become an important adjunct to the comprehensive cardiac MR examination in combination with dobutamine stress testing and perfusion imaging. At the present time, coronary MRA cannot replace conventional coronary angiography.

12.3.2 Cardiomyopathies

12.3.2.1 Introduction

Echocardiography is the primary technique used for the evaluation of cardiomyopathies; however, MR imaging may also be used for the diagnosis of various kinds of cardiomyopathy, such as congestive cardiomyopathy, hypertrophic cardiomyopathy, and restrictive cardiomyopathy. MR imaging is able to demonstrate morphological abnormalities associated with these diseases. Cine MR imaging demonstrates abnormal systolic and diastolic function of the left and right ventricles. Furthermore, the ventricular volume and global ventricular function in cardiomyopathy may be visualized and quantified, and the effectiveness of drug treatment in patients with congestive cardiomyopathy may be monitored.

Congestive (dilated) cardiomyopathy is a pathophysiological, not an etiological classification; it is characterized by ventricular dilatation, systolic dysfunction, and congestive heart failure. Alcohol, peripartum cardiomyopathy, various toxins, ischemia, diabetes, hypertension, obesity, viral disease, and hereditary factors may all lead to a dilated left ventricle with reduced pumping function and heart failure. This disease is the most common of the three forms of cardiomyopathy.

Hypertrophic cardiomyopathy is probably a genetic disorder, characterized by inappropriate left ventricular hypertrophy, often with left ventricular outflow tract obstruction and myocardial cellular disorganization. Restrictive cardiomyopathy is also a pathophysiological and not an etiological classification; it is characterized by impaired ventricular diastolic filling due to myocardial disease. It is a relatively rare condition.

12.3.2.2 MR Imaging Protocol

Table 12.8 shows a MR imaging protocol recommended for morphological and functional studies of patients with known or suspected cardiomyopathy.

12.3.2.3 MR Findings

12.3.2.3.1 Congestive (Dilated) Cardiomyopathy

In patients with congestive cardiomyopathy, the left ventricle is grossly dilated and may be globular in shape, with a smooth endocardial surface. The left ventricular wall thickness is usually within the normal range but is sometimes surprisingly hypertrophied, thus resulting in an overall substantial increase in the left ventricular mass (weighing up to 1000 g). Even with hypertrophy, the ventricular walls are often thinned, but the thickness is uniform around the circumference of the left ventricle (Fig. 12.18). Patients with ischemic cardiomyopathy generally show a nonuniform pattern. Regions of wall thinning exist in these patients as a consequence of myocardial infarction.

The primary value of morphological MR imaging in patients with congestive cardiomyopathy lies in the exclusion of pathological causes of the dilatation, such as infarction or the formation of local aneurysms. MR imaging can differentiate these causes from the global dilatation of congestive cardiomyopathy. Patients with congestive heart failure frequently present with mural thrombi in the left ventricular cavity (with a mass adhering to the ventricular wall), usually located at the septum or apex of the ventricle.

Cine MR imaging in a short-axis view, however, can provide functional information about the left ventricular cavity that is useful in the diagnosis and management of patients with congestive cardiomyopathy. It

Table 12.8. MR imaging protocol recommended for cardiomyopathy

Sequence	WI	Plane	No. of slices	TR (ms)	TE (ms)	Flip angle	TI (ms)	Echo train length	Slice thickness (mm)	Matrix	FOV	recFOV (%)	No. of acq.	Acq. time (min:s)
TSE	T1	Long	11	600	12	180		3	6	160×256	320	75	5	>2:39
FL2D[b]	T1	Long	1	167	6.2	30			6	160×256	280	100	1	>0:10
TSE[b]	T1	Short	1	700	32	160		9	6	160×256	320	75	1	>0:10
TSE[b]	T2	Short	1	800	57	160		15	6	160×256	320	75	1	>0:11
HASTE	T2	Short	21	800	43	150			6	160×256	320	75	1	>0:31
FL2D[a]	T1	Short	1	30	4.8	30			6	128×256	320	75	1	>0:19

[a] Cine mode; [b] Breath-hold

Abbreviations: *WI* weighting of images; *TR* repetition time; *TI* inversion time; *TE* echo time; *Matrix* phase × frequency matrix; *FOV* field of view (mm); *recFOV* % rectangular field of view; *Acq.* acquisition(s)

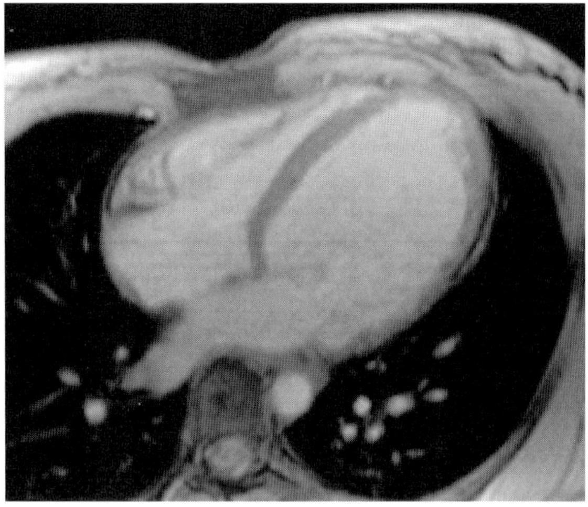

Fig. 12.18. Congestive cardiomyopathy. Long-axis view. T1-weighted FLASH 2D sequence (repetition time 1056 ms, echo time 6.2 ms). The left ventricle is grossly dilated, the ventricular walls are thinned, most uniform around the circumference of the left ventricle

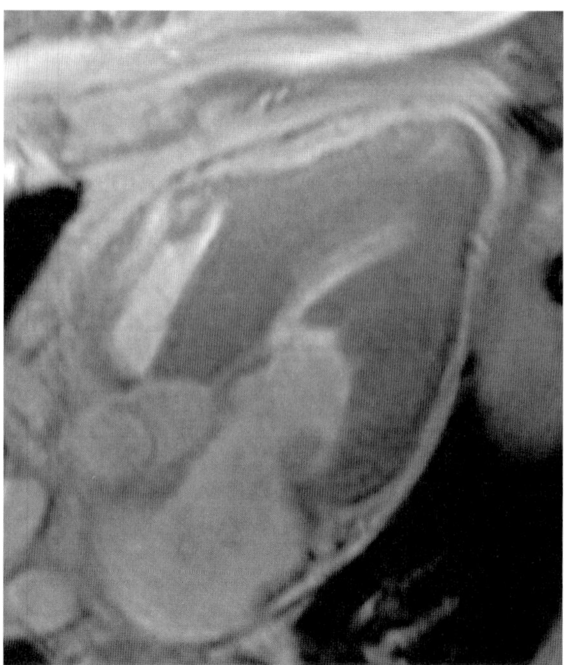

Fig. 12.19. Hypertrophic cardiomyopathy. Long-axis view. T1-weighted FLASH 2D sequence (repetition time 815 ms, echo time 6.2 ms). Marked and uniform hypertrophy of the left ventricular myocardium. Homogeneous signal intensity, isointense to the normal myocardium

may be used to demonstrate left ventricular wall thickening during the cardiac cycle and to calculate the stroke volume and ejection fraction. The ejection fraction is the most commonly used clinical parameter in these patients, and changes of the ejection fraction give the most reliable information about the therapeutic response or nonresponse. Furthermore, the presence of valvular regurgitation may be evaluated. The regurgitation is seen as a signal void, e.g., projecting into the left atrium during ventricular systole in patients with mitral regurgitation.

12.3.2.3.2
Hypertrophic Cardiomyopathy

Morphological MR imaging provides an accurate evaluation of the extent, location, and severity of hypertrophy in patients with hypertrophic cardiomyopathy. In some cases, hypertrophy exists only in the outflow portion of the septum (hypertrophic obstructive cardiomyopathy); in other cases, there is asymmetric septal hypertrophy or hypertrophy of the entire septum (Figs. 12.19–12.21). There are cases of focal or global hypertrophy in either the midventricular or apical myocardial regions of the left ventricle. MR imaging provides additional information in patients with known hypertrophic cardiomyopathy. Assessing the distribu-

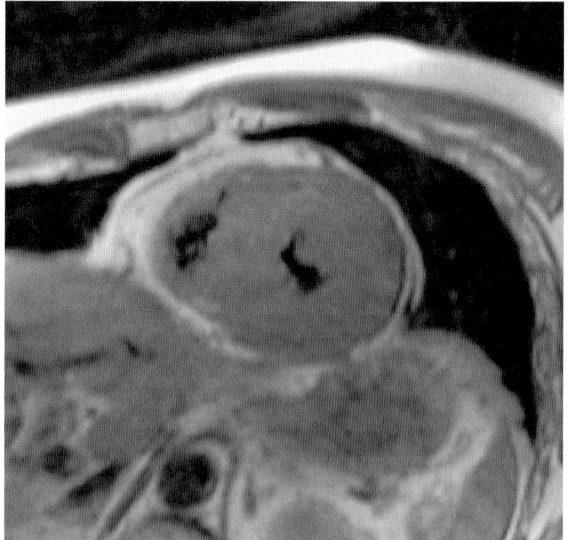

Fig. 12.20. Hypertrophic cardiomyopathy. Short-axis view. T1-weighted SE sequence (repetition time 715 ms, echo time 20 ms). Marked and uniform hypertrophy of the left ventricular myocardium. Homogeneous signal intensity. Small right ventricle

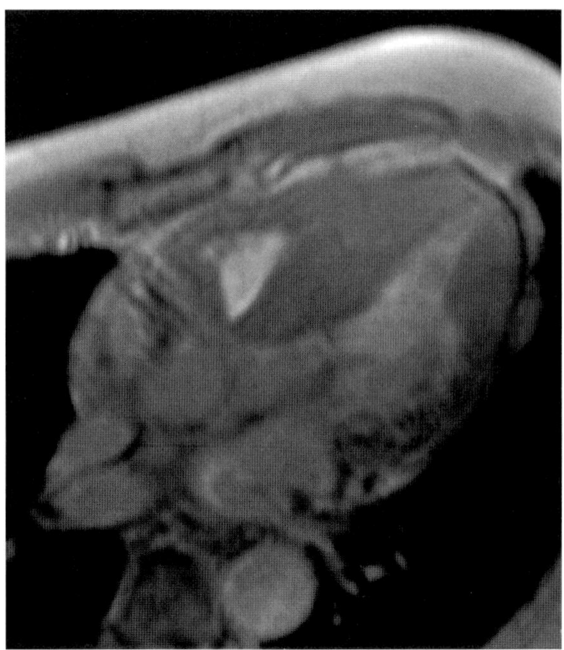

Fig. 12.21. Hypertrophic obstructive cardiomyopathy. Long-axis view. T1-weighted FLASH 2D sequence (repetition time 1205 ms, echo time 6.2 ms). Hypertrophy of the left ventricular myocardium with severe asymmetric hypertrophy of the septum. Obstruction of the left ventricular outflow tract. Homogeneous signal intensity, isointense to the normal myocardium

tion of hypertrophy (without chamber enlargement) is essential for diagnosing the pattern of hypertrophic cardiomyopathy, each of which is associated with a different prognosis and treatment strategy. In order to assess the wall thickness, two orthogonal plane views (short and long axis) are usually necessary. MR imaging is able to demonstrate the true distribution of hypertrophy with equal confidence for the anterior and inferior walls, as well as for the apex (areas that are associated with uncertainty using echocardiography). Finally, assessment of the right ventricular myocardium and demonstration of hypertrophy at this site are possible with MR imaging.

In most cases, hypertrophic myocardium shows homogeneous signal intensity (i.e., is isointense to the normal myocardium) in MR images. There is some evidence that the perfusion is altered in hypertrophied segments, which may result in regions of decreased signal intensity in T1-WI and T2-WI of the left ventricle (representing areas of focal fibrosis).

Functional MR imaging (cine GRE technique) has been used to evaluate the dynamics of global and regional wall thickening. Impairment of left ventricular relaxation results in decreased early diastolic filling. It is useful to demonstrate regional asymmetric ventricular function. Hypertrophic cardiomyopathy is often associated with decreased left ventricular volume and an increased ejection fraction. These parameters can be measured noninvasively by means of MR imaging, and the data correlate very well with invasive left ventriculography.

Mitral regurgitation is a common feature in patients with hypertrophic cardiomyopathy. The regurgitation is seen as a signal void projecting into the left atrium during ventricular systole, and its severity may be assessed by comparing right and left ventricular stroke volumes. This valvular dysfunction is due to the abnormal relationship of the interventricular septum and the anterior mitral leaflet, which also causes the systolic anterior motion of this leaflet.

12.3.2.3.3 Restrictive Cardiomyopathy

Restrictive cardiomyopathy is characterized by a restriction of diastolic ventricular filling due to abnormalities of the endocardium and/or the myocardium itself. MR imaging is of little use in the diagnosis of restrictive cardiomyopathy, but may demonstrate anatomical changes associated with infiltrative myocardial disease (Figs. 12.22 and 12.23). The characteristics of restrictive cardiomyopathy are enlargement of the atria combined with relatively normal-sized ventricles and prominent intracavity signal caused by stasis and slow movement of the blood through the chambers. It is helpful to use MR imaging to discriminate between restrictive cardiomyopathy and constrictive pericarditis, especially given that the treatment of constrictive pericarditis is surgical. These two entities show essentially the same clinical picture, but the treatment differs. Typical findings of constrictive pericarditis are a thickened pericardium with right ventricular narrowing, a disproportionally dilated right atrium and caval veins, and pericardial calcification.

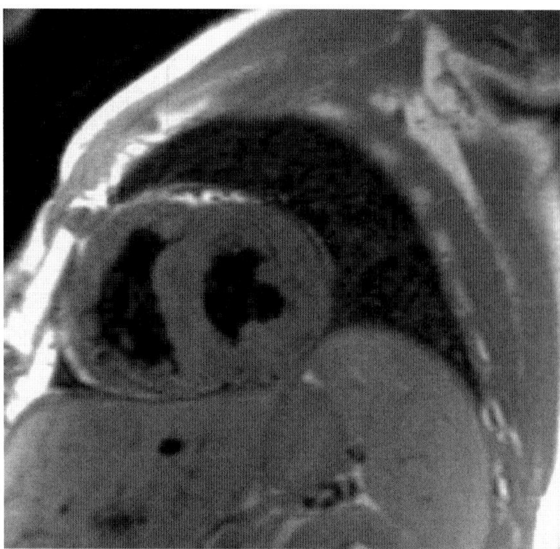

Fig. 12.22. Restrictive cardiomyopathy. Short-axis view. T1-weighted TSE sequence (repetition time 900 ms, echo time 32 ms) with dark-blood preparation, single-slice technique, breath-hold. Uniform thickening of the right and left ventricular walls, caused by amyloidosis. Restriction of the diastolic ventricular filling in functional MR studies, ejection fraction 40%

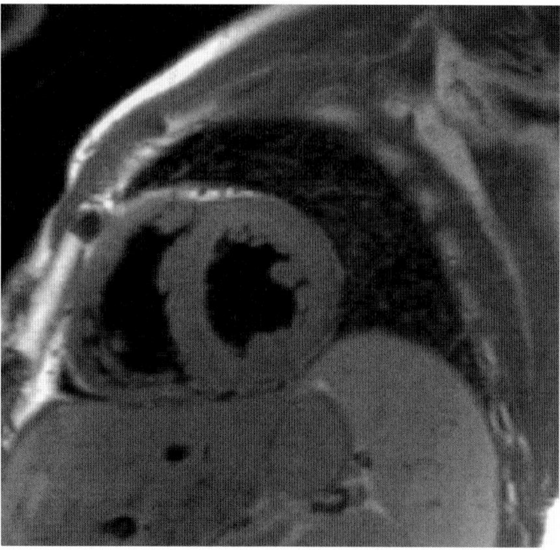

Fig. 12.23. Restrictive cardiomyopathy. Short-axis view. T2-weighted TSE sequence (repetition time 1763 ms, echo time 76 ms) with dark-blood preparation, single-slice technique, breath-hold. Uniform thickening of the right and left ventricular wall, caused by amyloidosis. Homogeneous signal intensity of the myocardium

12.3.3 Arrhythmogenic Right Ventricular Dysplasia/ Cardiomyopathy

12.3.3.1 Introduction

Arrhythmogenic right ventricular cardiomyopathy/ dysplasia (ARVC/ARVD) is a common cause of sudden death in patients with ventricular tachyarrhythmias. Unless anatomical proof can be obtained from autopsy, surgery, or endomyocardial biopsy, the diagnosis of ARVC/ARVD is based on the presence of ventricular arrhythmia with the left bundle branch block pattern (LBBB), often induced by exercise and by morphological changes or motion abnormalities, particularly those localized in the free wall of the right ventricle. These abnormalities are usually associated with right ventricular enlargement and segmental or diffuse hypokinesia that has no identifiable etiology. Different techniques are used to detect these abnormalities: angiocardiography, 2D echocardiography, radionuclide angiography, endomyocardial biopsy, electrocardiographic or invasive electrophysiological studies, and MR imaging. A congenital disposition towards infiltration of the right ventricular myocardium by progressive fibrous and lipomatous tissue, combined with hypertrophy and degeneration of surviving myocytes, is the pathogenetic factor that leads to changes in conduction and the resulting development of arrhythmogenic zones.

Given that there is no imaging modality commonly regarded as the standard of reference in the diagnosis of ARVC/ARVD, MR imaging is considered an accurate and reliable technique for evaluating ARVC/ARVD. MR imaging is the only method that depicts the morphology, structural changes, and function of the right ventricle.

12.3.3.2 MR Imaging Protocol

Table 12.9 demonstrates a combined MR imaging protocol to assess morphological and functional abnormalities in patients with ARVC/ARVD.

Table 12.9. MR imaging protocol recommended for arrhythmogenic right ventricular dysplasis/cardiomyopathy

Sequence	WI	Plane	No. of slices	TR (ms)	TE (ms)	Flip angle	TI (ms)	Echo train length	Slice thickness (mm)	Matrix	FOV	recFOV (%)	No. of acq.	Acq. time (min:s)
TSE	T1	Long	11	600	12	180		3	6	160×256	320	75	5	>2:39
TSE [b]	T1	Short	1	700	32	160		9	6	160×256	320	75	1	>0:10
TSE [b]	T2	Short	1	800	57	160		15	6	160×256	320	75	1	>0:11
FL2D [a]	T1	Short	1	30	4.8	30			6	132×256	320	75	1	>0:19

[a] Cine mode; [b] Breath-hold
Abbreviations: *WI* weighting of images; *TR* repetition time; *TI* inversion time; *TE* echo time; *Matrix* phase × frequency matrix; *FOV* field of view (mm); *recFOV* % rectangular field of view; *Acq.* acquisition(s)

12.3.3.3
MR Findings

MR imaging allows for the localization, characterization, and quantification of morphological alterations of the right ventricular myocardium. MR imaging can be used to detect enlargement of the right ventricle and allows for localization of structural changes of the right ventricular wall in patients with ARVC/ARVD.

Structural alterations in areas of the right ventricular myocardium are described in three different ways:

1. Morphological abnormalities, such as wall thinning, bulging, or outpouching (Fig. 12.24).
2. Signal intensity changes of the myocardium due to fatty or fibrous replacement (Figs. 12.25–12.27). Adipose infiltration of the right ventricular myocardium is characterized by an increase in signal intensity in T1-WI and T2-WI, whereas fibrous replacement is characterized by myocardial thinning and a decrease in signal intensity in T1-WI and T2-WI.
3. Regional or global hypokinesia or dyskinesia, as revealed by cine MR imaging.

Regional myocardial changes can be observed in all parts of the right ventricle. Typical locations are the right ventricular apex, outflow tract, and inferior sub-

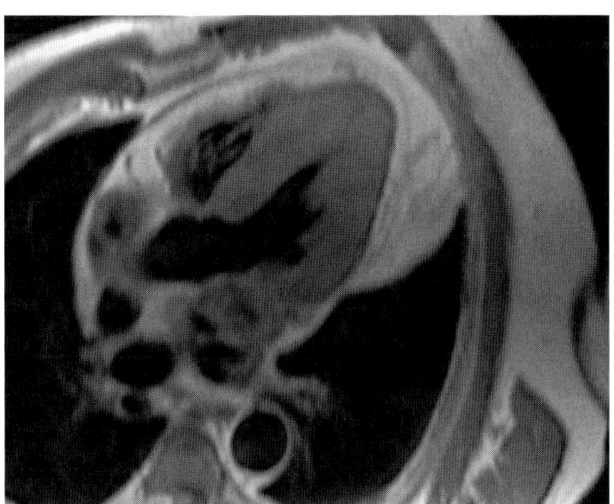

Fig. 12.24. Arrhythmogenic right ventricular cardiomyopathy. Long-axis view. T1-weighted SE sequence (repetition time 884 ms, echo time 20 ms). High signal intensity of the free right ventricular wall due to fatty replacement of the normal myocardial cells, no thinning

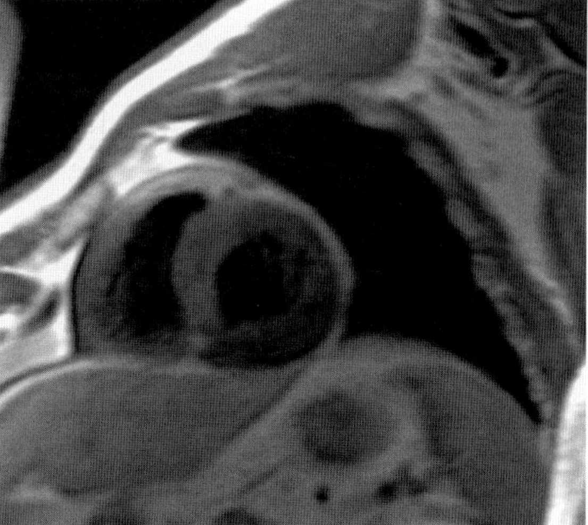

Fig. 12.25. Arrhythmogenic right ventricular cardiomyopathy. Short-axis view. T1-weighted SE sequence (repetition time 863 ms, echo time 20 ms). High signal intensity of the free right ventricular wall and the right ventricular outflow tract due to adipose infiltration of the right ventricular myocardium

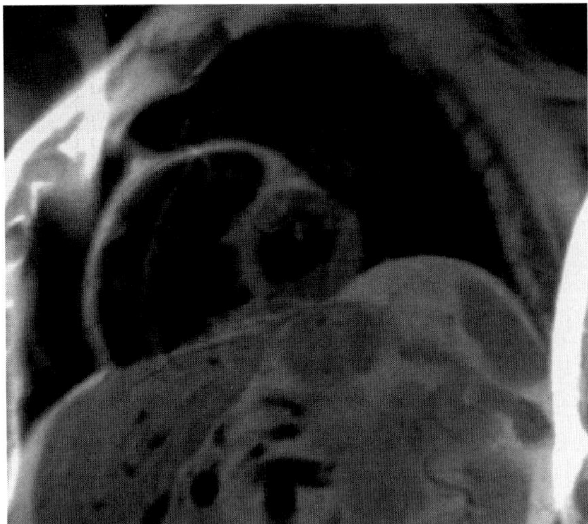

Fig. 12.26. Arrhythmogenic right ventricular cardiomyopathy. Short-axis view. T1-weighted TSE sequence (repetition time 775 ms, echo time 32 ms) with dark-blood preparation, single-slice technique, breath-hold. Marked dilatation of the right ventricle, extreme right ventricular wall thinning. Global hypokinesia revealed by cine MR imaging. Normal left ventricle

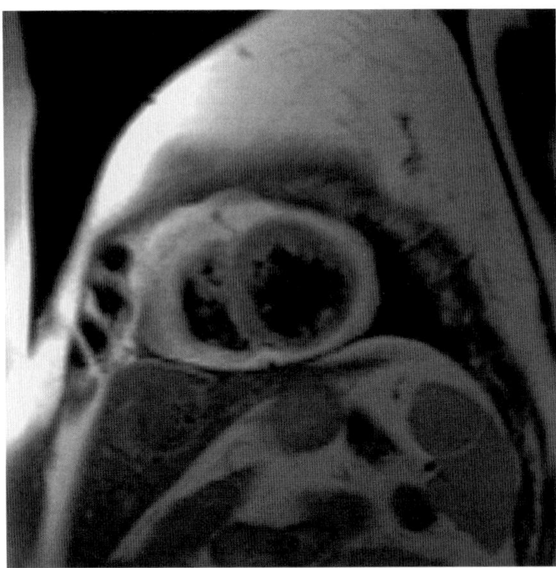

Fig. 12.27. Arrhythmogenic right ventricular cardiomyopathy. Short-axis view. T2-weighted TSE sequence (repetition time 2245 ms, echo time 76 ms) with dark-blood preparation, single-slice technique, breath-hold. High signal intensity myocardium of the right ventricular outflow tract and the apex due to fatty replacement of the normal myocardial cells, no fibrosis. Functional MR imaging shows regional hypokinesia

tricuspid wall, known as the triangle of dysplasia. When the disease is limited to portions of the right ventricle (localized disease), global right ventricular function may be normal.

12.3.4 Cardiac Masses

12.3.4.1 Introduction

Primary tumors of the heart are rare, whereas secondary tumors are somewhat more common. Primary tumors include benign and malignant entities. Despite their low incidence (0.002%–0.03%), it is important to diagnose and treat cardiac tumors promptly, because up to 80% are benign and are treatable by resection.

Myxoma accounts for nearly 50% of benign tumors. Other benign primary cardiac tumors include rhabdomyoma, fibroma, mesothelioma, hemangioma, teratoma, paraganglioma, pheochromocytoma, and lipoma. Some 20%–25% of primary cardiac tumors are malignant; the vast majority are sarcomas. Angiosarcoma, rhabdomyosarcoma, and malignant fibrous histiocytoma are the most common ones. Primary cardiac lymphomas are rare.

Secondary cardiac tumors are substantially more common and are found in up to 20% of patients with malignant disease. The most common primary sites are the lung, breast, and lymphatic system, which can reach the heart by hematogenous, lymphatic, or contiguous spread.

Although tumors are often diagnosed with echocardiography, MR imaging appears to be the modality of choice because of its capabilities. These include multiplanar imaging for excellent anatomical definition of the heart, pericardium, and mediastinum, improved morphological differentiation of tumorous and normal heart tissue, assessment of tissue perfusion, and dynamic imaging. The use of gadolinium chelates is helpful for enhancing tumors in MR images.

12.3.4.2 MR Imaging Protocol

To examine patients with primary or secondary cardiac neoplasms, we recommend plain and contrast-enhanced morphological MR studies (Table 12.10).

Table 12.10. MR imaging protocol recommended for cardiac masses

Sequence	WI	Plane	No. of slices	TR (ms)	TE (ms)	Flip angle	TI (ms)	Echo train length	Slice thickness (mm)	Matrix	FOV	recFOV (%)	No. of acq.	Acq. time (min:s)
TSE	T1	Long	11	600	12	180		3	6	160×256	320	75	5	>2:39
TSE[b]	T1	Short	1	700	32	160		9	6	160×256	320	75	1	>0:10
TSE[b] or	T2	Short	1	800	57	160		15	6	160×256	320	75	1	>0:11
HASTE	T2	Short	21	800	43	150			6	160×256	320	75	1	>0:31
STIR[b] or	T2	Short	1	800	57	160	170	15	6	160×256	320	75	1	>0:11
HASTEIRM	T2	Short	21	800	43	150	170		6	160×256	320	75	1	>0:31
TSE[a]	T1	Long	11	600	12	180		3	6	160×256	320	75	5	>2:39
TSE[a]	T1	Short	1	700	32	160		9	6	160×256	320	75	1	>0:10

[a] Post gadolinium; [b] Breath-hold
Abbreviations: *WI* weighting of images; *TR* repetition time; *TI* inversion time; *TE* echo time; *Matrix* phase × frequency matrix; *FOV* field of view (mm); *recFOV* % rectangular field of view; *Acq.* acquisition(s)

12.3.4.3 MR Findings

12.3.4.3.1 Myxoma

Left atrial myxomas are more common (75%) than right atrial myxomas (which account for the majority of remaining myxomas). Ventricular myxomas are rare. The tumor has its highest incidence in the sixth decade, with a predominance in women (up to 70%). MR imaging often shows the tumor better than echocardiography. Atrial myxomas are characterized by intermediate signal intensity on T1-W and T2-W SE images. Contrast-enhanced studies may show an intermediate tumor enhancement (Figs. 12.28–12.32).

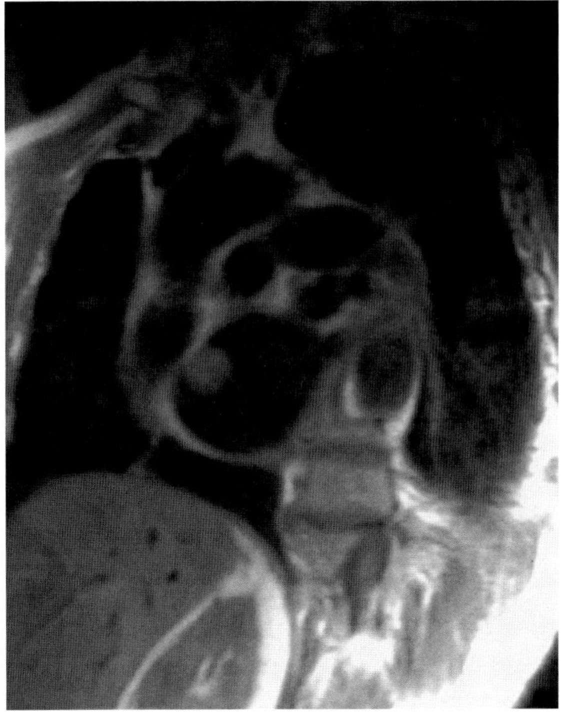

Fig. 12.28. Left atrial myxoma. Short-axis view. T1-weighted TSE sequence (repetition time 1069 ms, echo time 32 ms) with dark-blood preparation, single-slice technique, breath-hold. Round, well-shaped mass with low signal intensity arising from the atrial wall

12.3.4.3.2 Rhabdomyoma

Rhabdomyoma, the most common primary pediatric cardiac tumor, is a hamartomatous lesion occurring in early childhood and associated with tuberous sclerosis in 50%. The tumors are often multiple and are typically located intramurally. Tumors that deform the myocardial wall are likely to be detected by MR imaging, but tumors that are confined to the myocardial wall may not be identified. They are usually isointense to the myocardium in T1-WI and T2-WI. Contrast-enhanced studies may show greater enhancement of the tumors than of normal myocardium (Figs. 12.33–12.35).

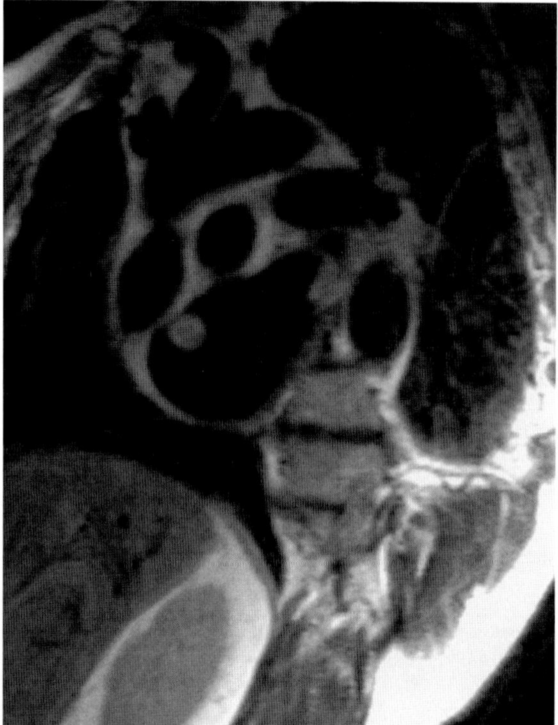

Fig. 12.29. Left atrial myxoma. Short-axis view. T2-weighted TSE sequence (repetition time 2114 ms, echo time 76 ms) with dark-blood preparation, single-slice technique, breath-hold. Intermediate signal intensity of the round left atrial mass

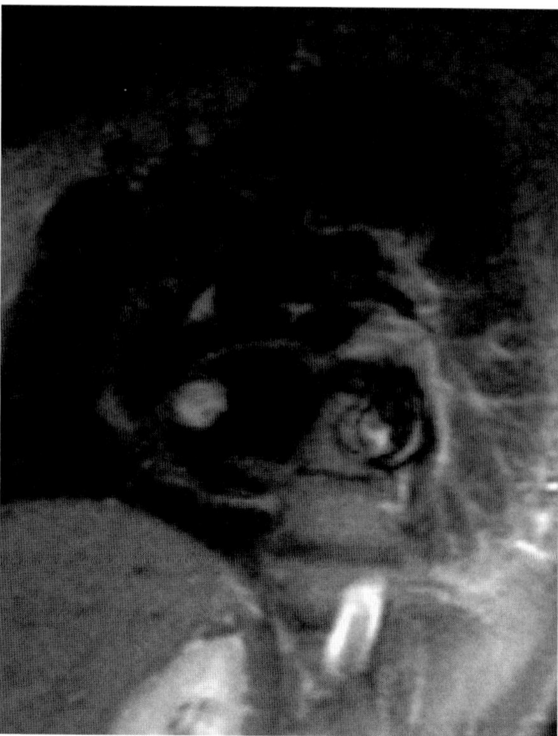

Fig. 12.30. Left atrial myxoma. Short-axis view. HASTE sequence (repetition time 800 ms, echo time 43 ms) with dark-blood preparation. High signal intensity of the well-shaped left atrial mass

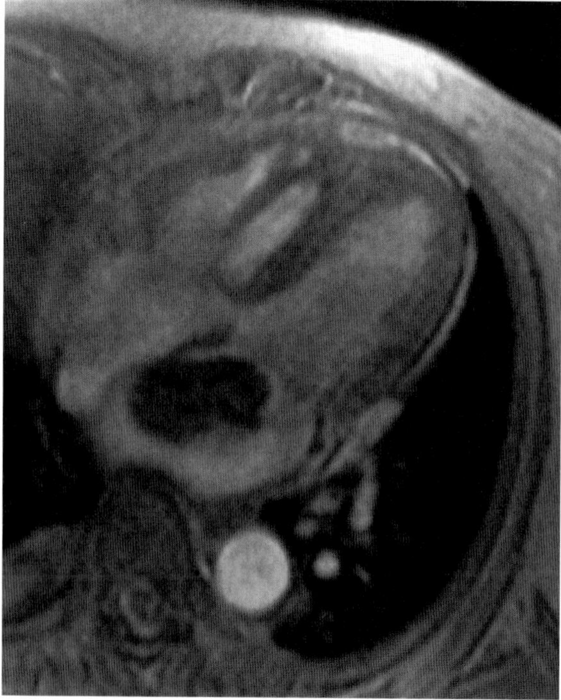

Fig. 12.31. Left atrial myxoma. Long-axis view. FLASH 2D sequence (repetition time 60 ms, echo time 4.8 ms), breath-hold technique. Low signal intensity of the large left atrial mass, acquisition in mid-systole

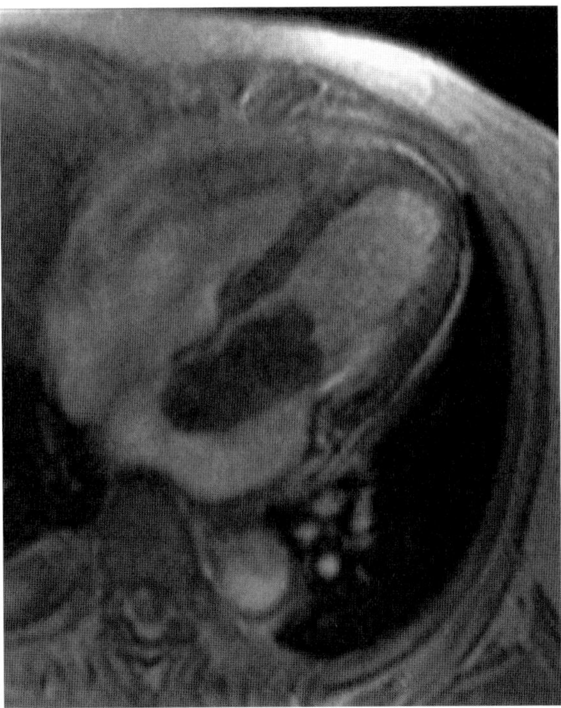

Fig. 12.32. Left atrial myxoma. Long-axis view. FLASH 2D sequence (repetition time 60 ms, echo time 4.8 ms), breath-hold technique. Low signal intensity of the large left atrial mass, end-diastolic acquisition. Herniation of the mass through the mitral valve into the left ventricle

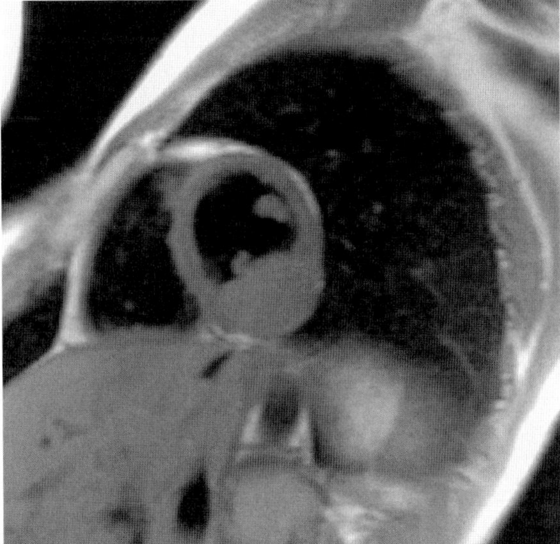

Fig. 12.33. Rhabdomyoma of the left ventricle. Short-axis view. T1-weighted TSE sequence (repetition time 809 ms, echo time 32 ms) with dark-blood preparation, single-slice technique, breath-hold. Large mass arising from the inferior wall of the left ventricle with isointense signal to the myocardium

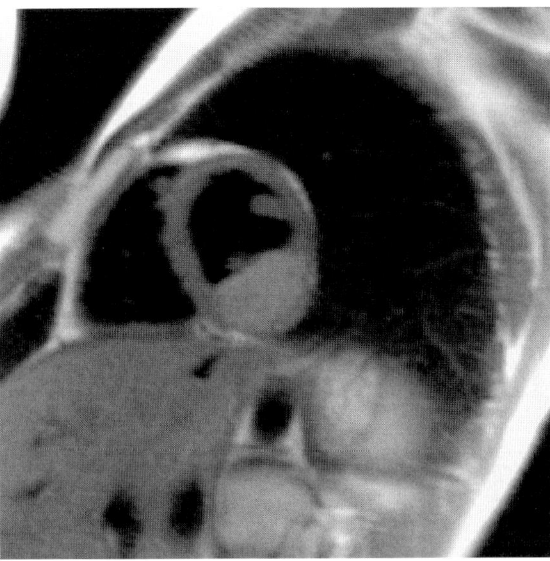

Fig. 12.34. Rhabdomyoma of the left ventricle. Short-axis view. HASTE sequence (repetition time 800 ms, echo time 43 ms) with dark-blood preparation. Large left ventricular wall mass with intermediate signal intensity

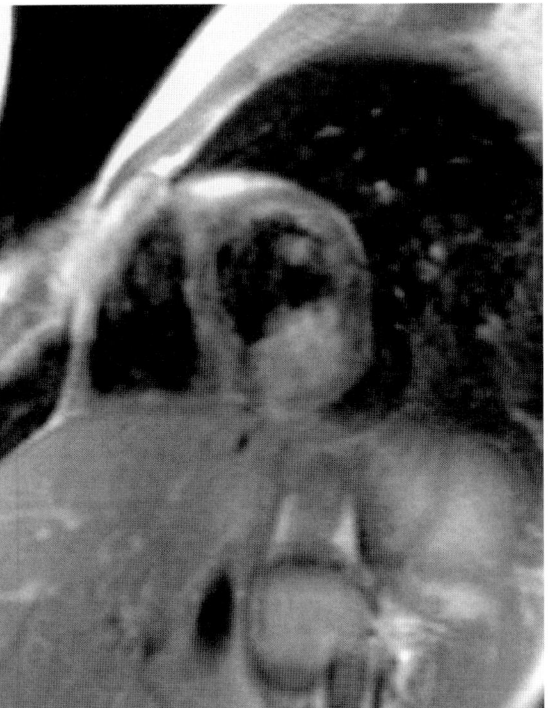

Fig. 12.35. Rhabdomyoma of the left ventricle. Short-axis view. T1-weighted TSE sequence (repetition time 809 ms, echo time 32 ms) after application of gadolinium chelate, 0.1 mmol/kg body weight, with dark-blood preparation, single-slice technique, breath-hold. Contrast enhancement of the tumor, higher than the enhancement of the normal myocardium

12.3.4.3.3 *Lipoma*

Lipomas are the second most common, primary, benign, cardiac tumors. They are typically located in the right atrium, but also in the left atrium and the ventricles. These tumors show a high signal in T1-WI and T2-WI, similar to epicardial or subcutaneous fat. Fat suppression or STIR techniques may contribute to establishing a diagnosis (Figs. 12.36–12.38).

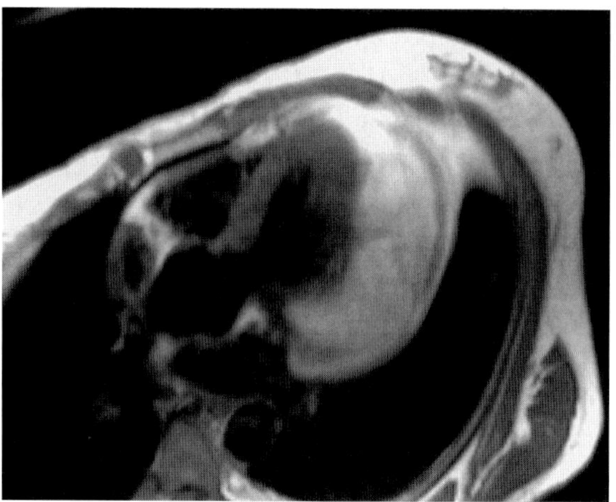

Fig. 12.36. Left ventricular lipoma. Long-axis view. T1-weighted TSE sequence (repetition time 688 ms, echo time 12 ms). Large left ventricular wall mass with high signal intensity, isointense to the epicardial fat

12.3.4.3.4 *Fibroma*

Fibromas are the second most common, benign, pediatric cardiac tumors, which primarily affect children but are detected occasionally in infants or in utero. They are often associated with cardiac arrhythmias, although up to 35% are asymptomatic. Patients with nevoid basal cell carcinoma syndrome (Gorlin syndrome) have an increased prevalence of cardiac fibromas. They arise most commonly from the interventricular septum or the free left ventricular wall. The signal intensity of the tumor is usually homogenous and hypointense on T2-WI and isointense to the myocardium on T1-WI with no or very little contrast enhancement after the application of gadolinium chelates.

12.3.4.3.5 *Angiosarcoma*

Angiosarcomas account for approximately one-third of primary malignant cardiac tumors and show a predilec-

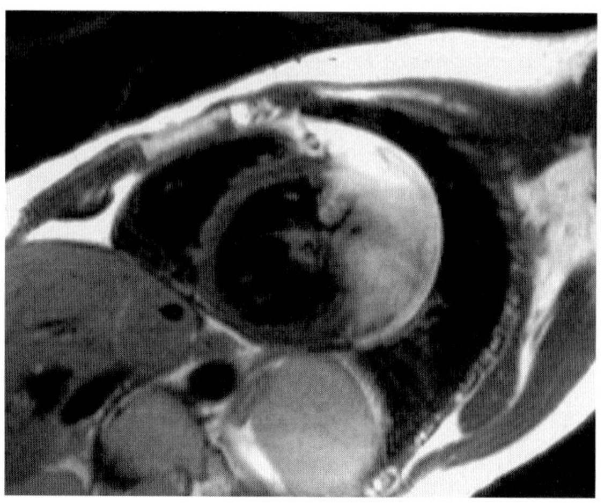

Fig. 12.37. Left ventricular lipoma. Short-axis view. T2-weighted TSE sequence (repetition time 1530 ms, echo time 76 ms) with dark-blood preparation, single-slice technique, breath-hold. The tumor shows a high signal, similar to the epicardial or subcutaneous fat

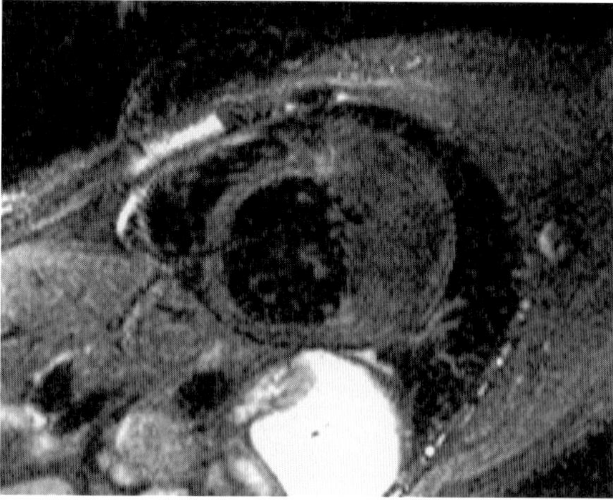

Fig. 12.38. Left ventricular lipoma. Short-axis view. Short tau inversion-recovery sequence (repetition time 1776 ms, echo time 76 ms) with dark-blood preparation, single-slice technique, breath-hold. Complete (fat) suppression of the signal of the tumor, establishing the diagnosis

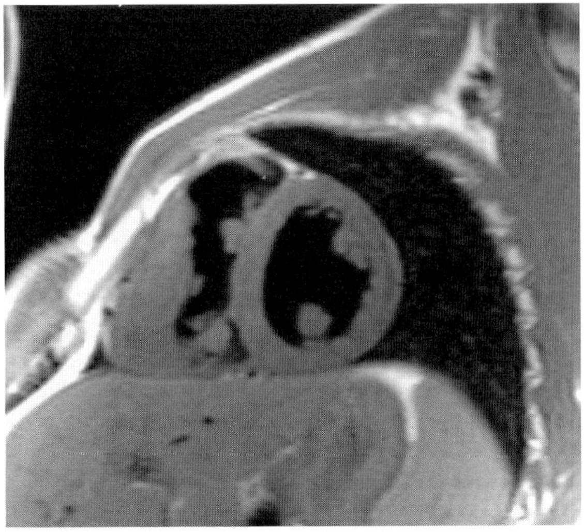

Fig. 12.39. Angiosarcoma of the right ventricle. Short-axis view. T1-weighted TSE sequence (repetition time 995 ms, echo time 32 ms) with dark-blood preparation, single-slice technique, breath-hold. Large right ventricular mass, arising from the free and subtricuspid right ventricular wall with intermediate signal intensity

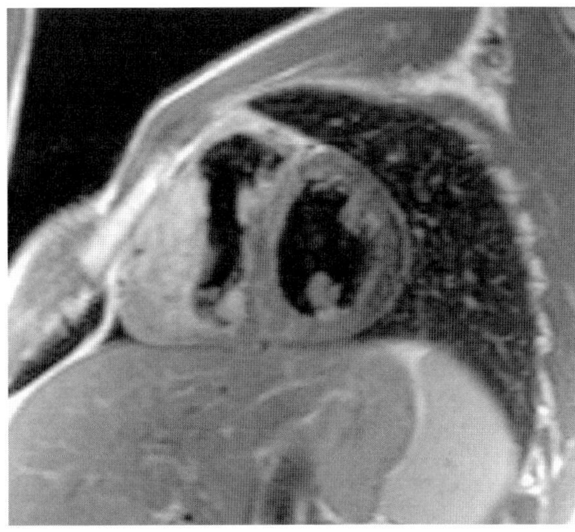

Fig. 12.40. Angiosarcoma of the right ventricle. Short-axis view. T1-weighted TSE sequence (repetition time 960 ms, echo time 32 ms) after application of gadolinium chelate, 0.1 mmol/kg body weight, with dark-blood preparation, single-slice technique, breath-hold. Large intramural mass of the right ventricle shows an increase in signal intensity after the application of contrast agent

tion for the right atrium. They have a propensity to involve the pericardium. Because of their vascular nature and site of origin, tamponade and right-sided heart failure are the most common clinical signs of angiosarcoma.

MR imaging of cardiac angiosarcomas most often reveals a cardiac mass arising from the right atrium. The signal intensity of the tumor is heterogeneous in T1-WI and T2-WI, with areas of high signal intensity representing blood-filled spaces that may also contain clots. Hemorrhagic pericardial effusion is frequently present due to pericardial involvement of the tumor (Figs. 12.39 and 12.40).

12.3.4.3.6 Leiomyosarcoma

Leiomyosarcoma is a rare malignant cardiac tumor (8%–9% of cardiac sarcomas) and often affects the left atrium in adults. Dyspnea is the most common symptom. MRI shows a large heterogeneous mass, often with pericardial or extracardiac invasion, and heterogeneous enhancement with central nonenhancing areas corresponding to tumor necrosis.

12.3.4.3.7 Lymphoma

Primary cardiac lymphoma (typically non-Hodgkin lymphomas) are very rare, although up to 30% of the patients with disseminated lymphoma have cardiac involvement. Often patients with acquired immunodeficiency syndrome are affected.

12.3.4.3.8 Secondary Cardiac Tumors

Secondary cardiac tumors are much more frequent (20–40 times more) than primary cardiac neoplasms and are found in up to 20% of patients with malignant tumors. They spread by direct extension, hematogenous or venous extension, or lymphatic extension. Bronchial carcinomas often invade the mediastinum and or the heart directly. Hematogenous extension was found with an incidence of up to 20% in autopsy studies of patients with malignant diseases, most commonly in patients with bronchial or breast carcinoma, melanomas, lymphomas, and leukemia. Isolated cardiac metastases are very unusual. Venous, intracaval extension is a very rare condition in patients with benign tumors, like leiomyomatosis of the uterus, or with malignant entities like hepatocellular carcinoma of the liver, renal-cell carcinoma, Wilms' tumor, pheochromocytoma, adrenocortical carcinoma, and thyroid carcinoma. Retrograde spread by lymphatic extension is found most commonly in patients with lymphoma and breast or bronchial carcinoma (Fig. 12.41).

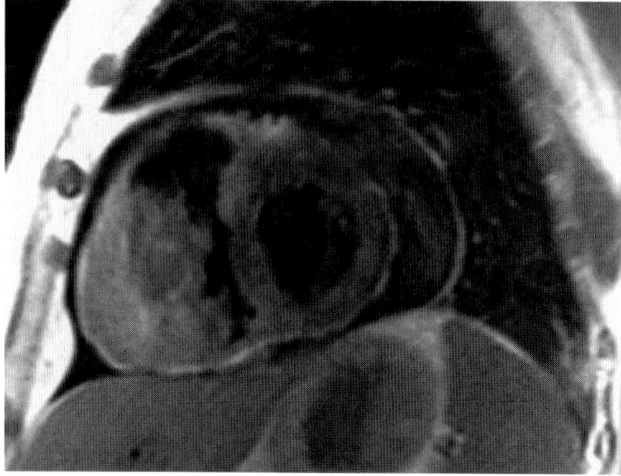

Fig. 12.41. Metastatic tumor (cervix carcinoma) of the right ventricle. Short-axis view. T1-weighted TSE sequence (repetition time 960 ms, echo time 32 ms) after application of gadolinium chelate, 0.1 mmol/kg body weight, with dark-blood preparation, single-slice technique, breath-hold. Large intramural mass of the right ventricle, pericardial effusion.

12.3.5 Valvular Diseases

12.3.5.1 Introduction

It was initially thought that MR imaging would be of little use in the evaluation of valvular heart disease. With advances in pulse sequence design and coil development, however, MR imaging now can be used to assess the pathoanatomy and pathophysiology associated with cardiac valvular diseases. Using MR imaging, it is possible to identify and quantify the severity of valvular disease and to monitor the effects of therapeutic interventions. Qualitative assessment of the severity of valvular stenosis and regurgitation is possible with cine MR imaging.

12.3.5.2 MR Imaging Protocol

Table 12.11 shows the protocol recommended for the assessment of patients with valvular heart disease.

Quantification of valvular regurgitation or valvular stenosis has become possible by employing phase-velocity mapping. Using this technique, phase shifts of protons within different voxels of the image are displayed at different gray levels, corresponding to the degree of phase shift. Motion is the major factor causing phase shift; phase shift is directly proportional to the degree of motion.

Table 12.11. MR imaging protocol recommended for valvular diseases

Sequence	WI	Plane	No. of slices	TR (ms)	TE (ms)	Flip angle	TI (ms)	Echo train length	Slice thickness (mm)	Matrix	FOV	recFOV (%)	No. of acq.	Acq. time (min:s)
TSE	T1	Long	11	600	12	180		3	6	160×256	320	75	5	>2:39
FL2D[b]	T1	Long	1	167	6.2	30			6	160×256	280	100	1	>0:10
TSE[b]	T1	Short	1	700	32	160		9	6	160×256	320	75	1	>0:10
FL2D[a]	T1	Short	1	60	4.8	20			6	128×256	320	75	1	>0:19

[a] Breath-hold, cine mode; [b] Breath-hold

Abbreviations: *WI* weighting of images; *TR* repetition time; *TI* inversion time; *TE* echo time; *Matrix* phase × frequency matrix; *FOV* field of view (mm); *recFOV* % rectangular field of view; *Acq.* acquisition(s)

12.3.5.3
MR Findings

12.3.5.3.1
Regurgitation

The volume of regurgitation across an incompetent valve is determined by the cross-sectional orifice, time, pressure difference, and total left ventricular stroke volume. Cine GRE techniques are sensitive for detecting regurgitant jets, because the signal intensity of the blood flow is altered by abnormal flow characteristics. The high velocity of regurgitant jets produces a signal void, thus demonstrating the presence of these lesions. High velocity with flow turbulence causes spin dephasing, which results in signal loss.

Valvular regurgitation is recognized by a signal void visible retrograde of the incompetent valve. With mitral and tricuspid regurgitation, the signal void jet appears during ventricular systole (Fig. 12.42). In patients with aortic or pulmonary regurgitation, the signal void jet appears during ventricular diastole (Fig. 12.43).

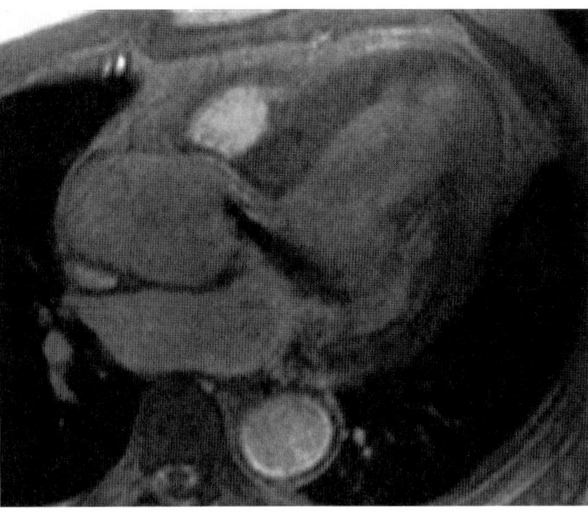

Fig. 12.43. Aortal regurgitation. Long-axis view. FLASH) 2D sequence (repetition time 60 ms, echo time 4.8 ms), breath-hold technique. Valvular regurgitation is recognized by a signal void visible retrograde of the aortic valve, appearing during ventricular diastole

12.3.5.3.2
Stenosis

In valvular stenosis, turbulent flow causes a signal void in the downstream great artery or ventricle. Estimation of the gradient across stenotic valves depends on the accurate measurement of the peak velocity in the central vena contracta region of the stenotic jet using velocity-encoded GRE techniques.

Evaluation of valvular heart diseases is incomplete without an assessment of the degree of left ventricular dysfunction. Therefore, it is necessary to acquire short-axis cine MR imaging from the base to the apex, which provides a 3D data set. This data set is used to measure left ventricular volumes (end-systolic and end-diastolic), ejection fraction, stroke volume, and ventricular mass. These parameters show variable sizes in the different valvular diseases of the heart.

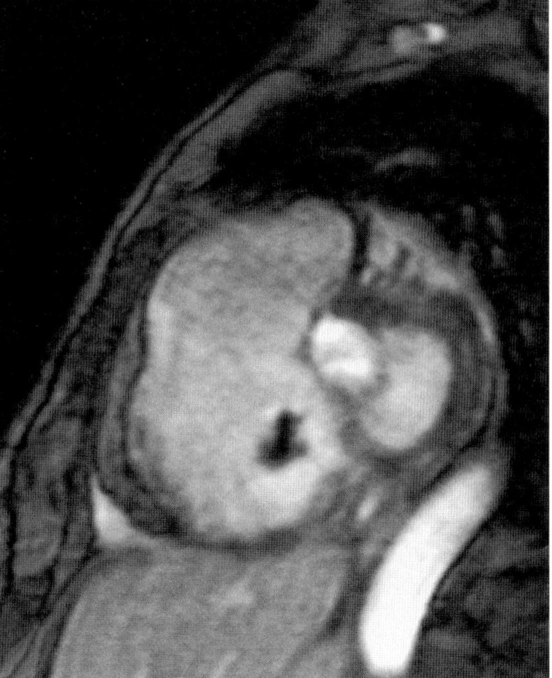

Fig. 12.42. Tricuspid regurgitation. Short-axis view. FLASH 2D sequence (repetition time 60 ms, echo time 4.8 ms), breath-hold technique. Valvular regurgitation is recognized by a signal void visible retrograde of the tricuspid valve, appearing during ventricular systole

12.3.6 Pericardial Diseases

12.3.6.1 Introduction

The pericardium is a fibroserous structure that consists of internal serous and external fibrous components. The serous component includes visceral and parietal layers. The fibrous component adheres to the diaphragm, and adipose tissue separates the outer pericardium from the sternum anteriorly. The pericardial space normally contains 15–50 ml of fluid.

12.3.6.2 MR Imaging Protocol

Table 12.12 demonstrates the recommended protocol (only morphological studies). If neoplastic pericardial disease is suspected, T1-W TSE are useful for pathological differentiation.

12.3.6.3 MR Findings

12.3.6.3.1 Normal Pericardium

The normal pericardium appears as a curvilinear line of low signal intensity between the high or medium signal intensity of the external pericardial fat and the internal epicardial fat. Its normal thickness ranges >from 1 mm to 2 mm; however, a width of up to 4 mm is not necessarily pathological. Some parts of the pericardium may not be visible because of a lack of epicardial fat in some regions.

12.3.6.3.2 Pericardial Effusion

Common causes of pericardial effusion are viral or idiopathic pericarditis, neoplasia, uremia, trauma, collagen vascular diseases, postpericardectomy or postinfarction (Dressler) syndromes, and acquired immunodeficiency syndrome (AIDS). The distribution of pericardial fluid is frequently asymmetrical. The signal characteristics are fluid-like with low signal intensity in T1-WI and high signal intensity in T2-WI (Fig. 12.44). In cases of hemorrhagic or proteinaceous pericardial effusion, T1-WI often show areas of medium or high signal intensity.

12.3.6.3.3 Constrictive Pericarditis

Constrictive pericarditis limits diastolic filling of the heart due to thickening and fibrosis of the pericardium (Fig. 12.45). Presenting symptoms are often similar to those of restrictive cardiomyopathy, but the differentiation between these two conditions is essential, because the treatment of choice for patients with constrictive pericarditis is surgical pericardectomy.

MR imaging effectively demonstrates pericardial thickening (greater than 4 mm). Patients with a history of cardiac surgery or postpericardectomy syndrome may have significant pericardial thickening without

Table 12.12. MR imaging protocol recommended for pericardial diseases

Sequence	WI	Plane	No. of slices	TR (ms)	TE (ms)	Flip angle	TI (ms)	Echo train length	Slice thickness (mm)	Matrix	FOV	recFOV (%)	No. of acq.	Acq. time (min:s)
TSE	T1	Long	11	600	12	180		3	6	160×256	320	75	5	>2:39
TSE [b]	T1	Short	1	700	32	160		9	6	160×256	320	75	1	>0:10
TSE [b]	T2	Short	1	800	57	160		15	6	160×256	320	75	1	>0:11
or														
HASTE	T2	Short	21	800	43	150			6	160×256	320	75	1	>0:31
TSE [a]	T1	Long	11	600	12	180		3	6	160×256	320	75	5	>2:39
TSE [a,b]	T1	Short	1	700	32	160		9	6	160×256	320	75	1	>0:10

[a] Post gadolinium, only if neoplatic pericardial is suspected; [b] Breath-hold

Abbreviations: *WI* weighting of images; *TR* repetition time; *TI* inversion time; *TE* echo time; *Matrix* phase × frequency matrix; *FOV* field of view (mm); *recFOV* % rectangular field of view; *Acq.* acquisition(s)

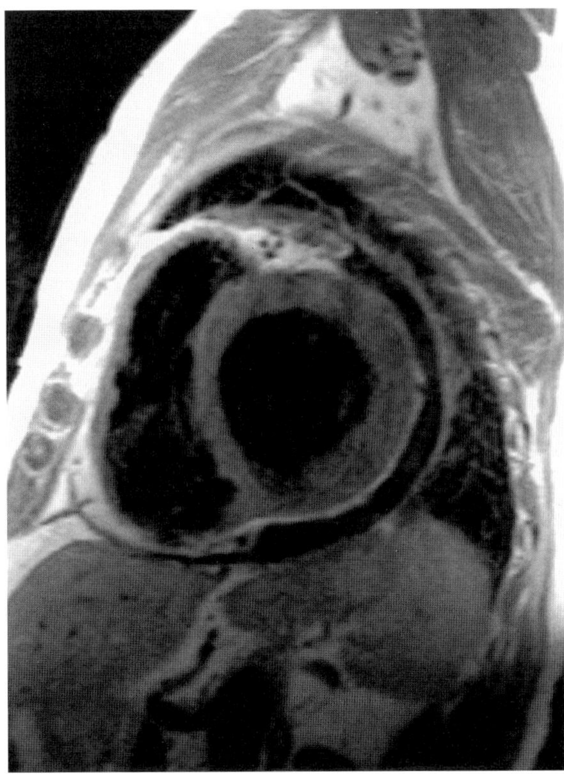

Fig. 12.44. Pericardial effusion. Short-axis view. T1-weighted TSE sequence (repetition time 1076 ms, echo time 32 ms) with dark-blood preparation, single-slice technique, breath-hold. Fluid-like signal characteristics with low signal intensity. Asymmetric distribution of the pericardial fluid

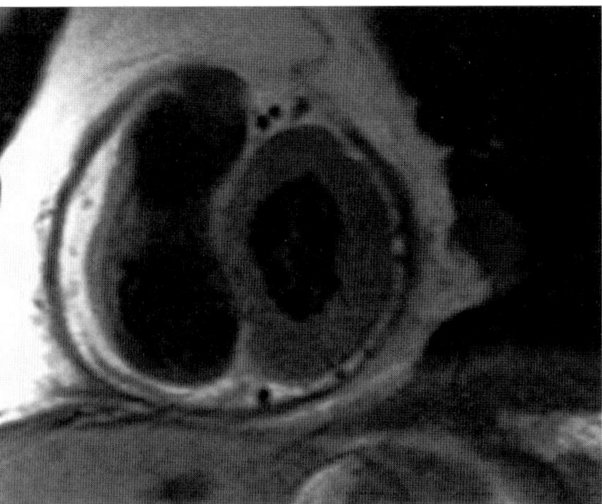

Fig. 12.45. Constrictive pericarditis. Short-axis view. T1-weighted TSE sequence (repetition time 972 ms, echo time 32 ms) with dark-blood preparation, single-slice technique, breath-hold. Thickening of the pericardium up to 6 mm

underlying constrictive pericarditis. Other MR imaging findings include narrow, tubular-shaped ventricles, dilatation of the right atrium, inferior vena cava, and hepatic veins. Ascites and pleural effusion may be present.

12.3.6.3.4 Pericardial Cyst

Pericardial cysts are benign developmental lesions formed within the embryonic pericardium. Most cysts are well-marginated and contain clear fluid. They are typically located in the right anterior cardiophrenic angle and occur less often in the left cardiophrenic angle. Most patients are asymptomatic. The cysts typically have a round or ovoid appearance and demonstrate low signal intensity on T1-WI and high signal intensity in T2-WI. This may be different for complicated cysts (hemorrhagic or proteinaceous).

12.3.6.3.5 Neoplastic Pericardial Disease

Primary neoplasms are very rare; secondary involvement is much more frequent and commonly results from lung and breast carcinoma, melanoma, lymphoma, and leukemia. Neoplastic pericardial involvement may present different signal characteristics on MR imaging. It may demonstrate pericardial effusion and regional pericardial thickening.

12.3.7 Congenital Heart Disease

12.3.7.1 Introduction

MR imaging can be applied to assess the cardiac anatomy and cardiovascular function, and to measure volumetric flow both before and after the treatment of patients with congenital heart disease. ECG-gated SE and ultra-fast TSE (HASTE) sequences are very useful in the evaluation of the complex anatomy (in variable

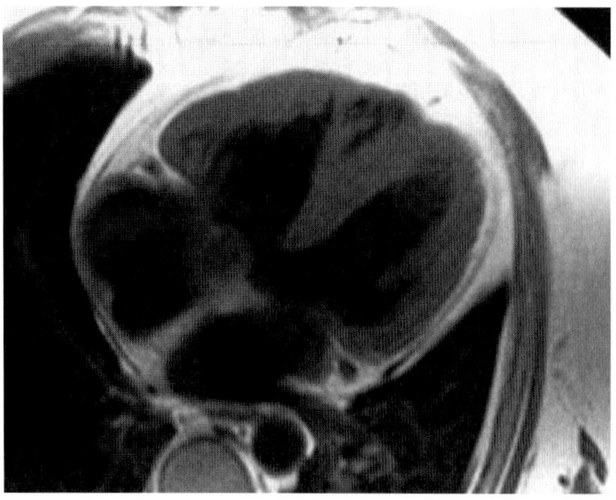

Fig. 12.46. Ventricular septal defect (VSD). Long-axis view. T1-weighted TSE sequence (repetition time 972 ms, echo time 32 ms) with dark-blood preparation, single-slice technique, breath-hold. Subvalvular defect of the ventricular septum

axes) of these patients. Cine mode studies (GRE images) are applied to detect stenosis, regurgitation, and left-to-right shunts and to visualize surgical anastomoses and conduits following treatment. With multisection cine mode MR imaging, it is possible to measure global left and right ventricular function. MR velocity-encoded GRE techniques measure peak blood flow velocities and are therefore useful for the quantitative assessment of hemodynamics. These possibilities make MR imaging a useful comprehensive tool for the follow-up of congenital heart disease (Figs. 12.46–12.48).

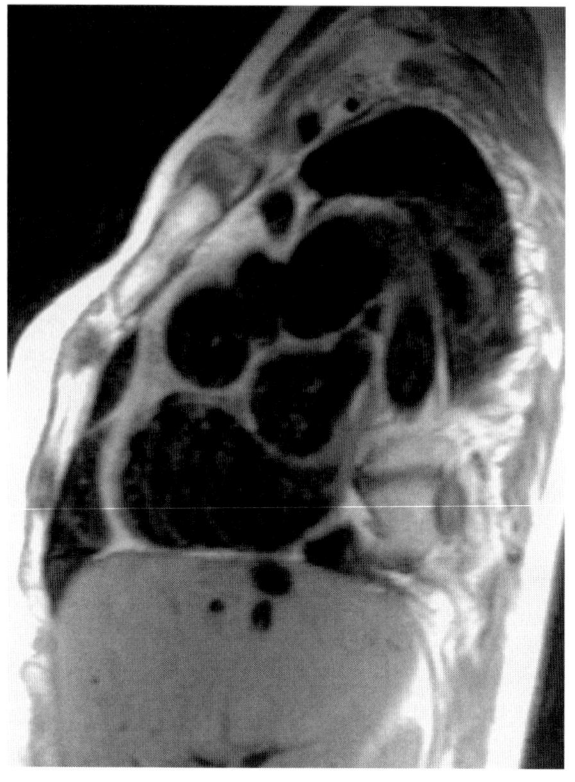

Fig. 12.47. Correction of Fallot's tetralogy. Short-axis view. T1-weighted TSE sequence (repetition time 1030 ms, echo time 32 ms) with dark-blood preparation, single-slice technique, breath-hold. Postoperative evaluation after correction of Fallot's tetralogy with ASD and VSD patch and reconstruction of the right ventricular outflow tract. Enlargement of the right atrium and the pulmonary arteries

12.3.7.2 MR Imaging Protocol

Table 12.13 shows a combined MR imaging protocol with morphological studies, cine-mode studies, flow quantification, and gadolinium-enhanced MR angiography studies. The usefulness of these different techniques depends on the clinical question.

12.3.7.3 MR Findings

Analysis of complex anatomical details in patients with congenital heart disease and complex cardiovascular malformation is best done using step-by-step analysis of the segmental anatomy. This approach is based on the premise that the three cardiac segments (atria, ventricles, and great arteries) develop independently of one another and includes the assessment of atrial situs, ventricular morphology, atrioventricular connections, position and morphology of the great vessels, ventriculoarterial connections, and associated defects or post-surgical findings.

The normal atrial situs situation is atrial situs solitus. The morphological left atrium is located on the left side of the patient; the morphological right atrium is located on the right side. The morphological right atrium receives the hepatic venous drainage and the vena cava. It contains an appendage with a triangular configuration and has a wide base of implantation into the atrial chamber. The left atrium contains an appendage

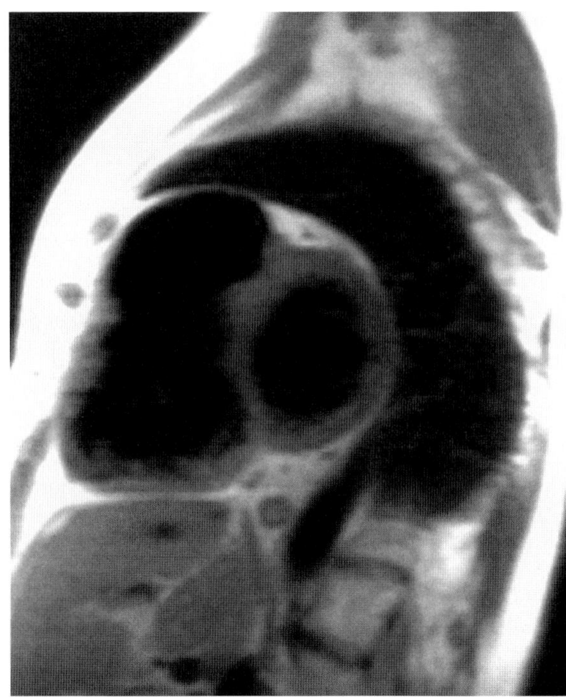

Fig. 12.48. Correction of Fallot's tetralogy. Short-axis view. Half-Fourier acquired single-shot TSE sequence (repetition time 800 ms, echo time 43 ms) with dark-blood preparation. Postoperative evaluation after correction of Fallot's tetralogy with ASD and VSD patch and reconstruction of the right ventricular outflow tract. Severe enlargement of the right ventricle

that is usually longer and thinner than the right atrium appendage and receives the pulmonary veins. In atrial situs inversus, one can find a mirror-image of the normal morphological arrangement.

The morphological right and left ventricles can be distinguished in MR images by observing their different characteristics. Short-axis MR images usually reveal a landmark moderator band in the morphological right ventricle. The trabecular pattern of the right ventricle is coarse, whereas the interior of the left ventricle is smooth. The septal attachment of the atrioventricular valve is closer to the apex in the right ventricle. An important morphological characteristic of the morphological right ventricle is an infundibulum that separates the tricuspid and pulmonary valves. The left ventricle has no infundibulum; there is fibrous continuity between the mitral and aortic valve.

Following evaluation of atrial situs and ventricular morphology, atrioventricular connections are identified. If blood flows from the morphological right atrium through the tricuspid valve into the right ventricle, and from the left atrium through the mitral valve into the left ventricle, there is atrioventricular concordance. Ventriculoarterial concordance exists when the right ventricle supports the pulmonary valve and pulmonary artery, and the left morphological ventricle contains the aortic valve and aorta. Transposition of the great arteries is visualized in various MR imaging planes. Ventriculoarterial discordance occurs in two important lesions, D-transposition and congenitally corrected transposition of the great arteries. This results in parallel pulmonary and systemic circulation in the absence of a shunt, and is not compatible with life.

Table 12.13. MR imaging protocol recommended for congenital heart diseases

Sequence	WI	Plane	No. of slices	TR (ms)	TE (ms)	Flip angle	TI (ms)	Echo train length	Slice thickness (mm)	Matrix	FOV	recFOV (%)	No. of acq.	Acq. time (min:s)
TSE	T1	Var	11	600	12	180		3	6	160×256	320	75	5	>2:39
HASTE	T2	Var	21	800	43	150			6	160×256	320	75	1	>0:31
FL2D[d]	T1	Long	1	167	6.2	30			6	160×256	280	100	1	>0:10
FL2D[a,d]	T1	Short	1	60	4.8	20			6	160×256	320	75	1	>0:19
FL2D[b]	T1	Var	1	25	6	30			6	160×256	300	75	2	>3:00
FISP3D[c,d]	T1	Var	Slab	5.0	2.0				2	160×256	320	100	1	>0:26

[a] Cine mode; [b] Flow quantification, in plane; [c] Angiography, gadolinium enhanced; [d] Breath-hold
Abbreviations: *WI* weighting of images; *TR* repetition time; *TI* inversion time; *TE* echo time; *Matrix* phase × frequency matrix; *FOV* field of view (mm); *recFOV* % rectangular field of view; *Acq.* acquisition(s)

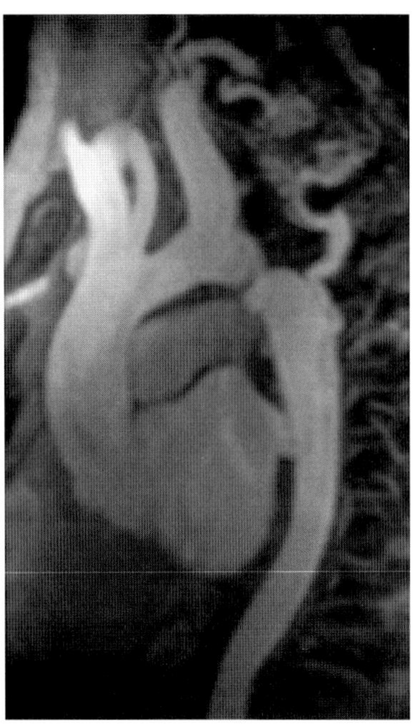

Fig. 12.49. Coarctation of the aorta. Oblique view, maximum intensity projection. Fast imaging into steady precession (FISP) 3D sequence (repetition time 5.0 ms, echo time 2.0 ms) after application of gadolinium chelate, 0.1 mmol/kg body weight. Postductal coarctation of the aorta with marked caliber difference. Collaterals from the left subclavian artery and the intercostal arteries

The aorta and pulmonary artery are defined by their usual branching pattern. Anomalies of the aortic arch are common, and the most common symptomatic congenital lesion is coarctation (Fig. 12.49). This is defined as a constriction of the aorta near the junction of the ductus arteriosus and the aortic arch. In aortic coarctation, MR velocity-encoded GRE images may show the functional significance of this anomaly.

MR imaging is useful for detecting pulmonary artery malformations. The pulmonary valve is normally supported by the right ventricular infundibulum and lies anterior, superior, and to the left of the aortic arch. Pulmonary arterial abnormalities, including pulmonary artery sling and origin from the ductus arteriosus, can be demonstrated directly. Marked dilatation of the pulmonary artery may be seen in patients with valvular stenosis or in pulmonary insufficiency. The final step in MR imaging is to identify and characterize any associated defect (e.g., atrial or ventricular septal defects) and to assess the postoperative situation.

Further Reading

Arlart IP, Bongartz GM, Marchal G (eds) (2002) Magnetic Resonance Angiography – 2nd Revised Edition, Springer, Berlin Heidelberg New York

Boxt LM (ed) (1996) Cardiac MR Imaging. In: Magnetic resonance imaging clinics of North America. Saunders, Philadelphia, pp 4

Braunwald E, Zipes DP, Libby P (eds) (2001) Heart Disease. A textbook of cardiovascular medicine – 6th ed., W.B. Saunders Company, Philadelphia

Duerinckx AJ (ed) (2002) Coronary magnetic resonance angiography, Springer, Berlin Heidelberg New York

Higgins CB, Ingwall JS, Pohost GM (eds) (1998) Current and future applications of magnetic resonance in cardiovascular disease (American Heart Association monograph series), Futura Publishing Company, New York

Manning WJ, Pennell DJ (eds) (2002) Cardiovascular magnetic resonance, Churchill Livingstone, Philadelphia

Skorton DJ, Schelbert HR, Wolf GL, Brundage BH (1996) Marcus Cardiac imaging: a companion to Braunwald's heart disease, 2nd edn. Saunders, Philadelphia

Large Vessels and Peripheral Vessels

13

M. Boos, J. M. Meaney

Contents

13.1 Introduction

Magnetic resonance angiography (MRA) is a noninvasive method which provides images similar to those obtained by digital subtraction angiography (DSA). Blood motion causes two phenomena that change longitudinal and transverse spin magnetization, both of which can be exploited to generate angiographic images. Firstly, time-of-flight (TOF) effects arise from the movement of longitudinal magnetization during a relatively long period. Secondly, a flow phenomenon occurs when transverse magnetization moves in the direction of a magnetic field gradient. These effects can be exploited to generate 'time-of-flight' and 'phase-contrast' angiographic images, respectively, without the use of contrast medium, and their use in clinical practice reflects the state-of-the-art technology available at the time (see also Chap. 1).

Non-contrast techniques, although accurate in clinical practice for many indications, have many limitations such as intravoxel dephasing, saturation-effects, high reliance on appropriate choice of the velocity-encoding (Venc) gradient, and long scan times. Contrast-enhanced techniques overcome most of these problems associated with non-contrast-techniques. Although intracranial MRA still relies heavily on non-contrast techniques, contrast-enhanced techniques have supplanted non-contrast techniques for almost all applications within the body since their introduction by Prince in 1994 due to their high spatial resolution, high contrast-to-noise ratios, ease of performance and short scan times.

13.1.1 Patient Preparation for MRA

No special patient preparation and no special positioning are necessary for MRA. If echocardiogram (ECG) gating is used for two-dimensional (2D) PC MRA or sequential (2D) TOF MRA, electrodes must be appropriately placed on the patient. For thoracic and abdominal imaging where breath-holding is required, the patient should be instructed and coached in breath-holding. Use of oxygen via nasal prongs and hyperventilation prior to the breath-hold scan may be appropriate, especially for contrast-enhanced MRA. It is helpful to exercise breath-holding with the patient using slight hyperventilation prior to a moderate inspiration.

13.1.2 Coils

All available coils are suitable for MRA. The integral body coil is used for signal transmission, and either the standard body or, preferably, phased-array (wrap-around) coils are used for signal reception. Dedicated neck and peripheral coils are useful for selective MR angiograms of the carotid arteries and peripheral arteries, respectively.

13.2 MRA Techniques

13.2.1 Time-of-Flight MRA

For neuro-MRA applications, the most widely employed method of performing TOF angiograms is a 3D acquisition, mainly used to visualize the intracranial vessels and carotid bifurcation. A big advantage of the 3D technique is that thin slices can be acquired. This results in diminished intravoxel phase dispersions and fewer signal voids. In addition, 3D acquisitions give high resolution and sufficient signal-to-noise ratio (SNR), ideal for visualizing the small peripheral intracranial vessels (Figs. 13.1 and 13.2). Finally, because of thick slab excitation, radiofrequency (RF) pulses of short duration can be used, thus allowing shorter echo times (TE), with resultant less dephasing. In comparison with 3D techniques, 2D (sequential-slice) techniques are more useful for visualizing slow flow (e.g. the venous circulation) and for acquiring data over a long segment where 3D techniques are inappropriate due to progressive saturation within the imaging slab as a result of the flowing spins experiencing multiple excitations during the 3D acquisition (Fig. 13.2D). Therefore, the 2D technique and not the 3D technique can be applied to imaging of vessels over large distances (such as the complete carotid arteries and peripheral arteries).

Prior to introduction of contrast-enhanced MRA, the 2D sequential-slice MRA technique was the most commonly used technique for evaluation of the large vessels of the abdomen, thorax and peripheries. However, the larger voxel size (2D slices are typically 2–4 mm thick compared with the effective slice thickness of 1 mm or less of 3D volumes) combined with a longer TE results in an increased intravoxel phase dispersion and, as a result, saturation effects. Saturation effects lead to diminished intravascular SNR and, in severe cases, signal voids, which cause exaggeration of the degree of stenosis and artefactual stenosis and occlusions. These are most marked in vessels with slow flow and in those which run in the plane of image acquisition.

Additional flow voids and artifacts occur due to the arterial blood flow pulsation resulting from reverse flow during diastole of the cardiac cycle, an effect which is particularly marked in the peripheral arteries, where reversal of flow during diastole is frequent in patients with severe arterio-occlusive disease. This effect can be partially overcome by use of ECG gating; however, one of the main disadvantages of the 2D-TOF technique is the long scan time of about 40–60 min to screen the pelvis and lower extremities, which is prolonged further by ECG gating. Additionally, bone marrow and subcutaneous fat present a relatively bright signal intensity on TOF MRA. This can be addressed by use of fat-saturation techniques, although this incurs a further time penalty. Because of the relatively long TE, severe intravascular signal loss is encountered around prosthetic hip and knee replacements, an effect that cannot be easily minimized (this artifact is minimal with CE MRA because of the shorter TE used). Despite the many limitations of 2D TOF MRA, which limit its usefulness in many instances, it remains widely available and is used for selective indications in many institutions. For example, substantially more distal run-off vessels can be shown with TOF MRA compared with conventional

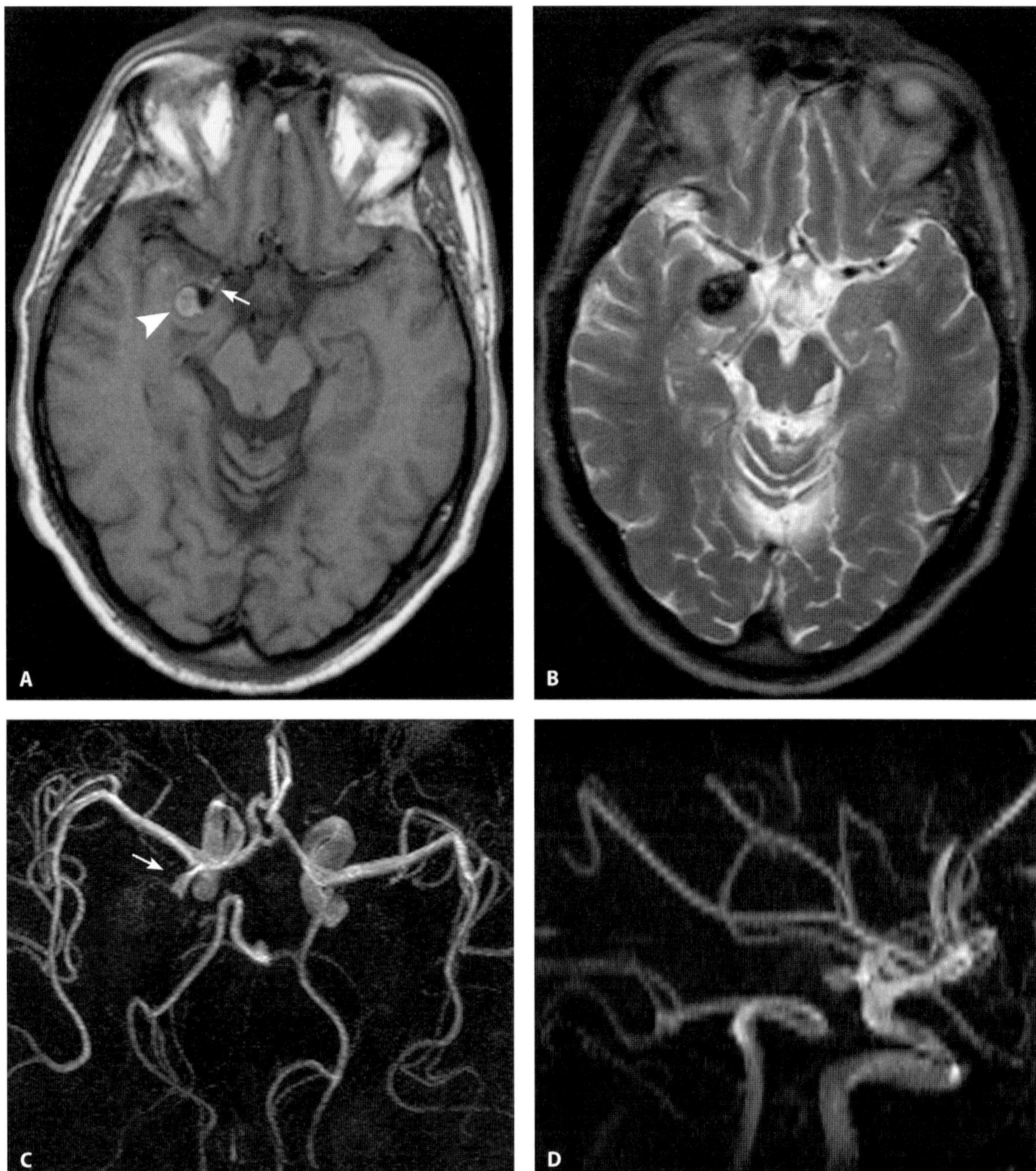

Fig. 13.1A–E. Patient with large aneurysm of the right middle cerebral artery which was treated by coiling. Follow-up MRI study was performed first as standard T1-weighted and T2-W SE and TSE technique (**A**,**B**). The aneurysm filled with the coil material gave susceptibility artifacts. It was not clear whether the aneurysm sac was patent or not. MIP of the 3D TOF MRA (MTS) showed no signal from flowing blood within the aneurysm (**C**,**D**). However, in order to improve diagnostic confidence, the TOF source images (**E**) should be evaluated. No perfusion was detected (*large arrow* neck of coiled aneurysm). The slightly increased signal within the aneurysm was due to thrombus (*arrowheads*)

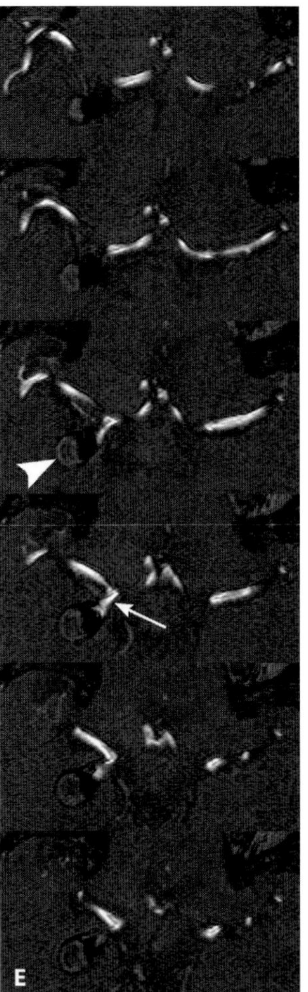

Fig. 13.1E.

angiography, because of its exquisite sensitivity to slow flow. However, because of the long scan times, this technique is restricted in most institutions to evaluation of the distal thigh, calf, and foot vessels.

13.2.1.1
Optimization Strategies in Time-of-Flight MRA

Flow-related enhancement can be improved by using gradient-motion rephasing (GMR or flow compensation), in which an additional gradient pulse is used to eliminate flow-related phase shifts. Use of gadolinium (Gd)-chelates improves visualization of distal vessels within the brain, but also results in overlay of venous structures and a higher signal from surrounding tissue (Fig. 13.2B). An appropriate balance between repetition time (TR) and flip-angle is necessary to decrease the relative signal intensity of stationary tissue and, conversely, increase the signal intensities of flowing blood. A reasonable compromise is to use a moderate flip-angle (30–60°) in conjunction with a shorter TR in instances where vessel orientation ensures good through-plane flow, and a somewhat longer TR and smaller flip-angle for vessels where slow flow or in-plane flow is anticipated (Table 13.1).

In conclusion, there are six ways to reduce saturation effects and increase the inflow-related signal intensity in TOF MRA:

1. Ensure that images are acquired orthogonal to the direction of flow
2. Increasing TR
3. Decreasing flip-angle

Table 13.1. Effect of changing various sequence parameters

Parameter		2D TOF MRA		Parameter		3D TOF MRA	
Change	Action	Effect		Change	Action	Effect	
TE	↓	Dephasing, flow voids	↓	TE	↓	Dephasing (higher order motion)	↓
TR	↓	Background suppression, measurement time	↓	TR	↓	Intraluminal signal, measurement time	↑ ↓
FA	↑	Intraluminal signal, background suppression	↑ ↑	FA	↑	Inflow saturation, background suppression	↓ ↑
Slice thickness	↓	Intraluminal signal (slow flow)	↑	Slice thickness	↓	Resolution dephasing	↑ ↓
No. of slices	↑	FOV in flow direction	↑	No. of slices	↑	Resolution, measurement time	↑ ↑
FOV	↓	Resolution dephasing	↑ ↓	FOV	↓	Resolution dephasing	↑ ↓

TOF, time-of-flight; D, dimension; MRA, magnetic resonance angiography; TE, echo time; TR, repetition time; FOV, field-of-view

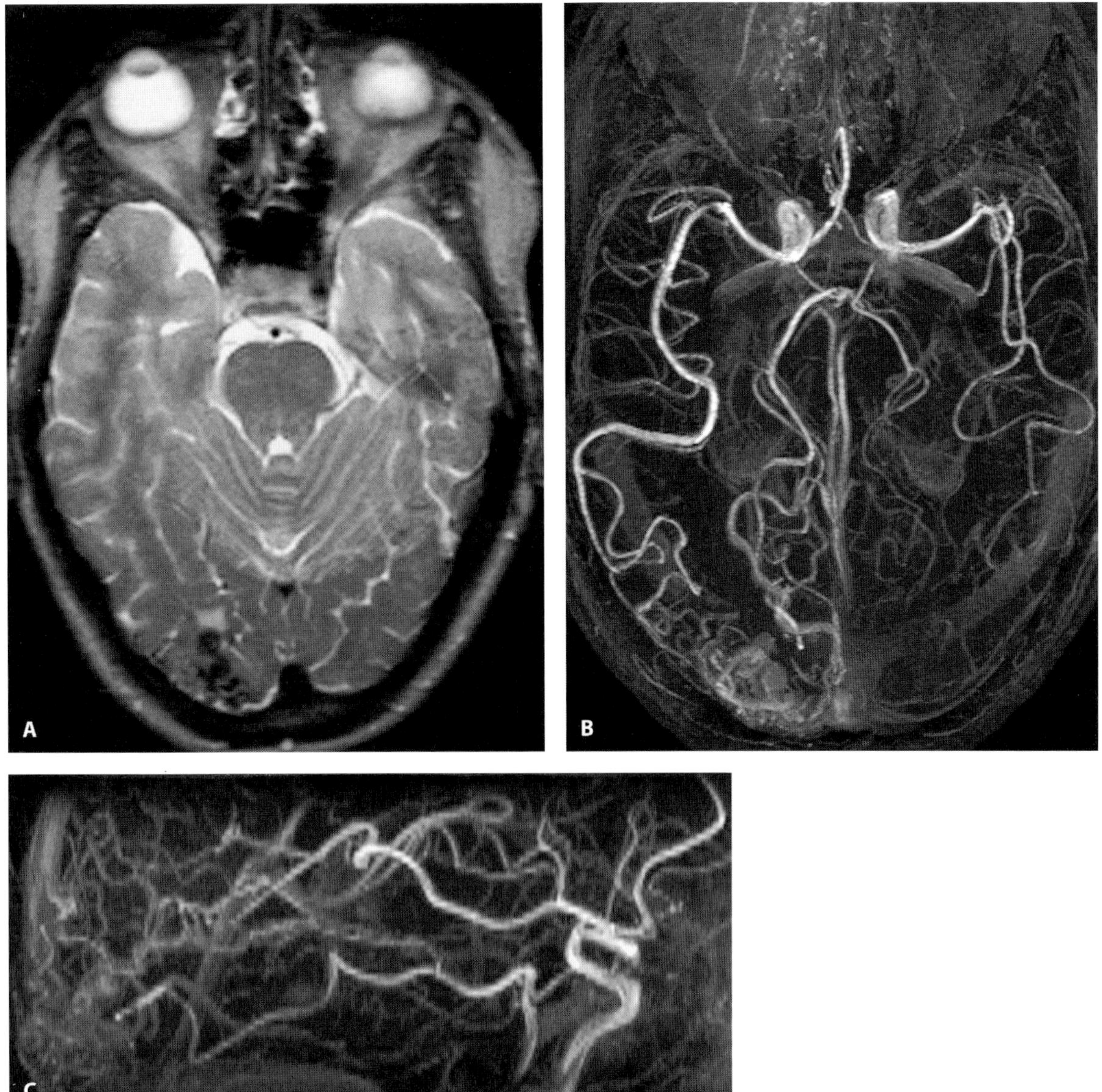

Fig. 13.2A–D. Patient with a vascular malformation of the right posterior hemisphere. On conventional T2-W image (**A**), multiple areas with signal loss (flow voids) suspicious of a vascular lesion were identified. Therefore, a contrast-enhanced 3D TOF MRA was performed (**B**,**C** show the MIP). The peripheral cerebral vessels were much better visualized using contrast agent at the cost of higher signal intensity of background compared with non-contrast TOF MRA (see Fig. 13.1). The middle and posterior cerebral arteries were well demonstrated. The 2D TOF MR angiogram (**D**) was sufficient to visualize the slow flow within the venous draining vessels

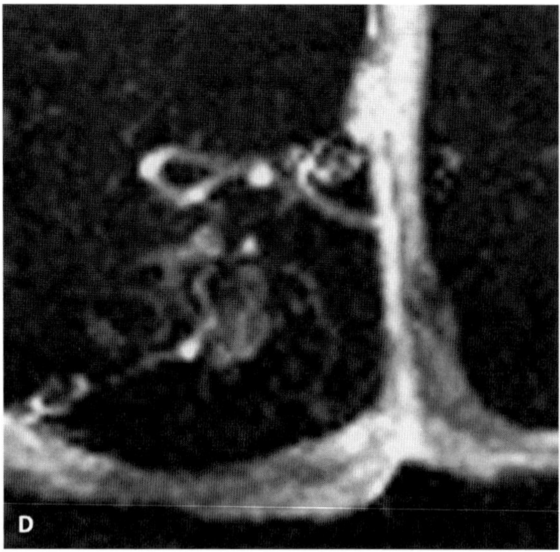

Fig. 13.2D

Table 13.2. Tools to reduce the effects causing stenosis overestimation on MRA images

Stenosis overestimation by	Effects	Reduce the effects by
Flow acceleration	Dephasing during TE	↓ TE (TOF)
Turbulent flow Vortex flow		↑ VENC (PC)
Stream separation distal to stenosis		↑ Resolution, dose (CE MRA)
Vessel tortuosity	Dose	CE MRA
Overlay of vessels within one voxel (PC MRA)	Dephasing → signal loss	Small volume TOF or CE MRA

CE, contrast enhanced; PC, phase contrast; VENC, velocity encoding gradient determining the sensitivity to flow velocity; TOF, time-of-flight; MRA, magnetic resonance angiography; TE, echo time

4. Multiple, overlapping, thin-slab acquisition (MOTSA)
5. Tilted, optimized, non-saturating excitation (TONE)
6. Use contrast medium (CM) (not commonly implemented for TOF MRA because of increased venous signal)

TOF-MRA can be further optimized by reducing pixel size and using magnetization transfer (MT) pulses; protons bound to macromolecules become saturated by applying a RF pulse, shifted 1500 Hz from water. The bound protons interact with the surrounding water, and the saturation is transferred to nearby water, resulting in improved suppression of the brain or muscle signal (Fig. 13.1B).

MOTSA (multiple, overlapping, thin-slice acquisition) is a combination of the 2D-TOF and 3D-TOF techniques to reduce the saturation effects associated with a thick slab. Multiple thin 3D slabs are used which overlap by approximately 30%. The MOTSA technique allows the use of higher flip-angles, providing both higher signal intensities and increased background suppression. The final imaging volume is created by extracting the central slices of each slab and discarding the slices at the top and bottom of the volume (which are more affected by saturation effects). The main drawback of this technique is the 'Venetian-blind' artifact due to differences in signal intensity between adjacent 3D volumes at the points where the slabs overlap.

Saturation of intraluminal signal additionally occurs as the blood flows into the excitation slab. By applying a specially designed ramped RF pulse (TONE), which produces a progressively higher flip-angle during movement across the slice, the saturation effects can be minimized. This allows better visualization of distal vessels and those with slow flow.

13.2.1.2
Reasons for Overestimation of Stenosis

It is well-known that stenosis can be overestimated by MRA. The main reasons for this are listed in Table 13.2, along with some features that reduce this effect.

13.2.1.3
Black-Blood MRA

Black-blood MRA is not just a photo negative of bright-blood MRA. Rapidly flowing blood (arterial flow) demonstrates flow-related signal loss, whereas slow-flowing blood (venous flow) has a higher signal intensity. A longer TE is used (20–30 ms) compared with standard T1-W imaging to maximize the black-blood effect. This TE is similar to the TR used to maximize intravascular signal loss for TOF MRA, as both techniques rely on the same phenomenon of movement of excited protons out of the imaging volume. Various presaturation and dephasing pulses can be employed in this technique to render flowing blood black.

The advantages of this method include absence of any dephasing artifact (this is the goal of black-blood MRA). which leads to less overestimation of the degree of stenosis. However, a significant disadvantage is that calcified plaques and other black materials may also be isointense with flowing blood, thus leading to underestimation of the degree of stenosis.

13.2.1.4 Postprocessing of the 3D Time-of-Flight MRA Data Set

The maximum-intensity projection (MIP) is the standard-bearer of postprocessing techniques for all types of bright-blood MRA. However, MIP has substantial drawbacks. Areas of diminished flow, including the edges of blood vessels and small vessels with slow flow, result in poor contrast between flowing blood and stationary tissues and thus poor or absent depiction on the reprojected image. Whole vessels or vessel segments may be obscured by overlap of brighter stationary tissue, especially fat. As a result, the apparent vessel lumen may be falsely narrowed and stenoses exaggerated (Fig. 13.3). As the MIP is non-selective, all bright objects are reprojected into the final image if sufficiently bright. Therefore, fresh extraluminal blood which appears bright on TOF MRA due to its short T1 (e.g. in patients with intraparenchymal brain hemorrhage) may obscure detail of vessels; clearly this is not a limitation for PC MRA as the stationary blood appears dark. Therefore, it is essential to view the individual partitions to determine the true diameter of the lumen or restrict the volume of interest for processing (target MIP; see also Fig. 13.3 C).

13.2.2 Phase-Contrast MRA

PC-MRA is widely available with sequences allowing the visualization of a particular range of flow velocities, both with 2D and 3D techniques using current scanner hardware and software. A thick slab is typically acquired with 2D PC MRA and displayed as a projection, while 3D PC MRA offers all of the advantages of a volumetric technique, including video display and subvolume reformatting.

Flow-related signal occurs when transverse magnetization moves in the direction of a magnetic field gradient, resulting in phase shifts. These phase shifts can be compensated for by applying a second gradient pulse of equal duration but opposite polarity. If the protons move during the interval between these two gradient pulses, a movement or flow-related phase shift will remain. This phase shift is directly proportional to the flow velocity and can be displayed in an angiographic image where pixel brightness is proportional to blood flow velocity. Using this approach, the amplitude and duration of the flow-velocity encoding gradient determine the sensitivity to flow velocity (*Venc*). In the case of phase shifts larger than 180°, aliasing occurs, and the MR signal does not reflect real velocity information. For this reason, the expected maximum velocity either has to be estimated before the measurement is started by prior knowledge of the range of velocities that typically exist in the vessel-of-interest (for 2D imaging) or calculated by applying a series of 2D phase-contrast images using a range of *Vencs* for 3D PCA. All methods require the acquisition of a flow-compensated data set and then additional flow-encoded data sets in different directions. The differences of these two data sets are used to calculate angiographic images. For 3D PCA, the scan times are very long as four measurements must be made: a flow-compensated image and additionally a flow-encoded image acquired in each of the three orthogonal planes.

PC methods can be applied with both small and large fields-of-view (FOVs) and typically provide complete suppression of signals from stationary tissue. Unlike inflow (TOF) techniques, PC methods directly measure flow and thus are not hindered by the artificial appearance of tissues having short T1, such as fresh thrombi. This ability to measure flow directly can be exploited to determine flow rates within individual arteries, using a 2D ECG-triggered technique.

The 2D acquisition slabs are comparable to projections achieved with intra-arterial (i.a.) DSA. Compared with sequential inflow MRA, this technique is more efficient; nonetheless, it has some disadvantages: (1) a *Venc* parameter has to be prospectively selected for the acquisition, (2) the necessity for subtraction of flow-compensated from flow-encoded image sets can result in artifacts from pulsatile flow, (3) breathing and peris-

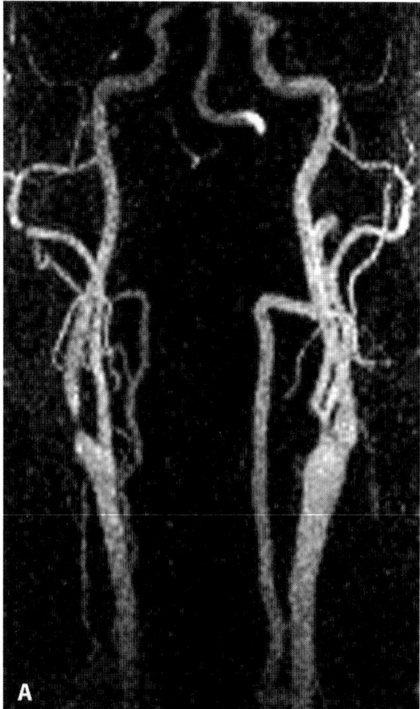

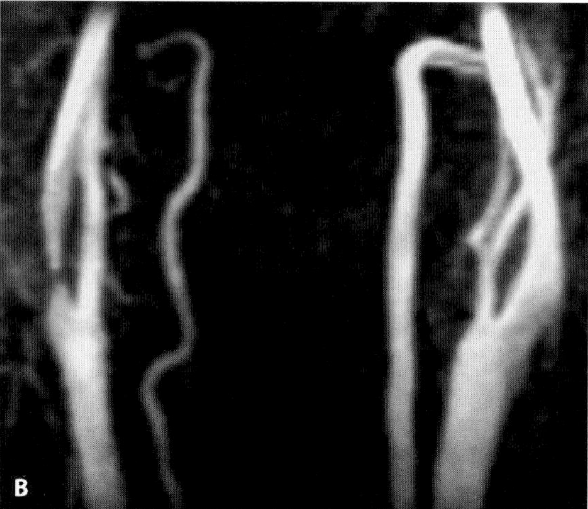

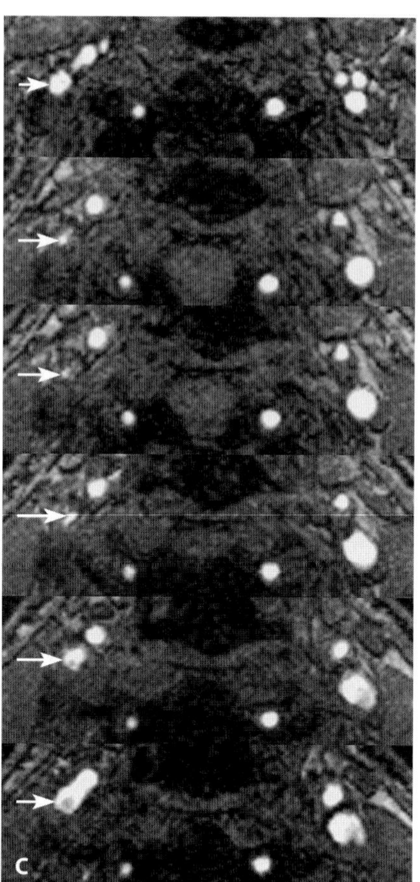

Fig. 13.3A–C. High-grade stenosis of right carotid artery: On CE MRA images a nearly complete flow void was visualized due to turbulence, related dephasing effects (**A**). However, TOF MRA showed a slight intraluminal inflow enhancement (*arrow*) which was only detected with source images (**C**). Note also the lower quality of the CE MRA image performed with single-dose technique (flow rate 2 ml/s) compared with CE MRA shown in Fig. 13.6A (double-dose technique)

talsis within the abdomen and pelvis impair image quality, (4) the highly anisotropic image voxel of this projection technique may result in destructive phase interference in the case of overlapping vessels. For these reasons, PCA is not widely used within the thorax and abdomen and, although accurate for evaluating the peripheral arteries, has few proponents (primarily due to the success of CE-MRA). However, the ability to measure flow within individual vessels, e.g. renal arteries in patients with renal artery stenosis, may stimulate further interest in this technique in the future.

13.2.3
Contrast-Enhanced MRA

13.2.3.1
Basics and System Requirements

13.2.3.1.1
Basics

All CE-MRA techniques are based on the same principle: a 10- to 25-fold shortening of the blood T1-relaxation time by an injection of a paramagnetic contrast medium (CM). This results in large signal-intensity differences between the brightest background tissue, fat (which has a T1 of approx. 200 ms) and contrast-enriched arteries (blood T1<50 ms after injection of an appropriate volume of contrast agent) on images acquired with a heavily T1-W sequence. Because images must be acquired *during* the relatively short first arterial passage of contrast agent *and* prior to onset of venous enhancement (the so-called 'arteriovenous window'), an ultrafast gradient-echo (GRE) sequence is used. The acquired 3D data set can be postprocessed using both MIP and MPR format to get different projections of the vessels, which the highest 3D signal-intensity structures is usually used on the image.

Because intravascular vessel contrast is generated by a T1 shortening effect of an injection of exogenous contrast agent and is not typically dependent on inherent flow effects, the images are said to be 'flow-independent'. SNR limitations are not a result of faster imaging (usually larger voxels) but higher resolution. Reduction of SNR can be addressed by injecting more contrast agent per unit time (increasing the flow rate). A huge additional benefit of CE-MRA is that data acquisition can be performed in whatever plane best suits the anatomy, without any reference to inflow or other flow-related effects.

13.2.3.1.2
System Requirements

In order to generate a sufficiently high resolution 3D data set within either the arteriovenous transit time or the breath-hold capability of the patient for imaging of the thoracic and abdominal vasculature, CE MRA is best performed on a high-performance MR system with short TR and TE. Strong gradients (>/= 20 mT/m), short rise times (</= 600 µs/mT/m) and 1.0 or 1.5 T field strength are currently required.

13.2.3.2
Vessel Contrast and K-Space

In a typical measurement sequence consisting of a linear phase encoding profile, k-space data are acquired line by line following the most basic format starting at one periphery of k-space, progressing in an incremental linear fashion through the center, and ending with the last line at the other edge of k-space. Using this algorithm, the center lines of k-space are acquired at the middle of the acquisition, and the k-space sampling strategy is referred to as 'linear'. However, k-space lines can be filled in any order, and the unique characteristics of k-space can be exploited to improve the quality of CE MRA. While the higher k-space frequencies, which determine the spatial resolution of the resulting image, are represented by the outer lines of k-space, the center of k-space (low spatial frequencies, central lines) determine the image contrast. Therefore, the central part (20% or so) of k-space is most crucial for vessel contrast in CE MRA; and CM must be present during the imaging field before the contrast-defining center lines are measured, otherwise severe 'ringing' artifacts will ensue which will impair the diagnostic quality (Figs. 13.4). On the other hand, image sharpness at the vessel contours depends on the presence of CM during sampling of the peripheral lines of k-space (high spatial frequencies). Optimal image quality can be expected therefore when CM persists throughout the entire measurement at the maximal concentration in the vessels under investigation. However, as the arteriovenous (AV) window (the time between the onset of arterial enhancement and the onset of venous enhancement) may be shorter than the acquisition time, venous overlay can cause difficulties in interpretation. Therefore, for improved arterial/venous differentiation it is essential to acquire the central k-space during the arterial peak prior to onset of venous enhancement. This can be achieved by either: (1) extremely short imaging times (shorter than the arteriovenous window) and/or (2) acquisition of the central k-space lines coincident with the arterial peak before venous enhancement occurs. This latter method requires accurate timing of the contrast bolus (see later) and typically employs a method where the central lines of k-space are acquired at the start of the 3D acquisition. This second method ('centric' acquisition) allows acquisition of higher resolution images by use of longer measurement times, but as the scan times in this instance greatly exceed the AV transit time, an accurate

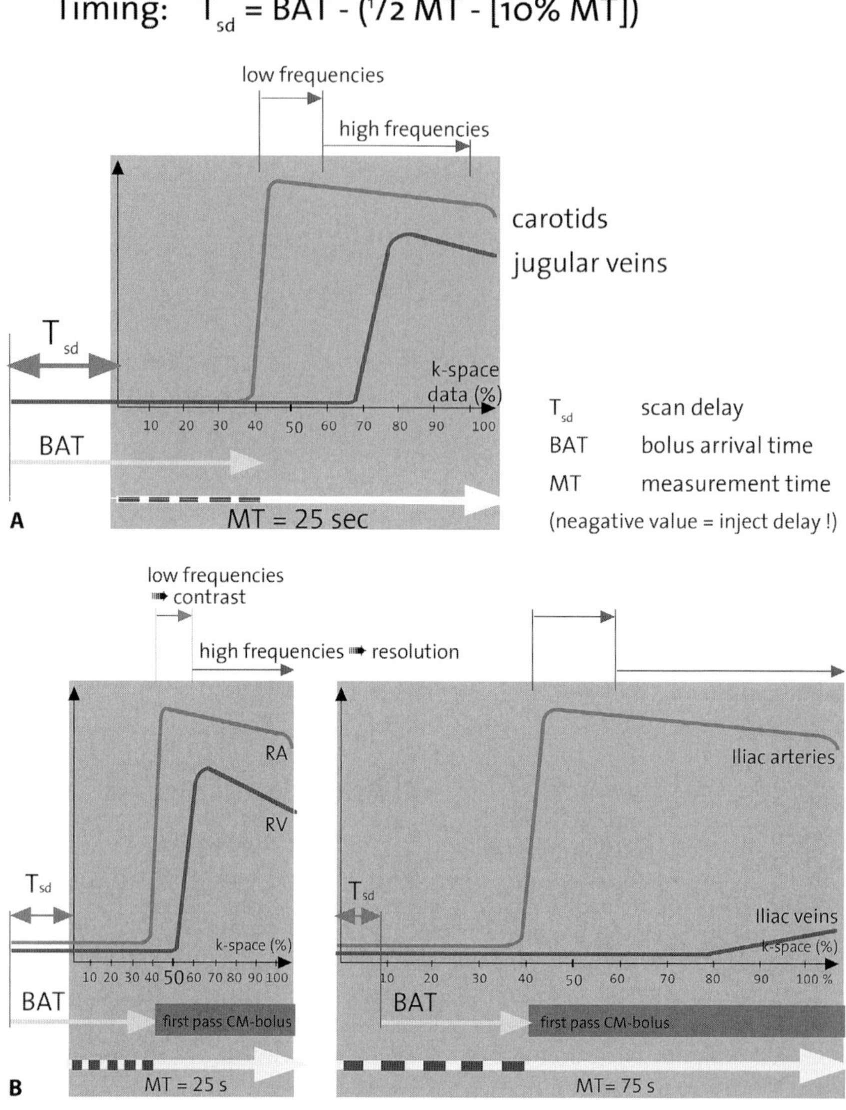

Fig. 13.4A,B. Adjustment of contrast administration and 3D CE MRA measurement: Bolus timing demonstrated at CE MRA of the carotids (**A**) renal and iliac arteries (**B**). The length of center k-space interval is different with respect to the acquisition time, influencing the available spatial resolution

method of bolus timing (e.g. fluoroscopic bolus detection) must be incorporated. This approach is widely used for imaging of the carotid arteries where high resolution is required in the face of an extremely short circulation time from carotid artery to jugular vein (see later). The approach is also used for imaging of the small arteries of the thighs and feet.

13.2.3.3 Measurement Parameters

The measurement parameters are tailored to cover the entire region of interest (ROI) related to the clinical requirement (Fig. 13.5). Any scan data orientation can be used; typically, the coronal plane is chosen due to optimal coverage for any combination of field-of-view and slab depth. In principle, the shortest TR (gives shortest scan time) and TE possible (to minimize

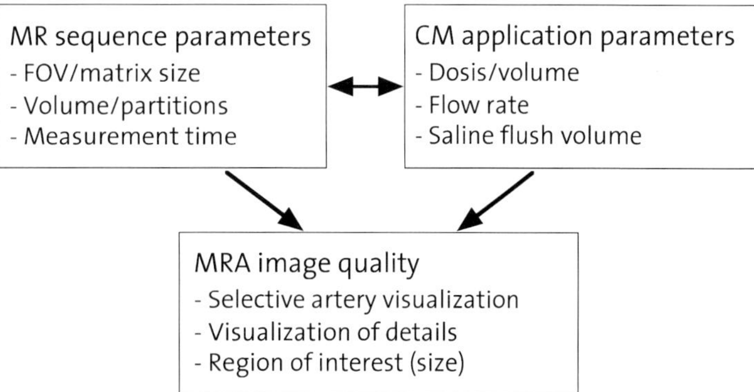

Fig. 13.5. Influence of measurement parameters and contrast administration parameter on image quality

dephasing) should be used. To increase spatial resolution, whenever possible 512 resolution is used in the read (frequency-encoding) direction with no time penalty, the slight disadvantages being reduced SNR (smaller voxel size) and slightly increased TE (more dephasing). In order to achieve higher resolution in the phase-encode and slice-select directions, more phase-encoding steps and thinner slices are needed, respectively, both of which lengthen the scan time. However, the scan time is limited by either the AV window or, more commonly, by the breath-holding capability of the patient for imaging within the thorax and abdomen. It is important to appreciate that a lower resolution breath-hold scan is infinitely superior to a higher resolution non-breath-hold scan for imaging of the aortic branches. Therefore, the best resolution possible given the breath-hold capability of the patient is used to ensure accurate stenosis grading. The choice of flip-angle is not critical but should be as close as possible to the range of 35°–50°.

Because of the unique structure of k-space, it is not always essential to acquire all lines of k-space. Providing that more than half (including the central lines) of k-space lines are measured, the remainder (40% or so) can be reconstructed from the measured data due to the symmetric nature of k-space, a technique referred to as partial Fourier imaging. This gives a reduction in scan time proportional to the amount of data that is reconstructed rather than measured, a huge benefit considering the stringent requirement for a short scan time.

Currently, sufficiently short scan times are possible with current state-of-the-art equipment. However, shorter scan times can also be achieved by using lower in-plane resolution and lower spatial resolution in the slice select direction (thicker slices). Slice interpolation, a technique to improve the quality of 'off-plane' MIP images that is widely exploited in the design of 3D MRA sequences by all manufacturers, does not overcome this problem because the calculated resolution cannot be considered as real spatial resolution.

13.2.3.4 Vessel Contrast and CM Bolus Geometry

T1-shortening within blood depends on the intravascular CM concentration. The aim of CM administration is to obtain the highest concentration in the arteries of interest during the acquisition of the central lines of k-space (as described above). The bolus geometry depends on the parameters of the i.v. bolus injection [flow rate (FR), CM dose and NaCl flush volume] and additionally on individual physiological and pathophysiological parameters such as blood flow rate, blood volume and physiological status (e.g. impaired cardiac function, anxiety, etc.).

- ⇑ FR (within the range of 1–3 ml/s) → bolus length ↓ (vessel contrast ↑)
- ⇑ Saline flush (NaCl volume) → bolus length ⇑
- ⇑ Quantity CM → bolus length ⇑

Studies have demonstrated that improved vascular contrast may be achieved by increasing the flow rate to 1–2 ml/s. Faster injections will shorten the bolus, and although increased contrast is anticipated, image quality may be unchanged or even worse if the bolus is so short that it is not present throughout the whole of the acquisition. The prolongation of the saline flush volume evidently causes a lengthening of the bolus by wash-out of contrast that otherwise might remain within the brachial and subclavian veins due to stasis. The bolus is physiologically diluted by the CM passage through the heart and lungs, but a susceptibility effect can be seen in the subclavian and brachiocephalic arteries on the side of injection due to the extremely high concentration of contrast agent within the adjacent vein. CM bolus dilution effects are identical for all systemic vessels, but despite this some vessels may be less conspicuous due to resolution constraints and proximity to overlap of subcutaneous or bone-marrow fat, if fat is not eliminated by subtraction or saturation effects. Additionally, segments distal to severe stenosis or distal segments reconstituted via collaterals may be poorly visible due to delayed arrival of CM (Fig. 13.22A).

However, it does not make sense to prescribe a high resolution scan if the bolus is not long enough to be present during acquisition of the high spatial frequencies at the outer k-space which define the resolution of the image. Therefore, the bolus geometry must be tailored to predefined parameters (specifically the scan duration) to optimize vessel contrast.

13.2.3.5 Bolus Timing and Contrast Medium Considerations for Contrast-Enhanced MRA

The scan time and the CM administration parameters have to be matched to each other to ensure optimal image quality.

For example, it is possible to perform a CE MRA of renal arteries using single (0.1 mmol/kg) or double (0.2 mmol/kg) doses of CM using an identical flow rate. By applying the same CE MRA sequence parameters, the single-dose examination predictably results in lower resolution, less edge detail and poorer depiction of more peripheral branches than the double-dose technique (see Fig. 13.16).

Although CE-MRA is 'flow-independent' in that there is little dependence on 'inflow' or 'phase' effects, high image quality relies on accurate timing of the bolus, which depends on the circulation time from peripheral vein to artery-of-interest. As this varies widely between individuals, the scan delay time (time from start of infusion to start of scanning) must be carefully selected. The following methods are used in practice:

1. Empiric timing (best guess): The scan delay time is set by the operator, taking into account several factors such as the patient's physical status and the knowledge that circulation times are predictable to a certain degree and fall within a certain range in most patients. This technique is rarely used nowadays.
2. Use of a timing bolus: The bolus arrival time (BAT) is measured prior to the 3D CE MRA. A test dose of 1–2 ml CM, followed by a volume of NaCl flush equal to the contrast volume for the 3D MRA (e.g. 30 ml), is injected. Time-resolved single-slice (2D GRE) imaging with a temporal resolution of 1 image/s) is used to visualize the arrival of the bolus. After first circulating through the cardiopulmonary circulation, the bolus arrives in the arteries of the ROI. The scan delay (T_{sd}) of the subsequent 3D CE MRA can then be calculated using the following formula (provided that a linear phase-encoding table is applied):

$$T_{sd} = \text{BAT} - \left(\frac{1}{2}\,\text{MT} - [10\%\text{MT}]\right)$$

(MT = measurement time).

■ **Automated Bolus Detection.** Two methods are used:

- 'Black-box' detection (SMARTPREP): a tracker volume is placed within the region-of-interest, and the signal intensity within the voxel is measured continuously. Increase in the signal intensity above a certain threshold signifies arrival of the contrast agent, and the 3D scan is 'triggered'.
- Fluoroscopic detection (CAREBOLUS, BOLUSTRAK): 2D single-slice images with a temporal resolution of 1image/s are dynamically acquired and reconstructed in real-time on the scan monitor. The operator aborts the 2D scan and then initiates the 3D scan once contrast is visualized within the imaging field.

■ **Multiphase MRA.** This approach does not use a timing sequence, rather several short 3D data sets are acquired in rapid succession, and the appropriate data set chosen. The disadvantage of this technique is the requirement for very high performance gradients and the need for several breath-holds, which precludes its use in many patients.

13.2.3.6
Contrast-Enhanced MRA: Tips and Tricks

- Use an automated mechanical injection pump to standardize the CM administration.
- Use the highest dose of CM possible if high resolution is required.
- Perform breath-hold exercises with the patient.
- Acquire a non-contrast 3D-MRA data set ('mask') before administration of CM to allow subtraction.

13.3
Summary of Basic Advantages and Disadvantages Associated with Different MRA Techniques

MRA, especially CE MRA, is a dynamically evolving technique. Each method suffers from limitations and artifacts, some of which are summarized in Table 13.3. With each new generation of software and hardware the limitations are becoming less and less.

■ **Contrast-Enhanced MR Venography (MRV):** A Special Case? Because i.v. injected commercial strength contrast agent shortens not only the T1 of the contrast-enriched blood, but also T2*, a susceptibility effect occurs. This results in severe signal dropout within the veins on the side of injection, which precludes acquisition of contrast-enhanced MR venograms with undiluted contrast. However, brightly enhancing arteries result

Table 13.3. Advantages, disadvantagses and special features of various MRA techniques

Technique	Advantages	Disadvantages	Special features
2D TOF	↑ Flow/Background contrast ↑ Visualization of slow flow Low saturation effects ↓ Measurement time	↓ SNR ↓ Visualization of in-plane flow Sensitive to short T1 species Flow voids due to diastolic back flow	ECG-gating: improves inflow signal during systole
3D TOF	↑ SNR ↑ Resolution	Slow flow saturation ↓ Background suppression Sensitive to short T1 species	MOTSA TONE MT-saturation
2D PC	↓ Measurement time ↑ Background suppression ↓ Saturation effects Intensive to short T1 species Sensitive to slow flow	Projection technique (single thick slice) Dephasing artifacts due to vessel overlap Aliasing (VENC to low) Requires experiences in interpretation and input by the operator	ECG-gating: Flow measurement Different flow images within cardiac cycle (diastolic and systolic images) Multiple VENC along main flow direction Use as fast vessel localizer
3D PC	↓ Dephasing artifacts ↑ SNR ↑ Background suppression Insensitive to short T1 species ↑ Resolution	↑↑ Measurement time Aliasing (VENC to low) Requires experiences in interpretation and input by the operator	
3D CE	↑ SNR ↑ Resolution, FOV ↓ Measurement time (breth-hold is possible) Relative flow independent Relative robust technique	Bolus timing is necessary Dephasing artifacts occur Contrast agents have to be applied	Time-resolved technique Digital subtaction (measure native and CE) Future special coils, blood pool agents

PC phase contrast; *CE* contrast enhanced; *FOV* flied-of-fiew; *D* dimension; *TOF* time-of-flight; *ECG* electrocardiogram; *SNR* sound-to-noise ratio; *MOTSA* multiple overlapping thin-slab acquisition; *TONE* tilted optimized non-saturating excitation; *VENC* velocity encoding gradient determining the sensitivity to flow velocity from injection of contrast medium due to dilution of the injected contrast volume during passage through the heart and pulmonary circulation, which prolongs the T2*, thus minimizing or eliminating the artifact. This consideration gives rise to two different ways to perform contrast-enhanced MRV:

1. 'Indirect' MRV: After completion of arterial phase imaging, a second acquisition is acquired during the 'venous' phase. This approach can be used for any venous territory and is commonly used to evaluate the splenoportal axis.
2. 'Direct' MRV: Contrast medium is diluted with saline (3%–6%) prior to injection and MR venograms acquired during the first pass. This approach can only be used in territories where CM can be injected 'upstream' of the region-of-interest (e.g. evaluation of the superior vena cava following injection into both upper extremities).

13.4 Sequence Protocols and Clinical Application

13.4.1 Intracranial Vessels

3D TOF MRA is the most effective technique for imaging of the intracranial arteries (Table 13.4). Stenoses of the primary branches of the circle of Willis are well depicted. Unfortunately, the technique is less reliable for evaluating small, distal vessels. The use of Gd-chelates may improve the visualization of peripheral vessels, but at the cost of a more enhanced surrounding tissue, reducing vessel contrast, and increased venous enhancement (Fig. 13.2B). Collateral flow can be determined using specially placed presaturation pulses that suppress signal within the vascular territory supplied by the presaturated vessel. The grading of vertebrobasilar stenoses is reliable, thereby influencing treatment strategies (anticoagulation). Anatomic variations such as the termination of the vertebral artery at the posterior inferior cerebellar artery or hypoplastic vessels (fetal or hypoplastic posterior cerebral artery of) are well visualized (Fig. 13.2D).

3D TOF MRA high-resolution imaging provides a high accuracy of detection of small (>3 mm) aneurysms. The source images of the 3D data set should be carefully evaluated (Fig. 13.1E). MIP reconstruction of subvolumes (targeted MIP) is also helpful to eliminate the overlay of several different vessels. This technique can also be used to determine a persistent nidus after radio-surgery in the case of intracranial vascular malformations but cannot substitute for conventional catheter angiography in defining feeder vessels and shunting. Sometimes, 3D or 2D PC MRA may improve the visualization of such vessel structures.

MRA of intracranial veins can be obtained by several means, including 2D TOF with arterial presaturation and the PC-MRA technique and CE techniques. Thrombosis involving the major venous sinuses can be depicted.

13.4.2 Carotid Arteries

Traditional non-contrast MRA sequences are 2D TOF or MOTSA 3D TOF of the whole carotid artery, or 3D TOF of the bifurcation only (Table 13.5). Because of its sensitivity to slow flow, 2D TOF MRA is more accurate for differentiating near from complete occlusion than 3D TOF MRA. Signal loss in areas of turbulence may occur with both 2D and 3D techniques, but 3D techniques give superior evaluation of the carotid bifurcation than 2D techniques for both severity and length of stenosis. MOTSA techniques overcome many of the limitations of 3D TOF MRA but suffer from movement artifacts

Table 13.4. Magnetic resonance (MR) angiography protocol recommendations for intracranial vessels

Sequence	WI	Plane	TR (ms)	TE (ms)	Flip angle	Slice thickness (mm)	No part	Effth	Matrix	FOV	recFOV (%)	BW	No. of acq.	Acq. time (min:s)
3D GRE	T1	tra	40–60	5–6	20–30	56	64	0,8–1	512	200	62,5	390	1	8
2D GRE	T1	tra	30	5–9	60	2	50		256	180	75	195	1	5:40

Abbreviations: *WI* weighted image; *TR* repetition time; *TI* inversion time; *TE* echo time; *No part* number of partitions; *Effth* effective thickness (mm); *Matrix* matrix (phase × frequency matrix); *FOV* field of view (mm); *recFOV* % rectangular field of view, *BW* bandwidth (Hz); *Acq* number of acquisitions

Table 13.5. Magnetic resonance angiography sequene parameters recommendations for extracranial carotid vessels

Sequence	WI	Plane	TR (ms)	TE (ms)	Flip angle	Slice thickness (mm)	No part	Effth	Matrix	FOV	recFOV (%)	BW	No. of acq.	Acq. time (min:s)
3D GRE (CE)	T1	cor	4.2	1.9	35	50	50	1	256	260	50	390	1	0:25
3D GRE MOTSA	T1	ax	30	6	25	132	132	1	256	220	75	390	1	12:40

Abbreviations: *WI* weighted image; *TR* repetition time; *TI* inversion time; *TE* echo time; *No part* number of partitions; *Effth* effective thickness (mm); *Matrix* matrix (phase × frequency matrix); *FOV* field of view (mm); *recFOV* % rectangular field of view; *BW* bandwidth (Hz); *Acq* number of acquisitions

due to the long acquisition times (10–12 min) (Fig. 13.7B) compared with 3D CE MRA (25 s).

The entire region of the carotids and the vertebral system can easily be depicted by CE MRA. Images can be acquired from the aortic arch to the base of the skull using a phase-array neck coil (Fig. 13.6A). Since the normal mean ICA diameter measures approximately 6 mm, accurate visualization of a residual diameter of approximately 1.8 mm is necessary to allow the detection of stenosis at the 70% cut-off. Therefore, high resolution that increases the scan time substantially beyond the AV window must be used. Nevertheless, arterial phase images without venous contamination can be acquired by using centric phase-encoding in association with fluoroscopic bolus detection to allow completion of central k-space imaging during the arterial peak prior to the onset of jugular venous enhancement, despite the fact that the AV transit time is typically 8–12 s only. Using state-of-the-art technology, a voxel size of 1×1×1 mm or less can easily be achieved, but further improvements in resolution are required to satisfy the stringent resolution requirements within the carotid system. Optimal vessel contrast is achieved by a double-dose injection at a rate of 1–2 ml/s (compare Figs. 13.3 and 13.6). Breath-hold acquisitions may improve visualization of the aortic arch vessels.

Artifacts caused by swallowing can be avoided by instructing the patient not to swallow during the 3D MRA (typically less than 40 s duration) prior to scan initiation.

13.4.3 Thoracic and Abdominal Aorta, Subclavian and Brachial Arteries

Congenital and acquired diseases of aortic arch vessels, thoracic and abdominal aorta can lead to aneurysm formation, stenosis and occlusion. Such diverse etiologies as atherosclerosis, trauma, infection, radiation, connective tissue disorders, fibrodysplasia and dissection may be encountered. All of these pathologies, including treatment planning and follow-up, are well depicted by CE MRA (Table 13.6). The measurement time should be decreased at the cost of resolution to facilitate breath-holding. To supplement information from the CE scan, it may be appropriate to orientate the timing sequence or 2D fluoroscopic technique in a sagittal plane in order to obtain information such as the blood supply to the two lumina in case of aortic dissection (Fig. 13.8A).

The evaluation of steno-occlusive disease in the subclavian or brachial region, such as thoracic outlet syn-

Table 13.6. Magnetic resonance angiography sequene parameters recommendations for aorta, subclavian and brachial arteries

Sequence	WI	Plane	TR (ms)	TE (ms)	Flip angle	Slice thickness (mm)	No part	Effth	Matrix	FOV	recFOV (%)	BW	No. of acq.	Acq. time (min:s)
3D GRE	T1	par-sag	3.85	1.5	35	90	58	1.55	256	400	75	650	1	0:43
3D GRE (ip)	T1	par-sag	4.6	1.8	35	100	32 (64)	3.12 (2.3)	256	400	75	390	1	0:28

Abbreviations: *WI* weighted image; *TR* repetition time; *TI* inversion time; *TE* echo time; *No part* number of partitions; *Effth* effective thickness (mm); *Matrix* matrix (phase × frequency matrix); *FOV* field of view (mm); *recFOV* % rectangular field of view; *BW* bandwidth (Hz); *Acq* number of acquisitions

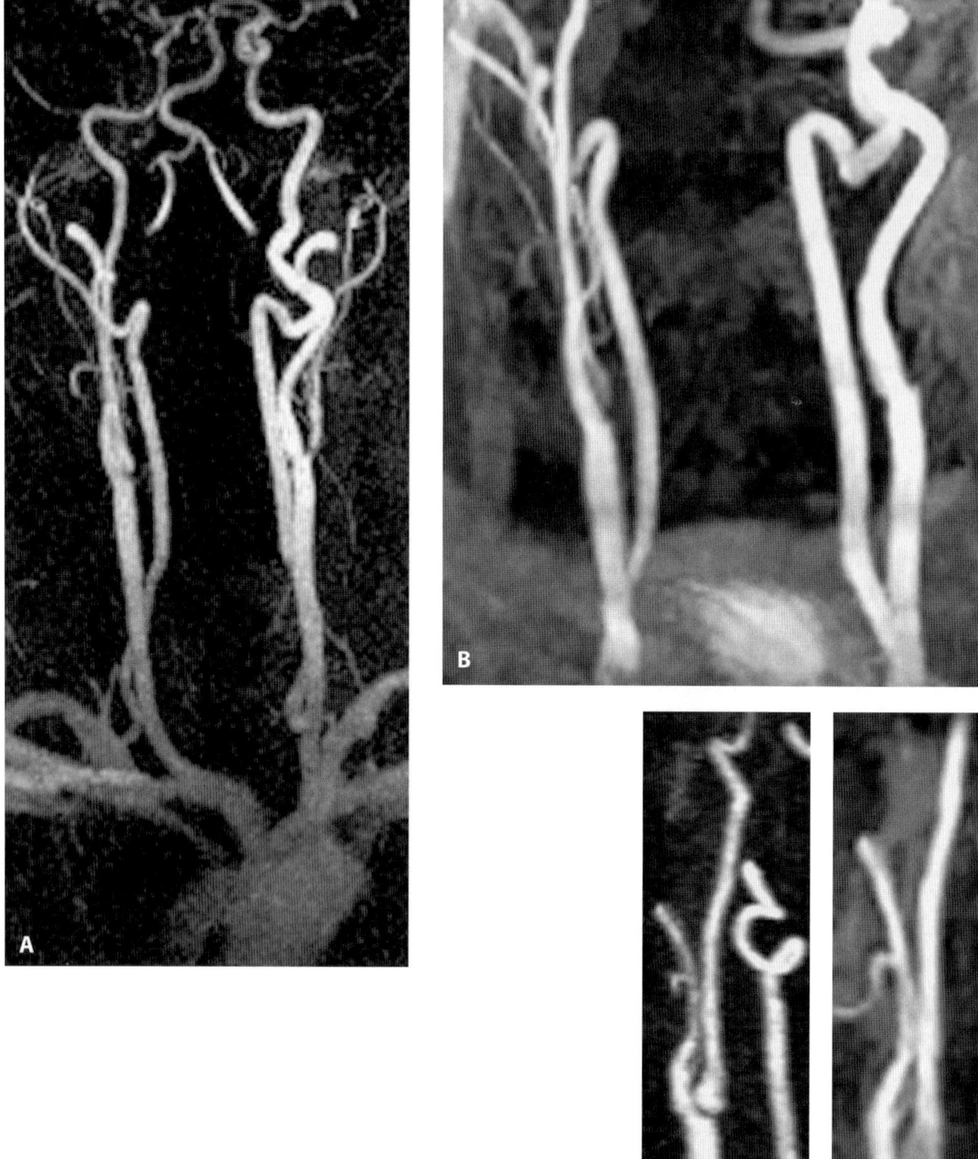

Fig. 13.6A–D. Patient with carotid disease: high-grade (>70%) stenosis of right internal and left external carotid artery. With CE MRA images (double-dose technique, 3 ml/s flow rate) the entire length of the carotid artery from the aortic arch up to the circle of Willis is visualized, whereas the TOF angiogram covered only 10 cm of the carotid vessel tree (**A**,**B**). MIP reconstruction software allows selective reprojection of the carotid stenosis at the bifurcation (**C**,**D**). Note the signal loss distal to the left external carotid stenosis on TOF images due to slow flow and overlay of fat

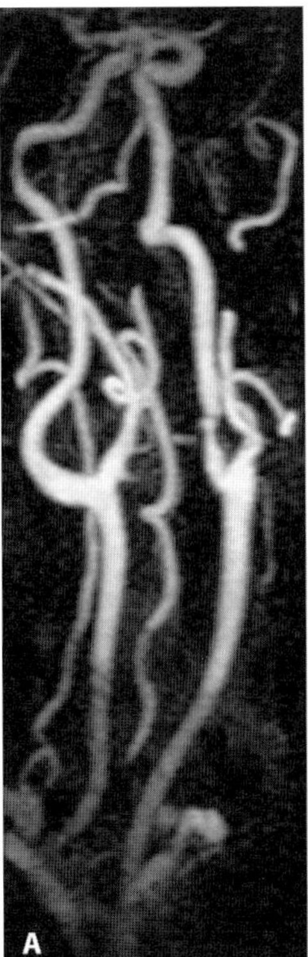

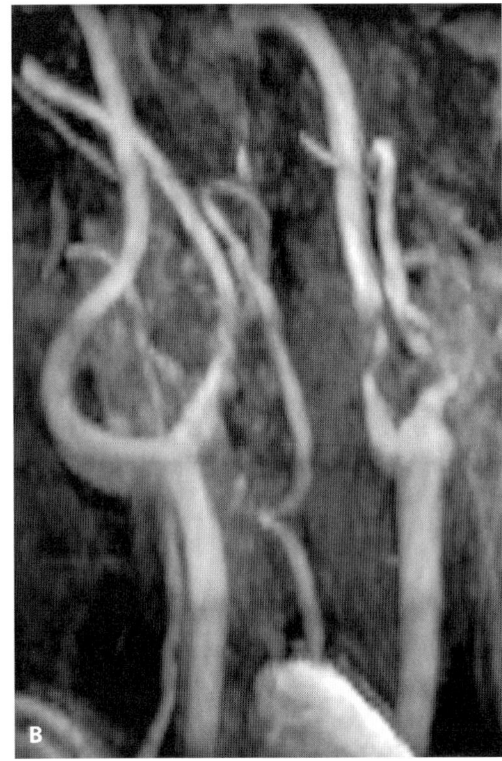

Fig. 13.7A,B. The approximately 70% stenosis of the left internal carotid artery was shown correctly by CE MRA (**A**). The stenosis was slightly overestimated by TOF MRA (**B**) due to poststenotic turbulence resulting in an intraluminal signal void. In addition, the image quality of TOF MRA is decreased by overlay of fat (**B**)

drome, is possible by CE MRA by performing two measurements in normal and abducted arm positions (Fig. 13.9). Because of contrast-induced susceptibility, contrast agent should always be injected on the asymptomatic side to avoid overinterpretation due to artefactual stenosis where the subclavian artery and vein lie adjacent to one another; in patients with bilateral symptoms, the right side should be used due to the more favorable anatomy. The subclavian and proximal brachial arteries require a moderately thick volume of approximately 60–90 mm (FOV=350–400 mm) during breath-holding, which dictates use of moderate resolution (voxel size $=0.7\times1.5\times1.7$ mm^3). A phased-array body coil is preferred because of the improved SNR. When performing selective CE MRA of subclavian and brachial arteries, a flexible wrap-around coil (FOV= 300 mm, double-dose technique, FR 2 ml/s) or an eccentrically placed body phased-array coil can be used (Fig. 13.10).

13.4.4 Pulmonary Arteries

CE MRA gives high CNR between brightly enhancing, contrast-enriched blood and emboli which appear dark. Although fifth- to seventh-order branches of the pulmonary artery can be visualized, a reliable diagnosis of acute pulmonary embolism can be made to the 4th order (segmental arteries) only. This technique is also suitable for treatment planning and follow-up studies in chronic pulmonary embolic disease. Although MIP provide a complete overview of the pulmonary vasculature, partially occluding emboli may be completely masked. These emboli are better visualized by viewing the individual slices and performing subvolume MIP and MPR images. At the subsegmental level, MIPs may improve the review process (see also targeted MIP of Fig. 13.13 C).

Because of the limited breath-hold capability of most patients with suspected pulmonary embolism, it may be necessary to sacrifice resolution in favor of a

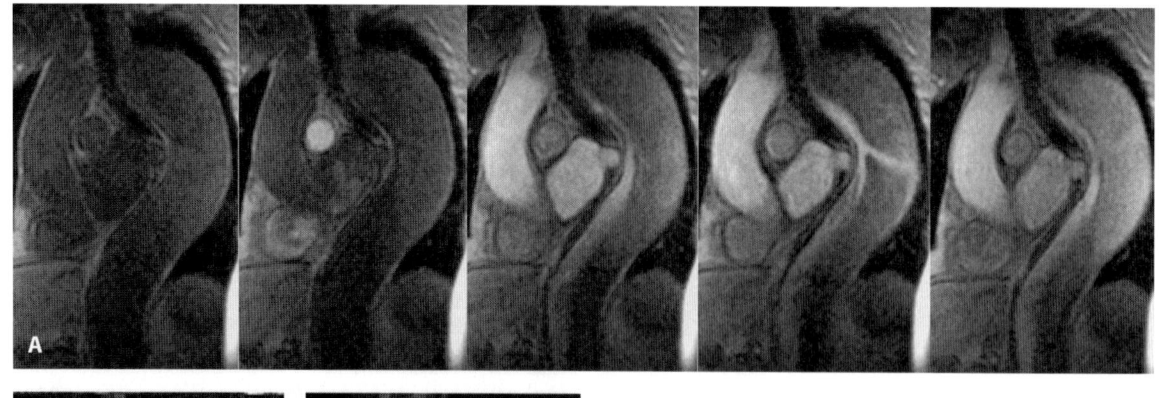

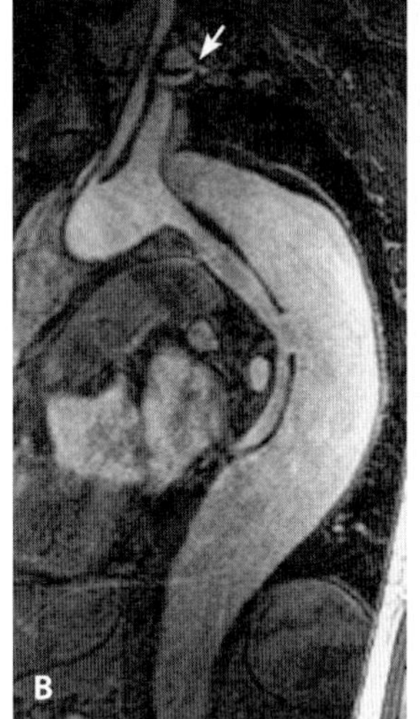

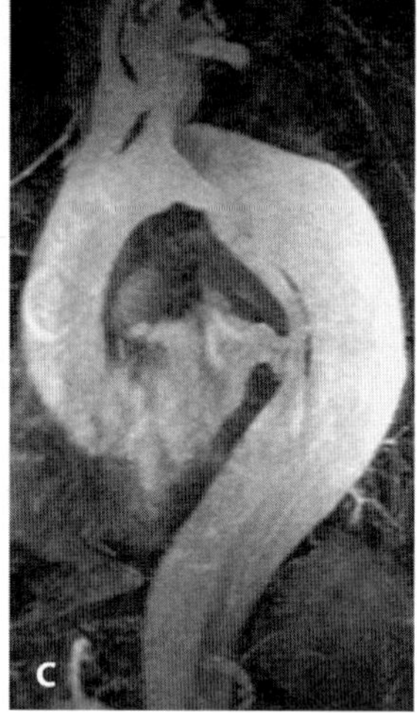

Fig. 13.8A–C. Patient with an aortic dissection type B: First, a 3D CE MRA (0.2 mmol Gd/kg, 2 ml/s) of the abdominal aorta was performed (Fig. 13.14A shows the MIP) to avoid overlay of venous signal. Subsequently, the patient and coil were repositioned to allow evaluation of the thoracic aorta. The BAT sequence (**A**) was acquired in the sagittal orientation (often results in a cut view of the dissection membrane). In this case, the jet of the contrast medium into the false lumen (entry) was very well depicted. (3D CE MRA images from the thoracic aorta were taken (0.1 mmol Gd/kg). The dissection flap can be better evaluated on the source images of the 3D CE MRA data set (**B**) than on the MIP images (**C**)

shorter scan that is within the patient's breath-hold capability. This, however, impairs the ability to diagnose small subsegmental emboli, although the significance of such emboli remains uncertain (Table 13.7) (Fig. 13.11). Both lungs can be evaluated in a single acquisition in the coronal plane, but scan times are relatively long. In order to shorten the acquisition, each lung can be evaluated separately in the sagittal plane, with the use of separate injections. Alternatively, in patients with reasonable breath-hold capability, images with increased resolution can be acquired by employing the sagittal plane. The use of a body phased-array coil is preferable to boost SNR within small peripheral vessels where resolution constraints are most marked.

Table 13.7. Magnetic resonance angiography sequene parameters recommendations for pulmonary vessels

Sequence	WI	Plane	TR (ms)	TE (ms)	Flip angle	3D Slice thickness (mm)	No part	Effth	Matrix	FOV	recFOV (%)	BW	No. of acq.	Acq. time (min:s)
3D GRE	T1	cor	3.85	1.5	40	96	48	2	256	350	75	650	1	0:35

Abbreviations: *WI* weighted image; *TR* repetition time; *TI* inversion time; *TE* echo time; *No part* number of partitions; *Effth* effective thickness (mm); *Matrix* matrix (phase × frequency matrix); *FOV* field of view (mm); *recFOV* % rectangular field of view; *BW* bandwidth (Hz); *Acq* number of acquisitions

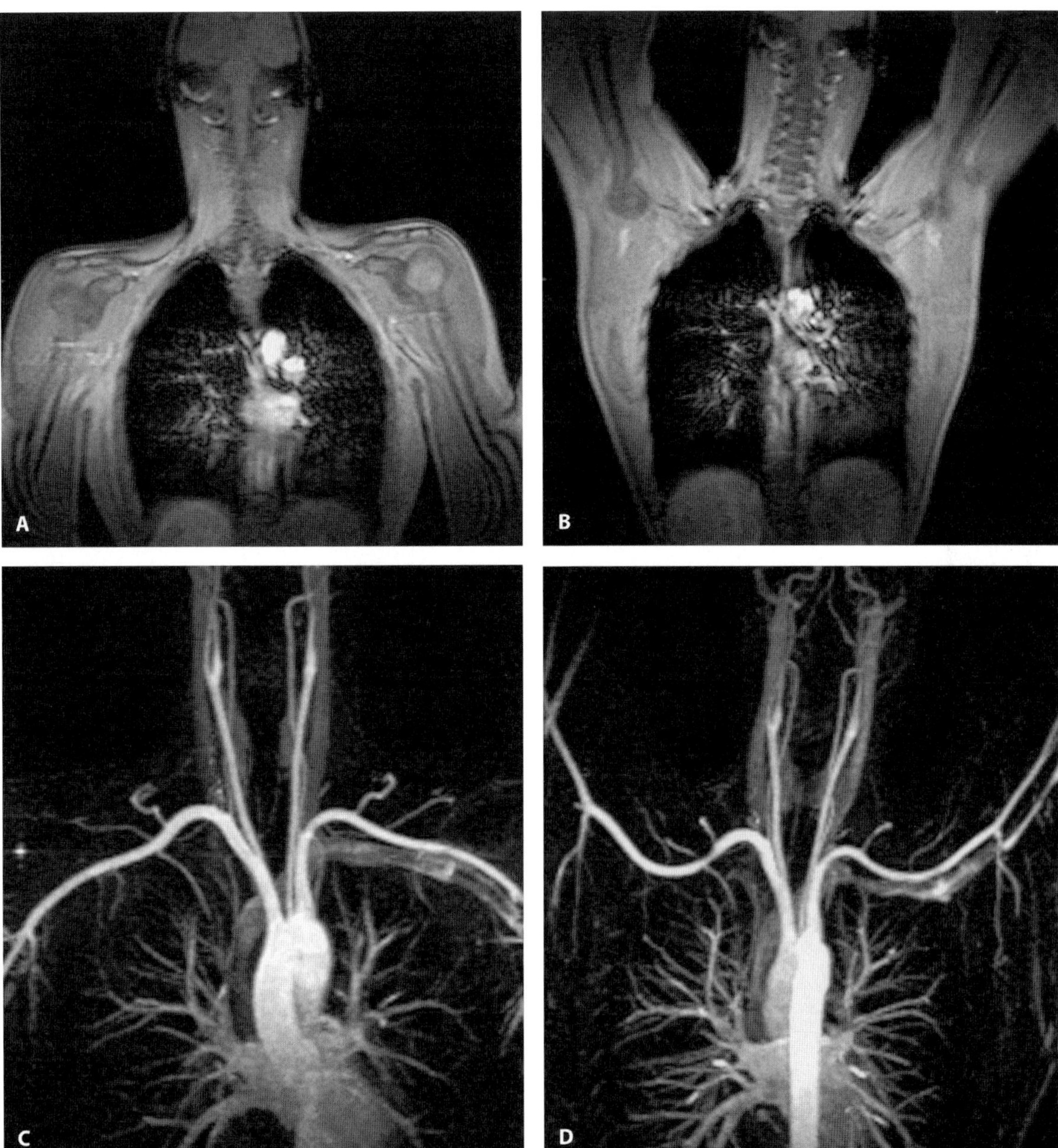

Fig. 13.9A–D. Patient with thoracic outlet syndrome: Moderate stenosis of the right subclavian artery was clearly shown when the arms were elevated during the second CE MRA measurement (**B,D**). The maximal CM dosage (0.3 mmol/kg) was divided into two rates for each CEMRA measurement [0.15 mmol/kg at normal (**A,C**) and elevated (**B,D**) position] using the same measurement parameters. The measurement time was about 50% longer than for the carotid CE MRA technique. Therefore, a slight venous overlay was seen

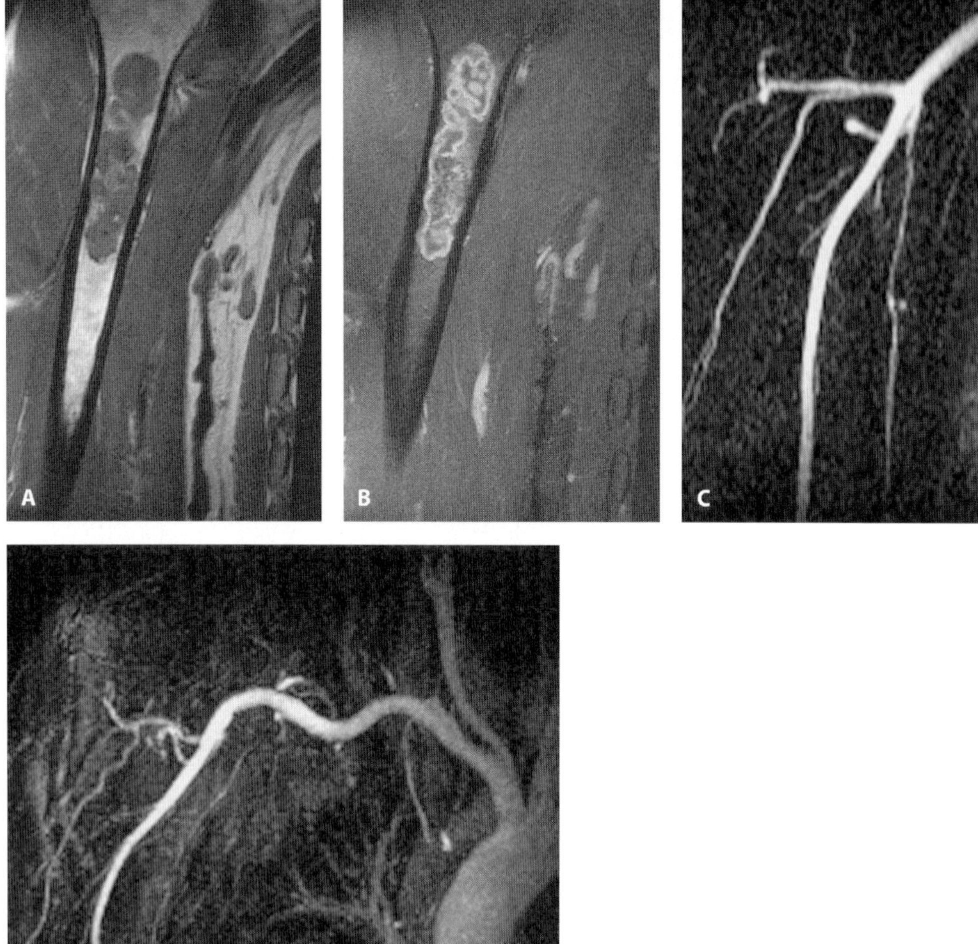

Fig. 13.10A–D. Bone infarction at the proximal humerus was detected on T1-W images before (**A**) and after CM (**B**; including fat saturation). CE MRA (**C**) was performed using a flexible wrap-around coil. A vascular malformation was excluded by CE MRA. **D** Normal findings of subclavian and brachial arteries (0.2 mmol Gd/kg). Note the body phased-array coil provides better depiction of the aortic branches (Fig. 13.9)

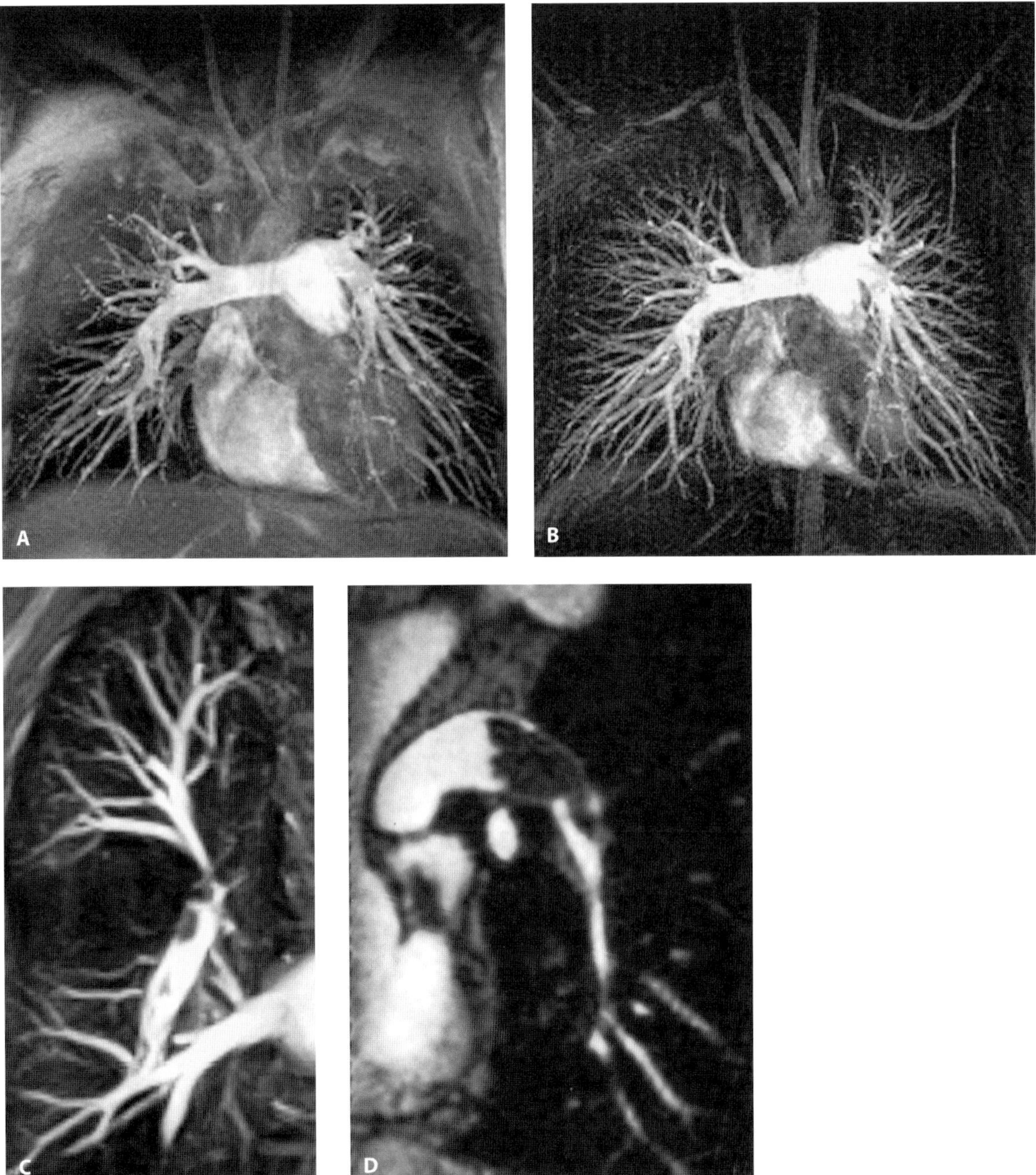

Fig. 13.11A–D. Highly selective CE MRA of normal pulmonary arteries with optimal bolus timing (**A**,**B**; 0.1 mmol Gd/kg, 3 ml/s flow rate). Note that MIP of non-subtracted data set (**A**) showed fewer peripheral vessels than MIP of the subtracted data set (**B**). The subtracted MRA technique improves the image quality due to elimination of background structures. Targeted MIP image and MPR image of another patient visualize multiple emboli within the right lower lobe artery (**C**) and a large embolus within the main left pulmonary artery (**D**)

Another method currently under scrutiny to evaluate the pulmonary arteries relies on the use of 'blood-pool' contrast agents. High resolution images can be acquired during free-breathing, using either respiratory triggering or navigator echoes to compensate for breathing artifacts. As high-resolution selective pulmonary arterial imaging cannot currently be performed using first-pass CE MRA due to the fast capillary passage and rapid onset of venous enhancement, the venous overlay seen on blood-pool images is not as problematic as in other territories where venous enhancement can substantially impair the image quality.

As the technique gives a 'road map', other pathologies affecting the pulmonary vasculature such as arteriovenous malformations (Fig. 13.12), pulmonary artery and vein stenosis or occlusion due to bronchogenic tumors, and sequestration can also be diagnosed using this technique.

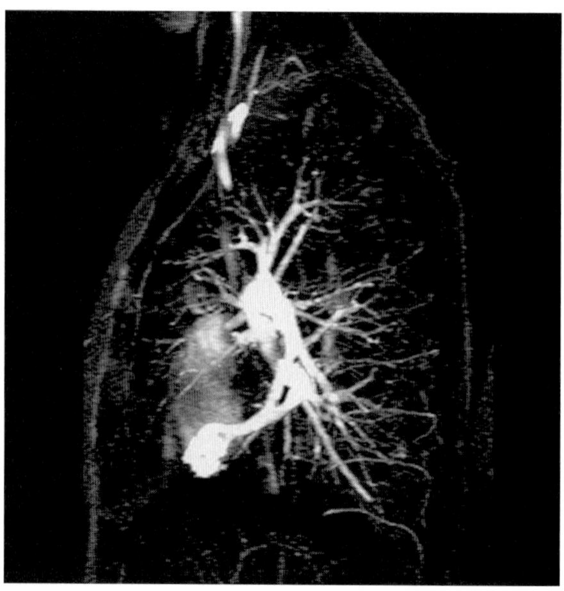

Fig. 13.12. Lateral MIP shows a pulmonary AV malformation within the right lower lobe. Images acquired in the sagittal plane with a single dose of contrast agent (0.1 mmol/kg)

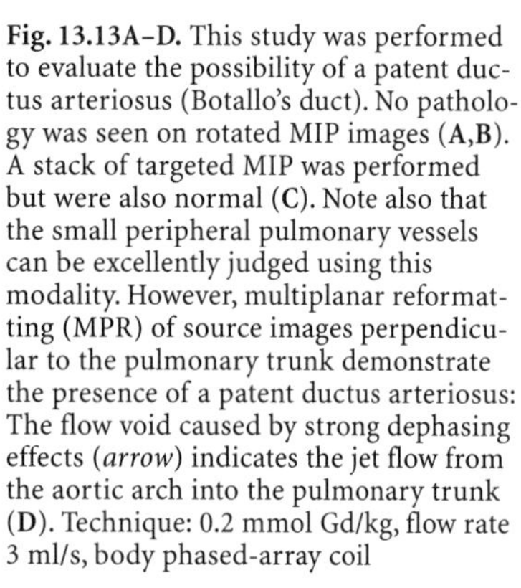

Fig. 13.13A–D. This study was performed to evaluate the possibility of a patent ductus arteriosus (Botallo's duct). No pathology was seen on rotated MIP images (**A**,**B**). A stack of targeted MIP was performed but were also normal (**C**). Note also that the small peripheral pulmonary vessels can be excellently judged using this modality. However, multiplanar reformatting (MPR) of source images perpendicular to the pulmonary trunk demonstrate the presence of a patent ductus arteriosus: The flow void caused by strong dephasing effects (*arrow*) indicates the jet flow from the aortic arch into the pulmonary trunk (**D**). Technique: 0.2 mmol Gd/kg, flow rate 3 ml/s, body phased-array coil

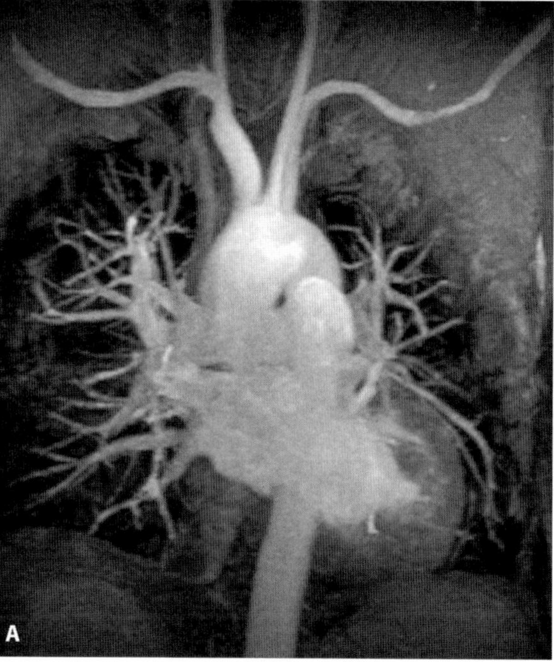

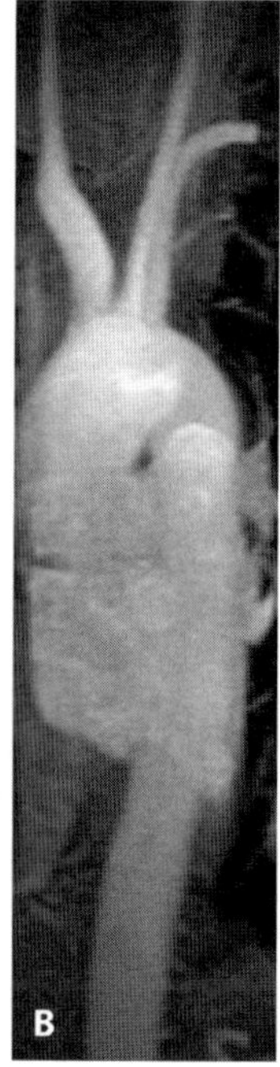

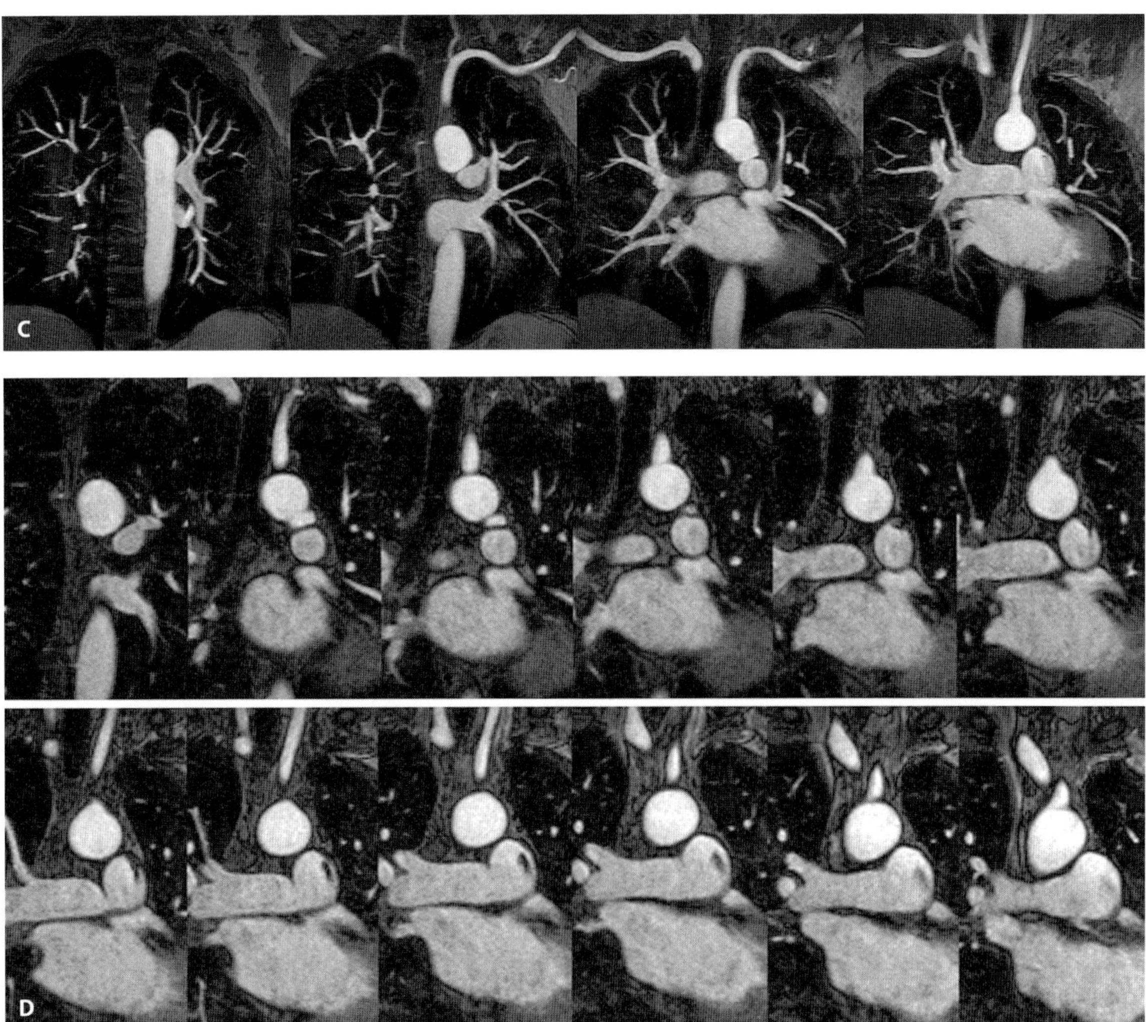

Fig. 13.13C, D.

13.4.5 Renal and Mesenteric Arteries

Breath-hold 3D CE MRA of the medium-sized renal arteries has been one of the enormous success stories of the last decade (Table 13.8) (Fig. 13.14). In institutions with access to high-quality CE MRA, catheter arteriography has now been completely supplanted for screening patients with suspected renal artery stenosis. High spatial resolution can be achieved by a 30 s measurement, resulting in an isotropic voxel size of 1.25 mm^3 (Figs. 13.15 and 13.17). However, in many patients with suspected renovascular disease, co-existent cardiopulmonary disease limits the breath-hold capability, and lower resolution must be accepted to allow a shorter scan time. The renal artery to renal veins transit time is even shorter than in the carotids (approximately 4–5 s), signal superposition caused by renal veins (especially on the left) can be avoided by exact bolus timing and the use of short breath-hold scans. In order to improve SNR, a body phased-array coil is superior to the standard body coil. A double dose (0.2 mmol/kg) is suffi-

Table 13.8. Magnetic resonance (MR) angiography sequene parameters recommendations for renal and mesenteric arteries

Sequence	WI	Plane	TR (ms)	TE (ms)	Flip angle	3D Slice thickness (mm)	No part	Effth	Matrix	FOV	recFOV (%)	BW	No. of acq.	Acq. time (min:s)
3D GRE	T1	cor	3.85	1.5	35	70	56	1.25	256	320	75	650	1	0:40

Abbreviations: *WI* weighted image; *TR* repetition time; *TI* inversion time; *TE* echo time; *No part* number of partitions; *Effth* effective thickness (mm); *Matrix* matrix (phase × frequency matrix); *FOV* field of view (mm); *recFOV* % rectangular field of view; *BW* bandwidth (Hz); *Acq* number of acquisitions

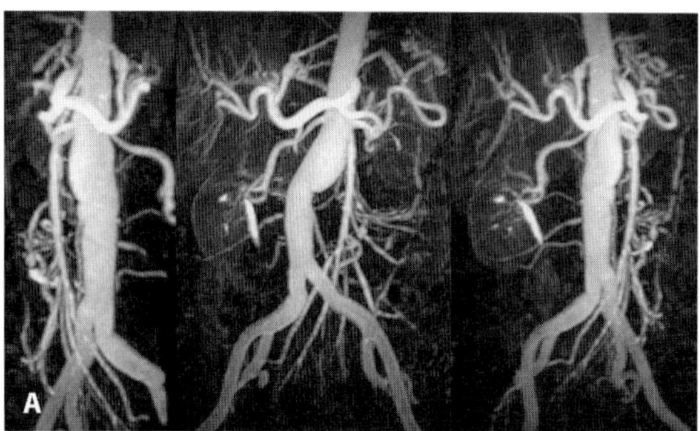

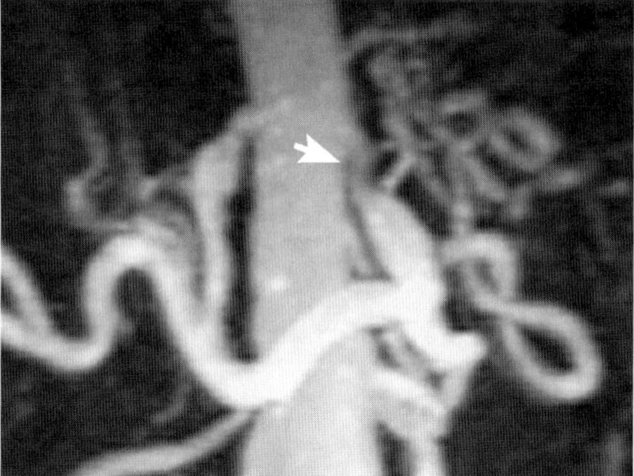

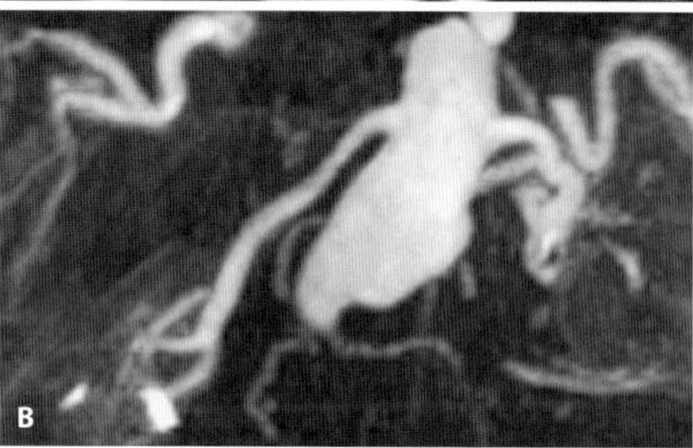

Fig. 13.14A,B. Patient with an aortic kinking and a small infrarenal aneurysm. Double dose injection of Gd is necessary to visualize all mesenteric vessels (flow rate 2 ml/s). Sometimes the whole-volume MIP gives confusing information (**A**), and therefore, selective MIPs (**B**) are helpful. The stenosis of the celiac artery (*arrow*) and the normal but elongated renal arteries were well identified by selective MIPs

cient and superior to the single-dose approach (Fig. 13.16). Assuming optimal image quality is achieved, small accessory renal arteries can be depicted, which is important for surgery treatment planning (Fig. 13.18). Intrarenal arteries are poorly visualized due to a combination of resolution constraints, venous overlap and brightly enhancing renal parenchyma.

Numerous studies attest to the accuracy of this technique for the detection of renovascular disease, with sensitivities and specificities over 90% in almost all studies. Few patients with fibromuscular dysplasia have been included in reported studies, and the exclusion value for FMD is uncertain, although likely to be high (Fig. 13.19). Although the severity of renal artery stenosis is usually assessed visually, secondary signs such as reduction in the intensity of the contrast nephrogram and shrunken kidneys are valuable secondary signs. Evaluation of flow rates within the renal arteries using a cardiac-triggered 2D PC acquisition offers enormous promise for determining both the appropriateness of revascularisation and response to treatment. A somewhat cruder method of determining significance can be implemented by using a 3D PCA acquisition, with the severity and length of signal drop-off within the proximal renal artery distal to the stenosis correlating with increasingly severe grades of stenosis.

Although conventional renal artery stents give an extensive susceptibility artifact that precludes evaluation of the vessel lumen within the stent, stents manufactured from platinum which give little artifact are

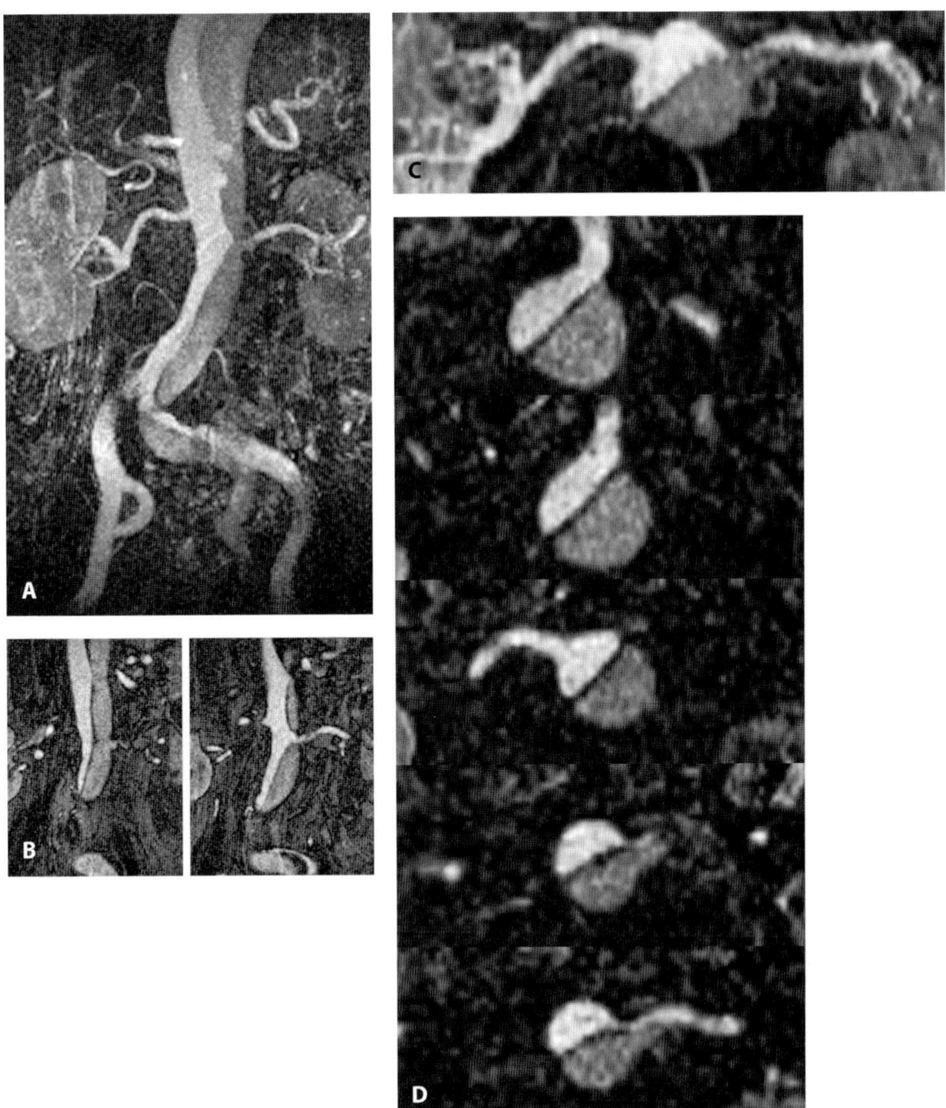

Fig. 13.15A–D. The dissection membrane shown in Fig. 13.8 extends into the iliac arteries. High resolution images may be necessary to clarify whether the dissection involves the renal arteries, resulting in a stenosis. Coronal MIP (**A**) and the source (**B**) images were suspicious of a left renal artery stenosis. The findings were confirmed by selective axial rotated MIP (**C**) and MPR images (**D**). The blood supply for the celiac, mesenteric and the right renal arteries came from the right lumen of the dissection

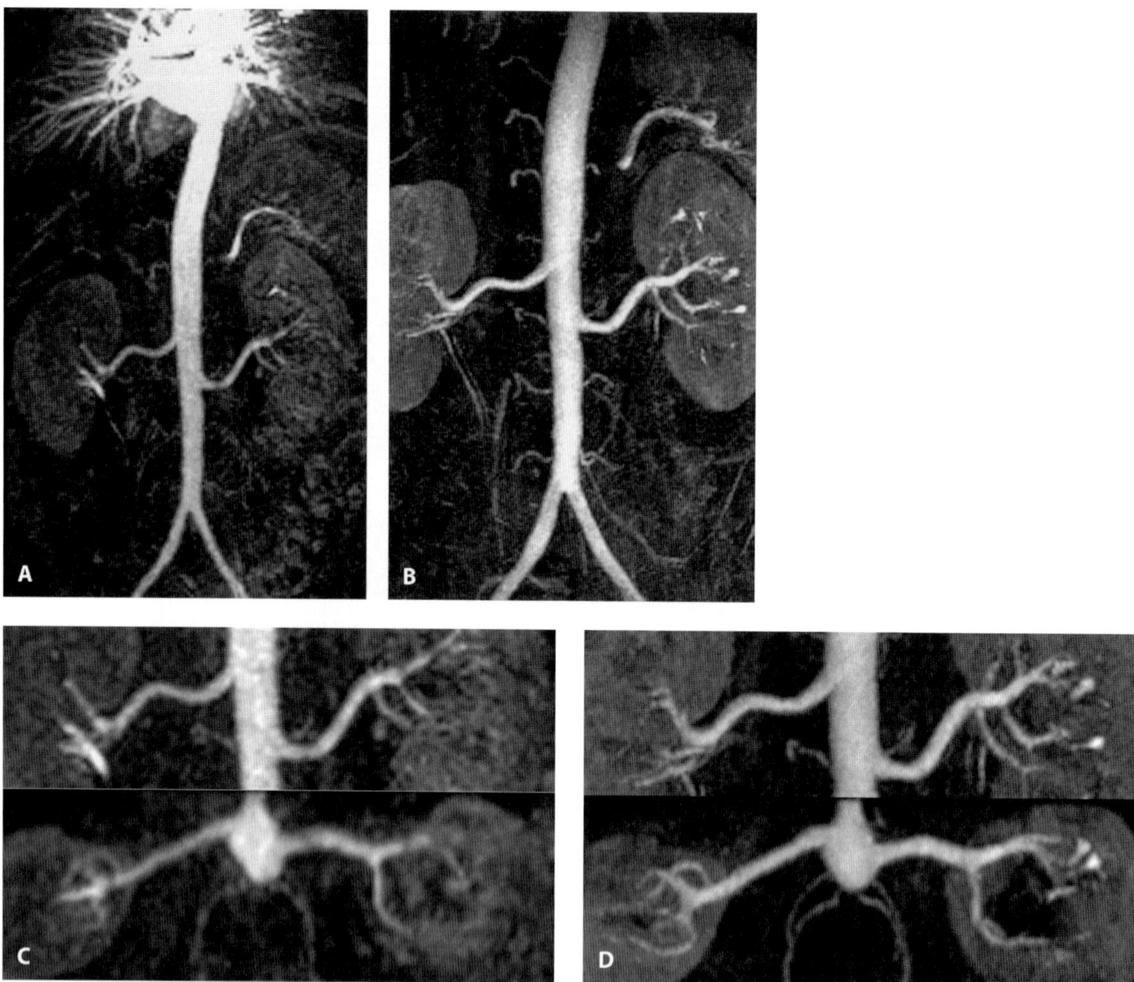

Fig. 13.16A–D. CE MRA studies of renal arteries: comparison of standard body coil with body phased-array coil measurements in the same patient using the same (double) dose of contrast agent. A larger FOV (500 mm) can be obtained by using the standard body coil but at the cost of both reduced resolution and reduced SNR (**A,C**). The smaller peripheral vessel branches can only be visualized by phased-array coil study (**B,D**). Note also the sharper delineated vessel edges in **D** as compared with **C**

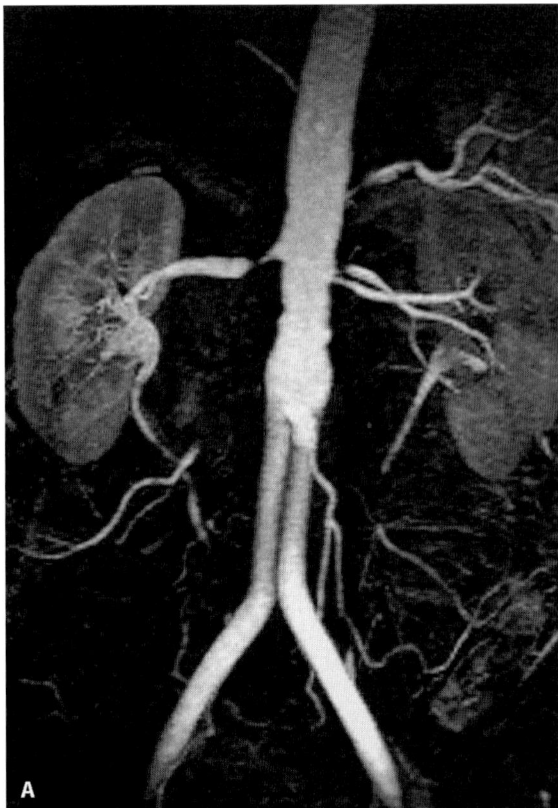

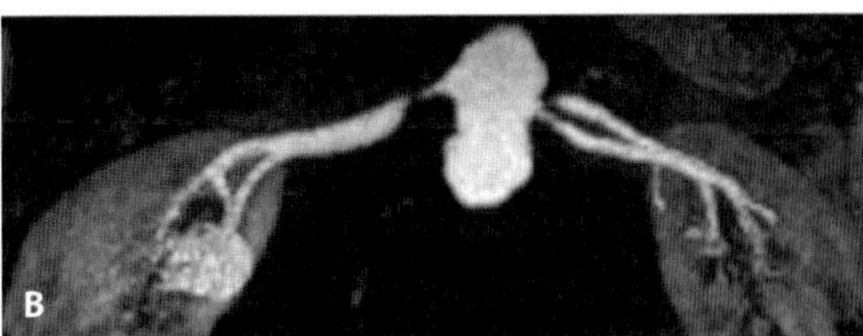

Fig. 13.17A,B. Double-dose Gd and high resolution technique enable high-quality images of renal arteries: The clearly eccentric high-grade stenosis of the right renal artery with poststenotic dilatation is visualized on transverse MIP images (**B**) providing high resolution is also obtained in the slice select direction (decrease the partition thickness to <1.5 mm). However, this is only possible in patients with good breath-hold capability. In addition, the high-grade stenosis of the left main renal artery and the 50%–75% stenosis of the accessory left renal artery can be well depicted (the patient had an aorto-bifemoral bypass graft)

currently under investigation. Use of minimum TE and use of extremely high flip-angles (70°) are necessary in such cases.

The mesenteric arteries are also medium-sized arteries that are ideally evaluated with CE MRA. Although subclinical stenosis within any of the three mesenteric arteries is common, symptomatic mesenteric ischaemia which only occurs with severe stenosis or occlusion of at least two of the three mesenteric arteries is rare. CE MRA is now the investigation of choice for the evaluation of patients with suspected chronic mesenteric ischaemia (Table 13.8) (Fig. 13.14, Fig. 13.21).

13.4.6 Vessels of Lower Extremities

13.4.6.1 Arteries of the Pelvis, Thigh, Leg and Foot

13.4.6.1.1 TOF MRA

Although CE MRA has supplanted TOF MRA for most applications, TOF MRA remains a useful technique for the evaluation of the lower extremity arteries (Table 13.9). Better results have been achieved within the relatively straight arteries of the thighs and legs, where the sensitivity of TOF MRA to slow flow offers substantial advantages. However, the main problem of inflow techniques is the unacceptably long examination times, because of the requirement to acquire data in the axial plane. Additionally, despite the proliferation of fast gradient technology that offers short scan times (secondary to short TRs), this rapid scanning approach cannot be implemented because of the requirement to maintain a relatively long TR of >30 ms to maximize the inflow effects. Therefore, TOF MRA, although accurate, is extremely inefficient in terms of scan time, a limitation that cannot easily be overcome. As a result TOF MRA is limited in most centers to the evaluation of the arteries of the calf and leg, where CE MRA may be suboptimal in some instances and where occult vessels (i.e. those not visualized by conventional DSA onto which bypass grafts can be placed) may be identified.

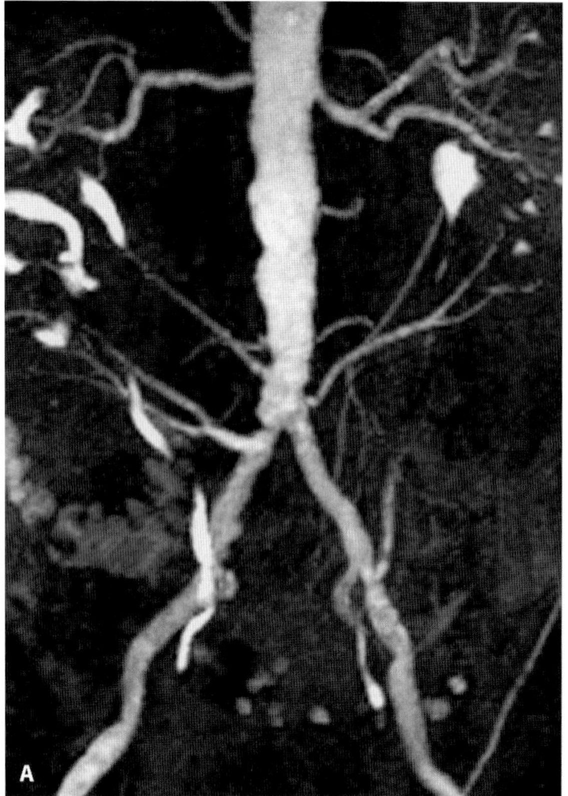

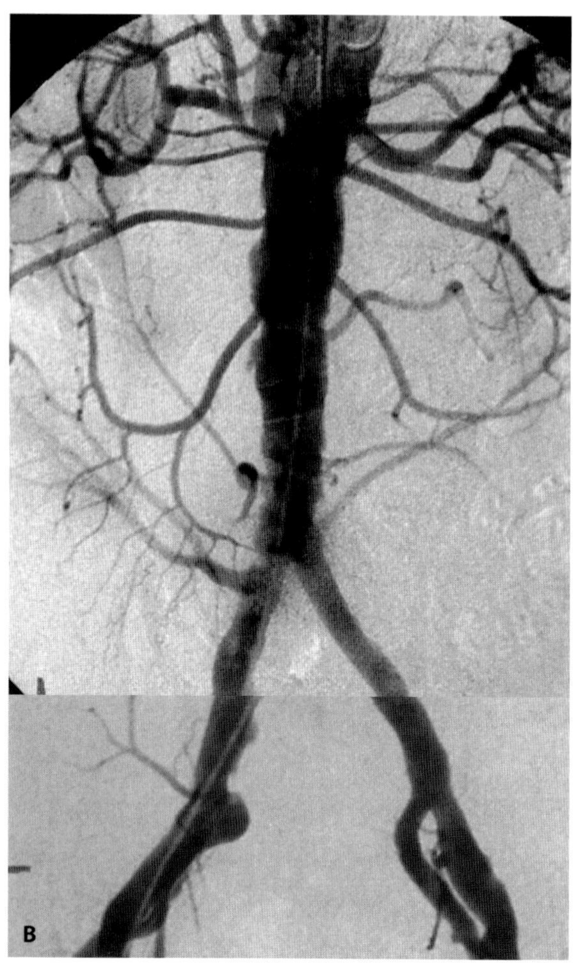

Fig. 13.18A,B. High-grade right common iliac artery stenosis that might be referred for angioplasty after color-duplex ultrasound examination. The double accessory artery at the origin of the stenotic plaque was misidentified as a lumbar artery. The additional accessory renal arteries branching from the distal aorta at both sides were clearly depicted by CE MRA (**A**). DSA is also shown (**B**)

Table 13.9. Magnetic resonance angiography sequene parameters recommendations for iliac, femoral, and lower leg arteries

Sequence	WI	Plane	TR (ms)	TE (ms)	Flip angle	Slice thickness (mm)	No part	Effth	Matrix	FOV	recFOV (%)	BW	No. of acq.	Acq. time (min:s)
3D GRE LR	T1	cor	3.85	1.5	35	90 3D	58	1.55	256	350	75	650	1	0:43
3D GRE HR	T1	cor	4.57	1.95	35	70 3D	70	1	512	400	75	650	1	1:07
2D FL PC	Ph	cor	83	9	11	80 3D	–	–	512	400	75		1	2:30
2D FL TOF	T1	ax	8	5	30	3	160	2	256	270	75		1	5

Abbreviations: *WI* weighted image; *TR* repetition time; *TI* inversion time; *TE* echo time; *No part* number of partitions; *Effth* effective thickness (mm); *Matrix* matrix (phase × frequency matrix); *FOV* field of view (mm); *recFOV* % rectangular field of view; *BW* bandwidth (Hz); *Acq* number of acquisitions; *LR* low resolution; *HR* high resolution

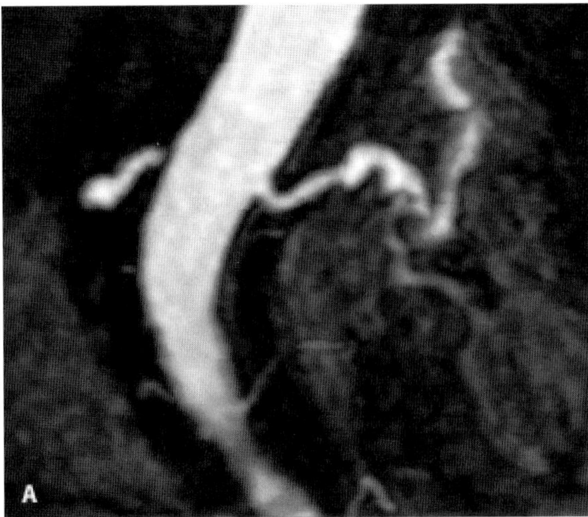

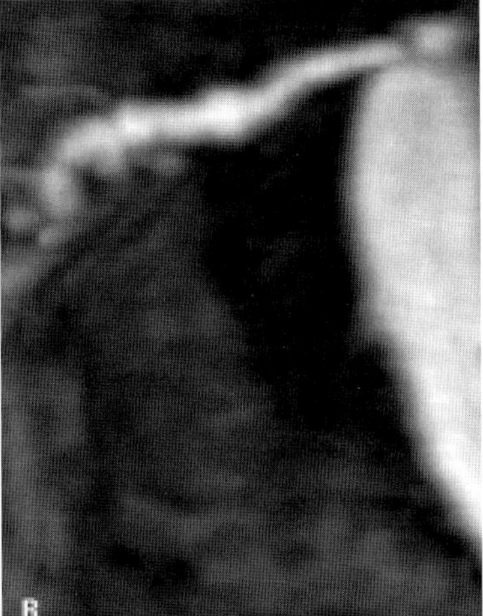

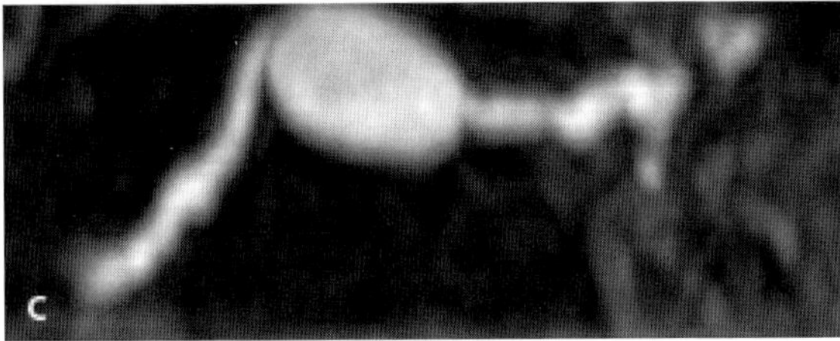

Fig. 13.19A–C. Woman with severe hypertension resistant to drug therapy. Selective oblique MIPs of the left (**A**) and right (**B**) renal arteries show the typical appearance of severe bilateral fibromuscular dysplasia. The craniocaudal MIP (**C**) confirms the findings of FMD

13.4.6.1.2 PC MRA

PC MRA permits coronal slice orientation using a larger FOV along the flow direction. Although 3D PCA scan times are long, a single flow-encoding gradient (rather than the customary three) can be applied in the head-foot direction due to the predominant craniocaudal direction of flow within the peripheral arteries, which substantially reduces the scan time (2D technique). However, as several velocities may be encountered within the imaging field, multiple *Venc* gradients must be applied for optimal imaging. Although this technique is reasonably accurate, there are few proponents of the approach, firstly due to difficulties in appropriately selecting the *Venc*, and secondly to the success of CE MRA.

13.4.6.1.3 CE MRA

CE MRA can be performed as a single location examination (as dictated by the clinical scenario), consecutive scans can be acquired at different imaging locations using separate injections for each location, or a moving table approach can be used that allows imaging at successive locations during a single injection.

13.4.6.1.4 Single-Location MRA

Using CE MRA, high-resolution images with high SNR can be acquired (Fig. 13.20). Images over a 40–50 cm FOV, targeted to the anatomically relevant area, can be acquired using a standard approach. The scan delay time can be determined using either a timing bolus or, preferably, a fluoroscopic technique.

13.4.6.1.5 Multi-location, Multi-injection MRA

The limitation of poor spatial coverage in the head-foot direction (requirement for coverage of a distance of more than 100 cm compared with a maximum permissible FOV of <50 cm on all commercially available systems) was initially overcome by performing successive imaging of the arteries of the pelvis, thighs and legs with separate injections. However, background and venous signal from earlier injections hampered evaluation of the arteries of the thighs and especially the legs.

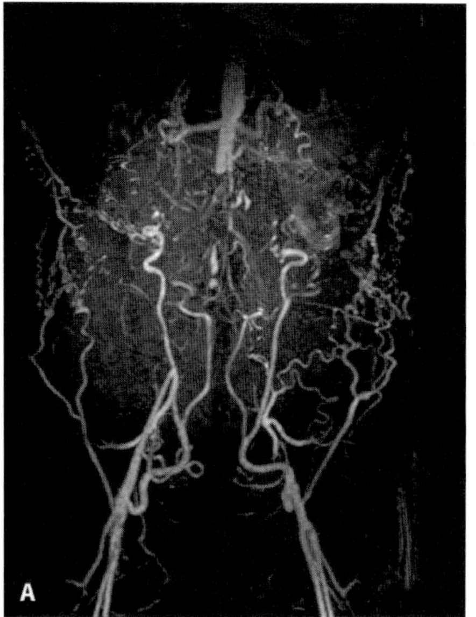

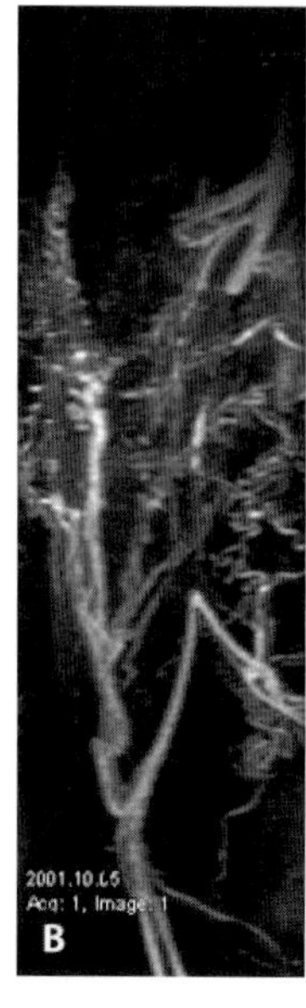

Fig. 13.20A–D. **A** Contrast-enhanced MRA of the abdominal arteries in a 20-year-old patient with a previous history of surgically corrected thoracic coarctation. Whole-volume MIP shows occlusion of the abdominal aorta just below the level of the renal arteries. **B** Lateral MIP shows extensive anterior abdominal wall collaterals. **C** Selective AP MIP shows the extensive collaterals (inferior and superficial epigastric) that reconstitute distal flow. **D** Selective AP MIP of the posterior thoracic wall showing multiple dilated intercostal channels, typical of this condition

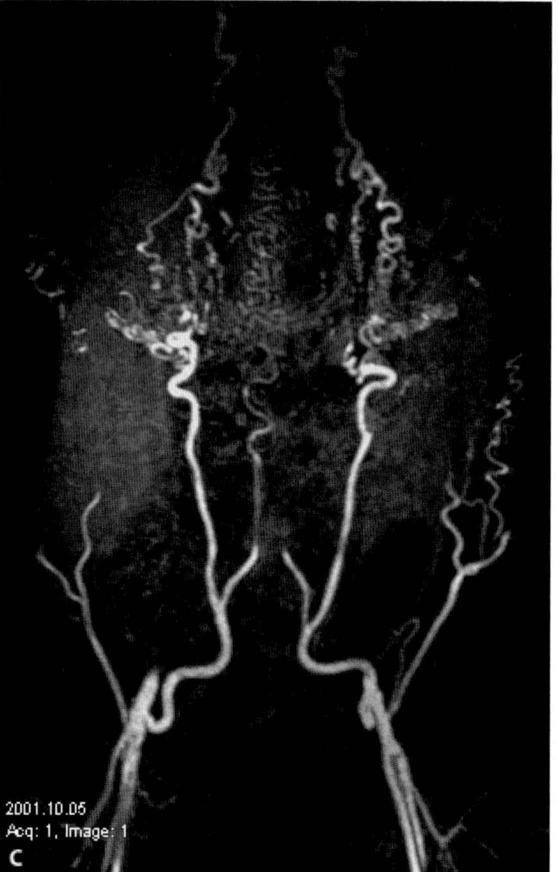

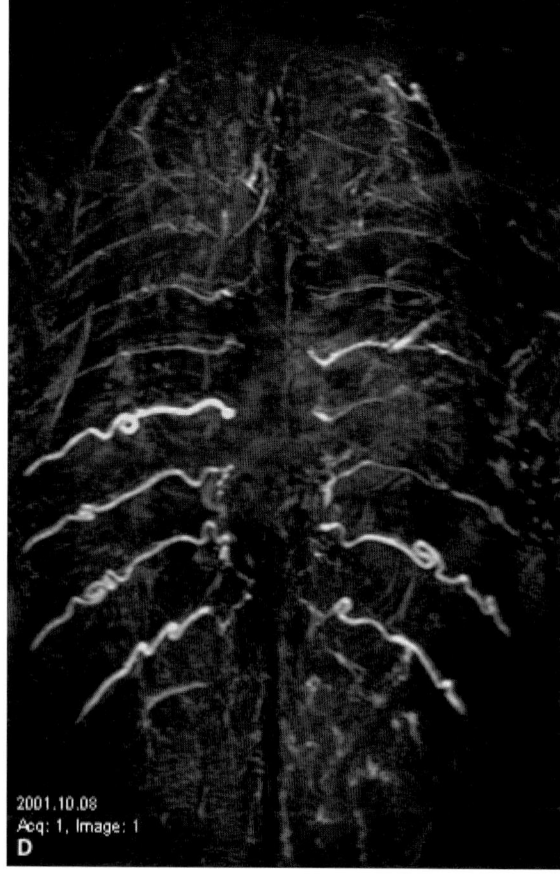

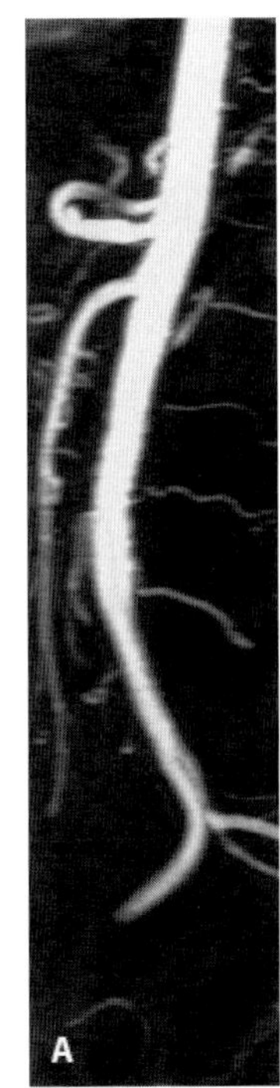

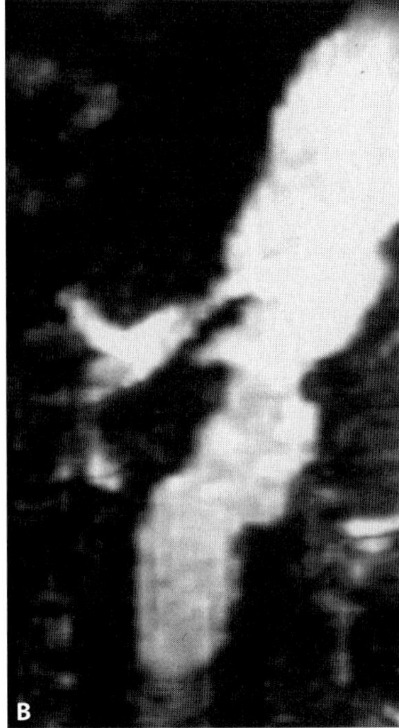

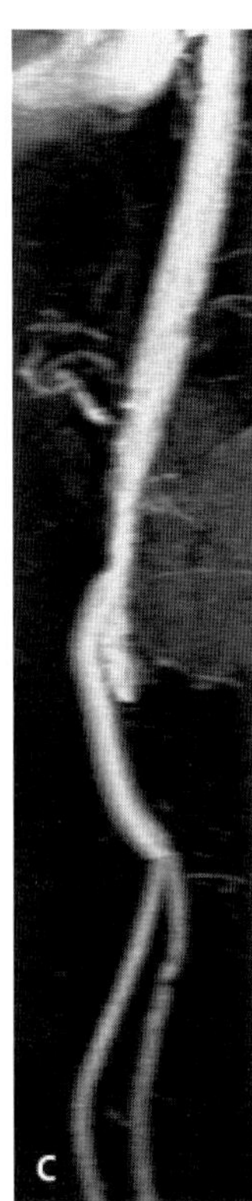

Fig 13.21A–C. A Lateral MIP of the abdominal aorta shows normal appearance of the celiac, superior and inferior mesenteric arteries in a normal subject. **B** Lateral MIP of the abdominal aorta shows >50% stenosis of the celiac axis and occlusion of the superior mesenteric artery. Additionally, the inferior mesenteric artery was occluded. These findings fulfil the criteria for chronic mesenteric ischaemia in a patient with a compatible history. **C** Lateral MIP of the abdominal aorta in another patient who had undergone aorto-bifemoral bypass grafting, with a history of chronic mesenteric ischaemia. The image shows severe stenosis of the celiac axis and occlusion of both the superior and inferior mesenteric arteries, confirming the suspected diagnosis of chronic mesenteric ischaemia

Using this approach, we recommend using 0.1 mmol/kg for each of the three measurements, with the body phased-array coil if possible (the coil position has to be changed twice) as it gives higher SNR for all regions. Either the pelvic arteries or the tibial vessels should be evaluated first, otherwise overlay by the bladder and other enhancing structures may complicate image evaluation.

The more distal run-off in the foot area can either be evaluated by a TOF MRA acquired prior to the CE MRA or by a separate CE MRA measurement with at least 0.2 mmol/kg/body weight (BW) enabling high resolution (Fig. 13.30B). The head coil should be used regardless of the technique. Evaluation of the foot arteries may not be necessary in all patients, but it is important in cases where distal bypass surgery is considered.

13.4.6.1.6 Moving Table MRA

More recently, the spatial limitation has been overcome by using a moving-table approach with rapid table translation between successive scans centered over the pelvis, thighs and legs in association with a single contrast injection. Because the scan time for three consecutive 3D scans is longer than the transit time from aorta to thigh and leg veins, several trade-offs must be implemented to ensure completion of imaging prior to onset of venous enhancement within the second and third stations. For example, the contrast injection rate must be reduced (with subsequent reduced SNR) due to the long scan times, and therefore, phase-array coils that boost SNR should be used whenever possible. A precontrast mask can overcome some of the limitations of the lower infusion rate by eliminating fat from the image after digital subtraction of the pre-contrast images. This technology has only recently been implemented in the design of MR systems, and further refine-

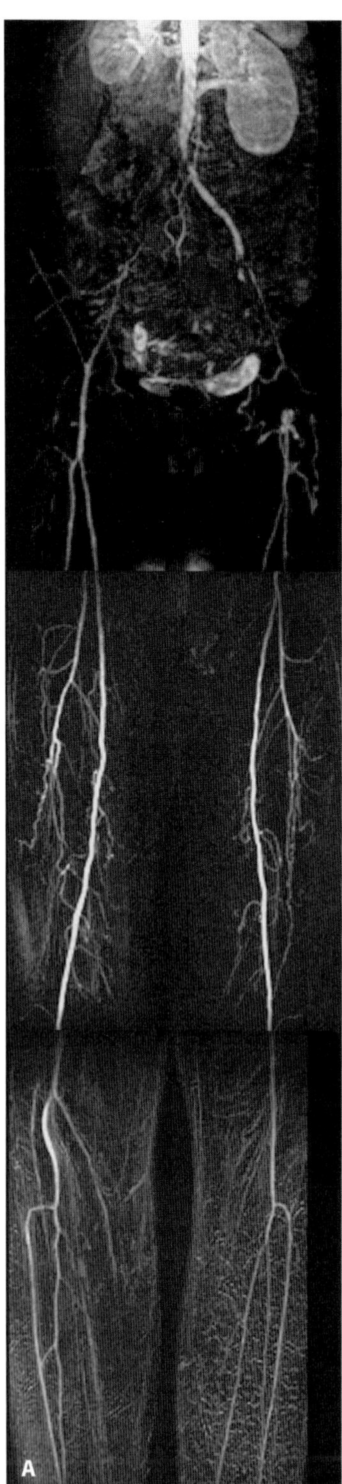
A

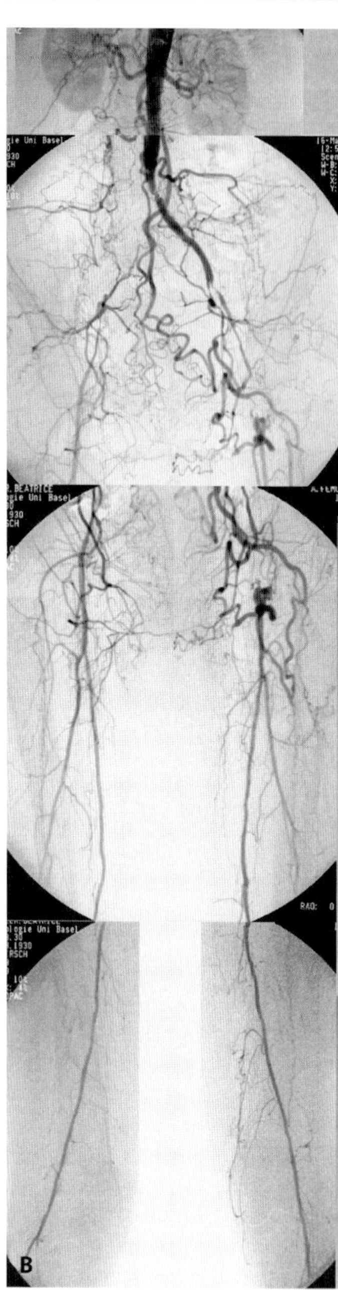
B

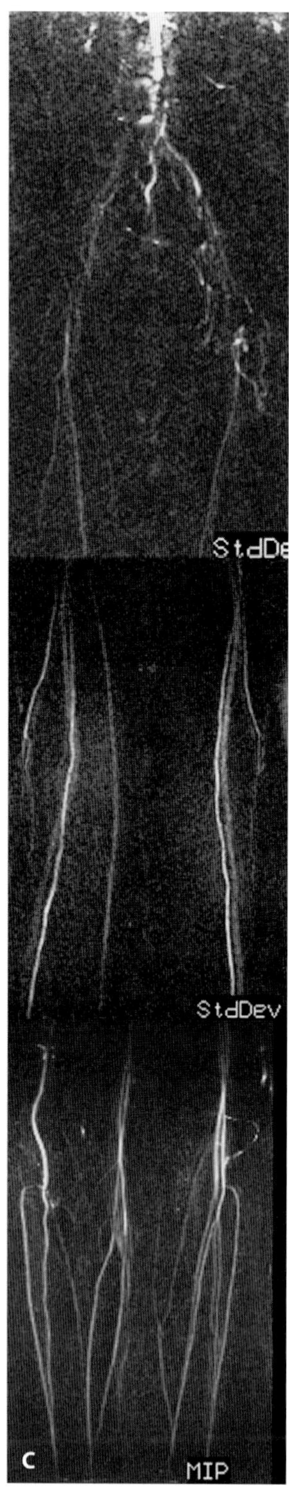
StdDev
MIP
C

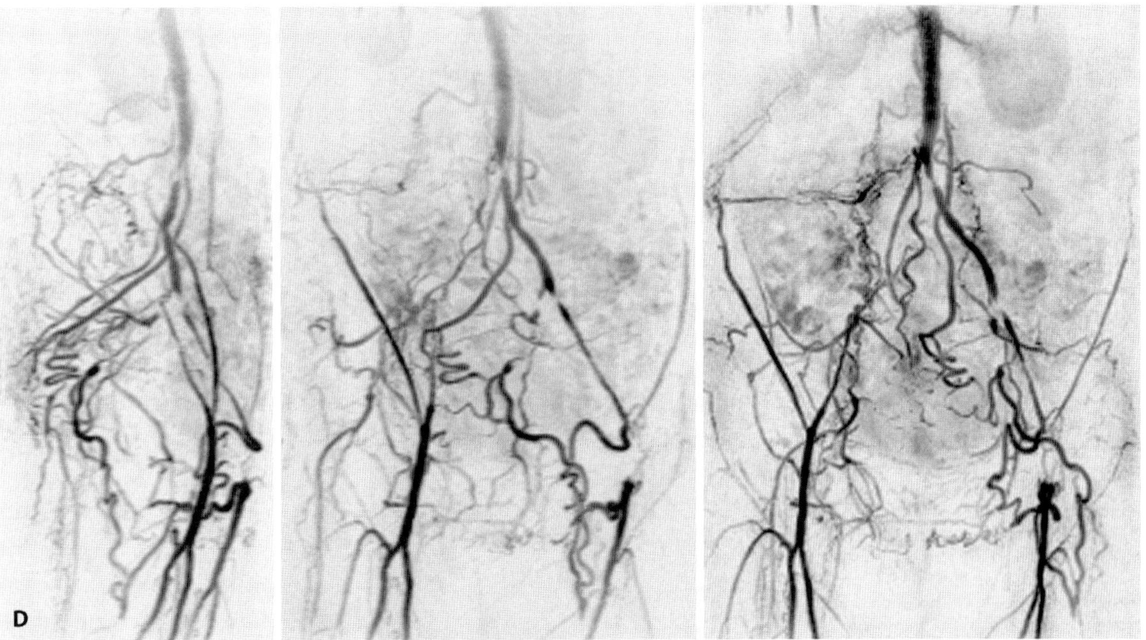

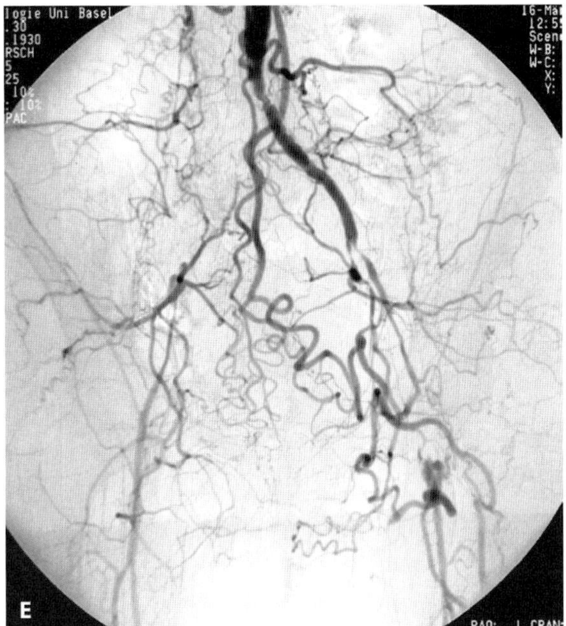

Fig. 13.22A–E. 3D CE MRA low (**A**) and high resolution (**D**); selective e.g. DSA (**B**); 2D PC MRA (**C**). Note the body weight of only 50 kg; therefore, 3×10 ml Gd (3×single dose) was applied. The long occlusion of the right common iliac artery, the high-grade proximal left common iliac artery stenosis, and the occlusion of the external iliac artery were correctly identified. The 2D PC MRA images are of poor diagnostic quality due to slow flow. A second high-resolution CE MRA (**D**) was performed 5 days later using the triple-dose technique (0.3 mmol Gd/kg, flow rate 1.5 ml/s, 150-mm slab thickness, 120 partitions; body phased-array coil). This CE MRA images gives better evaluation of collateral flow than the i.a. DSA (**E**) due to its multidirectional projection modality. Note the increased quality of this approach over the single-dose technique (**A**)

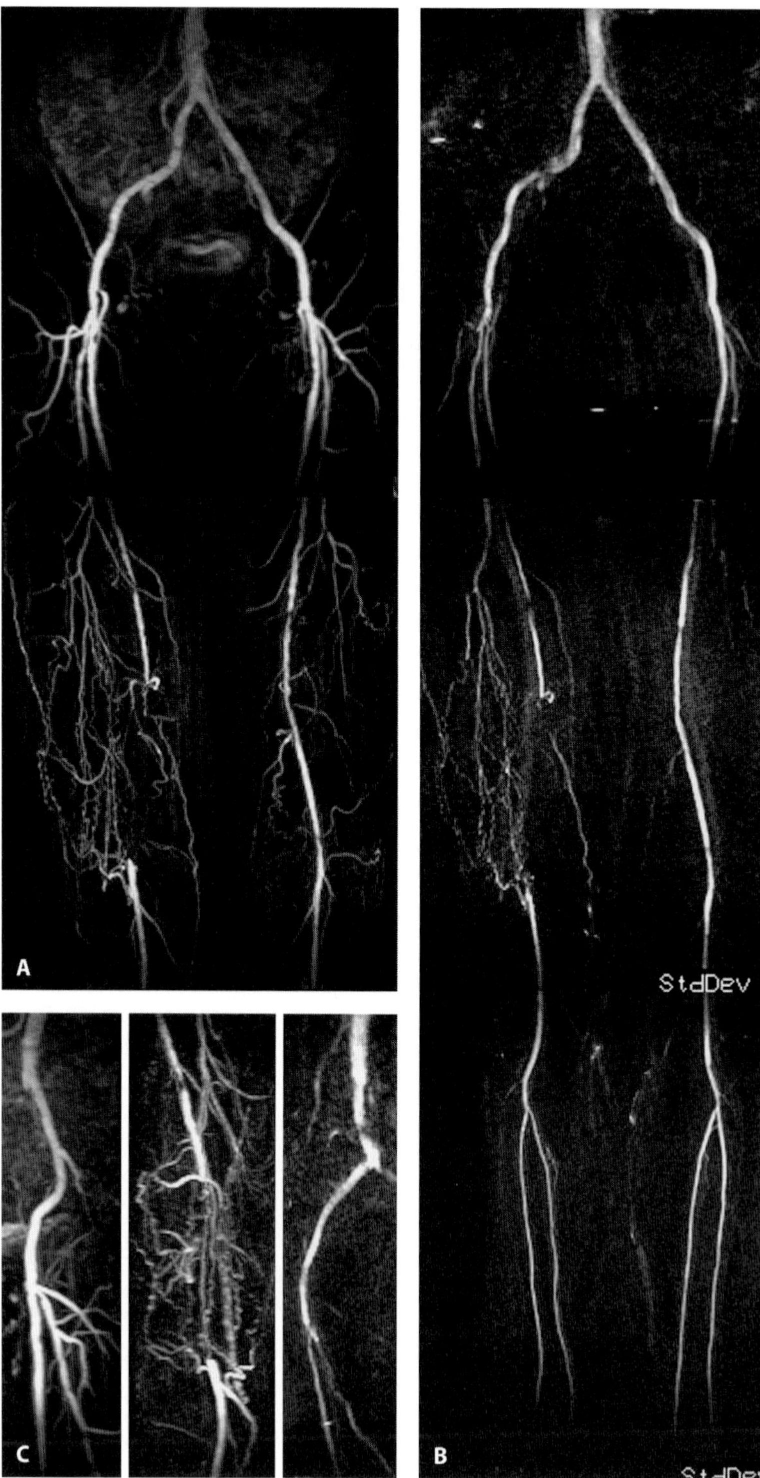

Fig. 13.23A–C. Patient with a 10-cm-long occlusion, two proximal and a middle-third high-grade stenosis of the right superficial femoral artery (SFA) and a high-grade stenosis of the left SFA. CE MRA (**A**) technique: (1) Iliac arteries, single-dose Gd; therefore, lower resolution parameters were obtained. (2) Femoral arteries, double-dose Gd after moving the patient: high-resolution measurement parameters were applied (voxel size 1×1×1.4 mm^3, 512 matrix, body phase-array coil was used for all measurements). 2D PC MRA (**B**) for all three localizations (*Venc* 90/60/30, 45/30/20 and 30/20/10 cm/s; multiple *Venc* values were defined for read-out gradient in head-foot direction). Note that the occlusion was identified by both modalities, but 3D CE MRA clearly shows more details of smaller and collateral vessels. Dephasing artifacts seemed to indicate a high-grade stenosis of the right external iliac artery on the PC MRA image, CE MRA clearly showed no stenosis. Another advantage of CE MRA is that it provides multidirectional MIP views (**C**), which made it possible to identify the high-grade stenosis of the deep femoral artery (**C**; *left image*)

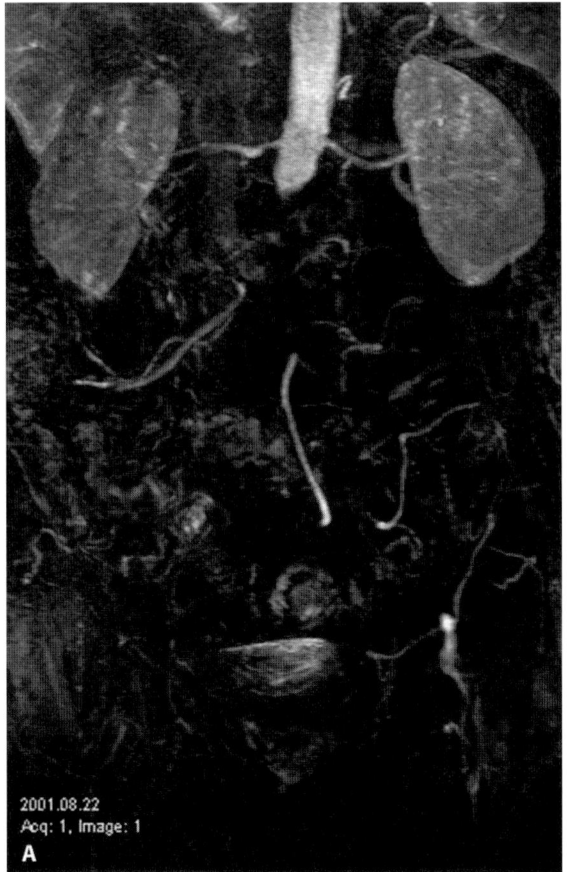

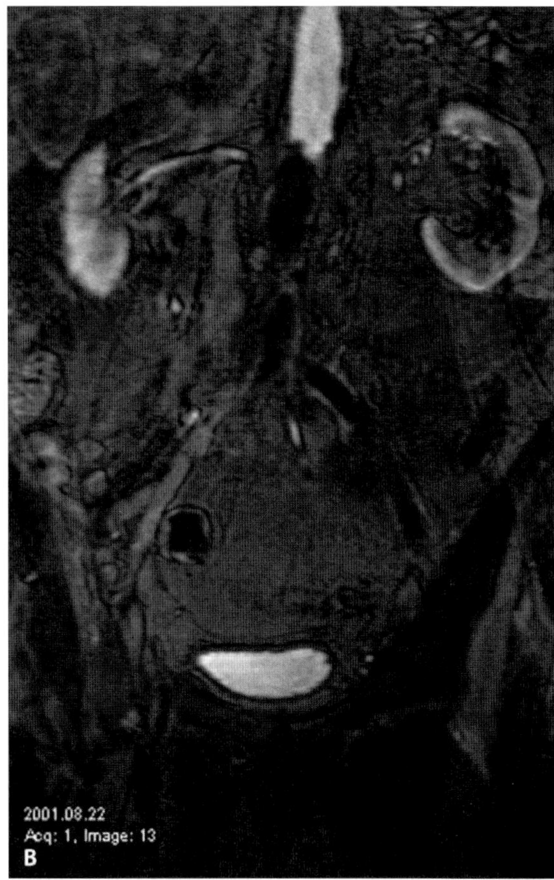

Fig. 13.24A–C. A Elderly male patient with sudden onset of severe left lower limb ischaemic pain, several months following an aorto-bifemoral graft. The right limb of the graft had previously occluded. Moving-table approach used. The whole volume MIP shows occlusion of the aorta below the renal arteries, and occlusion of the common and external iliac arteries bilaterally. Note a small enhancing segment of the left common femoral artery. **B** Individual partition shows intraluminal thrombus within the distal aorta and iliac arteries on the left side, consistent with a saddle embolus. Because the MIP is a 'projection' technique, the presence of intravascular thrombus/embolus can be masked unless the source images are evaluated. **C** Repeat MRA following surgical thrombectomy. The distal aorta and left iliac arteries are now patent. Note irregularity within the aorta due to clot adherent to the wall

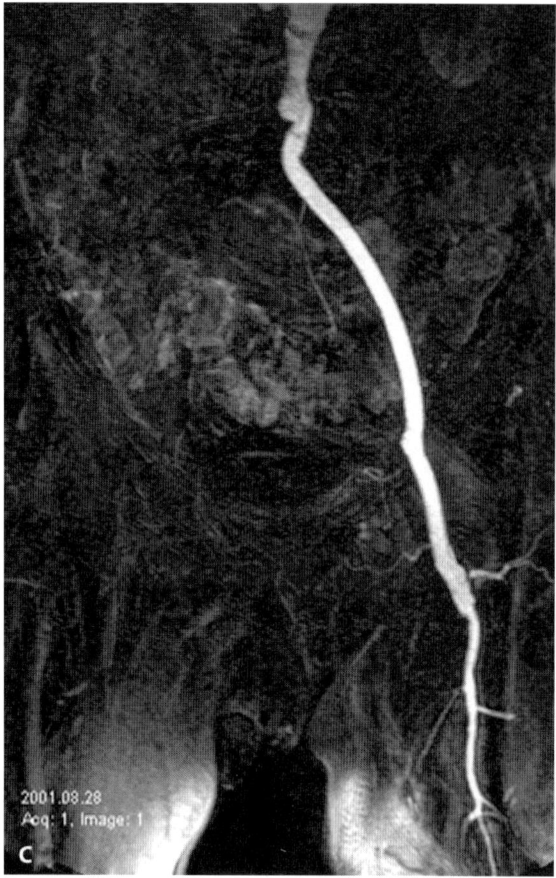

Fig. 13.24C.

ment of the technique is essential. Nonetheless, the results of 3D CE MRA compared with DSA are excellent regardless of the exact technique used.

For evaluation of the iliac arteries, breath-holding is not strictly necessary, but because of the frequent association (20%–45%) of renal artery stenosis with peripheral vascular disease, the slab volume should include the renal arteries if possible, and in this instance breath holding is essential. Thick 3D volumes (approximately 60–100 mm) in coronal orientation are required for the iliac region because of the superficial anterior course of the common femoral artery, the more posteriorly placed aorta, and tortuosity of the iliac arteries in between. The partition thickness must optimally be reduced to 1.5 mm. In our experience, isotropic resolution of 1.5 mm is sufficient to estimate the therapeutic relevance of iliac artery stenosis using a 256 (frequency-encoding direction) matrix. However, use of a 512 matrix doubles the resolution in the head-foot direction without increasing the scan time, with the minor penalties of reduced SNR and slightly increased echo time.

For evaluation of the thighs, similar parameters to those for the pelvic arteries can be used, but because of the smaller vessel size, higher resolution is preferable.

However, for evaluation of the arteries of the calf, higher resolution is essential due to the smaller size of the leg arteries. At the time of writing this chapter, a flexible parameter choice for each of the imaging locations is possible with only the minority of moving tables, although this modification is expected on all imaging systems in the near future. Clearly, in instances where separate examinations of the three regions of interest are performed in association with separate contrast injections, scan parameters can be individually optimized for each location.

13.4.6.1.7
Role of 2D Imaging?

Although the 3D technique has been exploited by most authors, contrast enhanced 2D imaging (using complex subtraction if possible) offers substantial advantages in terms of improved temporal resolution. Dynamic 2D CE MRA of the calf and foot (MR DSA) has been shown to be superior to 2D TOF MRA (which in turn is superior to DSA). Some authors advocate the use of hybrid 2D/3D techniques, which are currently being evaluated (Fig. 13.30A).

Table 13.10. Different spatial resolution of images can be obtained using various coils, Gd dosage, and slab volume thickness

Spatial resolution	Coil	Dose	Slab-volume thickness (mm)
Low	Standard body	0.1 mmol Gd/kg bw	70–120
Moderate	Standard body	0.1 mmol Gd/kg bw	70– 90
Moderate	Body phased array	0.1 mmol Gd/kg bw	70–120
High	Body phased array	0.2 mmol Gd/kg bw	70–120
High	Body phased array	0.3 mmol Gd/kg bw	120–170

The spatial resolution regarding the setting of coil, CM dose and slab-volume thickness is defined in Table 13.10.

13.4.6.2 Special CM-Application Features for CE MRA of Renal and Peripheral Arteries

The CM bolus will be much more diluted at the more peripheral site of the peripheral arteries. Therefore, our preliminary study results suggest varying the flow rate in relation to the dilution factor of CM. This dilution factor (Table 13.11) depends on the way the blood flows into the more peripheral vessel region. The flow rate (FR) than can be calculated as follows:

$$FR = \frac{BW \cdot D_{appl} \cdot BDF}{(5\,s{+}60\%\,MT) \cdot C_{Gd}}$$

$$V_{Gd} = \frac{BW \cdot D_{appl}}{C_{Gd}}$$

$$BL_{periph} = 5\ s + 60\ MT$$

$$BL_{inj} = \frac{BL_{periph}}{BDF}$$

$$BL_{inj} = \frac{(5\ s{+}60\%\,MT)}{BDF}$$

$$FR = \frac{V_{Gd}}{BL_{inj}}$$

(*) 5 s should be added because of time delay of CM running from main arteries to more peripheral vessels (small branching vessel, collateral circulation).

Abbreviations:

FR	flow rate (ml/s)
V_{Gd}	volume of applied GD (ml)
BW	body weight (kg)
D_{appl}	applied dosage (mmol/kg[bw])
sd	0.1 mmol/kg(bw)
dd	0.2 mmol/kg(bw)
td	0.3 mmol/kg(bw)
C_{Gd}	Concentration of applied Gd (usually 0.5 mmol/ml)
BL_{periph}	bolus length peripheral (s) (at vessel region of interest)
MT	measurement time (s)
BL_{inj}	bolus length of injection (s)

Table 13.11. Vessel regions and bolus dilution factor (regarding to our preliminary study results)

Vessel region	BDF
Renal arteries	2.0
Iliac arteries	2.1
Femoral arteries	2.4
Tibial arteries	2.7
Feet arteries	3.0

Example calculation for CE MRA of the entire peripheral circulation of a patient (Fig. 13.25).

Patient data: body weight: 83 kg; height: 176 cm; BAT: 33 s.

The useful dosage was 0.3 mmol Gd/kg bw because the MRA had to be finished during one investigation. Regarding the clinical question, it was sufficient to visualize the proximal third of the tibial vessels. Therefore, for all three measurement steps the body phased-array coil (CP-body array; FOV=370 mm) was used, and the measurement parameters were set to moderate spatial resolution.

Calculation of flow rate for CE MRA of iliac arteries:

$$BL_{inj} = \frac{83\ kg \cdot 0.1\ mmol\ Gd/kg \cdot 2.0}{(5\,s{+}60\% \cdot 29\,s) \cdot 0.5\ mmol/ml}$$

$$FR_{iliac} = 1.56\ ml/s$$

The measurement time of this example remained unchanged for all three CE MRA (BDF=2.4 and 2.7 for femoral and tibial region, respectively, was used). Therefore, the FR for femoral and tibial region was calculated as

$$FR_{femoral} = 1.8\ ml/s$$

$$FR_{tibial} = 2\ ml/s$$

13.4.6.3 Arteries of the Lower Leg and Feet

Motion artifact does not typically occur in this region. Venous overlay may occur especially in cases of AV shunts (Fig. 13.30A), but the acquisition time may be prolonged by use of centric or elliptic-centric phase-encoding (in association with bolus detection if images of the leg only are being acquired), which allows improved spatial resolution, an important considera-

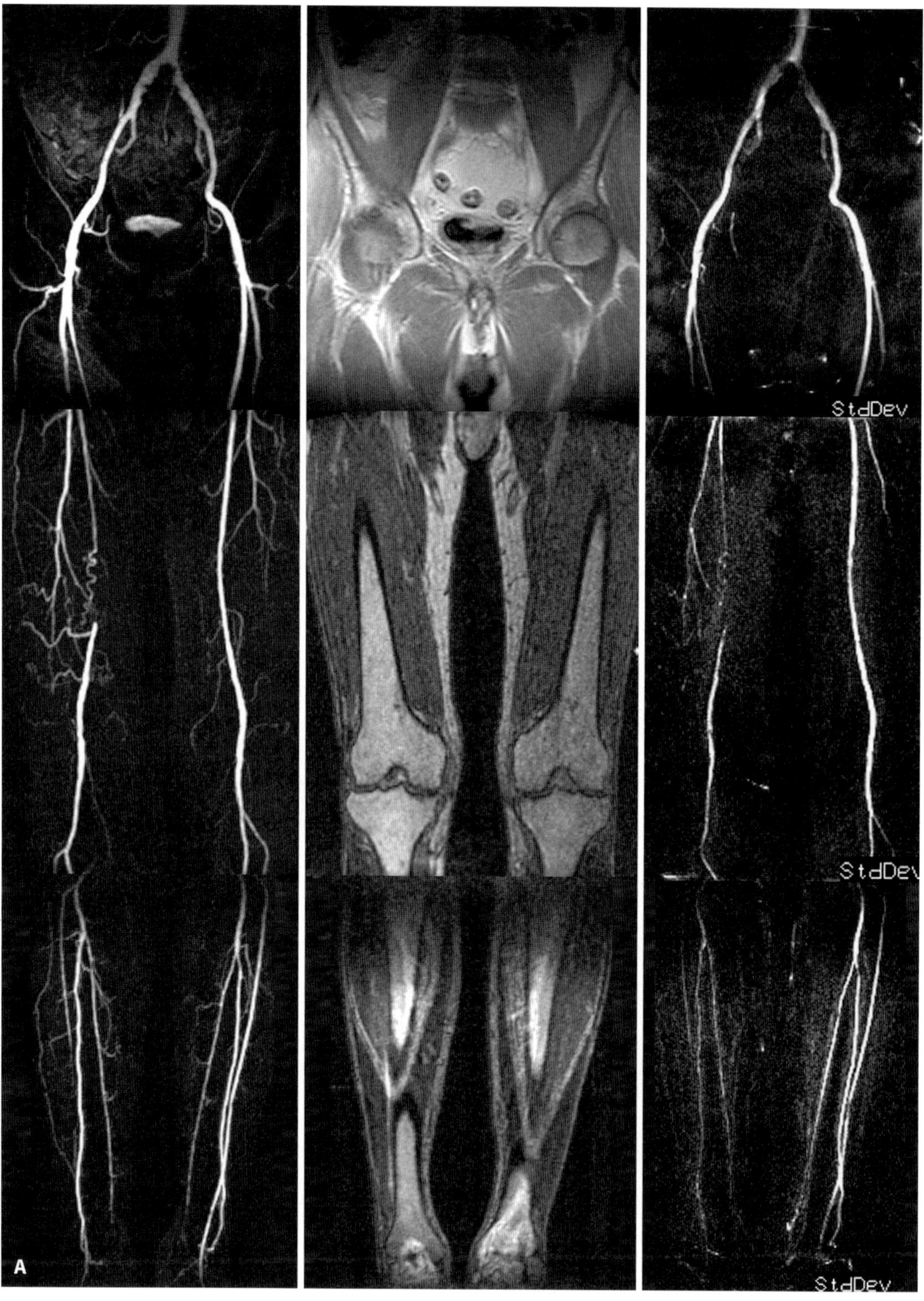
StdDev
StdDev
StdDev
A

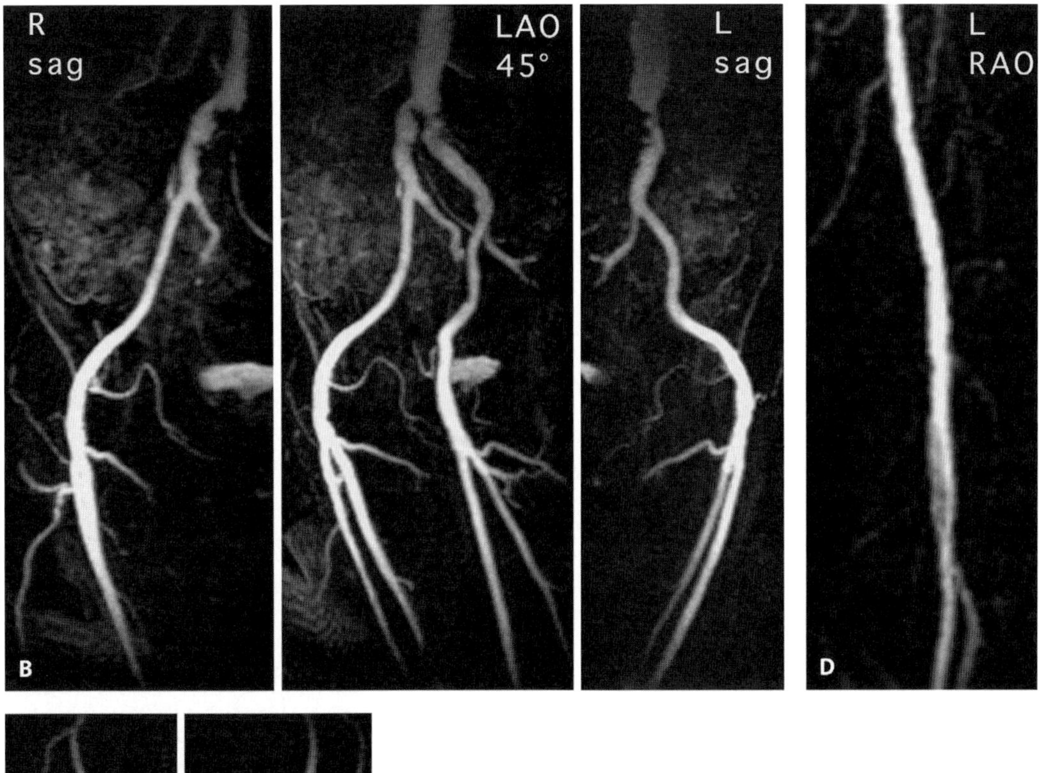

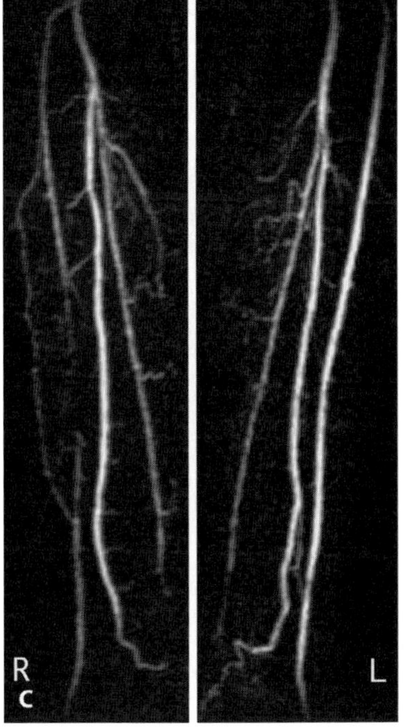

Fig. 13.25A–D. CE MRA (**A1**): 3× single-dose Gd, different flow rates, iliac arteries and lower leg arteries were scanned with body phased-array coil. The femoral region was measured with standard body coil. Anatomical scout (**A2**). 2D PC MRA (**A3**; technique same as in Fig. 13.19B). Patient with 5-cm-long occlusion of right SFA and multiple long proximal stenoses which are not suitable for angioplasty. The collateral circulation is well established. This finding was only depicted at CE MRA (**A1**). The quality of the 2D PC MRA images was not sufficient. Moderate resolution was applied for all three CE MRA scans which produced sufficient quality sagittal images and 45° projections to judge the eccentric high-grade stenoses of common iliac artery stenoses on both sides (**B**; performance of these selective MIP is recommended for each). Note that using this moderate- or high-resolution technique, 30° or 45° projections of lower leg arteries are available (**C**; the segmental occlusion of the right anterior tibial artery can be identified as well as the multiple stenoses of fibular arteries on both sides and the left proximal posterior tibial artery stenosis). The atypical proximal branching of left anterior tibial artery (**D**) was visualized by selective MIP of the middle 3D data set (lower resolution results in lower quality due to the use of a standard body coil)

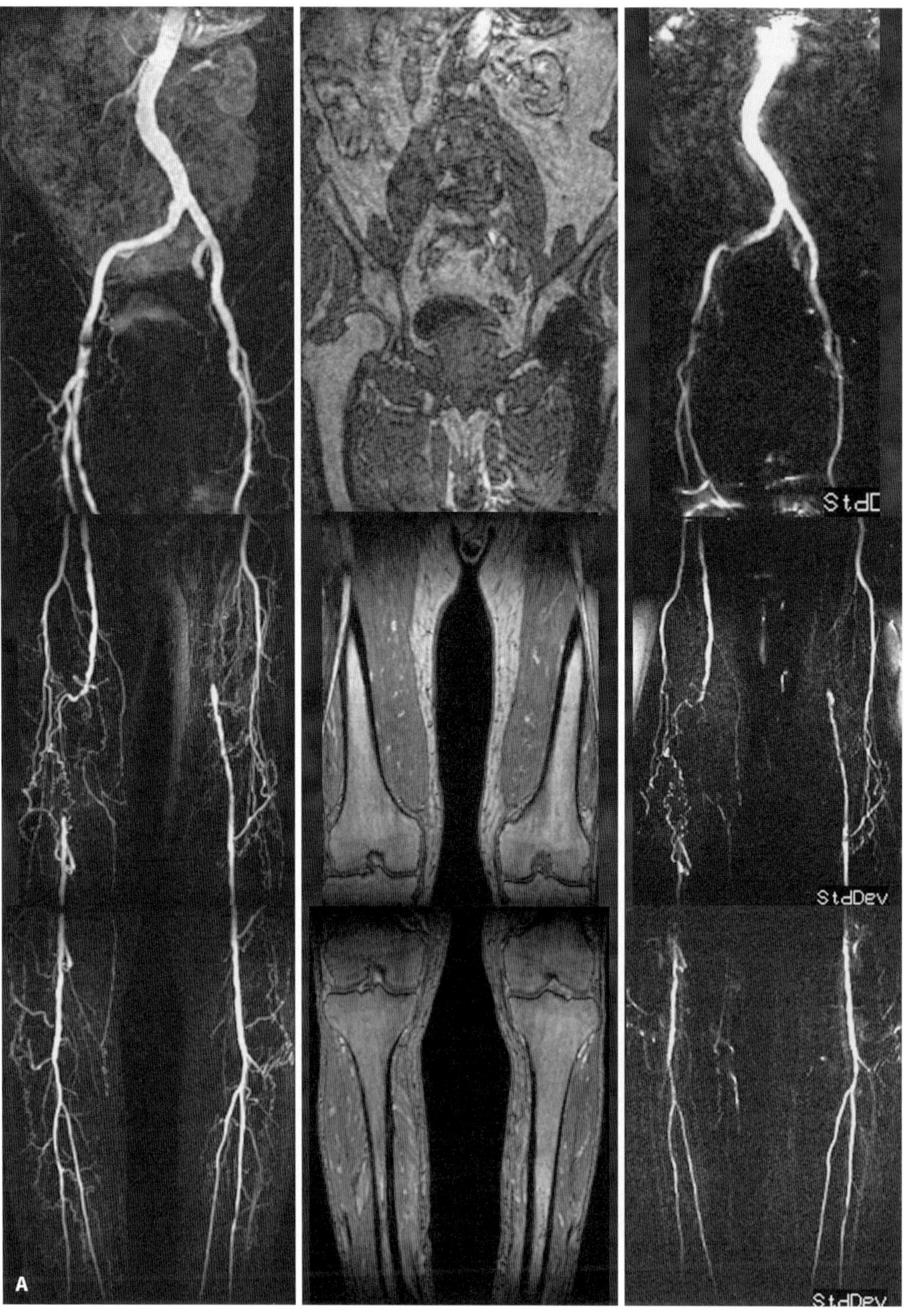
StdD
StdDev
StdDev
A

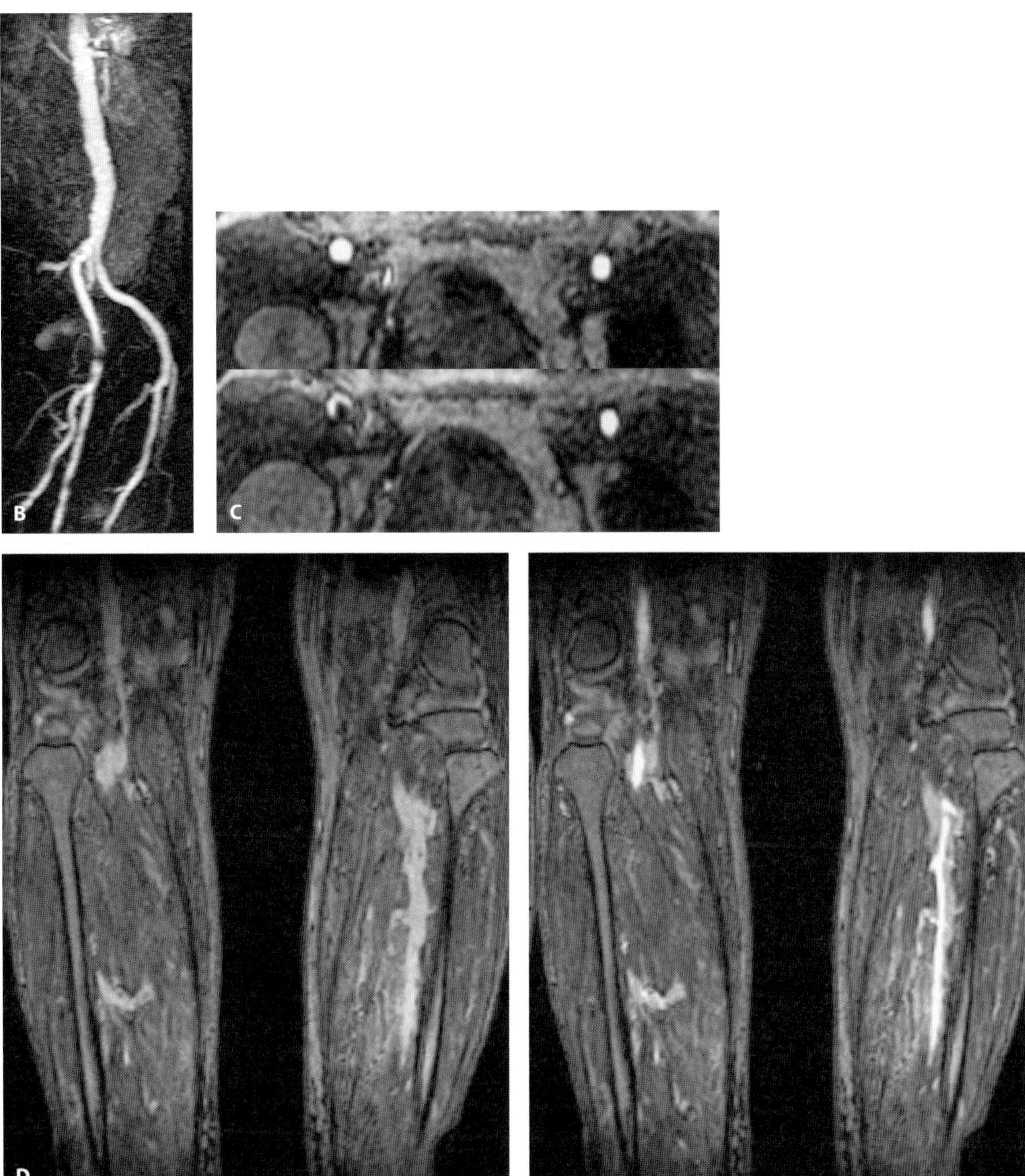

Fig. 13.26A–D. Legende see page 438

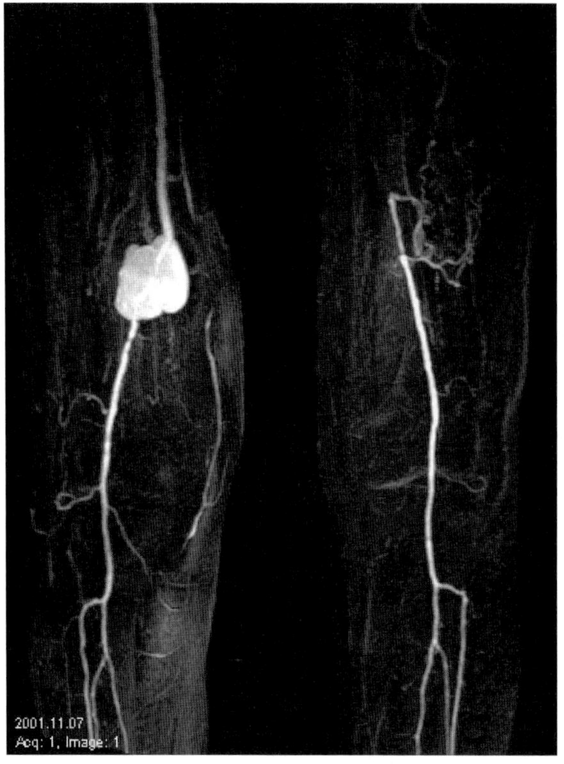

Fig. 13.27. Moving-table contrast-enhanced MRA (0.2 mmol/kg, infusion rate 1 ml/s, images acquired with a dedicated peripheral coil). Whole volume MIP shows a popliteal artery aneurysm on the right. On the left there is occlusion of the superficial femoral artery, with reconstitution of flow within the popliteal artery via collaterals. There is good run-off bilaterally into the calf arteries

tion as the diameter of the three main arteries of the calf varies between 1 mm and 3 mm. Therefore, voxel dimensions in all three directions should be tailored appropriately to 1 mm to achieve optimal results. To compensate for reduced SNR as a result of the small voxel size, the use of surface coils similar to the body phased-array coils is required. The more distal run-off in the feet area can be evaluated by a second scan, possibly best performed by a 2D technique prior to the moving table scan, using either a single (0.1 mmol/kg) or double (0.2 mmol/kg) dose. An in-plane spatial resolution of 1×1 mm is required for a 2D scan (slice thickness 60–100 mm) or 1×1×1 mm if a 3D scan is used (Fig. 13.30B).

13.4.7 Arteries of the Hand

MRA of the hand is rarely performed. Because of the small vessel size, high spatial resolution may be necessary. The scan volume thickness must be tailored appropriately, but a slab depth of approximately 50 mm will cover the anatomy adequately. Rapid venous return requires either short acquisition times or longer acquisition times with centric phase-encoding and bolus detection (Figs. 13.31A,B). Again, flexible wrap-around coils or extremity coils should be used depending on the FOV requirement.

13.5 Future Prospects

CE MRA is a dynamically evolving modality, with improvements in image quality occurring at a rapid rate. In-depth knowledge of contrast dynamics, approximate contrast arrival times, AV transit times, k-space filling order, parameter choice, image resolution and SNR is necessary to ensure the highest standard of practice.

Improvements in pulse sequences design (including parallel imaging techniques), improved contrast agents, more efficient k-space filling algorithms, better coil

◄

Fig. 13.26A–D. CE MRA (**A**; *left image*): 3× single-dose Gd injection; iliac region: standard body coil, femoral and lower leg region: body phased-array coil. 2D PC MRA (**A**; *right image*), a 92-year-old patient with peripheral occlusive disease (Fontaine IIb) due to high-grade stenosis of the right proximal femoral artery. The long occlusions of SFA on both sides are well collateralized by the deep femoral artery. The run-off is sufficient (occlusions of anterior tibial arteries at both sides). 2D PC MRA indicated a high-grade stenosis of the right external iliac artery, but this was not confirmed by 3D CE MRA. **B** Slightly blurred vessel edges at 45° MIP due to lower resolution using a standard body coil. An eccentric calcified plaque was well depicted on MPR images of the 3D CE MRA data set (**C**), which suggested surgical treatment rather than angioplasty. The finding was confirmed at operation. **D** (*left image*) The native data set (lower legs) measured after iliac and femoral regions were scanned. Enhancement of veins is visible (also at CM data set, *right image*) but does not produce overlay of veins if subtraction is performed (see Fig. 13.21A, left image, DS MRA of lower legs)

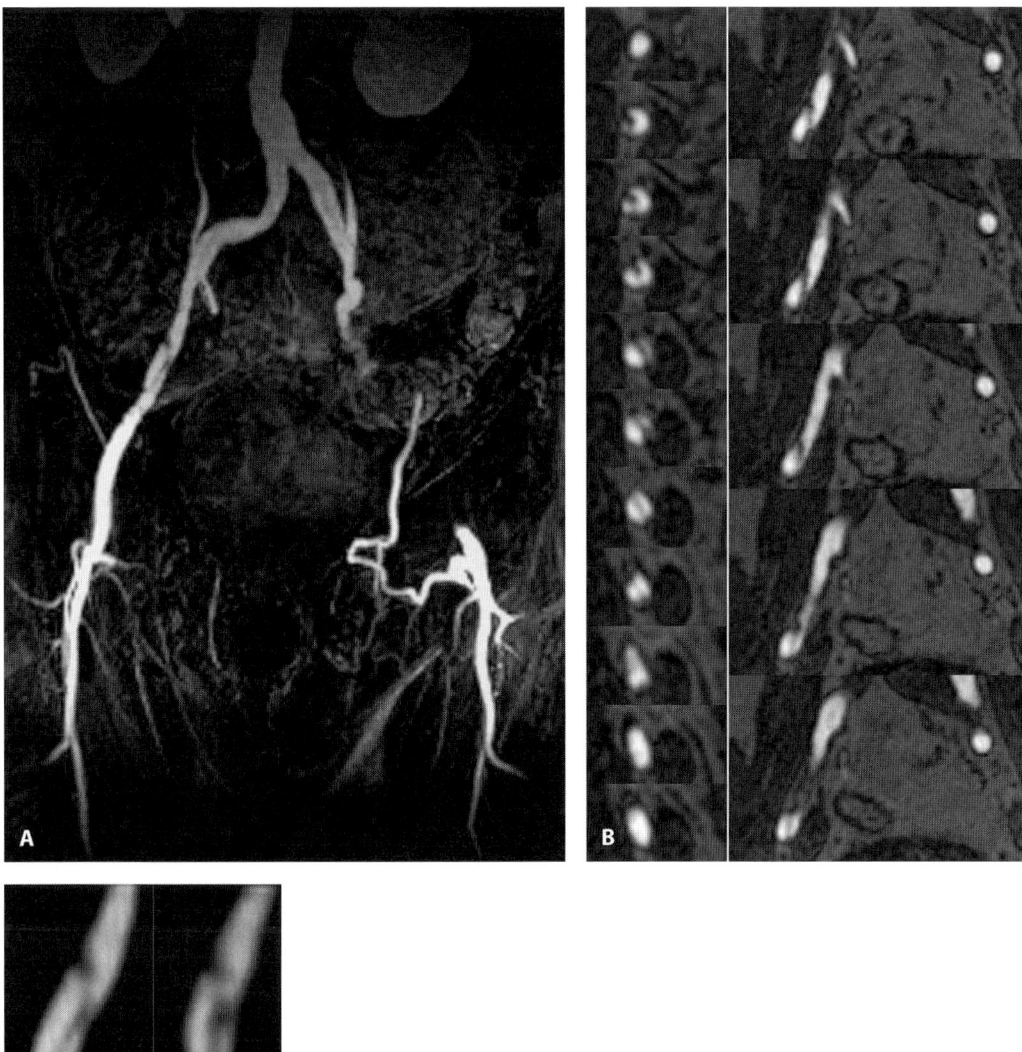

Fig. 13.28A–C. CE MRA at iliac region with moderate resolution (double-dose Gd injection, 2 ml flow rate). The coronal MIP (**A**) showed a long occlusion of left external iliac region with prominent internal iliac to femoral artery collateral flow. On the right side a large dissection flap (after PTA) was visualized. The findings have been selectively reconstructed by MIP (**B**). The MPR and source images (**C**) demonstrated the large dissection flap

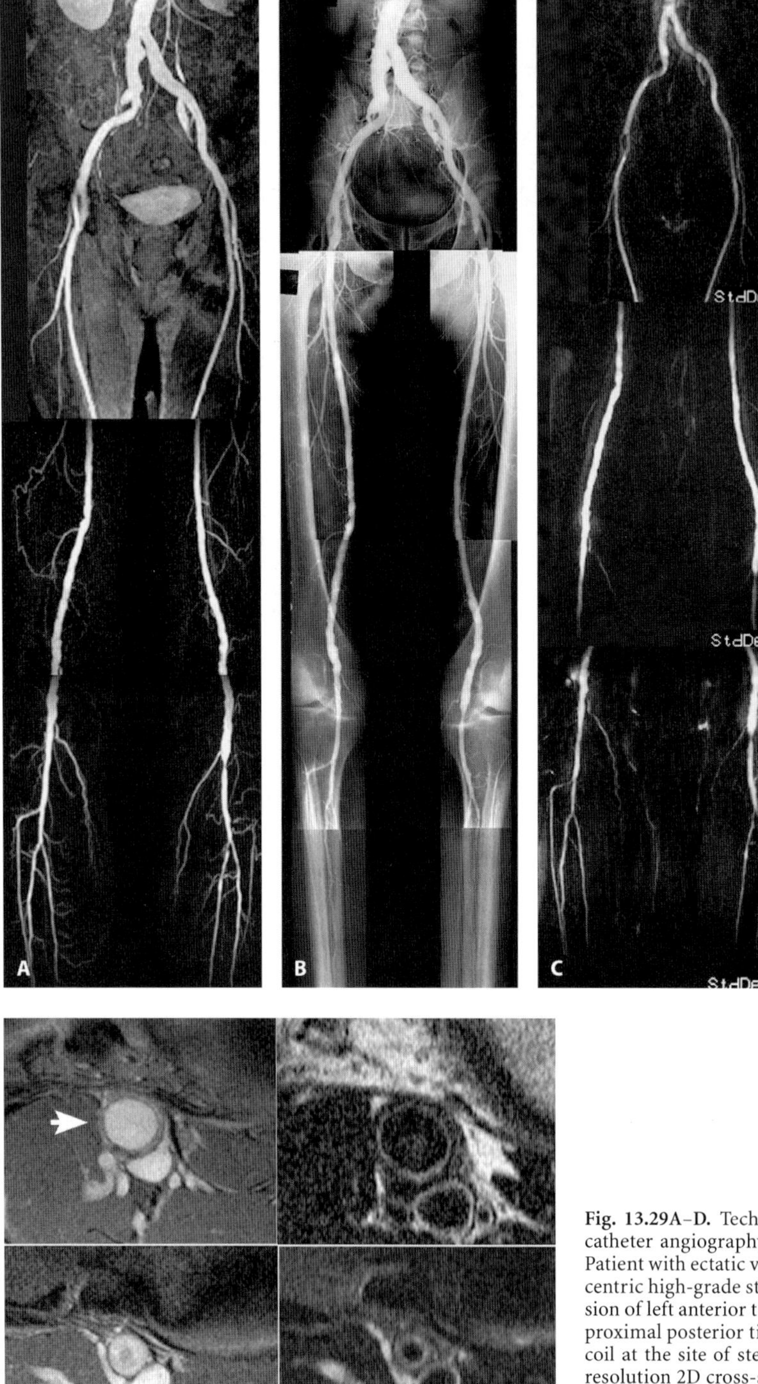

Fig. 13.29A–D. Technique: see Fig. 13.21. **A** CE-MRA (*left*), i.a. catheter angiography (*middle*), and PCA with identical findings. Patient with ectatic vessels secondary to atherosclerosis and a concentric high-grade stenosis of left popliteal artery, proximal occlusion of left anterior tibial artery and high-grade stenosis of the left proximal posterior tibial artery. **D** The use of a body phased-array coil at the site of stenosis offers the possibility to perform high-resolution 2D cross-sectional images (**C**). The *upper right* (T1-W) and *left* (T2-W) images showed the slightly atherosclerotic and dilated popliteal artery proximal of the stenosis. The images at the bottom demonstrated the thickened vessel wall at the site of the stenosis

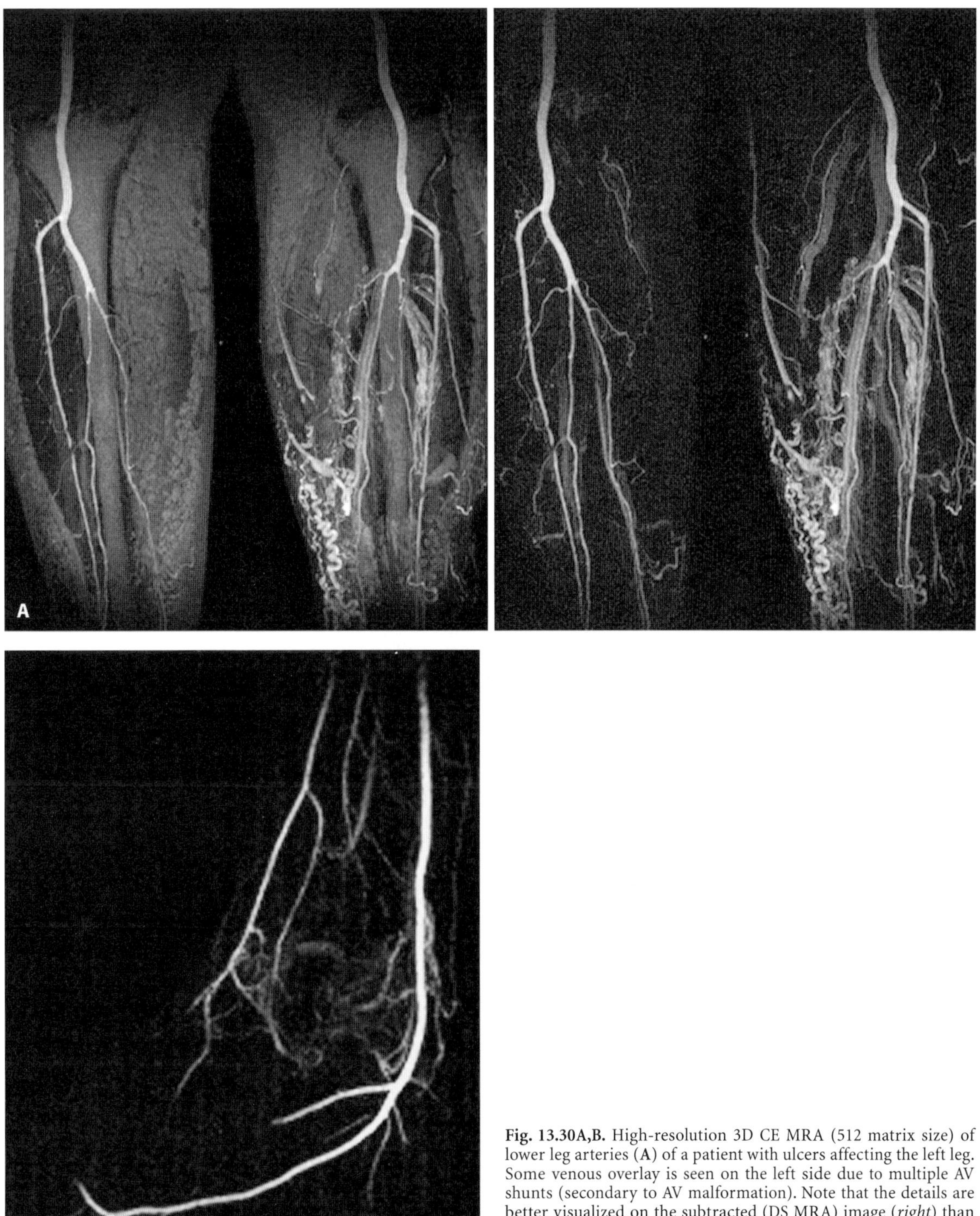

Fig. 13.30A,B. High-resolution 3D CE MRA (512 matrix size) of lower leg arteries (**A**) of a patient with ulcers affecting the left leg. Some venous overlay is seen on the left side due to multiple AV shunts (secondary to AV malformation). Note that the details are better visualized on the subtracted (DS MRA) image (*right*) than on the non-subtracted MIP image (*left*). 3D CE MRA of the feet (**B**): Normal finding, double-dose Gd injection

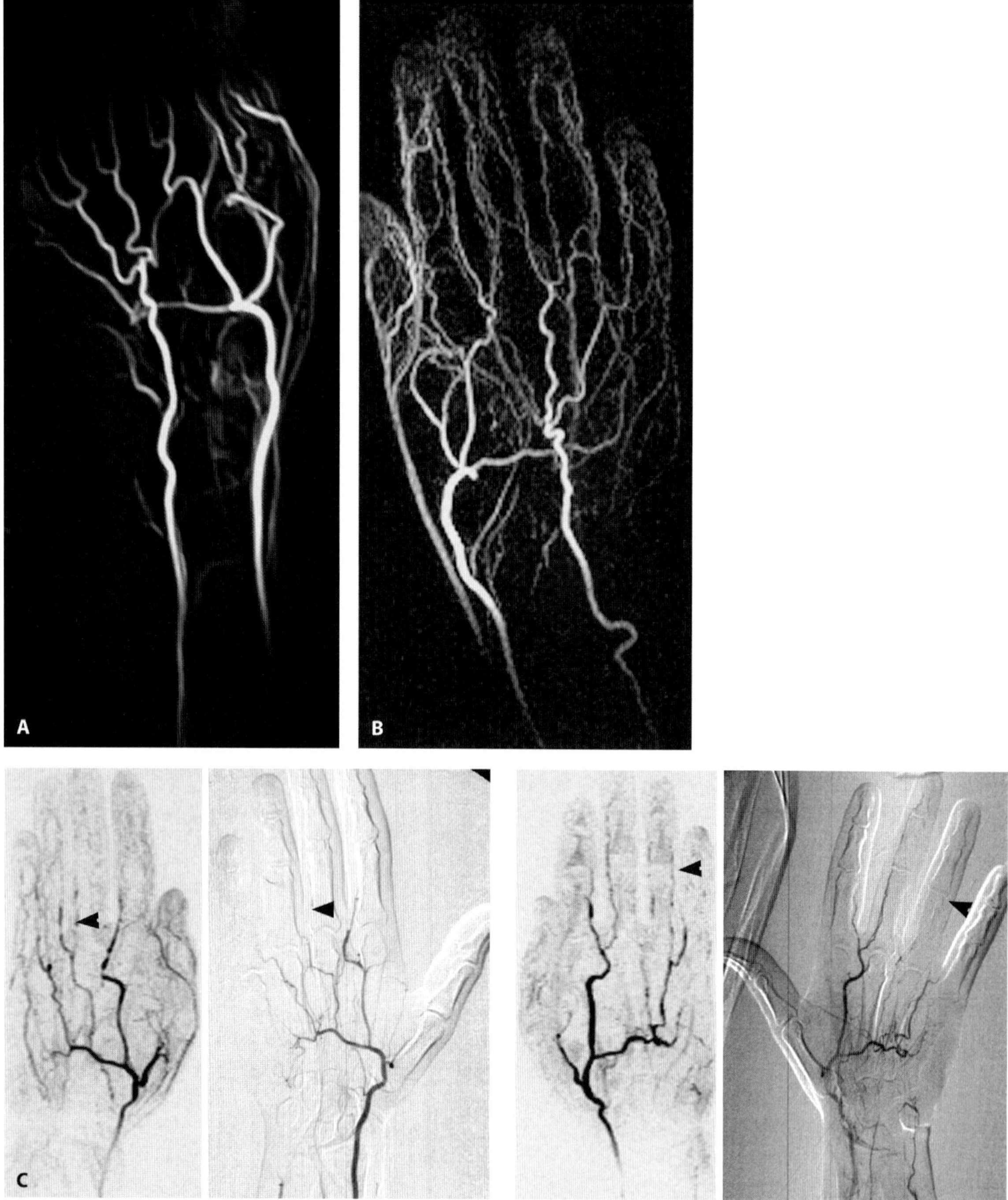

Fig. 13.31A–C. 3D CE MRA of the hand; **A,B** normal findings. Selective visualization of arteries (**A**). Venous overlay (**B**) due to incorrect timing. **C** 3D CE MRA of the hand arteries of a patient with Raynaud's disease in comparison with i.a. DSA. Some digital arteries are better visualized by CE MRA (*arrows*)

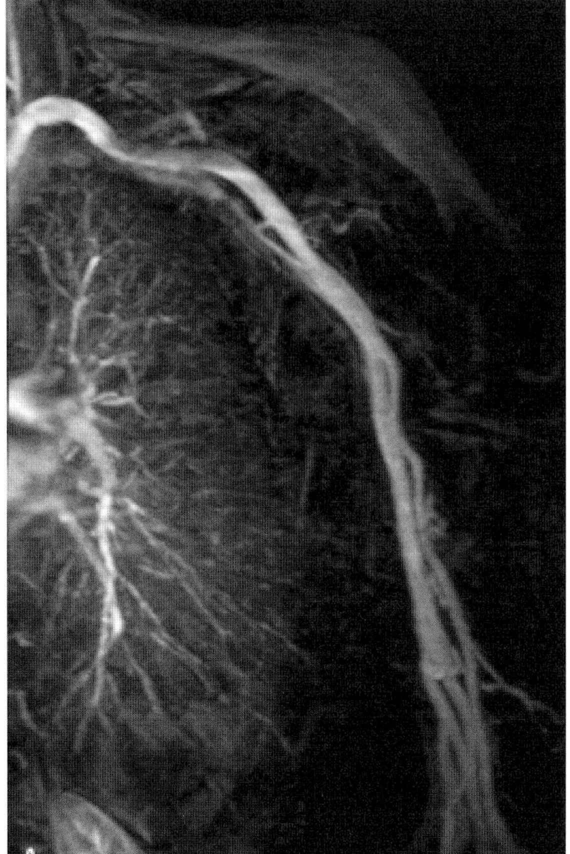

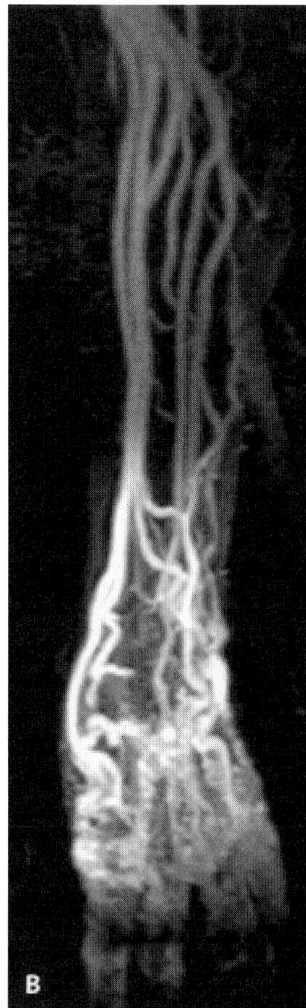

Fig. 13.32A,B. Young woman with an upper-limb AV malformation. 'Moving-table' contrast-enhanced MRA of the left upper limb during a single contrast injection. Whole volume MIP showing dilated subclavian and brachial arteries (**A**) and arteries of the forearm and hand (**B**), consistent with an extensive vascular malformation

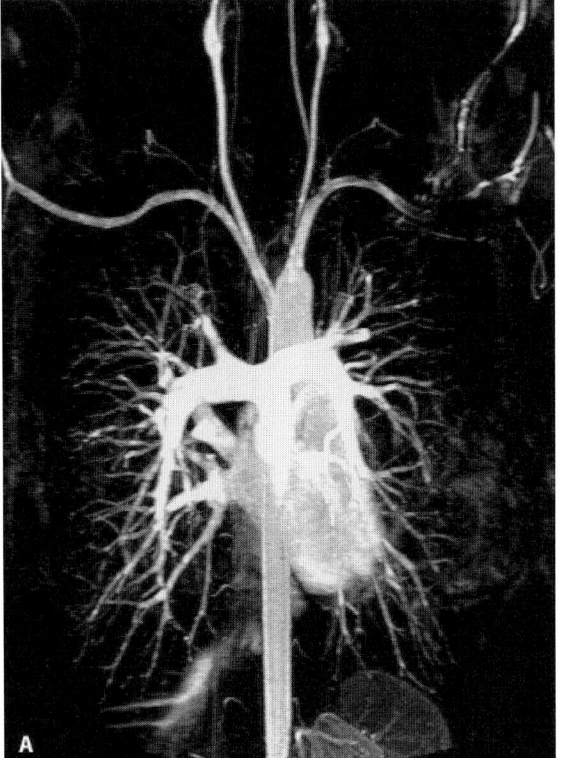

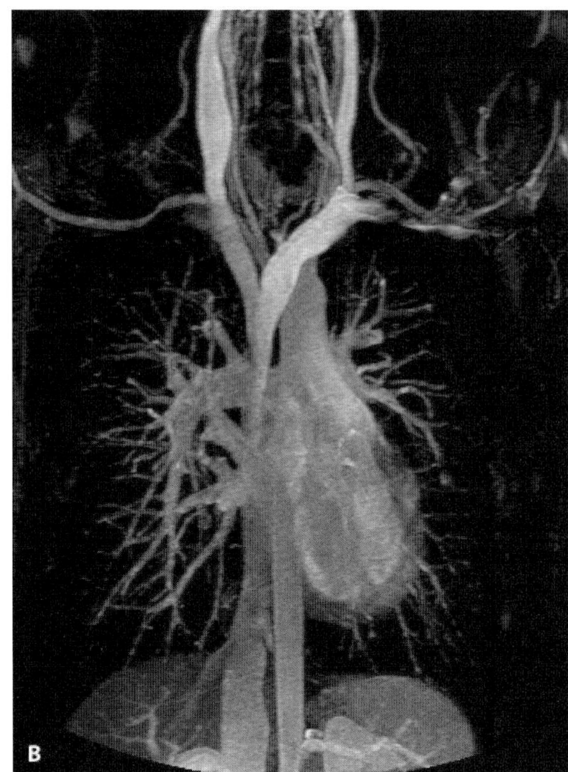

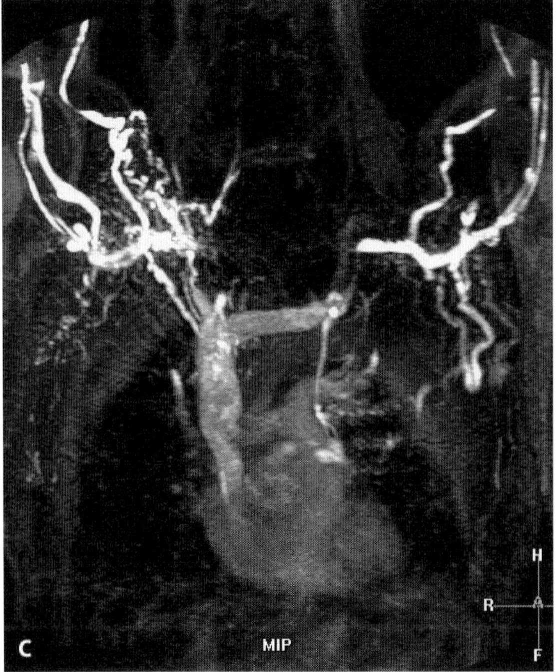

Fig. 13.33A. MRA of the thoracic vasculature showing severe signal drop-off within the left subclavian artery. This is because of the presence of highly concentrated contrast agent within the subclavian vein which makes the subclavian vein invisible due to susceptibility artifact and which causes severe artefactual signal loss within the adjacent subclavian artery secondary to T2* effect. **B** 'Indirect' contrast-enhanced MRV acquired during the venous phase (typically 45–60 s after start of injection). Note excellent depiction of the great veins of the thorax and of the inferior vena cava. No susceptibility effect is visible as the intravenously injected contrast agent is substantially diluted (by a factor of approximately 100-fold) by mixing in the blood pool. The susceptibility effect seen in **A** is therefore eliminated as a result of prolongation of the T2*. **C** 'Direct' contrast-enhanced MRV acquired during first pass of dilute contrast agent (3 ml of contrast agent in 50 ml of saline) injected into each arm. The susceptibility effect seen in **A** is overcome by dilution of the contrast agent prior to injection

design, improved fat suppression techniques and better postprocessing will further revolutionize MRA, especially CE MRA, which promises to revolutionize non-invasive imaging of patients with suspected vascular disease without the use of ionizing radiation, arterial puncture or nephrotoxic contrast agents.

Further Reading

Anderson CM, Edelman RR, Turski PA (1993) Clinical MRA. Raven, New York

Arlart IP, Bongartz GM, Marchal G (2001) MRA. Springer, Berlin Heidelberg New York

Graves MJ (1997) MRA. Br J Radiol 70:6–28

Hashemi RH, Bradley WG Jr (1997) MRI: the basics. In: Mitchell CW (ed) Williams and Wilkins, Baltimore

Hendrick RE, Russ PD, Simon JH (1993) MRI: principles and artifacts. In: Lufkin RB (ed) The Raven MRI teaching file. Raven, New York

Huston J et al (2001) Carotid artery: elliptic centric contrast-enhanced MR angiography compared with conventional angiography. Radiology 218:138

Ho KY, Leiner T, de Haan MW, Kessels AG, Kitslaar PJ, van Engelshoven JM (1998) Peripheral vascular tree stenoses: evaluation with moving-bed infusion-tracking MR angiography. Radiology 206:683–692

Lee HM et al (1998) Distal lower extremity arteries: evaluation with two-dimensional MR digital subtraction angiography. Radiology 207:505

Meaney JFM, Prince MR, Nostrant TT, Stanley JC (1997a) Gadolinium-enhanced MR angiography of visceral arteries in patients with suspected chronic mesenteric ischemia. J Magn Reson Imaging 7:171–176

Meaney JFM, Weg JG, Chenevert TL, Stafford-Johnson D, Hamilton BH, Prince MR (1997b) Diagnosis of pulmonary embolism with MRA. N Engl J Med 336:1422–1427

Meaney FM, Ridgway JP, Chakraverty S, Robertson I, Kessel D, Radjenovic A, Kouwenhoven M, Kasner A, Smith MA (1999) Stepping-table gadolinium-enhanced digital substraction MR angiography of the Aorta and lower extremity arteries: preliminary experience. Radiology 211:59–67

Nelemans PJ, Leiner T, de Vet HCW, van Engelshoven JMA (2000) Peripheral arterial disease: meta-analysis of the diagnostic performence of MR Angiography. Radiology 217:105–114

Oudkerk M, Edelman RR (1997) High-power gradient MR-imaging. Advances in MRI II. Blackwell Science, Oxford

Owen RS, Carpenter JP, Baum RA et al (1992) Magnetic Resonance Imaging of angiographically occult runoff vessels in peripheral arterial occlusive disease. N Engl J Med 326:157–1581

Prince MR (1998) Contrast-enhanced MR angiography: theory and optimisation. MRI Clin North Am 6:257

Prince MR, Grist TM, Debatin JF (1997a) 3D contrast MR angiography. Springer, Berlin Heidelberg, New York

Prince MR et al (1997b) Hemodynamically significant atherosclerotic renal artery stenosis: MR angiographic features. Radiology 205:128

Reimer P, Boos M (1999) Phase-contrast MR angiography of peripheral arteries: technique and clinical application. Eur Radiol 9:122

Rofsky NM, Johnson G, Adelman MA, Rosen RJ, Krinsky GA, Weinreb JC (1997) Peripheral vascular disease evaluated with reduced-dose gadolinium-enhanced MR angiography. Radiology 205:163–169

Wallner B (1993) MR angiography. Thieme, Stuttgart

Weiger M, Pruessmann KP, Kassner A, Rodite G, Reid A, Boesiger P (2000) Contrast-enhanced 3D MRA using SENSE. J Magn Reson Imaging 12:671–677

MRI of the Chest

14

H.-U. Kauczor, E. J. R van Beek

Contents

Traditionally, chest MRI was limited by motion artefacts of both lungs and heart and the low number of protons. Furthermore, the susceptibility artefacts due to air were a limiting factor. More recently, the development of fast (breath-hold) sequences and the introduction of novel contrast agents and mechanisms has caused chest MRI to gain ground in the imaging of an increasing range of chest pathologies. In this chapter, we will discuss the technical requirements, current clinical indications and ongoing developments of chest MRI.

14.1 Technical Demands

14.1.1 Coils, Planes and Positioning

Chest MR imaging relies on positioning radiofrequency (RF) coils in close proximity to the body. This requires advanced coil design, which has to take into account both the body size and shape as well as the changing diameters due to respiration. This generally implies that coils are made of at least two parts or are made of flexible material. Thus, most RF coils used consist of phased-array design, albeit that some modifications (such as wrap-around coils) are also increasingly used. Additionally, high-resolution imaging of the chest wall sometimes requires dedicated surface coils, e.g. spine coil, or the selective use of individual arrays of the phased-array body coil.

The traditional imaging methods relied heavily on axial planes (computed tomography, CT, and high resolution CT), albeit the introduction of multi-slice CT makes reconstruction in other planes possible. For MRI, axial images remain useful, especially when comparison with CT has to be made. However, the coronal plane has a major advantage in that it covers the entire chest and can show delineation of structures such as the diaphragm more clearly. For possible chest wall involvement one may have to rely on the sagittal plane, and this is also true for superior sulcus masses where vascular or brachial plexus involvement is suspected. Furthermore, MRI has the inherent advantage of not employing ionising radiation, which is a current topic in view of (European) legal requirements.

The patient is generally positioned supine and will enter the MR system head first. In most situations, patients will be requested to keep the arms down along the body. However, for high-resolution imaging of the mediastinum or blood vessels, it is usually better to have the arms up as this reduces wrap-around artefacts.

14.1.2 Factors Affecting Image Quality

The visualisation of the normal lung parenchyma using MRI is extremely difficult. The spatial resolution which can be obtained by MRI is inherently lower than that obtained with CT. CT, performed either as spiral CT with high-resolution CT or as multi-slice CT, is generally accepted as the radiological gold standard for visualisation of the morphology of the lung parenchyma. It yields excellent results of almost isotropic voxels at 1 mm.

Several technical challenges need to be addressed in order to obtain diagnostic quality MR images of the chest. These are discussed in the following paragraphs.

14.1.2.1 Signal Loss Due to Physiological Motion

Physiological motion comes from several sources. The main contributors are: (1) the lungs, (2) the heart and large blood vessels, and (3) blood motion.

14.1.2.1.1 Respiratory Motion

Respiratory motion is the most important influence on image quality in chest MRI. It leads to blurring, loss of delineation and decreased resolution. The simplest technique which is very effective in reducing motion artefact is breath-hold imaging. This requires sequences with acquisition times well below 30 s. For this purpose sequences such as FLASH or HASTE have been used successfully. As a result of its simplicity and good results, it has gained wide acceptance and application.

Other methods to reduce respiratory artefacts are gating procedures, which may comprise navigator pulses, a respiratory gating belt or reordering of phase encoding. The navigator pulses track the location of the diaphragm, allowing for maintenance of a constant position of the diaphragm and the lung volumes during the imaging periods. Respiratory gating using a belt has also shown marked improvement in image quality, as has respiratory compensation using reordering of phase encoding. Of these techniques, navigator pulses and reordered phase encoding seem to be most useful.

A higher number of acquisitions will also reduce the severity of breathing artefacts by averaging. A weakness of these methods is the fact that it prolongs the data acquisition time, thus resulting in extended overall imaging time. This can be especially problematic in dyspnoeic patients.

14.1.2.1.2
Cardiac and Large Blood-Vessel Motion

Electrocardiogram (ECG) triggering has been widely advocated to reduce cardiac and vascular pulsation artefacts, such as ghosting artefacts in the phase-encoding direction and blurring. Triggering in diastole allows more time to obtain data, whereas triggering in systole has the advantage of a more constant time profile. Reordering of phase encoding is mainly employed to reduce blurring of the lung parenchyma adjacent to the heart and great vessels. Similarly to respiratory gating methods, ECG triggering will prolong the imaging time.

14.1.2.1.3
Blood Motion

ECG triggering in systole can be used to obtain images during higher blood flow velocity, thus resulting in a greater flow void effect (black blood imaging). However, a disadvantage is the reduction in data acquisition time, thus leading to longer imaging intervals. Increasing the number of RF pulses can also be used to reduce blood motion effects, although this can interfere with the technique one wishes to employ.

14.1.2.2
Susceptibility Artefacts

Susceptibility artefacts are very closely related to the specific morphology of the ventilated lung. The unique combination of air and soft tissue that constitutes inflated lung is the cause for significant susceptibility artefacts since air-tissue interfaces induce local gradients. These gradients lead to inhomogeneities of the magnetic field, producing a complex spectrum of frequencies, which are spread across up to 9 ppm. They also lead to signal loss from intravoxel phase dispersion reflected by a short T2*. Whereas imaging of the normal parenchyma is rather difficult due to susceptibility artefacts, it is much easier to image consolidations within the lung. The loss of air and concomitant increase of tissue, cells or fluid significantly reduce the number of air-tissue interfaces and subsequently the degree of susceptibility artefacts. T2* increases from 7 ms in normal lungs to 35 ms in atelectatic lung and to more than 140 ms in lung tumours. This very short T2* in the normal parenchyma has an important impact on gradient recalled echo (GRE) sequences where they lead to blurring of pulmonary structures which is much more obvious than when using spin-echo (SE) sequences. At the same time, the short T2 relaxation time of the pulmonary parenchyma influences GRE and SE sequences in the same way.

Different strategies have been proposed to reduce susceptibility artefacts. Use of short echo times (TE) for T1-W SE or GRE sequences have been employed. Ultrashort echo times (50–250 μs) as part of projection-reconstruction techniques have been successfully applied to the lung parenchyma. They result in a significant improvement of the signal-to-noise ratio (SNR). Alternatively, one can apply T2-W turbo spin-echo (TSE) sequences or T2-W ultra-fast TSE sequences with high turbo factors. Furthermore, one can minimise susceptibility artefacts by using multiple 180° RF refocusing pulses.

14.1.2.3
Signal-to-Noise Ratio

Since about two-thirds of the lung consists of air and only one-third is tissue and blood, the density of spins is markedly lower than in any other organ. The low spin density is the major drawback in MRI of the lung, especially for the visualisation of lung diseases with loss of tissue such as emphysema. In other lung diseases, however, the amount of tissue, fluid and/or cells is increased by the pathological process. Thus, a higher number of protons (spins) becomes available, and significant improvements of the SNR can be achieved. To benefit from the higher number of spins, T1-W SE sequences with short TE (<7 ms), T1-W GRE sequences, like fast, low-angle, single-shot, half-Fourier (FLASH), with short TE (3 ms), or a higher number of acquisitions are recommended. The short echo times are particularly important to avoid signal loss from T2 relaxation, resulting in a significant increase of the SNR. For this purpose GRE sequences are superior to SE sequences.

14.2 Pulse Sequences and Contrast Mechanisms

14.2.1 Pulse Sequences

When imaging the chest, the pulse sequences used are relatively limited due to constraints of motion and susceptibility artefacts. Generally, fast imaging sequences using short TR and short TE have been applied with the most success. Fat-suppressed imaging, using inversion recovery (IR) techniques, is useful to assess mediastinal and chest wall masses. It will also yield relative signal enhancement from the lung. Furthermore, gadolinium (Gd) chelates have been used for vascular and mass enhancement. Postcontrast images should include fat-suppression techniques in the assessment of masses. Dynamic contrast techniques may be used for vascular studies and in the assessment of pulmonary masses or nodules. Newer contrast agents are also undergoing clinical trials, which are described elsewhere.

Table 14.1 gives an overview of the sequences that are most commonly employed. Some variation may exist between the various MR systems, and they should be seen as a rough guide to successful MR imaging of the chest.

14.2.2 Contrast Mechanisms

14.2.2.1 Natural Contrast

In all lung diseases with an increase of the amount of tissue, fluid and/or cells, the number of protons is

Table 14.1. Pulse sequences used in MRI of the chest

Sequence	WI	Plane	No. of slices	TR	TE	Flip angle	TI	Slice thickness	Matrix	No. of acq.	Acq. time TA
SE	T1	Transverse/ coronal	8	ECG 600–1100	20		50	5	≥128×256	4	
2D GRE (FLASH)	T1	Transverse/ coronal	11	129	2.2	80		6	≥128×256	1	21
	T1			140–165	4.5			8	≥128×256		18–21
3D GRE (FLASH)	T1	Transverse/ coronal/ sagittal	Slab	4.6–6.7	1.8–2.2	15–30		4–10	≥128×256	1	10–21
TruFi	T2	Transverse/ coronal	10	<7.5	<3.5	<80		10	≥128×256	1	20
2D HASTE	T2	Transverse/ coronal	8	ECG 800	25	160	Turbo factor 164	6	256×256	1	
SE	T2	Transverse/ coronal	10	2200–2700	80			8	≥128×256	2	
UFTSE respiration triggered	T2	Transverse/ coronal	10	3000–5000	120			6	270×512	2	
STIR	T2	Transverse/ coronal	8	2200	43		160	8	128×256	2	
3D VIBE breath-hold	T1	Coronal	3 slabs	4.5	1.9	12		Eff. 2.5	502×512	1	20
3D FLASH	T1	Coronal	Slab	3.65–6.5	1.6–1.8	25–40		1.25–3	106×512 128×256	1	17–27
FAIR/FAIRER		Transverse/ coronal	1	ECG	36		100–1800	8	128×256	3–5	20–27
TONE/VUSE		Coronal	Slab	6.7	1.9	6–35		1.2	64×256	1	28

Abbreviations: *WI* weighting of images, *Matrix* phase × frequency matrix, *Acq.* acquisition(s)

increased, and a higher signal can be obtained. This is referred to as the disease-related contrast mechanism leading to a higher SNR. However, in many cases such a disease-related increase of spin density is not sufficient for accurate delineation, characterisation and diagnosis of the disease process. For this purpose, different contrast agents and more advanced contrast mechanisms can be used.

14.2.2.2 Contrast Agents

The most common technique is the intravenous administration of contrast agents, like Gd chelates, which lead to an iatrogenic increase of the relaxivity of existent spins. These contrast agents are used for the enhancement of nodules or opacifications, MR angiography or perfusion imaging. Newer contrast agents, such as Gd-based blood-pool agents and ultra-small super-paramagnetic iron oxide (USPIO) particles, are also under development. Gadolinium in the form of a diethylene triamine penta-acetate (DTPA) chelate has also been applied in aerosolised form to assess the airways. Finally, the application of inhaled oxygen has been investigated for ventilation imaging.

14.2.2.2.1 Gadolinium Chelates: Intravenous Administration

The basic principles of Gd contrast are described in Chapter 2. Paramagnetic contrast agents enable better characterisation and delineation of pathological processes, such as identification of benign versus malignant nodules and in the definition of tumours from essential structures. Finally, it is possible to investigate disease activity, such as pulmonary fibrosis and alveolitis. The standard Gd chelates have the disadvantage that they are rapidly excreted and leave the blood compartment. So-called blood-pool agents remain in the blood compartment and offer advantages in terms of sequence design for MR angiography.

14.2.2.2.2 Gadolinium Chelates: Inhaled Administration

Commercially available Gd-DTPA can be diluted, aerosolised and applied using a nebuliser. This method has only been tried in animal models, but did show a 70%–120% increase in signal intensity of the lung parenchyma. This technology offers good potential for future use in the assessment of small airway diseases.

14.2.2.2.3 Oxygen Enhancement

Higher oxygen concentrations administered via inhalation will induce different paramagnetic effects and lead to a dose-dependent increase of signal intensity. Scans acquired after breathing normal room air (20% oxygen) are subtracted from scans acquired after breathing 100% oxygen using an inhalation mask. Subtraction is indispensable because the increase in signal intensity is rather low. The increase of signal intensity is explained by an enhancement of the lung parenchyma due to the presence of dissolved molecular oxygen. The highest increase of signal is found in the pulmonary veins. This technique seems to be applicable in clinical routine if adequate post-processing tools are available. It might be a complementary technique in the diagnosis of pulmonary embolism and in the assessment of oxygen uptake in obstructive and interstitial lung disease.

14.2.2.2.4 Iron Compounds

A number of agents which are based on USPIO crystals or particles are under development and undergoing preclinical and clinical trials. They are kept in solution by means of a coating. They can be applied for MR lymphography (as discussed below) or as blood-pool agents for MR angiography.

14.2.2.3 Non-proton MRI

The use of hyperpolarised noble gases (He-3 and Xe-129) is a new approach to overcome the low spin density in the airspaces when administered as an 'inhaled contrast agent'. The spin density of the noble gases which represents the source of the MR signal is significantly increased by optical pumping (five magnitudes above thermal equilibrium), which compensates for the 2500 times lower density of the gas as compared with proton concentrations in tissue. The decay of the hyperpolarisation as given by the T1 relaxation time is dependent on the environment. For MRI of pulmonary ventilation, 300–1500 ml of hyperpolarised He-3 are inhaled. Normal ventilation corresponds to a homogeneous high signal intensity visualisation of the airways and airspaces with rapid filling and distribution of He-3 gas within the trachea and lungs. This technology is currently undergoing clinical trials with the use of hyperpolarised He-3 for ventilation imaging. The main disadvantages are the limited availability of He-3 gas, the complexity of producing hyperpolarisation and the need for multi-nuclear MR capabilities. However, there are great expectations for this technology, as shown below.

14.2.3 MR Angiography

In general, 3D techniques with a minimum repetition time (TR) of less than 5 ms and TE of less than 2 ms are used for contrast-enhanced MRA (CEMRA) of the pulmonary arteries. A short TR allows for short breath-hold acquisitions. A short TE minimises background signal and susceptibility artefacts. The use of time-resolved CEMRA may be helpful. Subtraction of the data sets, such as in digital subtraction angiography leads to selective pulmonary arteriograms and venograms. Different flip-angles were proposed ranging from 15° to 40°, and up to 70°. Even linearly (tilted optimised N excitation; TONE) or non-linearly (variable angle uniform signal excitation; VUSE) increasing flip-angles, which have been used for non-enhanced, non-breath-hold acquisitions, can be applied for CEMRA to improve the detection of vessels in the lung periphery.

Adequate timing of the contrast agent (0.1–0.2 mmol/kg) administered by an automatic power injector is essential to achieve high contrast between the pulmonary artery branches and surrounding structures. In general, arterial opacification should be predominant since the pulmonary veins are of minor diagnostic importance. Since the time gap between opacification of pulmonary arteries and veins is very short, selective visualisation of vascular territories is difficult. To achieve a compact bolus, flow rates between 2 and 5 ml/s followed by a saline flush (20 ml) are recommended. The saline flush will ensure that the whole amount of contrast medium contributes to vessel opacification.

Contrast-enhanced MRA is especially useful for imaging complex and slow flow with different spatial orientations, which is rather common in the pulmonary vascular system. In the clinical setting, shortening of the acquisition time is of paramount importance for dyspnoeic patients suspected of pulmonary embolism. This holds particularly true since breath-holding in deep inspiration is strongly recommended for CEMRA. In adults, breath-hold periods of 18 s are achieved commonly. Only in severe pulmonary disease will breath-hold periods be significantly shorter. If breath-holding is not possible, imaging during shallow breathing will still be diagnostic in many cases despite a significant deterioration of image quality. The quality criteria for pulmonary CEMRA are (in decreasing importance): (1) complete visualisation of the central (pulmonary trunk, main and lobar arteries) and segmental pulmonary arteries with high signal; (2) high signal visualisation of peripheral pulmonary arteries (subsegmental branches); (3) virtually selective visualisation of the pulmonary arteries without significant superimposition by lung veins or the aorta and its side-branches. Several strategies have been advised to differentiate arteries and veins in case of superimposition: (1) cine or stackmode viewing, (2) continuous rotation, (3) multiplanar reformation (MPR) or (4) maximum intensity projection (MIP). These strategies will help to identify the arteries and veins according to their particular anatomical course (arteries have a steeper course, whereas veins have a more horizontal course within the chest).

14.3 Lung and Pleura

14.3.1 Anatomy

The airways are made up of large central airways, which contain cartilage in their walls. These airways subsequently branch down to three lobes on the right and two lobes on the left. Following these lobar divisions, the lobes are further divided into segments and continue to divide down to the 16th order, which is the alveolar space itself. The airways are surrounded by connective tissue, and there are distinct neurovascular, lymphatic and airway bundles within this lung structure.

The lung is surrounded by the visceral pleura, which has areas of invagination to give rise to the interlobar fissures. The chest wall is covered by the parietal pleura. Between the pleural surfaces, a small amount of fluid allows for smooth sliding of the lung during inspiration and expiration.

Proton MRI is capable of visualising the central tracheobronchial tree, the pleura and the interlobar fissures. Furthermore, the respiratory motion during inspiration and expiration can be visualised. The more distal airways and the alveolar space can be visualised using different technologies for ventilation imaging, such as hyperpolarised He-3 MRI.

14.3.2 Pathology

14.3.2.1 Bronchogenic Carcinoma and Nodules

14.3.2.1.1 Bronchogenic Carcinoma

Imaging techniques have to detect, characterise and stage malignant masses. Staging is based on the Tumour, Nodes, Metastases (TNM) classification (Table 14.2). MRI seems more or less equivalent to CT in the staging of bronchogenic carcinoma. The primary tumour will appear hypo- to isointense as compared with paravertebral muscle (Fig. 14.1). After the administration of Gd, a strong enhancement is observed. It will be homogeneous in tumours smaller than 3 cm in diameter (T1 tumours), whereas larger carcinomas will also exhibit central necrosis. T2 tumours (>3 cm in diameter) are easily depicted on MRI, as they are on both chest radiography and CT, when they are located in the periphery of the lungs. Delineation and staging are affected in case of poststenotic atelectasis. Here, MRI has some clear advantages (see below). Other particular advantages of MRI include the assessment of infiltration of adjacent structures, such as the mediastinum, chest wall and great vessels, which is relevant for staging (T3 and T4). The infiltration of the parietal pleura is one of the criteria for a T3 tumour. T2-W images in coronal or sagittal orientation yield the best results in the evaluation of pleural thickening, extent of contact between tumour and pleura, and differentiation between visceral and parietal pleura. The high signal intensity of the tumour on T2-WI is in clear contrast to the muscles of the chest wall. MRI is well suited to study the direct infiltration of the mediastinum (T3 tumour). The expectation that MRI might be superior to CT has not been proven. Although changes within the mediastinal fat are easily depicted due to the high contrast resolution, the dignity of these changes, whether malignant or inflammatory, frequently remains unclear. Obviously, broad infiltrations are easily delineated, whereas small infiltrations are more difficult. The direct contact between tumour and mediastinum is not a reliable sign of infiltration. Additionally, the loss of the regular fatty demarcation is not specific. Signs for resectable infiltrations of the mediastinum are (1) contact between tumour and mediastinum <3 cm, (2) contact

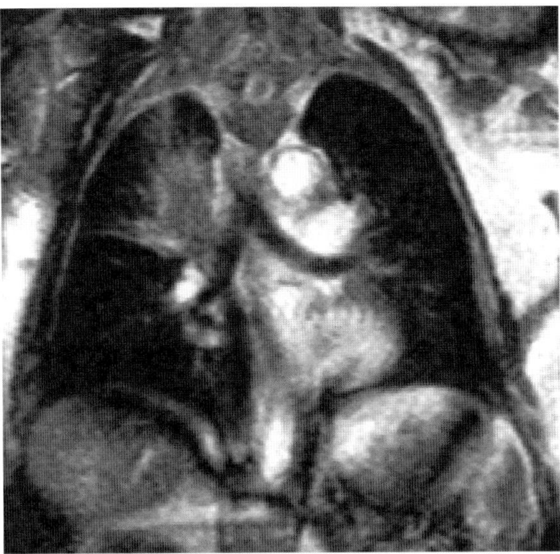

Fig. 14.1. Bronchogenic carcinoma of the right upper lobe. Coronal GRE T1-WI at 0.2 T with an irregular hypointense mass

Table 14.2. Tumour, Nodes, Metastases (TNM) Classification

T1	≤3 cm in greatest dimension
T2	>3 cm in greatest dimension, or extension to the hilar region, or invasion of the visceral pleura, or a tumour that has caused partial atelectasis
T3	Extension to the chest wall, diaphragm, mediastinal pleura, or pericardium, etc., or a tumour that has caused complete atelectasis
T4	Invasion of the mediastinum, heart, great vessels, trachea, oesophagus, etc., or the presence of malignant pleural effusion
N1	Metastasis to peribronchial or ipsilateral hilar lymph nodes
N2	Metastasis to ipsilateral mediastinal lymph nodes
N3	Metastasis to contralateral mediastinal lymph nodes

with the aorta <90° of the circumference, and (3) visible fat layer between tumour and adjacent structures. Definitive signs for non-resectability of large tumours (T4) are more difficult to define, as the management is dependent on the surgeon and the patient's individual circumstances. The use of contrast does not seem to improve the evaluation. The direct acquisition of coronal or sagittal sections facilitates the delineation of infiltrations of the aorto-pulmonary window and the sub-carinal space. This is also valid for the evaluation of a direct infiltration of the carina and the main bronchi, which requires distance measurements between the tumour and the carina.

MRI has some inherent advantages in the evaluation of the infiltrations of the chest wall. Definite proof, however, can only be derived from osseous destruction of a huge soft-tissue mass invading the chest wall. In addition, pain is a very specific sign. The loss of the extrapleural fat layer is often caused by reactive fibrotic or inflammatory changes. They can lead to false-positive results. The more extensive the changes, the more likely the infiltration. On the other hand, the presence of a fat layer is a good indicator that no infiltration is present. Compared to CT, MRI seems to be at least equal if not superior in the evaluation of an infiltration of the chest wall, with a sensitivity rising to 90% and an accuracy of 88%. T1-W images pre- and post-contrast will show the best resolution and a clear delineation. Tumour-identical changes within the extrapleural fat have a sensitivity of 85% and a specificity of 100% for an infiltration of the chest wall.

MRI is regarded as the modality of choice for the investigation of superior sulcus tumours (Pancoast). Direct coronal and sagittal acquisitions using fat suppression and T1-WI after contrast are recommended (Fig. 14.2). The infiltration through the lung apex is diagnosed on the basis of direct extension of the tumour into the extrapleural fat and the cervicothoracic junction. These direct infiltrations and involvement of the main blood vessels and the brachial plexus are far better observed on MRI than on CT.

With CT, the great vessels can only be evaluated after the application of a contrast agent. If there are contraindications for iodinated contrast, MRI is the method of

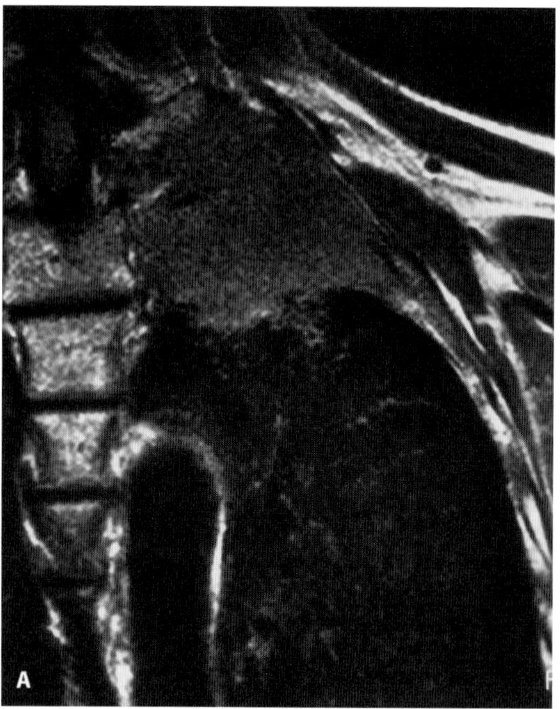

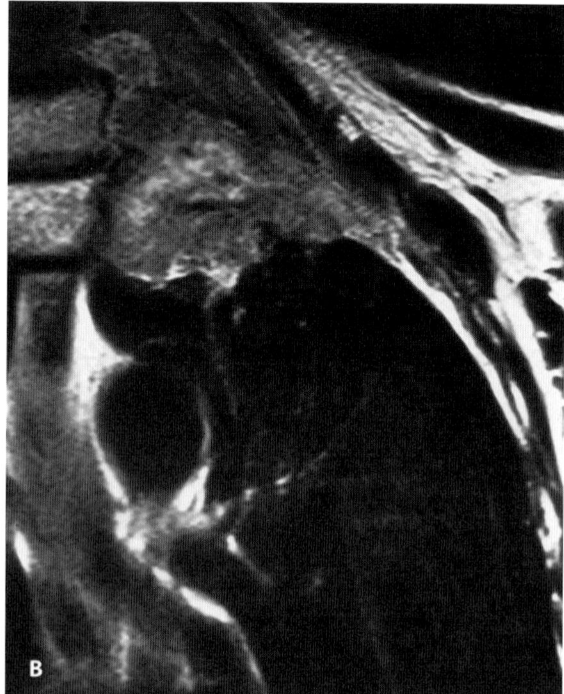

Fig. 14.2A,B. Superior sulcus tumour (Pancoast) tumour with infiltration of the cervicothoracic junction

choice. Infiltration of the great vessels can even be achieved on non-enhanced MR images with high contrast between the flow void within the vessels and the tumours exhibiting relatively high signal. Alternatively, MR contrast agent is much better tolerated than iodinated contrast media. The involvement of central pulmonary artery branches by tumour can be accurately evaluated using CEMRA with a sensitivity of 80% and a specificity of 95%. Source images and MIP are used to recognise irregularities of the vascular wall or lumen as well as cut-offs of peripheral vessels. MRI is also superior to CT for the demonstration of endoluminal tumour spread within the superior vena cava, the pulmonary veins and the heart chambers. Cine-images are useful to separate slow-flowing blood from tumour infiltrations.

In summary, MRI and CT are equivalent in the T-staging of bronchogenic carcinoma with regards to a surgical or conservative therapeutic approach with the sensitivity ranging between 43%–63% for CT and 52%–81% for MRI and the specificity between 94%–97% for CT and 80%–96% for MRI, respectively.

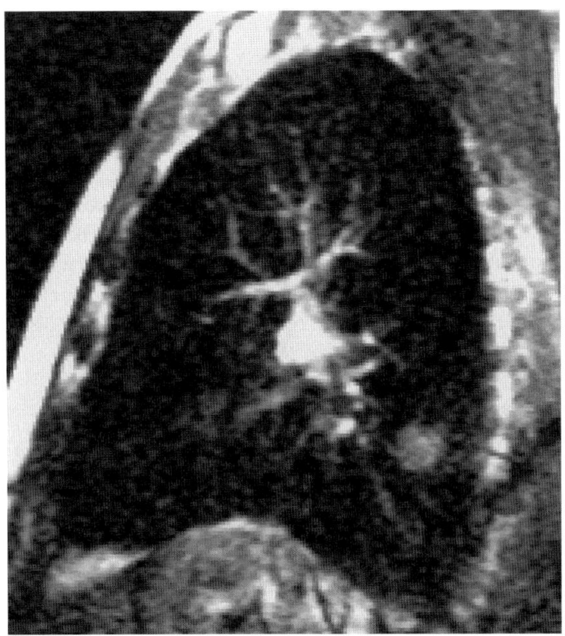

Fig. 14.3. Peripheral bronchogenic carcinoma (T1). Sagittal GRE T1-WI shows a hypointense lung nodule

14.3.2.1.2
Pulmonary Nodules

High contrast between nodules and the underlying parenchyma is an inherent advantage of MRI, which might compensate for the relatively low spatial resolution (Fig. 14.3). Different techniques are available for the detection of pulmonary nodules. In general, joint assessment of signal intensities and contrast enhancement is used to categorise nodules as malignant or benign. T2-W TSE images detected pulmonary metastases with an overall sensitivity of 84% as compared to CT, which served as the gold standard. The sensitivity is clearly size-dependent. It was as low as 36% for tiny nodules (<5 mm) and increased steadily to 100% for nodules >15 mm. The combination of T1-W and T2*-W turboFLASH sequences without using contrast yielded similar results: sensitivity 82%, specificity 67%. A wide variety of different sequences has been applied in the detection of pulmonary nodules. Generally, fat-suppressed short tau inversion recovery (STIR), T2-W SE or GRE, such as ultra-fast TSE, and T1-W GRE, such as FLASH, should be done pre- and post-contrast. The precontrast images are generally sufficient for the detection of nodules. Dynamic acquisitions during and after the administration of contrast are advised for the characterisation of the nodules. Malignant nodules are characterised by a fast increase in signal intensity during the first pass of the contrast agent. When smaller than 3 cm, they show a strong and homogeneous enhancement without significant necrosis. Granulomas, however, exhibit a significant lower enhancement. Cysts typically do not enhance.

14.3.2.2
Atelectasis and Pneumonia

14.3.2.2.1
Atelectasis

MRI is successful in the differentiation of different types of atelectasis as well as of central tumours from poststenotic atelectasis. Non-enhanced T1-WI show nearly identical low signal intensity as tumour and atelectasis. On T2-WI, obstructive atelectasis exhibits high signal, whereas non-obstructive atelectasis is hypointense. This is explained by the accumulation of secretions and fluid in obstructive atelectasis. For the same reason, poststenotic atelectasis in lung cancer also appears hyperintense on T2-WI and can be separated from central tumour, which appears hypointense.

Contrast-enhanced T1-WI images are also helpful. In most cases, the tumour will only enhance moderately together with a strong enhancement within the atelectasis. The tumour will be iso- or hyperintense with regards to the poststenotic changes after contrast administration in only a minority of cases. As in the characterisation of pulmonary nodules, dynamic investigations are helpful in the differentiation. The poststenotic atelectasis will exhibit a fast enhancement (within the first 3 min) with a slow decrease thereafter, whereas the lung cancer will show a slow enhancement with a peak after about 10 min followed by a slow decrease of signal intensity.

14.3.2.2.2 Pneumonia

MRI is also used for the detection and characterisation of inflammatory pulmonary infiltrates (Fig. 14.4), particularly in immunocompromised patients. Invasive pulmonary aspergillosis (IPA) belongs to the most dangerous complications in these patients. The early detection and diagnosis of IPA are of great importance to introduce or continue antifungal therapy. In the early stages, IPA infections exhibit nodular or patchy infiltrates in the upper lobes. Enlargement of the infiltrates and/or development of segmental/lobar consolidations are typical for later stages, when they show their characteristic signs: (1) target sign on T1-WI with peripheral high signal due to haemorrhage and a hypointense centre caused by central necrosis. After contrast administration a strong rim enhancement reflects active inflammation and central necrosis; (2) hyperintense angiotropic consolidations on T1-WI indicating haemorrhagic infarcts due to vascular invasion; (3) reverse target sign on T2-WI with high signal intensity in the centre indicating necrosis and a peripheral rim with low signal intensity. MRI is at least as sensitive as conventional chest X-ray in the detection of round infiltrates and more specific than CT in the characterisation of IPA and the depiction of central necrosis and pulmonary abscesses in different settings of pneumonia.

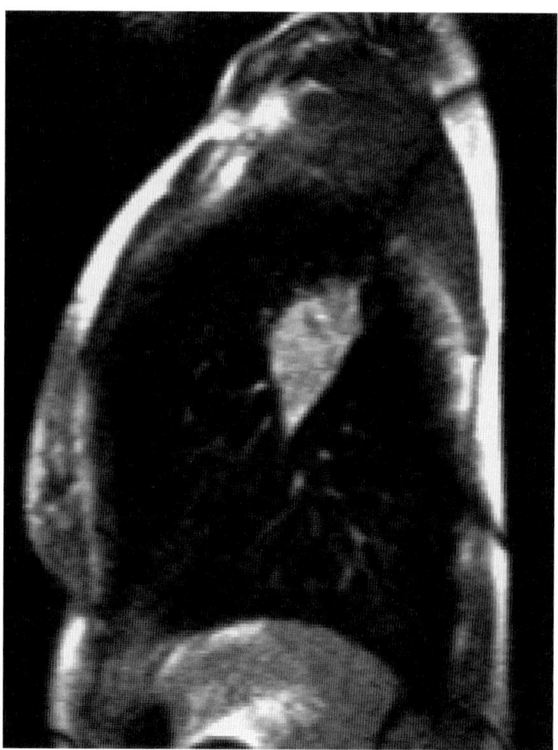

Fig. 14.4. Pneumonia in the right upper lobe. Sagittal GRE T1-WI at 0.2 T

Lipoid pneumonia is a rather rare condition, induced by mineral oil aspiration in most cases. MRI has a high sensitivity for the detection of fat, which will exhibit high signal intensity on T1-WI and T2-WI, characteristic for lipoid pneumonia.

Infarcts due to pulmonary embolism are either triangular or nodular in shape. Nodular infarcts are often seen as a sessile mass on the pleura and appear as humps. They often exhibit high signal intensity on T1-WI due to haemorrhage. The high signal is attributed to methaemoglobin formation in subacute haemorrhage. This appearance is also present in different diseases with pulmonary haemorrhage, such as Goodpasture's syndrome or IPA. Thus, MRI will differentiate infarctions and haemorrhage from pneumonia or atelectasis without haemorrhage more easily than CT. The detection and characterisation of infarction are included in the work-up protocol for pulmonary embolism.

14.3.2.3 Fibrosis and Alveolitis

In fibrotic lung disease, the disease itself is associated with an increase in spin density and a reduction of susceptibility artefacts. This increase in signal intensity is highly unspecific and is not successful in the differentiation of various causes of airspace disease, because there is considerable overlap in the measured T1 and T2 values between different underlying diseases. The extent and distribution of fibrotic lung disease is represented by parenchymal bands and reticulation, nodules and interlobular septal thickening on proton density and T1-weighting. The extent and distribution of airspace disease give helpful hints towards the final diagnosis. It has to be stated that MRI is inferior to CT regarding the anatomic assessment of fibrosis. Concomitant alveolitis (active inflammation) is represented by parenchymal opacification and ground glass opacities. It exhibits even higher signal intensity on T1-WI and T2-WI than fibrosis. The signal intensity is related to the clinical severity of the disease and a potential indicator for the response to therapy. Due to the active inflammatory process it also shows marked enhancement after contrast administration. Subsequently, successful anti-inflammatory treatment, which reduces the activity of alveolitis and the development of fibrosis, is associated with a marked decrease in signal intensity. This has been demonstrated for radiation pneumonitis in patients with bronchogenic carcinoma and in bleomycin-induced lung damage. Again, the reduction of active inflammation can be observed either on T2-WI or on T1-WI after contrast administration. Although there are no clinical studies thus far, it may be useful to employ this technique for the staging of sarcoidosis.

In areas of progressive massive fibrosis in silicosis and silicotuberculosis, marked contrast enhancement of the inflammatory process within is observed by MRI. It is hypointense on T2-WI compared with skeletal muscle, with some high signal areas centrally. These areas most likely correspond to necrosis. Precontrast, the consolidations are isointense to skeletal muscle in 70% of cases. Postcontrast, about 50% of the consolidations show rim enhancement, whereas the central areas, which most likely correspond to necrosis, will not enhance. Since the signal intensities are different in fibrotic and neoplastic tissue, lung cancer can be differentiated as a lesion with high signal on T2-WI.

The findings encountered in Wegener's granulomatosis, which is characterised by solid and cavitated intrapulmonary nodules, are similar to progressive massive fibrosis. The walls of larger nodules show marked enhancement after contrast administration whereas the central, necrotic areas do not enhance.

14.3.2.4
Airway Diseases and Emphysema

Due to the loss of tissue in emphysema, it is not an attractive candidate for proton MRI. The low signal from emphysematous lung, however, yields high contrast compared with the surrounding chest wall and mediastinum. Thus, segmentation of the lung volume is relatively easy to perform. The MR-based determination of lung volumes can be complemented by measurements of thoracic dimensions and the movement of the diaphragm during the respiratory cycle. The respiratory mechanics can be assessed using dynamic T1-WI. These parameters may be important in the preoperative work-up and postoperative follow-up of patients who are candidates for, or have undergone, lung volume reduction surgery for emphysema. Airway disease with bronchial wall thickening and mucus plugging, such as in cystic fibrosis and other bronchiectatic diseases, can be visualised by MRI. The direct visualisation of the bronchial wall is inferior to CT, but mucus and inflammatory changes are shown with high signal and sensitivity.

He-3 MRI demonstrates severe, localised and diffuse, nodular or wedge-shaped signal heterogeneities in airway diseases, such as in chronic obstructive pulmonary disease (COPD), asthma, bronchiectasis, and emphysema (Fig. 14.5). The different findings are attributed to

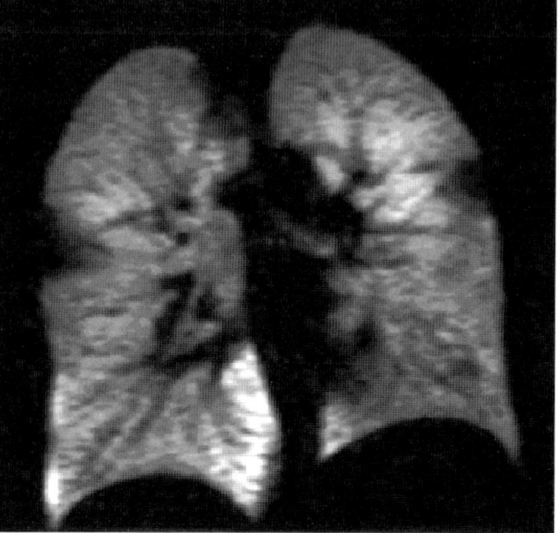

Fig. 14.5. Peripheral wedge-shaped ventilation defects in a smoker seen with coronal He-3 MRI

airway obstructions or the increased size of airspaces at different levels. Obviously, He-3 MRI is a highly sensitive modality for the detection and visualisation of airway disease. However, the low specificity still has to be improved. Furthermore, the interpretation of the imaging findings needs refinements, and the results of ongoing clinical trials are eagerly awaited.

14.3.2.5 Pleural Disease

14.3.2.5.1 Pleural Effusion

Pleural effusion is easily depicted by MRI, showing low signal intensity on T1-WI and high signal intensity on T2-WI, reflecting its water content. Compared with conventional chest radiography, MRI is more sensitive to the detection of pleural fluid collections. Compared with CT, however, MRI might be slightly superior in the characterisation of the fluid collection with exudates showing higher signal intensity on T1-WI and T2-WI than transudates, with T2-WI being more discriminatory. Septa are also more easily demonstrated on T2-WI. Subacute or chronic haemorrhages exhibit high signal intensity on T1-WI and T2-WI. Often they have a bright centre due to methaemoglobin and a dark periphery caused by the haemosiderin. A differentiation between benign and malignant effusions, is not possible, however. Nevertheless, in patients with bronchogenic carcinoma, the presence of pleural effusion alone is a strong indicator for malignant involvement and a poor prognosis.

14.3.2.5.2 Benign Masses

Benign masses of the pleura include lipoma, fibroma and round atelectasis. Lipoma typically shows the signal characteristics of subcutaneous fat on all sequences. Pleural fibromas are isointense to muscle on T1-WI and iso- to hyperintense on T2-WI: They will enhance after the administration of contrast.

Rounded atelectasis has a typical morphological appearance: the classical comet-tail sign, which describes the course of the vessels and bronchi into the ovoid or wedge-shaped mass. It will appear isointense on T1-WI, hyperintense on T2-WI and enhance strongly after the administration of contrast.

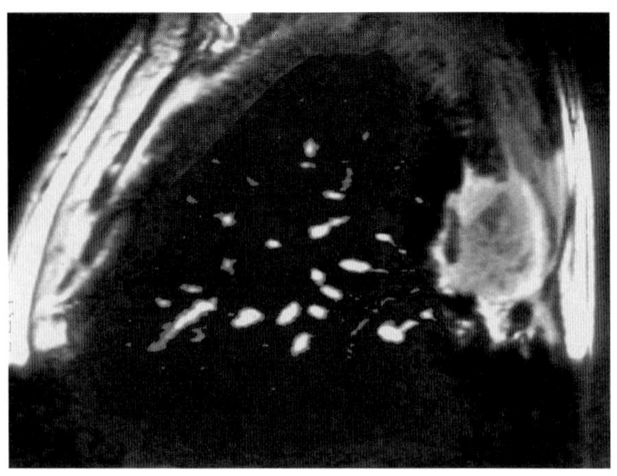

Fig. 14.6. Pleural metastasis with infiltration of the chest wall seen with contrast-enhanced sagittal GRE T1-WI

14.3.2.5.3 Malignant Masses

The primary malignancy of the pleura is the malignant mesothelioma, which is frequently associated with pleural effusion. Many are related to previous asbestos exposure, and calcified pleural plaques are a hallmark of this aetiology. MRI is less sensitive than CT for the demonstration of these calcifications. Generally, mesothelioma is a diffuse pleural process with the signal intensity slightly increased on T1-WI and moderately increased on T2-WI. Most mesotheliomas will enhance after the administration of contrast. MRI is superior to CT in the assessment of the extent of multiple pleural foci and infiltration of the chest wall, diaphragm and peritoneum. Pleural metastases secondary to carcinomas of the breast, lung, stomach, kidneys and ovaries are far more common. They often appear as diffuse nodular pleural thickening or as a large solid mass (Fig. 14.6) with pulmonary encasement and effusion mimicking mesothelioma.

14.4 Mediastinum

14.4.1 Anatomy

The mediastinum consists of fatty tissue. Apart from the heart, it contains multiple different anatomical structures: arteries, veins, nerves and lymphatics as well as the oesophagus belonging to the gastrointestinal tract, and the tracheobronchial tree belonging to the respiratory tract, and finally a primary mediastinal organ, the thymus. All of them can be the origin for disease spreading throughout the mediastinum and involving the other structures. Additionally, adjacent structures, such lungs, pleura, pericardium, thyroid and spine can afflict the mediastinum by means of continuous infiltration. We will not deal with the heart and pericardium, as this is described elsewhere. The thymus is a particularly relevant structure, as it changes appearances from childhood to adulthood. Its size will decrease and the fat content will increase, but there is great variability in these appearances.

14.4.2 Pathology

Mediastinal masses are differentiated into primary and secondary tumours, which also include lymphadenopathy. Additionally, benign diseases arising from one of the numerous structures within the mediastinum, e.g. aortic aneurysm, have to be differentiated. The location of masses often indicates the type of tumour one can encounter (Table 14.3). MRI plays an important role in the delineation and characterisation of mediastinal tumours where localisation, tissue composition, growth pattern as well as the patient's age and tumour markers are important for the differential diagnosis. Due to its superiority in tissue characterisation with regard to CT and the high number of young people affected by mediastinal tumours, MRI should be regarded as the first-line imaging modality in this population.

14.4.2.1 Primary Mediastinal Tumours

14.4.2.1.1 Thymus

Thymus masses are among the most frequent primary tumours in the mediastinum. The majority of thymus masses are benign, including thymoma, thymolipoma and (reactive) hyperplasia. More infrequently, malignant tumours may arise in the thymus, and this is almost invariably thymic carcinoma (although up to 30% of thymomas may invade surrounding structures). Thymoma typically shows low signal intensity on T1-WI and increased signal intensity on T2-WI. There may be inhomogeneous signal on T2-WI (which favours a benign nature), and cysts may also be present. Encapsulated thymomas exhibit a complete tumour capsule on MRI, whereas invasive thymomas will penetrate the capsule and diffusely infiltrate the mediastinal fat and the adjacent structures, e.g. pericardium, great vessels. Furthermore, invasive thymomas more commonly show multi-nodularity with low intensity fibrous septa.

Thymolipoma is a relatively rare mass, showing high amounts of fat, but also some thymic tissue. This is easily demonstrated on T1-W sequences. The mass may arise from the thymus or be connected by a pedicle, and can often be large with compression of surrounding structures.

Thymus hyperplasia is indistinguishable from normal signal intensities. The thymus will be enlarged, however. Rebound thymus hyperplasia has to be suspected in those patients who are undergoing treatment for lymphoma or leukaemia.

Thymic carcinoma is less common than thymoma. It shows high signal intensity on both T1-WI and T2-WI and may exhibit inhomogeneity due to necrosis, cyst formation or haemorrhage. Although MRI is not capable of differentiating invasive thymoma from thymic carcinoma, it has been suggested that invasive thymoma is more frequently lobulated.

14.4.2.1.2 Germ-Cell Tumours

Germ-cell tumours also have a predilection for the anterior mediastinum. They account for approximately 15% of mediastinal masses. These masses are benign in 80%, and are mainly teratomas. Teratomas may consist of different types of tissue, which is reflected in the signal intensity pattern (Fig. 14.7). Thus, fat tissue, cysts and solid component may all be demonstrated, and fat-fluid levels are thought to be highly pathognomonic. Different classifications exist according to maturity of differentiation, with most mature teratomas presenting early in life.

Malignant germ-cell tumours are almost exclusively seen in men, with seminoma as the most common type. These masses are usually very large at presentation, and may be inhomogeneous due to necrosis and haemorrhage.

Table 14.3. Differential diagnosis of common mediastinal masses

Origin	Type	Typical Location	Features			
			Morphology	T1-W	Enhancement	T2-W
Thymus	Thymoma	Anterior	Encapsulated, inhomogeneous invasive, lobulated, septa	Low	Intermediate	High
	Thymolipoma	Anterior	Large	High	Low	Intermediate
	Hyperplasia	Anterior	Homogeneous, large	Intermediate	Intermediate	High
	Carcinoma	Anterior	Inhomogeneous	Intermediate	Strong	High
Germ-Cell Tumours	Teratoma	Anterior	Inhomogeneous, cystic and solid, fat-fluid levels	Variable	Strong	High
	Seminoma	Anterior	Large, lobulated, inhomogeneous	Variable	Strong	High
	Non-seminoma	Anterior	Large, irregular, inhomogeneous	Variable	Strong	High
Thyroid	Grave's disease	Anterior	Band-like	High	Strong	High
	Goitre	Anterior	Multinodular, inhomogeneous	Low	Strong	High
			Haemorrhage	High		
			Cystic	Low		
Neurogenic Tumours	Nerve sheath benign	Posterior	Sharply marginated	Variable	Uniform	Periphery high
			Spherical			Centre low
			Lobular			Target sign
	Nerve sheath malignant	Posterior	Large, inhomogeneous	Low	Inhomogeneous	High
	Sympathetic ganglia	Posterior				
	Ganglioneuroma		Well marginated, homogeneous irregular, inhomogeneous	Intermediate variable	Variable	Intermediate variable
	Neuroblastoma				Inhomogeneous	
Lymphatics	Lymphoma untreated	Anywhere	Homogeneous	Low	Strong	High
	Early response phase		Inhomogeneous	Low	Variable	Variable
	Complete response		Inhomogeneous	Variable	Minor	Variable
	Inactive residual fibrosis		Homogeneous	Low	None	Low
	Metastatic disease	Anywhere	Homogeneous	Low	Strong	Intermediate
	Infectious disease	Anywhere	Homogeneous	Low	Variable	Intermediate
Mediastinal Cysts	Thymic	Anterior	Well circumscribed	Low	None	High
	Bronchogenic	Middle	Well circumscribed	Low	None	High
	Oesophageal	Posterior	Well circumscribed	Low	None	High
	Neurenteric	Posterior	Well circumscribed	Low	None	High
	Pericardial	Middle	Well circumscribed	Low	None	High

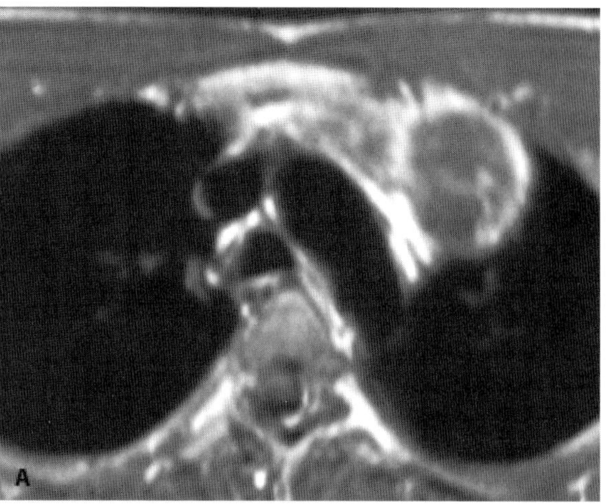
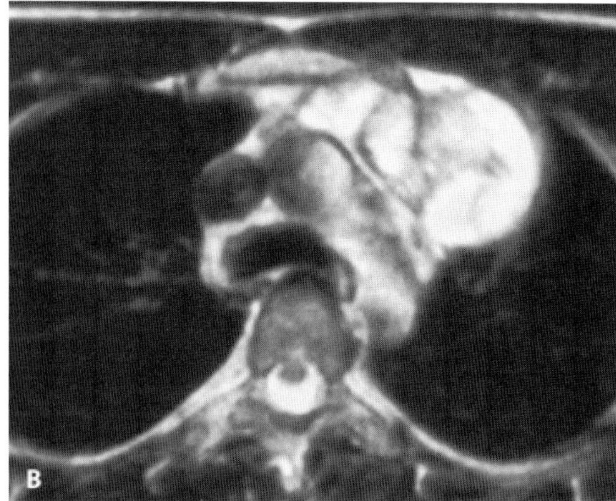

Fig. 14.7A,B. Teratoma in the anterior mediastinum. **A** Axial SE T1-WI inhomogeneous hypointense mass, **B** axial GRE T2-WI inhomogeneous hyperintense mass

14.4.2.2 Secondary Mediastinal Tumours

14.4.2.2.1 Thyroid

The most frequently encountered secondary mediastinal tumour is the goitre, extending through the cervicothoracic junction into the mediastinum. Mainly, the anterior mediastinum is affected with the goitre extending into the retrosternal supra-aortic space. However, different ways are also possible, and include the middle mediastinum with the thyroid tissue extending in between the trachea and the oesophagus as well as into the posterior mediastinum.

The normal thyroid gland is isointense with muscle on T1-WI and hyperintense on T2-WI. Multi-nodular goitre shows a relatively low signal on T1-WI and inhomogeneous high signal on T2-WI due to haemorrhage, necrosis and cyst formation. In patients with hypothyroidism (Graves' disease), the features change, and the signal intensity is high on both T1-WI and T2-WI. Furthermore, there are the appearances of band-like structures and dilated vascular structures throughout the thyroid gland.

14.4.2.2.2 Neurogenic Tumours

Neurogenic tumours are typically positioned in the posterior mediastinum. There is a close relationship with the vertebral column, and frequently there is a relationship with the nerve root canal. Three main subgroups can be distinguished: peripheral nerve tumours (neurofibroma and schwannoma), malignant nerve sheath tumours (malignant neurofibroma, malignant schwannoma and neurofibrosarcoma) and tumours arising from the sympathetic ganglia (ganglioneuroma, ganglioneuroblastoma and neuroblastoma). The benign tumours arising from the nerve sheath present themselves as well-defined, spherical or lobulated masses (Fig. 14.8). They always show variable T1-W signal and high signal on T2-WI, characteristically with low central T2-W signal as a result of fibrosis ('target sign'). The malignant nerve sheath tumours present themselves as large masses with inhomogeneous signal due to haemorrhage and necrosis. Finally, ganglioneuromas and ganglioneuroblastomas, which take their origin from the sympathetic ganglia, present as well-demarcated, homogeneous masses of intermediate signal intensity on T1-WI and T2-WI. Conversely, neuroblastomas show inhomogeneous signal on both T1-WI and T2-WI due to haemorrhage, necrosis, cystic generation and calcium deposition. Neuroblastoma shows inhomogeneous enhancement following Gd. Malignant

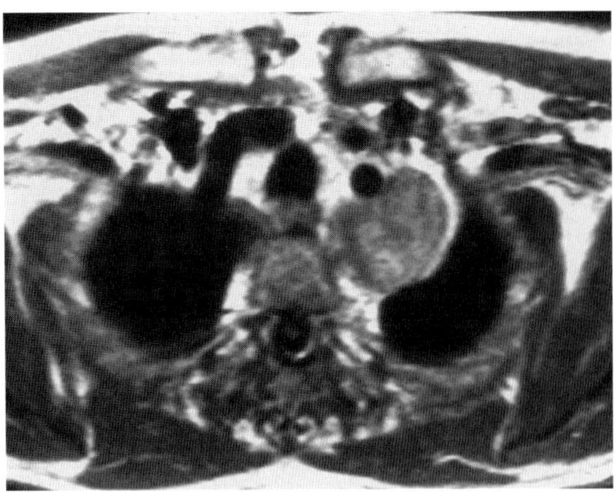

Fig. 14.8. Neurofibroma in the posterior mediastinum. Axial SE T1-WI shows inhomogeneous hypointense mass

neuroblastomas usually present early in childhood. The level of malignancy is often reflected in the amount of necrosis and haemorrhage. In this setting, MRI is clearly the imaging modality of choice and superior to CT since it can better illustrate the relationship of the tumour with regard to neural foramina, spinal cord and bone.

14.4.2.2.3
Oesophagus

Oesophageal tumours are the second most frequently encountered masses in the posterior mediastinum. However, MRI plays an insignificant role in the staging and diagnosis of these malignancies since it does not offer any essential advantages over CT.

14.4.2.3
Lymphatic Tissues

Lymphadenopathy is a common feature of both benign and malignant diseases. MRI is capable of demonstrating lymph nodes with accuracy and can also show the effects of lymph node enlargement on adjacent structures. MRI is less capable of demonstrating calcification, although a decrease in signal on T2-WI may be appreciated.

14.4.2.3.1
Lymphoma

Malignant lymphoma is the most common primary mediastinal neoplasm. Mediastinal manifestations occur either in isolation or as a part of generalised disease. Hodgkin's disease is the most common and often presents as a huge mediastinal bulk. Although MRI is superior to CT in displaying the extent of the mass, it does not lead to a change in the clinical management. MRI can be employed in monitoring treatment effects in patients with lymphoma. Four different signal patterns can be defined, which may help (to some extent) to determine these effects:

1. Homogeneous, hyperintense pattern of untreated lymphoma, which shows low signal T1-W and high signal T2-W. This is never encountered in inactive residual masses.
2. Heterogeneous, active pattern of post-treatment response phase, which exhibits homogeneous low signal on T1-W and inhomogeneous high and low signal on T2-WI. This pattern can also be present in untreated nodular sclerosing Hodgkin's disease.
3. Heterogeneous, inactive pattern of early complete response phase. During this phase there is mixed high and low intensity on both T1-WI and T2-WI.
4. Homogeneous, hypointense pattern of inactive residual fibrosis, which shows low signal on both T1-WI and T2-WI.

However, the potential of MRI to separate vital from non-vital lymphoma tissue is not reliable enough to provide conclusive prognostic information or to detect recurrent disease early. Thus, it has not been generally established as the first-line imaging modality in mediastinal lymphoma to replace CT. Positron emission tomography (PET) offers clear advantages over both technologies, as it is more sensitive in detecting metabolically active cells.

14.4.2.3.2
Metastatic Disease

Malignant involvement of the lymph nodes is mainly determined by size. Similarly to CT, a short axis diameter of more than 1 cm is generally considered suggestive for malignancy, which carries a negative predictive value of approximately 85% (Fig. 14.9). The lymph node size should also be regarded with respect to the ana-

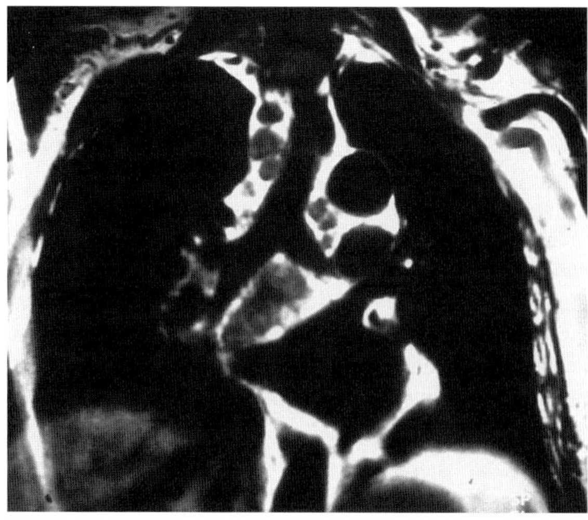

Fig. 14.9. Mediastinal lymphadenopathy due to bronchogenic carcinoma. Coronal SE T1-WI showing multiple, enlarged, hypointense lymph nodes

tomical location, e.g. lymph nodes in the paratracheal region are often bigger without being malignant. Thus, comparing lymph node size between the right and left sides might be helpful, with a difference of more than 5 mm suggesting malignancy. Calcifications, which are an important sign of benign lymphadenopathy, are difficult to appreciate on MRI. The differentiation between lymph nodes and blood vessels is straightforward – even on non-enhanced scans – if fast-flowing blood leads to a flow void. In the case of slow-flowing blood or turbulence, the differentiation can be difficult. The addition of CEMRA or bright-blood techniques may offer useful information in this setting.

Although some early indications suggested that differences in signal intensities could differentiate between benign and malignant nodes, this has not proven to be clinically useful. However, current ongoing clinical trials are evaluating new contrast agents with a main focus on lymphography and decreased uptake of contrast in malignant lymph nodes. MR lymphography is based on T2-W and T2*-W GRE images taken 24–48 h after the intravenous administration of ultra-small super-paramagnetic iron particles (USPIO). The effect is based on the fact that macrophages take up iron oxide much more avidly than tumour cells. Thus, normal lymph nodes will show a decrease in signal intensity, whereas the contrast effect is absent or less pro-

Table 14.4. Advantages and disadvantages of CT versus MRI

Criteria	CT	MRI
Independence from motion artefacts	+	–
Spatial resolution	++	+
Detection of calcifications	++	–
Cost	+	+
Need for contrast agents	–	++
Multiplanar capabilities	+	++
Soft-tissue contrast	+	++
Tissue characterisation	+	++
Vascular studies	+	++

nounced in neoplastic nodes. In preliminary clinical studies MR lymphography in patients with bronchogenic carcinoma yielded a sensitivity of 100%, and a specificity of 38%.

In clinical routine, CT and MRI are more or less equivalent regarding the N-staging (see Table 14.2), especially N2. Both can be used to stratify the patient for invasive procedures, such as mediastinoscopy or thoracotomy with mediastinal lymph node dissection. The advantages and disadvantages of CT and MRI in this context are given in Table 14.4. Although MRI seems to have some capability to distinguish between normal and invaded lymph nodes, PET has a greater diagnostic accuracy for the identification of mediastinal metastatic lymph nodes.

14.4.2.3.3 Benign Disease

A wide range of benign causes of lymphadenopathy exists, and differentiation between these is very difficult. Some aetiologies more commonly give rise to calcifications, which will result in more inhomogeneous signal (especially on T2-WI). The poor spatial resolution can lead to blending together of numerous small lymph nodes and appearing like a single enlarged lymph node, resulting in a false-positive finding.

14.4.2.4 Mediastinal Cysts

Five different types of cystic masses can be identified, and these are usually classified based on their primary location. Thus, thymic cysts are found in the anterior mediastinum, bronchogenic cysts and pericardial cysts are mainly present in the middle mediastinum (Fig. 14.10), while oesophageal duplication cysts and neurogenic cysts are found in the posterior mediastinum. All cysts have characteristically well-defined margins and show low signal on T1-WI and high signal on T2-WI. Typically, no enhancement is observed after the administration of contrast. In the case of multiple cysts and the presence of cysts below the diaphragm, pancreatic pseudocysts or hydatid disease are likely differential diagnoses.

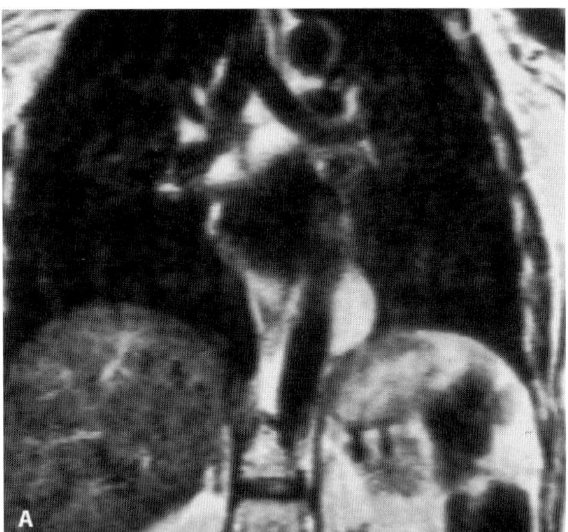

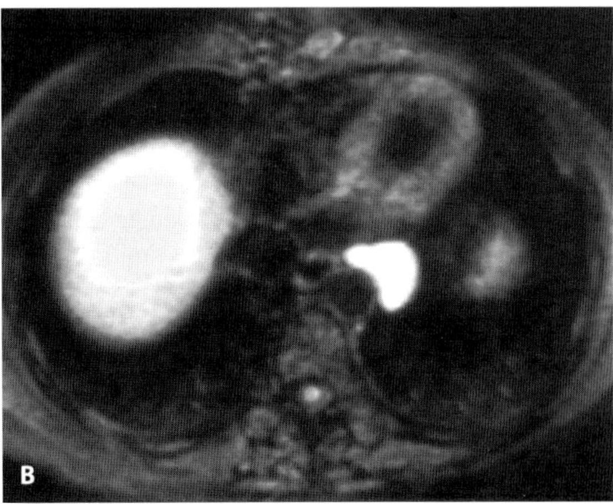

Fig. 14.10A,B. Bronchogenic cyst in the posterior mediastinum. **A** Coronal GRE T2-WI, **B** axial GRE T2-WI showing a homogenous, lobulated hyperintense cyst

14.5 Pulmonary Arteries

14.5.1 Anatomy

Using state-of-the-art techniques (see above) and breath-holding, the central and lobar arteries can be completely visualised on a routine basis (Fig. 14.11). Furthermore, more than 90% of segmental arteries and more than 80% of subsegmental 4th order arteries can be depicted. Some of the congenital abnormalities of the heart also involve the pulmonary arteries, but these are dealt with elsewhere.

14.5.2 Pathology

14.5.2.1 Pulmonary Embolism

Pulmonary embolism is an extremely common and potentially life-threatening disorder. Its clinical signs, history, clinical examination and chest radiograph are

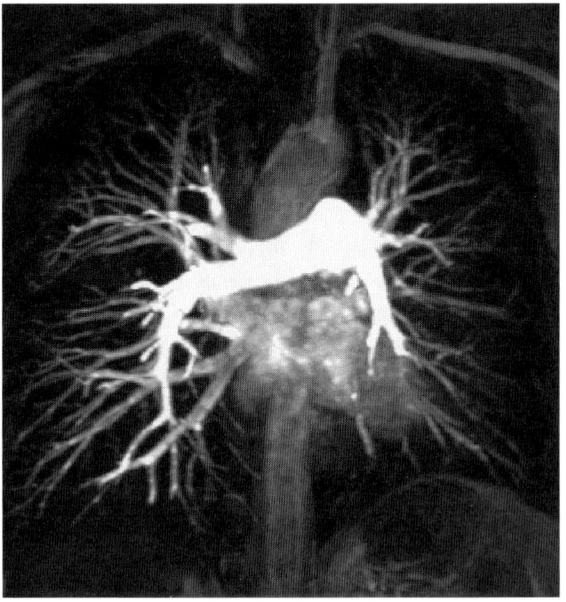

Fig. 14.11. Normal pulmonary MR angiogram. Coronal maximum intensity projection

generally unspecific. Pulmonary angiography is generally regarded as the gold standard modality but is invasive. Therefore, accurate, highly sensitive, highly specific, easy and fast to perform, cost-effective and widely available, non-invasive alternatives are required. Spiral CT meets a lot of these expectations with an average sensitivity >80% and specificity >90%. In parallel, encouraging results have been observed using CEMRA, which may become a competitive alternative in the future. Several findings can indicate the presence of acute pulmonary embolism (Table 14.5). In CEMRA, a homogeneous intravascular high signal intensity is reliably obtained. Slow or turbulent flow does not mimic pulmonary emboli, which are diagnosed as constant intraluminal filling defects (Fig. 14.12) or abrupt vascular cut-offs. Multi-planar reformats are frequently used to depict wall-adherent, segmental or subsegmental emboli with a high level of confidence. From the beginning, CEMRA was superior to non-enhanced MRA for the central pulmonary artery branches. Using state-of-the-art techniques (see above), CEMRA achieves a sensitivity >85% and a specificity >95% for the diagnosis of pulmonary embolism on a per patient basis. On a per-embolus basis the sensitivity is >65%. Furthermore, isolated subsegmental emboli cannot be reliably excluded, but this is a problem of most (if not all) diagnostic modalities. Secondary signs of pulmonary embolism may include pleural effusions and lung consolidation (including pulmonary infarction). These are usually easily identifiable on MRI, as discussed above, as this will result in a high signal on T2-WI. Haemorrhagic infarction will also show high signal on T1-WI.

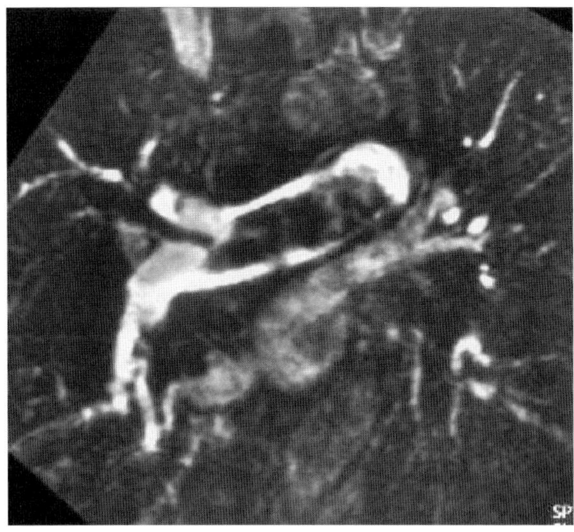

Fig. 14.12. Acute pulmonary embolism. Coronal, contrast-enhanced GRE T1-WI showing a central thrombus in the right pulmonary artery

Table 14.5. Criteria for the MRI diagnosis of pulmonary embolism

Criteria	Acute embolism	Chronic thromboembolic pulmonary hypertension (CTEPH)
Direct – filling defects	Central, intraluminal, convex	Wall-adherent, concave
	Lack of opacification	Lack of opacification
		Intraluminal webs
Direct -vascular wall		Irregular wall thickening
		Abnormal proximal-to-distal tapering
		Variations in size of segmental vessel
		Absence of segmental vessels (cut-off)
Indirect – parenchyma	Infarction	Infarction
	Pleural-based, round	Mosaic perfusion
	Pleural effusion	Pleural effusion
Indirect – pulmonary hypertension	Cardiomegaly	Cardiomegaly
	Paradoxical movement of interventricular septum	Negative axis of interventricular septum
		Dilation of central pulmonary arteries
		Pericardial effusion, ascites

14.5.2.2
Chronic Thromboembolic Pulmonary Hypertension

Chronic Thromboembolic Pulmonary Hypertension (CTEPH) is a long-term outcome following acute pulmonary embolism in approximately 3%–7% of patients. Although this represents a minority of patients with acute pulmonary embolism, it is being diagnosed with increasing frequency. The differentiation between acute or chronic pulmonary embolism is possible by CEMRA in most patients (Table 14.5). A diagnosis of CTEPH can be confidently made with the following criteria: dilated central pulmonary arteries, direct visualisation of wall-adherent thrombotic material and thickening of the vessel wall, absence of segmental vessels (cut-off), abnormal proximal-to-distal tapering of pulmonary vessels, variations in size of segmental vessel, intraluminal webs, and heterogeneous contrast enhancement within the lung parenchyma.

The main differential diagnosis of CTEPH is primary pulmonary hypertension (PPH). This disorder gives similar findings in general, but without the signs of (previous) pulmonary embolism. More than 90% of patients with PPH can be differentiated from those with CTEPH and normal subjects on the basis of CEMRA.

14.5.2.3
Primary and Metastatic Tumours Involving the Pulmonary Arteries

Tumours involving the pulmonary artery (sarcomas or metastases) are depicted as filling defects at CEMRA. In patients who are suspected of a mass involving the pulmonary arteries, delayed scans after contrast administration are advised to demonstrate enhancement, indicating neoplasms instead of pulmonary embolism. Care has to be taken since neoplasms have different degrees of vascularity, and they may be associated with secondary thrombus formation or necrosis.

14.5.2.4
Pulmonary Artery Aneurysms

Aneurysms of the pulmonary arteries are rare and may be associated with a wide variety of conditions, such as congenital heart disease, hereditary telangiectasia and trauma. Multiple aneurysms may be observed in patients with Behçet's disease or Hughes-Stovin syndrome. A non-invasive diagnosis, which is particularly important in these patients, is easily obtained by CEMRA. The imaging data can be used as the basis for surgical planning. Finally, false aneurysms can be caused by interventions, such as the introduction of Swan-Ganz catheters.

14.5.2.5
Pulmonary Arteriovenous Malformations

They consist of a racemose convolute of vascular structures. Flow within the malformation can be highly variable. Patent vessels will show flow void, whereas slow flow will exhibit low signal, and thrombosed vessels and haemorrhage will show high signal. After contrast administration, malformations enhance strongly, while high calibre feeding arteries and draining veins are easily depicted with CEMRA. The differentiation of arteriovenous malformations from other pulmonary nodules or masses is obvious.

14.5.2.6
Pulmonary Sequestrations

These consist of non-functioning lung tissue, which is not in continuity with the tracheobronchial tree. They contain mucus, inflammatory, granulomatous and fibrotic tissue, and they exhibit high signal intensity on T2-WI and intermediate to high signal intensity on non-enhanced T1-WI. After contrast administration, the lesion demonstrates strong enhancement. The atypical systemic arteries arise from the descending or abdominal aorta in most cases. They are visualised by MRI, including CEMRA, with a high degree of confidence, thus avoiding conventional angiography in most cases.

14.5.2.7
Anomalous Pulmonary Venous Return

MRI and MRA can be successfully used for the accurate identification of pulmonary venous confluence and total or partial anomalous pulmonary venous return, such as seen in scimitar syndrome (Fig. 14.13). Additional information of concomitant bronchial and visceral abnormalities can be obtained. Flow measurements will allow for quantitation of shunt volumes. The limitations of echocardiography and the invasiveness of angiography make CEMRA the modality of choice for the assessment of anomalies of the pulmonary veins.

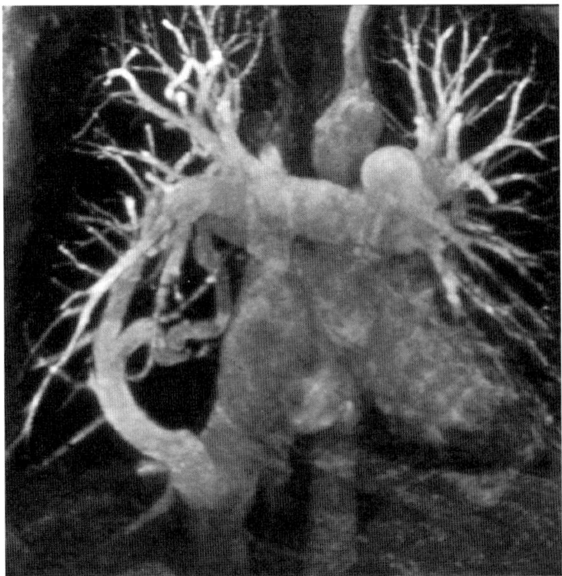

Fig. 14.13. Scimitar syndrome. Coronal maximum intensity projection showing an anomalous venous drainage of the right lower lobe into the inferior vena cava

14.6 Future Prospects

MRI of the chest is increasingly used for a variety of disorders. The introduction of fast and ultra-fast sequences, allowing breath-hold techniques, has paved the way for improved visualisation of the main structures in the chest. Thus, MRI of the mediastinum, chest wall and superior sulcus is now commonly regarded as the modality of choice. Contrast-enhanced MRA is now routinely employed in the assessment of vascular pathology, and progress is being made in the assessment of patients with suspected acute pulmonary embolism. Airway imaging is becoming available by the application of fast imaging techniques in the presence of pathological changes in the lung parenchyma, such as consolidations and masses. Finally, dynamic processes of the lung, including airway dynamics and oxygen exchange mechanisms are currently being investigated.

Further Reading

Bergin CJ, Hauschildt J, Rios G, Belezzuoli EV, Huynh T, Channick RN (1997) Accuracy of MR angiography compared with radionuclide scanning in identifying the cause of pulmonary arterial hypertension. AJR 168:1549–1555

Kauczor H-U, Kreitner K-F (1999) MRI of the pulmonary parenchyma. Eur Radiol 9:1755–1764

Kauczor H-U, Chen XJ, van Beek EJR, Schreiber WG (2001) Pulmonary ventilation imaged by magnetic resonance: at the doorstep of clinical application. Eur Respir J 17:1–16

Landwehr P, Schulte O, Lackner K (1999) MR imaging of the chest: mediastinum and chest wall. Eur Radiol 9:1737–1744

Lange S, Walsh G (1998) Radiology of chest diseases, 2nd edn. Thieme, Stuttgart

Naidich DP, Webb WR, Müller NL, Krisky GA, Zerhouni EA, Siegelman SS (1999) Computed tomography and Magnetic Resonance of the Thorax, 3rd edn. Lippincott-Raven, Philadelphia

Oudkerk M, van Beek EJ, Wielopolski P, van Ooijen PM, Brouwers-Kuyper EM, Bongaerts AH, Berghout A (2002) Comparison of contrast-enhanced magnetic resonance angiography and conventional pulmonary angiography for the diagnosis of pulmonary embolism: a prospective study. Lancet 359 (9318): 1643–1647

White CS (2000) MR imaging of the thorax. Magn Reson Imaging Clin North Am 8:1–219

Wielopolski PA, Oudkerk M, van Ooijen PMA (1999) Magnetic resonance imaging and angiography of the pulmonary vascular system. In: Oudkerk M, van Beek EJR, ten Cate JW (eds) Pulmonary embolism, 1st edn. Blackwell Science, Berlin, pp 250–331

Magnetic Resonance of the Breast

15

C. Kuhl

Contents

15.1 Before Getting Started

For successful breast magnetic resonance imaging (MRI), one of the most important steps is to interview the patient before she proceeds to the magnet. This serves two important purposes: (1) to obtain patient history data, which are indispensable for adequate image interpretation, and (2) to explain to the patient what is going to happen, to ensure her cooperation (particularly to reduce motion, thus, subtraction artifacts). Typically, this part of the exam takes longer than the part in the magnet. A thorough patient history should focus on issues related to breast diseases and physiology. Questions to be answered are:

1. Previous breast cancer, including stage, age at diagnosis
2. If applicable, type of breast cancer treatment: breast conservation or mastectomy; previous radiation therapy, reconstructive surgery, chemotherapy, antihormonal therapy
3. Family history of breast or ovarian cancer, including age at diagnosis
4. Previous fine-needle aspiration cytology/core biopsy/excisional biopsy of benign lesions
5. Menstrual/menopausal state
6. Hormonal-replacement therapy
7. Pregnancy or lactation (if yes, do not do breast MR)
8. Present complaints, in particular:
9. Nipple discharge (note texture/color)
10. Mastodynia (cycle phase dependency?)
11. Palpable abnormalities

Inspect the breast to check for any nipple discharge or skin changes. Note any inflammatory changes, because they may cause substantial differential diagnostic difficulties. If there is any inflammation, consider postponing the imaging until this has resolved. A clinical examination of the breasts is an integral part of any breast MR imaging studies and needs to be performed thoroughly to identify any palpable abnormalities.

It is necessary to have previous conventional imaging studies (mammograms, US studies) available before beginning. If the patient's case is unknown, be sure that the problem that is to be explored by breast MR is well understood. In particular, if there is an equivocal mammographic finding, identify it on the mammograms, because the MR exam may have to be tailored accordingly, e.g., in case the finding is in the axillary tail, this may require a change of image orientation to rotate the heart-pulsation artifact band out of the way.

It is important to check the indications for breast MR. Many diagnostic difficulties can be avoided by proper indication and patient selection. Appropriate indications for breast MR can be divided into two main categories.

1. Clarification of equivocal clinical or conventional imaging findings (mammography, breast ultrasound), particularly in the post-treatment breast, or in high-risk patients with very dense breasts. This includes cases for follow-up after breast conservation surgery and radiation therapy (differentiation of scar versus recurrent tumor), follow-up after reconstructive or implant surgery, monitoring of primary or adjuvant chemotherapy, and search for primary breast cancer in patients with axillary lymphadenopathy.
2. Preoperative breast MR in patients scheduled for excisional biopsy of a suspicious focus (BI-RADS 4 or 5). This serves to improve the preoperative local staging to assess the true tumor extent, to demonstrate an extensive intraductal component (EIC) or infiltration of the chest wall or the nipple, and to rule out multifocal, multicentric or contralateral disease before a breast-conserving therapy is initiated. According to a recent study by Fischer and co-workers, systematic preoperative breast MRI in patients with presumed solitary BI-RADS category 4 or 5 lesions will reveal additional multicentric breast cancer foci in 14% of patients.

It should be kept in mind that, for clarification of palpable or conventional imaging abnormalities (mammography or ultrasound guided), core biopsy is a safe and inexpensive alternative to breast MR. It should go without saying that breast MR cannot be used to spare a patient a mammogram. A mammogram must accompany the reading of any breast MR study – this is not a formal requirement, but it is necessary to check the indication, to ensure the sensitive diagnosis of in-situ cancers, and to avoid diagnostic errors secondary to breast cancers with atypical MR imaging presentation (e.g., cancers with shallow enhancement).

15.2 Hardware Requirements

To image the breast, a dedicated breast surface coil is an indispensable prerequisite. Usually, this is a double-breast surface coil that allows imaging of both entire breasts simultaneously. It is not important to extend the range of the surface coil to include the axilla. Diagnosis of lymph-node involvement is not necessarily an integral part of breast imaging with MR, because there are no criteria to distinguish involved from normal lymph nodes anyway. If the radiologist still wishes to screen for enlarged lymph nodes, this can be done with the body coil.

Concerning the MR system used for breast MR, a simple rule of thumb applies: the higher the field and the stronger the gradients, the better. The higher signal-to-noise ratio (SNR) offered by magnets with 1.5 T is better able to fulfill the specific technical requirements of breast MR. However, if suitable pulse sequences and strong gradients are available, breast MR is feasible with 1.0-T or 0.5-T systems.

15.3 Patient Positioning

Imaging must be performed with the patient in the prone position. The arms should be placed alongside the body. Raising them up above the head does have advantages in terms of reducing fold-over artifacts; however, in this position, the blood circulation tends to become restricted, which in turn may lead to patient movements. Moreover, with her arms over her head, the patient is more likely to push herself out of the coil.

A venous line (18–20 G) is placed into an antecubital vein and kept patent via a saline infusion. Before moving her into the bore, explain to the patient again that she must lie perfectly still – also in between scans (when the scanner noise stops) – and explain to her why this is so important. Explicitly instruct her not to turn her head from side to side, and not to move her arms, particularly during the injection of contrast material. Movements of the upper extremities are almost always associated with pectoral muscle contractions, which in turn translate into changes of the cross-sectional aspect of the entire breast, thus giving rise to severe motion and subtraction artifacts.

15.4 Imaging: Pulse Sequence Parameters and Documentation

In the past, two different 'schools' evolved in breast MRI. The 'European approach' was to perform dynamic imaging to assess the lesions contrast-enhancement characteristics. The 'US approach' favored static, high-spatial-resolution imaging to characterize lesion morphology. As a consequence, the two different schools advocated completely different imaging techniques. Depending only on the diagnostic criterion that was given priority, and given the limitations of the MR equipment, the proposed imaging sequences were designed to allow optimal spatial or optimal temporal resolution.

To date, among those who perform breast MR clinically, there is broad agreement that both concepts should be integrated. This means that MRI of the breast must consider both lesion morphology and lesion contrast-enhancement kinetics. However, as yet, with current MR systems and pulse-sequence software, any proposed pulse sequence is only a compromise on the diverging demands of temporal and spatial resolution. Accordingly, there is no such thing like an 'optimal pulse sequence'. All parameters given here are suggestions and should be understood as such. We perform breast MRI with 1.5-T systems with pulse sequences that provide adequate temporal and high spatial resolution.

Before discussing the various technical issues, it is important to realize that personal practical experience with breast MR should be considered an absolute prerequisite for using breast MR imaging clinically, and this has most definitively more impact on the technique's accuracy rates than any other single factor, including choice of imaging technique. Also, in this respect, breast MR is in no way different from conventional breast imaging techniques. All pulse sequences recommended for breast MRI are heavily T1-weighted (T1-W), two-dimensional (2D) or 3D, gradient-echo (GRE) sequences (Table 15.1). As the echo times (TEs) are more or less given by field-dependent in-phase settings of fat and water resonance frequencies, improving the sequences' T1-contrast is only possible by reducing the repetition time (TR). The flip-angle has then to be adapted to the TR; in general, it must be set smaller with shorter TRs.

At 1.5 T, we use a transaxial (2D GRE pulse sequence with TR/TE/FA 290/4.6/90°, with a 512×400 imaging matrix. The field of view (FOV) should be adjusted to

Table 15.1. Pulse sequence parameters recommendations for diagnostic breast magnetic resonance

Sequence	WI	Plane	No. of slices	TR (ms)	TE (ms)	Flip angle	Echo train length	Slice thickness (mm)	Matrix	FOV	recFOV	No. of acq.	Acq. time (min)
TSE[a]	T2	Axial	20–35	2500–4000	90–110	90	12–15	3–4	512×512	270–320	100	2	4
TSE[b]	T2	Axial	25–35	2500–4000	90–110	90	12–15	3–4	512×512	270–320	100	2	4
SE[c]	T1	Coronal	25–35	300–500	10–15	90		3–4	256×256	350	60	2	2
2D or 3D dynamic GRE[d]	T1	Axial	20–35	250 (2D) or 15 (3D) (always as short as possible)	in phase (4.6 ms at 1.5 T) (6.9 ms at 1.0 T) (3.0 ms at 0.5 T)	90 (2D) or 25 (3D)		3–4	512×5400	270–320	100	1	1:50 per dynamic scan

[a] Standard sequence to use without fat suppression
[b] Optional sequence to use with spectral-selective fat suppression
[c] Optional sequence to cover the chest wall including axilla with cranio-caudal phase encoding direction
[d] Standard sequence to use as a dynamic study pre- and 5–8 times postcontrast (Gadolinium)

Abbreviations: *WI* weighting of images; *TR* repetition time (ms); *TE* echo time (ms); *Matrix* phase × frequency matrix; *FOV* field of view (mm); *recFOV* rectangular field of view (%); *Acq.* acquisition(s)

the size of the breast (not chest), typically 280–300 mm (for bilateral acquisition). The section thickness should be 3 mm or less without gaps between sections. With this parameter setting, about 30–35 sections are needed to cover the entire breast parenchyma. A total of 5–7 dynamic scans are obtained in a series, i.e., one precontrast and 4–6 times after bolus injection of 0.1 mmol/kg gadopentetate dimeglumine. The temporal resolution should be kept at 1–2 min per dynamic scan; we do not recommend improving the temporal resolution beyond the 1-min margin, because there is no additional diagnostic information to be expected. Instead, the temporal resolution should be set at 1–2 min, and all remaining scanner capacity should be invested to improve the spatial resolution.

If breast MRI has to be performed at 0.5 T, the shorter tissue T1-relaxation times need to be compensated for by use of a pulse sequence with a substantially shorter TR. This is why a 3D pulse sequence is mandatory for breast MR at this field strength. At 0.5 T, in-phase TE for fat and water resonance frequencies is 14 ms; however, this is too long to maintain an adequate temporal resolution, and, moreover, the long TE would introduce some T2-contrast. Therefore, a TE of 3.0 ms is recommended to reduce phase-cancellation effects while preserving dynamic imaging capabilities. At 1.0 T, in-phase imaging settings dictate a TE of 7.0 ms, a necessity that limits the image acquisition speed considerably.

Concerning the choice of image orientation, the following facts are important. With current magnets, sagittal imaging is feasible only in single breast protocols. For bilateral protocols, one needs to decide between the axial or coronal image orientation. We prefer the axial orientation because we believe that it is easier to assess the retro-areolar and pre-pectoral region in these images, and because fewer sections are needed to cover the parenchyma. Coronal imaging may be advantageous, especially to compensate for the limited temporal resolution secondary to the long in-phase TE settings at 1.0 T: With coronal imaging, with the feet-head phase-encoding direction, a rectangular field-of-view can be used to reduce the number of phase-encoding steps at a given spatial resolution.

In all protocols for breast MR, the signal from fatty tissue must be suppressed to improve the detection and delineation of contrast-enhancing lesions. In principle, fat suppression can be achieved by active (frequency- or spectral-selective prepulses) or passive (subtraction) techniques. For dynamic breast MR imaging, fat suppression must be obtained via image subtraction, which is done off-line and, as such, does not affect the temporal resolution. A spectral- or frequency-selective fat suppression takes too much time to allow image acquisition in a rapid, dynamic pattern.

We do not recommend obtaining images in complementary orientations after the dynamic series, because the lesion-to-parenchyma contrast deteriorates rapidly in the intermediate and late postcontrast period, such that it would be difficult to detect the lesion in question in these images. To elucidate the lesion's location in, for example, the sagittal and coronal planes, it is much more useful to obtain maximum intensity projection (MIP) or multiplanar reconstruction (MPR) views of the early postcontrast subtracted images.

Prior to the dynamic series, we regularly obtain a T2-W turbo spin-echo (TSE) pulse sequence (TR/TE/TF 2800/110/16) with geometric parameters corresponding to those of the subsequent dynamic series. The T2-W images are obtained to improve the detection of (residual) interstitial edema after, for example, radiation therapy or the diagnosis of inflammatory changes, to improve the delineation of lymphangiosis or cystic lesions, and also to help categorize solid enhancing tumors.

If regional (axillary, internal mammary) or remote (supraclavicular) lymph node involvement or osseous metastases are to be evaluated, we use the built-in body coil to acquire coronal T1-W SE images prior to the dynamic series. This should be done before the contrast-enhanced study, because lymph nodes or bone-marrow metastases are visible only on the precontrast image as hypointense lesions against the adjacent hyperintense subcutaneous or bone-marrow fatty tissue.

Documentation should at least include hard copies of early, intermediate, and late postcontrast fat-suppressed (subtracted) images and nonsubtracted, precontrast and postcontrast images. In addition, any time/intensity curves (see below) should be documented together with the corresponding lesion.

15.5 Kinetic Analysis

For analysis of lesion-enhancement kinetics, a small region of interest (ROI) should be placed in the lesion to obtain the time course of signal intensity over the dynamic series. The ROI must be placed selectively into vital tumor components, because only here can meaningful time courses be obtained. Vital tumor should be identified by searching for the area where enhancement appears first on the early postcontrast image, i.e., by identifying the area with the fastest and strongest enhancement, at wide window settings. Parametric images may be helpful in identifying tumor areas with the most rapid enhancement. It is *not* useful to include the entire lesion in a ROI or to place a large region that encircles most of a lesion, because then necrotic or hypovascular tumor areas are averaged together with the vital parts. Two different kinetic parameters may be derived from the ROI-based signal intensity (SI) curves:

1. The initial SI rise in the early postcontrast period ('upstroke' of the curve) provides the lesion's enhancement rate (quantified as 'enhancement velocity').
2. The behavior of SI in the intermediate and late postcontrast period (time course or shape of the time course) is visually assessed and classified as type I–III.

Regarding the enhancement rate: the SI increase in the early postcontrast period may be used to quantify the early phase-enhancement rate (or 'enhancement velocity'); to do this, SI increase is given relative to baseline SI.

The rationale of calculating enhancement rates is based on the observation that malignant lesions tend to have enhancement kinetics that differ from those of benign lesions. On average, malignant lesions exhibit higher enhancement velocities and a different time course kinetic (see below) than benign ones. However, the concept of an 'enhancement threshold' to separate benign from malignant lesions, which was propagated in early studies in the field of dynamic breast MR, cannot be maintained any more (see below). Still, enhancement should be quantified routinely in all enhancing lesions in order to be used as one diagnostic criterion among others.

Regarding the shape of the time course, according to the SI changes in the intermediate and late postcontrast period, the time courses may be visually classified as type I–III:

1. Type I: straight or curved type. Signal continues to increase over the entire dynamic period. In the curved type, the time course is flattened in the late postcontrast period due to saturation effects.
2. Type II: plateau type. After initial upstroke, enhancement is abruptly cut off, and the signal plateaus in the intermediate and late postcontrast period.
3. Type III: wash-out type. After the initial upstroke, enhancement is abruptly cut off, and the signal decreases (washes out) in the intermediate postcontrast period (2–3 min post injection).

The rationale of evaluating the lesions' SI time courses is in terms of the differential diagnosis of enhancing solid lesions. A type I time course indicates the presence of a benign lesion, as it is mostly found in benign tissues (9:1 benign versus malignant), such as normal breast tissue, fibrocystic disease, and fibroadenomas. A type-I course may rarely occur in malignant lesions with poor angiogenetic activity, such as some lobular or scirrhotic ductal cancers or ductal carcinoma-in-situ (DCIS). A type-II time course increases the suspicion of malignancy of a lesion, as it is obtained more often in malignant than in benign tissues (3:2 malignant versus benign). A type-III time course is highly suspicious, because it is seen much more often in breast cancers than in benign lesions (6:1 malignant versus benign). A type-III time course in benign lesions may occur in hypervascularized tissues such as inflammatory lesions and, rarely, in hypervascular fibroadenomas, papillomas, or focal adenosis. It is important to understand that the diagnostic information provided by the kinetic analysis may only be used for the differential diagnosis in lesions with strong enhancement. Lesions with slow or gradual enhancement, i.e., those that lack significant angiogenic activity, including slow-enhancing breast cancers, will almost always exhibit 'benign', steady signal time courses. A wash-out or plateau time course will be obtained only in lesions with extensive hypervascularity and arteriovenous shunts. So while absence of a plateau or wash-out time course can be used to support the diagnosis of a benign lesion in cases with rapid and strong enhancement, it cannot be used to do the same in a lesion with slow and shallow enhancement.

15.6 Reading the Breast Magnetic Resonance Study

15.6.1 Diagnostic Criteria in Dynamic Breast Magnetic Resonance

When a contrast-enhancing lesion is identified on the postcontrast subtracted images, the process of the lesion differential diagnosis is initiated. To distinguish benign and malignant enhancing lesions, the following diagnostic criteria may be considered: morphology (configuration, borders, internal architecture); enhancement kinetics (early-phase enhancement rate, degree of enhancement, shape of time/signal intensity curve, spatial progression of enhancement); and lesion SI in T2-W TSE images.

15.6.2 The Normal Breast

Because the breast is a hormone-reactive organ that responds to endogenous (ovarian hormones) or exogenous (replacement therapy) hormonal stimuli, what is looked upon as 'the normal breast' changes steadily, depending on the patient's age, menstrual/menopausal state, and hormone/antihormone intake. When starting with breast MR in general, it is of the utmost importance to be familiar with the variable aspect of the breast parenchyma in MRI.

Particularly in the very young premenopausal patient (at or below the age of 35 years), strong, spontaneous, focal contrast enhancement may be found which can mimic benign and malignant lesions. These 'lesions' correspond to the hormone-reactive part of the parenchyma and should not be mixed up with true lesions requiring biopsy (Fig. 15.1). According to a

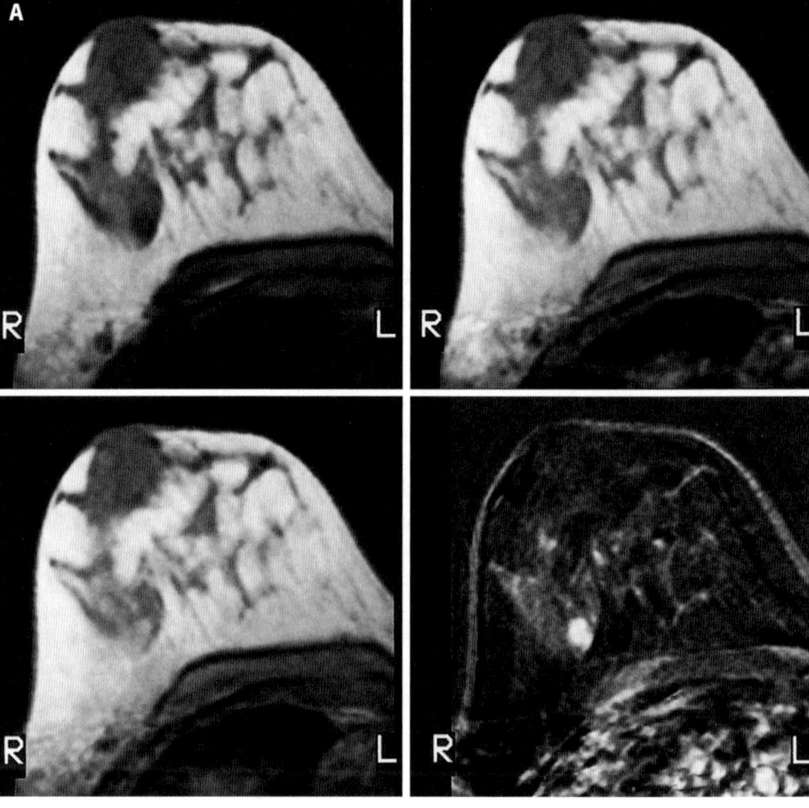

Fig. 15.1. A Young premenopausal volunteer underwent breast magnetic resonance (MR) during the first week of her menstrual cycle (day 3). **B** Same volunteer 1 week later (day 10). *Upper left* precontrast; *upper right* first postcontrast; *bottom left* second postcontrast; *bottom right* early postcontrast subtracted image of her dynamic series. Note the focal, nodular lesion with rapid enhancement visible during the first week of the menstrual cycle (**A**), which completely resolves by the second week (**B**). This is what we would call an 'unidentified breast object' (UBO). No biopsy indicated or required

Fig. 15.1B

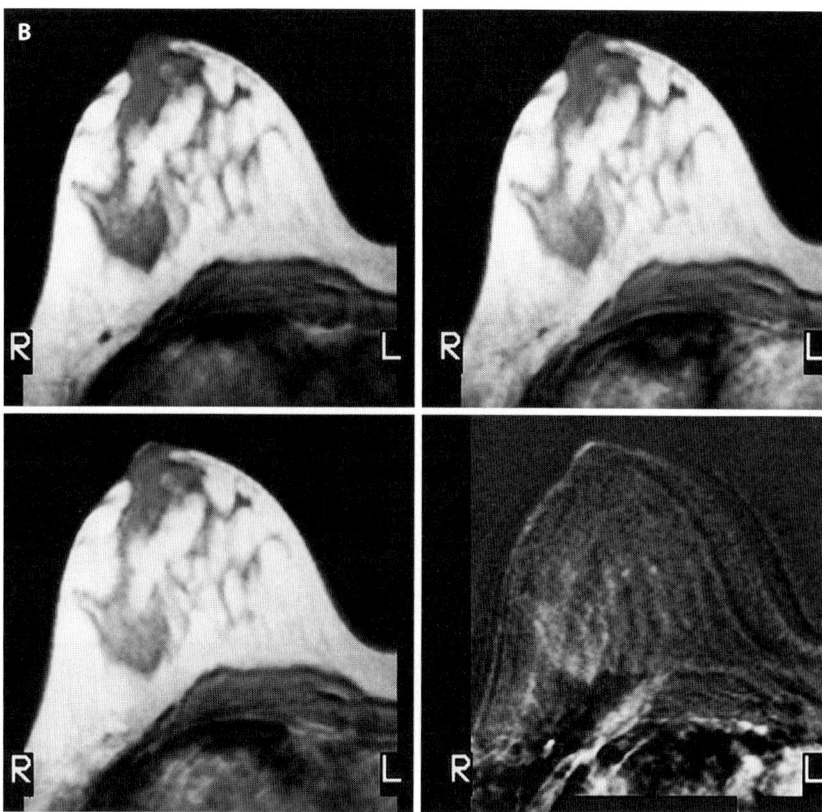

recent series, the incidence of spontaneous contrast-enhancing 'lesions' or 'unidentified breast objects' (UBOs) is highest in weeks 1 and 4 of a menstrual cycle, whereas significantly less enhancement is encountered in week 2.

A distinction of UBOs and serious pathology is often difficult enough, because the morphology of these 'lesions' may appear quite suspicious. Enhancement rates may also be well beyond any 'enhancement threshold'. To solve this problem, we recommend the following:

1. Avoid MRI of very young premenopausal patients, because here, diagnostic difficulties can be predicted to occur.
2. Be conservative with the indication to biopsy a young patient with 'MR-only' lesion. Our rationale is that if, in a premenopausal patient, a contrast-enhancing lesion has no correlate on conventional imaging and has no wash-out time course (type-III TIC), we recommend follow-up after 2–4 menstrual cycles, during the second week of her menstrual period.

Fortunately, these very young patients are not routinely subjected to breast MR; yet, they are increasingly seen owing to the increasing number of patients who are BRCA1/BRCA2 gene carriers or who, on the basis of their family history, are identified as high-risk patients.

Moreover, evidence exists that with exogenous hormone-substitution therapy, the premenopausal situation is restored (as is intended by the medication). Accordingly, in patients receiving replacement therapy, if contrast enhancement is seen that is not clearly suspicious, it is dealt with like the 'UBOs' in premenopausal patients. We ask the patients to discontinue hormone medication for at least 6 weeks and schedule a follow-up exam.

In many patients, a streak of (early) contrast enhancement is seen in the parenchyma just adjacent to the subcutaneous fat, i.e., in the most peripheral parts of the parenchymal volume. This is a normal finding – probably due to the centripetal vascular supply of the parenchyma – and should not be confused with regional or segmental enhancement (see below).

15.6.3 Breast Cancer

Histologically, biologically, prognostically, and also in terms of breast MR, breast cancers are not all alike. First, a fundamental histologic and, thus, diagnostic difference exists between DCIS and invasive breast cancers (IBCs). Among the invasive cancers, many different histologic subtypes exist, including ductal invasive cancers not otherwise specified (NOS; about 80% of invasive cancers), lobular invasive cancers (10%–15% of cancers), and rare invasive cancers, such as medullary, mucinous, or tubular cancers (5%–10% altogether).

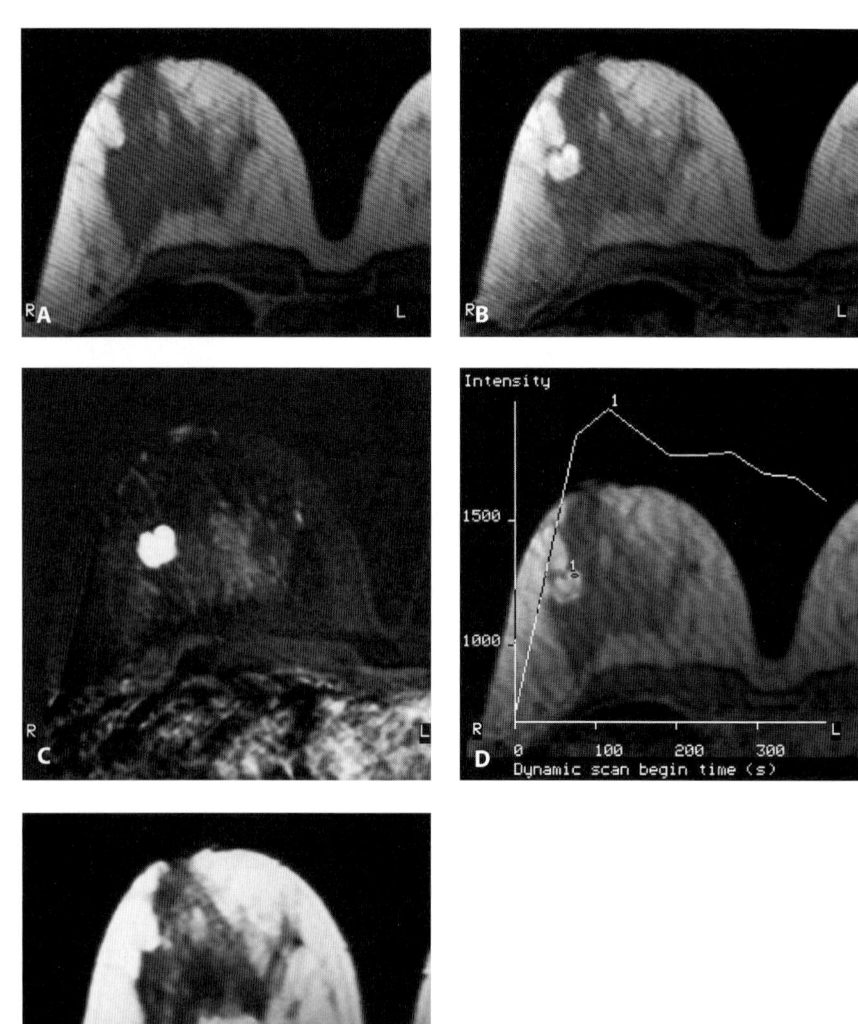

Fig. 15.2A–E. Breast MR appearance of ductal invasive breast cancer in a 52-year-old patient. **A** Precontrast, **B** early postcontrast, **C** early postcontrast subtracted, **D** time/intensity curve, **E** T2-weighted (T2-W) TSE image. There is a focal lesion with rapid and strong enhancement, lobulated shape, partly indistinct borders, homogeneous enhancement. Time course of signal intensity (SI) shows a clear wash-out phenomenon (type III). In the T2-W TSE image, the lesion is about iso- to hypointense to the remainder of the parenchyma. Although the lobulated shape and the homogeneous enhancement might suggest fibroadenoma, the wash-out time course clinches the diagnosis. Moreover, the somewhat indistinct margin and the low SI on T2-WI clearly support the diagnosis of a malignant lesion

15.6.3.1 Invasive Breast Cancer

Owing to their high neo-angiogenetic activity, IBCs induce capillary sprouting and the formation of new vessels, mostly with leaky vessel linings. Accordingly, in IBCs, an increased vessel density is associated with an increased vessel permeability. Both effects account for the rapid and strong SI increase observable on breast MR of IBCs.

In the 'typical' ductal invasive breast cancer, enhancement is usually well beyond 80% signal increase in the early postcontrast period, followed by a type-II (plateau) or type-III (wash-out) SI time course (Figs. 15.2–15.5). Concerning lesion morphology, everything that has been found useful in mammography or ultrasound also applies for breast MR; IBCs tend to appear as a focal mass with irregular morphology, indistinct margins, and an inhomogeneous internal architecture. In about 15%–20% of cases, a rim enhancement is seen – a finding that is almost pathognomonic for breast cancer. The rim corresponds to the vital tumor periphery around a more or less fibrotic or necrotic tumor center. If a dynamic imaging technique is used with good temporal resolution, it is possible to monitor the progression of enhancement, starting in the tumor periphery in a centripetal fashion (Fig. 15.3). In T2-W TSE images, IBCs tend to exhibit a low SI, isointense or even hypointense, with respect to the adjacent parenchyma (Fig. 15.2).

Lobular breast cancers tend not to form focal nodules, but to grow more or less diffusely, with gradual replacement of the preexisting breast parenchyma (Fig. 15.6). This is also the reason why lobular invasive cancers may go undetected by mammography until they become very large: they often do not form masses or nodules, and in the vast majority, they do not exhibit microcalcifications. One should be prepared to see lobular breast cancer more often on MR than one would expect based on its natural prevalence – this tumor is

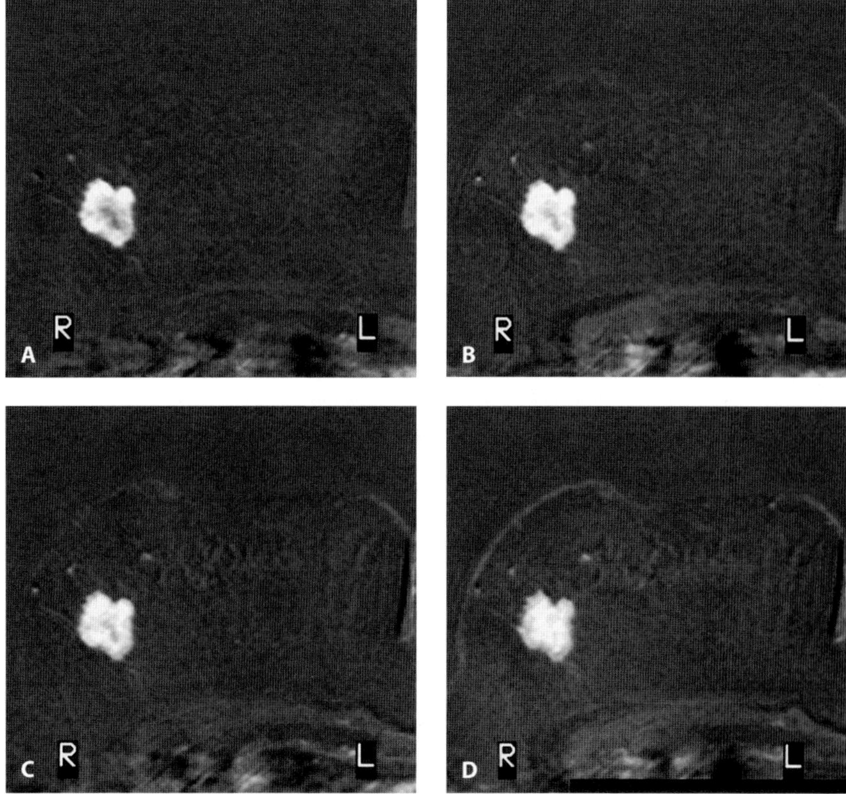

Fig. 15.3A–D. Progression of enhancement in a ductal invasive breast cancer. First, second, third, and fourth postcontrast subtracted image (at 40, 80, 120 and 160 s postbolus injection of gadopentetate dimeglumine). Note the irregular morphology and the ring enhancement, which is particularly evident in the earliest postcontrast image. Note the centripetal progression of enhancement, with filling-in of the central fibrotic tumor parts in the intermediate and late postcontrast period

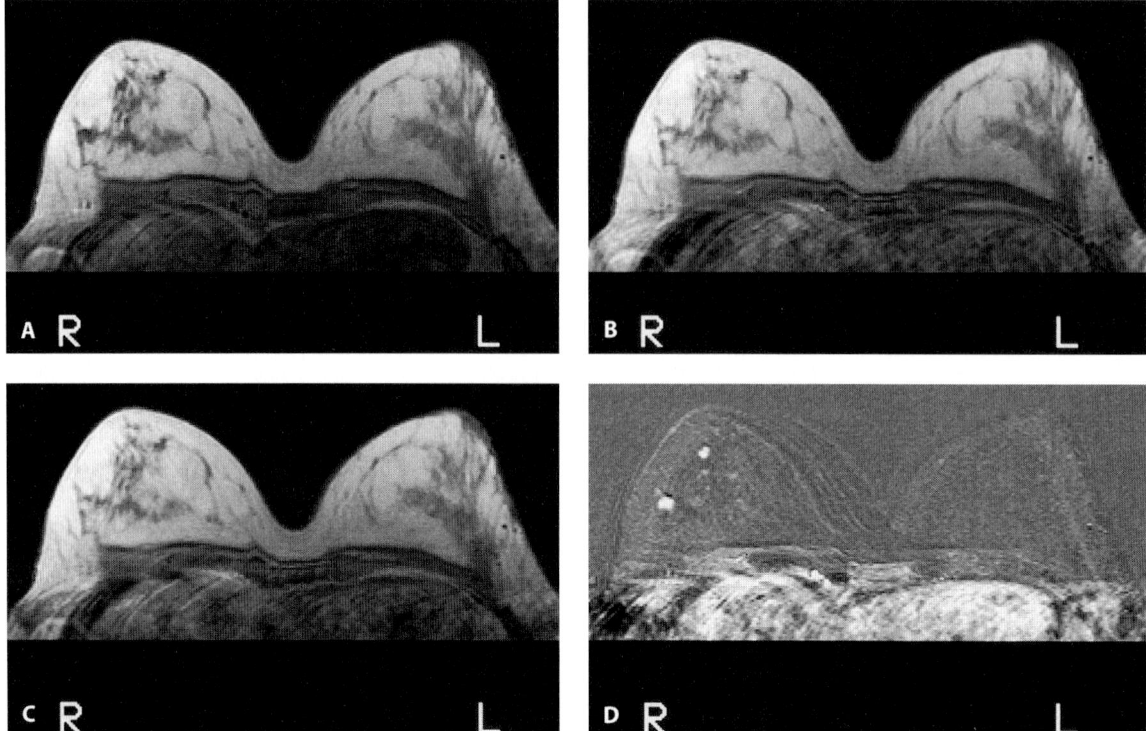

Fig. 15.4A–D. A 51-year-old woman referred for preoperative breast MR. She was scheduled for excisional biopsy of microcalcifications in her upper outer quadrant that were suspicious of breast cancer. She underwent breast MR to check whether she would be a candidate for possible breast conservation therapy. **A** Precontrast, **B** early postcontrast, **C** late postcontrast, **D** early postcontrast subtracted image. Breast MR confirms the presence of a malignant lesion in her upper outer quadrant, but detects a second tumor manifestation between both upper quadrants. Histology confirmed a multicentric invasive breast cancer, 8 mm and 6 mm in size. Mastectomy was performed

difficult to diagnose mammographically and may cause nonspecific mammographic changes, which may prompt a referral to breast MR. Accordingly, in our series of breast cancers detected by breast MR, lobular cancers make up as many as 27% of cases. In breast MR, more than 80% of lobular invasive cancers enhance rapidly and strongly – as one would expect a breast cancer to enhance. In these cases, the diagnosis is quite straightforward and simple. However, due to their particular 'Indian-path-like', diffuse growth pattern, some 20% of lobular IBCs are not particularly hypervascular. Accordingly, this fraction of lobular invasive cancers may enhance gradually – well below any 'enhancement threshold'. For the same reason (lack of hypervascularity), time course assessment tends to be of little use for a correct classification in these cases, because they usually exhibit a steady (type I) or a plateau (type II) time course. However, other diagnostic criteria, particularly morphologic features, should still allow the correct diagnosis to be reached.

Medullar IBCs, an uncommon entity with a relatively favorable prognosis, is the most important differential diagnosis of myxoid fibroadenomas. Medullary cancer is seen in younger patients (Fig. 15.7), it is a roundish, very well circumscribed tumor, with intermediate but usually heterogeneous enhancement, and high SI in T2-W TSE images. Fortunately, it is rather rare, accounting for less than 7% of all IBCs. It is important, however, to consider this diagnosis in patients with a strong family history of breast cancer (in particular patients with family members who were diagnosed with breast cancer at age 35 or younger), or patients in whom a genetic predisposition has been identified (BRCA1 or BRCA2 mutation carriers).

Inflammatory breast cancer is a clinical rather than a distinct pathologic entity. It is diagnosed in cases where an invasive breast cancer (usually of ductal origin) is associated with clinical findings of inflammation, i.e., cutaneous edema and erythema. On histopathology, there is extensive tumor lymphangiosis. The MR findings are as variable as the clinical presentation. What is visible clinically appears as dermal thickening and edema, interstitial edema (best appreciated on T2-WI), and variable cutaneous enhancement. The underlying cancer usually enhances strongly, but there are also reports of nonenhancing or very slowly enhancing inflammatory cancers. In addition, abscess formation does occur in inflammatory cancer. To conclude, in no way can MR be used to distinguish (puerperal or nonpuerperal) mastitis from inflammatory breast cancer. The only role of MR (if any) is to demonstrate the extent of the disease and to monitor the response to chemotherapy.

15.6.3.2 Ductal Carcinoma-In-Situ

Although there are reports in the current literature stating that microcalcifications can be visualized by high-resolution breast MR, for current clinical practice, there is ample evidence confirming that microcalcifications (particularly the relevant, tiny ductal calcifications) are

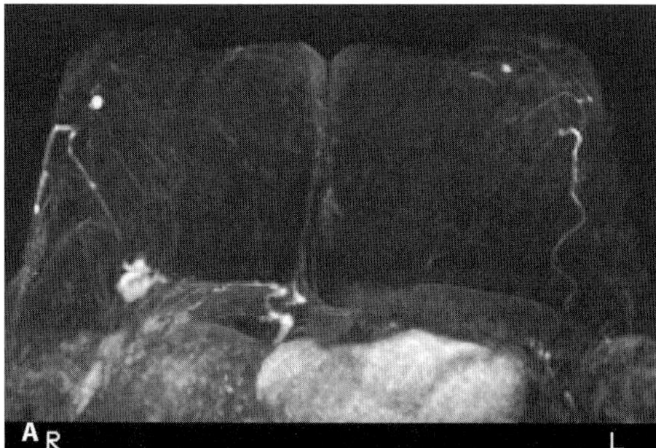

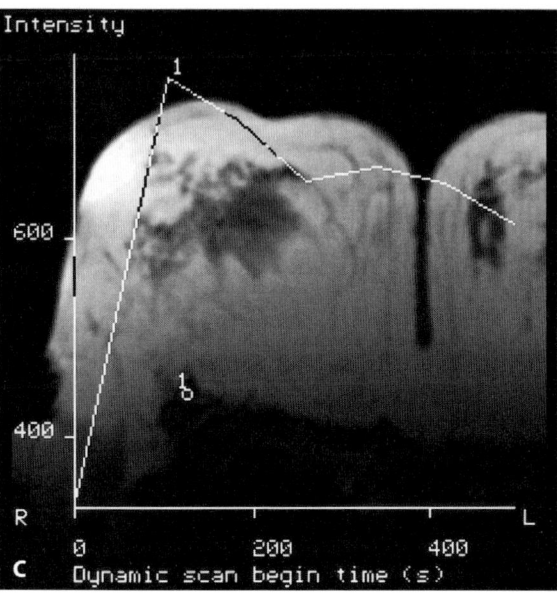

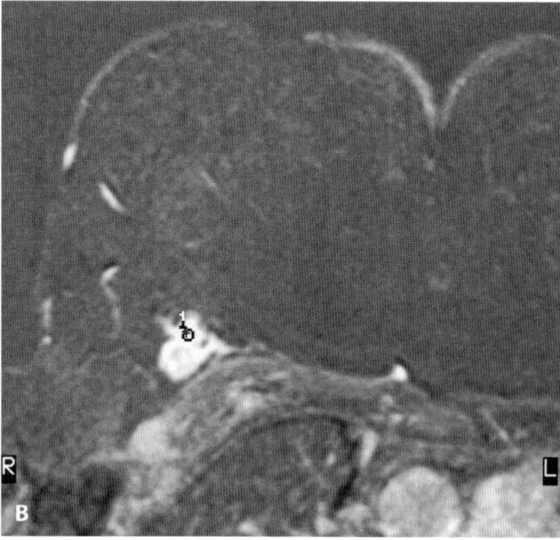

Fig. 15.5A–E. A 61-year-old woman with right axillary lymphadenopathy, unknown primary. **A** The maximum intensity projection (MIP) image of the early postcontrast subtracted images of her dynamic series reveals three lesions. In her right breast, there is an irregular lesion immediately adjacent to the chest wall and another lesion in her upper outer quadrant. In her left breast, there is a small lesion in the retro-areolar region. **B** Early postcontrast subtracted image of the prepectoral lesion, **C** corresponding time/intensity curve. **D** Dynamic series over the small lesion in the upper outer quadrant of her right breast (*upper left* precontrast; *upper right* early postcontrast; *bottom left* late postcontrast; and *bottom right* early postcontrast subtracted image). **E** Signal intensity time course of the lesion in **D**. There is a multicentric invasive breast cancer (IBC) in her right breast plus a contralateral small IBC in her left breast. With irregular morphology, rapid and strong enhancement and wash-out time course, the diagnosis is straightforward in the prepectoral lesion. The small additional foci in the same and the contralateral breast are well circumscribed, yet also here, the wash-out time course allows the correct diagnosis

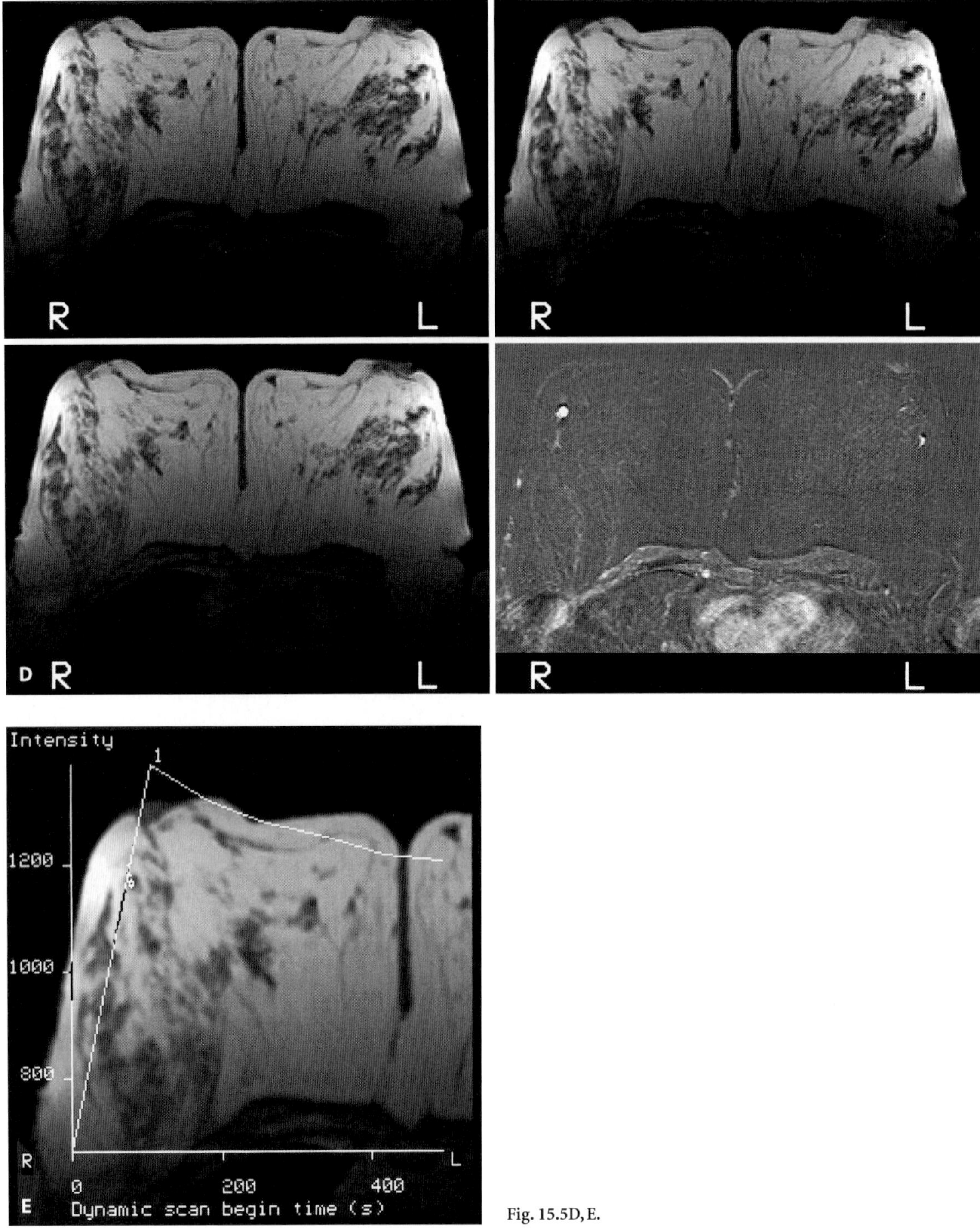
R
L
R
L
D
R
L
R
L
Intensity
1
1200
1000
800
R
L
0
200
400
E
Dynamic scan begin time (s)

Fig. 15.5D, E.

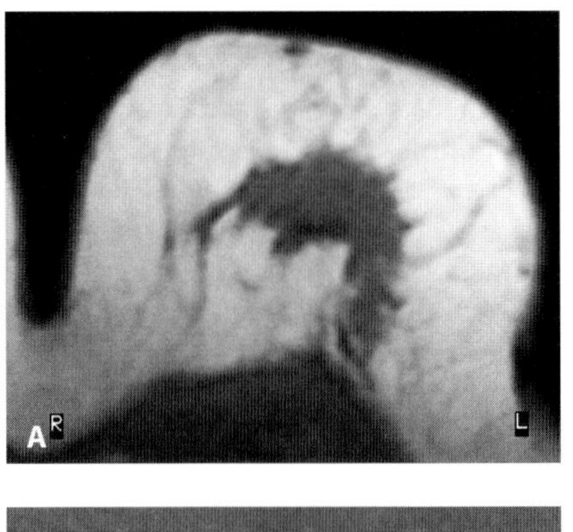

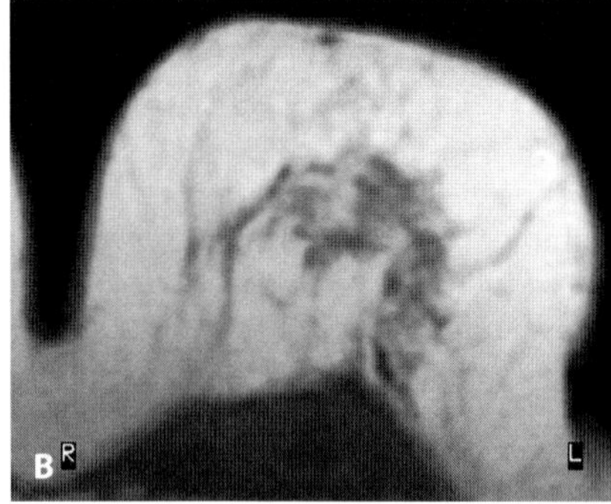

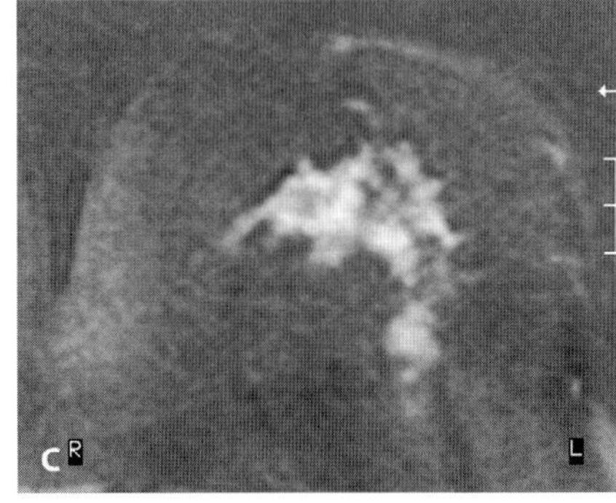

Fig. 15.6A–C. Lobular invasive cancer with slow and shallow enhancement in a 57-year-old woman. Precontrast (**A**), early postcontrast (**B**), early post-contrast subtracted images (**C**). Note that the tumor has replaced the entire residual parenchyma. On the precontrast image (**A**), there is homogeneous, low-signal-intensity tissue, no interspersed fatty tissue. In an otherwise involuted breast, this is suspicious. Note the shallow enhancement rate, not exceeding 50% in the early postcontrast period. However, the particularly irregular morphology and the very inhomogeneous enhancement do allow the correct diagnosis

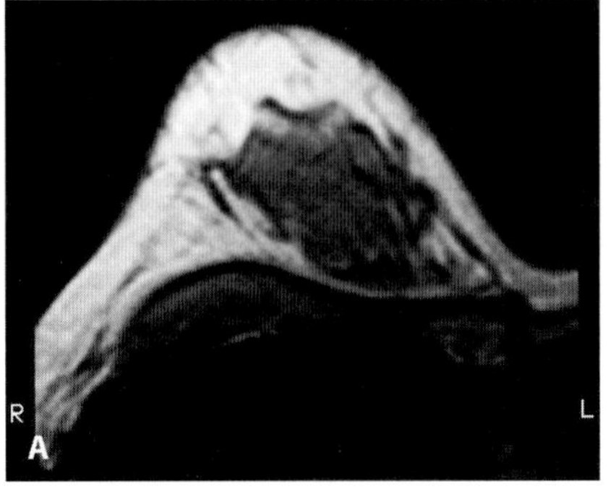

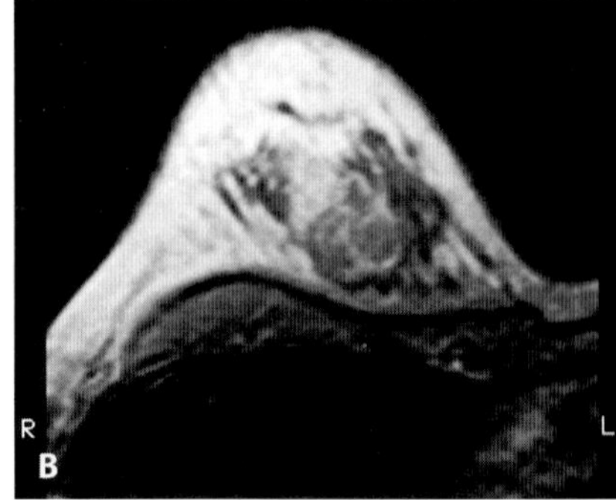

Fig. 15.7A,B. Precontrast (A) and early postcontrast (**B**) images. This is a 27-year-old woman who underwent preoperative breast MR. Note the well-circumscribed, nodular lesion in her upper quadrant. However, enhancement is inhomogeneous with peripheral rim. Excisional biopsy revealed medullary invasive cancer

not visible on MRI. One could even go beyond this and state that, as soon as a calcification is detected on an MRI, it cannot be a suspicious calcification. However, accordingly, while the in-situ cancers' propensity to form microcalcifications constitutes the basis of DCIS diagnosis in mammography, this feature cannot be exploited for MRI of DCIS. Moreover, the criteria pertinent to the diagnosis of IBC in dynamic MR may not be transferred to the diagnosis of DCIS (rather, the absence of these features may not be used to exclude DCIS). Probably due to the variable angiogenic activity of in-situ cancers, enhancement in breast MR can be anywhere between strong to moderate to even absent. Accordingly, diagnostic criteria based on contrast-enhancement kinetics are not reliable enough to exclude DCIS. Enhancement rate, degree of enhancement, and time course of SI may (but not necessarily will) be misleading. A recent study revealed that DCIS exhibits nonspecific or even delayed enhancement in about two-thirds of cases, and that in about 10% of cases, no enhancement is obtained at all – in our series, we found nonenhancing DICS less often, i.e., in 3% of all cases. So, unlike IBC, DCIS may be missed by breast MR. As a result, a recent state-of-the-art mammogram must be available when a breast MR study is read. If a mammogram shows suspicious microcalcifications, it is not possible to avoid biopsy due to a negative breast MR study. Accordingly, it is not useful to attempt a clarification of mammographically suspicious microcalcifications by an MR study. What can be done in this setting is to see whether there is multifocal or multicentric tumor growth before breast-conserving therapy is initiated (Figs. 15.4 and 15.5).

While enhancement kinetics may be misleading in DCIS, there are some morphological features that may be used to establish the diagnosis prospectively, even in cases where no specific findings suggest DCIS on mammography. In DCIS, tumor growth is confined to the distribution of a single duct or a ductal system; therefore, there are specific MR findings that are very suggestive of DCIS irrespective of the enhancement kinetics:

1. A segmental enhancement (isolated regional enhancement with triangular configuration, tip towards the mammilla, corresponding to the distribution of a ductal system) (Fig. 15.8).
2. A dendritic, branching enhancement, sometimes with arborizing configuration, corresponding to the enhancement within a single duct.
3. Any diffuse, regional enhancement around an invasive breast cancer is suggestive of an intraductal component.

DCIS may also present as a focal lesion with strong and rapid enhancement, with or without wash-out, indistinguishable from an invasive breast cancer.

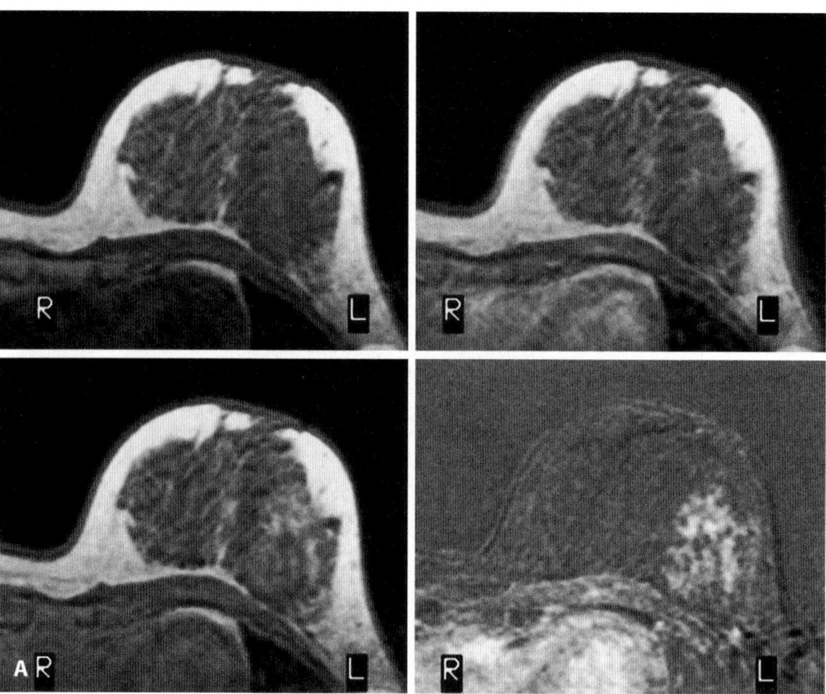

Fig. 15.8A–C. A 32-year-old woman who underwent mastectomy on her right breast 2 years previously due to invasive breast cancer. Routine follow-up breast MR was performed in this high-risk patient: no clinical or conventional imaging findings. **A** Dynamic series on her left breast (*upper left* precontrast; *upper right* early postcontrast; *bottom left* late postcontrast; and *bottom right* late postcontrast subtracted image). **B,C** Two other postcontrast subtracted sections obtained cephalad from the position of the section in **A** show that the enhancement occupies the entire lower outer quadrant. Note the extremely dense, homogeneous parenchyma in this very young patient. Note the slowly progressive enhancement in her lower outer quadrant. Enhancement rate is 30% in the early postcontrast period. However, the enhancement has an isolated regional, segmental configuration (tip towards mammilla). This is suspicious of a large ductal carcinoma in situ (DCIS), which was confirmed by excisional biopsy

Fig. 15.8B, C.

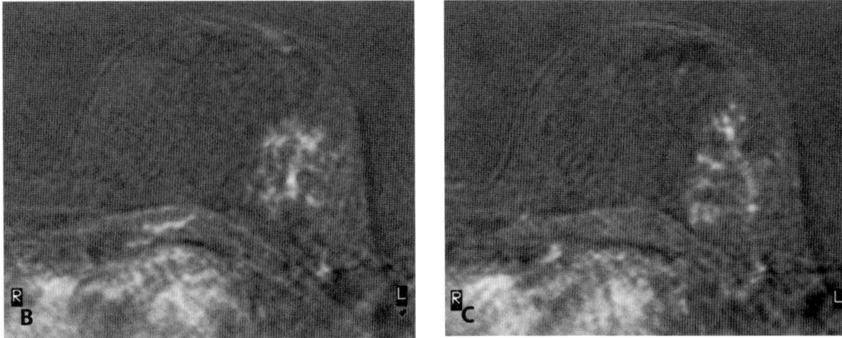

15.6.4
Cystosarcoma Phyllodes: Phyllodes Tumors

This is a rare fibroepithelial tumor that can have benign and malignant variants. The benign variant can behave in a semimalignant pattern owing to a local recurrence rate of up to 20%; the malignant version metastasizes as IBCs. Clinically, these are rapidly growing tumors, usually of considerable size at the time of presentation. Histologically, phyllodes tumors are hypercellular, hypervascular, with internal cystic (or necrotic) areas and with (macroscopically) expansive growth pattern. On MR, these tumors are well circumscribed, exhibit a very rapid and strong enhancement, and show (sometimes huge) internal cysts or central tumor necrosis (Fig. 15.9).

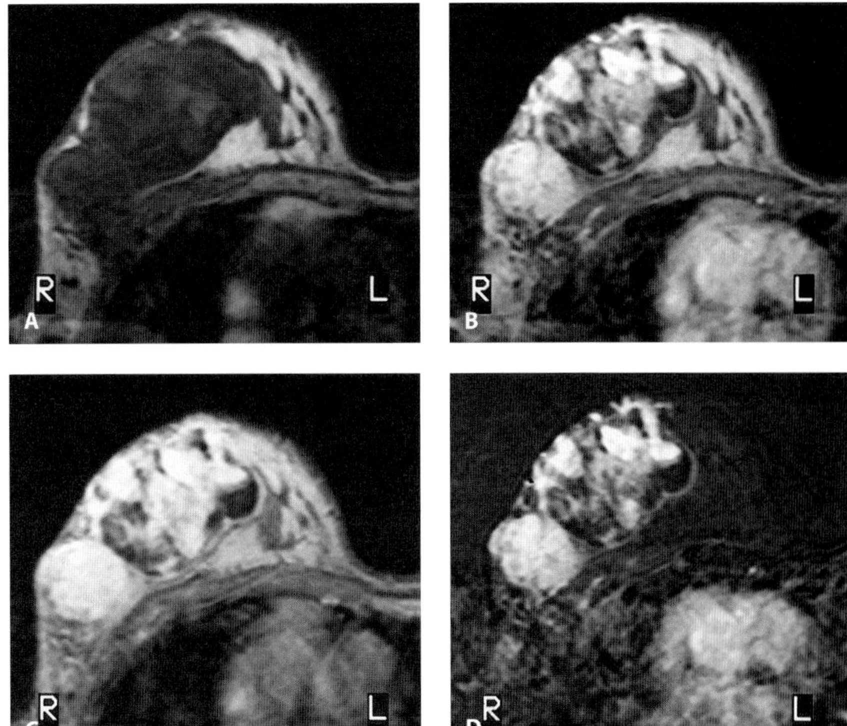

Fig. 15.9A–D. Malignant cystosarcoma phyllodes. A huge tumor affects virtually the entire right breast and bulges the breast contours. **A** Precontrast, **B** early postcontrast, **C** late postcontrast, **D** early postcontrast subtracted image. Note the strong, rapid, inhomogeneous enhancement with multifocal, nonenhancing, central necrosis

While it is already difficult to distinguish benign and malignant cystosarcoma histologically, breast MR cannot be expected to deliver this information. Moreover, if no internal cysts or necrosis have evolved yet in a small cystosarcoma, it cannot be distinguished from a fibroadenoma on the basis of MR.

15.6.5 Fibroadenoma

Fibroadenomas represent a frequent finding in breast MR – much more frequent than is detected on mammograms. Fibroadenomas constitute one of the major differential diagnostic problems for MRI, as they do in mammography or breast ultrasound. There are a variety of diagnostic criteria to distinguish fibroadenoma from breast cancer; however, none of them are 100% specific. Accordingly, it is up to the practical experience of each radiologist, to his or her degree of diagnostic confidence in the individual case, and to his or her personal preferences in terms of aggressiveness or conservativeness whether or not, eventually, a biopsy is recommended.

In general, the MR appearance of fibroadenomas varies strongly with the degree of fibrosis; there are myxoid fibroadenomas with a large extracellular/interstitial fraction filled with a gelatinous matrix. With increasing age, regressive changes take place, the interstitial matrix undergoes fibrosis, resulting in a sclerotic fibroadenoma.

Typically, a myxoid fibroadenoma is a well-circumscribed lesion with rapid and strong, 'carcinoma-type' enhancement and type-I time course of SI (steady increase or bowing of TIC, Fig. 15.10). Ideally, it has low-SI internal septations (often best seen on T2-WI) (Fig. 15.11). However, with the limited spatial resolution available with double-breast imaging techniques, these are only visible in about 15% of cases; if seen, they are almost pathognomonic for fibroadenoma. Otherwise, fibroadenomas show a homogeneous internal enhancement. The enhancement starts in the center of the lesion and progresses from there to the tumor periphery, such that the lesion seems to grow from one dynamic scan to the other ('blooming fibroadenoma', Fig. 15.10). In T2-W TSE images, the lesion has a hyperintense signal with respect to parenchyma.

In sclerotic fibroadenomas, the enhancement is reduced or even absent, and the SI in T2-WI is low. As a consequence, internal septations are hardly visible. If enhancement is present, the time course of SI corresponds to a type-I shape. Enhancement may be somewhat heterogeneous due to regressive clumps of calcifications and the slow progression of enhancement.

According to our experience, the diagnosis can be established with sufficient confidence if all criteria support the diagnosis of either myxoid or sclerotic fibroadenoma.

An important differential diagnosis of myxoid fibroadenoma, however, is medullary breast cancer, and breast MR may not be useful to distinguish these two entities further. The same holds true for the differentiation of fibroadenoma and a (small) phyllodes tumor.

15.6.6 So-called 'Mastopathic' or Fibrocystic Changes

In breast MRI, so-called 'mastopathic' or fibrocystic changes appear as diffuse, bilateral, patchy, and heterogeneous enhancement. The histopathological correlate of the small enhancing dots has been shown to be focal adenosis, i.e., proliferation of the glandular epithelium. It is important to realize that there is no correlation of the presence of enhancement with the presence or absence of atypias. Accordingly, it is not possible to distinguish ductal hyperplasia from atypical ductal hyperplasia (ADH) by breast MRI.

The heterogeneity of enhancement that is seen in patients with fibrocystic disease is due to the presence of areas with predominant epithelial proliferation next to areas with predominant regressive changes (fibrosis) and associated cysts. The enhancement is usually steady (type-I curve) but may become rapid and strong. Often, there are small dots of rapidly enhancing foci interspersed within the diffusely enhancing parenchymal tissue, owing to small fibroadenomas or nodes of focal adenosis. Hence, it may be difficult, if not impossible, to distinguish fibrocystic changes from 'serious pathology', such as DCIS or invasive cancer. In turn, small foci of cancer or DCIS may be masked by enhancement secondary to focal adenosis. The following hints have emerged from clinical practice and may prove helpful.

First, if diffuse spotty enhancement is present, it is not useful to attempt quantification or time-course analysis of each and every enhancing spot. However, note that as opposed to DCIS, mastopathic changes are diffuse, usually more or less symmetric on both breasts;

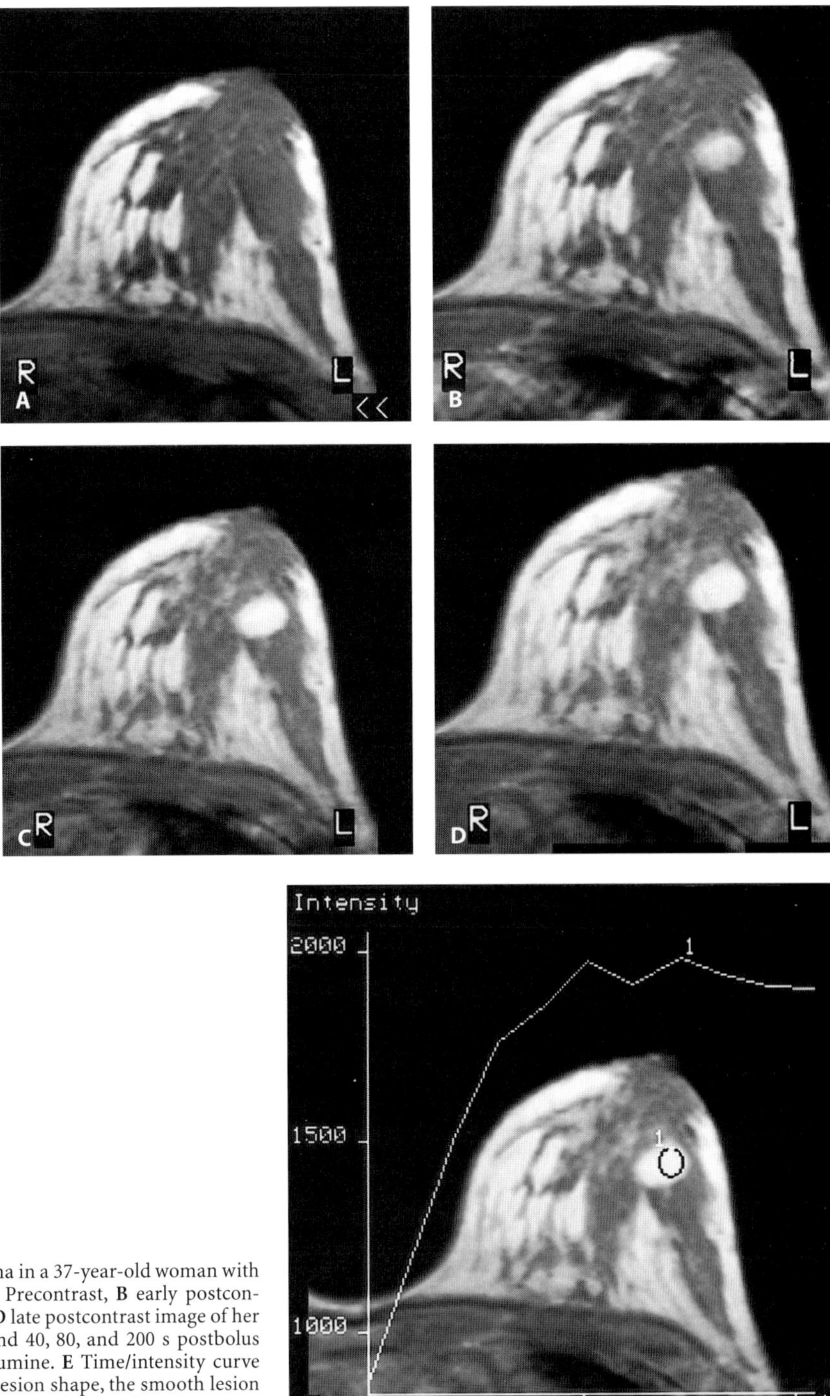

Fig. 15.10A–E. Myxoid fibroadenoma in a 37-year-old woman with typical breast MR presentation. **A** Precontrast, **B** early postcontrast, **C** intermediate postcontrast, **D** late postcontrast image of her dynamic series, obtained before and 40, 80, and 200 s postbolus injection of gadopentetate dimeglumine. **E** Time/intensity curve of the same lesion. Note the ovoid lesion shape, the smooth lesion borders, the homogeneous enhancement, the centrifugal progression of enhancement ('blooming' fibroadenoma; it seems to grow between the dynamic scans). Note the rapid and strong enhancement, followed by a type-I time course of signal intensity

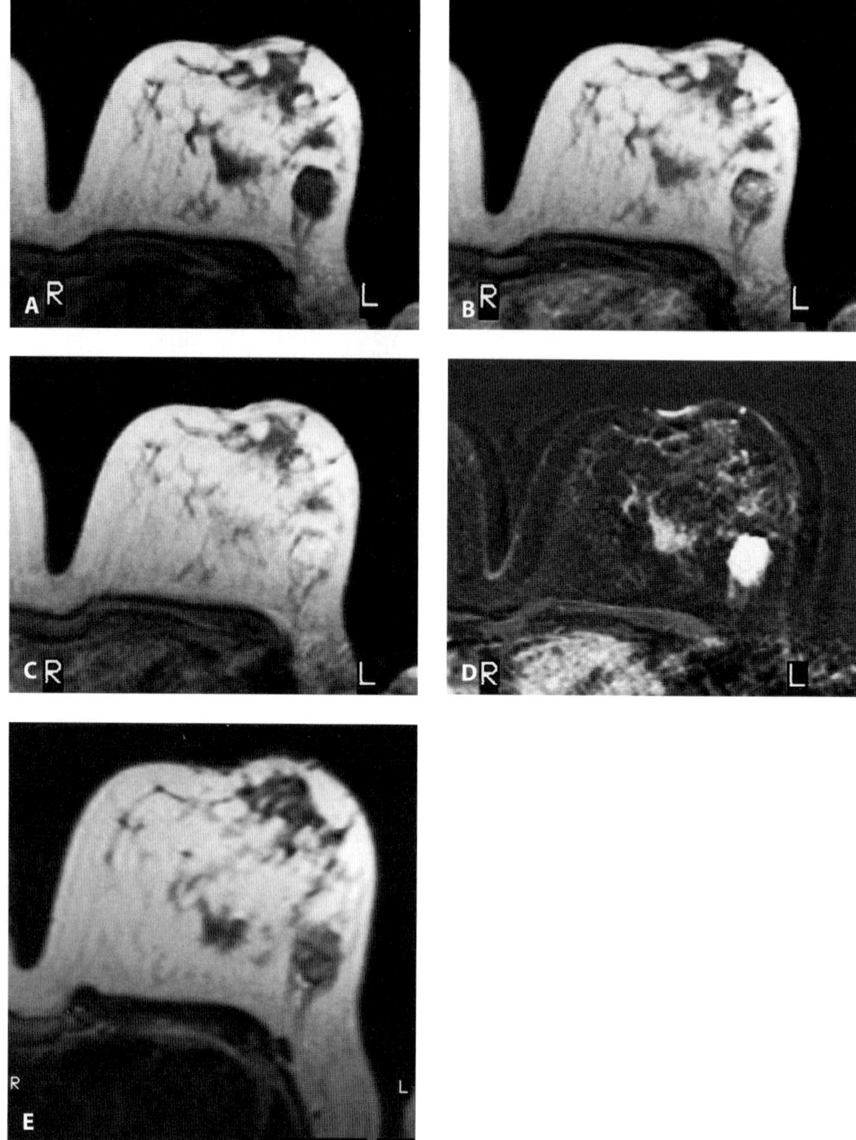

Fig. 15.11A–E. Myxoid fibroadenoma in a 39-year-old woman with chronic renal failure. **A** Precontrast, **B** early postcontrast, **C** late postcontrast, **D** early postcontrast subtracted image of her dynamic series. **E** T2-weighted turbo spin-echo (TSE) image of the lesion. Note the somewhat inhomogeneous, rapid and strong enhancement. However, there is a type-I time course, the lesion's signal on the T2-weighted TSE image is increased, and there are internal low signal-intensity septations visible on the T2-weighted TSE image. The diagnosis '-fibroadenoma' was confirmed by sonographic follow-up over the past 4 years

they are not confined to the territory of a distinct duct. Symmetry is the clue to the diagnosis. As opposed to invasive cancer, mastopathic changes tend to exhibit a gradual and steady SI increase. On follow-ups, mastopathic changes, in fact, change their appearance and location, reflecting the cyclical rebuilding of the breast parenchyma. Last, always remember that bilateral, diffuse, multifocal breast cancer is rare; fibrocystic disease is not. So, if in doubt, follow-up examinations should be performed.

Concerning the clinical use of the term 'mastopathic' or 'fibrocystic disease', it is important to understand that according to biopsy results, what is histologically called a 'mastopathy' or a 'fibrocystic disease' seems to be so ubiquitous that the terms easily qualify as a misnomer. Similarly, in imaging studies, it is a frequent habit that almost anything that is apparently benign but does not correspond to a 'completely negative study' is generously (and somewhat thoughtlessly) categorized as 'mastopathic' or 'fibrocystic'. However, it should be well understood that contrast enhancement – to a variable degree – may be one facet of normal, healthy breast parenchyma and is by no means necessarily a sign of ('mastopathic' or 'fibrocystic') disease. The diagnosis of 'mastopathic changes' should be avoided or reserved for cases where cysts and diffuse, spotty enhancement suggest a true imbalance of tissue formation and regeneration.

15.6.7 Guidelines for Diagnostic Problem Cases

It is important to note that, of course, not every breast cancer behaves as expected in every aspect. The following guidelines can be used to help make decisions in cases where the diagnostic criteria point in different directions.

1. A wash-out (type III) time course overrides any other diagnostic criterion and should prompt biopsy. Make sure that no 'fake wash-out' is produced by motion; make sure that the 'lesion' is not a vessel.
2. An irregular morphology (stellate lesion shape) overrides any other diagnostic criterion, as long as there is at least intermediate enhancement; in our setting, 30%–40% early postcontrast. Make sure that the lesion is not, in fact, an island of residual normal parenchyma – with normal enhancement – that is entirely surrounded by fatty tissue, producing a 'pseudo-mass' on subtracted images.
3. Rim enhancement overrides any other diagnostic criterion and should prompt biopsy. Make sure that the 'rim' is within the lesion. A 'fake rim enhancement' may be seen on subtracted images of complicated cysts; however, on the nonsubtracted images, it is readily obvious that the 'rim', in fact, corresponds to reactive enhancement in the parenchyma adjacent to the cyst.
4. In a lesion with well-circumscribed morphology and rapid enhancement, a low SI on the T2-W TSE image should increase suspicion.
5. If no enhancement is seen in the location of a presumed lesion, the presence of IBC can be definitely excluded, because non-enhancing IBCs are too rare to be mentioned as a reasonable differential diagnosis. However, make sure that contrast material reached the arterial circulation in a timely manner by checking the enhancement of parenchymal vessels. Please note that the absence of enhancement does not exclude the presence of DCIS.
6. An isolated regional segmental enhancement or a linear-branching enhancement overrides any other diagnostic criteria; a biopsy to rule out DCIS is indicated. However, make sure by checking the nonsubtracted images that no subtraction artifacts at fat/parenchyma interfaces produce a 'fake' linear enhancement.

Further Reading

Fischer U (1999) Lehratlas der MR-Mammographie. Thieme Verlag. ISBN 3131185813
Fischer U, Kopka L, Grabbe E (1999) Breast carcinoma: effect of pre-operative contrast-enhanced MR imaging on the therapeutic approach. Radiology 213:881–888
Ikeda D, et al. ACR-Imaging and Reporting System-Magnetic Resonance Imaging™: Illustrated BI-RADS®-MRI™. American College of Radiology, in press
Kuhl CK (2000) MRI of breast tumors. European Radiology 10(1):46–58
Kuhl CK, Schild HH (2000) Dynamic image interpretation of MRI of the breast. J Magn Reson Imaging 12:965–974
Orel SG (2001) MR imaging of the breast. Magn Reson Imaging Clin N Am 9:273–288

Magnetic Resonance Imaging of Pediatric Patients

16

B. Kammer, T. Pfluger, M. I. Schubert, C. M. Keser, K. Schneider

Contents

16.1 General Considerations and Remarks for MR Imaging of Pediatric Patients

The lack of radiation exposure, the possibility of multiplanar imaging, and the wide range of tissue contrast has made magnetic resonance (MR) imaging an important tool in the evaluation of pediatric diseases. In general, ultrasonography, conventional radiography, and fluoroscopy remain the primary imaging modalities for the majority of clinical requests. If there is a need for further evaluation and the diagnostic information from both computed tomography (CT) and MR are comparable, then MR should be the next step. Common indications for MR imaging in children include developmental abnormalities of the brain and spine, neurodegenerative disorders, tumors, infections, and inflammations.

16.1.1 Patient Preparation, Sedation, and Monitoring

It is essential for any successful pediatric examination to achieve sufficient immobilization of the frequently uncooperative pediatric patients during the long acquisition times. In the first 3 months of life, an examination after feeding and immobilization by wrapping in blankets may be sufficient. The age group between 3 months and 5 years requires sedation or even general anesthesia, thus necessitating the assistance of anesthesiologists. By the age of 5 years, a simple explanation of the examination and the attendance of the parents or nursing staff often enables a successful examination. If administration of intravenous paramagnetic contrast is necessary or planned, the referring colleagues should place a peripheral line in advance to avoid excitement immediately before the examination.

Numerous protocols for sedation and general anesthesia have been developed in different hospitals; the choice of the protocol strongly depends on the radiologists' training and the availability of anesthesiologists. In our institution, the common practice includes monitored conscious sedation, deep sedation, or general anesthesia. For any sedation procedure, children should not eat or drink anything for at least 4 h prior to the examination. Monitoring of vital functions is fundamental and easily achieved by the use of a pulse oximeter. A nurse remains in the procedure area for the imaging time and periodically records vital signs (oxygenation, ventilation, circulation, and temperature). When conscious sedation is the method selected, the radiologist applying sedative drugs should be familiar with those agents, aware of their possible complications, and must have some training in pediatric advanced life support. Drugs for conscious sedation include: (1) chlorprothixene 1–2 mg/kg orally, (2) chloral hydrate 50–100 mg/kg rectally, or (3) diazepam 0.2–0.5 mg/kg rectally. Alternatively, children can receive oral midazolam 0.2–0.5 mg/kg in a specially flavored preparation. Sufficient time should be allowed for drug administration before the onset of the procedure (0.5–1.5 h). For optimal sedation, it is often helpful to move the child and parents into a dark, quiet room after drug administration and wait until the patient is asleep. Monitored conscious sedation is most appropriate for healthy children and short diagnostic examinations. If deeper levels of sedation are necessary, a pediatric anesthesiologist must be in charge of the intravenous drug administration and monitoring. One intravenous regimen in our institution includes midazolam 0.1–0.15 mg/kg supplemented with small doses of thiopental, if necessary. Another efficient sedation method for children is the titrated intravenous application of propofol 0.5–1.5 mg/kg until the child is asleep. Sedation is maintained by a continuous infusion of propofol 3–5 mg/kg/h during imaging time. After the procedure is completed, all sedated children should be transferred to a recovery room close to the examination area. Monitoring should be continued until the patient is alert and able to drink. For many examinations, general anesthesia with tracheal intubation is the best choice.

16.1.2 Contrast Media

Administration of paramagnetic contrast is necessary in many clinical requests. For children, 0.2 ml/kg of gadolinium diethylene triaminopentaacetic acid (Gd-DTPA) for intravenous application is used. Oral contrast media and organ-specific contrast agents are not approved in children.

16.2 Pediatric Brain Imaging

16.2.1 Coils and Patient Positioning

The standard head coil is used for examination of the pediatric brain. In very small infants, the knee coil (an extremity coil, which functions as both a receiving and transmitting coil) may be used. Optimal positioning in the center of the coil and immobilization with vacuum beds, sponges, sand bags, and blankets are mandatory for the patients.

16.2.2 Sequence Protocol

Sequences used in pediatric brain imaging are spin-echo (SE), inversion recovery (IR), and gradient-echo (GRE) sequences (Table 16.1). SE sequences are commonly used because of their accurate anatomical depiction of brain tissue and representation of tissue characteristics based on T1- and T2-relaxation. However, to maximize T2 differences between the normal unmyelinated brain tissue and abnormal tissue in the first 18 months of life, it is necessary to use longer repetition times (TR). A repetition time of 3000 ms and echo times (TE) for the first and second echo of 40/120 ms should be chosen in children from birth to 3 months of age. TR of 3000 ms and TE of 30/100 ms are recommended in children from 3 to 6 months. For children older than 6 months, TR of 2500 ms and TE of 30/100 ms should be used.

IR sequences are most commonly used for one of two reasons: to improve T1 contrast or to eliminate the signal from one tissue. IR sequences significantly improve T1-weighted (T1-W) contrast by doubling the distance that spins have to recover. Thus, these sequences are ideal to evaluate myelination and subtle lesions such as cortical dysplasia. Fluid attenuated IR (FLAIR) sequences eliminate the signal from cerebrospinal fluid (CSF) by using a TI around 2000 ms and allow images of the brain with no fluid signal for heavily T2-W. Therefore, a T2-W TSE sequence in combination with a FLAIR sequence can be used alternatively to a multi-echo turbo spin-echo (TSE) sequence.

Three-dimensional (3D) GRE, especially magnetization prepared rapid acquisition GRE (MP-RAGE), can also be used to obtain T1-W images with excellent gray/white matter differentiation. This technique also has the ability to acquire very thin contiguous images and can be reformated in any plane. The main drawback of GRE sequences is that they are more sensitive to susceptibility artifacts. These sequences are recommended for the evaluation of complex malformations, tumors, and subtle lesions.

For studies of the intracranial vasculature, 3D time-of-flight (TOF), multislice 2D phase contrast (PC), 2D TOF or contrast-enhanced 3D-GRE (FISP 3D) sequences should also be performed. In addition to the transverse plane, a sagittal plane is mandatory for the evaluation of the corpus callosum, midline structural development, and tumors. In elucidation of schizencephaly, holoprosencephaly, septo-optic dysplasia, and periventricular leukomalacia, coronal planes are helpful. Furthermore, in patients with seizures, evaluation of the hippocampus in the coronal plane in thin slices is

Table 16.1. Sequence protocol recommendations for children older than 18 months

Sequence	WI	Plane	No. of slices	TR (ms)	TE (ms)	Flip angle	TI (ms)	Echo train length	Slice thickness (mm)	Matrix	FOV	recFOV (%)	Bandwidth (Hz)	No. of acq.	Acq. time (min:s)
TSE	T2	tra	19	3579	96	180		7	6	226×512	230	87.5	65	1	3:01
FLAIR	T2	tra	15	5000	105	180	1755	7	6	168×512	230	87.5	130	1	4:55
SE	T1	tra	19	570	14	70			6	224×512	230	87.5	89	2	4:19
3D-GRE	T1	sag/cor	128	11.6	4.9	12			1.25	200×256	230	100	130	1	5:59
IR	T1	tra/cor	25	9975	60	180	223	11	2	220×256	230	87.5	130	1	3:29

Abbreviations: *WI* weighting of images, *TR* repetition time (ms), *TE* echo time (ms), *TI* inversion time (ms), *Matrix* phase × frequency matrix, *recFOV* rectangular field of view (%), *acq.* acquisition(s)

necessary. Another important thing to keep in mind is that the examination must be performed within the time frame of either allowable sedation or patience of the little patients. The order of sequences should be chosen so that the essential information is acquired first.

16.2.3 Common Findings in Pediatric Brain Imaging

16.2.3.1 Developmental Abnormalities

The development of the brain is a complex process beginning with the closure of the neural tube during the fourth week of gestation. Developmental abnormalities can be classified into two main types. The first category consists of disorders of organogenesis in which genetic defects or any ischemic, metabolic, toxic, or infectious insult to the developing brain can cause malformation. These malformations result from abnormal neuronal and glial proliferation and from anomalies of neuronal migration and/or cortical organization. They may be supra- and/or infratentorial and/or may involve gray and white matter. When dealing with these kinds of abnormalities, the examiner should keep in mind that, as soon as one anomaly is found, expanded scrutiny of the whole brain for further anomalies is required. The second category of congenital brain abnormalities is disorders of histogenesis, which result from abnormal cell differentiation with a relatively normal brain appearance. The neurocutaneous abnormalities (phakomatosis) fall into this group.

16.2.3.1.1 Anomalies of Organogenesis

■ **Anomalies of the Corpus Callosum.** Formation of the corpus callosum occurs during weeks 8 to 20 of gestational age. The corpus callosum is composed of four sections: the rostrum, the genu, the body, and the splenium. The corpus callosum forms anteriorly from the genu, progressing posteriorly through the body to the splenium. The rostrum (anterior) forms last. The normal corpus callosum appears thin at birth and thickens as myelination of its fibers occurs, a process that develops from posterior to anterior. Any insult occurring during formation always affects the posterior aspect of the callosum and the rostrum, which results in partial agenesis. If insult occurs very early, complete agenesis may be the result. Sagittal images clearly show the exact extent of callosal dysgenesis. Loss of supporting function of the corpus callosum leads to a high riding third ventricle, occasionally extending between the interhemispheric fissure to form an interhemispheric cyst. Axons usually crossing the interhemispheric fissure within the corpus instead extend medially to the medial walls of the lateral ventricles, parallel to the interhemispheric fissure. These so-called bundles of Probst invaginate the medial borders of the lateral ventricles to give them a crescent shape in the coronal plane. The anterior commissure is usually present, whereas the hippocampal commissure is usually absent or hypoplastic. A further consequence of an absent corpus callosum is an everted cingulate gyrus and an absent cingulate sulcus, as normal inversion of the cingulate gyrus and consecutive formation of the cingulate sulcus do not take place. As a result, the mesial hemispheric sulci course uninterrupted in a radial manner into the third ventricle. The shape and the size of the normal ventricular system, especially posteriorly, are maintained by the presence of an intact corpus callosum. When the genu is absent, the frontal horns are prominent and are laterally convex instead of concave. In case of an absent body, the bodies of the lateral ventricles are straight and parallel. In the absence of the splenium, the trigones and the occipital horns dilate more and may be strikingly distended, a condition referred to as colpocephaly. Associated anomalies are Arnold-Chiari II, neuronal migration disorders, Dandy-Walker complex, and interhemispheric lipoma. Most patients have mental retardation, seizures or a large head; only a small proportion remains asymptomatic (see Chapter 4, Fig. 4.7).

■ **Encephaloceles.** Encephaloceles may be occipital, frontoethmoidal, and, rarely, parietal or sphenoidal. This condition is not a result of brain maldevelopment, but rather a calvarial defect, which allows extracranial herniation of the brain and the meninges (see Chapter 4, Fig. 4.2).

■ **Gray Matter Heterotopia.** An insult to the germinal matrix during neuronal migration can cause migrational arrest, resulting in heterotopic gray matter (normal gray matter in an abnormal location other than the cortex). Heterotopia can be divided into subependymal, focal subcortical, and band heterotopia (double cortex). Subependymal heterotopia are usually seen along the lateral ventricles, either subependymal or within the periventricular white matter (Fig. 16.1). Because they represent foci of normal gray matter, they will be isointense with gray matter on all sequences and will not enhance with contrast. The major differential diagnostic consideration is tuberous sclerosis; however, in the latter condition the subependymal hamartomas are typically isointense with white matter rather than gray matter. Focal subcortical heterotopia appear as multinodular or swirling, curvilinear gray matter masses, and the overlying cortex is thin with shallow sulci (see Chapter 4, Fig. 4.8). Band heterotopia are uncommon and present as a band of gray matter between the cortex and the periventricular white matter. Patients with heterotopic gray matter usually have seizures.

■ **Lissencephaly and Pachygyria.** In these conditions, the neuronal migration is subcortically stopped, involving a large area of the brain. In lissencephaly (agyria), the brain shows a smooth surface with no sulcations and the so-called 'figure-of-eight' brain configuration with shallow sylvian fissures. In pachygyria, there are some cortical sulci present (Fig. 16.2). In both conditions, imaging reveals thickened gray matter and enlargement of the ventricular trigones and occipital horns. The brainstem often appears hypoplastic. The cerebellum is only rarely involved. Clinically, patients present with hypotonia at birth and develop spasticity, seizures, and mental retardation.

■ **Cortical Dysplasia and Polymicrogyria.** Cortical dysplasia and polymicrogyria are two different subtypes of cerebral cortical dysgenesis, which is defined as a heterogeneous disorder of cortical development and organization commonly associated with seizures. Both disorders can be exactly differentiated by histology, but on MR imaging, they may be indistinguishable from each other and may be overt or subtle. In more obvious

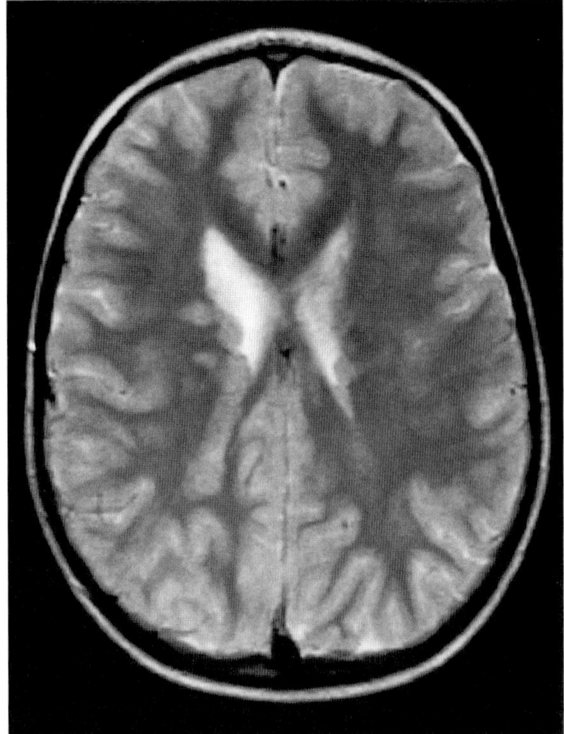

Fig. 16.1. Gray matter heterotopia. Transverse T2-WI shows multiple nodular gray matter heterotopia along the borders of the lateral ventricles

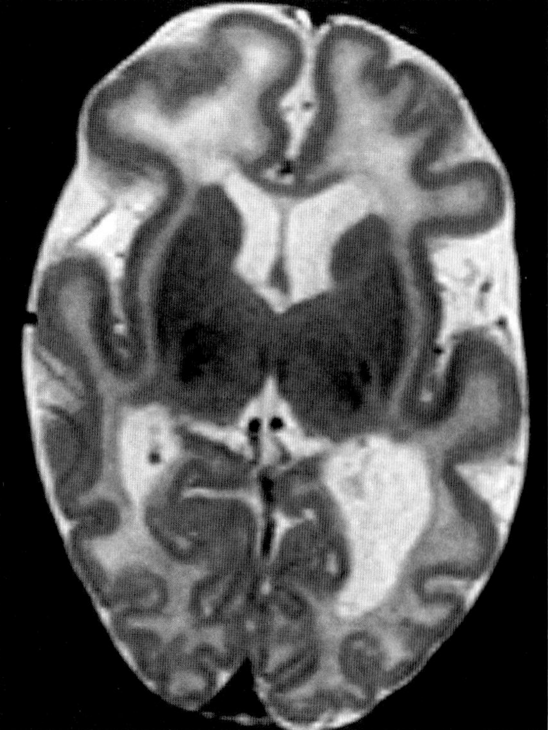

Fig. 16.2. Pachygyria. Transverse T2-WI shows some cortical sulci, thickened cortex, and widened sylvian fissures

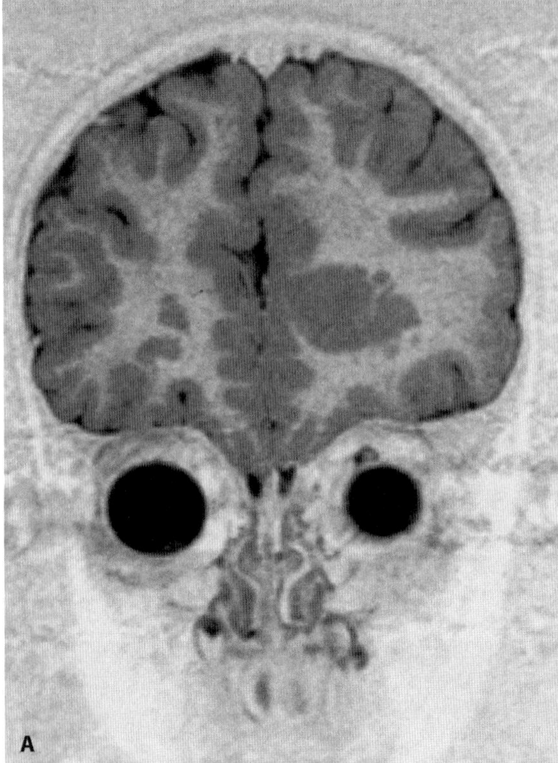

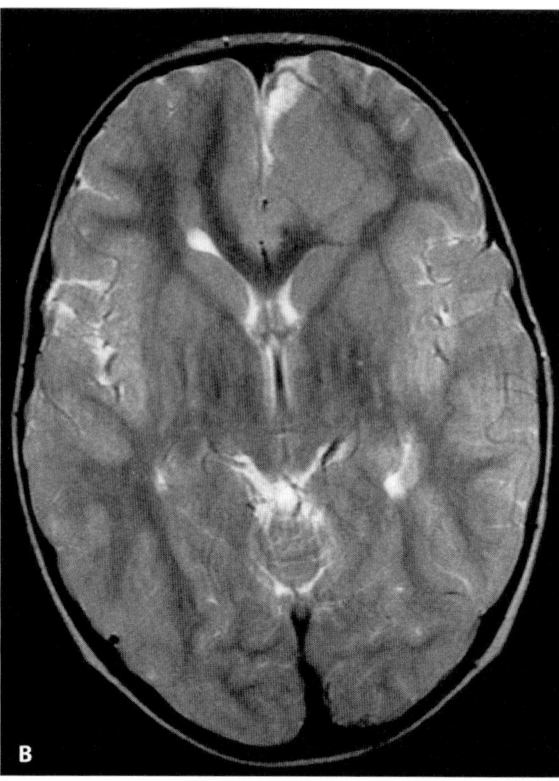

Fig. 16.3A, B. Cortical dysplasia. Coronal inversion recovery image (**A**) and transverse T2-WI (**B**) show thickened gray matter in the left frontal lobe

cases, a thickened, poorly sulcated band of cortex may be recognized (Fig. 16.3), often mimicking pachygyria. In more subtle cases, IR sequences with 2 mm slice thickness or volume 3D gradient-echo acquisitions with thin partition size (1.5 mm or less) and evaluation in three planes are more revealing. Small or large portions of the hemispheres can be involved, with the posterior aspect of the sylvian fissure being the most common location. Dysplastic cortex is isointense to normal cortex, but in 20%–25% of the patients, MRI shows an abnormally high signal intensity of the underlying white matter on T2-W sequences, probably reflecting gliosis. Anomalous draining veins can help differentiate this condition from pachygyria. Cortical dysplasia is a common manifestation of congenital cytomegalovirus (CMV) infection and is clinically less severe than agyria or pachygyria. In addition to seizures, patients present with motor dysfunction, and some exhibit developmental delay.

■ **Holoprosencephaly.** Holoprosencephalies are a group of disorders with a failure of diverticulation and cleavage of the prosencephalon. Facial dysmorphism, such as hypotelorism and midline facial clefts, is seen in severe forms. Holoprosencephaly is divided into three subgroups: alobar, semilobar, and lobar holoprosencephaly.

The alobar form is the severest type and presents with an anteriorly located pancake of brain with fused thalami and a huge monoventricle leading into a large dorsal cyst. No septum pellucidum, falx cerebri, or interhemispheric fissure can be delineated. These patients are rarely imaged, as they are stillborn or have a very short life span.

The semilobar form (Fig. 16.4) presents with underdeveloped and fused frontal regions of the brain and a monoventricle, which shows rudimentary occipital and temporal horns and an absence of the septum pellucidum. A small third ventricle can be recognized because

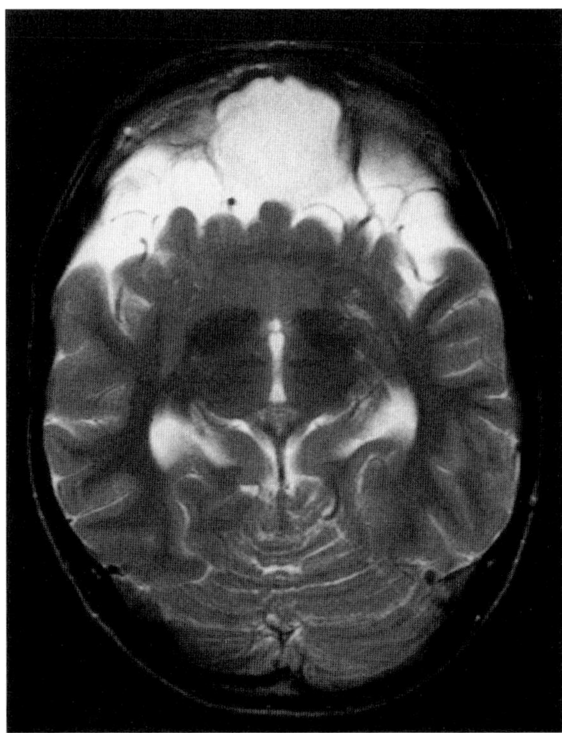

Fig. 16.4. Semilobar holoprosencephaly. Transverse T2-WI shows fused frontal lobes with abnormal gyral configuration

the thalami are partially separated. The falx cerebri and the interhemispheric fissure are usually partially formed posteriorly. The callosal splenium is present without the body or genu in many patients with holoprosencephaly. Therefore, holoprosencephaly is the only disorder in which the posterior corpus callosum forms in the absence of the anterior corpus callosum.

In lobar holoprosencephaly, the frontal lobes and the frontal horns are hypoplastic, and the septum pellucidum is absent. The third ventricle is fully formed, and the thalami are normal. The falx cerebri and the interhemispheric fissure extend into the frontal area of the brain, although the anterior falx may be hypoplastic. Patients with lobar holoprosencephaly present with visual problems, mild to moderate developmental delay, and hypothalamic-pituitary dysfunction. The mild form of lobar holoprosencephaly may be indistinguishable from septo-optic dysplasia, as these entities present a continuum of developmental abnormalities.

■ **Septo-optic Dysplasia.** Septo-optic dysplasia is characterized by an absent or hypoplastic septum pellucidum and by hypoplastic anterior optic pathways. Hypoplasia of the optic chiasm and the hypothalamus often results in dilatation of the anterior recess of the third ventricle and a large suprasellar cistern. Mild hypoplasia of the optic tract may be difficult to recognize. Clinical presentations of patients with septo-optic dysplasia are variable, but the main symptoms are visual problems and hypothalamic-pituitary dysfunction. There are at least three subsets of patients with septo-optic dysplasia, which can be distinguished by MRI. One group has schizencephaly, gray-matter heterotopia, a remnant of the septum pellucidum, an almost normal visual apparatus, and classically suffers from seizures. A second subset of patients presents with hypoplasia of white matter, consecutive enlarged ventricles, and an absent septum pellucidum, but otherwise normal cortex. This form is believed to be a mild form of lobar holoprosencephaly. The third subset of patients demonstrates a hypoplastic or absent septum pellucidum along with a sometimes mild hypoplasia of the optic nerves and suffers from endocrine dysfunction secondary to either hypoplastic or ectopic pituitary gland (Fig. 16.5).

■ **Aplasia/Hypoplasia of the Pituitary Gland.** The pituitary gland develops between 28 and 48 days of embryonic life. The posterior lobe forms from a downward extension of the embryonic hypothalamus, known as the neurohypophysis, whereas the anterior lobe and pars intermedia form from Rathke's pouch, which appears on the roof of the foregut and grows dorsally toward the infundibulum. Rathke's pouch detaches from the buccal cavity and becomes associated with the developing posterior pituitary lobe.

The normal appearance of the pituitary gland in a newborn is convex with a uniform high signal on T1-WI (Fig. 16.34). By the age of 2 months, the adenohypophysis loses its high SI, while the neurohypophysis still shows a high signal on T1-WI. During infancy and childhood, the superior margin flattens, and the gland grows normally, showing a height between 2 and 6 mm in the sagittal plane. During puberty, the gland increases dramatically in size in girls and demonstrates an upward convexity with a height up to 10 mm. The normal height in boys during puberty is 7–8 mm. After puberty, the pituitary gland diminishes slightly in size, evolving to adult appearance.

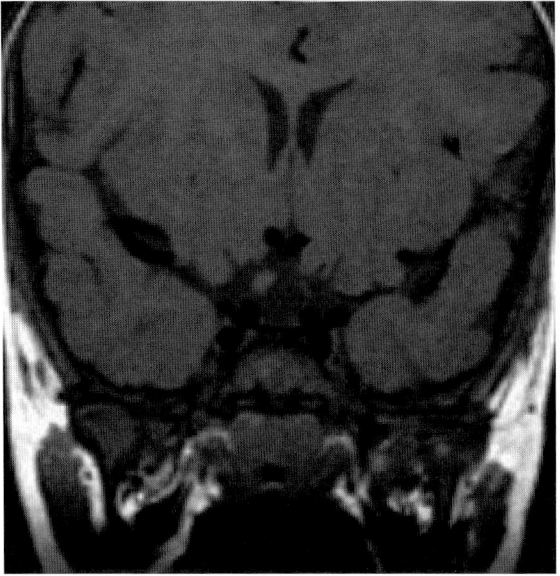

Fig. 16.5. Septo-optic dysplasia. Coronal T1-WI shows a normal right and a hypoplastic left optic nerve. Septum pellucidum is present. Clinically, this patient suffered from growth hormone deficiency (GDH) and TSH deficiency and was blind in the left eye. Other images demonstrated a hypoplasia of the anterior lobe of the pituitary gland and an ectopic posterior pituitary lobe

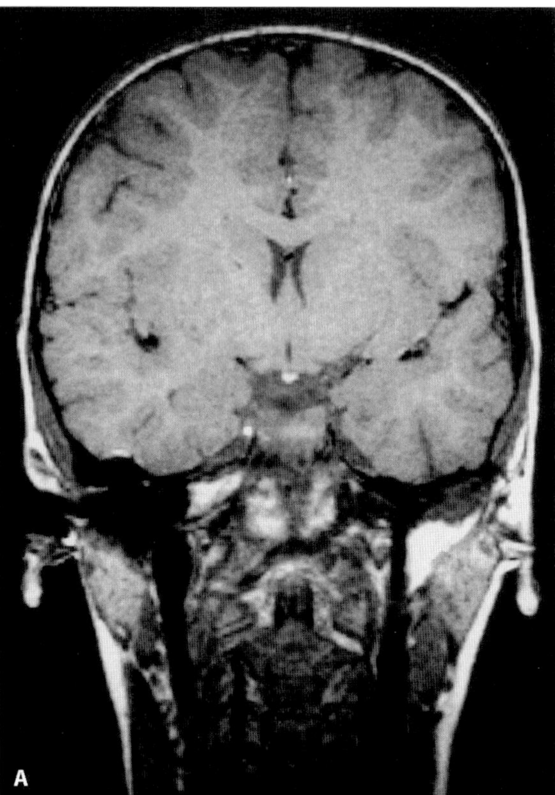

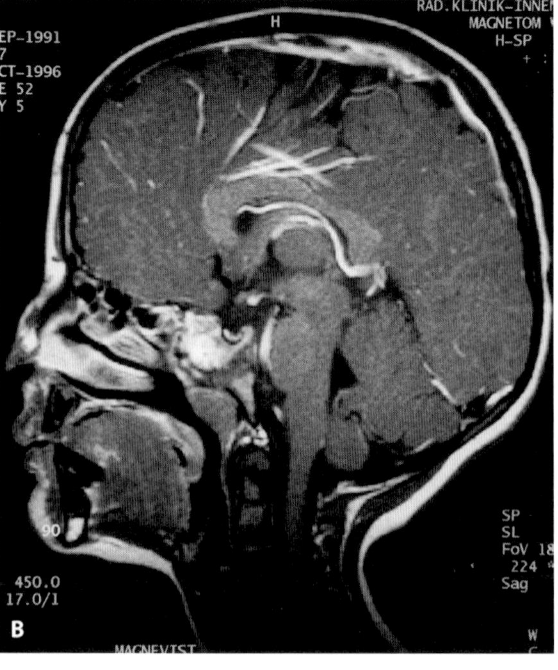

Patients with aplasia or hypoplasia of the pituitary gland either suffer from growth failure due to growth hormone deficiency (GHD) and/or symptoms of anterior pituitary hormone deficiencies (MPHD, multiple pituitary hormone deficiencies). Imaging findings consist of one or more of the following: small shallow sella, small anterior pituitary gland, absence of the usually high SI from the posterior pituitary gland, absence or hypoplasia of the distal pituitary stalk, and an anomalous high signal area in the proximal pituitary stalk. Three patterns are frequently encountered: one subset of patients presents with posterior lobe ectopia (high signal area in the proximal pituitary stalk), aplasia of the stalk, aplasia or hypoplasia of the anterior lobe (small sella), and almost always suffers from MPHD ▶

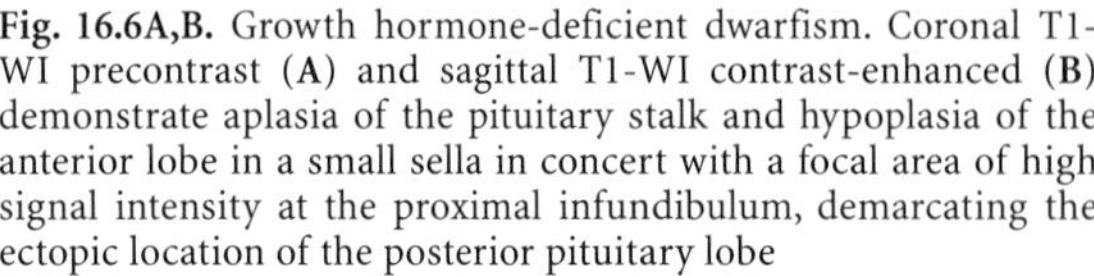

Fig. 16.6A,B. Growth hormone-deficient dwarfism. Coronal T1-WI precontrast (**A**) and sagittal T1-WI contrast-enhanced (**B**) demonstrate aplasia of the pituitary stalk and hypoplasia of the anterior lobe in a small sella in concert with a focal area of high signal intensity at the proximal infundibulum, demarcating the ectopic location of the posterior pituitary lobe

(Fig. 16.6). The second subset of patients demonstrates only anterior lobe hypoplasia (small sella and loss of high signal in the posterior pituitary gland) and suffers from GHD. The third subset of patients clinically presents only with mild endocrine dysfunction and has a normal-appearing pituitary gland. These anomalies are often associated with other midline anomalies, and both developmental anomalies and 'trauma' secondary to breech delivery have been accused of being responsible for this entity.

■ **Unilateral Megalencephaly (Hemimegalencephaly).** Unilateral megalencephaly is defined as a localized or complete hamartomatous overgrowth of one hemisphere due to neuronal migrational defects. Pathologically, the affected hemisphere contains areas of cortical dysplasia, pachygyria, heterotopia, and gliosis of the underlying white matter. The affected hemisphere is enlarged on imaging studies, with the sulci appearing shallow and the gyri broad. The dysplastic cortex appears thickened, and the margin between the cortex and underlying white matter may be indistinct. Areas of gliosis in the white matter show high signal on T2-WI and low signal on T1-WI. There is a characteristic appearance of the enlarged lateral ventricle on the affected side with a straight, superiorly and anteriorly pointing frontal horn. However, the changes can be subtler, and the cerebrum appears grossly normal. Patients with this anomaly usually present with intractable seizures, often starting within the first month of life, as well as developmental delay and hemiplegia. There are indications for partial or complete resection of the affected hemisphere in selected cases. Unilateral megalencephaly is associated with neurofibromatosis type 1 (NF-1), epidermal nevus syndrome, tuberous sclerosis, and unilateral hypomelanosis of Ito.

■ **Schizencephaly.** Schizencephaly is defined as a cleft extending from the lateral ventricles to the cortical surface lined by abnormal gray matter. Schizencephaly is divided into clefts with open and fused lips. In open-lip schizencephaly (Fig. 16.7), the cleft contains CSF, and in closed-lip schizencephaly, the walls of the cleft are in apposition to each other and therefore may be difficult to detect. The dimple usually seen in the wall of the lateral ventricle and a linear hyperintense signal intensity representing the pial and arachnoid lining of the cleft in T2-WI are helpful signs in depicting this condition. Bilateral clefts are not uncommon, and in about half of the patients, there are other neuronal migration anomalies. The septum pellucidum is absent in 80%–90% of patients with schizencephaly. Clinical symptoms, usually seizures and hemiparesis, are proportional to the size of the clefts.

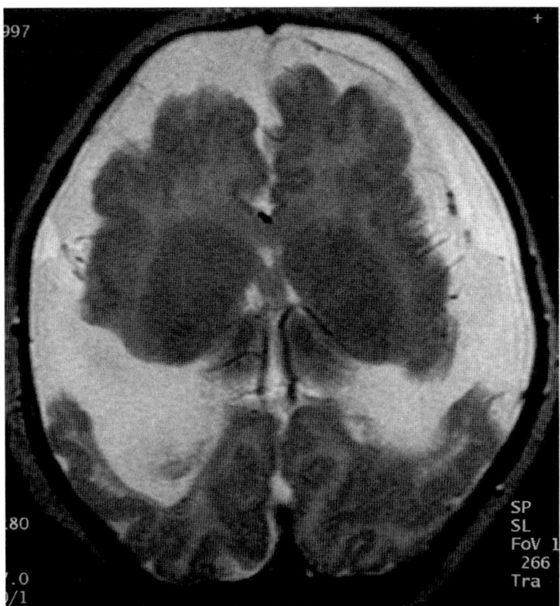

Fig. 16.7. Schizencephaly. Transverse T2-WI shows bilateral open-lip schizencephaly

■ **Arnold-Chiari Malformations.** The Arnold-Chiari I malformation is more often found in adults than children and is defined as displacement of 6 mm or more of the cerebellar tonsils below the foramen magnum (see Chapter 4, Fig. 4.4). Displacement of the tonsils between 3 and 6 mm is indeterminate; in the age group between 5 and 15 years, displacement of 6 mm should not be considered pathological. When the cerebellar tonsils extend more than 5–6 mm below the foramen magnum, clinical symptoms are more likely to occur. Midline sagittal MR images reveal peg-like cerebellar tonsils displaced inferiorly to the foramen magnum. Concurrent findings are hydrocephalus, syringohydromyelia, osseous malformations of the craniocervical junction, or acquired deformities of the foramen magnum.

The Arnold-Chiari II malformation is always associated with a meningomyelocele, inferior tentorial attachment, and small posterior fossa. The cerebellar tonsils and often both the vermis and medulla are displaced inferiorly into the cervical canal, frequently causing a cervicomedullary kink. The cerebellar hemispheres may extend anterolaterally, wrapping around the brainstem. The fourth ventricle is narrow and low in position, and beaking of the tectum occurs. Supratentorially, callosal dysgenesis and, subsequently, colpocephaly is seen in 80%–90% of the patients. The falx is hypoplastic, often fenestrated, and interdigitation of the gyri occurs. Most patients show further anomalies, such as stenogyria, which is defined as an abnormal pattern in the medial aspect of the occipital lobes due to dysplasia, resembling multiple small gyri. About 90% of patients have concurrent hydrocephalus and/or spinal-cord cysts. Segmentation anomalies of the upper cervical spine are seen in 10% of cases (see Chapter 4, Fig. 4.5).

The Arnold-Chiari III malformation is an extremely rare malformation, which combines the intracranial features of Arnold-Chiari II with a herniation of the posterior fossa contents through a posterior spina bifida C1–C2. This encephalocele may contain the cerebellum, and sometimes the brainstem and aberrant venous structures. Spinal-cord cysts may be present.

■ **The Dandy-Walker Complex.** The Dandy-Walker complex represents a spectrum of malformations, varying from the mega cisterna magna to the Dandy-Walker malformation. This malformation (Fig. 16.8) is characterized by a superior attachment of the tentorium, resulting in a large posterior fossa, a cystic dilatation of the fourth ventricle filling the posterior fossa, and concurrent hypoplasia or aplasia of the cerebellar vermis. The cerebellar hemispheres are almost always hypoplastic. Hydrocephalus develops in 75% of patients by the age of 3 months; there are associations with corpus callosum agenesis, neuronal migration anomalies, and occipital cephaloceles.

The Dandy-Walker variant may show unilateral or bilateral hypoplasia of the cerebellar hemispheres, mild hypoplasia of the vermis, and a slightly enlarged fourth ventricle. The posterior fossa is normal or near normal

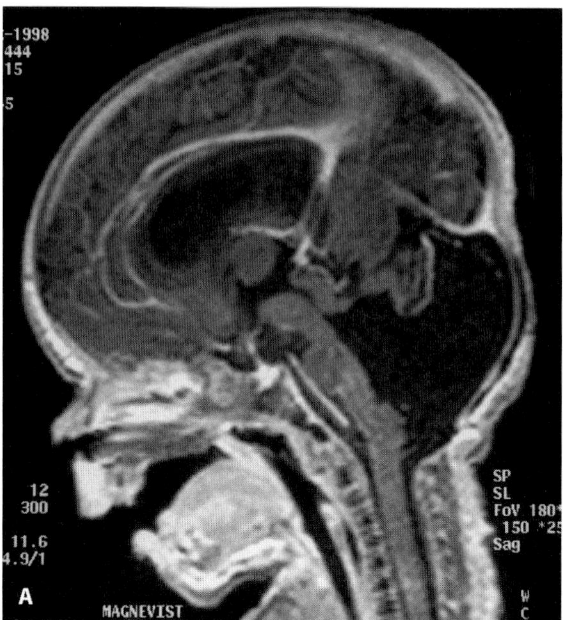

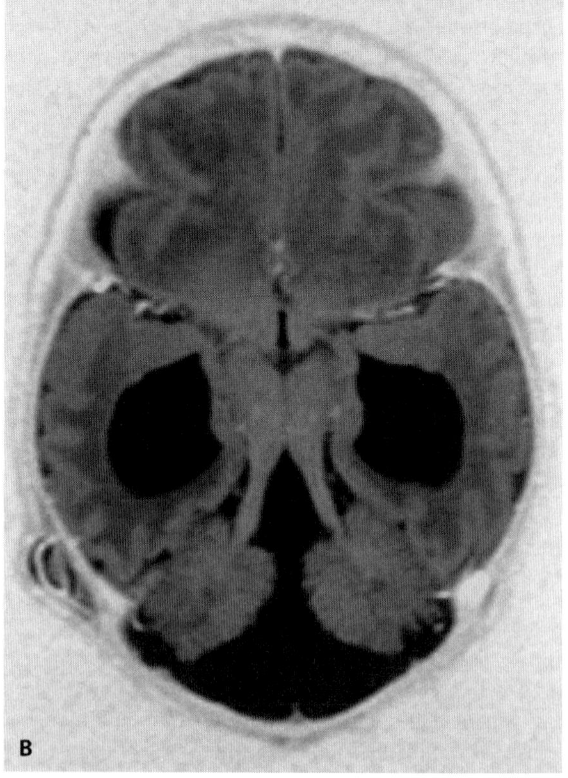

▶

Fig. 16.8A,B. Dandy-Walker malformation. Sagittal T1-WI (**A**) and transverse inversion recovery (**B**) contrast-enhanced image show dilatation of the fourth ventricle, expanded posterior fossa, high insertion of venous torcular, and absence of the inferior vermis

in size, and hydrocephalus may develop during infancy or early childhood.

Mega cisterna magna is characterized by expansion of the cisterna magna and both a morphological normal vermis and fourth ventricle. Whether this entity represents a true malformation or a normal variant is subject to debate.

Patients with these anomalies may present with developmental delay and enlarged head circumference due to hydrocephalus or mass effect by the enlarged fourth ventricle sometimes scalloping the inner table. The degree of developmental delay correlates with the extent of supratentorial anomalies and the level of control of the hydrocephalus.

■ **Blake's Pouch.** Blake's pouch is an arachnoid cyst of the posterior fossa and an important differential diagnosis to the aforementioned posterior fossa malformations. The cyst is located posterior to the inferior vermis. Arachnoid cysts are benign lesions developing between the layers of the arachnoid membrane and do not communicate freely with the subarachnoid or ventricular spaces. Depending on the location and size of Blake's pouch, children may develop hydrocephalus and present with an increased head circumference and signs of increased intracranial pressure. MR imaging demonstrates a well marginated, mostly unilocular, nonenhancing lesion compressing adjacent structures with CSF signal characteristics on all sequences. Due to mass effect, there may be scalloping of the inner table (see Chapter 4, Fig. 4.6).

16.2.3.1.2
Anomalies of Histogenesis: Phakomatoses

■ **Neurofibromatosis Type 1.** NF is an autosomal dominant disorder and is classified as type 1 (NF-1) and type 2 (NF-2). NF-1 is ten times more common than NF-2 and inherited via a genetic defect located on chromosome 17. The most reliable diagnostic criteria are the demonstration of six or more 'cafe-au-lait' spots of 1.5 cm in size, Lisch spots, and a family history. Central nervous system (CNS) abnormalities include true neoplasms, usually optic nerve (in 10%–20% bilateral) and parenchymal gliomas, as well as dysplastic, hamartomatous lesions, and multifocal signal changes with bright signal on T2-WI. These signal alterations probably represent either abnormal myelination or hamartomatous change (Fig. 16.9A).

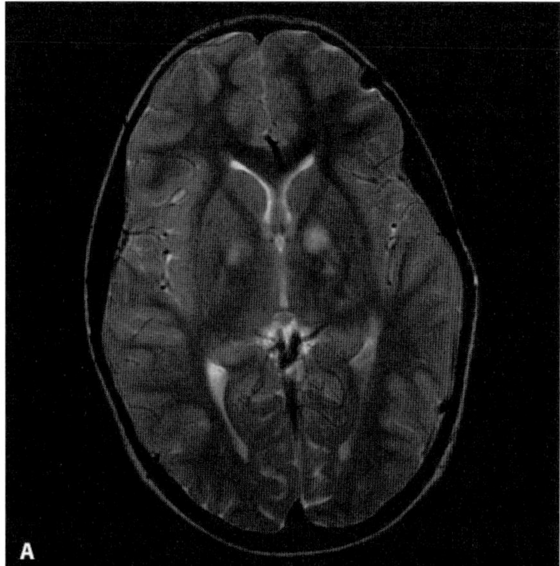

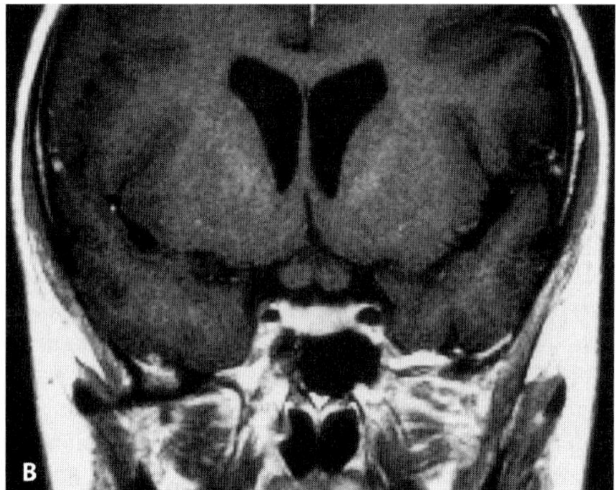

Fig. 16.9A,B. Neurofibromatosis type 1. Axial T2-WI (**A**) shows bright signal changes in the pallidum on both sides consistent with abnormal myelination or hamartomatous change. Coronal contrast-enhanced T1-WI (**B**) of another patient shows bilateral optic nerve gliomas (**B**, courtesy of G. Schuierer MD, Radiologie, Westfälische-Wilhelms Universität, Münster)

The gliomas extend from the optic nerves (Fig. 16.9B) along the optic pathway, or primarily arise from the optic chiasm, hypothalamus, thalamus, basal ganglia, brainstem, occipital lobe, or brainstem. Gliomas are hyperintense on T2-WI, isointense or hyperintense to gray or white matter on T1-WI, and enhance after administration of contrast.

Furthermore, hamartomas, predominantly occurring in the basal ganglia, optic radiations, brainstem, and cerebellar and cerebral peduncles are frequently encountered in NF-1. On MR, these lesions show no mass effect, are hyperintense on T2-WI and isointense with gray or white matter on T1-WI, and do not enhance with paramagnetic contrast. If these lesions show contrast enhancement and mass effect, they are considered to be low-grade gliomas. However, one exception to this rule are the lesions in the globus pallidus, which demonstrate abnormally high signal on T1-WI in more than 50% of affected patients and are often associated with mild mass effect.

In one-third of patients with NF-1, there will be neurofibromas affecting the intraorbital and facial branches of the cranial nerves III–VI and/or diffuse plexiform neurofibromas of the face and the eyelids (Fig. 16.10). Plexiform neurofibromas are hyperintense on T2-WI and hypointense or heterogeneous on T1-WI and demonstrate a variable enhancement. In 5%–10% of the patients, there is a proptosis of the globe because of dehiscence and dysplasia of the sphenoid bone. Dysplasia of the greater wing of sphenoid is a diagnostic feature for NF-1.

Vascular dysplasia of the proximal cerebral vessels can also occur and lead to moya-moya syndrome.

Hydrocephalus occurs in NF-1 due to aqueduct stenosis or secondary to mass effects by hamartomatous or neoplastic lesions. Spine abnormalities are present in more than 60% of NF-1 patients and consist of acute angle kyphoscoliosis, expansion of neuroforamina, and widening of the spinal canal due to neurofibromas arising from the spinal and paraspinal nerves, or due to arachnoid cysts, dural ectasia, or dysplastic neuronal foramina. Additionally, lateral thoracic meningoceles are strongly suggestive of NF-1.

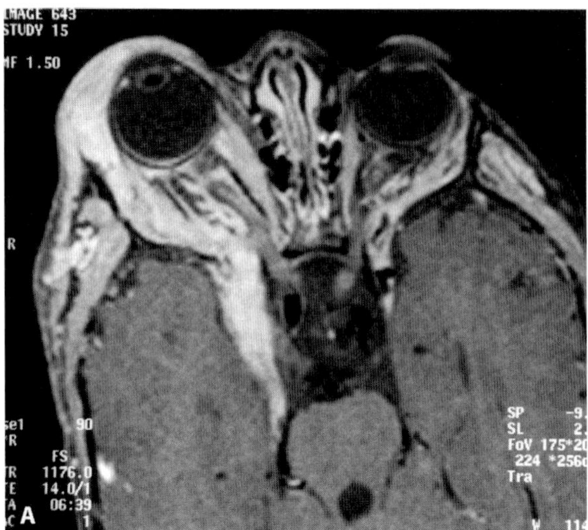

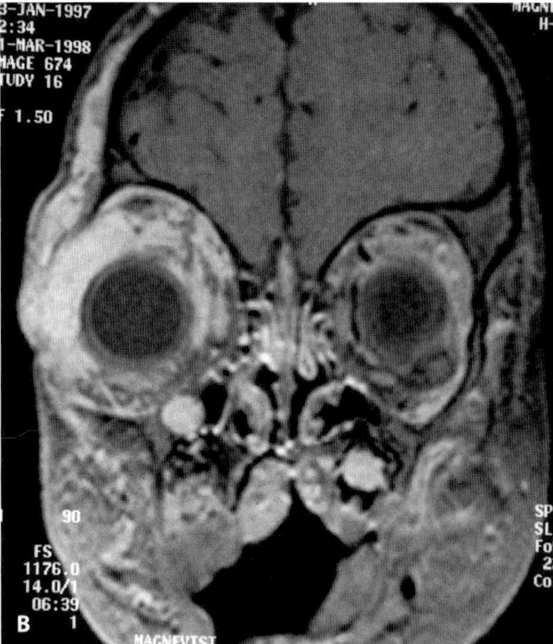

Fig. 16.10A,B. Neurofibromatosis type 1. Transverse (**A**) and coronal (**B**) FS contrast-enhanced T1-WI show plexiform neurofibromas of the cranial nerves (N III–IV), eyelids, and face

■ **Neurofibromatosis Type 2.** NF-2 is a dominant disease with the abnormality located on chromosome 22. The diagnostic criteria for NF-2 are unilateral or bilateral presence of vestibular nerve schwannomas (Fig. 16.11), plus two of the following: neurofibroma or schwannoma in other locations, meningioma, glioma, juvenile posterior subcapsular lens opacity, or a first-degree relative with NF-2. Therefore, a meningioma in a child should always raise suspicion for NF-2. Cutaneous lesions in NF-2 are rare. Patients with NF-2 develop multiple schwannomas of the cranial and spinal nerves (Fig. 16.47), meningiomas occurring in atypical locations, and spinal cord ependymomas. On MRI, schwannomas show high signal on T2-WI and low signal on

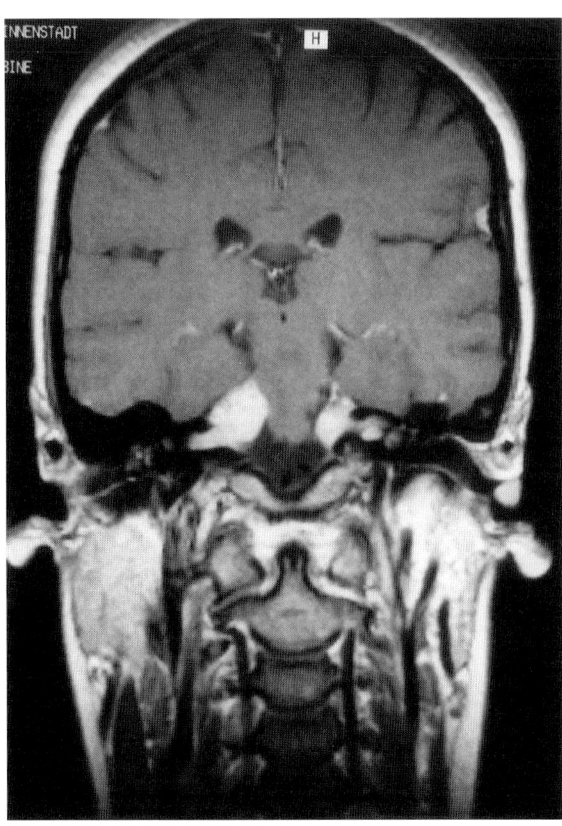

Fig. 16.11. Neurofibromatosis type 2. Coronal T1-WI shows bilateral enhancing vestibular nerve schwannomas

T1-WI with prominent enhancement after the administration of Gd-DTPA. As they enlarge and age, schwannomas tend to become heterogeneous masses with heterogeneous enhancement because of cystic degeneration and hemorrhage.

■ **Tuberous Sclerosis.** Tuberous sclerosis is an autosomal dominant disorder and related to abnormalities in chromosomes 9 and 16. The classic triad includes facial angiofibromas, seizures, and mental retardation. The diagnosis of tuberous sclerosis should be considered in any child with infantile spasms and seizures. The estimated incidence was revised from about 1 in 100,000 to 1 in 6000 live births. Depigmented nevi occurring on the trunk and the extremities are often present at birth and are as common as angiofibromas, which appear between the ages of 1 and 5 years.

About 95% of patients present with hamartomas, with and without calcifications, which occur in the periventricular regions, subependymal or anywhere in the white matter or cortical regions. Cerebellar lesions are occasionally seen. The cortical hamartomas (Fig. 16.12A) flatten the gyri, giving them a more pachygyric appearance. Gross calcification within these hamartomas is extremely rare in infants but can be commonly seen in children 2 years and older and in adults. Hamartomas can be solitary or multiple; they are isointense or hypointense on T1-WI and hyperintense on T2-WI. Subependymal hamartomas (Fig. 16.12B) most commonly occur at the head of the caudate nucleus and/or the lateral bodies of the ventricles. They are usually multiple and bilateral and contain calcification more often than cortical or white-matter hamartomas. They are usually hyperintense on T2-WI and isointense with, or slightly hyperintense to, gray matter on T1-WI and show a variable enhancement after administration of Gd-DTPA. Although MRI lacks sensitivity and specificity for the detection of calcifications, large calcium deposits may be seen as hypointensity or hyperintensity on T1-WI and hypointensity on T2-WI. Hamartomas can degenerate to giant-cell astrocytoma. Most commonly, subependymal hamartomas at the level of the foramen of Monro (Fig. 16.12C) degenerate to subependymal giant-cell astrocytomas. These lesions do grow slowly on sequential studies, lead to unilateral and/or bilateral dilatation of the lateral ventricles, and show contrast enhancement.

■ **Sturge-Weber Syndrome.** Sturge-Weber syndrome is characterized by angiomatous malformation of the skin, eyes, and brain. Although patients are normal at birth, over 90% develop seizures, dementia, hemiparesis, hemianopsia, and glaucoma during their lifetime. The main manifestation consists of a port-wine nevi in a trigeminal nerve distribution and angiomatosis of the pia mater in the ipsilateral occipitoparietal region. Cortical veins do not develop in the area of the pial angioma, and this leads to blood stasis with secondary calcification of the cortex. After contrast administration, the pial angioma may be clearly delineated by MRI (Fig. 16.13). Occasionally, the involved cerebral hemisphere becomes atrophic.

■ **Von Hippel-Lindau Syndrome.** Von Hippel-Lindau syndrome (VHL) is an autosomal dominant disorder and is linked to a defect in chromosome 3. The associa-

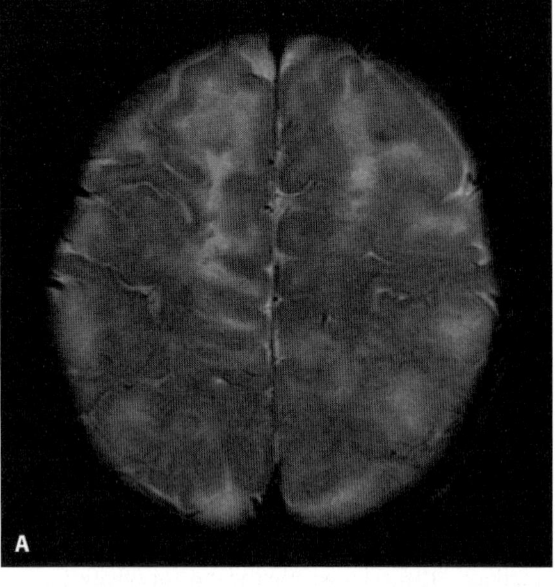

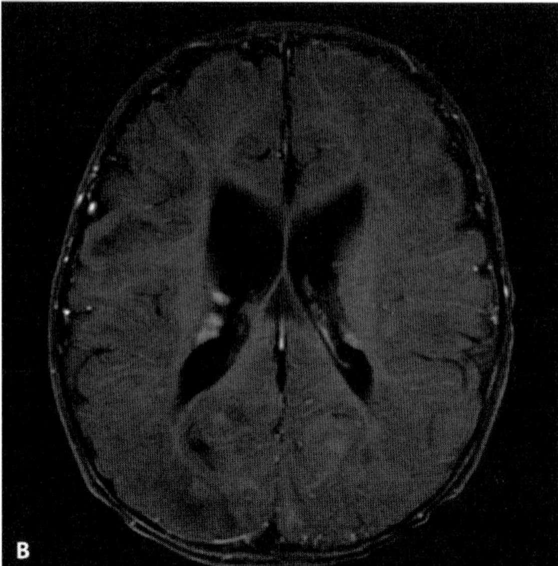

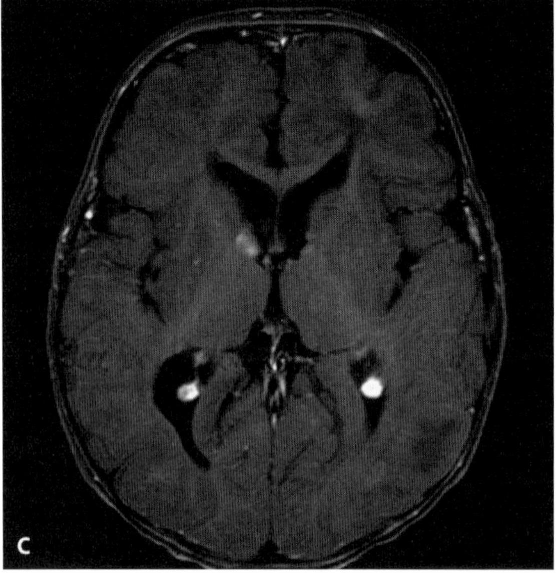

Fig. 16.12A–C. Tuberous sclerosis. Transverse T2-WI (**A**) shows multiple hyperintense cortical tubers. Transverse contrast-enhanced T1-WI demonstrate multiple subependymal hamartomas at the lateral bodies of the ventricles (**B**) and at the foramen of Monro (**C**) on both sides that enhance after administration of contrast

tion of angiomatous retinal tumors and angiomatous tumors of the CNS characterizes this syndrome. About 75% of hemangioblastomas are located in the cerebellum, and the remaining 25% in either the brainstem or the spinal cord. About 20% are solid, but the majority are typically cystic with a mural nodule. Retinal angiomas are present in half of the patients and are the only prepubertal manifestation. VHL syndrome is commonly associated with retinal and cerebellar hemangioblastomas, cysts, angiomas of the liver and kidneys, renal cell carcinomas, and pheochromocytomas.

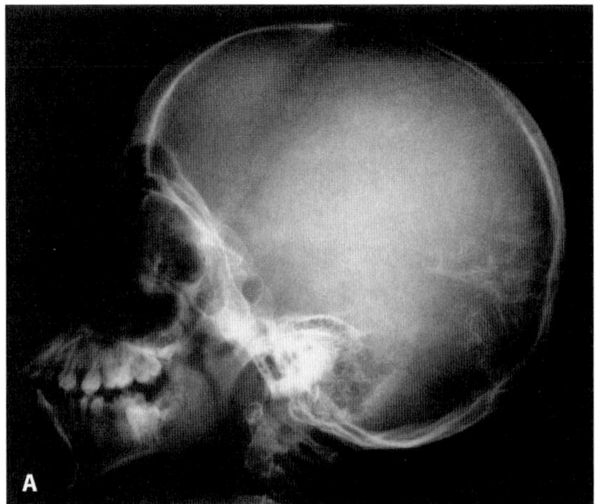

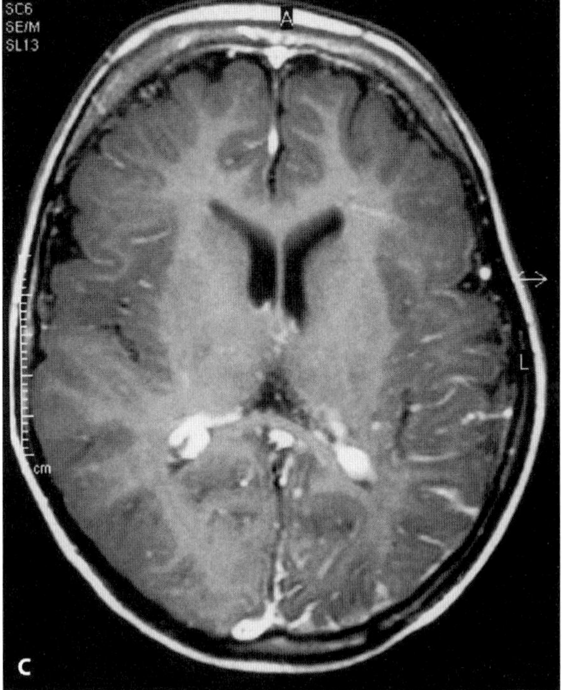

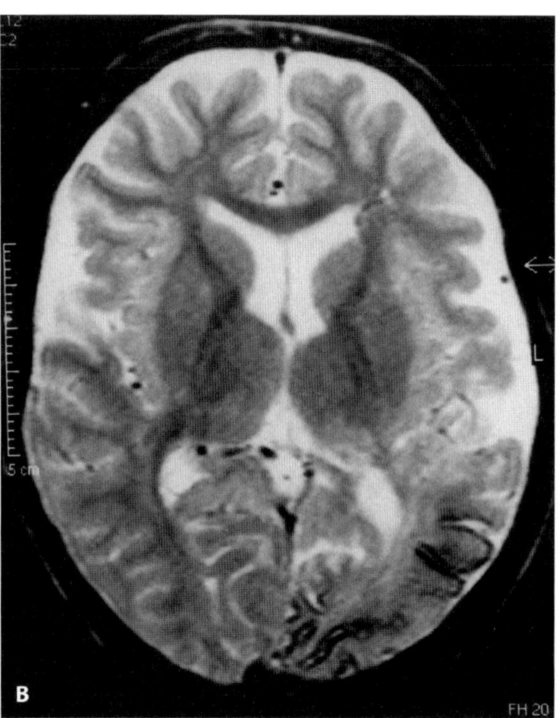

Fig. 16.13A–C. Sturge-Weber syndrome. Lateral skull film (**A**) and transverse T2-WI (**B**) demonstrate calcification of left occipital cortex. Transverse contrast-enhanced T1-WI (**C**) reveals marked pial enhancement, representing pial angioma involving the left parieto-occipital region (courtesy of W. Michl, MD, Institut für Röntgendiagnostik des Krankenhauszweckverbandes, Kinderradiologie, Augsburg)

16.2.3.2 Myelination

Familiarity with the normal process and appearance of myelination is important in pediatric MRI of the brain. The appearance of myelination varies with magnet field strength and imaging sequence used. Myelination changes seem to appear earlier at lower field strengths and on IR sequences.

Myelination begins in utero and continues after birth. By the age of 2 years, the degree of myelination is close to that of an adult. The process of deposition of

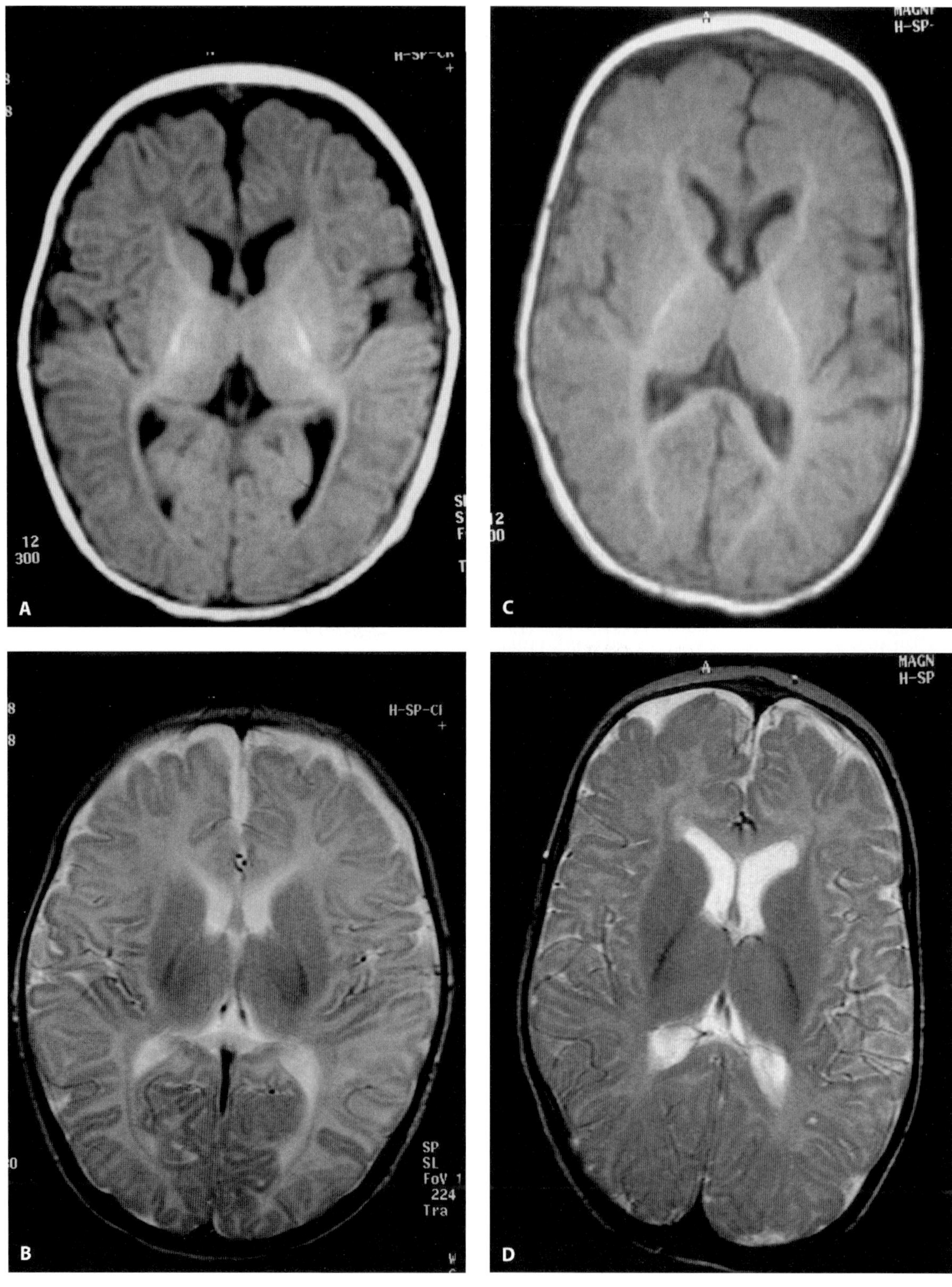
A
12
300
C
B
H-SP-CI
SP
SL
224
Tra
D
MAGN
H-SP

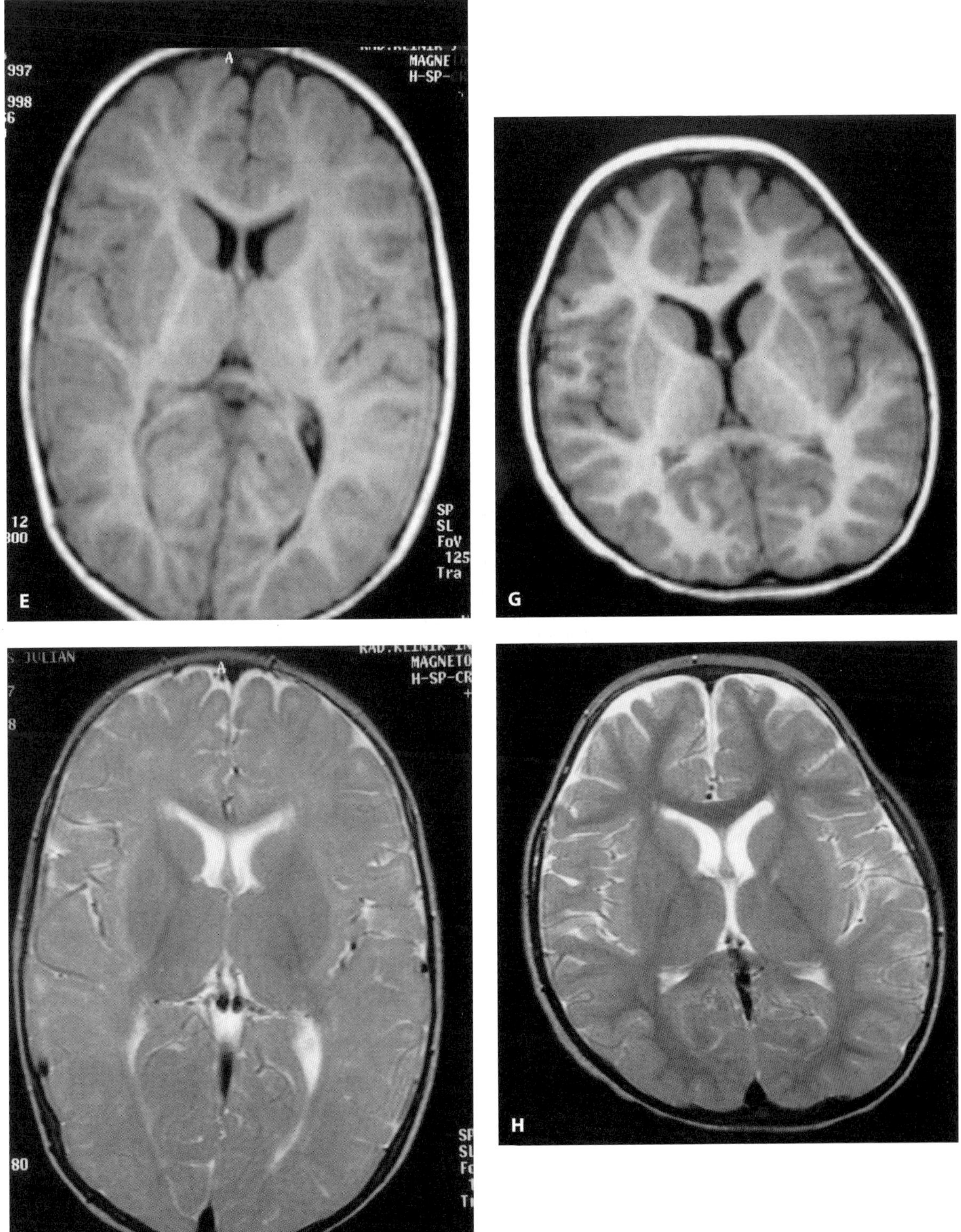

Fig. 16.14A–H. Legend see page 506

Fig. 16.14A–H. Normal myelination according to age. Transverse T1-W (**A**) and T2-W (**B**) images of a 2-month-old infant. Unmyelinated deep white matter tracts are hypointense on T1-W and hyperintense on T2-W. Myelination of the posterior horns of the internal capsule is seen on both T1-WI and T2-WI. Transverse T1-W (**C**) and T2-W (**D**) images of a 6-month-old infant. Myelination of the deep white-matter tracts has further progressed. Both the splenium and the genu of the corpus callosum are of high signal intensity on T1-WI. On T2-WI, the splenium of the corpus callosum is of low signal intensity. Transverse T1-W and T2-W images of a 10-month-old infant. T1-WI (**E**) shows myelination of the external capsule, and the hyperintensity extends far more peripherally into a branching pattern in the occipital, parietal, and frontal lobes. T2-WI (**F**) shows decreasing signal intensity of the white matter throughout the brain. The cortex and the underlying white matter are isointense throughout most of the brain. The anterior limbs of the internal capsule are hypointense compared with the surrounding structures in essentially all patients of this age. Compare this with the mature brain of a 2.5-year-old child (**G**,**H**)

myelin, which is a hydrophobic glycolipoprotein, can be followed by MRI. On one hand, deposition of myelin can be followed in T1-WI, as fat is hyperintense on T1-WI. The accumulating lipid content results in a relatively increased signal in the white matter. This change is greatest on T1 in the first 6 months of life. On the other hand, deposition of myelin results in a decrease of the water content of the white matter. A transition on T2-WI from hyperintense, unmyelinated white matter to hypointense, myelinated white matter can be seen with the development of myelination. T1-WI demonstrate signal change related to the presence of myelin approximately 2 months prior to T2-WI, because the quantity of myelin deposition required to change SI is smaller in T1-WI than in T2-WI. However, the final assembly of myelin is better reflected on T2-WI. Therefore, to study the process of myelination, it is recommended to use T1-WI in children under 6 months of age and subsequently to use T2-WI.

In general, myelination progresses from caudal to cranial and from posterior to anterior. Central structures are myelinated first, with more peripheral areas following. Central sensory pathways tend to myelinate before the central motor pathways. It is, therefore, possible to establish a series of milestones in myelination. At 40 weeks' gestational age, myelin can be seen on T1-WI in the medulla oblongata, the middle cerebellar peduncle, the tegmentum pontis, and especially the medial lemniscus and the colliculus inferior. Additionally, myelination is seen in the central tegmental part of the mesencephalon, the optic tracts, the posterior limb of the capsula interna, the white-matter tracts in each of the basal ganglia, the ascending tracts towards the postrolandic gyrus, and the primary sensory cortex.

By 3 months of age, high SI (myelination) should appear in the anterior limbs of the internal capsule and should extend distally from the deep cerebellar white matter into the cerebral folia. By the age of 4 months, the splenium of the corpus callosum should be of moderately high SI. By the age of 6 months, the genu of the corpus callosum should be of high SI. As stated earlier, after the age of 6 months, T2-WI are recommended to assess normal brain maturation. On T2-WI, the splenium of the corpus callosum should be of low SI by 6 months, like the genu of the corpus callosum by 8 months and the anterior limb of the internal capsule by 11 months of age. By the age of 14 months, the deep frontal white matter should be of low SI with the temporal lobes being the last to myelinate. The entire brain should have an adult appearance, except for the most peripheral arcuate fibers, by 18 months (Fig. 16.14) (Table 16.2).

A delayed or abnormal myelination pattern is an important finding in the pediatric brain. It may reflect failure in myelin formation or dysmyelination; it may

Table 16.2. Normal myelination of the brain

Anatomic region	Myelination changes with age in months	
	T1-WI Bright signal	T2-WI Dark signal
Middle cerebellar peduncle	0	0–2
Cerebellar white matter	0–4	3–5
Posterior limb of internal capsule		
Anterior portion	0	4–7
Posterior portion	0	0–2
Anterior limb internal capsule	2–3	7–11
Genu of corpus callosum	4–6	5–8
Splenium corpus callosum	3–4	4–6
Occipital white matter		
Central	3–5	9–14
Peripheral	4–7	11–15
Frontal white matter		
Central	3–6	11–16
Peripheral	7–11	14–18
Centrum semiovale	2–4	7–11

Adapted from Barkovich; WI, weighted image

be a consequence of white-matter injury in utero or at the time of birth; or it may simply be seen in children with delayed development without obvious cause. Sometimes an abnormal myelination pattern is found in asymptomatic children, or occasionally, both clinical development and myelination fall behind expected milestones, only to show a later recovery to normal in both parameters.

16.2.3.3 Metabolic and Neurodegenerative Disorders and Disorders with Abnormal Myelination

Normal brain maturation can be severely disturbed by alterations in the cellular metabolism, which can primarily affect either gray matter, white matter, or both. The principal effect of neurodegeneration and altered cellular metabolism in gray matter is the loss of the neuron, whereas metabolic anomalies affecting the white matter mainly involve the formation and structure of myelin. When both gray and white matter are involved, the primary injury may be to the gray matter with secondary degeneration of the axons in the white matter or vice versa. The diagnosis of metabolic and neurodegenerative disorders and disorders with abnormal myelination is often based on the clinical history, symptoms, and subsequent metabolic and pathologic testing. Patients with affection of the deep gray matter clinically present with athetosis, chorea, and dystonia, whereas those with involvement of the cortical gray matter suffer from seizures, visual loss, and dementia. In contrast, patients with white matter disorders present with ataxia, hyperreflexia, and spasticity. If an imaging study is to have a role in the diagnosis of these entities, the study should be performed early in the course of the disease, since most disorders have a similar imaging appearance in the late stages of the disease. By proper analysis of the early pattern of brain involvement, many disorders may be diagnosed or excluded. Symmetry, spread pattern, involvement of the subcortical or the deep white matter, the basal ganglia, the brainstem, and associated cortical infarctions are clues to the diagnosis. For the following, all common entities are listed in two tables using the cellular organelle classification, and important diseases are elucidated (Tables 16.3, 16.4).

Table 16.3. Common metabolic disorders based on involved organelle

Disorers of the lysosome
Predominant white matter involvement
Metachromatic leukodystrophy[a]
Krabbe disease (Globoid cell leukodystrophy)[a]
Predominant gray matter involvement
GM_1-Gangliosidosis
Neuronal ceroid lipofuscinosis
Mucolipidosis
Both gray and white matter involvement
GM_2-Gangliosidosis
Mucopolysaccharidosis
Mannosidosis
Disorders of the peroxisome
Predominant white matter involvement
Zellweger's syndrome
Pseudo-Zellweger's syndrome
Neonatal adrenoleukodystrophy[a]
X-linked (classic) adrenoleukodystrophy[a]
Adrenomyeloneuropathy
Infantile Refsum's disease
Disorders of the mitochondria
Leigh disease (subacute necrotizing encephalopathy)[a]
MELAS (myopathy, encephalopathy, lactat acidosis, stroke)[a]
MERRF (myopathy, encephalopathy with ragged red fibers)
Kearns-Sayre syndrome
Alper's disease

Adapted from Ball
[a] Diseases discussed in the text

16.2.3.3.1 Metachromatic Leukodystrophy

Metachromatic leukodystrophy (MLD) is inherited as a recessive disorder with a deficiency of arylsulfatase A, resulting in the accumulation of sulfatides that are toxic to white matter. Most patients will present between 14 months and 4 years of life with gait disturbances, ataxia, spasticity of the lower limbs, strabismus dysarthria, and mental retardation. Death usually occurs 1–4 years after the onset of symptoms. Imaging studies show diffuse white-matter disease with high SI on T2-WI with sparing of subcortical U-fibers and areas of increased SI on T2-WI in the cerebellum. The endstage of the disease shows generalized cerebral and spinal-cord atrophy.

Table 16.4. Common metabolic disorders without specific organelle involved

Disorders of amino acid metabolism
Lowe's disease (Oculocerebral syndrome)
Phenylketonuria
Maple syrup urine disease
Homocystinuria
Nonketotic hypoerglycinemia
Urea acid cycle defects
Organic acidurias
Methylmelonic aciduria
Proprionic aciduria
Glutaric aciduria type I[a]
Primary disorders in myelin formation
Cockayne's syndrome
Pelizaeus-Merzbacher disease[a]
Trichothiodystrophy
Disorders with macrocrania
Canavan disease[a]
Alexander disease[a]
Hepatic disorders with neurodegeneration
Wilson's disease
Galactosemia
Chronic hepatic encephalopathy
Carnitine deficiency
Miscellaneous disorders
Neuroaxonal dystrophy
Hallervorden-Spatz disease
Seitelberger's disease
Neuronal ceroid lipofuscinosis
Congenital muscular dystrophy with white matter changes
Encephalitis disseminata

Adapted from ball
[a] Disease discussed in the text

16.2.3.3.2 Globoid Cell Leukodystrophy: Krabbe Disease

Krabbe disease is an autosomal recessive disorder characterized by a deficiency of the enzyme galactocerebroside β-galactosidase. This lysosomal enzyme degrades cerebroside to galactose and ceramide; thus, the globoid cells found within the white matter contain cerebroside. The brain may be initially enlarged, but later becomes atrophic. Onset of symptoms occurs between 3 and 6 months of life, with irritability, progressive stiffness in conjunction with opisthotonic spasms, and atypical seizures. This disease is rapidly progressive and fatal. MR shows nonspecific white-matter hyperintensity in T2-WI, especially in the periventricular regions. Changes in the cerebellar white matter may sometimes also be seen. Noncontrast CT may show calcifications in the basal ganglia and corona radiata.

16.2.3.3.3 Adrenoleukodystrophy

Adrenoleukodystrophy (ALD) is a peroxisomal disorder, causing an impaired capacity to degrade very-long-chain fatty acids. There are two types: the X-linked type, which is inherited by a single enzyme defect, and the neonatal type, which is caused by multiple enzyme defects. The neonatal type involves the white matter diffusely, resulting in a nearly complete absence of myelin in the cerebral white matter, which causes severe volume loss and small head size. Patients with the X-linked type typically present between 5 and 10 years of age, with homonymous hemianopsia, behavioral changes progressing to mental retardation, and gait disturbances. Rarely, adrenal insufficiency may occur without neurologic involvement. A vegetative state or death usually occurs 2 years after the onset of symptoms. On T2-WI, the X-linked type shows bilateral and symmetrical

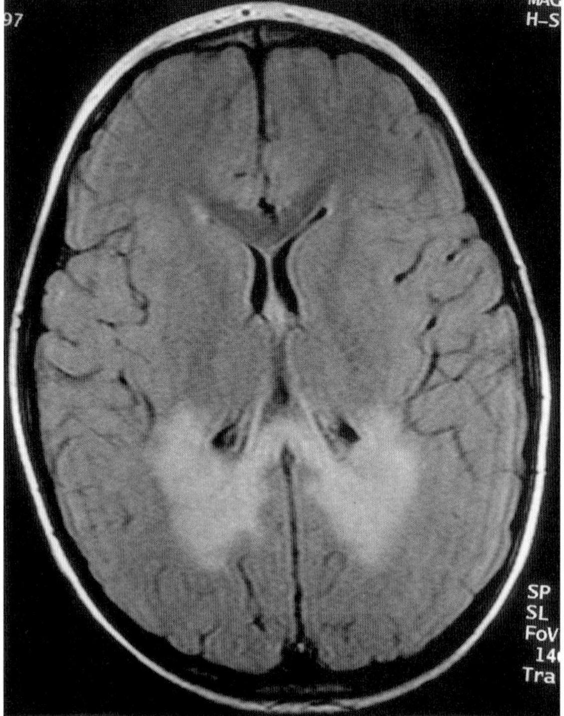

Fig. 16.15. Adrenoleukodystrophy. Transverse fluid-attenuated inversion recovery image shows high signal intensity in the occipital white matter

increased hyperintensity in the occipitoparietal regions along the occipital horns, with an enhancing margin at the front due to demyelination (Fig. 16.15). There may be an involvement of the auditory pathways and the corpus callosum.

16.2.3.3.4 Leigh Disease: Subacute Necrotizing Encephalopathy

Leigh syndrome is observed in a number of different enzyme deficiencies, such as cytochrome *c* oxidase, pyruvate dehydrogenase, and, less frequently, NADH coenzyme Q reductase deficiency. In some patients, elevation of lactate and pyruvate in the blood and CSF are observed. The clinical presentation of Leigh disease is that of a multisystemic disorder dominated by the signs of CNS dysfunction, such as hypotonia, psychomotor deterioration, ophthalmoplegia, and respiratory and/or swallowing problems. The disease typically starts towards the end of the first year of life and leads to death within months or years. The putamen and the caudate nucleus are usually hypointense on T1-WI and hyperintense on T2-WI on MR examinations. In addition, the globus pallidus, dentate nucleus, substantia nigra, brain stem, tegmentum, and red nuclei are also frequently affected. Involvement of the thalamus, hypothalamus, subthalamic nucleus and cortex, and enlargement of the ventricular system due to polycystic white-matter changes may be present. In young children, delay of myelination may be observed (Fig. 16.16).

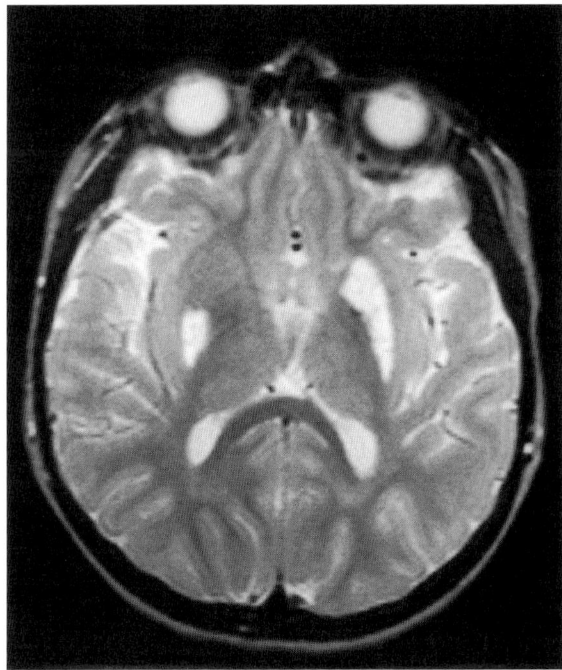

Fig. 16.16. Leigh disease. Transverse T2-WI demonstrates increased signal intensity in the putamina

16.2.3.3.5 Mitochondrial Encephalomyopathy with Lactic Acidosis and Stroke

In mitochondrial encephalomyopathy with lactic acidosis and stroke (MELAS), patients most commonly present in the second decade of life with signs of mitochondrial disease, stroke-like events, and episodes of nausea and vomiting. Typical imaging findings include calcium deposits in the globus pallidus and the caudate nucleus due to basal ganglia involvement, which are more easily depicted on CT than MR. MR precisely delineates the increased water content in areas affected by the stroke-like episodes. Interestingly, these infarcts do not follow vascular border zones and usually affect the cortex of the parietal and occipital lobes more severely than the underlying white matter. Follow-up studies reveal migrating infarcts and progressive atrophy.

16.2.3.3.6 Glutaric Aciduria Type I

Glutaric aciduria type I is an autosomal recessive aminoacidopathy resulting from a defect in glutaryl-CoA dehydrogenase. Patients present with progressive hypotonia, dystonia, tetraplegia, and encephalopathy, usually beginning in the first year of life. MR imaging reveals delayed myelination, degeneration of the basal ganglia with low SI on T1-WI, high SI on T2-WI, and frontotemporal atrophy with widening of the sylvian fissure (Fig. 16.17).

16.2.3.3.7 Pelizaeus-Merzbacher Disease

Pelizaeus-Merzbacher disease is an X-linked recessive disorder characterized by an impaired function of oligodendrocytes leading to hypomyelination. There are two types: the neonatal form, which is rapidly fatal, and

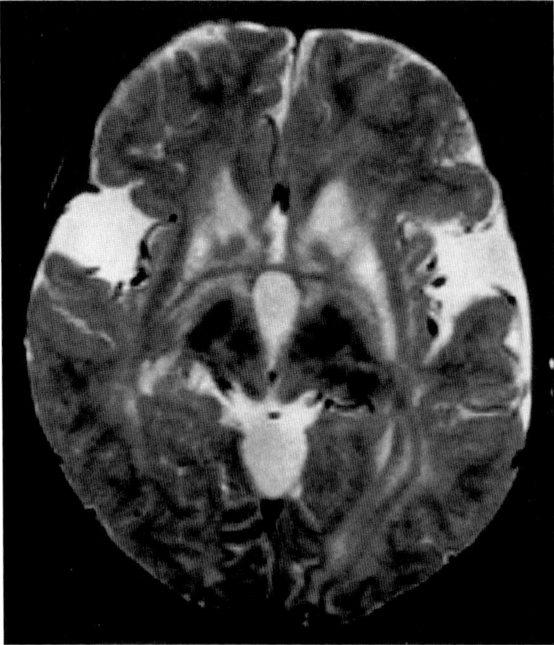

Fig. 16.17. Glutaric aciduria type I. Transverse T2-WI shows abnormal hyperintensity in the putamina with widening of the sylvian fissures due to atrophy

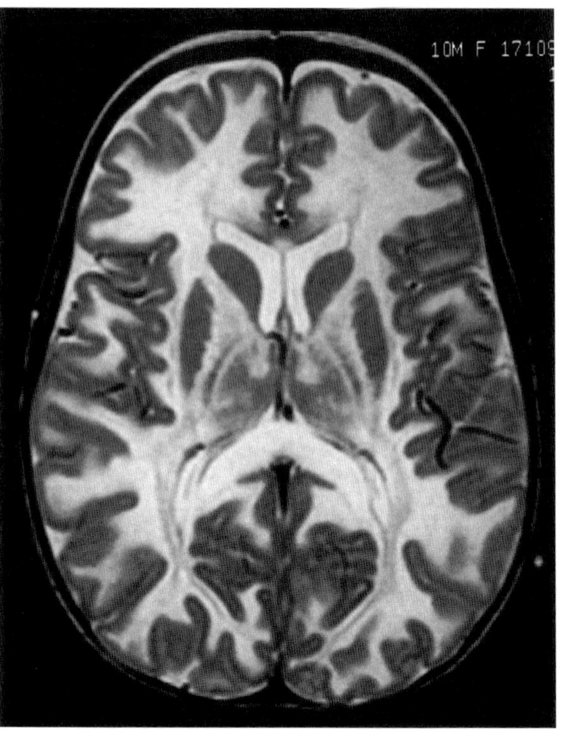

Fig. 16.18. Canavan disease. Transverse T2-WI shows hyperintense signal intensity in the white matter with involvement of the internal and external capsules and the subcortical U-fibers

the classic form, which has a progressive course. The classic form presents in young boys with pendular eye movements, failure to develop normal head control, spasticity, choreoathetoid movements, cerebellar ataxia, and mental retardation. The lack of mature myelin manifests as diffuse high SI on T2-WI, involving both cerebral and cerebellar hemispheres, including the long white-matter fiber tracts of the brainstem and spinal cord. The basal ganglia may have low SI on T2-WI, presumably due to increased iron deposition (see Chapter 4, Fig. 4.30).

16.2.3.3.8 Canavan Disease

Canavan disease is an autosomal recessive disorder characterized by a deficiency of *N*-acetylaspartylase and is also referred to as spongy degeneration of the CNS. The most common infantile type appears within the first 6 months of life. Patients present with hypotonia, spasticity, blindness, myoclonic seizures, irritability, and enlarging head size. The disease usually has a rapid and fatal course. Demyelination typically begins in the peripheral subcortical U-fibers, and only involves all white matter of the brain in the later stages, causing atrophy. Therefore, MR demonstrates high SI on T2-WI of the white matter (Fig. 16.18). Usually, proton MR spectroscopy shows a large *N*-acetylaspartate peak.

16.2.3.3.9 Alexander Disease

This disease requires brain biopsy for diagnosis, as it has no detectable biochemical defect and indeterminate etiology. Three clinical types exist: infantile, juvenile, and adult. The infantile type is the most common, with symptoms starting from birth, with developmental delay, pyramidal tract signs, seizures, and progressive macrocephaly. Death occurs 2–3 years after birth. The adult form may simulate multiple sclerosis (MS). Macrocephaly results from increased astrocytic eosinophilic Rosenthal's fibers within the white matter, lead-

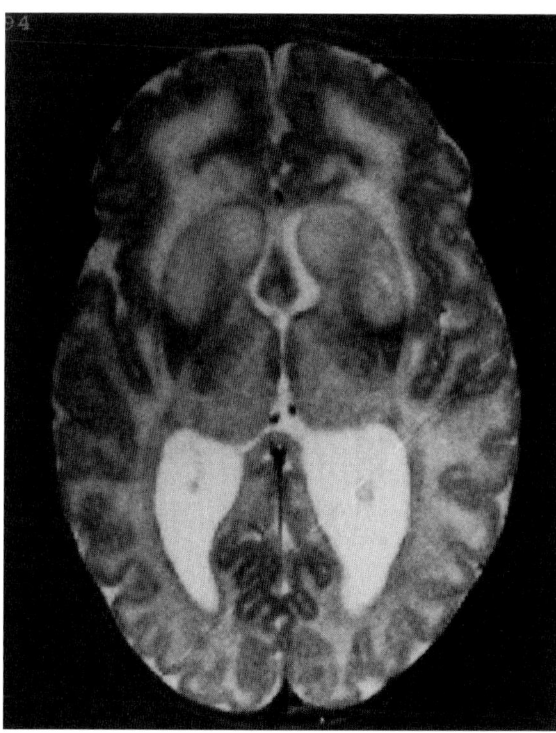

Fig. 16.19. Alexander disease. Transverse T2-WI shows high signal intensity in the frontal white matter involving the U-fibers and extending posteriorly into the external capsules and affection of the head of the caudate nuclei and putamina

ing to increased weight and size of the brain. Most commonly, the disease shows high SI on T2-WI, occurring in the periventricular region of the frontal lobes and later extending to entire cerebral hemispheres, due to demyelination. The lateral parts of the basal ganglia may also be affected (Fig. 16.19). Contrast enhancement may be present at the leading edges.

16.2.3.4 Infections and Inflammation

16.2.3.4.1 Congenital Infections

Congenital infections of the CNS are most commonly due to toxoplasma, rubella, CMV, and herpes simplex organisms (TORCH), human immunodeficiency virus (HIV), and bacteria. The developing fetal brain and the immature fetal immune system have a limited ability to respond to an inflammatory insult. Depending on the time point of infection, in-utero infections can cause either developmental brain anomalies (hydranencephaly, schizencephaly, neuronal proliferation alterations) or focal or multifocal destructive changes (necrotizing encephalitis, vasculitis, and meningitis).

■ **Toxoplasmosis.** Toxoplasmosis is the second most common congenital CNS infection after CMV infection. The principal CNS findings are bilateral chorioretinitis (85% of the patients), seizures, hydrocephalus, microcephaly, and intracranial calcifications. The calcifications vary with the extent of disease and typically occur in a periventricular or basal-ganglia distribution, but may involve the cerebral cortex in severe cases with near-total destruction. Hydrocephalus is due to ependymitis, leading to aqueductal stenosis. An important differentiating feature is the absence of cortical dysplasia, which is a common finding in congenital CMV infection. CT is the best modality to depict calcifications, whereas MR is primarily performed to prove the absence of cortical dysplasia.

■ **Cytomegalovirus.** CMV is the most common congenital infection among newborns. The most common clinical features of symptomatic CMV infection include: hepatosplenomegaly, jaundice, chorioretinitis, microcephaly, and optic atrophy. Approximately 10%–15% of infected infants develop neurological and developmental deficits in the first year of life. Patients infected in the beginning of the second trimester have complete lissencephaly with a thin cortex, hypoplastic cerebellum, delayed myelination, ventriculomegaly, and significant periventricular calcifications. Those infected later will present with cortical dysplasia, less ventricular dilatation, and less cerebellar hypoplasia. Patients infected perinatally have normal gyral patterns, mild atrophy, periventricular calcifications, and hemorrhage. CT is the best modality to evaluate calcifications, whereas MRI best demonstrates cortical dysplasia, myelination delay, and gliosis (Fig. 16.20).

■ **Herpes Simplex Virus.** Approximately 75% of congenital herpes simplex infections are caused by type II. Infection can either spread from the mother to the fetus transplacentally or during vaginal delivery. If the infection occurs in the first trimester, it may produce microcephaly, atrophy, hydranencephaly, and intracranial calcifications. Perinatally infected newborns present with

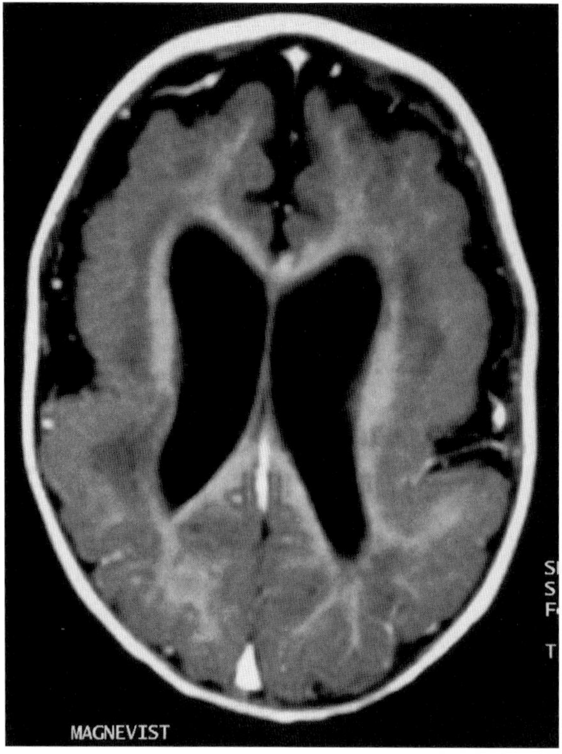

Fig. 16.20. Congenital cytomegalovirus infection. Transverse T1-WI shows pachygyria with cortical thickening and irregularity of the gray-matter/white-matter border

meningoencephalitis, seizures, and fever as well as other symptoms. Patchy areas of low SI on T1-WI and high SI on T2-WI in the white matter can be delineated on MR examinations. Meningeal contrast enhancement may be observed, as well as areas of hemorrhagic infarction. Cortical gray matter is involved with progressing disease. The end stage of severe herpes simplex virus (HSV) infection is cystic encephalomalacia and atrophy. Dystrophic calcifications in a periventricular and basal-ganglia distribution or in the cortex are more easily evaluated by CT.

■ **Human Immunodeficiency Virus.** Maternal transmission of HIV occurs in up to 30% of cases. The manifestation of neurological symptoms in children with congenital acquired immunodeficiency syndrome (AIDS) generally occurs between the ages of 2 months and 5 years. Intracranial imaging shows calcifications of the basal ganglia and subcortical white matter, most commonly in the frontal lobes, as well as atrophy and microcephaly.

16.2.3.4.2 Postnatal Infections

■ **Meningitis.** Meningitis is the most common CNS infection in children and may be either bacterial or viral. It is most commonly caused by hematogenous spread and primarily diagnosed by clinical symptoms and lumbar puncture. Neuroimaging is only performed if the diagnosis is unclear or if complications such as focal neurologic deficits or signs of increased intracranial pressure occur. Cerebral infections can have severe sequelae in newborns due to the immature immune system. Imaging reveals edema with or without ischemic or hemorrhagic infarction due to vessel occlusion. Intense contrast enhancement of the ependyma and meninges, reflecting ventriculitis and arachnoiditis, is observed; the latter two frequently lead to hydrocephalus. Abscess formation is relatively rare.

Imaging is often negative in older children in the acute stage. Later stages present similar imaging findings, although more often, subdural effusions, dilated subarachnoid spaces, and ventricular enlargement are present with contrast-enhancing meninges.

■ **Cerebritis, Abscess, and Empyema.** Bacterial infection of the brain produces cerebritis and meningitis and, if not sufficiently treated, abscess or empyema. It usually results from hematogenous spread, penetrating trauma, postoperatively, or from contiguous spread of mastoiditis and sinusitis. In newborns and small infants, the most common organisms involved are *Escherichia coli*, *Proteus*, *Klebsiella*, followed by group B-streptococci, *Pseudomonas* and *Listeria*. In infants and older children, *Meningococcus* and *Pneumococcus* prevail. In early cerebritis, edema may be present, demonstrating low SI on T1-WI, high SI on T2-WI, and patchy contrast enhancement. When abscess formation develops, the center of the abscess and the surrounding edema are hypointense on T1-WI and hyperintense on T2-WI. The rim of an abscess is isointense on T1-WI and hypointense on T2-WI and will enhance intensely with paramagnetic contrast (see Chapter 4, Fig. 4.36). Subdural and epidural empyema occur more frequently in adolescents and usually follow sinusitis . Imaging reveals crescent- or lens-shaped extracerebral fluid accumulations with peripheral contrast enhancement.

■ **Lyme Disease.** Children are frequently affected by this multisystemic disorder caused by *Borrelia burgdorferi*, which is a tick-borne disease. In children, the typical triphasic course, comparable to that of lues, is not always observed. In 10%–20% of cases, a neurologic involvement with lymphocytic meningitis, meningoencephalitis, facial palsy, or palsy of other cranial nerves is present. On MRI, different patterns of manifestation can be found. Either focal lesions of the cerebral white matter with high SI on T2-WI and enhancement after paramagnetic contrast can be detected or meningitis with leptomeningeal enhancement. In patients with cranial neuropathy, enhancement of the affected cranial nerve may be found.

■ **Encephalitis.** Encephalitis is a nonsuppurative inflammation of the brain, sometimes accompanied by meningitis. Encephalitis can be due to autoimmune processes or to viral infections.

■ **Herpes Simplex I.** In older children, herpes simplex type I produces a more focal, localized meningoencephalitis, with swelling and mass effect displaying low SI on T1-WI and high SI on T2-WI involving the frontal and temporal lobes (see Chapter 4, Fig. 4.37). However, in children younger than 10 years of age, a generalized involvement of the brain is typically encountered. Because the virus has a predilection for the limbic system, the hippocampus and the amygdala are frequently involved. Encephalitis may be bilateral, and hemorrhage or hemorrhagic infarction may occur. Gyriform enhancement after administration of paramagnetic contrast may be present by the end of the first week. Calcifications occur as late sequelae in the following weeks. End-stage findings include volume loss and cystic encephalomalacia.

■ **Progressive Multifocal Leukencephalopathy.** Progressive multifocal leukencephalopathy is an inflammation caused by a papovavirus in immunocompromised patients. The disease has a fatal course with death occurring within 1 year after onset of symptoms, commonly consisting of hemiparesis, visual impairment, and dementia. On MRI, initially multifocal, later in the course confluent lesions in the periventricular and/or subcortical white matter are detected with increased SI on T2-WI. Mass effect is uncommon, and contrast enhancement is rarely seen.

■ **Subacute Sclerosing Panencephalitis.** Subacute sclerosing panencephalitis is probably the result of a slow, progressive measles infection, typically affecting those children between the ages of 5 and 12 years who had clinical measles before the age of 3 years. There is a relentless progression of the disease, with death occurring within 2–6 years. MRI shows nonspecific imaging findings with atrophy and diffuse bilateral areas of increased SI on T2-WI in the periventricular white matter and basal ganglia; these will not enhance with paramagnetic contrast or show mass effect. Occasionally, MRI will demonstrate involvement of the cerebellar white matter and pons.

■ **Rasmussen Encephalitis.** Rasmussen encephalitis is a chronic focal encephalitis tending to affect one hemisphere and can only be diagnosed by brain biopsy or postmortem. Children suffer from intractable focal seizures and progressive neurologic deficits. Initial MR examinations may be normal. In the course of the disease, MR demonstrates areas of increased SI on T2-WI in the white matter and/or in the putamen. On follow-up studies, progressive focal or hemispheric atrophy is revealed. Therefore, Rasmussen encephalitis is an important differential diagnosis of atrophies affecting one hemisphere, including congenital aplasia of the common carotid artery and atrophy secondary to infarction.

■ **Acute Disseminated Encephalomyelitis.** Children may develop acute disseminated encephalitis (ADEM) late in the course of a viral infection or after vaccination. This is caused by an autoimmune response; it is postulated that the precipitating illness induces a host-antibody response against a central-nervous antigen. Common clinical presentations are seizures and focal neurologic signs 4–7 days after the clinical onset of the viral infection. Less severe cases present with headache, fever, and myelopathy. The neurological symptoms resolve over a period of weeks, although 10%–20% of patients will have some permanent neurological damage. On MRI, the lesions presenting inflammation and demyelination are asymmetric hyperintensities on T2-WI in the subcortical white matter, either unilateral or bilateral, with no mass effect and may show occasional enhancement with paramagnetic contrast on T1-WI. Cortical and deep gray matter, particularly the thalami, may be involved. The brainstem, spinal cord, and the cerebellar white matter may also be affected (Fig. 16.21).

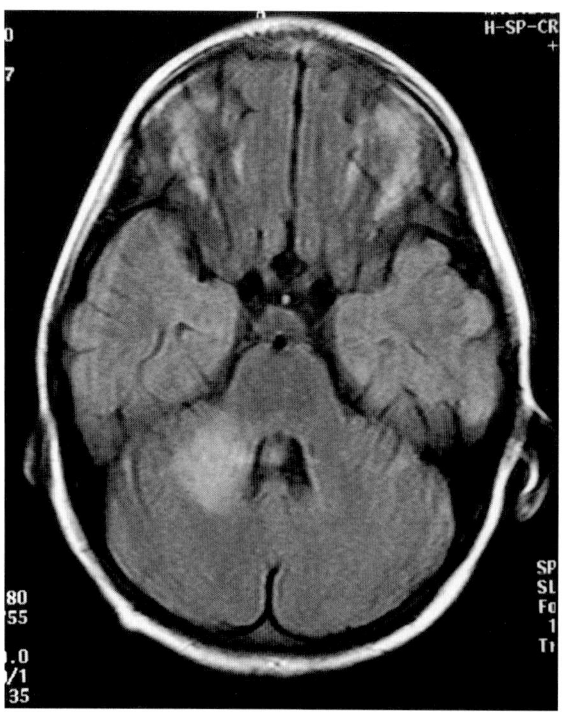

Fig. 16.21. Acute disseminated encephalitis. T2-W transverse image reveals hyperintensity in the right cerebellum

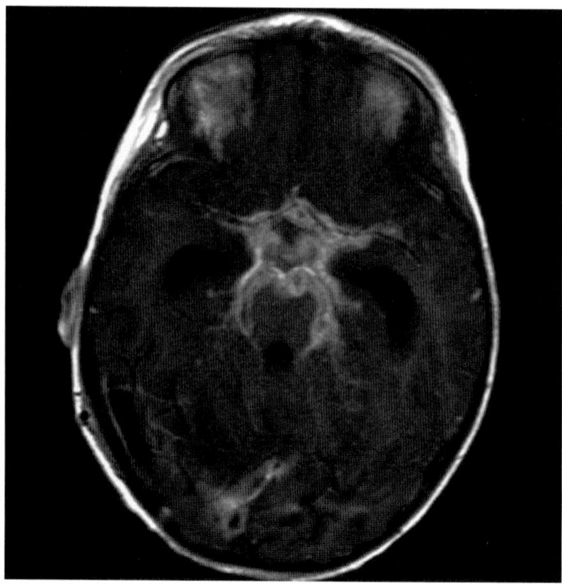

Fig. 16.22. Tuberculosis. Transverse contrast-enhanced T1-WI shows a basal meningitis

■ **Multiple Sclerosis: Encephalitis Disseminata.** MS is usually considered an adult disease, but occasionally manifests in childhood. MS is indistinguishable from ADEM by imaging findings; only labor findings, clinical history, and follow-up confirm the diagnosis. Imaging findings in children with MS do not differ from those in adults (see Chapter 4).

■ **Tuberculosis.** Tuberculosis typically causes basal meningitis with marked contrast enhancement of the basal leptomeninges (Fig. 16.22). Basal meningitis is very often complicated by hydrocephalus. It may cause vasculitis of the lenticulostriate and thalamoperforate vessels, leading to infarctions of the basal ganglia and thalami displaying low SI on T1-WI and high SI on T2-WI. Parenchymal tuberculomas will present as nodular or ring-enhancing lesions, often located at the gray/white matter junction and may calcify.

■ **Fungal Infections.** Fungal diseases of the CNS are less common in children than in adults. The most common fungi involved are *Cryptococcus neoformans*, *Candida*, *Aspergillus*, *Coccidioides immitis*, *Histoplasma capsulatum* and *Mucor*. They typically produce granulomatous basal meningitis similar to that seen in tuberculosis. Parenchymal abscesses, granulomas, and infarction due to vasculitis may also be present, depending on the species of fungi.

16.2.3.5 Brain Tumors in Childhood

CNS neoplasms during childhood are the second most common pediatric tumors, being exceeded only by leukemia (Fig. 16.23). In newborns, infratentorial and supratentorial tumors occur with almost the same frequency; germ-cell tumors, teratomas, gliomas, neuroepithelial tumors (PNETs), and choroid plexus papillomas are observed. In older children, posterior fossa neoplasms predominate, and therefore, primitive neuroepithelial tumors (PNETs, called medulloblastomas in most classifications), ependymomas, astrocytomas, and hemangioblastomas are frequently encountered. In general, the most common tumors in the pediatric age group are gliomas, ependymomas, medulloblastomas (PNETs), craniopharyngiomas, and pinealomas (Fig. 16.24).

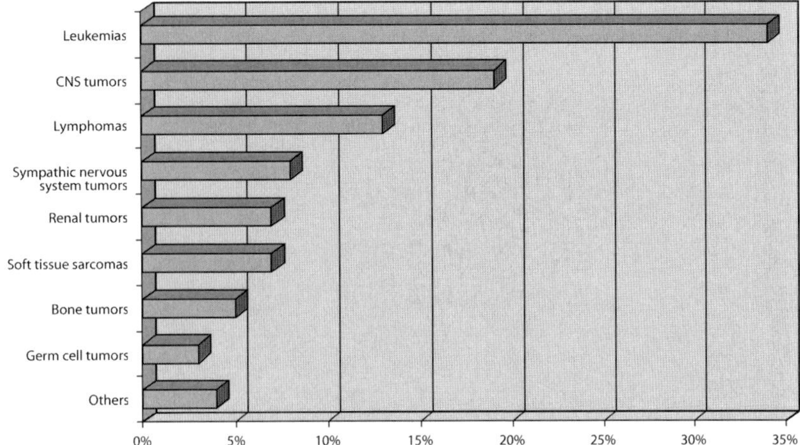

Fig. 16.23. Relative frequencies of the most common pediatric tumors in Germany (1990–1999). Adapted from Kaatsch et al. (2000)

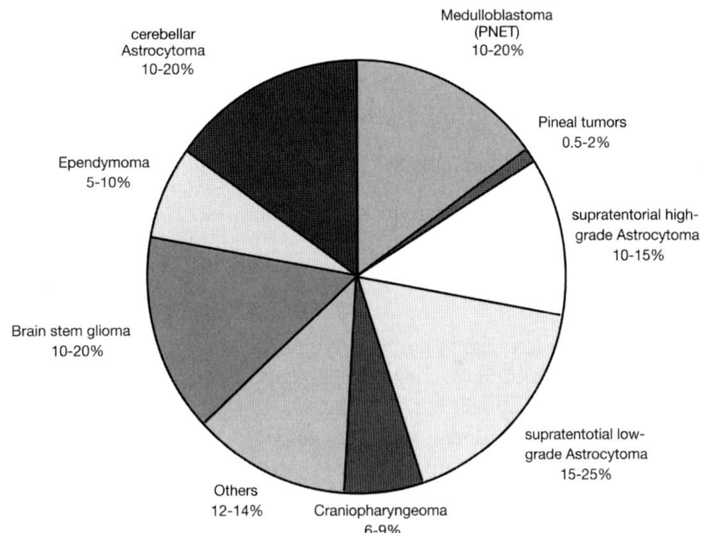

Fig. 16.24. Approximate incidence of common central nervous system tumors in children. Adapted from Heidemann et al. (1997)

For MR imaging of CNS neoplasms, T2-WI and T1-WI should be obtained in two planes, before and after the administration of paramagnetic contrast, preoperatively and postoperatively to analyze the neoplasm and its possible recurrence. Early postoperative imaging (in the first 72 h) is important, as the surgically induced contrast enhancement at the operative margins directly increases postoperatively. It will decrease on sequential exams after about 6 weeks and will generally disappear within 12 months. Meningeal enhancement is almost always seen on follow-up examinations and may persist, especially in patients with shunt tubes or subdural hygromas. A focus on the most common infratentorial and supratentorial tumors in children follows.

16.2.3.5.1 Intra-axial Infratentorial Tumors

■ **Medulloblastomas: PNETs.** Medulloblastomas (PNETs) are highly malignant tumors composed of very primitive, undifferentiated, small, round cells and account for approximately 10%–20% of common CNS tumors in children (Fig. 16.24). Classically, medulloblastomas present as hypointense tumors of the vermis

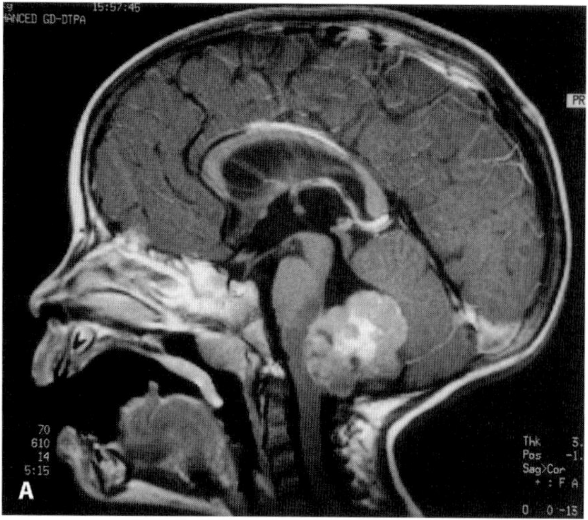

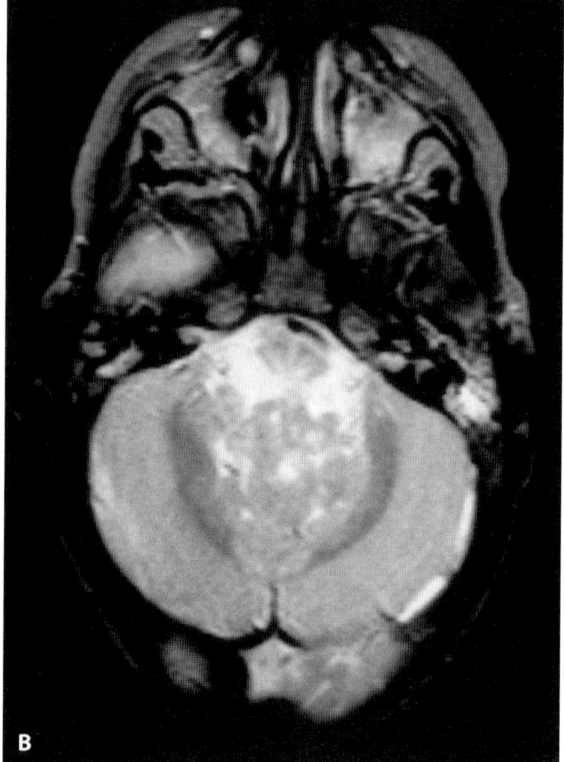

Fig. 16.25A,B. Medulloblastoma (primitive neuroepithelial tumors). Sagittal contrast-enhanced T1-WI (**A**) shows an inhomogeneously enhancing mass sitting in the fourth ventricle. Transverse T2-WI (**B**) shows the tumor to be of slightly mixed signal intensity, probably reflecting necrosis and solid tumor

on T1-WI with a variable contrast-enhancement pattern ranging from homogeneous to patchy. On T2-WI, medulloblastomas appear heterogeneously hypointense or isointense compared with gray matter. Cystic components may be present in up to 80% of medulloblastomas. Because of the location of this lesion, consecutive hydrocephalus is often observed. Medulloblastomas readily spread and develop subarachnoid metastasis. Therefore, precontrast and postcontrast studies of the brain and spine are recommended before surgery and for follow-up (Fig. 16.25 and 16.48; Table 16.6).

Table 16.5. Classification of astrocytic brain tumors

Diffuse or infiltrative type	Localized or non-infiltrative type
Astrocytoma	Pilocytic astrocytoma
Anaplastic astrocytoma	Pleomorpohic xanthoastrocytoma
Glioblastoma multiforme	Subependymal giant cell astrocytoma

Adapted from Atlas

■ **Astrocytomas.** Cerebellar astrocytomas account for 10%–20% of common CNS tumors in children (Fig. 16.24). About 60% of astrocytomas are located in the posterior fossa (40% in the cerebellum, 20% in the brainstem). Astrocytomas are glial tumors that arise from astrocytes and can be divided into two major groups: the infiltrative or diffuse astrocytomas and the localized, noninfiltrative astrocytomas (Table 16.5). In children, 85% of cerebellar astrocytomas are juvenile pilocytic astrocytomas (JPAs), which are of the localized type and considered relatively benign with a 90% survival rate at 10 years after total resection. About 15% of cerebellar astrocytomas are of the infiltrating type, similar to cerebral astrocytoma of the adult. Usually, the MR appearance of JPAs is virtually diagnostic. JPAs appear as well-demarcated cysts with a contrast-enhancing mural nodule (Fig. 16.26). On T1-WI, the cystic component is usually hypointense, but may be isointense to hyperintense due to hemorrhage or proteinaceous content. The infiltrating astrocytomas are solid lesions, frequently associated with hemorrhage

Table 16.6. Posterior fossa tumors in childhood

	JPA	Medulloblastoma (PNET)	Ependymoma	Brainstem astrocytoma
SI characteristics on T2	Cystic, sharply demarcated	Homogenous, low to moderate SI	Markedly heterogenous	Ill-defined, high SI
Contrast enhancement	Common in solid portion	Common, dense	Common, irregular	Common
Calcification	Uncommon	Uncommon	Common	Rare
Hemorrhage	Rare	Uncommon	Common	Uncommon
Tendency to seed via CSF	Extremely low	High	Low to moderate	Low
Prognosis (estimated survival)	>90% 10-year survival	50% 5-year survival	50% 5-year survival	20% 5-year survival

Adapted from Atlas PNET, primitive neuroepithelial tumors; JPA, juvenile pilocytic astrocytoma; SI, signal intensity; CSF, cerebrospinal fluid

and necrosis with variable presentation on MR imaging (Table 16.6).

■ **Brainstem Gliomas.** Astrocytomas account for 95% of brainstem neoplasms, which may be located in the pons, the midbrain extending to the thalami, or the medulla (see Chapter 4, Fig. 4.18). The vast majority of brainstem astrocytomas are of the infiltrative type. Less than 20% resemble the more benign JPAs on histology. MR appearance of brainstem astrocytomas is somewhat variable; they may be totally or partly solid with a cystic, necrotic, or hemorraghic component. Contrast enhancement is present in approximately half of the cases and is often focal and nodular. Pilocytic brain-

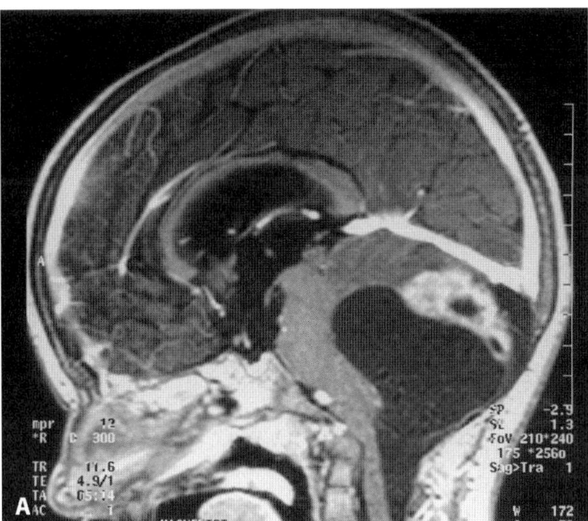

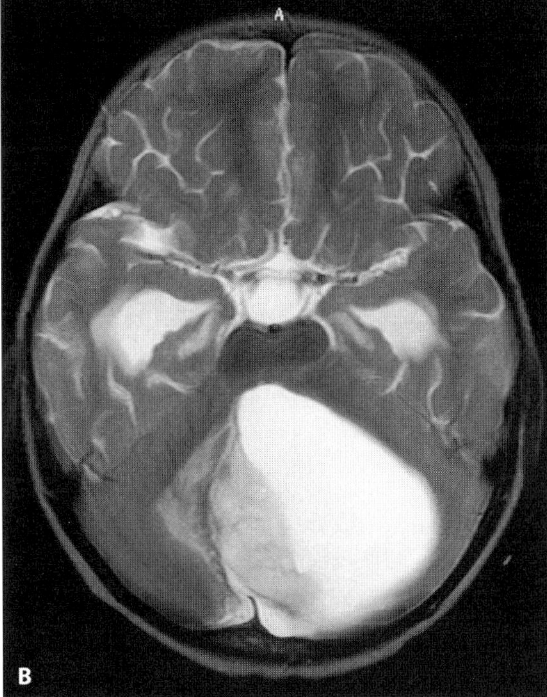

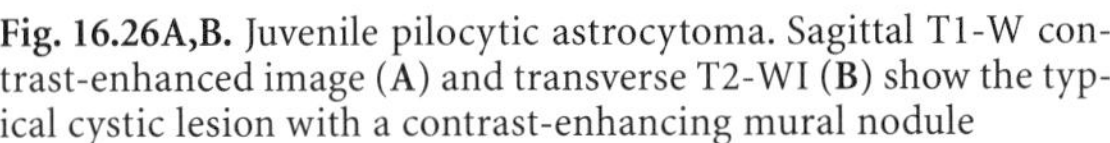
Fig. 16.26A,B. Juvenile pilocytic astrocytoma. Sagittal T1-W contrast-enhanced image (**A**) and transverse T2-WI (**B**) show the typical cystic lesion with a contrast-enhancing mural nodule

stem gliomas are often better circumscribed, markedly exophytic, and present as cerebellopontine angle lesions. These dorsally exophytic lesions, often being of the pilocytic type, enhance intensely after intravenous contrast and are grossly multicystic. Brainstem gliomas may spread by infiltrating to other portions of the brain, spinal cord, or outside the brain parenchyma via a CSF-leptomeningeal route to other parts of the brain and the spinal canal.

■ **Ependymomas.** Ependymomas account for 5%–10% of pediatric brain tumors, and 95% arise from the ependyma of the fourth ventricle. They present as intraventricular masses with calcifications. Ependymomas within the supratentorial region arise from ependymal rests of cells within the cerebral hemispheres. MRI reveals foci of high intensity (necrotic areas and cysts) and low intensity (calcifications or hemorrhage) within the tumors on T2-WI. On T1-WI, they may present as slightly hypointense masses with foci of marked hypointensity, with the solid portion of the tumors showing either a homogeneous or inhomogeneous enhancement after the administration of Gd-DTPA. However, ependymomas may be homogeneous on all imaging sequences; therefore, the pattern of growth is a major hint to the diagnosis. Ependymomas grow directly along an ependymal surface, particularly through the foramen of Luschka and the foramen of Magendie into the upper cervical canal (Fig. 16.27). In addition, they are the second most common brain tumor to metastasize outside the CNS; medulloblastoma is the most common one (Table 16.6).

16.2.3.5.2 *Intra-axial Supratentorial Tumors*

■ **Astrocytomas.** Supratentorial astrocytomas account for 25%–40% of brain tumors in children (Fig. 16.24). As already stated, astrocytomas can be divided into two major groups: the infiltrative or diffuse forms and the localized, noninfiltrative forms (Table 16.5). Of the latter, the pilocytic type arises in the optic chiasm and hypothalamus and is seen with a higher frequency in patients with NF-1. Pleomorphic xanthoastrocytomas are most often located on the surface of the temporal or occipital lobes. Subependymal giant-cell astrocytomas are lateral ventricular masses, particularly in young adults with tuberous sclerosis. Presently, the most wide-

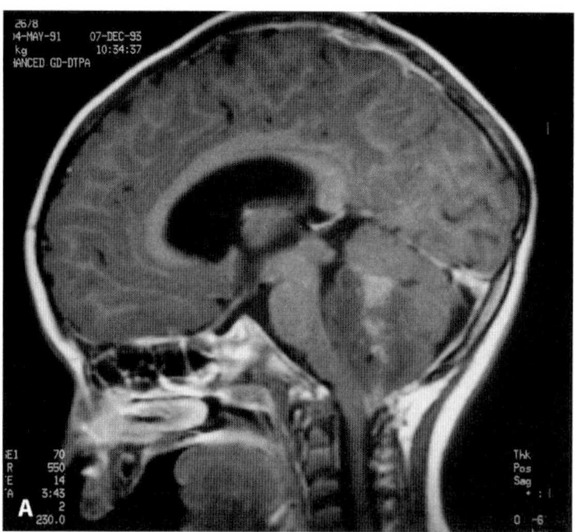

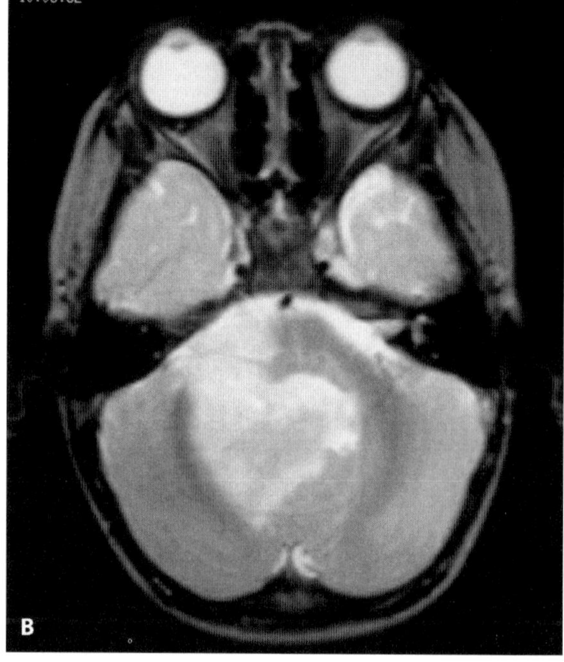

Fig. 16.27A,B. Ependymoma. Sagittal T1-W contrast-enhanced image (**A**) and transverse T2-WI (**B**) show a heterogeneously enhancing mass within the fourth ventricle extending down below the foramen magnum

ly accepted approach to grading of infiltrating astrocytomas derives from the World Health Organization's (WHO) classification of brain tumors, which separates these tumors into astrocytoma, anaplastic astrocytoma, and glioblastoma multiforme. These infiltrating lesions can arise in any part of the hemispheres, as well as in the infratentorial locations. On MR imaging, astrocytomas have very variable imaging features, and the tumors may be solid, cystic, or both. The absence or presence and pattern of contrast enhancement are key factors in evaluating the grade of astrocytoma. With the exception of JPAs, most low-grade astrocytomas show little or no contrast enhancement, whereas higher grade tumors will show enhancement after administration of paramagnetic contrast (see Chapter 4, Fig. 4.11, 4.12).

■ **Gangliogliomas, Gangliocytomas, and Dysembryoplastic Neuroepithelial Tumors.** Gangliogliomas, gangliocytomas, and dysembryoplastic neuroepithelial tumors (DNETs) are relatively benign tumors most commonly seen in children. They typically arise in the supratentorial space within the cerebral hemispheres. Frequent locations are the temporal lobes and the frontoparietal region but also the deep parts of the cerebral hemisphere . These slow-growing tumors are important because they are almost always associated with a long history of seizures without other neurologic findings, due to their site of occurrence in the region between the frontal and parietal lobes, and may be found in concert with mesial temporal sclerosis (see Chapter 4, Fig. 4.41). Therefore, resection of both is necessary for symptomatic relief. Gangliogliomas and gangliocytomas are typically hypodense on CT; approximately one-third appears cystic, one-third contains calcifications, and half of the tumors show contrast enhancement. The tumor signal is, therefore, variable on MRI. The solid tumors are usual hypointense on T1-WI and hyperintense on T2-WI. Cystic areas are higher in signal than surrounding CSF, and calcifications may cause mixed SI on T1-WI and hypointense signal on T2-WI.

■ **Primitive Neuroectodermal Tumors.** The category of PNETs represents a spectrum of primitive tumors, which may arise from a common neuroepithelial precursor. The PNET group includes medulloblastomas, cerebral neuroblastomas, retinoblastomas, pineoblastomas, ependymoblastomas, and medulloepitheliomas. Of the various subcategories, the cerebral neuroblastomas are considered prototypical. Cerebral neuroblastomas are tumors of younger children, comprising 15%–20% of neonatal brain tumors. Neuroblastomas may originate as primary brain tumors, or they may metastasize from neuroblastomas within the adrenal gland or the sympathetic paraspinal ganglionic chain. Primary neuroblastomas commonly occur in the frontal and parietal lobes. PNETs are usually quite large at the time of presentation and have an extraordinary variability. MR appearance ranges from homogeneous to markedly heterogeneous to a rim of solid tumor surrounding a central necrosis. Punctate calcifications may be apparent as foci of low SI. Cystic areas may present with or without hemorrhage. After administration of Gd-DTPA, there is always some enhancement, which varies from homogeneous to inhomogeneous, or may be ring-like, depending on the size and number of cysts and necrotic areas. When a large, sharply marginated, and markedly heterogeneous mass inducing only minimal edema is seen in a young child, the diagnosis of PNET should be made (Fig. 16.28). Seeding of tumor through the CSF pathways and metastases to the spinal cord, lungs, liver, and bone marrow have been reported.

■ **Germ-Cell Tumors.** Germ-cell tumors, including germinomas, embryonal carcinomas, endodermal sinus tumors, choriocarcinomas, and teratomas frequently arise from the pineal or hypothalamic region or both. With the exception of mature teratomas, all germ-cell tumors are classified as malignant tumors and possibly seed along CSF pathways. Germinomas demonstrate variable SI, ranging from hypointense to isointense on T1-WI and isointense to hyperintense on T2-WI. Contrast enhancement is seen after injection of Gd-DTPA. If a pineal lesion is discovered in concert with a suprasellar lesion in a child, the diagnosis germinoma (Fig. 16.29) is practically assured.

Embryonal carcinomas, yolk-sac tumors, and choriocarcinomas may produce α-feto-protein or β-human chorionic gonadotrophin (HCG) in CSF and usually have even more variable tumor intensity and contrast-enhancement characteristics.

Teratomas contain a mixture of differentiated tissue derived from all three embryonic germ layers and may be immature or mature. These tumors are usually lobulated, frequently cystic masses and may contain calcification, bone, teeth, or fat.

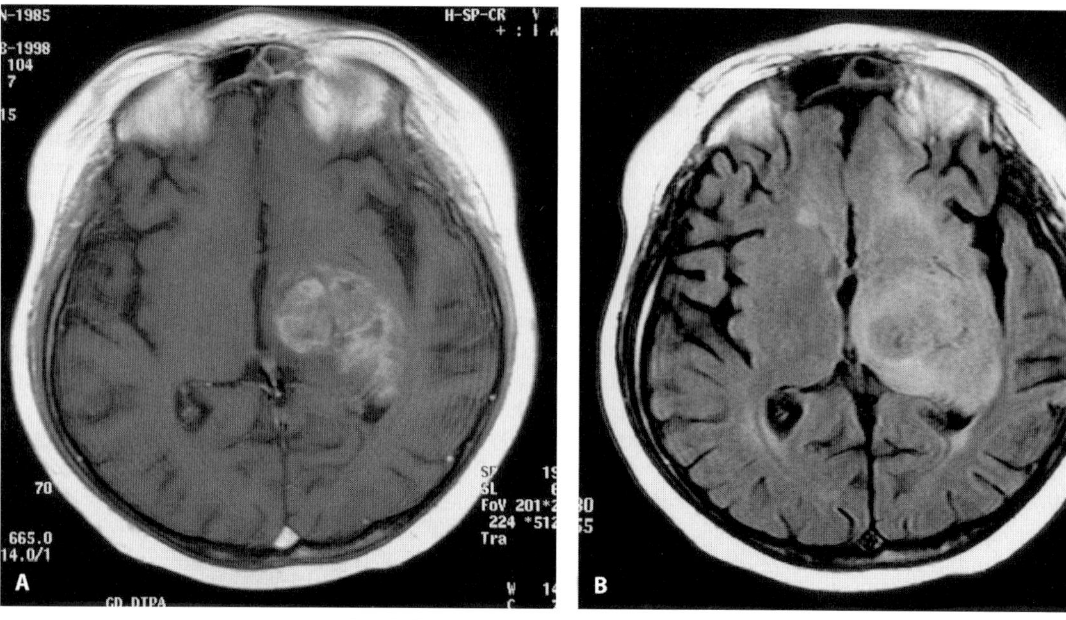

Fig. 16.28A,B. Primitive neuroepithelial tumor. Transverse T1-W contrast-enhanced image (**A**) and transverse fluid attenuated inversion recovery image (**B**) show heterogeneous enhancement of a large thalamic mass

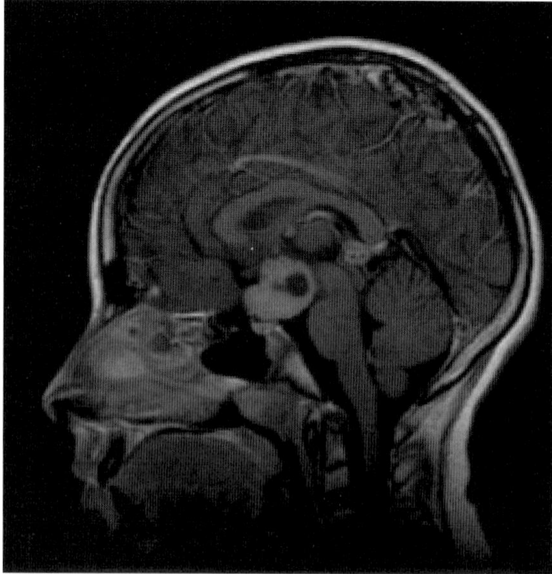

Fig. 16.29. Germinoma. T1-W contrast-enhanced image shows a pineal lesion in concert with a suprasellar lesion (courtesy of Prof. A. Heuck, MD, Radiologisches Zentrum Pippingerstrasse 25, Munich)

■ **Pinealomas.** Pineal parenchymal tumors include pineoblastomas, pineocytomas, and mixed pineal tumors. Pineoblastomas are highly malignant tumors readily metastasizing via CSF, demonstrating isointense signal on T2-WI and hypointense to isointense signal on T1-WI. They will show prominent enhancement with paramagnetic contrast. There is almost always ventricular enlargement due to obstruction. Pineocytomas are indistinguishable from pineoblastomas by CT and MRI.

16.2.3.5.3
Extra-Axial Supratentorial Tumors

■ **Craniopharyngiomas.** Craniopharyngiomas are among the most common parasellar mass lesions in children and account for 6%–9% of childhood intracranial tumors. Children with craniopharyngiomas will present with headache, nausea, vomiting, visual symptoms, and, in one-third of cases, endocrinological disturbances. Craniopharyngiomas may be entirely cystic or entirely solid, but most commonly are a combination of both. Calcifications are seen on CT in over 90% of the

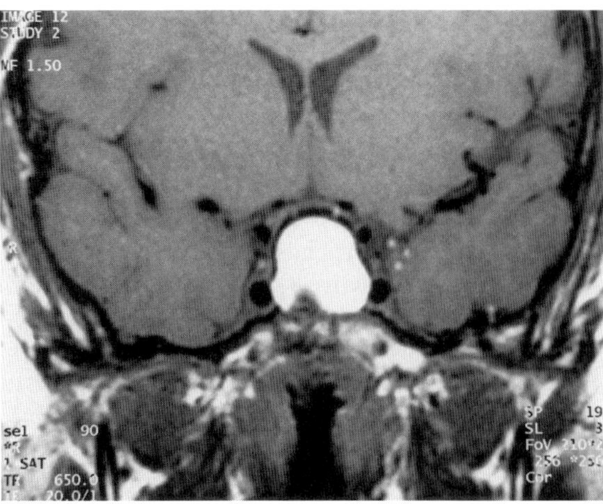

Fig. 16.30. Craniopharyngioma. Coronal T1-WI shows tumor with heterogeneous hypointense solid portion and hyperintense cystic portion

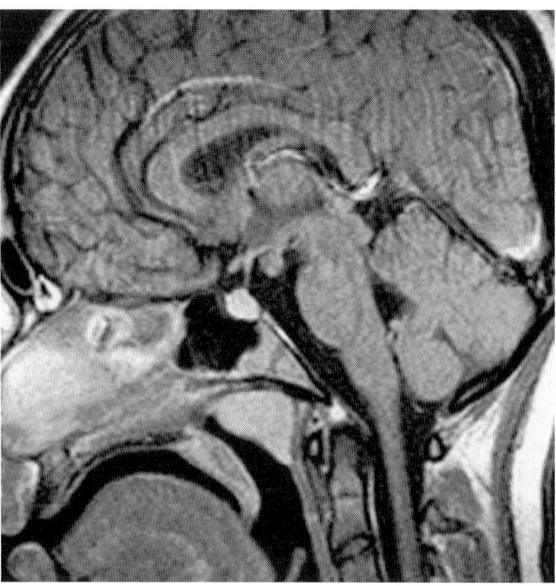

Fig. 16.31. Hamartoma of the tuber cinereum. T1-W sagittal contrast-enhanced image shows a sessile lesion originating from the tuber cinereum posterior to the stalk

cases but are less obvious on MRI; CT may, therefore, be necessary to prove their presence. The heterogeneous nature of craniopharyngiomas results in a variety of appearances on MR imaging. Solid tumors are usually isointense on T1-WI and hyperintense on T2-WI, but may be inhomogeneous due to tumor hemorrhage and/or calcifications. Cystic tumors are hyperintense on T2-WI and may be hypo-, iso-, or even hyperintense on T1-WI, depending on the presence of free methemoglobin or protein in the cysts (Fig. 16.30). Therefore, it is difficult to distinguish the cystic component from solid portions of the tumor without the administration of contrast.

■ **Hamartomas of the Tuber Cinereum.** Children with hamartomas of the tuber cinereum will present with precocious puberty and, more pathognomonically, with gelastic seizures characterized by fits of laughter-like outbursts. These either pedunculated or sessile lesions are located in the region of the mammillary bodies and demonstrate isointense SI to gray matter on T1-WI and isointense or slightly hyperintense SI on T2-WI. Hamartomas do not enhance after administration of Gd-DTPA (Fig. 16.31).

■ **Choroid Plexus Papillomas and Carcinomas.** Choroid plexus papillomas and carcinomas arise from the epithelium of the choroid plexus and account for 5% of supratentorial tumors in children. Most of these lesions are discovered within the first 5 years of life. Papillomas are most often found in the first year of life due to the resultant hydrocephalus. The most common sites of these lesions are the lateral ventricles, with the glomus being a frequent location. The diagnosis of papilloma is easily made on CT because of the location, punctate calcifications, and an occasional hemorrhage. The MR choroid plexus papillomas are lobulated intraventricular masses, mostly isointense in T1-WI, with uniform intense enhancement after the administration of Gd-DTPA. On T2-WI, these lesions are somewhat hypointense compared with gray matter. Approximately 5%–10% of papillomas degenerate to carcinomas.

Choroid plexus carcinomas are heterogeneous in appearance and invade the surrounding brain parenchyma. Due to hemorrhage and necrotic and cystic components, they often present with areas of high and low SI on T1-WI and T2-WI. These lesions have a poor prognosis because of their tendency to metastasize via the CSF.

16.2.3.6
Cerebrovascular Disease

Cerebrovascular disease in children is far more common than generally recognized. Cerebral infarctions, developmental vascular anomalies (persistent primitive arteries, hypoplasia/aplasia of the carotid arteries), fistulas, intracerebral vascular malformations, intracranial aneurysms, and the moyamoya syndrome are encountered in children.

As in adults, cerebral infarction can occur from intraluminal arterial or venous occlusion (thrombosis) or vasospasm induced by hypoxia or infection. Basically, imaging findings of basal-ganglia infarctions, arterial infarctions restricted to a typical territory, watershed, and venous infarctions do not differ from those encountered in adults. About 55% of strokes in children are ischemic, and 45% are hemorrhagic. Ischemic infarction may progress to a hemorrhagic stroke, or hemorrhagic infarction may be the initial presentation. Common causes for ischemic infarctions in children include cardiac disease, trauma, disorders of coagulation, primary dyslipoproteinemia, CNS infection, vascular disease associated with syndromes, primary or secondary CNS vasculitis, collagen-vascular disease, hemoglobinopathies, inborn errors of cerebral metabolism, and drug/irradiation-induced injury to the CNS. Hemorrhagic infarctions in children are frequently secondary to superficial and/or deep venous sinus occlusion. MR angiography should be additionally included in the sequence protocol for the evaluation of cerebrovascular disease in children.

16.2.3.6.1
Hypoxic-Ischemic Brain Injury in Preterm and Term Infants

Prolonged periods of hypoxia or anoxia result in severe damage to the brain, a problem commonly encountered perinatally. The pattern of destruction depends on three different factors:

1. severity of hypotension
2. duration of the event
3. maturity of the brain

In the case of mild to moderate reduction of blood flow, blood is shunted from the anterior to the posterior circulation in order to maintain sufficient perfusion of the brainstem, cerebellum, and basal ganglia. Therefore, the damaged areas are limited to vascular border zones between the major arterial territories. In profound hypotension with complete or near complete cessation of blood flow, the deep cerebral nuclei (thalami and basal ganglia) and the brainstem are initially affected. Damage to the cortex and white matter occurs later in the course of the hypotensive episode. The extent of the damage additionally depends on the duration of the event. Patients with relatively short arrests (10–15 min) have damage limited to the ventrolateral thalami, globus pallidus, posterior putamen, perirolandic cortex, and sometimes, hippocampi. With longer arrests (15–25 min), the superior vermis, the optic radiations, and the calcarine cortex are additionally affected. Finally, when arrest extends into the 25-min to 30-min range, nearly all of the gray matter is injured, and the child is left with diffuse multicystic encephalomalacia and shrunken basal ganglia (Fig. 16.32). The regions of the brain that are most susceptible to hypoxic-ischemic injury change with the postconceptional age of the child, as on one hand the vascular system is still under

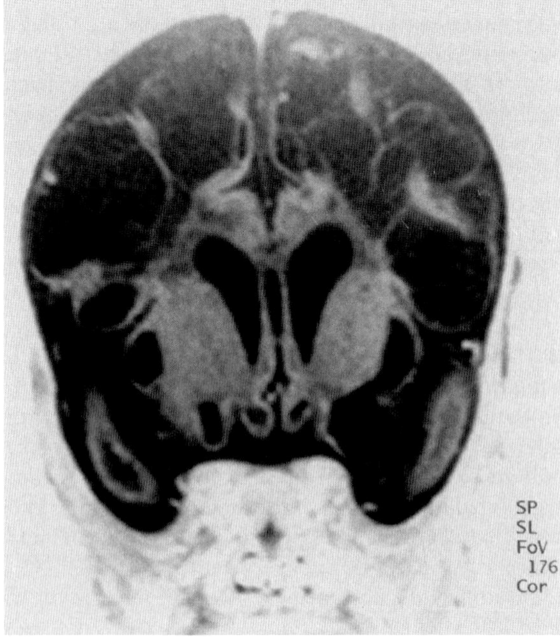

Fig. 16.32. Multicystic encephalomalacia. Coronal inversion recovery (IR) image shows enlargement of the lateral ventricles with multicystic encephalomalacia involving the hemispheric white matter and thinning of the cerebral cortex

Table 16.7. Patterns of hypoxic-ischemic brain injury

Age of child	Mild to moderate hypotension	Profound hypotension
Preterm newborn (<34 weeks postconception)	Periventricular white matter injury	Thalamic, basal ganglia, and brainstem injury
Term newborn (~36–56 weeks postconception)	Parasagittal watershed injury	Dorsal brainstem, thalamic, basal ganglia, and perirolandic cortex injury
Older child (>~6 months postnatally)	Parasagittal watershed injury	Basal ganglia and diffuse cortical injury

Adapted from Barkovich (2000)

development and on the other hand the relative energy requirements of various portions of the brain vary with state of maturity (Table 16.7).

In the preterm infant, most ischemic injury leads to germinal matrix bleeding, intraventricular hemorrhage, and periventricular leukomalacia (PVL). Prior to 35–36 weeks of gestational age, the border zone or watershed area between the major arterial territories (posterior choroidal branches and middle cerebral arteries) is in a periventricular location. Ischemic injury to the periventricular region produces necrosis of white matter, resulting in PVL and subsequent cystic degeneration. The two most common locations for PVL are the white matter adjacent to the foramen of Monro and the posterior periventricular white matter adjacent to the lateral aspect of the trigone of the lateral ventricles. MRI does not play a major role in the early diagnosis of PVL, as these sick premature neonates are primarily diagnosed and monitored by ultrasound in the neonatal intensive care unit. However, MR examinations are useful to determine the extent of damage in severely affected patients at a later time. MR findings of end-stage PVL (Fig. 16.33) are:

1. abnormally increased SI in the periventricular white matter on T2-WI, most commonly bilaterally observed in the peritrigonal regions,
2. ventriculomegaly with irregular outline of the body and trigone of the lateral ventricles,
3. reduced quantity of periventricular white matter, always at the trigones but, in severe cases, involving the whole centrum semiovale,
4. deep, prominent sulci that abut or nearly abut the ventricles with little or no interposed white matter,
5. delayed myelination,
6. thinning of the corpus callosum, most commonly the posterior body and splenium.

In term infants, the severity of an insult compared with that of a preterm infant must be significantly greater to lead to morphologic changes. The vascular border zones are typically in a parasagittal location high over the cerebral convexities between the anterior and middle cerebral arteries and the middle and posterior arteries. These border regions lie within the cortical mantle and the underlying white matter. Consequently, asphyxia produces a pattern referred to as ulegyria (mushroom-shaped gyri) with shrunken gyri and enlarged sulci. In the chronic phase, encephalomalacia is noted in the parasagittal regions.

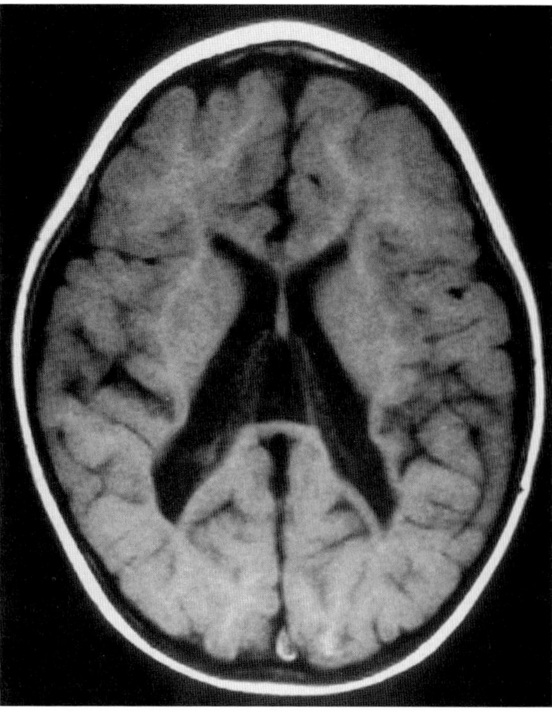

Fig. 16.33. End-stage periventricular leukomalacia. Transverse T1-WI shows enlarged ventricles with irregular borders. The cerebral cortex nearly abuts the ventricular surface because of the diminished volume of white matter

16.2.3.6.2 *Arterial Infarctions in Preterm and Term Infants*

Based on autopsy data, arterial infarctions in the term infant are far more common (17%) than in the preterm infant (3%–5%). Due to the normal appearance of the unmyelinated brain, it may be difficult to detect subtle edema and/or hypoperfusion of the involved brain. Cortical infarctions are best identified on T1-WI as areas of hypointensity, while adjacent white matter becomes slightly hyperintense. The gyri may be minimally hyperintense and appear swollen on T2-WI. There is a loss in the ability to distinguish between white and gray matter. Gyral enhancement with paramagnetic contrast is common within 5–10 days of the acute event.

16.2.3.6.3 *Venous Thrombosis*

Superficial and/or deep venous-sinus occlusion in children is frequently secondary to prematurity and germinal-matrix hemorrhage, dehydration, hypercoagulable states, infection, or trauma (Fig. 16.34). Hemorrhagic infarctions not corresponding to an arterial vascular territory should suggest venous thrombosis. Deep venous system occlusion is more common in children than in adults and presents with infarction and hemorrhage of the deep gray-matter nuclei and the thalami. The combination of infarction and hemorrhage of the thalamus associated with intraventricular bleeding should raise the suspicion of underlying deep-vein thrombosis, especially in full-term neonates.

16.2.3.6.4 *Vein of Galen Aneurysm*

A vein of Galen aneurysm is a rare congenital-vascular malformation demonstrating single or multiple fistulas between cerebral arteries and the vein of Galen. It is classified into choroidal and mural types. The choroidal type is more common (90%), usually presenting in the neonate with congestive heart failure, intracranial

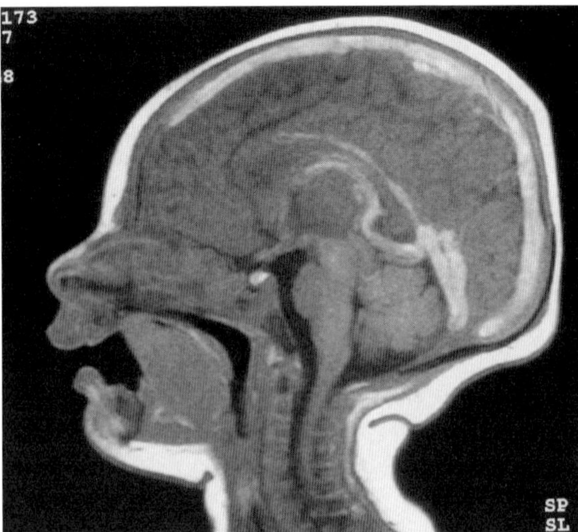

Fig. 16.34. Venous thrombosis. Sagittal T1-WI demonstrates high signal intensity in the superior sagittal sinus, straight sinus, inferior sagittal sinus, vein of Galen, and internal cerebral vein. Note that the pituitary gland is convex and demonstrates a uniform high signal; this is the normal appearance of the pituitary gland in newborns (courtesy of W. Michl, MD, Institut für Röntgendiagnostik des Krankenhauszweckverbandes, Kinderradiologie, Augsburg)

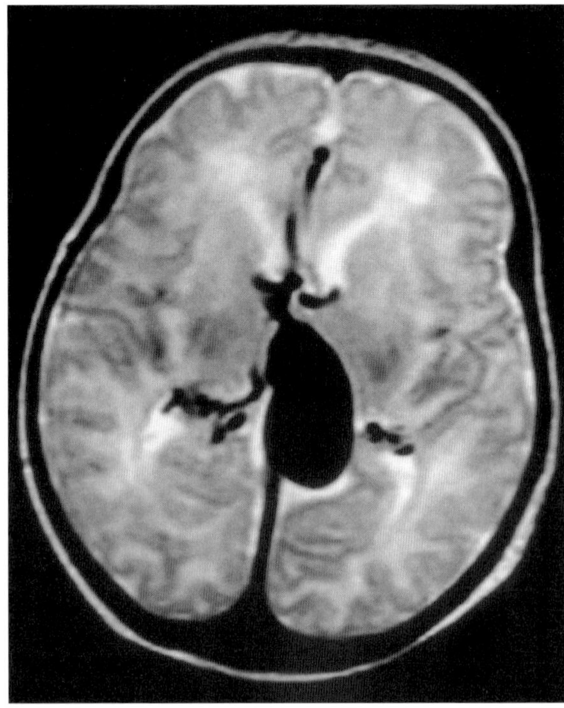

Fig. 16.35. Vein of Galen aneurysm. Transverse T2-WI of a 7-day-old newborn displays a huge rounded lesion with flow void in the midline (courtesy of W. Michl, MD, Institut für Röntgendiagnostik des Krankenhauszweckverbandes, Kinderradiologie, Augsburg)

bruit, and/or hydrocephalus (Fig. 16.35). The mural type of Galenic malformation presents later in infancy with developmental delay, seizures, and hydrocephalus. These two conditions must be differentiated from a parenchymal arteriovenous malformation (AVM) in the midbrain or thalamus with drainage into the deep venous system, including the vein of Galen and the straight sinus. These AVMs frequently present with hemorrhage in older children and adults. MR imaging of a vein of Galen aneurysm demonstrates a huge rounded lesion, dorsally located in the midline, which displays no signal on both T1-WI and T2-WI, due to flow void. Concurrent thrombosis can be depicted by T1-W sequences before contrast and by MR angiography. A 3D PC MR angiography should be performed to display feeding vessels and venous drainage of this lesion.

16.2.3.6.5 Moyamoya Disease

Moyamoya disease is a primary arterial disorder leading to occlusion of the intracranial internal carotid artery, accompanied by the development of collaterals. It is mainly encountered in Japan. Moyamoya is Japanese and means 'hazy, like a puff or cloud of smoke' and describes the angiographic appearance of this condition. Furthermore, the same radiographic pattern has been described in children with sickle-cell anemia, collagen-vascular disorders, NF-1, Down syndrome, as well as after radiation therapy. This condition is referred to as the moyamoya syndrome by some authors. MR reveals infarcts in up to 80% of cases and multiple flow voids corresponding to enlarged basal collateral arteries at the level of the middle cerebral artery and the basal ganglia.

16.2.3.7 Child Abuse

Intracranial injury is the main reason for death and disability in child abuse. If an inconclusive history is given for an injury in a young child or injuries of varying ages

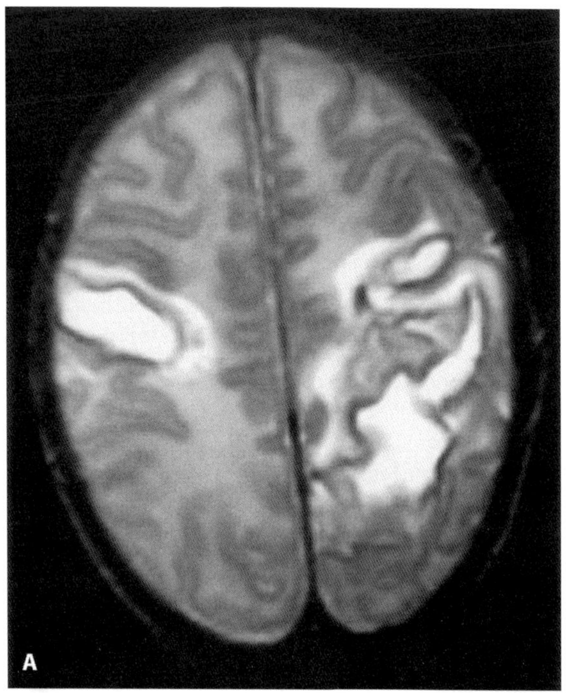

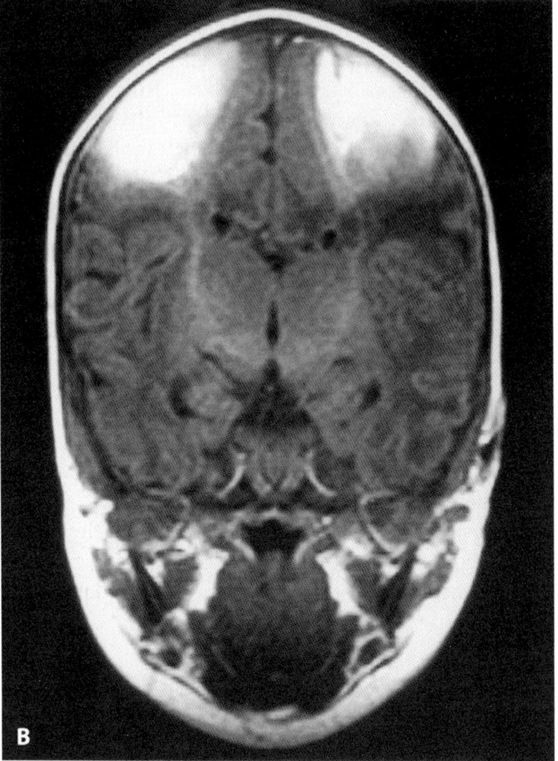

Fig. 16.36A,B. Child abuse. Transverse T2-WI (**A**) and coronal T1-WI (**B**) show huge bilateral parenchymal bleedings involving both hemispheres in a 5-week-old battered infant

Table 16.8. Sequence protocol recommendations for evaluation of pediatric spine

Sequence	WI	Plane	No. of slices	TR (ms)	TE (ms)	Flip angle	TI (ms)	Echo train length	Slice thickness (mm)	Matrix	FOV	recFOV (%)	Band-width (Hz)	No. of acq.	Acq. time (min:s)
TSE	T2	sag	11	4300	112	180		15	3	270×512	320	62.5	130	3	3:56
SE	T1	sag	11	473	20	90			3	160×512	320	62.5	65	1	2:34
with FS	T1	sag	11	660	20	90			3	160×512	320	62.5	65	1	3:34
SE	T1	tra	15	450	14	90			4	256×256	180	100	89	1	3:53
with FS	T1	tra	15	735	14	90			4	256×256	180	100	89	1	6:20

Abbreviations: *WI* weighting of images; *TR* repetition time (ms); *TE* echo time (ms); *TI* inversion time (ms); *Matrix* phase × frequency matrix; *recFOV* rectangular field of view (%); *Acq.* acquisition(s)

are present, child abuse should be considered. Approximately 40% of physically abused children are infants, and 80% of children are less than 5 years of age. Signs of child abuse in the CNS are spread sutures and bilateral skull fractures, subdural and subarachnoid hemorrhages, petechial hemorrhages of the parenchyma, shearing injuries, cortical contusions, cerebral edema, and infarctions. Intrahemispheric subdural hematoma (shaken-impact injury) and subdural hematoma associated with hypoxic-ischemic injury or infarction (strangulation/suffocation injury) make one particularly suspicious of child abuse. Noncontrast CT depicts acute hemorrhage with high sensitivity. Furthermore, contrast-enhanced MRI should be performed in order to date the timing of CNS injuries and to rule out other lesions causing the patient's symptoms (Fig. 16.36).

16.3 Pediatric Spine Imaging

16.3.1 Coils and Patient Positioning

The spine coil or the spine-array coil should be used for imaging of the spine. Optimal positioning in the center of the coil and immobilization with vacuum beds, sponges, sand bags, and blankets are mandatory for patients.

16.3.2 Sequence Protocol

The standard protocol for evaluation of the spine should include T2-WI and T1-WI in a sagittal plane and a T1-WI transverse plane through the region of interest (Table 16.8). For the evaluation of associated tumors in spinal dysraphism, tumors, infections, and inflammations, paramagnetic contrast agents should be administered, and FS T1-WI in sagittal and transverse planes should be additionally obtained. Coronal planes are useful in the evaluation of patients with paraspinal masses (NF, neuroblastoma), scoliosis, and split-cord malformation.

16.3.3 Common Findings in Pediatric Spine Imaging

16.3.3.1 Appearance of the Spine in the Neonate

The normal appearance of the spine can be difficult to interpret, especially in newborns and young infants. From birth to 1 month of age, T1-WI show hypointense ossified vertebral bodies adjacent to hyperintense nonossified cartilage with small hypointense disks. T2-WI are easier to interpret, as ossified and nonossified parts of the vertebrae are hypointense, while the disks are hyperintense (Fig. 16.37). From 1 to 6 months, conversion of the vertebrae start from the periphery to the center. Therefore, the periphery of the vertebrae is hyperintense on T1-WI, with the center of the vertebrae and the disks remaining hypointense. Appearance on

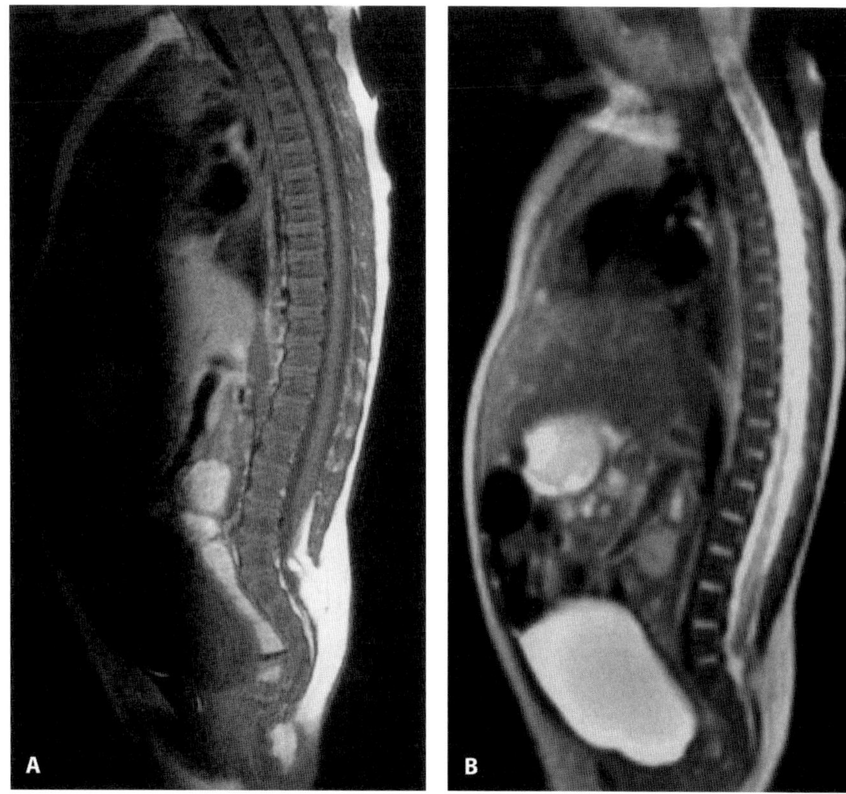

Fig. 16.37A,B. Normal appearance of the vertebral bodies and disks from birth to 3 months of age in an infant with lipomyelocele and tethered cord. Sagittal T1-WI (**A**) of a 4-week-old infant reveals the hypointense ossified vertebrae with the hyperintense, nonossified cartilage on each end. The hyperintense endplates of the vertebral bodies are separated by a thin, hypointense structure that represents the intervertebral disk. Sagittal T2-WI (**B**) demonstrates ossified and nonossified parts of the vertebrae as hypointense, while the disks are hyperintense. In addition, images display spina bifida aperta with a lipomyelocele and tethered cord

T2-WI remains the same. From 7 months on, vertebrae are hyperintense and disks hypointense on T1-WI. T2-WI remain the same and are easy to interpret.

16.3.3.2 Developmental Abnormalities

During the fourth week after gestation, the conversion of the neural plate into the neural tube takes place, by a process called neurulation (Fig. 16.38A–F). Neurulation begins in the occipitocervical region as the neural plate invaginates along its central axis to form a longitudinal median neural groove that has neural folds on both sides. The lateral edges of the neural folds meet in the midline and fuse, while simultaneously separating from the surface ectoderm. The free edges of the surface ectoderm then fuse with each other so that this layer becomes continuous over the neural tube. At the same time, the neural crest cells migrate ventrolaterally on each side of the neural tube and form a flattened mass, called the neural crest. The neural crest then separates into right and left parts and begins to migrate and give rise to dorsal-root ganglia, ganglia of the autonomic nervous system, and some other structures. Disturbance of this process may result in severe anomalies. In the case of premature separation of neural ectoderm from cutaneous ectoderm, mesenchyme cells gain access to the inner surface of the neural tube. Mesenchyme cells are believed to evolve into fat when mingling with primitive ependyma, thus giving rise to spinal lipomas. Complete nondysjunction of cutaneous ectoderm from neural ectoderm results in the forma-

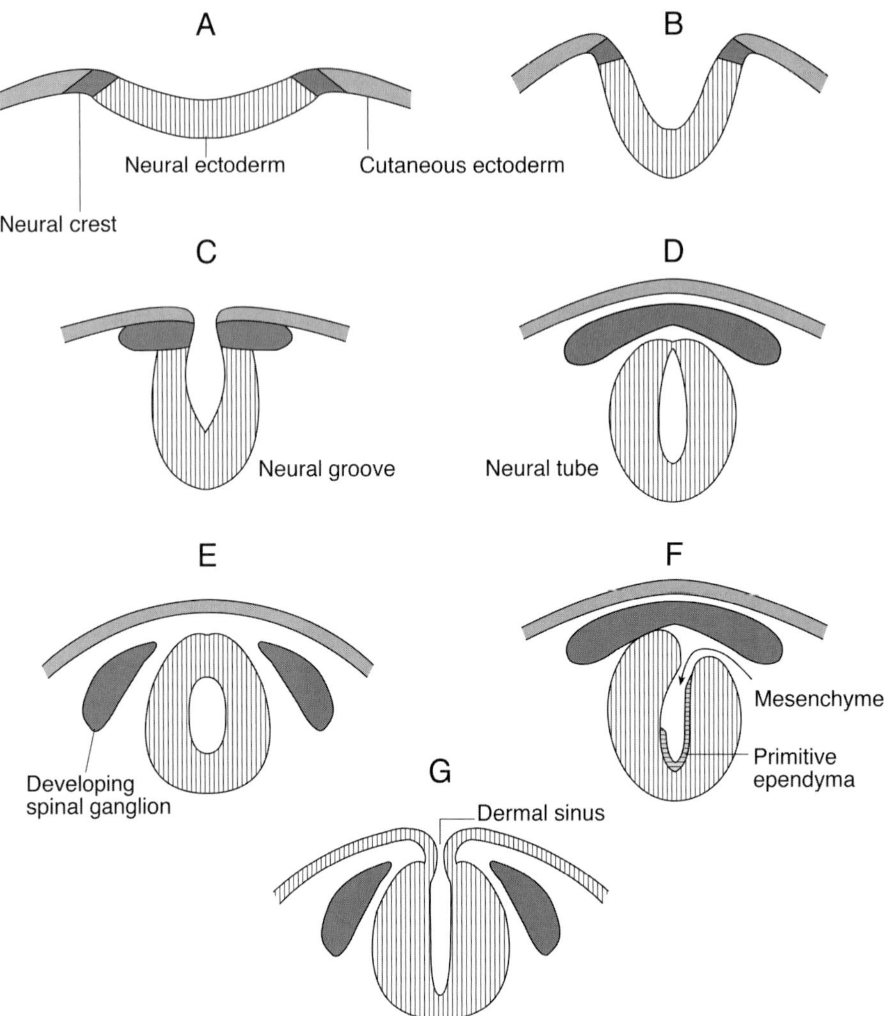

Fig. 16.38A–G. Normal and abnormal neurulation. **A–E** Normal neurulation. The neural plate is composed of neural ectoderm, neural crest, and cutaneous ectoderm. **B** During the third week of gestation, the neural plate begins to thicken and fold. **C** The neural plate invaginates along its central axis and forms the median neural groove. **D** Neurulation (closure of the neural tube) begins when the neural folds meet in the midline. The overlying ectoderm separates from the neural tissue and fuses in the midline and becomes continuous over the neural tube. At the same time, the neural crest cells migrate ventrolaterally and form a transient structure immediately dorsal to the tube. **E** The neural crest then separates into right and left parts and migrates to form root ganglia and multiple other structures. **F, G** Abnormal neurulation. **F** In case of premature disjunction of the neural ectoderm from the cutaneous ectoderm, the surrounding mesenchyme gains access to the inner surface of the neural tube and evolves to fat. This process is postulated to give rise to spinal lipomas. Complete nondysjunction of cutaneous ectoderm from neural ectoderm results in the formation of myelomeningoceles. **G** Focal nondysjunction results in the formation of a dorsal dermal sinus. Adapted from Barkovich (2000)

tion of myelomeningoceles, whereas focal nondysjunction results in the formation of a dermal sinus. Furthermore, multiple spine anomalies can be present in the same patient. A patient with myelomeningocele may have diastematomyelia, a tight filum terminale, and a dorsal sinus as well. Consequently, it is important to image the whole spine as soon as a cutaneous or vertebral body anomaly is discovered.

16.3.3.2.1 Spinal Dysraphism

Spinal dysraphism is a group of spinal column and neuroaxis disorders in which there is a defective midline closure of the neural, bony, and other mesenchymal tissues. In almost all cases of spinal dysraphism, there are vertebral body anomalies indicating the level of the lesion. The term spina bifida refers to incomplete posterior closure of the bony elements of the spine. Spina bifida aperta refers to an open neurulation defect, in which the neural tissue is exposed through a spina bifida without skin covering. Meningoceles, myelomeningoceles, and myeloceles belong to this group. Occult spinal dysraphism, in which the myelodysplasia lies beneath intact skin, includes lesions such as dermal sinus, spinal lipoma, lipomyelomeningoceles, myelocystoceles, tight filum terminale syndrome, diastematomyelia, and caudal-regression syndrome. Patients with occult spinal dysraphism almost always have cutaneous stigmata, such as a hairy patch, a nevus, a hemangioma, or a sinus tract.

16.3.3.2.2 Myelocele, Meningocele, and Myelomeningocele

Myelocele, meningocele, and myelomeningocele result from a lack of closure of the neural tube. In a myelocele, the neural tissue cannot separate from the cutaneous ectoderm, and therefore, the placode of reddish neural tissue is seen in the middle of the back. Myelomeningocele is almost identical to myelocele with the exception that there is an expansion of the ventral subarachnoid space, which posteriorly displaces the placode. A meningocele is characterized by the frequent presence of a complete skin covering and herniation of distended spinal meninges but not neural tissue through the dysraphic spine (Fig. 16.39). The Arnold Chiari II malformation is rarely present in patients with meningocele but is essentially always associated with myelomeningocele and myelocele. Due to the risk of infection, these entities are rarely imaged and are operated on within the first 24–48 h of life.

16.3.3.2.3 Hydrosyringomyelia/Syringohydromyelia

By definition, hydromyelia is the accumulation of fluid in the enlarged, ependymal-lined central canal of the spinal cord. Syringomyelia and syrinx are defined as diverticulation of the central canal with associated dissection of CSF into the cord parenchyma, resulting in glial-lined cysts, which may or may not communicate with the central canal. Because these two are difficult to distinguish by imaging, the terms hydrosyringomyelia or syringohydromyelia are used to describe these find-

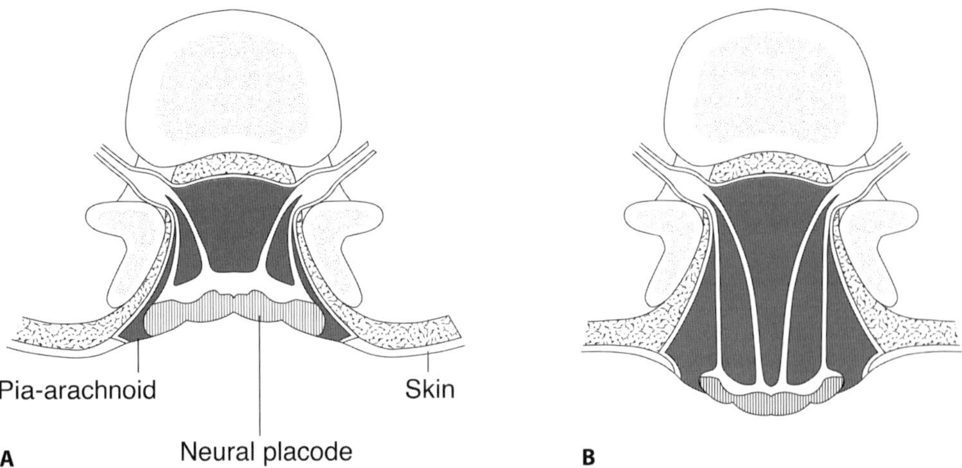

Fig. 16.39A,B. Myelocele and myelomeningocele. **A** Myelocele. The neural placode is a flat plaque of neural tissue that is exposed to air. The dura is deficient posteriorly, and the ventral surface of the placode and dura is lined by the pia and arachnoid, forming an arachnoid sac. Both the dorsal and ventral roots arise from the ventral surface of the placode. **B** Myelomeningocele. In this similar entity, the placode is posteriorly displaced due to expansion of the ventral subarachnoid space. Adapted from Barkovich (2000)

ings. Hydrosyringomyelia or syringohydromyelia are observed in multiple congenital anomalies, such as Arnold Chiari I and II (see Chapter 4, Fig. 4.5), lipomyelomeningocele, myelomeningocele, diastematomyelia (Fig. 16.43), Dandy-Walker cysts, or may occur secondary to intramedullary or extramedullary tumors, ischemia, inflammation, and trauma.

16.3.3.2.4 Congenital Dermal Sinus

Congenital dermal sinus is an epithelium-lined channel which extends from the skin to the spinal canal and may either reach the dura or pass through it (Fig. 16.38F). If the sinus tract passes the dura, it may end in, or traverse, the subarachnoid space and terminate within the conus medullaris, the filum terminale, a nerve root, or an epidermoid/dermoid cyst.

16.3.3.2.5 Lipomyelocele, Lipomyelomeningocele, Myelocystocele

Lipomyelocele and lipomyelomeningocele are very similar to myelocele and myelomeningocele with the following additional features: a symmetrical or asymmetrical lipoma is attached to the dorsal surface of the placode, which is continuous with the subcutaneous fat and covered by an intact layer of skin (Fig. 16.40B,C).

16.3.3.2.6 Intradural Lipoma

Intradural lipomas are a group of fatty tumors lying almost entirely within the bony spinal canal. They are typically subpial-juxtamedullary dorsal lesions, with the lipoma located between the central canal and the pia. Most commonly, intradural lipomas are found in the cervical or thoracic spine. The imaging characteristics of intradural lipomas are similar to those of subcutaneous fat (Fig. 16.41 and 16.40A).

16.3.3.2.7 Tight Filum Terminale and Tethered Cord

Tethered cord may occur alone or in association with other lower spinal anomalies and is defined as an abnormal low position of the conus terminalis. This tethering may either be primary due to a tight filum terminale or secondary to other dysraphic entities, such as diastematomyelia, lipo/myelomeningoceles, or after meningomyelocele repair. Patients will present with neurologic symptoms (bowel or bladder dysfunction,

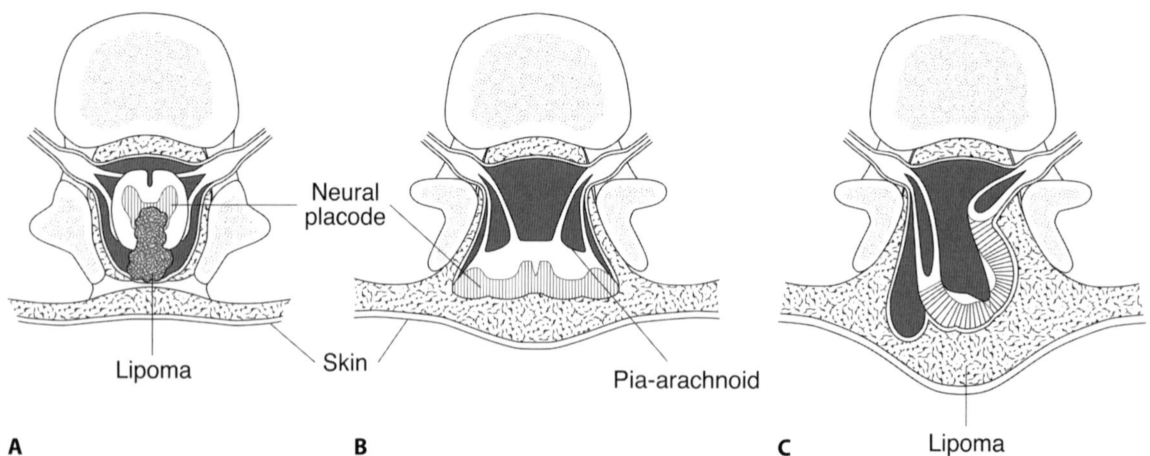

Fig. 16.40A–C. Illustration of spinal lipomas, lipomyelocele, and lipomyelomeningocele. **A** Intradural (subpial-juxtamedullary) lipoma. The spinal cord is open in the midline dorsally with the lipoma located between the unapposed lips of the placode. **B** Lipomyelocele. This lesion is very similar to a myelocele with two additional features: the lipoma is situated dorsally and attached to the surface of the placode. It is continuous with subcutaneous fat and covered by skin. **C** Lipomyelomeningocele with rotation of the neural placode. When the lipoma is asymmetric, it extends into the spinal canal and causes the ventral meningocele to herniate posteriorly and the dorsal surface of the placode to rotate to the side of the lipoma. Adapted from Barkovich (2000)

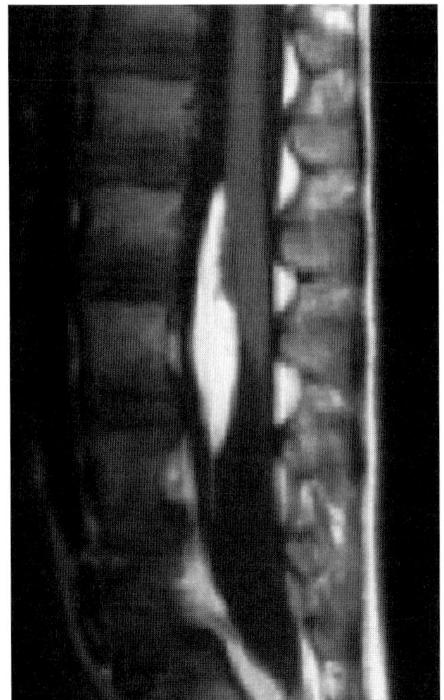

Fig. 16.41. Intradural lipoma: sagittal T1-WI demonstrates a hyperintense mass within the lumbar spinal canal and tethered cord (courtesy of G. Schuierer, MD, Radiologie, Westfälische-Wilhelms Universität, Münster)

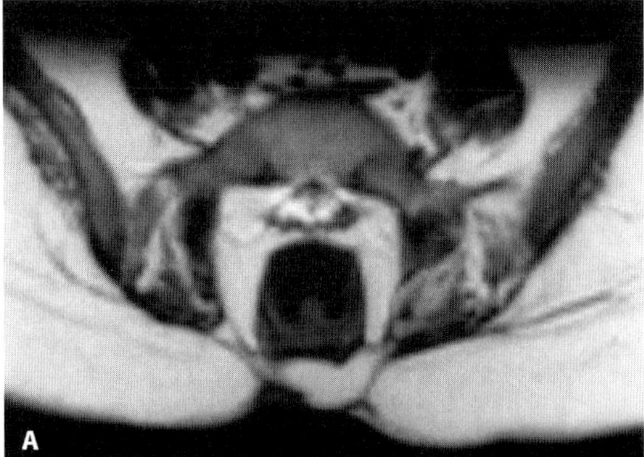

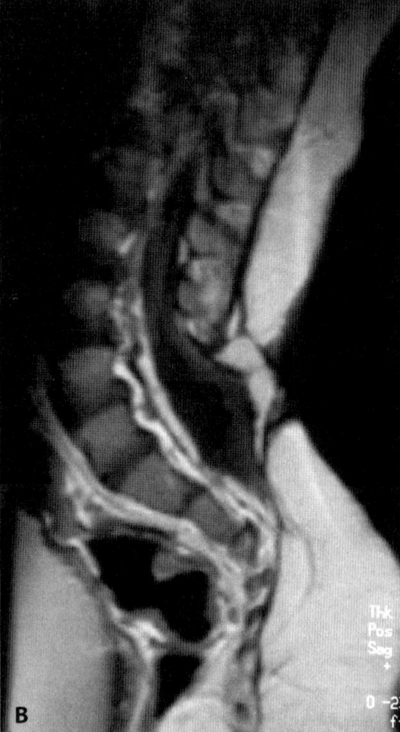

Fig. 16.42A,B. Lipomyelocele. Transverse (**A**) and sagittal (**B**) T1-WI display a typical example of a lipomyelocele with tethered cord. Compare with Fig. 16.40B

gait disturbances, weakness), orthopedic symptoms (scoliosis, foot deformities, back pain), or urologic symptoms (urinary incontinence, recurrent urinary-tract infections). The definitive diagnosis is made by demonstration of the conus medullaris below the L2/L3 interspace, associated with a short and thickened filum terminale, or termination of the conus or filum in a dysraphic lesion, such as a lipomyelocele (Fig. 16.42) or other developmental tumors, such as epidermoids/dermoids or lipomas (Fig. 16.41).

16.3.3.2.8 Diastematomyelia

Diastematomyelia is the most common anomaly of the split notochord syndrome spectrum. A bony or fibrous band coursing from the posterior elements to the vertebral body splits the spinal cord sagittally into two symmetric or asymmetric hemicords, each having the ventral and dorsal nerve roots for that side (Fig. 16.43). Diastematomyelia is commonly associated with thickened filum terminale, myeloceles, myelomeningoceles, hemimyeloceles, lipomas, dermal sinus, epidermoid/dermoid tumors, and tethering adhesions. Anomalies of the vertebral bodies are nearly always present in dia-

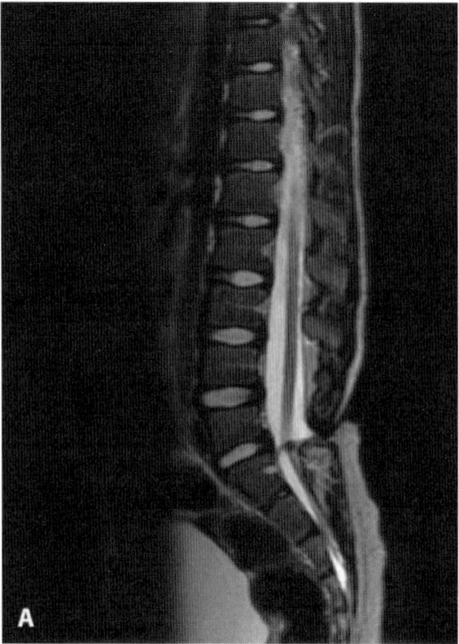

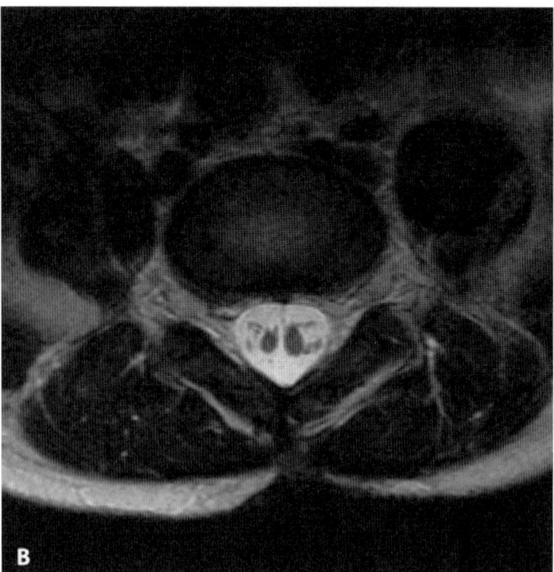

Fig. 16.43A,B. Diastematomyelia. Sagittal T2-WI (**A**) shows a tethered-cord syndrome in concert with a spur. Transverse T2-WI (**B**) displays diastematomyelia with two hemicords, each having the ventral and dorsal nerve roots for that side

stematomyelia, and kyphoscoliosis follows in more than 50% of the patients. For definition of the bony or fibrous septum by MRI, it is necessary to obtain transverse T1-WI and T2-WI. Since even osseous spurs can be missed on T1-WI, transverse SE T2-W or transverse T2* GRE sequences are recommended. The spur is hypointense compared with CSF on T1-WI if nonossified, and hyperintense, if ossified. On T2-WI, the spur is hypointense, whether it is bony, cartilaginous, or fibrous.

16.3.3.2.9 Hemimyelocele

In 31%–46% of patients with myelomeningocele or myelocele, there is an association with diastematomyelia. In some patients, only one of the hemicords is combined with a myelomeningocele. The term hemimyelocele is used to describe this anomaly. The other hemicord most commonly terminates in the filum terminale within the spinal canal and may or may not be associated with either a second small myelomeningocele at a lower level and/or tethered cord.

16.3.3.2.10 Caudal-Regression Syndrome

Caudal-regression syndrome is a part of the caudal-dysplasia spectrum and consists of one or more of the following: partial or total agenesis of the lumbar and sacral vertebrae, anal atresia, malformation of genitalia, renal abnormalities, pulmonary hypoplasia, and, rarely, fusion of the lower extremities (sirenomelia). Most patients present with neurogenic bladder, motor weakness, and foot deformities. There may be associations with other developmental abnormalities of the spine. MRI of the spinal canal demonstrates a high positioned and blunted or wedge-shaped conus, in addition to the aforementioned vertebral anomalies (Fig. 16.44).

16.3.3.2.11 Anterior Sacral Meningoceles

Anterior sacral meningoceles are diverticula of the intraspinal thecal sac, which protrude anteriorly into the extraperitoneal presacral space. They occur sporadically or in association with NF, Marfan's syndrome, or the Currarino triad. Patients with anterior sacral meningoceles may be asymptomatic or suffer from disturbances secondary to the mass effect, ranging from back pain, constipation, and genitourinary problems to neurological symptoms. The spinal canal is widened, and a minor or major sacrum defect is almost always

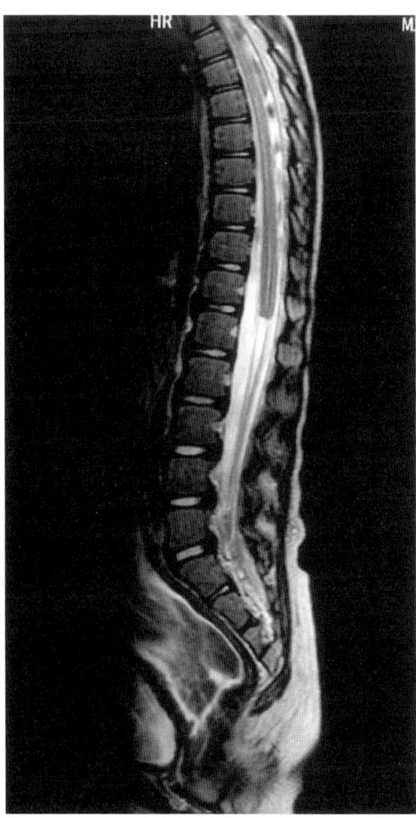

Fig. 16.44. Mild caudal regression. The spinal column is normal except for the sacrum. S3 and S4 are dysplastic. In addition, S5 and the coccyx are absent. The cord terminus is situated at the T12/L1 level and has the characteristic blunted shape of caudal regression

present. On MRI, these rounded masses may be unilocular or multilocular and demonstrate signal characteristics of CSF on all sequences, sometimes containing neural structures.

16.3.3.2.12 Currarino Triad

Currarino triad is an autosomal dominant inherited complex, consisting of an anorectal malformation, sacral defects, and a presacral mass. Patients suffer from constipation from birth, and plain films reveal a scimitar sacrum. MRI is necessary to evaluate patients for concurrent anterior sacral meningocele, lipoma, dermoid, teratoma, and tethered cord (Fig. 16.45).

16.3.3.3 Spinal Infections

Inflammatory processes during childhood include spondylitis, discitis, spondylodiscitis, sacroiliac pyarthrosis, epidural abscess, meningitis, arachnoiditis, myelitis, and, finally, spinal-cord abscess. All of these entities show the same appearance as in adults and should be examined with paramagnetic contrast. In this section, attention is paid to discitis and autoimmune demyelination due to MS.

16.3.3.3.1 Discitis and Spondylodiscitis

Discitis is an inflammatory process of the intervertebral disk space. The most common site is the lumbar region. Discitis occurs frequently in children from 6 months to 4 years of age, with a second peak from 10 years to 14 years of age. Cultures of blood or biopsy material are positive in up to 50% of the patients; the organism almost always involved is *Staphylococcus aureus*. At first, radiographs of the spine are normal; bone scintigraphy shows increased uptake as early as 1–2 days after the onset of symptoms. On T1-WI, disk-space infection demonstrates poor delineation of the involved disk, with hypointense signal in the adjacent vertebrae reflecting marrow edema. On T2-WI, the disk and the adjacent vertebrae show abnormally increased SI (see Chapter 5, Fig. 5.17). There may be contrast enhancement of the disk and the adjacent vertebral body, with or without disk extrusion, and epidural or paraspinal extension of the infection.

16.3.3.3.2 Multiple Sclerosis

MS is rare in the pediatric age group, but since the mean age of presentation in children is 13 years, a radiologist dealing with children should be aware of its presentation within the spine. Additionally, spinal-cord lesions due to MS in children may differ from the presentation in adults. MS in children tends to show more diffuse cord involvement (three or more vertebral levels) or even holocord involvement with increased T2-W signal and decreased T1-W signal reflecting demyelination and cord edema. Enhancement with paramagnetic contrast is variable and is associated with disease activity.

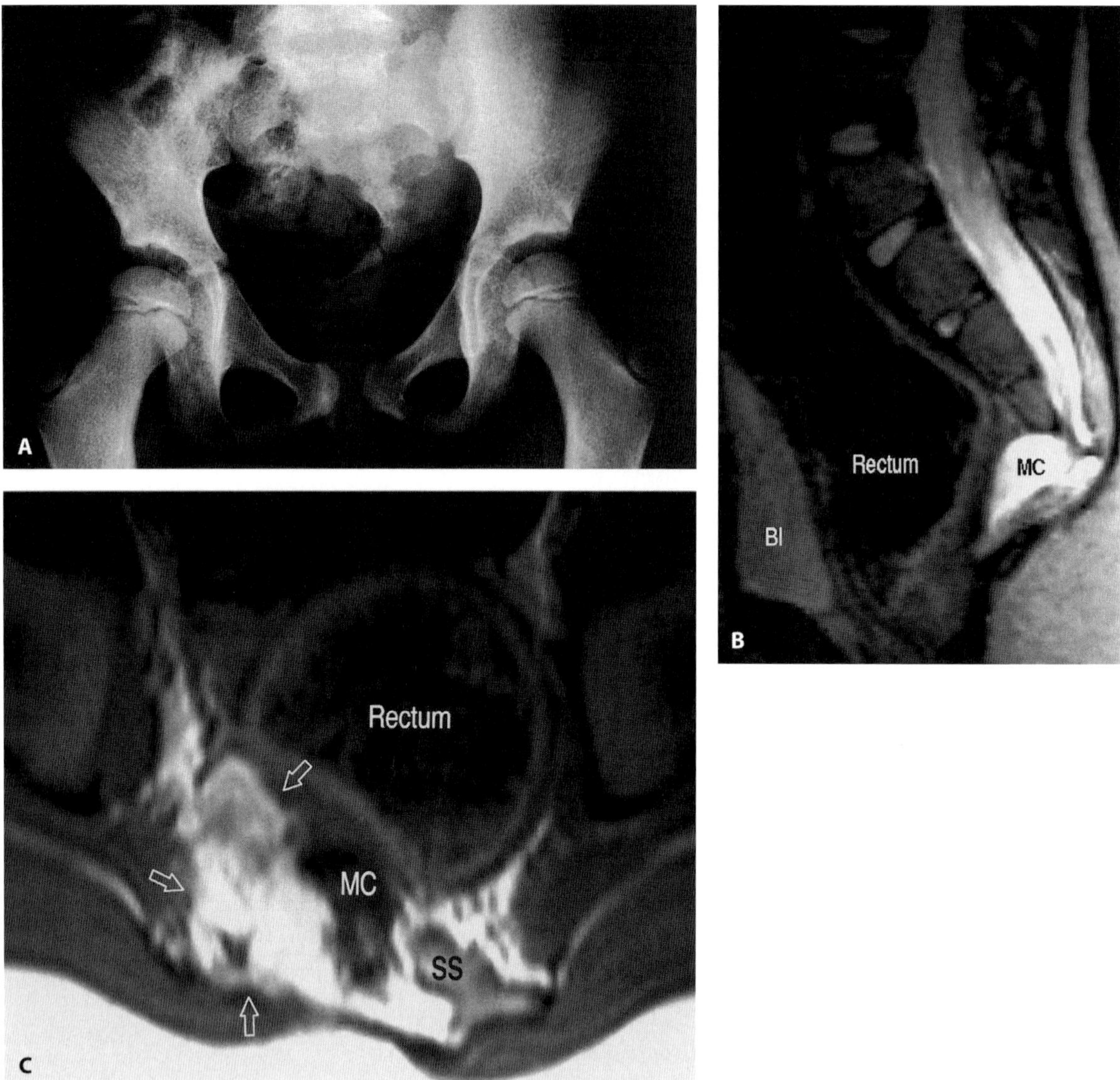

Fig. 16.45A–C. Currarino triad. Conventional radiograph (**A**) shows sacral dysplasia with a curved deviation to the left, a so-called scimitar sacrum. Sagittal T2-WI (**B**) and transverse T1-WI (**C**) show a presacral meningocele, a left-sided scimitar sacrum, and a predominately right-sided fatty mass

The differential diagnosis includes ADEM, transverse myelitis, cord infarct, AIDS-related myelopathy, and neoplasm.

16.3.3.4 Spinal Tumors in Childhood

16.3.3.4.1 Intradural-Intramedullary Tumors

■ **Astrocytoma.** Approximately 50%–60% of intramedullary tumors in children are astrocytomas which are frequently low grade (grade I or II) by histology. Occasionally, higher-grade malignancies occur, such as malignant glioma or glioblastoma multiforme. Astrocytomas are most often located in the thoracic spine. On MRI, astrocytomas present with spinal-cord enlargement and are most commonly hypointense on T1-WI and hyperintense on T2-WI. However, they can also appear as mixed signal-intensity lesions, rarely hemorrhagic, that have variable contrast enhancement. They may contain cysts, either representing tumor-lined or gliotic-lined cystic cavities or syringomyelia above or below the tumor (Fig. 16.46).

■ **Ependymoma.** Ependymomas constitute 20%–30% of intramedullary tumors in children. They typically arise in the lumbar region from ependymal cells within the spinal cord or filum terminale (see Chapter 5, Fig. 5.21). Ependymomas tend to be more sharply circumscribed hypointense or isointense masses, enhancing more heterogeneously on T1-W sequences than astrocytomas. Evidence of hemorrhage at their inferior and superior margins may be another helpful imaging finding in differentiating ependymoma from astrocytoma.

■ **Hemangioblastoma.** Hemangioblastomas may be associated with von Hippel-Lindau syndrome and occur anywhere along the spinal axis. They are difficult to distinguish from AVMs and present as well-demarcated, intense contrast-enhancing masses with cysts, areas of hemorrhage, and flow voids, due to draining and feeding vessels.

16.3.3.4.2 Intradural Extramedullary Tumors

The four most common intradural extramedullary tumors in childhood comprise neurofibroma/schwan-

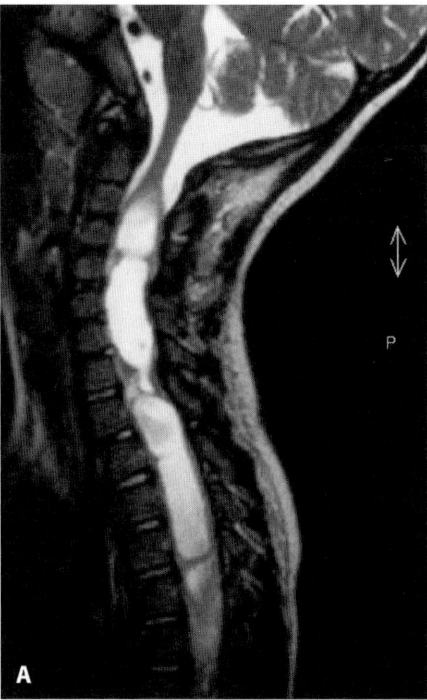

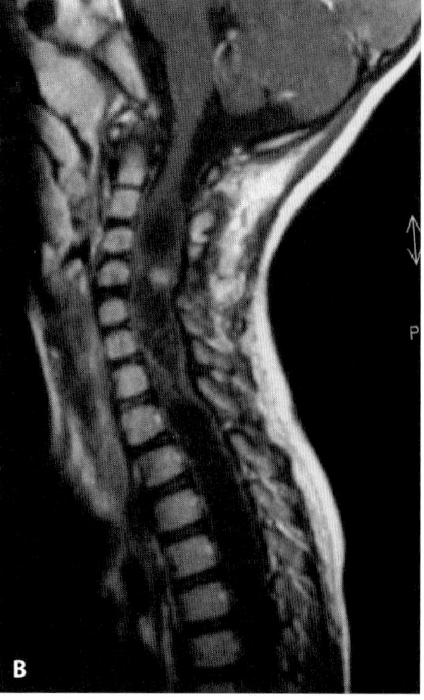

Fig. 16.46A,B. Spinal astrocytoma. Sagittal T2-WI (**A**) and sagittal T1-WI (**B**) after administration of contrast show an enhancing nodule of tumor at the C4 level within the cervical cord. The cystic areas presumably represent necrotic regions within the tumor and tumor-associated cysts (courtesy of W. Michl, MD, Institut für Röntgendiagnostik des Krankenhauszweckverbandes, Kinderradiologie, Augsburg)

noma, drop metastasis from primary intracranial tumors, congenital lipomas, and epidermoids/dermoids.

■ Neurofibroma and Schwannoma. Neurofibromas and plexiform neurofibromas are typically associated with NF-1, whereas schwannomas may occur in patients without NF. Neurofibroma and schwannoma of the spine originate from the nerve roots and typically present as well-demarcated, dumbbell-shaped, soft-tissue masses passing through a frequently enlarged neural foramen. Neurofibromas are commonly hypointense or isointense on both T1-WI and T2-WI, with variable enhancement after Gd-DTPA. They may be less frequently hyperintense on T2-WI. Plexiform neurofibromas are typically wavy, elongated masses, which are hyperintense on T2-WI and heterogeneous on T1-WI, with variable contrast enhancement.

In contrast, schwannomas are well-demarcated masses, typically hyperintense on T2-WI, and usually enhance homogeneously with paramagnetic contrast (Fig. 16.47).

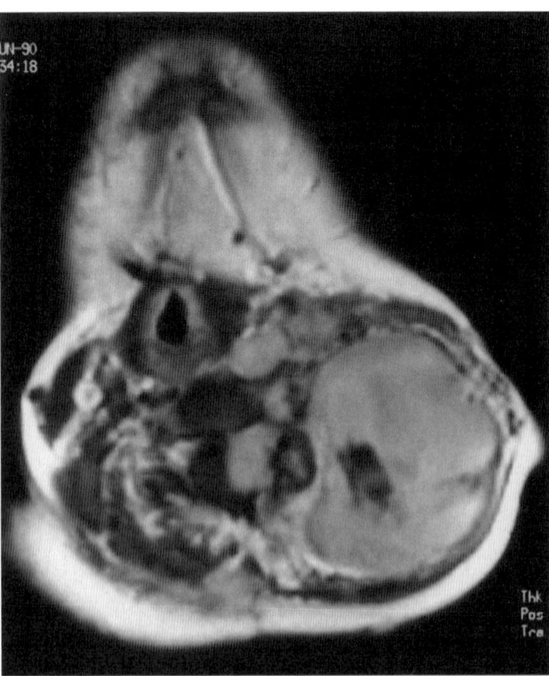

Fig. 16.47. Schwannoma. Transverse contrast-enhanced T1-WI demonstrates a huge, dumbbell-shaped mass with an area of tumor necrosis in the cervical spine and the left neck

■ Drop Metastasis from CNS Neoplasms. CSF seeding from other CNS neoplasms is more common in children than adults. The CNS neoplasms which most frequently metastasize in childhood are PNET and ependymoma. However, other tumors, such as germinomas, high-grade gliomas, lymphoma, choroid plexus tumors, and neuroblastoma may present with metastatic subarachnoid disease (Fig. 16.48).

■ Epidermoid/Dermoid. The MR appearance of dermoids is variable, sometimes showing high intensity on T1-WI, but more commonly having low to intermediate SI on T1-WI and high SI on T2-WI. Dermoids are more common in the lumbar region, whereas epidermoids are distributed uniformly along the spinal canal.

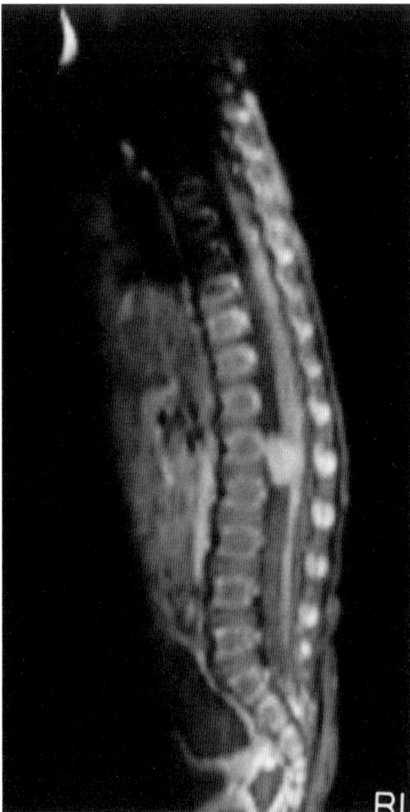

Fig. 16.48. Drop metastases. Sagittal FS contrast-enhanced T1-WI reveals drop metastases in the spinal canal from medulloblastoma (primitive neuroepithelial tumors) (courtesy of W. Michl, MD, Institut für Röntgendiagnostik des Krankenhauszweckverbandes, Kinderradiologie, Augsburg)

Epidermoids are most commonly isointense to CSF on both T1-WI and T2-WI. However, they are sometimes hyperintense on T1-WI and, consequently, difficult to distinguish from dermoid or lipomas without the use of FS T1-W sequences. Neither dermoids nor epidermoids enhance with paramagnetic contrast unless they are infected. Infection is much more common if these lesions have developed in association with dermal sinuses.

16.3.3.4.3
Extradural Tumors

Extradural tumors in children are most commonly metastatic lesions from paravertebral soft tissue with extension through the neural foramina into the spinal canal. Neuroblastoma is the most important extradural tumor in children (see 16.4.5.1).

■ **Primary Neoplasms of the Spinal Column.** Primary tumors of the spine are rare in children. Hemangioma, osteoid osteoma, osteoblastoma, aneurysmal bone cyst, osteochondroma, giant-cell tumor, osteosarcoma, Ewing's sarcoma, chondrosarcoma, and chordoma are included in this group. These lesions do not differ in radiographic and MR appearance from the same lesions in adults.

Secondary neoplasms of the spine in children comprise Langerhans cell histiocytosis, leukemia, lymphoma, rhabdomyosarcoma, neuroblastoma, Wilms' tumor, and PNET. The imaging findings of these tumors are discussed in Section 16.5 and Chapters 5 and 8.

16.4 Pediatric Abdominal Imaging

16.4.1 Coils and Patient Positioning

For abdominal MR examinations of neonates and young infants, the head or knee coil (sending and receiving coils are preferred) is used, as long as the coil is large enough for the child. Older children are positioned in the body phased-array coil, and the coil is fixed by a plastic tunnel to reduce artifacts caused by a moving coil due to breathing. In the head, knee, and body phased-array coil, the patients are in a supine position. A symmetric and comfortable posture should be arranged.

16.4.2 Sequence Protocol

A special localizer sequence for abdominal examinations is obtained. This localizer should consist of five images in all three orientations covering the region of interest. We prefer three images in frontal orientation and one image in both transverse and sagittal orientation. With regard to the imaging strategy, it is important to consider that breath-hold techniques generally cannot be used in children. Therefore, the sequence protocol differs from that of adults. If available, HASTE sequences in transverse orientation covering the entire abdomen should be performed next. Due to an acquisition time of 0.4 s/slice, the resulting images are free of motion artifacts, often enabling the clinically relevant diagnosis. This is of great advantage if the child

Table 16.9. Sequence protocol recommendations for abdominal imaging

Sequence	WI	Plane	No. of slices	TR (ms)	TE (ms)	Flip angle	TI (ms)	Echo train length	Slice thickness (mm)	Matrix	FOV	recFOV (%)	Band-width (Hz)	No. of acq.	Acq. time (min:s)
TSE	T2	tra	19	4450	96	180		7	5	224×512	250	75	65	1	3:03
SE	T1	tra	19	646	14	90			3	148×256	250	75	150	4	6:25
FL 2D	TOF	tra	40	27	9	50			2	192×256	210	75	195	1	4:08
FI 3D	TOF	tra	42	29	6	20			60	160×256	330	62.5	195	1	3:17

Abbreviations: *WI* weighting of images; *TR* repetition time (ms); *TE* echo time (ms); *TI* inversion time (ms); *Matrix* phase × frequency matrix; *recFOV* rectangular field of view (%); *Acq.* acquisition(s)

denies cooperation for other more time-consuming sequences.

The following imaging protocol is suggested (Table 16.9).

- Transverse T2-W TSE sequence: besides the soft-tissue classification of the lesion, this sequence is necessary for the detection of liver metastases.
- Transverse T1-W SE sequence.
- Transverse FLASH 2D TOF venous MR angiography (optional). Especially for Wilms' tumors, this sequence is recommended for the assessment of renal vein or inferior vena cava (IVC) involvement by tumor.
- FISP 3D tone down TOF arterial MR angiography (optional). This sequence should be used particularly in cases of unclear vessel displacement caused by abdominal masses.
- Intravenous application of contrast media.
- Transverse T1-W SE sequence.
- Coronal T1-W SE sequence.
- Thin slice (2–3 mm) T1-W SE sequence (optional). Thin slice sequences in sagittal or coronal orientation are necessary for the evaluation of small lesions in the kidney and spinal-canal involvement.

16.4.3 Common Findings in Pediatric Kidney Imaging

16.4.3.1 Normal Anatomy

Due to the retroperitoneal position and the surrounding perinephric fat, kidneys can be seen very well by MR imaging. They are predominantly marked by medium SI and are well defined by the high SI of the surrounding fat. The SI behavior of kidneys in different sequences is pointed out in the following:

- SE T1-W:
  - Cortex, higher SI than medulla
  - Pyramids, more prominent in neonates and young children than in older children and adults
  - Renal artery and vein, low SI due to the rapid blood flow (flow void)
  - Urine within the pelvocaliceal system and ureter, low SI
  - No high SI in the hilar region in young children because of lack of adipose tissue
  - SI of renal hilum increases with age (by puberty, kidneys have the same appearance as adults)
- TSE T2-W:
  - Cortex and medulla: high SI
  - Less corticomedullary differentiation
- SE T1-W plus Gd-DTPA:
  - Renal cortex: increasing SI
  - Renal medulla: decreasing SI, followed by gradual increase

16.4.3.2 Kidney Abnormalities

- Agenesis: unilateral agenesis may be associated with other abnormalities of the genitourinary tract, often discoid configuration of the ipsilateral adrenal gland.
- Renal hypoplasia and dysplasia.
- Ectopic kidney: intrathoracic or pelvic kidney.
- Fusion anomalies: crossed-fused ectopia or horseshoe kidney.

MR imaging is superior to ultrasonography because it gives an overall view of the abdominal and pelvic organs. It allows easy differentiation between renal agenesis and abnormal location of the kidney. MR imaging is not limited by bone or bowel-gas artifacts. T1-WI in coronal orientation is best to visualize kidney ectopia or anomalies, whereas T1-WI in transverse orientation allows visualization of a horseshoe kidney; as in coronal planes, the fusion of the lower poles across the midline can easily be missed.

16.4.3.3 Renal Cystic Lesions

- Simple cysts:
  - Solitary cysts
  - Multilocular cysts
- Multicystic kidneys:
  - Multicystic dysplastic kidney (MDK)
  - Multilocular cystic nephroma (MLCN)
- Polycystic kidneys
  - Infantile (recessive) polycystic disease (RPKD: Potter type I)
  - Adult (autosomal dominant) polycystic disease (ADPK: Potter type III)

Ultrasound is the imaging modality of choice with regard to renal cysts. Solitary cysts are uncommon in childhood. These asymptomatic cysts are incidental findings and must be differentiated from Wilms' tumor or multilocular cystic nephroma. MR imaging may help to clarify inconclusive cases, such as complicated cysts with hemorrhage. Small amounts of calcification in the wall of the cyst may not be identified by MR imaging, but larger amounts of calcifications may be seen as a rim of signal void. A reliable differentiation of hemorrhagic cysts, infected cysts, or neoplasms is not always possible.

MR Imaging Findings

Homogeneous, well-defined masses with clearly defined thin walls.

- Pure fluid in the cyst.
  - SE T1-W: low SI.
  - SE T2-W: medium to high SI.
- High protein fluid or subacute hemorrhage in the cyst.
  - SE T1-W and SE T2-WI: inhomogeneous high SI.
- Hemorrhagic cysts show a variable MR appearance, even within the same kidney.

16.4.3.4 Multilocular Cystic Nephroma

Multilocular cystic nephroma (MLCN) includes both the cystic nephroma and the partially differentiated cystic nephroblastoma. The latter shows cysts with blastemal tissue as septa, whereas the cystic nephroma does not have any blastemal tissue in its cysts. The MLCN is rare and is considered a benign tumor. There are two peak incidences: one in children at an age of 3 months to 4 years, the other in adults at an age of 40–70 years. Patients may present with a palpable mass in the abdomen and sometimes with hematuria and/or back pain. On MR imaging, a well-demarcated, septated, multiloculated cystic mass is observed. The septa of the cysts may enhance with paramagnetic contrast. MLCN must be distinguished from nephroblastomas, as the therapeutic management is completely different. Resection of the mass and preservation of the residual kidney is the therapy of choice. Preoperative chemotherapy as in Wilms' tumor must be avoided.

16.4.3.5 Infantile (Recessive) Polycystic Disease

RPKD is inherited as an autosomal recessive disorder which shows a spectrum of abnormalities, including both microcystic and macrocystic renal disease, and variable degrees of hepatic fibrosis and biliary ectasia. In infancy, the renal problems dominate, whereas in later childhood, portal hypertension and gastrointestinal bleeding due to liver cirrhosis are the problem. Numerous small cysts (1–2 mm in diameter) in both the cortex and the medulla and bilaterally enlarged kidneys are characteristic of infantile polycystic disease. MR imaging demonstrates enlarged, lobular kidneys with

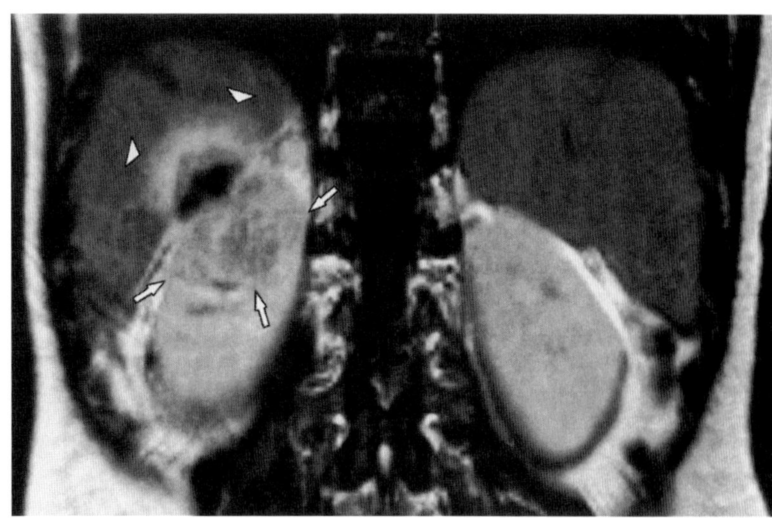

Fig. 16.49. Renal abscess. Coronal T1-W spin-echo gadolinium (Gd)-enhanced image shows an inhomogeneous mass in the upper part of the right kidney (*arrows*). The irregular border of the abscess demonstrates a strong enhancement of Gd-DTPA. Surrounding inflammatory reaction (*arrowheads*) may mimic a necrotic nephroblastoma with infiltration of the liver

dilated tubules and absence of corticomedullary differentiation.

16.4.3.6 Renal Abscess

Renal abscesses and carbuncles occur less frequently in children than in adults. However, they represent an important differential diagnosis to renal malignomas. Again, preoperative chemotherapy must be avoided in any case. On MR imaging, an abscess with a surrounding inflammatory reaction may mimic a necrotic malignoma with adjacent soft-tissue infiltration (Fig. 16.49). Therefore, exact analysis of the patient's history as well as clinical and laboratory findings (fever, other signs for inflammation) are mandatory. An irregular mass lesion with low to medium signal in the center is typical for a renal abscess on plain T1-WI. On corresponding T2-WI, the center shows high SI. The irregular border of the abscess enhances markedly with paramagnetic contrast. Perinephric abscesses may be caused by pyelonephritis or carbuncle rupture.

16.4.3.7 Tumors of the Kidneys

Wilms' tumor is the most common primary renal neoplasm, whereas renal rhabdomyosarcoma, primary renal lymphoma, renal cell carcinomas, and renal teratomas are extremely rare entities in children. Table 16.10 gives an overview of the most important abdominal tumors in children.

The initial diagnosis of renal masses is made by ultrasound. For further therapy planning, MR imaging should be performed as it provides:

- Precise definition of the tumor extent and its relationship to adjacent structures,
- Exact visualization of the tumor capsule,
- Assessment of the degree of vessel involvement,
- Visualization of lymph-node metastases,
- Visualization of liver and bone metastases,
- Detection of even small tumoral lesions in the contralateral kidney.

16.4.3.7.1 Wilms' Tumor: Nephroblastoma

Table 16.10. Incidence of abdominal tumors in children (percentage of all tumors in children)

Abdominal tumors	Incidence (%)
Wilms' tumors	6
Neuroblastomas	5
Rhabdomyosarcomas	1
Hepatoblastomas	0.6

Wilms' tumor shows its peak incidence at an age of 1–3 years, with 90% of patients younger than 7 years of age. An increased incidence is seen in children with syndromes, such as aniridia, hemihypertrophy, genitourinary anomalies (Drash syndrome), and Beckwith-Wiedemann syndrome. In 5%–10% of cases, Wilms' tumor occurs bilaterally. A triphasic histology with blastemal, epithelial, and stromal cells is characteristic. Metastatic spread depends on the histology, which is divided into classic or favorable and unfavorable histology:

- 90% classic or favorable histology
  - Invasion of local tissues, renal veins, inferior vena cava
  - Liver and lung metastases
  - Regional lymph-node metastases
- 10% unfavorable histology (several subtypes)
  - Rhabdoid tumor: brain metastases
  - Clear-cell sarcoma: bone metastases

Clinically, a large, unilateral, abdominal mass is usually found. Less common signs are abdominal pain or hematuria. Specific laboratory findings do not exist. According to the SIOP9 therapy protocol, Wilms' tumor is treated with preoperative chemotherapy. Due to the danger of tumor rupture and intraperitoneal tumor spread, biopsy is not performed in Wilms' tumor. Therefore, the diagnosis and indication for preoperative chemotherapy are primarily based on imaging. Wilms' tumor is staged according to the National Wilms' Tumor Study (NWTS) (Table 16.11). Benign masses and other malignant tumors, i.e., neuroblastoma, must be safely differentiated.

MR Imaging Findings

- Well-defined mass, pseudocapsule of compressed adjacent tissue (Fig. 16.50)
- Often areas of hemorrhage and/or necrosis resulting in an inhomogeneous internal structure

Table 16.11. Staging of Wilms' tumor according to the National Wilms' Tumor Study (NWTS)

Stage I	Tumor limited to the kidney and completely excised
Stage II	Tumor extended beyond the kidney, but completely excised
Stage III	Residual tumor after surgery confined to the abdomen
Stage IV	Hematogeneous metastases as in lung, liver, bone, brain
Stage V	Bilateral renal involvement

- Coronal images reveal decisive information about:
  - Identification of the tumor's origin (kidney: Wilms' tumor, adrenal gland: neuroblastoma)
  - Visualization of possible invasion of adjacent organs
  - Craniocaudal extension
  - Tumoral lesions in the contralateral kidney (nephroblastomatosis, Drash syndrome)
- Plain T1-W: low SI (lower than that of normal renal parenchyma)

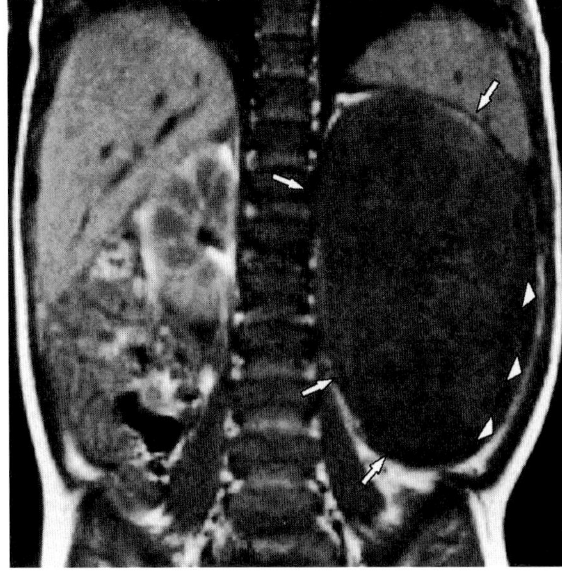

Fig. 16.50. Wilms' tumor. Plain coronal T1-W spin-echo image depicts a typical left-sided stage-1 nephroblastoma with an internal structure of low signal intensity. Visualization of the pseudocapsule (*arrows*) and delineation of peritumoral adipose tissue (*arrowheads*) allow for exclusion of an infiltration of adjacent structures

- Plain T1-W: lower SI in necrotic than in vital tumor areas
- Plain T1-W: high SI indicates focal hemorrhage
- T2-W: marked increase of SI
- T2-W: even more increase of SI in necrotic areas than in vital tumor areas (Fig. 16.51)
- Gd-DTPA helps to:
  - Differentiate between tumor and residual kidney (Fig. 16.52)

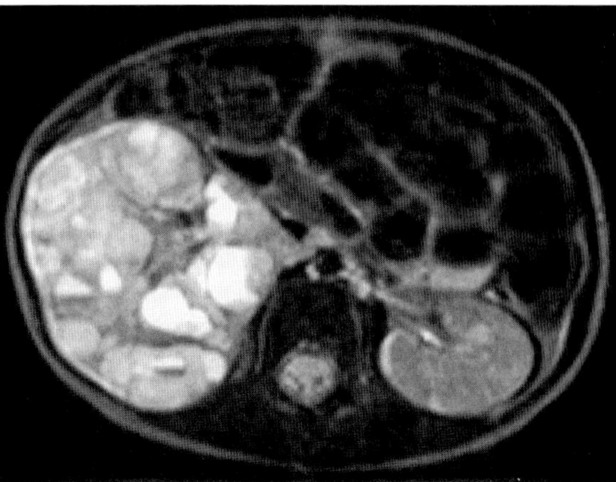

Fig. 16.51. Wilms' tumor. T2-W turbo spin-echo image shows a well-defined stage-2 nephroblastoma with typical high signal, inhomogeneous internal structure. Cystic and necrotic areas within the mass can be delineated

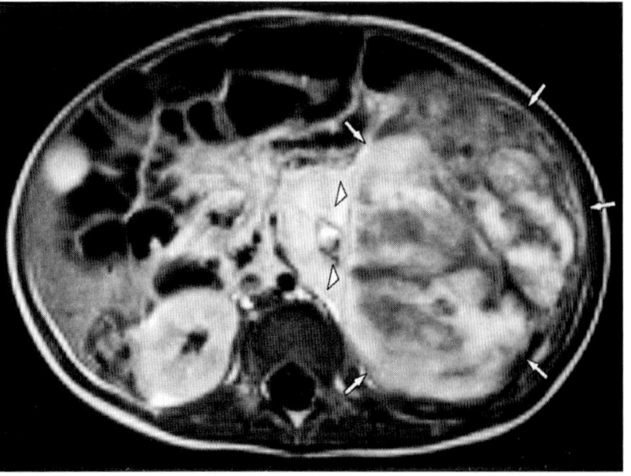

Fig. 16.52. Wilms' tumor. Axial T1-W spin-echo Gd-enhanced image shows a well-encapsulated (*arrows*) nephroblastoma. After application of Gd-DTPA, differentiation between residual kidney and tumor is possible (*arrowheads*)

- Identify cystic components
- Assess the tumor vascularity

- Lack of flow in venous MRA allows evaluation of possible tumor thrombus in the renal vein or IVC
- Wilms' tumor rather displaces than encases the abdominal aorta and IVC. Direction and position of displacement seen by MR imaging, and MRA is helpful in planning the surgical approach.

16.4.3.7.2 Nephroblastomatosis

In newborns, there are small rests of primitive metanephric epithelium. This nephrogenic blastema within the kidneys usually regresses by 4 months of age. If there is no regression, blastemic remnants become confluent, causing enlargement and distortion of the kidney with sparing of the renal pelvis. Nephroblastomatosis is a premalignant lesion, which may progress to Wilms' tumor. In up to 44% of cases, Wilms' tumor is associated with nephroblastomatosis. Nephroblastomatosis often affects both kidneys and shows different locations within the kidneys (Table 16.12). For the detection of nephroblastomatosis, T1-W sequences after application of Gd-DTPA are most important. Nephroblastomatosis lesions are nodules of varying size with a homogeneous low signal compared with normal renal tissue (Fig. 16.53). Due to the bilateral occurrence and malignant potential (Fig. 16.54) of nephroblastomatosis, careful evaluation (thin slices) of the contralateral kidney in all Wilms' tumor patients is necessary (Table 16.12).

16.4.3.7.3 Drash Syndrome

The Drash syndrome is defined by three symptoms: pseudohermaphroditism, nephropathy, and Wilms' tumor. The occurrence of bilateral Wilms' tumor is seen more often in patients with Drash syndrome. Patients

Table 16.12. Forms and location of nephroblastomatosis

Form	Location
Perilobular	Periphery of renal lobe and subcapsular
Intralobular	Deep cortcal or medullar lesion
Panlobular	Universal rest of immature blastemic cells

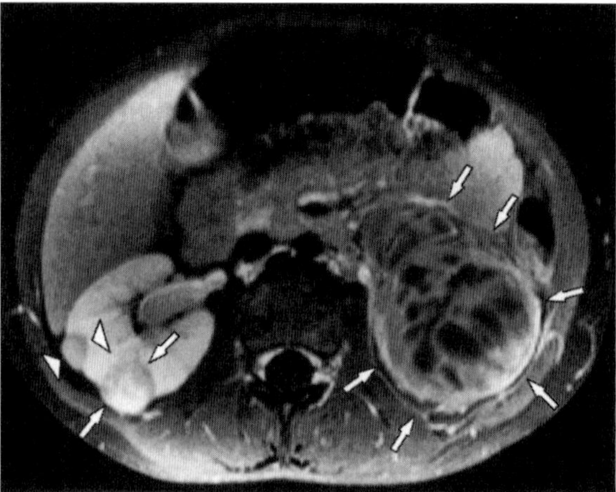

Fig. 16.53. Bilateral Wilms' tumor and nephroblastomatosis. Axial T1-W, fat-saturated, spin-echo, Gd-enhanced image demonstrates bilateral nephroblastoma (*arrows*) with typical inhomogeneous internal structure. The nodule of nephroblastomatosis (*arrowheads*) shows a homogeneous low signal

with Drash syndrome are younger than patients with Wilms' tumor alone. As in nephroblastomatosis, coronal T1-W sequences after the application of Gd-DTPA allow for the detection of even small dysplastic lesions in the contralateral kidney (Fig. 16.55A). As mentioned before, these dysplastic lesions have a malignant potential (Fig. 16.55B) and must be followed up carefully.

16.4.4 Lower Urinary Tract

Congenital abnormalities of the lower urinary tract in children are primarily diagnosed by ultrasound, voiding cystourethrography, and intravenous urography. Because of the precise anatomic resolution and the clear demonstration of adipose tissue, multiplanar T1-W sequences and, particularly, coronal images are helpful in depicting these abnormalities. However, MR imaging is more valuable in the evaluation of associated complex anomalies affecting the pelvic diaphragm, os sacrum, and spinal canal. Hence, caudal-regression syndrome, bladder exstrophy, all forms of sexual differentiation anomalies, anal atresia, hydrometrocolpos, and hematometrocolpos represent indications for MRI.

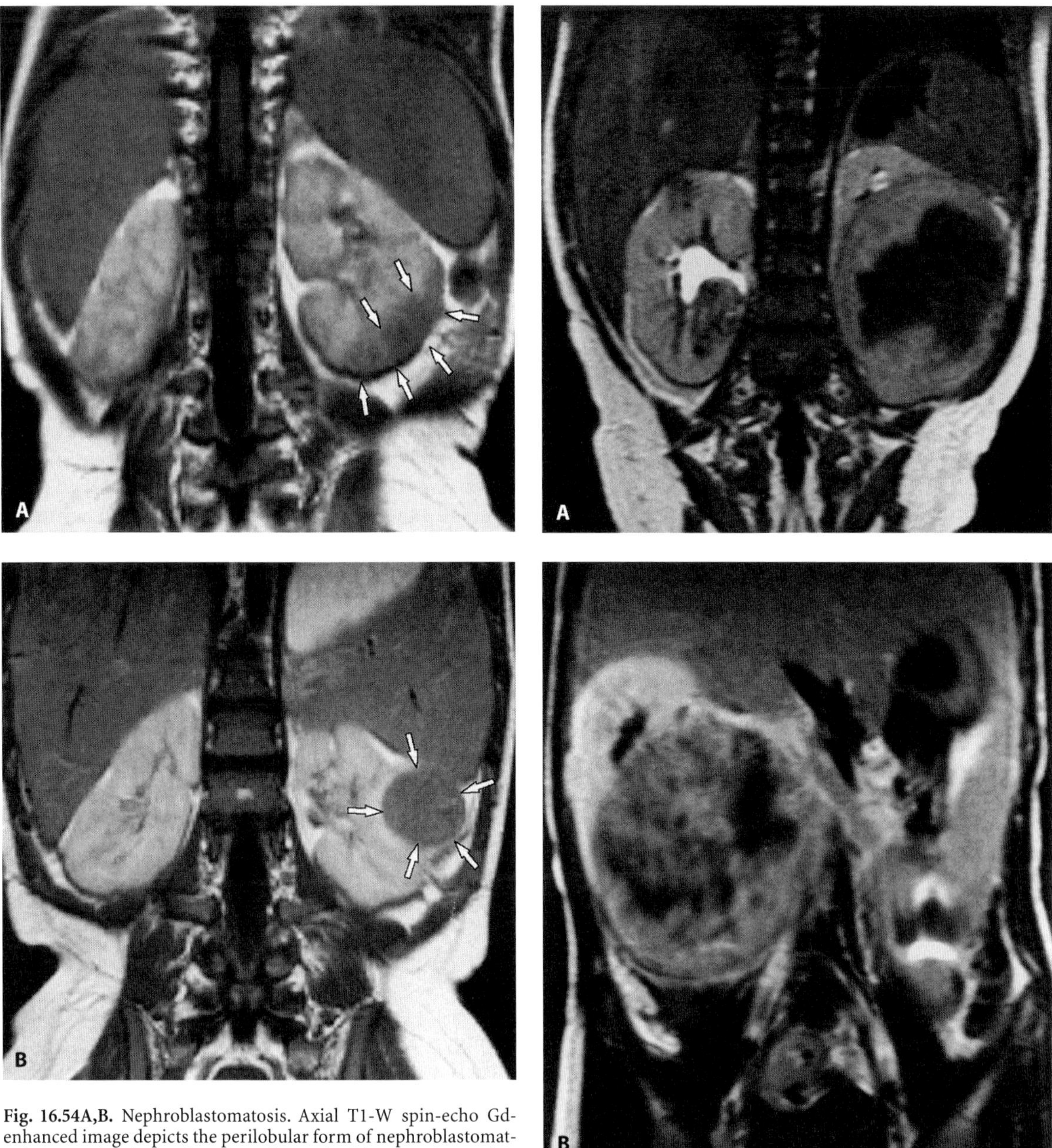

Fig. 16.54A,B. Nephroblastomatosis. Axial T1-W spin-echo Gd-enhanced image depicts the perilobular form of nephroblastomatosis (*arrows*) (**A**). Development of a nephroblastoma (*arrows*) is seen 1 year later (**B**), demonstrating the malignant potential of nephroblastomatosis

Fig. 16.55A,B. Drash syndrome. Coronal T1-W spin-echo Gd-enhanced image shows a necrotic, left-sided Wilms' tumor and cystic, dysplastic, right-sided lesions in the contralateral kidney (**A**) in a patient with Drash syndrome. As in nephroblastomatosis, these dysplastic lesions developed into a recurrent right-sided Wilms' tumor 6 months later (**B**)

16.4.5 Common Findings in Imaging of Adrenal Glands

16.4.5.1 Neuroblastoma

Neuroblastoma is the most common solid pediatric tumor, with an incidence of 5%–15% of all pediatric malignant neoplasias (Fig. 16.23). In the first year of life, neuroblastoma is the most common malignancy, and at the time of diagnosis, affected children are usually under 4 years of age. Neuroblastoma may arise anywhere along the sympathetic chain in the neck, in the thorax, in the abdomen and pelvis, or in the adrenal gland. In 60%–70% of cases, neuroblastoma has its origin in the adrenal gland. Neuroblastomas arising from the adrenal glands do not show involvement of the spinal canal in contrast to those arising from the sympathetic chain. Neuroblastoma has a tendency for direct spread, metastases to bone and liver (on initial presentation, 70% of neuroblastomas have already metastasized), and calcifications (60% gross, 90% microscopic). A spontaneous maturity into benign ganglioneuroma is possible. Although neuroblastoma shows the highest rate of spontaneous regression of any human malignancy, late recurrence is possible.

Patients often present late with large tumors and symptoms caused by invasion or compression of adjacent structures or metastatic disease. Despite the high frequency of increased catecholamine secretion by neuroblastomas, only 10% of children will present with hypertension. In addition, two paraneoplastic syndromes are observed in 4%: myoclonic encephalopathy of infancy (MEI) and intractable diarrhea caused by excessive secretion of vasoactive intestinal peptides. In contrast to Wilms' tumor, there exist specific laboratory (24-h urine catecholamine concentration) and nuclear medicine (I^{123}-MIBG scintigraphy) examinations that help in the differentiation of neuroblastoma. The Evans system is still widely used for the staging of neuroblastomas (Table 16.13). An important prognostic factor in neuroblastoma is the presence or absence of N-*myc*, which is a DNA fragment. Patients that are N-*myc*-positive have a poor prognosis. Although ultrasound detects the abdominal mass, and CT more sensitively depicts calcifications, MR imaging is clearly the modality of choice in the evaluation of abdominal neuroblastoma. The main reason is that MR imaging is the only imaging modality that allows sufficient assessment of any intraspinal involvement. In addition, MR imaging shows the extent of the mass, displacement and encasement of vessels, direct spread into adjacent tissue, and metastatic disease to lymph nodes, liver, bone marrow, and other organs, and exactly defines the tumor origin.

Table 16.13. Staging of neuroblastoma

Stage I	Tumor is limited to tissue of origin
Stage II	Local regional spread of tumor without any crossing of midline
Stage III	Tumor crosses midline
Stage IV	Tumors with metastases to skeleton, distant lymph nodes and other tissue
Stage IV-S	Children under the age of 1 year, metastases confined to liver, skin and bone marrow (frequently spontaneous regression, without any therapy)

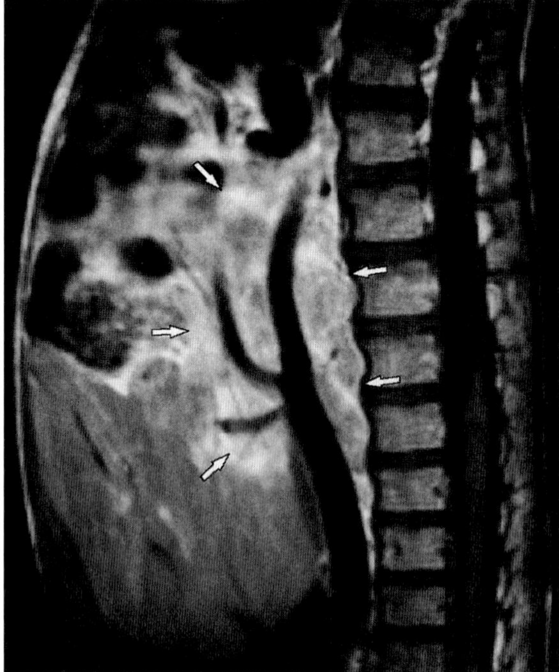

Fig. 16.56. Lymph-node metastases of neuroblastoma. Sagittal T1-W spin-echo Gd-enhanced image depicts multiple lymph-node metastases of a neuroblastoma with displacement of the abdominal aorta, superior mesenteric artery, and celiac trunk (*arrows*)

MR Imaging Findings

- Well-defined margins of the primary tumor in most cases
- Internal structure: homogenous or irregular due to hemorrhage (high SI on T1-W and T2-WI) or necrosis (low SI on T1-W, high SI in T2-WI) within tumor
- T1-W: SI equal to or less than muscle
- T2-W: higher SI than muscle
- Gd-DTPA helps to:
  - Differentiate between neuroblastoma and kidney
  - Identify necrotic components
  - Assess tumor vascularity
  - Identify lymph-node metastases
- Midline crossing and displacement of blood vessels primarily by lymph node metastases (Fig. 16.56)
- Inferior and lateral displacement of the kidney in adrenal neuroblastomas (Fig. 16.57)
- Frequent spread to local lymph nodes, involvement of spinal cord primarily by neuroblastomas deriving from the sympathetic trunk (Fig. 16.58)

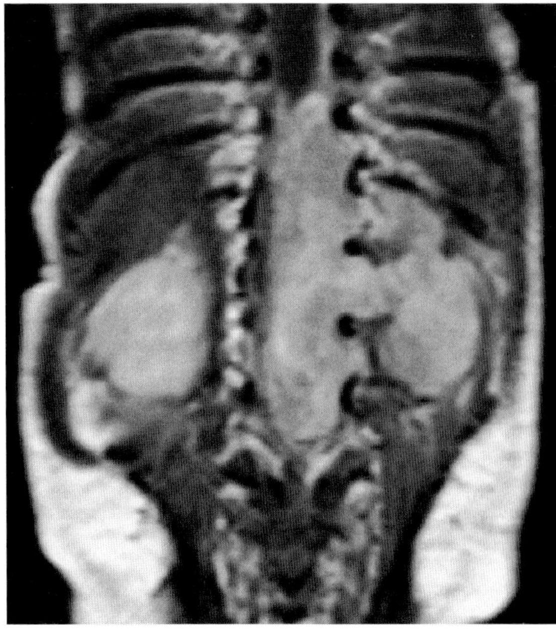

Fig. 16.58. Neuroblastoma. Coronal T1-W spin-echo Gd-enhanced image illustrates a left-sided paravertebral neuroblastoma of the sympathetic trunk with intraspinal infiltration and growth through intervertebral foramina

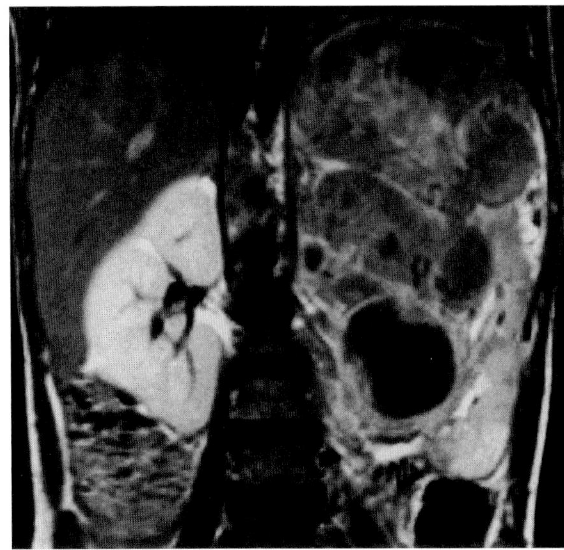

Fig. 16.57. Neuroblastoma. Coronal T1-W spin-echo Gd-enhanced image demonstrates a large, left-sided, inhomogeneous neuroblastoma with displacement of the kidney. The inhomogeneous internal structure of the kidney represents a histologically proven tumor infiltration

Differential Diagnoses

- Wilms' tumor: origin in the kidney, no increased catecholamines, no uptake of I^{123}-MIBG
- Ganglioneuroma: no distinction possible between low stage neuroblastoma (Fig. 16.59) and ganglioneuroma (Fig. 16.60)
- Adrenal hemorrhage (high SI on T1-W and T2-WI): hemorrhage and tumor shrink after 2–3 weeks, elevated catecholamines only in neuroblastoma
- Pheochromocytoma

16.4.5.2 Ganglioneuroma

In contrast to neuroblastoma, ganglioneuroma is a benign tumor and mainly affects patients under 10 years of age. Some 60% of patients are younger than 20 years of age. In 43% of patients, the tumor is located in the sympathetic ganglia in the posterior mediastinum, in 32% in the retroperitoneum, and in 8% in the neck. Symptoms depend on location, size, growth, and

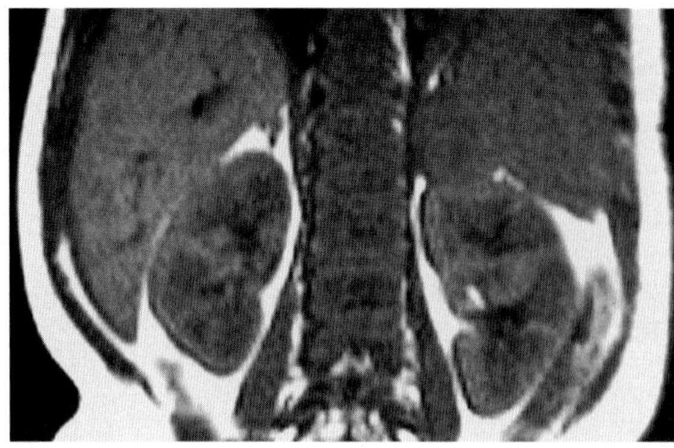

Fig. 16.59. Stage-1 neuroblastoma. Plain T1-W spin-echo image in coronal orientation shows a homogeneous, well-defined mass of the left adrenal gland without infiltration of the surrounding tissue

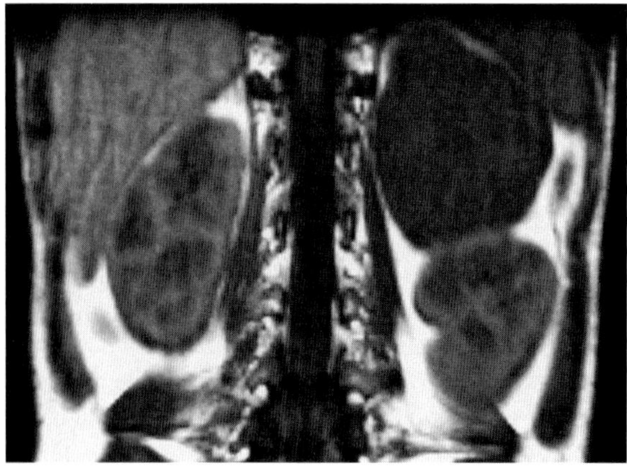

Fig. 16.60. Ganglioneuroma. Plain T1-W spin-echo image in coronal orientation demonstrates a large, left-sided, suprarenal tumor that displaces the left kidney. With respect to MR criteria, this mass is not distinguishable from a low stage neuroblastoma (Fig. 16.59)

displacement of adjacent structures. The prognosis is excellent after complete resection of the tumor. As mentioned before, clinical and imaging features can be identical to that of low-stage neuroblastoma. Differentiation can only be achieved by histology. Preoperative chemotherapy must be avoided in this benign lesion.

16.4.5.3 Pheochromocytoma

Pheochromocytoma is a very rare entity during childhood, with 80% located in the adrenal medulla and 20% extra-adrenally (aortic paraganglion, paravertebral sympathetic nervous ganglia). Multiple occurrence is found in up to 30% of cases. In 10% of cases, pheochromocytomas are situated bilaterally. Often, there is an association with MEN IIa and IIb, von Hippel-Lindau disease, and rarely von Recklinghausen's disease. Pheochromocytomas can turn into malignant in 5%–46% of cases. Clinically, patients present with hypertension, palpitation, chest pain, and impaired vision. Usually, the diagnosis is made by elevated catecholamine concentrations in urine and serum and by I^{123}-MIBG scintigraphy. Surgery is usually performed. Chemotherapy is another option, especially in malignant cases.

MR Imaging Findings

- Moderate size, about 2 cm in diameter at time of presentation
- Well defined
- T1-W: lower SI than liver
- T2-W: very high SI (so high that it may mimic a cyst), fairly characteristic for pheochromocytoma in contrast to other adrenal tumors (Fig. 16.61)
- Marked enhancement with Gd-DTPA

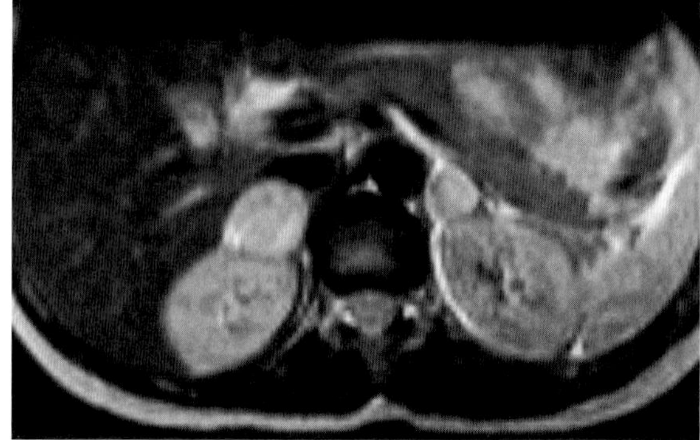

Fig. 16.61. Bilateral pheochromocytoma. Axial T2-W turbo spin-echo image illustrates bilateral pheochromocytoma with very high signal intensity

16.4.6 Common Findings in Pediatric Liver Imaging

16.4.6.1 Primary Liver Tumors

The liver is the third most common site of origin of abdominal malignancies in children after the kidney and adrenal glands. Approximately one-third of primary liver tumors in children are benign, and two-thirds are malignant. Table 16.14 shows a survey of liver tumors in children.

Table 16.14. Classification of liver tumors (Smith 1983)

Benign tumors	
Mesenchymal	Hemangioma Hemangioendothelioma Hamartoma
Congenital cysts	Solitary or multiple cysts in combination with cystic lesions of other organs
Focal nodular hyperplasia	
Adenomas	
Malignant tumors	
Primary	Hepatoblastoma Hepatocellular carcinoma Sarcoma
Secondary	Metastases

16.4.6.2 Liver Cysts

Liver cysts are usually discovered incidentally by ultrasound, CT, or MR imaging. They are benign tumors, which must be differentiated from parasitic or malignant lesions. The incidence in the whole population is less than 5%. Most commonly, the cysts are small and asymptomatic, or may be of varying size (Fig. 16.62). Occurrence can be solitary, multiple, or diffuse. Complications, such as intracystic hemorrhage, rupture, infection, and compression of surrounding tissue, are possible. Liver cysts can also result from a parasitic infection by *Echinococcus granulosus* or *multilocularis.* Cysts of *E. granulosus* or *cysticus* (Fig. 16.63) cause local displacement, whereas those of *E. multilocularis* or *alveolaris* grow in an infiltrative and destructive manner. Metastases similar to a malignant tumor are possible. The imaging features of liver cysts do not differ from those in adults.

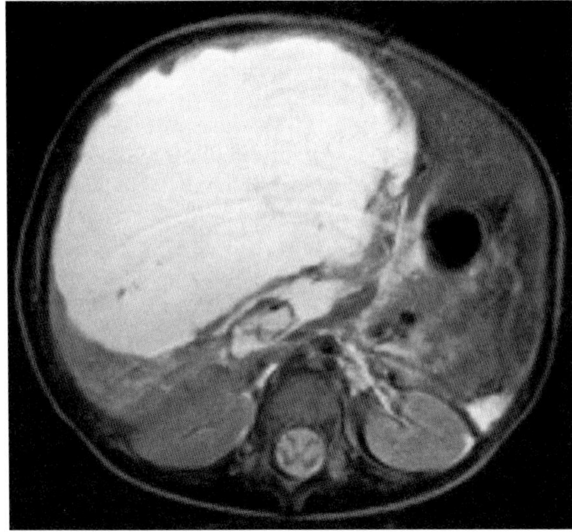

Fig. 16.62. Congenital liver cyst. Axial T2-W turbo spin-echo image depicts a benign, very large, nonseptate cyst in the right lobe of the liver with irregular borders

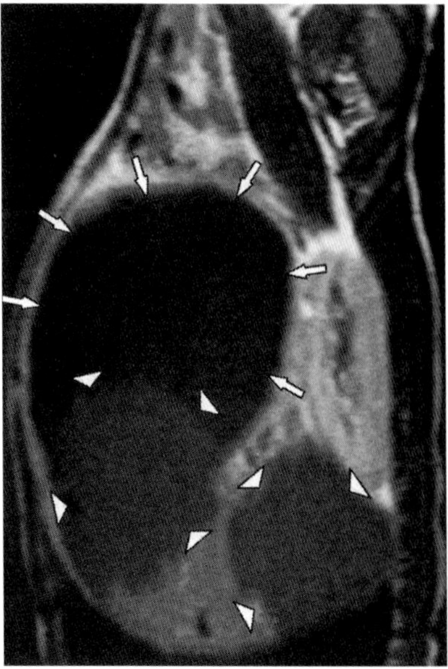

Fig. 16.63. *Echinococcus granulosus* cysts. Sagittal T1-W spin-echo Gd-enhanced image reveals two, well-circumscribed, large, predominantly cystic liver lesions (*arrows*) in a 5-year-old boy. In the upper part of these lesions, soft-tissue components without enhancement by Gd-DTPA can be seen (*arrowheads*)

16.4.6.3 Hemangioma and Hemangioendothelioma

Hemangiomas are very common benign liver tumors. Pathologically, they are endothelium-lined, cystic, blood-filled spaces. Cavernous hemangiomas are focal, well-defined lesions, whereas hemangioendothelioma are more diffuse lesions. Fibrosis or thrombosis is frequently seen in large lesions. Large hemangioendotheliomas, particularly in newborns, may cause congestive heart failure due to extensive shunting. MR imaging shows marked enlargement of the hepatic artery, whereas an abrupt narrowing of the aorta at the level of the celiac artery is seen. Slow blood flow through the enlarged vascular spaces is often noticed. MR findings of hemangiomas in children are the same as in adults. There is a high rate of spontaneous resolution of hemangiomas in childhood. Large focal hemangioendotheliomas in newborns with congestive heart failure are resected, whereas diffuse lesions can be treated with steroids, hepatic artery ligation, or embolization.

16.4.6.4 Hepatoblastoma and Hepatocellular Carcinoma

Hepatoblastomas comprise 54% of primary liver tumors and 15% of all pediatric abdominal tumors. The male:female ratio is 2.3:1. Children are usually affected under the age of 3 years. The exact etiology of hepatoblastoma is unknown. One theory is that hepatoblastoma arises from primitive hepatic blastema. Histologically, four groups are distinguished: fetal, embryonic, small cell undifferentiated, and macrotrabecular anaplastic type. The latter is the one with the worst prognosis. Risk factors for the tumor are biliary atresia, metabolic disorders involving the liver, such as cystinosis and Wilson's disease, hereditary polyposis of the colon, Beckwith-Wiedemann syndrome, trisomy 18, and fetal alcohol syndrome. Cirrhosis is not a risk factor. Hepatoblastoma is usually a solitary, well-defined mass, with a pseudocapsule with a tendency to invade the portal and hepatic veins. Occasionally, multifocal lesions do occur. Primarily nonresectable hepatoblastomas are found in 56% of cases. At the time of diagnosis, 8% of hepatoblastomas have already metastasized. Metastases are seen in the lungs, abdominal lymph nodes, CNS, and bones. Hepatoblastomas are more common in the right lobe of the liver and may produce hormones causing unusual clinical symptoms, such as osteoporosis, virilization, precocious puberty, and hypercalcemia. Other symptoms, such as weight loss, fever, diarrhea, vomiting, and, rarely, dyspnea and jaundice, are not specific. Hepatomegaly is often present on physical examination; an abdominal mass may be palpable. In 90% of cases, the serum levels of α-fetoprotein are elevated, which is useful for the diagnosis and monitoring therapy. Although hepatoblastoma is seen as a focal mass lesion within the liver in ultrasound, CT and MR imaging are better at defining the margins of the tumor. MR imaging seems to be better than CT for the detection of a pseudocapsule, identification of internal trabeculae, vessel involvement, and recurrence of the tumor. Planning of the surgical resection strategy depends on precise localization of the tumor within the liver segments. Therefore, demonstration of the hepatic veins is mandatory. Furthermore, thrombosis of the portal vein can be exactly assessed. Because of excellent vessel visualization on MR imaging, conventional angiography is no longer necessary.

MR Imaging Findings

- T1-W: low SI
- T2-W: varying SI
- Gd-DTPA: immediate enhancement on T1-WI: rim or center of tumor, patchy or diffuse
- Variable internal structure: from fairly homogeneous to very irregular
- Compression, displacement, possible tumor invasion of vessels

The therapy of choice for hepatoblastoma is surgery. Staging of hepatoblastoma is shown in Table 16.15. The 5-year survival rates for hepatoblastoma after surgery are: 100% for stage I, 75% for stage II, 67% for stage III, and 0% for stage IV. If multimodal therapeutic concepts

Table 16.15. Staging of hepatoblastoma

Stage I	Tumor resected completely
Stage II	Tumor resected completely macroscopically, microscopic tumor infiltration
Stage III	Large primary tumor, involvement of both hepatic lobes, no compolete tumor resection macroscopically
Stage IV	Distant metastases

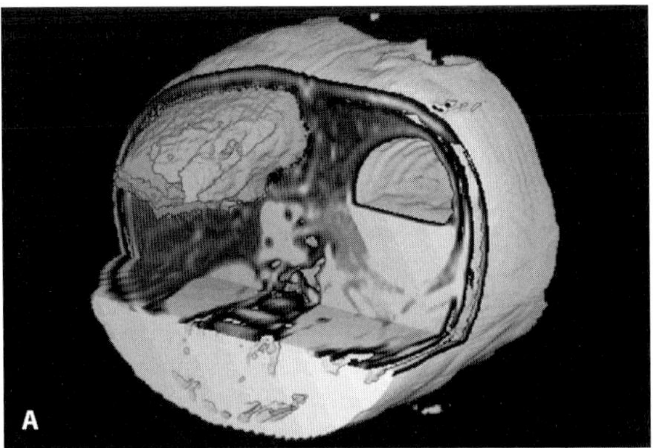

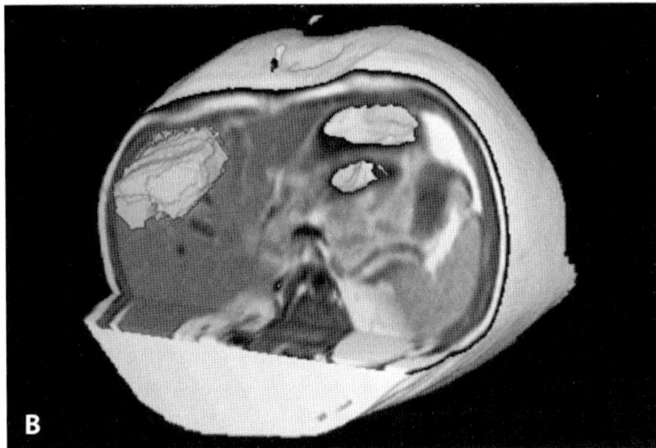

Fig. 16.64A,B. Hepatoblastoma. 3D reconstruction of an axial T2-W turbo spin-echo image (**A**) and axial T1-W spin-echo Gd-enhanced image (**B**) show a hepatoblastoma before (**A**) and after (**B**) preoperative chemotherapy. 3D reconstructed images allow for visualization of the size of the mass and, more importantly, exact calculation of the tumor volume

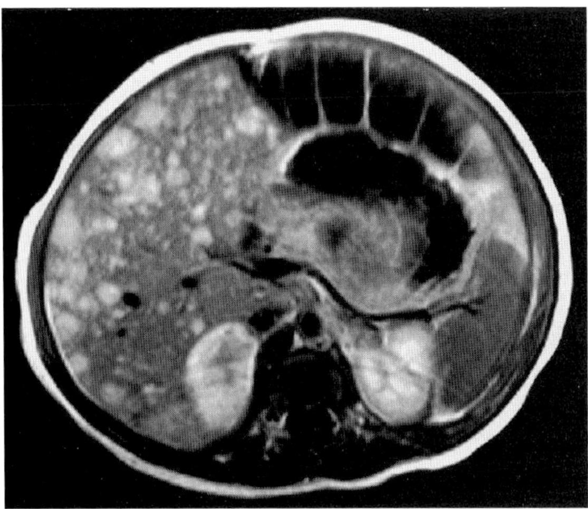

Fig. 16.65. Diffuse metastases of a neuroblastoma. Axial T1-W spin-echo Gd-enhanced image demonstrates multiple, strongly contrast-enhancing metastases all over the liver

are used, MR imaging is performed to evaluate the tumor response to neoadjuvant chemotherapy and to plan further surgical procedures (Fig. 16.64).

In contrast, hepatocellular carcinoma (HCC) is rare in children under the age of 5 years and is associated with chronic diseases such as tyrosinemia, glycogenosis, deficiency of α-1-antitrypsin, biliary atresia, cirrhosis, and hepatitis. HCC may present as a focal mass or a diffusely infiltrating process. Other features include a tumor capsule (40%), intratumoral septa, daughter nodules, tumor thrombi in large portal or hepatic veins, central scarring, and calcifications. Due to hemorrhage, necrosis, and cystic areas, HCC has a variable MR appearance. HCC cannot be distinguished from hepatoblastoma with imaging alone. One subtype of HCC, fibrolamellar carcinoma, which occurs in the later teenage years, is more benign than the classic HCC. The serum levels of α-fetoprotein are normal. The appearance of this unusual type of HCC displays characteristic signs on MR imaging, on both T1-WI and T2-WI, an area of low SI reflecting a central stellate scar in the middle of the tumor.

16.4.6.5 Hepatic Metastases

Many different tumors may metastasize to the liver, with neuroblastoma being the most common (Fig. 16.65). As in adults, the MR imaging appearance of hepatic metastases is variable.

16.4.7 Tumors of Different Origin

16.4.7.1 Mesenteric Cysts

Mesenteric cysts are relatively rare; 40% of mesenteric cysts are seen in children under 1 year of age, 80% in patients under 5 years of age. Mesenteric cysts are divided into embryonic cysts, pseudocysts, developmental cysts, traumatic cysts, neoplastic cysts, infectious cysts, and degenerative cysts. Among the neoplastic cysts are lymphangioma and lymphangioendothelioma. Lymphangiomas are rare, congenital, benign cystic lesions. Multiple and generalized occurrence is termed lymphangiomatosis. The diffuse form is a disease of children and juvenile patients. Lymphangiomas consist of multiseptate, proliferative, endothelial cysts, which are filled with lymph fluid. Of the intraabdominal lymphangiomas, 69% is located in the mesenterium, 15% in the omentum, 11% in the mesocolon, and 5% in the retroperitoneum, with 65% of the lymphangiomas already existing before birth. Spontaneous regression is seen in 10%–15% of cases. Patients may present with pain, fever, nausea, a palpable tumor, or with complications such as obstruction, hemorrhage, and infection. Rectal bleeding and hydronephrosis may be caused by large cysts. Complete resection is the therapy of choice.

Mesenteric cysts and lymphangiomas are characterized by a very high SI on T2-WI (Fig. 16.66). Depending on the fluid content, SI varies from low (simple fluid) to high (blood) on plain T1-WI. Cystic lesions usually do not enhance after the application of Gd-DTPA. Lymphangiomas and lymphangiomatosis, however, may demonstrate a moderate to high contrast enhancement. Therefore, differentiation from other tumors, i.e., neuroblastoma, may be difficult.

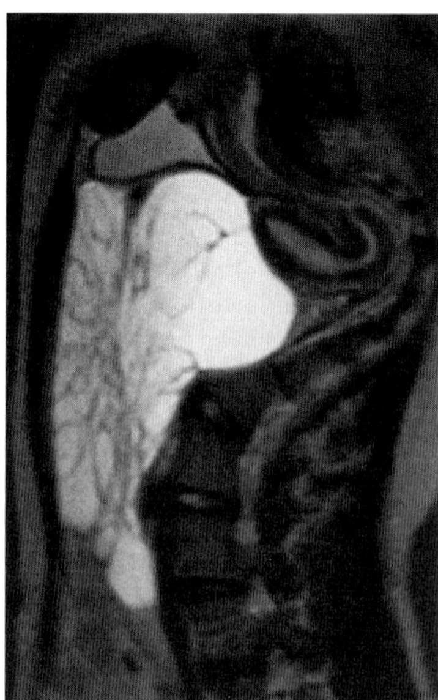

Fig. 16.66. Mesenteric cyst. Axial T2-W turbo spin-echo image depicts a large, multiseptate, prevertebral cyst with typical high signal intensity

16.4.7.2 Duplication Cysts

Duplication cysts can occur at any site in the gastrointestinal tract. They may contain ectopic, gastric, or pancreatic tissue. Usually, the cyst wall appears with low SI on T2-WI, unless the wall is infected, in which case high SI on T2 will be seen. The cyst fluid itself shows a very high SI on T2-WI. Depending on the fluid content, the SI on T1-WI varies from very low signal in simple fluid, slightly higher signal due to infection, and high SI due to hemorrhage. They are treated by surgical excision.

16.4.7.3 Choledochal Cysts

Although MR imaging has a limited role to play in the routine evaluation of patients with suspected choledochal cyst, it may be found incidentally on MR examinations. Choledochal cysts are focal areas of dilatation of the biliary duct system. Usually, the common bile duct is affected. MR imaging shows an elongated and oval-shaped cystic lesion. The SI of the cyst is the same as that from bile in the gall bladder on all pulse sequences. Recent technical developments offer the performance of MR cholangiography (MRC) for the depiction of anatomical and pathological bile-duct structures. Surgical excision is performed as therapy.

16.4.7.4 Lymphoma

For the staging of abdominal lymphoma in childhood, MR imaging should be used due to the lack of radiation dose exposure. Imaging features and findings are the same as in adults.

16.4.7.5 Rhabdomyosarcoma

Rhabdomyosarcoma is the most common tumor of the lower urinary tract in children. One-third of rhabdomyosarcomas are located in the abdomen, especially in the urogenital tract, one-third are found in the orbit, and one-fifth in the head and neck. The generalized form occurs in 4%. Rhabdomyosarcomas are embryonic tumors consisting of undifferentiated mesenchymal tissue, which has the ability to produce striated muscle cells and can affect almost every organ. Two peak incidences are seen, one between 1 and 3 years of age, particularly in the head and neck, the other one between 13 and 18 years of age, especially in the urogenital tract. Patients present with urinary retention and less commonly with hematuria. Unfortunately, abdominal rhabdomyosarcomas are very large in size (Figs. 16.67, 16.68) at the time of presentation. Therapy of rhabdomyosarcoma consists of a combination of operation, chemotherapy, and radiation therapy.

MR Imaging Findings

- Invasion of vagina and uterus or adjacent tissue
- Thickening of bladder wall
- T1-W: medium SI of solid mass
- T2-W: high SI
- Gd-DTPA: marked enhancement on T1-WI

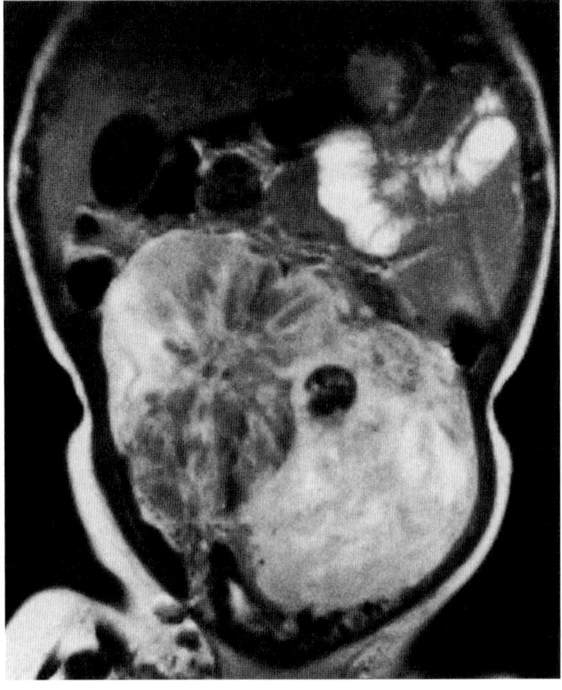

Fig. 16.67. Rhabdomyosarcoma. Coronal T1-W spin-echo Gd-enhanced image demonstrates a large, contrast-enhancing tumor with an inhomogeneous internal structure in a typical lower abdominal and pelvic location

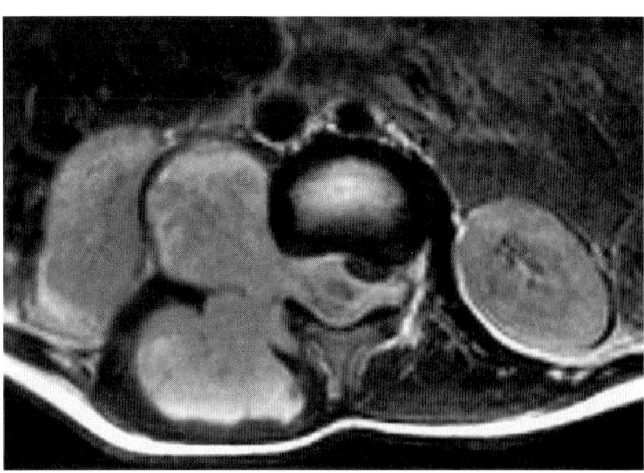

Fig. 16.68. Paravertebral rhabdomyosarcoma. Axial T2-W turbo spin-echo image depicts a histologically proven paravertebral rhabdomyosarcoma with a growth pattern like neuroblastoma and infiltration of the spinal canal through intervertebral foramina

16.4.8 Anorectal Anomalies

Anorectal anomalies include ectopic anus, imperforate anus, rectal atresia, and anal/rectal stenosis, with ectopic anus being the most common form (Table 16.16). In the latter condition, the hindgut fails to descend and

Table 16.16. Anorectal anomalies

Ectopic anus	The hindgut opens ectopically at an abnormal high location (i.e. perineum, vestibule, urethra, bladder or vagina). There is a failure of normal descent of the hindgut
Imperforate anus	The terminal bowel ends blindly and there is no opening or fistula. Two types are distinguished: (a) membranous imperforate anus; and (b) anorectal or anal atesia
Rectal atresia	The anus is present and open, but a variable segment of rectum is atretic. No fistula is present
Anal and rectal stenosis	Incomplete atresia of either structure
Cloacal anomalies	Only in females; urethra, vagina and uterus end in one opening tract. Often associated with hydrometrocolpos and duplication of vagina and/or uterus

Modified from Swischuk

opens ectopically through a fistula into the perineum, vestibule, vagina, urethra, or bladder. Furthermore, associated abnormalities of the genitourinary system and spine are frequently present. Arrest of the hindgut can be high, intermediate, or low. In the case of high arrest, the colon ends at or above the puborectalis sling, which is hypoplastic or even absent. In the case of low arrest, the ectopic hindgut passes through a usually well-developed puborectalis sling and demonstrates a superficial covering at the skin margin. Plain films and injection of contrast agent into the bladder, female genital tract, and male urethra are necessary for visualization of the rectum and fistulas. On MR imaging, fistulas are difficult to depict. However, MR imaging plays an important role in the evaluation of the associated anomalies and the preoperative and postoperative assessment. T1-WI in all three imaging planes are required for excellent anatomic resolution. The levator ani muscle and the residual external sphincter muscle mass can be demonstrated well by MR imaging. Specifically, the identification and location of the external sphincter-muscle mass are crucial for guiding the pull-through surgical procedure. High or intermediate ectopic anus is treated by decompression colostomy initially, with definite pull-through corrective surgery at an age of 1–2 years. Postoperatively, MR imaging may be necessary to prove malplacement of the rectum or inclusion of mesenteric fat within the sphincter ring.

16.5 Pediatric Musculoskeletal System and Bone Marrow Imaging

16.5.1 Coils and Patient Positioning

Depending on the scanner, there are different coil systems designed for adults that have to be used for children. Depending on the system and the available coils, it may be advisable to use the head coil not only for the head but also for the spine, pelvis, and extremities, as long as the coil is large enough for the infant. The spine coil and/or phased-array coils are recommended for evaluation of the upper and lower leg, especially if side-to-side comparison is useful. The pelvis and/or hips are examined with the body-array coil. The extremity coil is preferred to examine the knee, unless it is in a cast, in which case the head coil is used. Flexible surface coils should be used and selected based on the patient's size, because of an improved signal-to-noise ratio and better spatial resolution. In general, the coil which provides highest spatial resolution in concert with the smallest field-of-view is most appropriate for imaging small joints. Optimal positioning in the center of the coil and immobilization with vacuum beds, sponges, sand bags, and blankets are mandatory for the patients.

16.5.2 Sequence Protocol

Basically, the sequence protocols used in children for evaluation of the bone marrow and musculoskeletal system do not differ from those used in adults. Slice thickness, field-of-view, and rectangular field-of-view are adapted to the patient's size. The basic imaging protocol includes T2-W sequences, short tau IR (STIR) sequences, T1-W sequences, and FS T1-W sequences after the administration of paramagnetic contrast, if necessary. For imaging protocols of the different regions, the reader is referred to Chapters 7 and 8 and hints in the following text.

16.5.3 Common Findings in Pediatric Musculoskeletal and Bone Marrow Imaging

16.5.3.1 Normal Appearance of Bone Marrow in Children

Knowledge of the normal appearance and expected marrow distribution in each age group is important for the diagnosis of diseases affecting the bone marrow in children. Normal yellow or fatty marrow consists of 15% water, 5% protein, and 80% fat. It is less vascularized than red or hematopoietic marrow, which is composed of 40% water, 20% protein, and 40% fat. At birth, the entire skeleton contains hematopoietic marrow, and there is a progressive transformation from red to fatty marrow in a predictable pattern from infancy to early adulthood (Fig. 16.69). In the extremities, the conversion progresses distally (fingers, toes) to proximally (shoulder, hips) within each bone, starting in the epiphysis. In the tubular bones, marrow transformation starts in the diaphysis and moves toward the metaphyses,

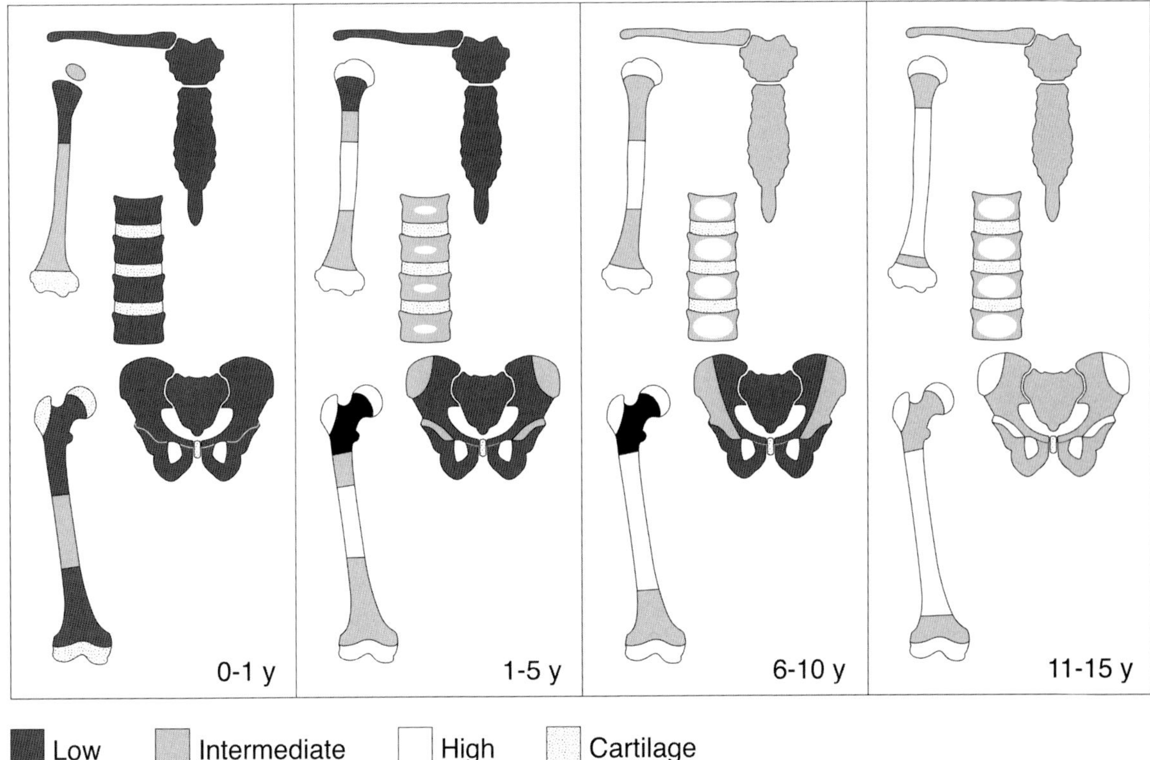

Fig. 16.69. Marrow transformation as depicted on T1-WI. In infants, most of the bones are of low signal intensity due to the presence of hematopoietic marrow. The vertebral bodies are hypointense compared with disks. In early childhood (1–5 years), the epiphysis and the diaphysis of the long bones are of high signal intensity, and the vertebral bodies are isointense with the disks. During late childhood (6–10 years) and early adolescence (11–15 years), the spine, iliac wings, and distal metaphyses become more and more hyperintense due to replacement of hematopoietic marrow by fatty marrow. Adapted from Kirks (1998)

which contain red marrow up to adulthood. This process is slower in the axial skeleton and the pelvis, where red marrow is present throughout life. On T1-WI, fatty marrow is of high SI, whereas red marrow is of low SI. On conventional T2-W SE sequences, fatty and red marrow are of intermediate SI. On STIR images, fatty marrow is of very low SI and red marrow is of intermediate to high SI. In general, coronal planes are most useful in the evaluation of the bone marrow. As a consequence of anemia or other processes that cause an elevation of the level of the circulating hormone erythropoietin, yellow marrow reconverts to red marrow. Marrow reconversion proceeds in the reverse order of conversion.

16.5.3.2 Bone-Marrow Disorders

16.5.3.2.1 Sickle Cell Anemia

Marrow abnormalities related to sickle cell disease include red-marrow expansion due to chronic hemolytic anemia, infarction or avascular necrosis secondary to erythrocyte abnormality, and secondary hemosiderosis due to multiple transfusions. Red-marrow expansion results in decreased marrow SI on T1-WI and mixed SI on T2-WI, whereas hemosiderosis leads to a marked decrease in SI on all pulse sequences. Bone infarcts typically present as sharply demarcated areas with irregular rims of low SI (Fig. 16.70).

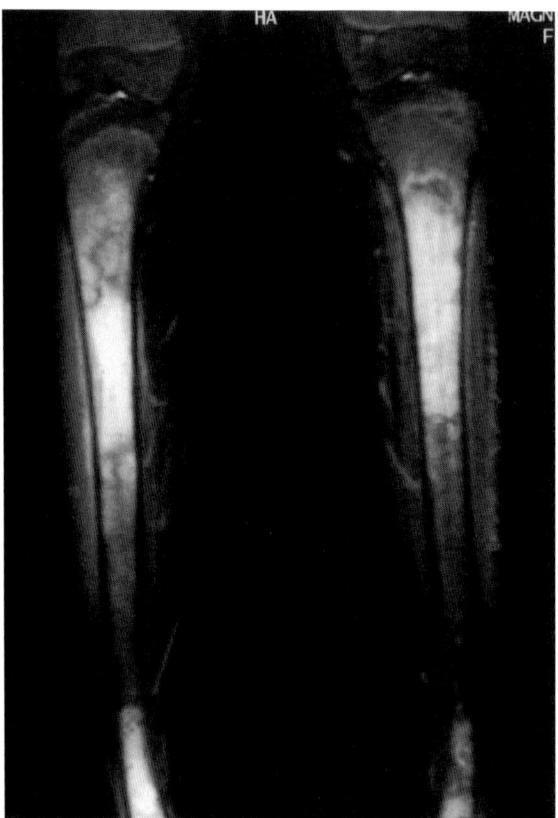

Fig. 16.70. Sickle cell anemia. Coronal short tau inversion recovery image of both lower legs reveals bone infarctions with serpiginous low signal intensity rim and associated edema

16.5.3.2.2
Aplastic Anemia

Aplastic anemia is simple to recognize by MRI, as the extensive replacement of normal red marrow with fat results in bright SI on T1-WI, often including the axial skeleton as well. Especially in the vertebral column, patchy areas of decreased SI develop with treatment, reflecting regeneration of red marrow.

16.5.3.2.3
Gaucher Disease

Storage of glucocerebrosides in the bone marrow, due to a relative deficiency of β-glucocerebrosidase, produces patchy, heterogeneous, decreased SI on T1-WI and T2-WI and increased signal on STIR images, frequently with sparing of the epiphyses. Typical involvement of the distal femurs causes the characteristic Erlenmeyer flask deformity. Patients may additionally suffer from bone infarctions and conditions that clinically and radiographically are indistinguishable from osteomyelitis.

16.5.3.2.4
Iron-Storage Disorders

Iron storage of ferritin and hemosiderin, due to repeated blood transfusions, anemias, hemoglobinopathies, and hemochromatosis, causes decreased SI in both T1-W and T2-W sequences.

16.5.3.2.5
Bone Infarction and Avascular Necrosis

Bone infarction and avascular necrosis are associated with conditions such as sickle cell anemia, Gaucher's disease, meningococcal infection, slipped capital epiphysis, steroid therapy, leukemia, and bone-marrow transplantation. The most common affected site in the pediatric age group is the femoral head. Otherwise, bone infarcts typically occur in the metaphysis and are characterized by a serpiginous low SI rim on both T1-WI and T2-WI (Fig. 16.70); this corresponds to the rim of sclerosis often detected on plain films. In acute and subacute stages, normal fat signal on all sequences of the central island of the infarct is preserved.

16.5.3.2.6
Legg-Calvé-Perthes Disease

Legg-Calvé-Perthes (LCP) disease is an idiopathic avascular necrosis of the immature proximal femoral epiphysis and affects children between the ages of 3 and 12 years. There is a boy-to-girl ratio of 4:1 and a striking retardation of skeletal maturation in both sexes. In 20% of cases, LCP may metachronously occur bilaterally. Children may present with groin, thigh, or knee pain and limitation of abduction and internal rotation. For the prognosis and treatment of LPC, it is necessary to perform a staging and a grading (extension of femoral head involvement). Probably the most commonly accepted classification based on radiographic findings is the one by Caterall, who divides patients into four prognostic groups based on seven radiographic findings. The prognosis depends on the stage at the time of presentation, the child's age, and the extent of femoral head, physeal, and metaphyseal involvement. Fortunately, 50% of children will do well without treatment. On plain-film radiography, four stages of LPC can be distinguished: initial, fragmentation, reparation, and healed stages. MRI has been used to identify both morphologic and signal characteristics of the proximal femur in early stages with negative plain-film findings. MRI delineates the extent of physeal and marrow involvement and, thus, helps with the prognosis and treatment planning. In advanced disease, MRI can help with preoperative assessment of femoral-head coverage and articular integrity.

For evaluation of the LCD, coronal T2-WI and T1-WI, precontrast and postcontrast, and additional T1-WI in sagittal orientation are necessary. Slice thickness should be 3–4 mm. MR findings vary with the stage and extent of the disease. In the initial stage, low SI within the epiphyseal marrow on T1-WI and high SI on T2-WI affecting either the subchondral region or the whole femoral epiphysis are observed, reflecting bone marrow edema. In the early beginnings of LCP, joint effusions are always present. In this stage, plain-film findings are negative or show subchondral lucency in the femoral head.

In the late initial and fragmentation stages, areas affected by avascular necrosis demonstrate complete loss of signal on T1-WI and T2-WI and show no enhancement after the administration of Gd-DTPA. Metaphyseal involvement with loss of signal on T1-WI may be observed as well. Plain-film radiography in these stages shows either increasing sclerosis, flattening of the femoral head, and/or fragmentation (Fig. 16.71).

During reparation, there is femoral and acetabular cartilaginous hypertrophy, and the normal SI of bone marrow reappears, first medially and laterally; the proximal femur remodels, and deformities of the femoral head become evident.

In the healed stage, the proximal femur is remodeled by trabecular bone, and residual shape alterations may or may not be seen. There may be complete restoration to a normal appearance or the final stage may be a physeal arrest, a flattened misshapen femoral head, a short femoral neck, or coxa magna. Important items in the differential diagnosis of LCP include normal variants (femoral head dysplasia of Meyer in patients less than 4 years of age) and other reasons for avascular necrosis such as treatment with steroids, trauma, osteomyelitis,

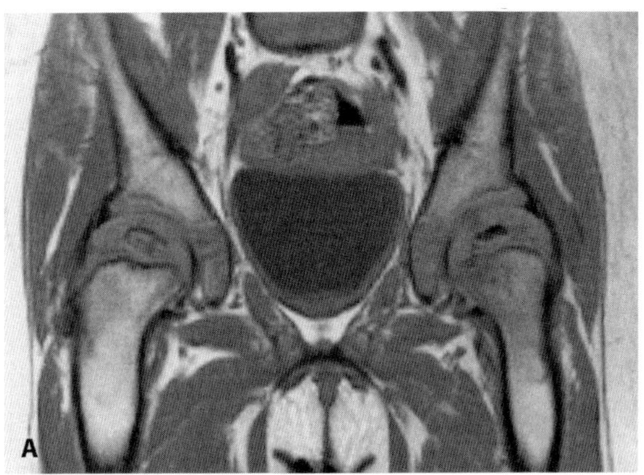

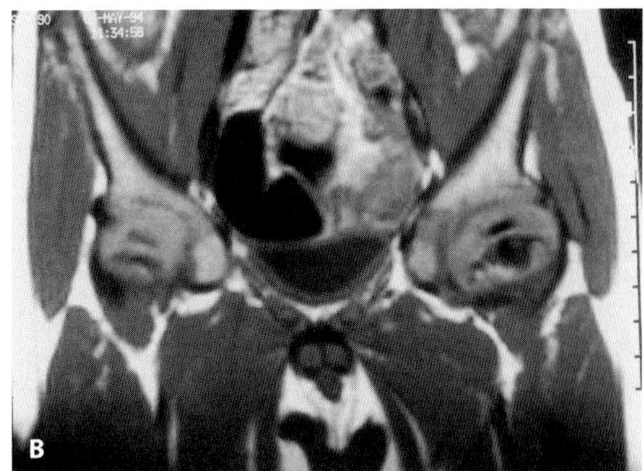

Fig. 16.71A,B. Legg-Calvé-Perthes disease. Coronal T1-WI (**A**) shows complete loss of signal in the left femoral epiphyses and less severe physeal and metaphyseal involvement. Coronal T1-WI (**B**) shows extensive avascular necroses involving epiphyses, physis, and metaphyses on the left side

hemoglobinopathies, and Gaucher disease. Femoral-head deformity is also seen in multiple epiphyseal dysplasias (Fairbank disease), mucopolysaccharidoses, and after developmental dysplasia of the hip. Coxitis fugax can be distinguished from LCD by ultrasound showing synovitis, joint effusion, and clinical course, as clinical symptoms of coxitis fugax resolve in less than 4 weeks.

16.5.3.2.7 Osteochondritis Dissecans

Osteochondritis dissecans (OD) most often involves the medial femoral condyle, but also occurs in children in the capitellum and the talus (see Chapter 7, Fig. 7.6).

Bilateral involvement of the knees is encountered in 20% of the cases. A staging system for OD has been developed based on the arthroscopic findings. An osseous lesion of 1–3 cm in size and an intact articular cartilage characterize stage 1. In stage 2, an articular cartilage defect without a loose body is present. Stage 3 is defined by a partially detached osteochondral fragment with or without interposition of fibrous tissue. In stage 4, a loose body and a defect filled with fibrous tissue is found. The focus of OD shows low SI on both T1-WI and T2-WI. STIR sequences or T2*-weighted images help to decide whether cartilage is intact or not. Areas of high SI on these sequences reflect subchondral fluid or cystic lesions secondary to fissuring of the overlying cartilage. These findings have a high correlation with lesion instability. Administration of Gd-DTPA provides information about the degree of vascularization of the focus. Healed lesions do not demonstrate a bright SI interface between the fragment and the bone and show return of normal fat-marrow signal.

16.5.3.3 Synovial Disorders

16.5.3.3.1 Juvenile Chronic Polyarthritis

Juvenile chronic polyarthritis (JPC) is a chronic inflammatory condition and often has its onset early in childhood. JCP may affect several organ systems (spleen, liver, serous membranes of pericardium and pleura), producing severe symptoms and high fever, but most commonly involves the joints. Some patients may have monarticular involvement. Chronic synovitis leads to synovial hypertrophy, pannus formation, followed by cartilage and bone destruction, eventually ending in ankylosis or joint instability. Localized hyperemia and disuse are the reasons for epiphyseal overgrowth associated with gracile diaphyses. On MRI, synovial hypertrophy and pannus formation will present as thickened areas of low SI on T1-WI and high SI on T2-WI. As it is difficult to distinguish synovial hypertrophy from joint fluid on both T1-WI and T2-WI, the administration of Gd-DTPA is recommended to delineate enhancing synovium (Fig. 16.72).

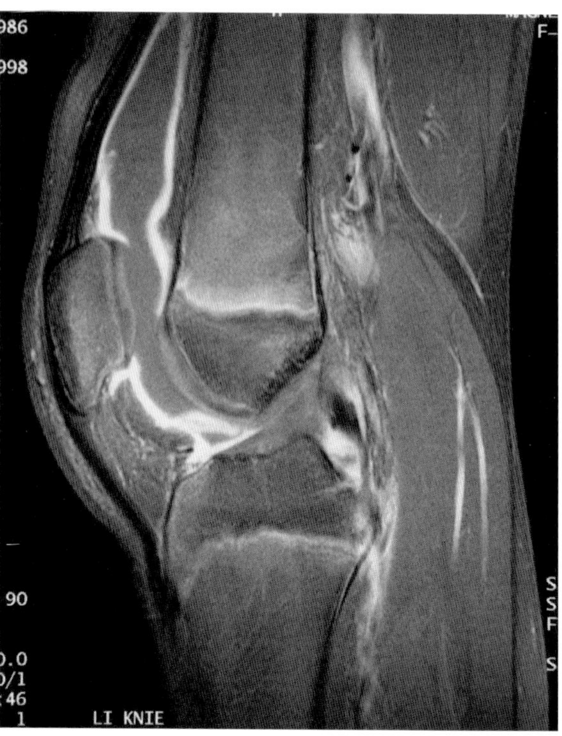

Fig. 16.72. Juvenile chronic polyarthritis. Sagittal FS T1-W contrast-enhanced image shows marked synovial enhancement and joint effusion

16.5.3.3.2 Hemophilia

In hemophilia, deficiency of factor VIII (hemophilia A) or factor IX (hemophilia B) causes repeated hemarthrosis, leading to synovial inflammation, pannus and fibrous-tissue formation, focal or diffuse cartilage destruction, and subchondral cysts with variable signal contents. Due to hemosiderin deposition, the hypertrophic synovium demonstrates low SI on T1-WI and T2-WI. Fibrous tissue also presents with low SI on T1-W and T2-W sequences. Additional typical findings are thickened, irregular fat pads and joint effusions with variable SI, depending on the presence of various blood breakdown products.

16.5.3.4 Acute Osteomyelitis and Septic Arthritis

The majority of pediatric cases of osteomyelitis are due to hematogenous spread from acute sepsis with bacterial, viral, or other infectious agents. *Staphylococcus aureus* is responsible for up to 70% of hematogenous osteomyelitis, and 30% of patients have a history of upper respiratory infection, otitis media, or other infections. Osteomyelitis may also result from a direct penetrating wound or spread to bone by extension from other adjacent structures. The majority of cases of hematogenous osteomyelitis involve the tubular bones and the metaphysis. In children younger than 18 months, transphyseal vessels still exist, and therefore, infection can spread to the physis, epiphysis, and the adjacent joint. In older children, avascular physeal cartilage acts as a relative barrier (Fig. 16.73). Spread to the medullary cavity and diaphysis easily occurs. In children, most cases of septic arthritis are due to spread from an adjacent focus of osteomyelitis, leading to synovitis and joint effusions, possibly being complicated by epiphyseal infarction and joint destruction. Osteomyelitis is difficult to diagnose in the first years of life, as it is usually silent and is often detected only 2–4 weeks after onset of infection. Plain-film radiographs obtained during the first week of disease may show nothing but soft-tissue swelling. Later on, destructive bone changes appear as focal or confluent radiolucencies in bone. After about 10 days, early periosteal new bone formation is observed. MRI is the method of choice to diagnose osteomyelitis, as differentiation between isolated periostitis, medullary infection, periosteal abscess, and involvement of joints can be excellently depicted. On MRI, osteomyelitis appears as a defined focal lesion in the metaphysis, with low SI on T1-WI and high SI on T2-WI, accompanied by edema extending into the marrow and adjacent soft tissues. After administration of Gd-DTPA, nonenhancing areas of necrosis can be detected (Fig. 16.74). Findings may naturally be much more pronounced, depending on the extent of the inflammatory process. Finally, osteomyelitis may be indistinguishable from Ewing sarcoma on radiographic and MR findings.

16.5.3.5 Tumors and Tumor-Like Conditions

The diagnosis of musculoskeletal tumors is still primarily based on plain-film radiographs and confirmed by biopsy. As a rule, MR examinations of tumors and tumor-like conditions should not be performed without

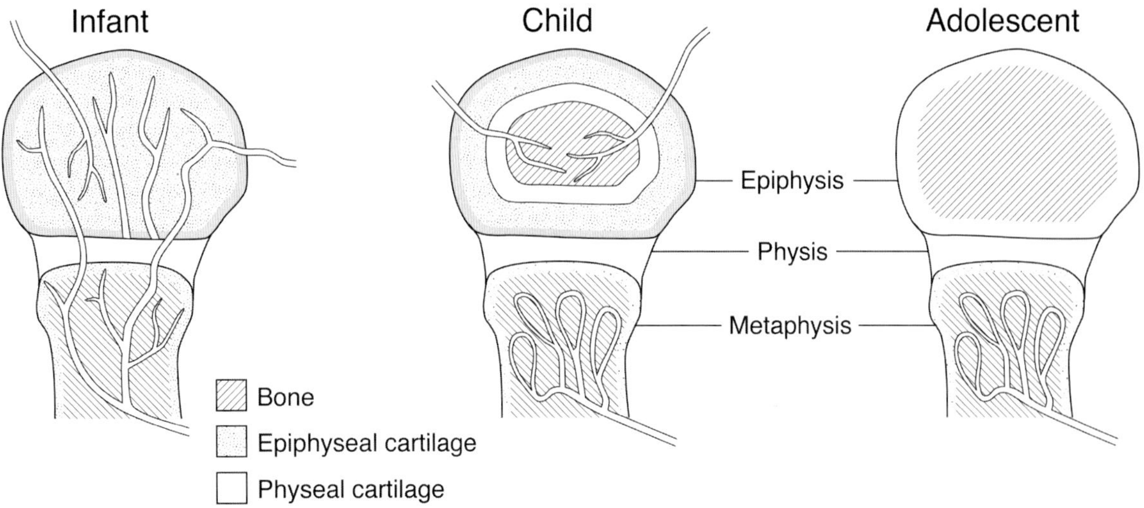

Fig. 16.73. Age-related changes in the anatomy of a growing long bone. *Infant*: the epiphysis is completely or almost completely cartilaginous. Epiphyseal and metaphyseal vessels communicate across the physis. *Child*: the ossification center in the epiphysis is well formed. The physis acts as a relative barrier between epiphyseal and metaphyseal vessels. *Adolescent*: the epiphysis is ossified, but the physis remains cartilaginous. The epiphysis has fewer vessels than the metaphysis. Adapted from Kirks (1998)

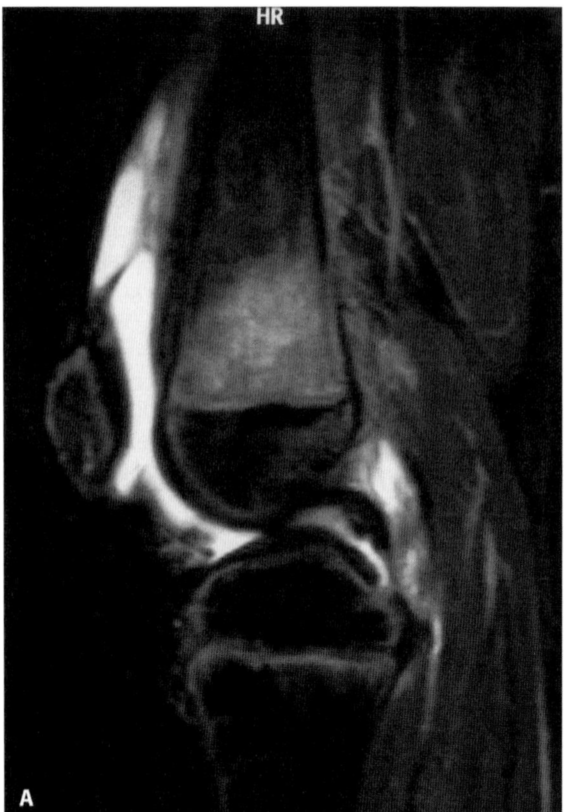

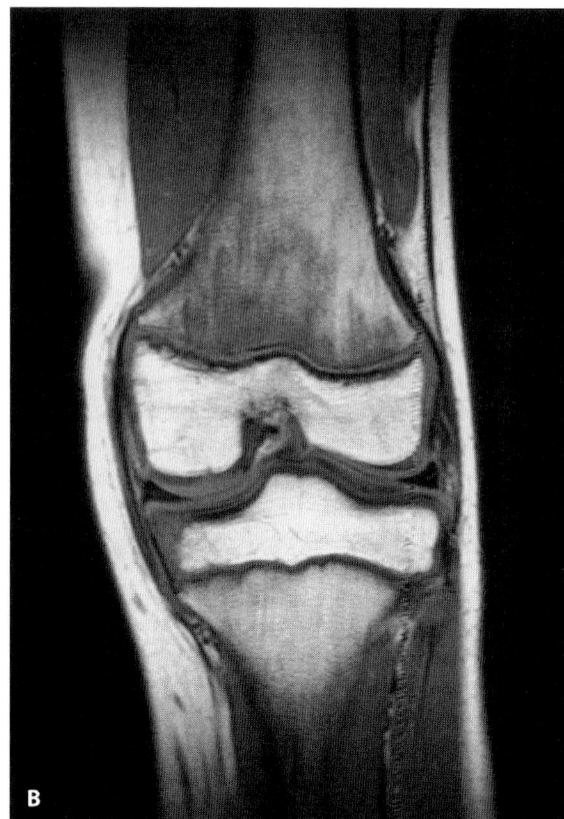

Fig. 16.74A,B. Osteomyelitis with joint empyema. Sagittal short tau inversion recovery image (**A**) demonstrates joint effusion and increased signal intensity in the metaphyses with destruction of the cortical bone dorsally and soft-tissue involvement. Coronal T1-WI (**B**) demonstrates corresponding low signal intensity in the metaphysis

plain-film radiography. Due to advances in neoadjuvant therapy and surgical techniques, approximately 80% of patients with malignant bone lesions are now potential candidates for limb-salvage procedures. Determination of the tumor extent, detection of skip lesions, and evaluation of vital structure involvement, such as neurovascular bundles, adjacent muscle groups, joint and transphyseal extension, is best accomplished by MRI. In addition, assessment of successful therapy, completeness or complications of surgery, and detection of recurrent disease can be monitored by MRI. Indicators suggesting a response to therapy include decrease of tumor size and peritumoral edema with better demarcation and recurrence of normal fatty marrow signal. However, in many cases, the presence or absence of vital tumor cells may only be proven by biopsy.

When evaluating an extremity tumor, obtaining a combination of transverse and coronal or sagittal images, including the entire length of an involved bone, is recommended. Whether coronal or sagittal planes should be obtained depends on the location of the lesion. A process located ventrally or dorsally should be examined in the sagittal plane, whereas a process located medially or laterally is better evaluated by coronal plane imaging. Contrast should be administered for better delineation of the tumor and for distinction between tumor and necrosis.

T1-W SE sequences in a coronal plane are best for judgment of intramedullary extent, whereas T2-W transverse images are suitable for the evaluation of invasion into adjacent musculature and neurovascular bundles. FS T1-WI after the administration of Gd-

DTPA are recommended to make a distinction between tumor, peritumoral edema, and necrosis. In the following paragraphs, attention is given to the most common pediatric tumors.

16.5.3.5.1
Benign Bone and Soft-Tissue Tumors

There are no generally accepted indications for the performance of MR imaging of benign bone tumors, such as unicameral bone cyst, osteochondroma, enchondroma, and chondroblastoma, as they show typical findings on conventional plain-film radiographs.

■ **Osteoid Osteoma.** Patients with osteoid osteoma typically present with a history of pain, especially at night, which is relieved by aspirin. There are four different types: cortical, medullary, subperiosteal, and intra-articular. The cortical type is the most frequent (80%–90%). The lesion is characterized by a central, often calcified, nidus surrounded by reactive bone sclerosis and cortical thickening. Osteoid osteomas may be visualized either by CT or MRI. On MRI, the nonossified nidus has high SI on T2-WI and is almost always invisible on T1-WI prior to the administration of paramagnetic contrast (Fig. 16.75). The ossified nidus is hypointense on both T1-WI and T2-WI but surrounded by a rim, which is hypointense on T1-WI and hyperintense on T2-WI. Associated bone marrow and soft-tissue edema enhancing with paramagnetic contrast are frequently observed. In the intraarticular type, synovitis and joint effusions are encountered.

■ **Aneurysmal Bone Cyst.** Aneurysmal bone cysts (ABCs) are most commonly found in the posterior osseous elements of the spine and in the long bones, where they appear as expansile, lytic, and eccentric metaphyseal lesions. On MRI, ABCs present as well-defined lesions with lobulated margins and areas of mixed SI on T1-W and T2-W sequences, reflecting chronicity of the associated hemorrhage. ABCs may have multiple cavities containing fluid-fluid levels, probably representing layering of uncoagulated blood within the lesion, separated by enhancing internal septations (Fig. 16.76). Fluid-fluid levels were initially believed to be highly suggestive of ABCs, but they have also been described in lesions such as simple bone cyst, fibrous dysplasia, giant cell tumor, chondroblastoma, telangiectatic osteosarcoma, vascular malformations, and malignant fibrous histiocytomas. One-third of ABCs are secondary to preexisting lesions, such as giant-cell tumor, osteoblastoma, chondroblastoma, fibrous dysplasia, nonossifying fibroma, chondromyxoid fibroma, and osteosarcoma. Because of the aforementioned association with osteosarcoma and the fact that the telangiectatic variant of osteosarcoma, in particular, may be indistinguishable from ABCs, close clinical follow-up and biopsy are mandatory in these lesions.

■ **Langerhans' Cell Histiocytosis.** Langerhans' cell histiocytosis (LCH) is a disease of unknown etiology and is characterized by an abnormal proliferation of LC with either focal or systemic manifestation. LCH clinically presents in three different types: eosinophilic granuloma (EG), Letterer-Siwe disease (LS), and Hand-Schüller-Christian disease (HSC) (Table 16.17). Many cases of LCH cannot be categorized into one of the aforementioned groups, as there is considerable overlap and evolution from one syndrome to the other. The prognosis of EG is excellent, whereas the prognosis of the disseminated forms strongly depends on the number of involved organs and extent of organ infiltration. The therapy of LCH depends on the histologic classifi-

Table 16.17. Manifestations of Langerhans' cell histiocytosis

	LS	HSC	EO
Type	Acute disseminated	Disseminated	Localized
Age range	<1 year	3–6 years	10–14 years
Frequency	10%	20%	80%
Involved organs	Skin, liver, spleen, lymph nodes, bone marrow	Classic triad: diabetes insipidus, exophthalmus, calvarial destruction	Bone or lung

LS, Letterer-Siwe; HSC, Hand-Schüller-Christian; EO Eosinophilic granuloma

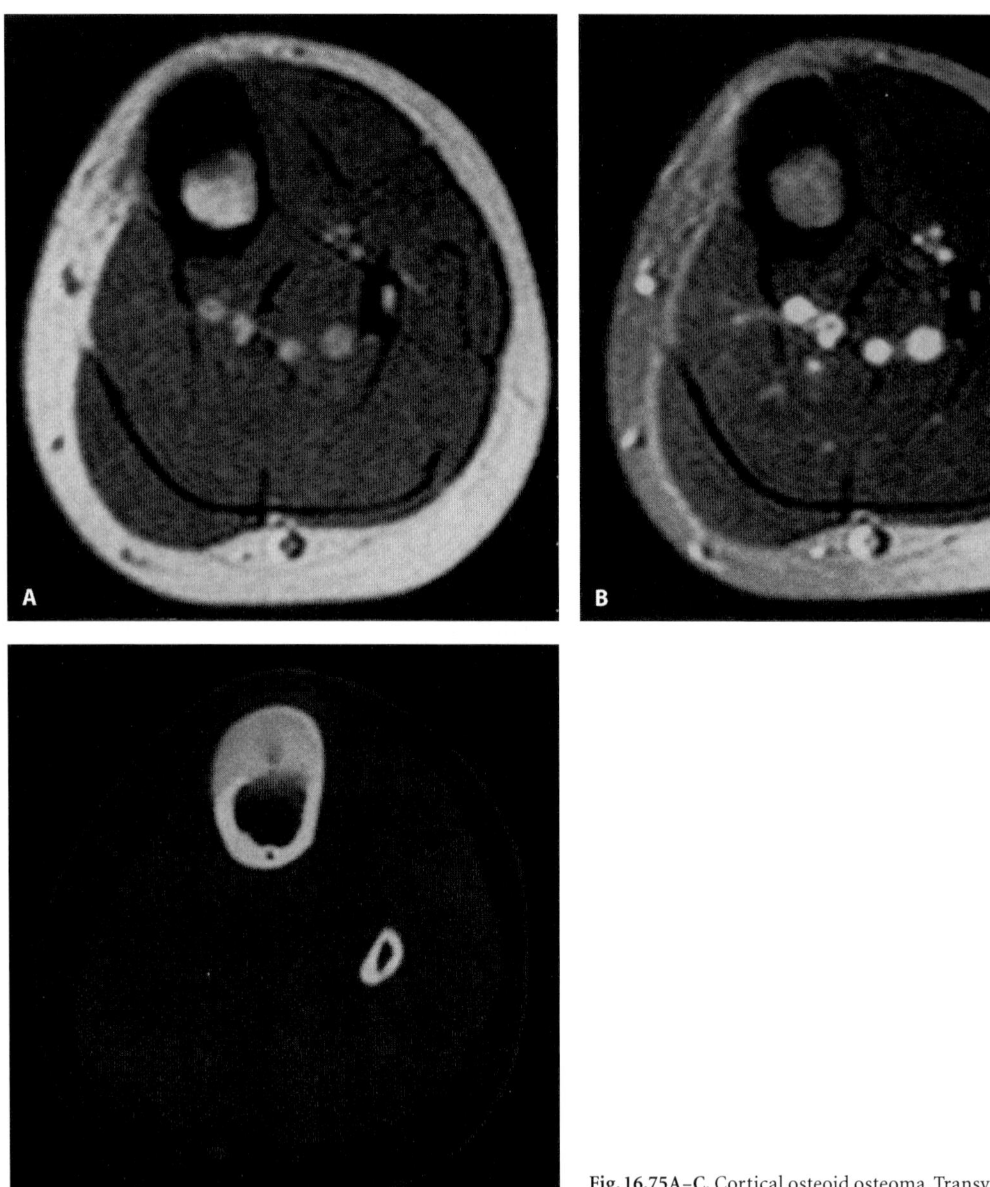

Fig. 16.75A–C. Cortical osteoid osteoma. Transverse T1-W precontrast (**A**) and postcontrast (**B**) images demonstrate enhancing nidus in the left tibia with marked reactive bone sclerosis. Corresponding transverse CT (**C**) depicts a nonossified nidus

cation and extent of disease. It may consist of observation without intervention, curettage of the involved bone in EG, or even chemotherapy.

The most common sites of skeletal involvement in LCH are the skull (28%) (Fig. 16.77), the ribs (14%), the femur (13%), the pelvis (10%), the spine (7%), the mandible (7%), and the humerus (6%). LCH can have many different radiographic appearances. Lesions in flat bones tend to be well-defined lytic lesions, whereas lesions in long bones more often present as lytic lesions

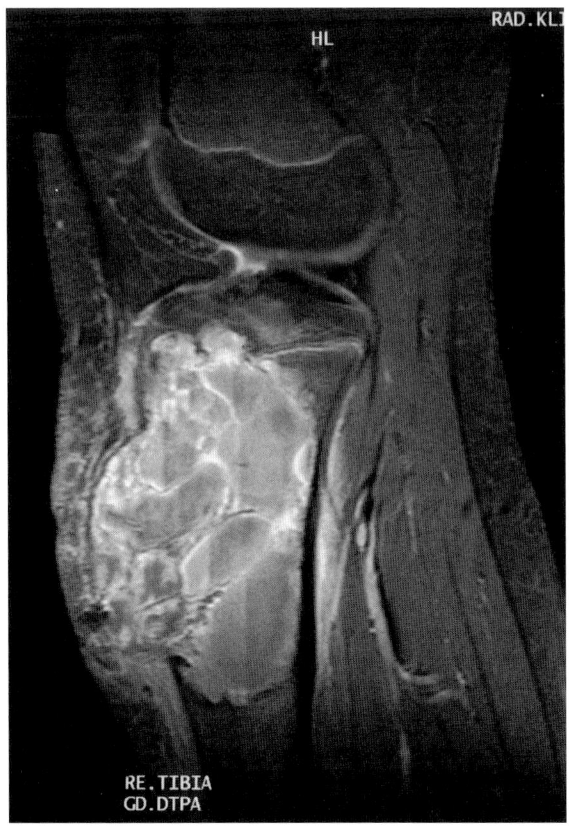

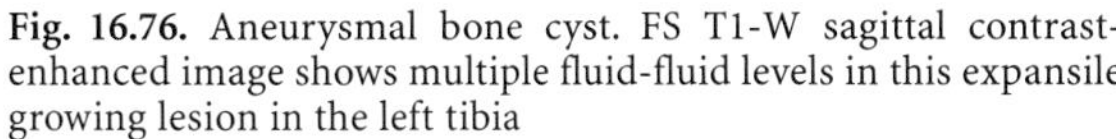
Fig. 16.76. Aneurysmal bone cyst. FS T1-W sagittal contrast-enhanced image shows multiple fluid-fluid levels in this expansile growing lesion in the left tibia

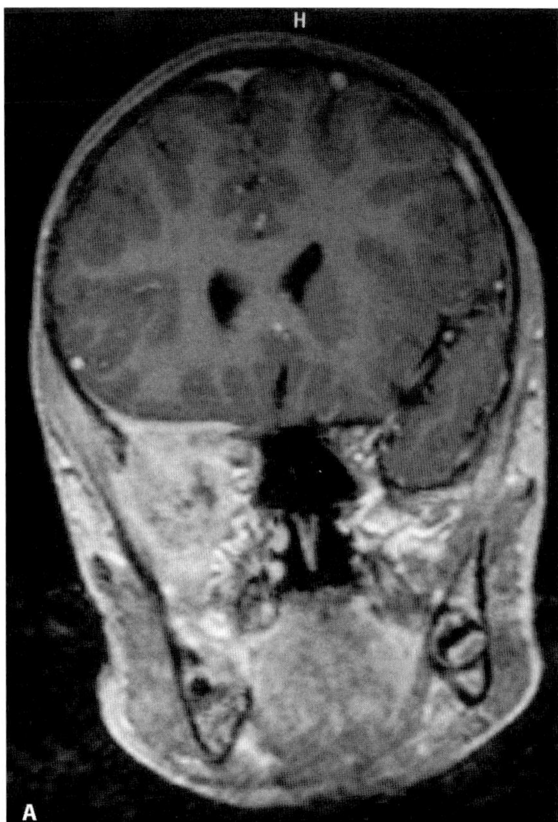

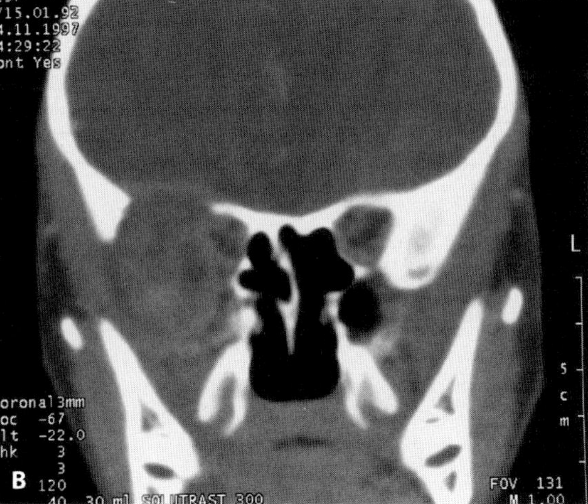

Fig. 16.77A,B. Langerhans' cell histiocytosis of the skull base. T1-W coronal contrast-enhanced image (**A**) shows a uniformly enhancing mass in the right orbit with a sharply demarcated defect in the sphenoid bone. Coronal CT (**B**) clearly depicts the osseous defect

with reactive sclerosis and periosteal reaction, most commonly located in the diaphysis. LCH of the skull presents with uneven destruction of the inner and outer tables or other peculiar calvarial lesions in children involving the sella turcica, mastoids, orbits, and mandible (floating teeth). Involvement of the spine typically manifests as vertebra plana (Fig. 16.78) and a soft-tissue paravertebral mass. On MRI, the area of abnormal SI is usually larger than suggested by plain-film radiography. The lesions are hyperintense on T2-WI and STIR images and hypointense on T1-WI with homogeneous enhancement after GD-DTPA. However, MRI cannot distinguish actual LCH involvement from edema in soft tissues and bone marrow.

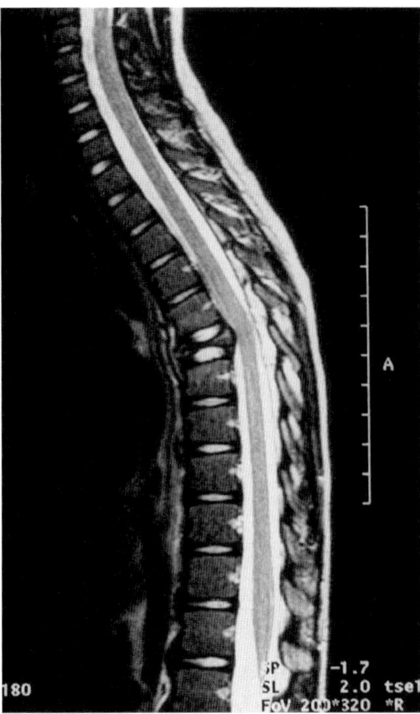

Fig. 16.78. Langerhans' cell histiocytosis of the spine. Sagittal T2-WI shows vertebra plana of Th6 with resulting gibbus

■ **Vascular Anomalies.** Vascular anomalies are classified into two major groups: hemangiomas and vascular malformations (Table 16.18). Hemangiomas are proliferative endothelial cell tumors, which typically present in infancy, grow rapidly in the first year of life and then slowly involute. Vascular malformations have a normal cellular turnover, grow commensurately with the child, and are further classified according to channel abnormalities (arteriovenous, capillary, venous, lymphatic, mixed) and flow characteristics (high-flow, low-flow). In contrast to hemangiomas, vascular malformations are always present at birth. For the MR appearance of hemangiomas, arteriovenous, venous and lymphatic (lymphangiomas) malformations, see Table 16.19 and Figs. 16.79 and 16.80.

Table 16.18. Classification of vascular anomalies

Hemangioma
Proliferating
Involuting
Involuted
Vascular malformation
High flow
Arteriovenous fistula
Arteriovenous malformation
Low flow
Capillary malformation
Venous malformation
Lymphatic malformation (=Lymphangiomas)
Macrocystic
Microcystic
Mixed

Adapted from Kirks

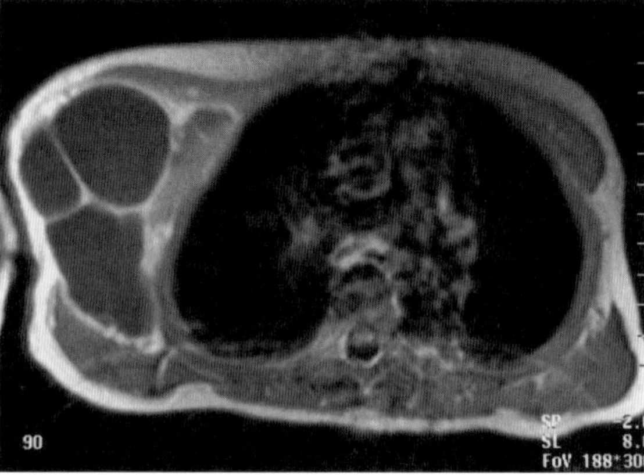

Fig. 16.79. Macrocystic lymphatic malformation. Transverse T1-WI postcontrast shows large, septated, cystic, soft-tissue mass with rim enhancement in the right axilla

■ **Dermatomyositis.** Dermatomyositis is an idiopathic inflammatory disorder of the skeletal muscle, which presents with increased SI on (FS) T2-WI in the affected muscle groups. The adductors, gluteus, and quadriceps groups are most commonly involved, and there may also be increased SI in the adjacent subcutaneous fat, reflecting edema. MRI is performed in transverse planes to determine the biopsy site selection.

16.5.3.5.2 Malignant Bone and Soft-Tissue Tumors

■ **Osteosarcoma.** Osteosarcoma is the most common primary malignant bone tumor of childhood. The peak incidence is between the ages of 10 and 20 years. Osteosarcoma may be either osteogenic, showing considerable new bone formation, or primarily osteolytic, especially in teleangiectatic osteosarcoma. Usually,

Table 16.19. Magnetic resonance imaging findings in pediatric vascular anomalies

Lesion	T1-WI	T1-W+contrast	T2-W	Gradient
Hemangioma				
Proliferating	STM iso- or hypo-intense to muscle, flow voids	Uniform intense enhancement	Increased SI	HFV within and around STM, flow voids
Involuting	Variable fat content	As above	Variable fat	As above
Involuted	High SI (fat)	No enhancement	Decreasd SI	No HFV
Vascular malformation				
Arteriovenous MF	STT, mixed SI, flow voids	Diffuse enhancement	Variable increased SI, flow voids	HFV throughout abnormal tissue
Venous MF	Septated STM, isointense to muscle, high signal thrombi	Diffuse or inhomogeneous enhancement	High SI, signal voids (phleboliths)	No HFV, signal voids (phleboliths)
Lymphatic MF, macrocystic	Septated STM, low SI	Rim or no enhancement	High SI, fluid-fluid levels	No HFV
Lymphatic MF, microcystic	STT, hypo – or isointense to muscle	No enhancement	Diffuse increased SI, subcutaneous stranding	No HFV

STM, soft tissue mass; STT, soft tissue thickening; SI, signal intensity; HFV, high flow vessels; MF, malformation; WI weighted image. Adapted from Kirks

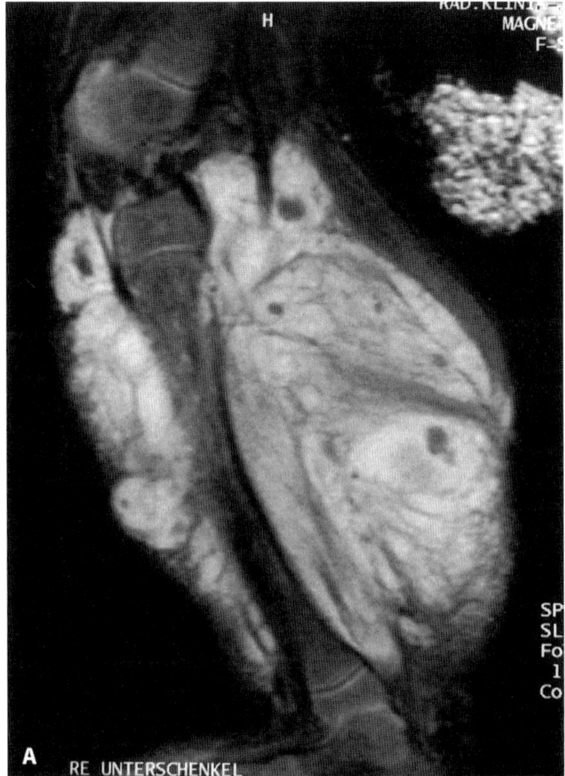

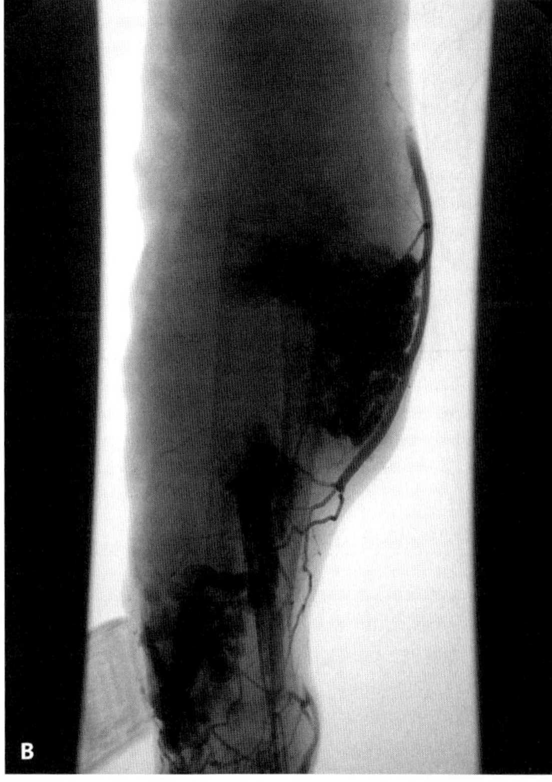

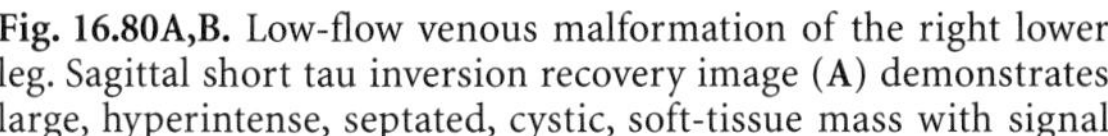

Fig. 16.80A,B. Low-flow venous malformation of the right lower leg. Sagittal short tau inversion recovery image (**A**) demonstrates large, hyperintense, septated, cystic, soft-tissue mass with signal voids due to phleboliths. Phlebography performed 2 years later (**B**) (early filling) shows complete infiltration of subcutaneous fat and muscles by anomalous veins in the lower leg

there is a considerable permeative bony destruction with various irregular periosteal reactions (layered periosteal new bone deposition, spicules, formation of a Codman triangle) and a soft-tissue mass. Osteosarcoma most commonly arises in decreasing order of frequency in the distal femur (40%), the proximal tibia (20%), and the proximal humerus (15%), often eccentrically in the metaphysis. Occasionally, osteosarcoma presents with uniform sclerosis of the affected bone, without periosteal reaction, a soft-tissue mass, or destruction of the cortex. On MRI, osteosarcoma presents with low SI on T1-WI and high SI in T2-WI. Areas of tumor osteoid formations are of low SI in all sequences (Fig. 16.81), whereas teleangiectatic osteosarcomas contain hemorrhagic components showing areas of high SI on T1-WI and T2-WI, resembling ABCs. For better distinction between tumor, necrosis, and peritumoral edema, Gd-DTPA should be administered, and FS T1-W sequences should be used in addition to conventional SE sequences. Tumor response to therapy results in decrease of soft-tissue mass and peritumoral edema and bone destruction.

■ **Ewing's Sarcoma.** Ewing's sarcoma is the second most common primary bone tumor in children, occurring between 5 and 25 years of age. With Ewing's sarcoma, the bone destruction is often extensive and lytic. Ewing's sarcoma may affect any bone in the body, but most commonly occurs in decreasing order of frequency in the femur, pelvis, tibia, and humerus; it is one of the malignant round-cell tumors involving bone. The tumor is located typically in the diaphysis, but more commonly occurs in the metaphysis. Lesions in the diaphysis are usually central, whereas those in the metaphysis are eccentric. Ewing's sarcoma demonstrates high SI on T2-WI and low SI on T1-WI, with prominent enhancement after contrast administration (Fig. 16.82). Ewing's sarcoma may be indistinguishable from osteomyelitis by radiographic and MR findings.

■ **Leukemia and Lymphoma.** Acute leukemias are aggressive disorders arising from the primitive stem-cell level and are basically classified as either lymphocytic or myelogenous. Of patients with acute lymphocytic leukemia, 80% are children, whereas 90% of patients with acute myelogenous leukemia are adults. Acute lymphoblastic leukemia infiltrates the marrow more diffusely, whereas acute myelocytic leukemia presents with a patchier pattern. If destruction of the cortex occurs, it is usually located in the metaphyseal region. Recognition of pediatric leukemias is complicated by two facts: (1) the signal characteristics of neoplastic infiltration is quite similar to red marrow, showing low SI on T1-WI and high SI on T2-WI; contrast enhancement may be moderate, and (2) these lesions arise typically in red-marrow locations; therefore, short TI IR sequences or FS sequences should be used to detect leukemic infiltrates.

■ **Metastatic Disease.** Metastatic skeletal lesions in children most commonly arise from small round-cell tumors, such as leukemia, lymphoma, or neuroblastoma, but may also be due to osteogenic sarcoma, Ewing's sarcoma, PNET, rhabdomyosarcoma, retinoblastoma, cerebellar medulloblastoma, and Wilms' tumor (5%). In general, metastatic disease appears as focal lesions, involving both cortical bone and marrow, demonstrating low SI on T1-W sequences and bright SI on STIR and T2-W sequences. However, diffuse metastatic disease may be difficult to distinguish from normal marrow on MR, especially in children.

■ **Juvenile Fibromatosis.** Juvenile fibromatosis is a locally invasive tumor and can involve subcutaneous tissues, muscles, nerves, and vessels, but rarely bone, and may recur after initial resection. Juvenile fibromatosis demonstrates low SI on T1-WI and enhances after the administration of Gd-DTPA. On T2-WI, hypointense to hyperintense SI is observed (Fig. 16.83).

■ **Fibrosarcoma and Rhabdomyosarcoma.** In the neonate and young infant, fibrosarcoma is the most common soft-tissue malignancy. This soft-tissue mass has large feeding vessels and shows low SI in T1-WI and high SI on T2-WI, with demarcation of areas of necrosis after the administration of Gd-DTPA. The adjacent bones are often splayed rather than destroyed.

In the older child, rhabdomyosarcomas are more common, and the prognosis is much better than in fibrosarcomas, because of their better response to chemotherapy. Rhabdomyosarcomas demonstrate low SI on T1-WI and high SI on T2-WI, but may appear heterogeneously and enhance inhomogeneously with paramagnetic contrast, due to hemorrhage and necrosis (Fig. 16.84).

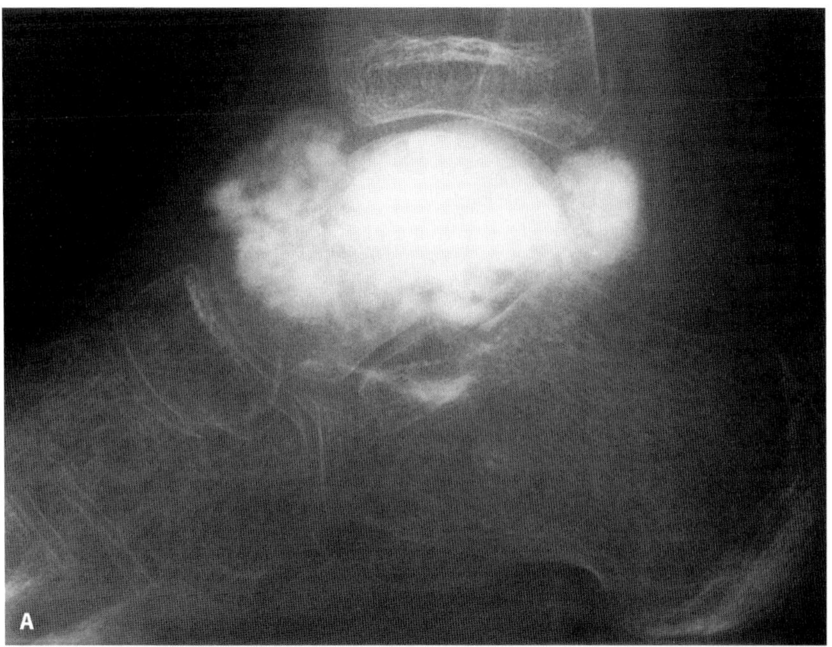

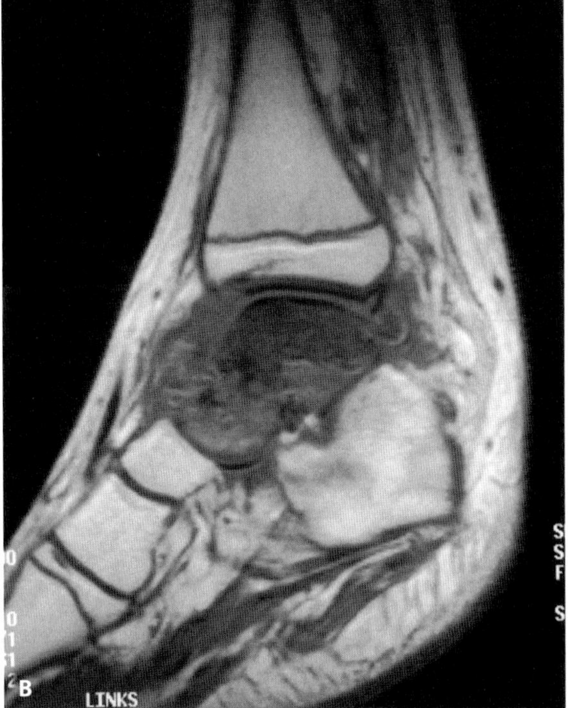

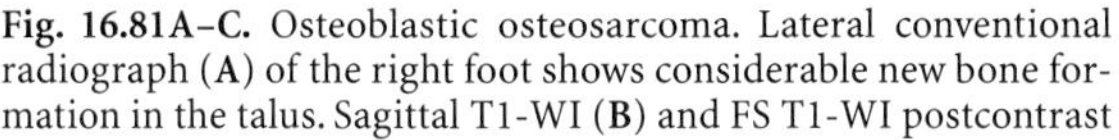

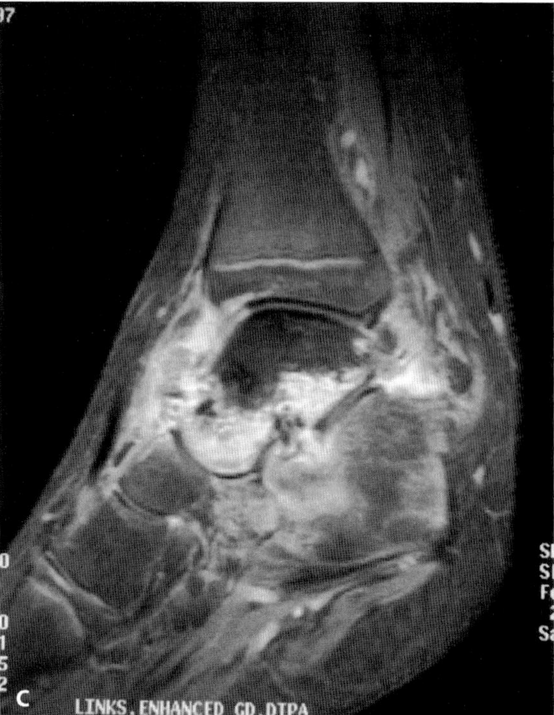

Fig. 16.81A–C. Osteoblastic osteosarcoma. Lateral conventional radiograph (**A**) of the right foot shows considerable new bone formation in the talus. Sagittal T1-WI (**B**) and FS T1-WI postcontrast (**C**) demonstrate markedly enhancing marrow involvement and soft-tissue component

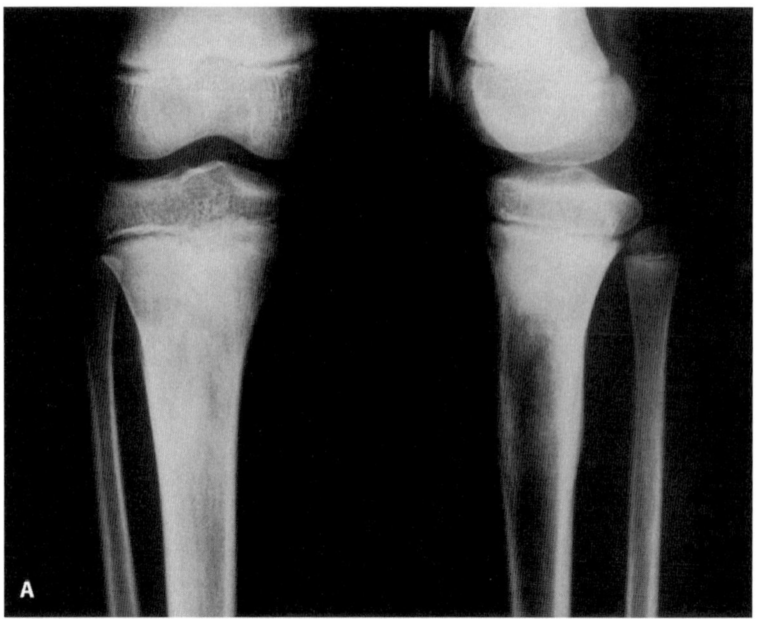

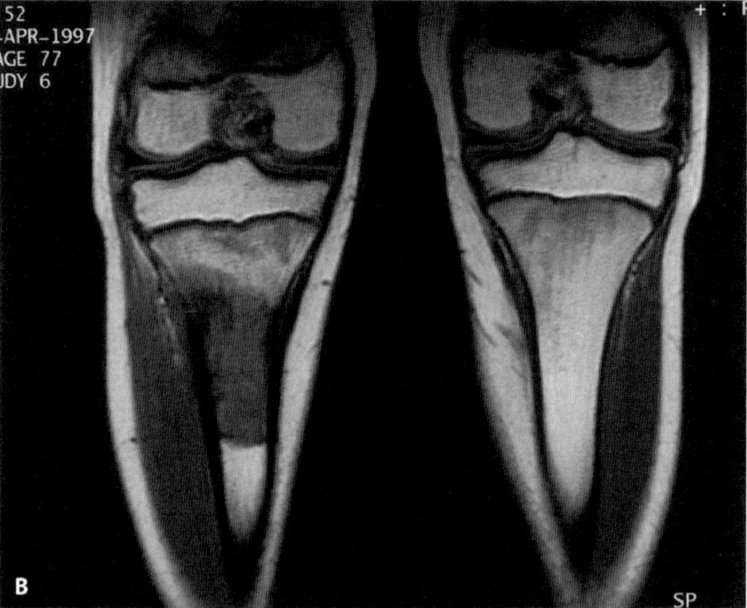

Fig. 16.82A–C. Ewing's sarcoma. Conventional radiographs (**A**) of the right lower leg show an irregular osteolytic area in the proximal tibia with a periosteal thickening dorsally. Coronal T1-WI (**B**) and FS T1-WI postcontrast (**C**) demonstrate markedly enhancing focus of involved marrow

Fig. 16.82C.

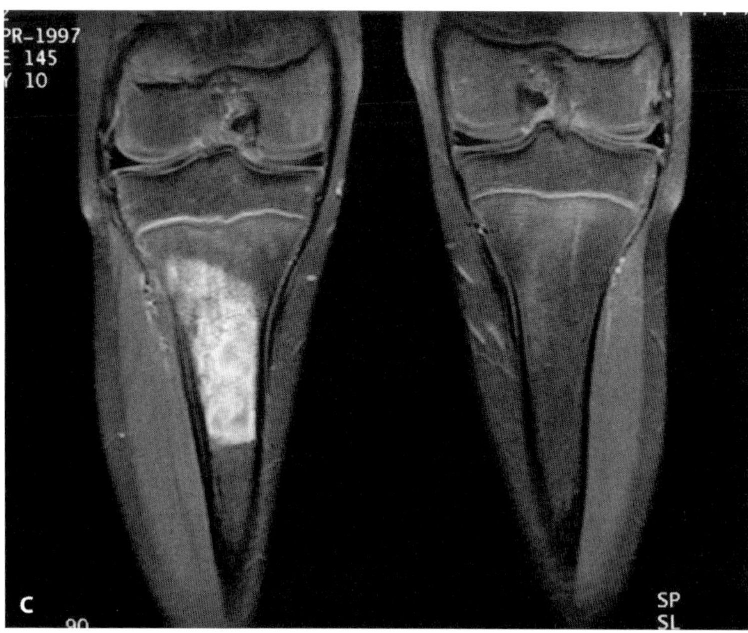

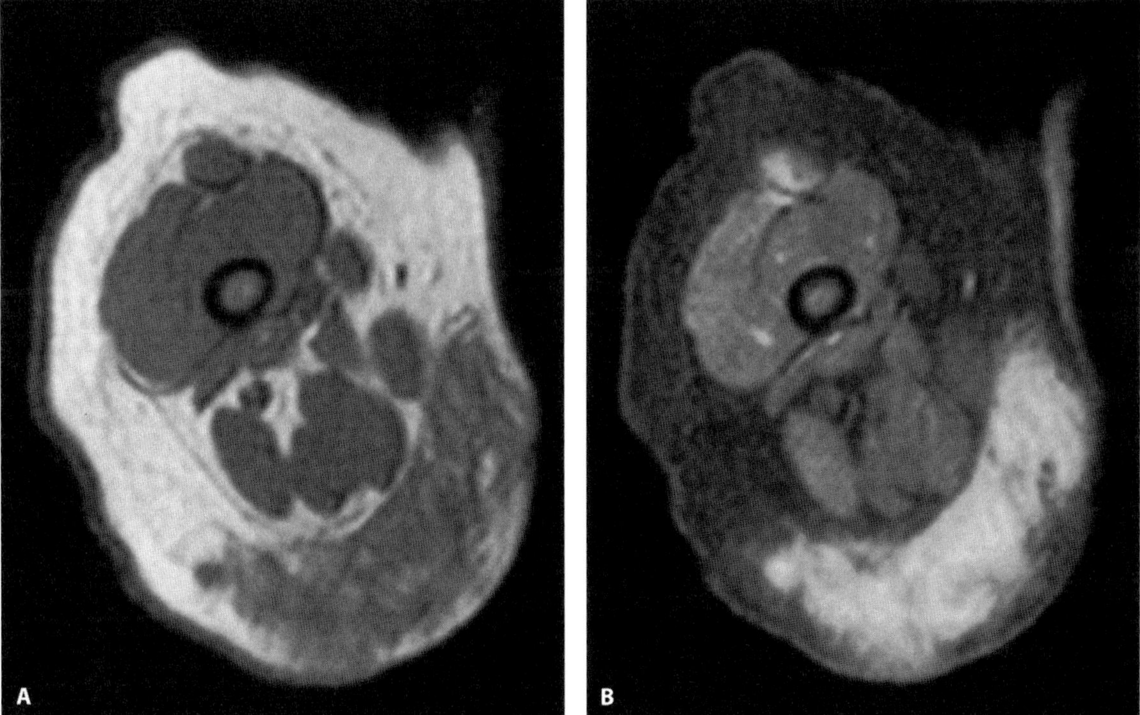

Fig. 16.83A,B. Juvenile fibromatosis. Transverse T1-W (**A**) and FS T1-W (**B**) images show homogeneously enhancing tissue within the subcutaneous fat dorsally and in the rectus femoris muscle of the right upper leg

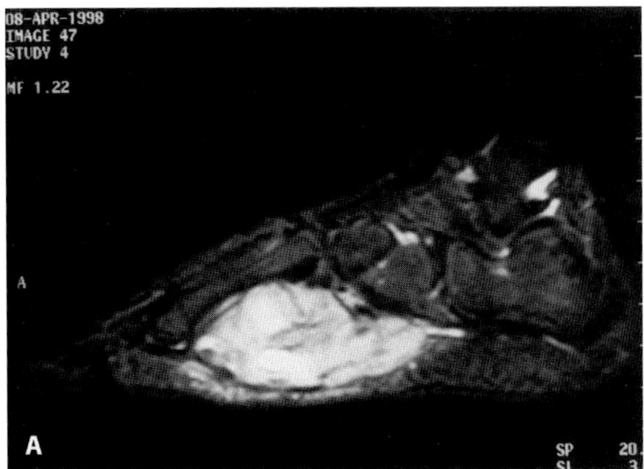

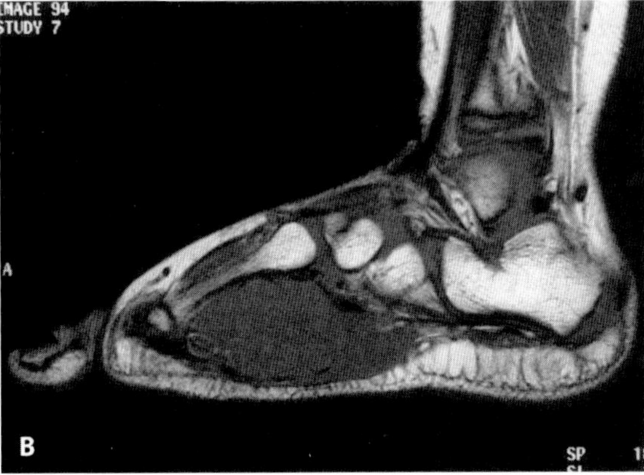

Fig. 16.84A,B. Rhabdomyosarcoma. Sagittal T2-W (**A**) and T1-W (**B**) images show a mass in the sole of the left foot

16.5.3.6
Trauma

Fractures in children differ from those in adults because, on the one hand, children's bones are more porous and can tolerate a greater deformation than the bone of an adult, and, on the other, the epiphysis is not fused. Typical childhood fractures are bowing fractures, torus fractures, greenstick fractures, and complete fractures, which can be easily diagnosed by plain-film radiographs. Stress fractures are rare and occur mostly in the proximal tibia in older children. They demonstrate a zone of sclerosis along a fracture line and periosteal new bone deposition, findings which should not be misinterpreted as a malignant process. With MRI, the area of sclerosis appears as an area of low SI on T1-WI and T2-WI.

More complex are those fractures involving the physis. The standard classification for physeal fractures is that of Salter and Harris. This classification categorizes injuries of the epiphyseal-metaphyseal complex according to the course of the fractures:

- SH I fracture: widened physis
- SH II fracture: widened physis with metaphyseal fragment
- SH III fracture: widened physis with epiphyseal fracture
- SH IV fracture: fracture extending through epiphysis and metaphysis
- SH V fracture: crush injury of the physis (rarely seen on plain-film radiographs)
- SH VI fracture: injury of the perichondral ring

In most cases, plain-film radiography is sufficient to diagnose these lesions. There are no generally established indications for the performance of MR examinations in the case of uncomplicated or physeal fractures, as immobilization and follow-up radiographs are sufficient for treatment. However, MRI can be helpful in selected cases, such as fractures of the femoral neck with risk of developing femoral-head necrosis, or complex injuries of the elbow and ankle, frequently necessitating surgery. On MRI, fracture lines can be identified as lines or zones of low SI in T1-WI, with high SI on T2-WI, reflecting concurrent bone bruise and edema. In contrast to CT, MR is appropriate to depict the area of bridging exactly in the case of premature closure of the epiphysis caused by physeal bridging.

Joint dislocations occur almost exclusively in older children, as the epiphyseal-metaphyseal junction is a weak zone and, therefore, physeal fractures are more frequently encountered than joint dislocation. In young children, the joint most commonly injured is the elbow, whereas in older children, the ankle and knee are frequently affected. A severely injured knee joint should be evaluated by MRI.

Acute or chronic avulsion fractures in older children occur along the crest of the iliac wing, the greater and lesser trochanters, along the inferior aspect of the ischium, the medial supracondylar ridge of the femur, and the medial epicondyle of the humerus. MRI is very helpful in evaluating the extent of avulsion fractures (Fig. 16.85). The bones can be strikingly irregular, and a pseudomalignant appearance can result in the course of healing.

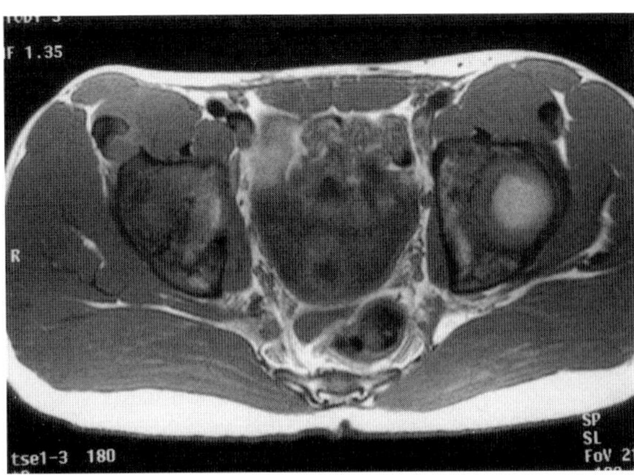

Fig. 16.85. Avulsion fracture. Transverse T1-WI shows avulsion of the rectus femoris tendon from the anterior inferior iliac spina on the right side

16.5.3.6.1
Slipped Femoral Capital Epiphysis

Slipped femoral capital epiphysis occurs in obese, marfanoid, or normal children between the ages 9 and 14 years and is bilateral in up to 40% of cases. Normally, both hips do not slip simultaneously, but if both hips are affected, this usually occurs within 2 years. In the acute form, the epiphysis slips within a short time span and, with this condition, there is a 10%–20% risk for avascular necrosis of the femoral head, whereas in the chronic form, the epiphysis slips slowly, and femoral head necrosis never occurs. Slipped femoral capital epiphysis is also associated with metabolic disorders such as rickets, renal osteodystrophy, hypothyroidism, and GHD. MRI is useful in evaluating a developing femoral-head necrosis in the acute form or postoperatively and may be used to illustrate the degree of slippage and femoral neck angulation prior to surgical treatment by pin fixation.

Further Reading

Atlas SW (1996) Magnetic resonance imaging of the brain and spine, 2nd edn. Lippincott-Raven, Philadelphia

Ball WS Jr (1997) Pediatric neuroradiology. Lippincott-Raven, Philadelphia

Barkovich AJ (2000) Pediatric neuroimaging, 3rd edn. Lippincott / Williams and Wilkins, Philadelphia

Edelmann RA, Hesselink JR, Zlatkin M (1996) Clinical magnetic resonance imaging, 2nd edn. Saunders, Philadelphia

Heidemann RL, Packer RJ, Albright LA et al (1997) In: Pizzo PA, Poplack DG (eds) Principles and practice of pediatric oncology, 3rd edn. Lippincott-Raven, Philadelphia, pp 633–697

Kaatsch P, Spix C, Michaelis J (2000) Jahresbericht 1999 des Deutschen Kinderkrebsregisters. IMSD Johannes-Gutenberg-Universität Institut für Med Statistik und Dokumentation. Mainz, Nov 2000

Kirks DR (1998) Practical pediatric imaging, 2nd edn. Lippincott-Raven, Philadelphia

Knaap MS, van der Valk J (1995) Magnetic resonance of myelin; myelination and myelin disorders, 2nd edn. Springer, Berlin Heidelberg New York

Osborn AG (1993) Diagnostic neuroradiology. Mosby, New York

Semelka RC, Ascher SM, Reinhold C (1997) MRI of the abdomen and pelvis. A text atlas, 1st edn. Wiley-Liss, New York

Stoller DW (1997) Magnetic resonance imaging in orthopaedics and sports medicine, 2nd edn. Lippincott-Raven, Philadelphia

Swischuk LE (1997) Imaging of the newborn, infant, and young child, 4th edn. Williams and Wilkins, Philadelphia

Interventional Magnetic Resonance

17

C. Bremer

Contents

17.1 General Considerations

Several attributes of magnetic resonance (MR) imaging make it very attractive for a potential use in interventional radiological procedures. The free choice of imaging planes, excellent soft-tissue contrast, plus simultaneous information on the vasculature while avoiding radiation exposure are particularly useful for many interventions. However, the capability of monitoring functional and physical changes of the tissue (fMRT, MR thermometry) is an even more striking tool, highly attractive for minimally invasive MR-guided therapies. Clinical experiences with interventional MRI (iMRI) are very promising, although there is still a lot of work to do in terms of hardware and software development to keep up with the current standard of conventional interventional radiology. This chapter intends to provide an overview of current and future applications of iMRI.

17.1.1 Magnets

A variety of procedures may be performed on conventional MR scanners, although limited patient accessibility might complicate some MR interventions. Different systems are available that offer more comfort concerning the degrees of freedom for iMRI.

Various ‘open’ magnets with a vertically oriented field between two horizontal poles, and thus offering a wide, lateral patient access, are commercially available from different vendors. Siemens (Erlangen, Germany) offers a 0.2-T low-field scanner (Magnetom Concerto) and a 1.0-T superconducting magnet (Magnetom Rhapsody); General Electric manufactures a 0.35-T (Signa Ovation) and a superconducting 0.7-T (Signa

OpenSpeed) open MRI; Phillips Medical Systems (Best, Netherlands) a 0.23-T (Panorama 0.23 T) and a 1.0 (Panorama 1.0 T) scanner; and Toshiba a 0.35-T (Opart) MR scanner. Generally speaking, a low field strength results in a lower signal-to-noise ratio, while instrument-related artifacts are less pronounced in these systems (see below).

Dedicated interventional systems are made by GE (Signa SP) and by Philips Medical Systems (Intera I/T). The Signa SP system consists of a cryogen-free, superconducting, mid-field magnet with two vertically oriented poles ('double donut', 0.5 T field strength) with a 58-cm vertical gap allowing a wide range of access to the patient. The Intera I/T system is a high-field (1.5 T field strength) interventional MR system with a short magnet and a flared opening of the magnet to allow better patient access. It can be combined with an X-ray fluoroscopy system through a floating table, offering an uncomplicated conversion between MRI and conventional X-ray fluoroscopy for angiographic procedures.

The systems are equipped with fast imaging techniques for MR fluoroscopy (see Chapter 1) and optional active tracking systems.

17.1.2 Instrument Visualization

Visualization of instruments is important in order to perform interventional procedures exactly. Passive and active visualization methods may be used for iMRI. While instruments are depicted as part of the normal imaging process during passive visualization, active visualization requires additional hardware and software to actively generate a signal of the device.

17.1.2.1 Passive Visualization

Passive visualization is based on signal void due to spin 'replacement' by the iMRI device, susceptibility artifacts, and labeling of the device with contrast agents (Debatin 1998).

17.1.2.1.1 Signal Void

Interventional MR devices do not contain protons that contribute to the imaging signal. They, moreover, displace spins of the surrounding tissue so that iMRI instruments will be seen by the resulting signal void. Visibility of the device is, in this regard, mainly determined by the image resolution. Signal void will work best in fairly large iMRI devices. Furthermore, it is mandatory that the iMRI device is surrounded by tissue generating a signal.

17.1.2.1.2 Susceptibility

Magnetic susceptibility describes the degree to which a substance, such as an iMRI device, becomes magnetized in response to an external magnetic field (see Chapter 2), resulting in local field disturbances, which can be used for the visualization of iMRI instruments.

Several factors influence the size of the susceptibility artifact. In general, stronger magnetic fields will result in severer artifacts. Gradient-echo (GRE) sequences are particularly sensitive to susceptibility artifacts, especially with increasing echo time (TE), while the 180° refocusing pulse of spin-echo (SE) sequences makes them less sensitive to susceptibility artifacts. Moreover, artifacts in SE sequences are less dependent on TE. Artifacts (i.e., the depicted width of the MR device) in SE sequences will be clearly attenuated with the frequency-encoding direction parallel to the iMRI device, while the tip of the instrument is slightly less accurately depicted in this case. Likewise, parallel orientation of the object to B_0 will decrease the susceptibility artifact of the iMRI device compared with perpendicular orientation to B_0, while again the parallel orientation slightly decreases the accuracy of the tip positioning. Finally, increasing the gradient strength or the receiver bandwidth will result in a reduction of the artifact seen on MRI (Fig. 17.1).

Due to the design of the standard MR scanner, biopsy needles will most likely be applied in an axial plane, i.e., almost perpendicular to B_0, so that SE or turbo spin-echo (TSE) sequences may have to be applied for localization of the iMRI devices. However, artifacts might still be too large on high-field scanners (1.5 T) and, therefore, obscure small targets. On the other hand, in low-field scanners (0.2–0.5 T), artifacts might be insufficient for visualization of the iMRI device if the angle to B_0 is $<20°$. In this case, GRE sequences should be chosen for positioning of the iMRI device (angle 10°–60°; Lewin et al. 1996).

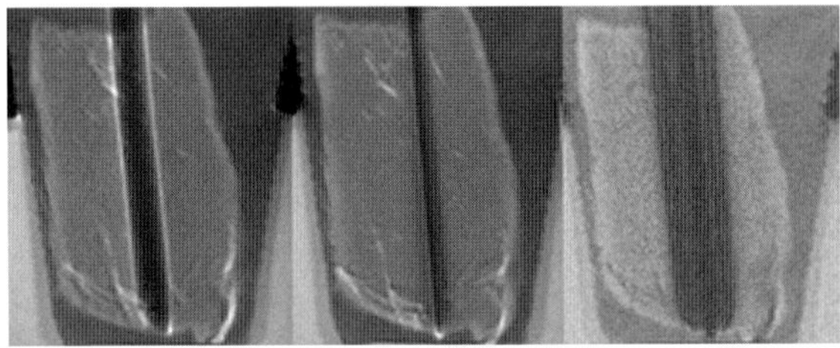

Fig. 17.1. Size of susceptibility artifact of a MR-compatible biopsy needle (Guerbet, Westbury, USA) perpendicular to B_0 in a muscle phantom at 1.5 T with frequency encoding perpendicular (*left*) or parallel (*middle*) to the needle using a spin-echo sequence [repetition time (TR)/echo time (TE) 500/14]. Artifact size of a spoiled gradient-echo sequence on the right (TR/TE/FA 24/12/30°)

17.1.2.1.3 Contrast Agents

Marking of the iMRI devices with paramagnetic contrast agents, such as gadolinium (Gd)-chelates, will deliver a signal from the iMRI instrument. Combination of a short repetition time (TR) and a high flip-angle saturates the surrounding spins of the tissue, resulting in a better contrast between the iMRI devices and the tissue. A drawback of this technique is the need for an extra lumen within the device, which increases its size.

17.1.2.1.4 Catheter Visualization

Intravascular catheters run in several curves within the vessels through the body, with changing orientation of the catheter to B_0. The resulting differences in susceptibility artifacts (see above) complicates the catheter visualization over its entire length for intravascular interventions. One solution to this problem is the fact that a dot-shaped deposit of paramagnetic (or superparamagnetic) material will always appear similarly on MR images, independent of the position within the imaged volume. For instance, intravascular catheters with integrated dysprosium rings, which reveal a constant, almost dot-shaped, artifact have been designed. Furthermore, field-inhomogeneity catheters, which are equipped with a thin copper wire wrapped around the catheter, are currently under investigation. A small current within the copper wire results in a local disturbance of B_0 and, therefore, intravoxel dephasing, which again results in visualization of the catheter over its entire length.

17.1.2.2 Active Visualization

Active visualization methods are based on additional hardware components actively creating a signal from the iMRI device, which enables exact localization of the device in the imaged volume. To date, MR tracking, MR profiling, and external flash-point tracking systems are under investigation.

Integration of a small radiofrequency (RF) receiver coil, either at the tip of the instrument (MR tracking) or over a length of several centimeters (MR profiling), is the one basic principle for active visualization. The receiver coils have a limited sensitive volume, so that only MR signals of the adjacent tissue are perceived, which allows for exact localization of the device within the volume of interest (Debatin and Adam 1998).

External flash-point tracking systems work with infrared light-emitting diodes (LED), which are mounted on a hand-held, custom-built device attached to the iMRI instrument. An integrated camera system determines the position and the angular orientation of the device in the scanning volume, so that the position of an attached rigid instrument can easily be calculated.

For precise anatomical correlation, the data obtained by active visualization methods are superimposed on a previously acquired image data set. These systems might prove to be advantageous for complex iMRI interventions, such as vascular procedures or brain biopsies.

17.1.3 Needles and Wires, Instruments

Ferromagnetic substances may not be used for iMRI devices since they induce strong translational forces within the magnet. Numerous MR-compatible iMRI instruments are currently available. They principally do not differ from conventional interventional devices, although they contain nickel, chrome, and titanium alloys to reduce susceptibility artifacts. However, hook-wires, for instance, will typically reveal artifacts of about 3–5 mm, while biopsy needles may exhibit artifacts of more than 1 cm (Fig. 17.1). A list of vendors for iMRI equipment is given by Debatin and Adam (1998).

17.2 Diagnostic Interventions

17.2.1 MR-Guided Localization and Biopsies of Breast Lesions

MR mammography has been shown to be a sensitive method for the detection of breast tumors (Chapter 15). While the majority of breast lesions will still be visualized with conventional mammography, lesions exclusively seen on MRI can only be localized or biopsied using the same imaging modality.

Freehand localization of breast lesions, similar to CT freehand biopsy procedures, can be performed if no breast biopsy device is available. A tube filled with MR-visible fluid should be attached parallel to the body axis and a reference transverse slice can be marked for instance with a vitamin-E capsule. However, this approach should not be applied for core biopsies of the breast.

To date, different approaches to MR-guided breast interventions using dedicated breast biopsy devices have been developed (Debatin and Adam 1998).

One approach uses a dedicated breast biopsy coil with a built-in stereotaxy system presented by Heywang-Köbrunner and co-workers in cooperation with Siemens (Erlangen, Germany). The first generation of this device consists of a circularly polarized surface coil with integrated compression plates that are perforated for biopsy devices. The patient is examined in a prone position. A further development of this device allows mediolateral breast compression with two independently moving compression plates and thus medial and lateral access to the breast. The compression plates now consist of flexible ribs so that there is no dead space between the entry points. This device allowed for successful MR-guided vacuum biopsies of the breast (Heywang-Köbrunner et al. 2000).

Fischer and co-workers developed an add-on stereotactic device, which can be used with a regular surface coil ('eye and ear coil'). It is built of two semicircular perforated plates with a hinge to allow angulation against each other and, thus, gentle breast compression. The plates fit into the coil mentioned above. In this setting, the patient is examined in the supine position.

Kuhl and co-workers (1997) developed a stereotactic device in cooperation with Philips Medical Systems, which consists of two parallel compression plates with an integrated stereotaxy system. A regular flexible circular surface coil is placed between the patient support and the chest wall around the breast. The patient is examined in a semiprone position, which combines the advantage of free-needle angulation and breast extension away from the chest wall as in the true-prone position (Fig. 17.2).

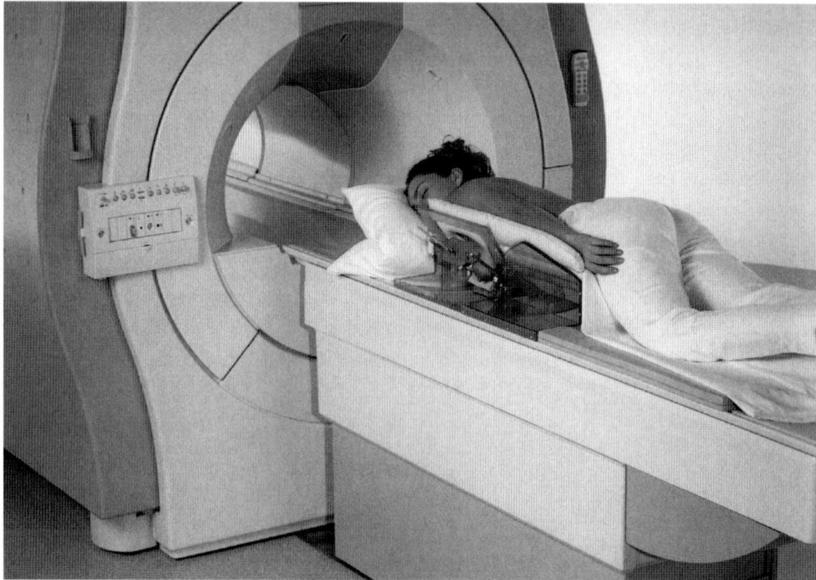

Fig. 17.2. Stereotaxy device for localization and biopsy of breast lesions in the semiprone position. Extension of the breast away from the thorax, as well as free angulation of the iMRI, are guaranteed in the semiprone position (courtesy of Dr. C. Kuhl, University of Bonn)

For pre-interventional lesion detection, the same imaging protocol as in MR mammography should be used (Chapter 15). Since the lesions do not need to be characterized, fewer dynamic postcontrast scans need to be performed in order to shorten the protocol (for example, three postcontrast scans).

The stereotactic coordinates are determined with reference to visible MR markers on the stereotactic device. In-plane coordinates are obtained by the system's distance function, while the third coordinate is given by the offset of the slice that best displays the lesion. After the bore hole of the stereotactic device has been chosen according to the calculated coordinates, it is recommended to repeat one-scan (2D-GRE) with a needle phantom in place to check for calculation errors. For rapid orientation of the needle position, a T1-weighted (T1-W) SE scan should be applied. After the needle reaches the correct position, the guide wire is released or the biopsy needle is advanced to take the samples. After release of the hook wire, a 2D-GRE sequence may be repeated to delineate the wire position for the surgeon more clearly (greater artifact, see Fig. 17.1). Finally, a T1-W SE sequence needs to be performed for subtle documentation of the hook-wire position (Fig. 17.3).

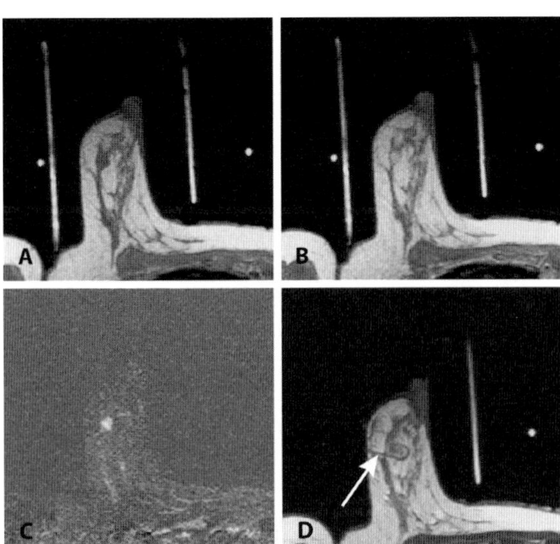

Fig. 17.3A–D. Magnetic resonance (MR)-guided lesion localization in the breast. MR images before and 40 s after gadolinium-DTPA injection [repetition time (TR)/echo time (TE)/FA 220/4.6/90°, **A+B**] reveal a highly suspicious lesion with strong contrast enhancement, easily visible on the corresponding subtracted image (**C**). Lesion localization was performed with a hook wire (**D**, see *arrow*; T1-W spin-echo, TR/TE 300/11), and postinterventional surgery revealed a T1N0M0 carcinoma of 7 mm in size (courtesy of Dr. C. Kuhl, University of Bonn)

17.2.1.1 Pitfalls

Contrast enhancement of the lesion is tapered over time, due to wash-out of contrast medium from the lesion into the surrounding tissue ('vanishing target phenomenon'). In this case, a second Gd bolus (0.1 mmol/kg bw) may be applied, and fat-suppressed MRI may be performed. Moreover, too strong a compression of the breast may interfere with contrast enhancement of the lesion, so that it might not be visualized.

17.2.1.2 Clinical Remarks

MR-guided biopsy of the breast should, at this stage, not be considered as a clinical routine modality for histopathological lesion determination, since the spatial accuracy and consistency of positioning are not yet high enough. Especially in lesions less than 1 cm in size, which can be completely obscured by the needle artifact, MR-guided breast biopsy should not be performed, but wire placement followed by lesion excision should be preferred. In cases of discrepancies between the histological and MR findings, early postoperative follow-up (within 3 days postoperatively) for the detection of residual tumor is recommended.

17.2.2 MR-Guided Abdominal and Pelvic Biopsies

Indications for MR-guided abdominal biopsies are, to date, limited since ultrasound and computed tomography (CT)-guided procedures sufficiently cover the vast majority of image-guided biopsies. However, some lesions might only be visible with MRI. Furthermore, the multiplanar imaging capability of MRI may be exploited especially well in long and intercostal approaches to tumors in the upper abdomen, such as subphrenic liver lesions or subdiaphragmatic fluid collections, which are difficult to reach with ultrasound (Fig. 17.4). Moreover, patients with a known allergy to

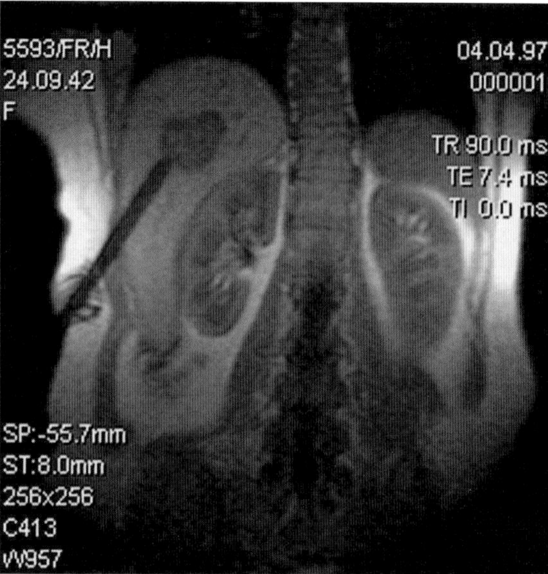

Fig. 17.4. MR-guided biopsy of a liver lesion with a 14-gauge biopsy needle. Note the highly angulated subcostal approach to reach the subphrenic mass (courtesy of Dr. H.B. Gehl, Lübeck Medical University)

iodinated contrast agents may preferentially be biopsied using MRI.

The patient is typically positioned supine, and an appropriate coil (e.g., flexible surface coil) is placed close to the probable puncture site. Sequence parameters for lesion detection should be chosen as given in the corresponding chapters. Instrument visualization may be realized using a 2D spoiled GRE or fast imaging with steady-state precession (FISP) sequence with acquisition of 5–7 slices in a breath-hold. Depending on the magnet strength, TSE sequences might have to be applied in order to reduce susceptibility artifacts (see above).

For determination of the entry point, MR visible markers (e.g., plastic grid filled with 1:200 diluted Gd-chelates) are attached to the patient's skin, and coordinates are obtained as pointed out earlier. Especially for difficult approaches, a 3D laser-guidance system can be very helpful to check for angulation of the instrument during needle advancement. In the case of a long needle pathway, intermittent scanning for needle localization is recommended. Before cutting or aspiration, the needle position should be documented in one or two planes. There are reports of MR-guided biopsies for liver lesions, adrenal masses, the prostate gland, and pelvic masses such as lymph-node biopsies in patients with bladder cancer. Lesion size should be at least 1.5 cm due to the size of susceptibility artifacts.

17.2.3 MR-Guided Biopsy of Bone

Bone marrow edema of unknown origin may reflect a clear indication for MR-guided bone biopsy since MR is the method of choice for detection of this pathology. For all other bone lesions, MRI does not provide additional information for guiding bone biopsies. However, younger patients with suspected benign lesions may benefit from this procedure with respect to radiation safety. MR-compatible biopsy needles for osteosclerotic or osteolytic lesions are currently available. The accessing procedures are similar to the interventions described above. A limited clinical series indicates that the accuracy of these procedures is comparable to CT-guided bone biopsies. However, for high-risk areas, such as the spine, CT guidance is still the imaging modality of choice (Debatin and Adam 1998).

17.2.4 MR-Guided Biopsy of the Head and Neck

The excellent soft-tissue contrast and possibility of active tracking could also turn out to be advantageous for biopsies in the head and neck area, where there are many critical anatomic structures. Most imaging protocols for lesion detection comprise multiplanar TSE and contrast-enhanced GRE sequences. Fat-saturation techniques may provide imaging quality superior to CT scanning and ultrasound. Biopsies of the thyroid, parathyroid, maxilla, and skull base have been described to date. The clinical relevance of MR-guided biopsy versus ultrasound remains to be shown (Debatin and Adam 1998).

17.3 Therapeutic Interventions

Due to its multiplanar imaging capacity and excellent soft-tissue contrast, as well as its temperature-monitoring capabilities, MRI is an important tool for the monitoring of minimal invasive ablation thermotherapies.

17.3.1 MR Thermometry (Müller and Roggan 1995)

Several MR parameters such as the T1 relaxation time, the diffusion coefficient and the chemical shift of the water peak are temperature dependent and can thus be exploited for noninvasive temperature mapping in vivo.

17.3.1.1 T1 Effects

For a temperature range of 37°–50°C, the T1 relaxation time correlates almost linearly with the temperature. Thus, T1-W images (T1-WI) show a constant decrease in signal intensity with increasing temperature (Fig. 17.5). It is obvious that the rate of signal change in T1-WI depends on the sequence (TE, TR, flip angle) and tissue parameters. Hence, only qualitative and not quantitative temperature changes may be evaluated. Availability and rapid data acquisition make this technique a widely used method for MR thermometry.

17.3.1.2 Proton Frequency Shift

The resonance frequency of the spins is determined by the local magnetic field at the proton. Increasing tissue temperature is associated with a decrease of hydrogen bonds of the water molecules, resulting in a decrease of the local magnetic field due to increased 'electronic screening' (quantified by the 'molecular screening constant' *r*). A decrease of the local magnetic field is responsible for the proton frequency shift (PFS). PFS is linearly correlated with the temperature and, thus, is an accurate method for 2D quantitative temperature mapping. A high linearity and temperature sensitivity make this technique a good choice for mid- to high-field scanners. Using radiofrequency spoiled gradient-echo imaging techniques, temperature maps with a standard deviation of less than 1°C at a high temporal resolution are feasible.

17.3.1.3 Diffusion Imaging

MRI is sensitive to thermal Brownian movement, which is characterized by the diffusion coefficient [D(x,y)]. Temperature and diffusion coefficients are exponentially related, so that temperature changes may be sensitively measured by diffusion WI. Long scanning time, diffusion changes due to microcirculatory regulations, and sensitivity to motion are factors that limit the clinical applicability of this technique.

17.3.2 Laser-Induced Interstitial Thermotherapy

17.3.2.1 Technical Principle

Laser-induced interstitial thermotherapy (LITT) is based on energy deposition into the tissue with laser light near the infrared spectrum, typically delivered by an Nd:YAG laser (1064 nm), which offers deep tissue penetration. An optical fiber that allows homogeneous light distribution within the tissue is percutaneously placed under CT or ultrasound guidance into the target.

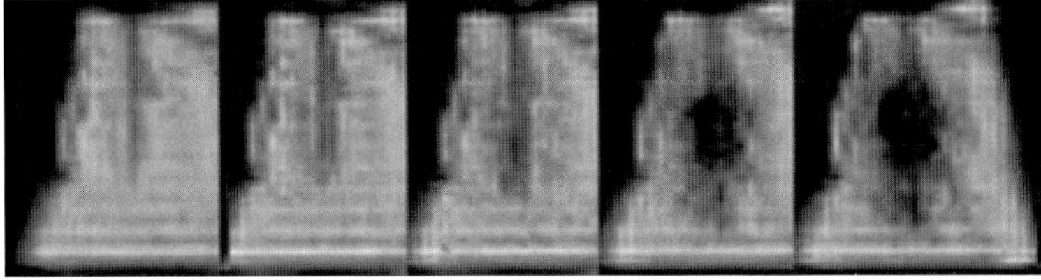

Fig. 17.5. MR thermometry ex vivo in a liver sample using a two-dimensional turbo FLASH sequence (echo time/repetition time/TI/FA 13/5/300/10°), images taken every other minute during application of 10 J/s laser power with an Nd:YAG laser at 1064 nm. Note the signal loss during application of laser energy due to temperature increase and protein denaturation

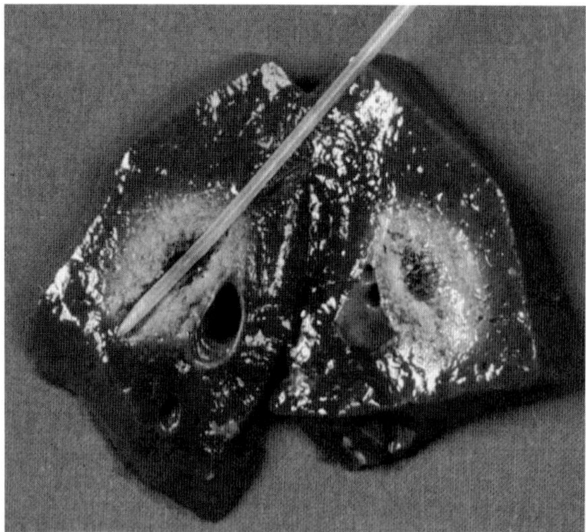

Fig. 17.6. Coagulation necrosis after laser-induced interstitial thermotherapy (LITT) in a liver sample after application of approximately 4200 J laser energy using an Nd:YAG laser at 1064 nm and a standard LITT applicator with an active length of 20 mm. Note the protective catheter in position at the puncture site

The majority of the laser energy is converted to heat, so that coagulation necrosis occurs (Fig. 17.6). The ablation capacity is critically dependent on the LITT-applicator design. While the standard LITT applicator with an active length of 2 cm only allows treatment of lesions <3 cm in diameter, multiple puncture techniques, pull-back approaches, or the use of an internally cooled LITT applicator system (Somatex/Hüttinger, Germany) allow for larger coagulation volumes.

For online thermometry, a T1-W spoiled GRE (TR 148 ms, TE 6 ms, FA 60°) or turbo FLASH (TR 13 ms, TE 5 ms, TI 300 ms, FA 10°) sequence may be applied. After the intervention, tissue necrosis is assessed by contrast-enhanced MRI using the same sequences (0.1 mmol/kg bw Gd-DTPA, optional dynamic scanning). Perfusion deficits within the lesion or rim enhancement around the treated area, respectively, help to estimate real tissue necrosis.

17.3.2.2 Clinical Applications

The use of LITT for the treatment of various tumor entities is currently under investigation. Overall, most tumor ablations have been performed on hepatic tumors. In a large series, 705 patients were treated with LITT for liver lesions from various primary tumors (colorectal, HCC, breast cancer). The mean survival time in this patient population ranged around 4 years. The survival rate was 92% at 1 year decreasing to 36% at 5 years after treatment (Mack et al. 2001), which is comparable to outcome data of surgical tumor resection (5-year survival rate of 20%–40%, Mack et al. 2001). However, the morbidity after surgical resection can be relatively high (15%–43%), while LITT is generally well tolerated, and patients can be discharged within 2–3 days after the procedure (Fig. 17.7) (Vogl et al. 1997; Bremer et al. 1998). Compared to untreated patients (mean survival of about 16 months), LITT provided a significant increase in survival and thus can be considered an attractive palliative tumor therapy (Mack et al. 2001).

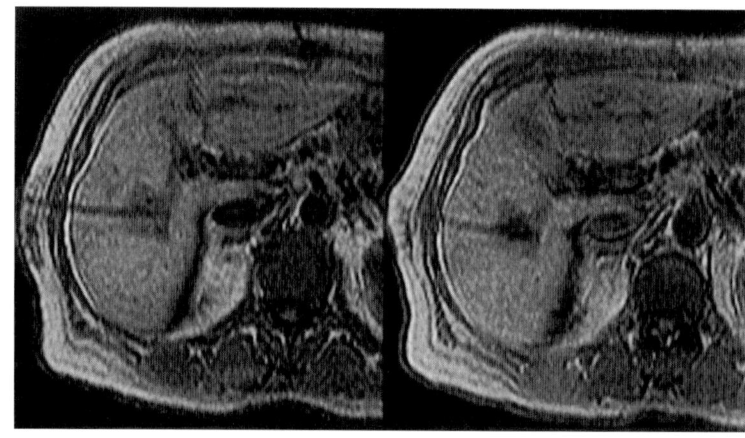

Fig. 17.7. Laser-induced interstitial thermotherapy (LITT) on a patient with hepatocellular carcinoma who was inoperable due to poor general medical condition. Note the decrease in signal intensity around the tip of the laser fiber during LITT in a T1-W spoiled gradient-echo sequence (echo time/repetition time/FA 146/6/60°). The lesion could be completely ablated, and the patient was discharged 2 days after the intervention

Furthermore, LITT has been applied to cerebral tumors (astrocytomas WHO II, anaplastic gliomas WHO III–IV, and metastases), head and neck tumors as well as malignant and benign breast lesions, suggesting that LITT has a good potential for palliative tumor treatment (Reimer et al. 1998). LITT has also been applied for the treatment of benign prostatic hyperplasia with considerable success (Müller and Roggan 1995).

17.3.3 MR-Guided Radiofrequency Thermal Ablation

In RF thermal ablation, a rapidly alternating current is guided through the tissue, resulting in a transfer of electrical energy. Due to the high tissue resistance, ionic agitation causes frictional heating, which finally leads to coagulation effects comparable to LITT. Most of the RF procedures are currently performed under ultrasound guidance. However, similar to LITT, MR thermometry can be exploited in RF ablation to monitor the therapy. Clinically, image-guided RF ablations have been used for a variety of lesions including hepatocellular carcinomas, renal cell carcinomas, hepatic, cerebral, and retroperitoneal metastases, as well as osteoid osteomas. From a larger series of RF ablation of liver tumors under ultrasound guidance, one would expect that the clinical potential for RF ablation is comparable to LITT (Debatin and Adam 1998).

17.3.4 MR-Guided Focused Ultrasound

A third way to induce tissue heating for tumor ablation is high-intensity focused ultrasound. A mechanical ultrasound wave (frequency 0.5–10 MHz) is absorbed within the target, according to the attenuation coefficient of the tissue. This results in a temperature increase, cavitation secondary to high pressure amplitudes with gas bubble formation, and mechanical disruption of the tissue. Furthermore, high-amplitude, focused ultrasound beams can be distorted into shock waves, leading to changes in membrane permeability.

A problem with this technique is the need for an acoustic window to avoid gaseous or bony obstructions to the beam path. Moreover, since tissue disruption is not as efficient as in LITT or RF, only small target volumes can be treated, which requires multiple sessions to ablate larger tumors. However, if applicable, this technique is completely noninvasive. The first clinical evaluations are in progress for the treatment of breast, liver, and prostate tumors. While most studies currently employ ultrasound for guidance and monitoring, MRI maybe helpful for thermomonitoring and to assess focused ultrasound-induced lesions (Debatin and Adam 1998).

17.3.5 MR-Guided Cryotherapy

Tissue ablation based on cooling, as opposed to heating, may also be excellently visualized by MRI since the T2 of frozen tissue is so short that there is effectively no RF signal from the frozen region. Ice formation within the tissue can thus be seen as a signal-free area in both T1-W and T2-W sequences. The cryoprobe, typically cooled with liquid nitrogen, is placed under MR guidance into the target. Cooling leads to ice formation, and subsequent thawing of the tissue is followed by inflammatory resorption and scar formation in the treated area. Total necrosis may be seen approximately 7 days after freezing. Clinical experiences are derived from the treatment of superficial organs (ophthalmology, dermatology), endoscopically treatable organs (pulmonology, gastroenterology) as well as intraoperative applications. Interstitial applications of cryotherapy are known from the treatment of prostate cancer under ultrasound guidance with good success (Debatin and Adam 1998). The first clinical applications of percutaneous cryotherapy of liver tumors under MR guidance show the feasibility of this concept for clinical use. The depiction of a clearly demarcated margin of the ice ball (and thus tissue necrosis) might be advantageous compared with the heating techniques discussed above. However, there are concerns about bleeding complications with this technique based on surgical cryotherapy experiences.

17.4 Further Perspectives

Minimally invasive diagnostic and therapeutic procedures are increasingly important for future patient care, since they enhance the patient's safety while decreasing the cost of medical treatment due to reduced hospitalization. The first clinical experiences with MR-guided diagnostic interventions have proved the feasibility of this method, and further technical developments might replace a wide range of CT-guided interventions and, therefore, promote radiation hygiene. The first reports on MR-guided intravascular angioplasty show the feasibility of this concept.

MR-guided intravascular interventions may be particularly helpful in complex interventions, such as transjugular intrahepatic portosystemic shunts (TIPS), to avoid excessive radiation exposure for the patient and the radiologist. Furthermore, minimally invasive interstitial thermotherapies offer a fascinating potential for the treatment of solitary tumors. MRI may, in this regard, serve in a threefold way: for tumor detection, online monitoring of the therapy, and postinterventional follow-up. Clinical studies are now warranted to exactly define the indication for MR-guided interstitial ablation therapies compared with surgery, radiation, and chemotherapy. Finally, the intraoperative use of MRI in combination with active visualization methods and fast imaging techniques will significantly increase the positional accuracy and decrease the time of surgery in specialties such as neurosurgery. MRI images may, for this purpose, be linked to functional MR images, MR angiographies, and other 3D data sets, such as positron emission tomography (PET) and CT, offering a new dimension of anatomical and functional neuronavigation for the surgeon.

References

Debatin JF, Adam G (1998) Interventional magnetic resonance imaging, 1st edn. Springer, Berlin Heidelberg New York

Heywang-Köhbrunner S H, Heinig A, Pickuth D, Alberich T, Spielmann RP (2000) Interventional MRI of the breast: lesion localisation and biopsy. Eur Radiol 10:36–45

JMRI, Volume 12 Issue 4 (2000) Special Issue: Interventional MRI, Part 1

JMRI, Volume 13 Issue 1 (2001) Special Issue: Interventional MRI, Part 2

Kuhl CK, Elevelt A, Leutner C, Gieseke J, Pakos E, Schild HH (1997) Clinical use of a stereotactic localization and biopsy device for interventional breast MRI. Radiology 204:667–676

Lewin JS, Duerk JL, Jain VR, Petersige CA, Chao CP, Haaga JR (1996) Needle localization in MR-guided biopsy and aspiration: effects of field strength, sequence design, and magnetic field orientation. AJR Am J Roentgenol 166:1337–1345

Liberman L (2002) Percutaneous image-guided core breast biopsy. Radiol Clin North Am 40(3):483–500

Mack MG, Straub R, Eichler K, Engelmann K, Zangos S, Roggan A, Woitaschek D, Böttger M, Vogl TJ (2001) Percutaneous MR imaging-guided laser-induced thermotherapy of hepatic metastases. Abdom Imaging 26:369–374

Müller G, Roggan A (1995) Laser induced interstitial thermotherapy. SPIE Press, Bellingham, Washington

Straube T, Kahn T (2001) Related Articles. Thermal therapies in interventional MR imaging. Laser. Neuroimaging Clin N Am 11(4):749–757

Viehweg P. Heinig A, Amaya B, Alberich T, Laniado M, Heywang-Kobrunner SH (2002) MR-guided interventional breast procedures considering vacuum biopsy in particular. Eur J Radiol 42(1):32–39. Review

Vogl TJ, Balzer JO, Mack MG, Bett G, Oppelt A (2002) Hybrid MR interventional imaging system: combined MR and angiography suites with single interactive table. Feasibility study in vascular liver tumor procedures. Eur Radiol 12(6):1394–1400

Vogl TJ, Mack MG, Straub R, Roggan A, Felix R (1997) Percutaneous MRI-guided laser-induced thermotherapy of hepatic metastases for colorectal cancer. Lancet 350:29

Yeung CJ, Susil RC, Atalar E (2002) RF safety of wires in interventional MRI: using a safety index. Magn Reson Med 47(1): 187–193

Subject Index

F

N